# Lecture Notes in Computer Science    11764

More information about this series at http://www.springer.com/series/7412

Dinggang Shen · Tianming Liu ·
Terry M. Peters · Lawrence H. Staib ·
Caroline Essert · Sean Zhou ·
Pew-Thian Yap · Ali Khan (Eds.)

# Medical Image Computing and Computer Assisted Intervention – MICCAI 2019

22nd International Conference
Shenzhen, China, October 13–17, 2019
Proceedings, Part I

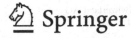

Springer

*Editors*
Dinggang Shen
University of North Carolina
at Chapel Hill
Chapel Hill, NC, USA

Terry M. Peters (iD)
Western University
London, ON, Canada

Caroline Essert (iD)
University of Strasbourg
Illkirch, France

Pew-Thian Yap
University of North Carolina
at Chapel Hill
Chapel Hill, NC, USA

Tianming Liu
University of Georgia
Athens, GA, USA

Lawrence H. Staib (iD)
Yale University
New Haven, CT, USA

Sean Zhou
United Imaging Intelligence
Shanghai, China

Ali Khan
Western University
London, ON, Canada

ISSN 0302-9743          ISSN 1611-3349 (electronic)
Lecture Notes in Computer Science
ISBN 978-3-030-32238-0          ISBN 978-3-030-32239-7 (eBook)
https://doi.org/10.1007/978-3-030-32239-7

LNCS Sublibrary: SL6 – Image Processing, Computer Vision, Pattern Recognition, and Graphics

This Springer imprint is published by the registered company Springer Nature Switzerland AG
The registered company address is: Gewerbestrasse 11, 6330 Cham, Switzerland

# Preface

We are pleased to present the proceedings for the 22nd International Conference on Medical Image Computing and Computer-Assisted Intervention (MICCAI), which was held at the InterContinental Hotel, Shenzhen, China, October 13–17, 2019. The conference also featured 34 workshops, 13 tutorials, and 22 challenges held on October 13 or 17. MICCAI 2019 had an approximately 63% increase in submissions and accepted papers compared with MICCAI 2018. These papers, which comprise six volumes of *Lecture Notes in Computer Science* (LNCS) proceedings, were selected after a thorough double-blind peer-review process. Following the example set by the previous program chairs of MICCAI 2018 and 2017, we employed Microsoft's Conference Managing Toolkit (CMT) for paper submissions and double-blind peer-reviews, and the Toronto Paper Matching System (TPMS) to assist with automatic paper assignment to area chairs and reviewers.

From 2625 original intentions to submit, 1809 full submissions were received and sent out to peer-review. Of these, 63% were considered as pure Medical Image Computing (MIC), 5% as pure Computer-Assisted Interventions (CAI), and 32% as both MIC and CAI. The MICCAI 2019 Program Committee (PC) comprised 69 area chairs, with 25 from the Americas, 21 from Europe, and 23 from Asia/Pacific/Middle East. Each area chair was assigned ∼ 25 manuscripts, with up to 15 suggested potential reviewers using TPMS scoring and self-declared research areas. Subsequently, over 1200 invited reviewers were asked to bid for the papers for which they had been suggested. Final reviewer allocations via CMT took account of PC suggestions, reviewer bidding, and TPMS scores, finally allocating 5–6 papers per reviewer. Based on the double-blinded reviews, 306 papers (17%) were accepted immediately, and 920 papers (51%) were rejected, with the remainder being sent for rebuttal. These decisions were confirmed by the area chairs. During the rebuttal phase, two additional area chairs were assigned to each rebuttal paper using CMT and TPMS scores, who then independently scored them to accept or reject, based on the reviews, rebuttal, and manuscript, resulting in clear paper decisions using majority voting. This process resulted in the acceptance of further 234 papers for an overall acceptance rate of 30%. Regional PC teleconferences were held in late June to confirm the final results and collect PC feedback on the peer-review process.

For the MICCAI 2019 proceedings, 538 accepted papers have been organized in six volumes as follows:

Part I, LNCS Volume 11764: Optical Imaging; Endoscopy; Microscopy
Part II, LNCS Volume 11765: Image Segmentation; Image Registration; Cardiovascular Imaging; Growth, Development, Atrophy, and Progression
Part III, LNCS Volume 11766: Neuroimage Reconstruction and Synthesis; Neuroimage Segmentation; Diffusion-Weighted Magnetic Resonance Imaging; Functional Neuroimaging (fMRI); Miscellaneous Neuroimaging

Part IV, LNCS Volume 11767: Shape; Prediction; Detection and Localization; Machine Learning; Computer-Aided Diagnosis; Image Reconstruction and Synthesis
Part V, LNCS Volume 11768: Computer-Assisted Interventions; MIC Meets CAI
Part VI, LNCS Volume 11769: Computed Tomography; X-ray Imaging

We would like to thank everyone who contributed to the success of MICCAI 2019 and the quality of its proceedings, particularly the MICCAI Society for support, insightful comments, and providing funding for Kitty Wong to be the ongoing Conference System Manager. Given the increase in workload for this year's meeting, the Program Committee simply could not have functioned effectively without her, and she will provide ongoing oversight of the review process for future MICCAI conferences. Without the dedication and support of all of the organizers of the workshops, tutorials, and challenges, under the guidance of Kenji Suzuki, together with satellite event chairs Hongen Liao, Qian Wang, Luping Zhou, Hayit Greenspan, and Bram van Ginneken, none of these peripheral events would have been feasible.

Also, the Industry Forum (led by Xiaodong Tao and Yiqiang Zhan), the Industry Session (led by Sean Zhou), as well as the Doctoral Symposium (led by Junzhou Huang and Dajiang Zhu) brought new events to MICCAI 2019. The publication chairs, Li Wang and Gang Li, undertook the onerous task of assembling the camera-ready proceedings for publication by Springer.

Behind the scenes, MICCAI secretariat personnel, Janette Wallace and Johanne Langford, kept a close eye on logistics and budgets, while Doris Lam and her team from Momentous Asia, this year's Professional Conference Organization, along with the Local Organizing Committee chair, Dong Ni (together with Jing Qin, Qianjin Feng, Dong Liang, Xiaoying Tang), handled the website and local organization. The Student Travel Award Committee chaired by Huiguang He, Jun Shi, and Xi Jiang evaluated numerous applications, including awards for undergraduate students, which is new in the history of MICCAI. We also thank our sponsors for their financial support and presence on site. We are especially grateful to all members of the Program Committee for their diligent work in the reviewer assignments and final paper selection, as well as the reviewers for their support during the entire process. Finally, and most importantly, we thank all authors, co-authors, students/postdocs, and supervisors, for submitting and presenting their high-quality work that made MICCAI 2019 a greatly enjoyable, informative, and successful event. We are indebted to those reviewers and PC members who helped us resolve issues relating to last-minute missing reviews. Overall, we thank all of the authors and attendees for making MICCAI 2019 a spectacular success. We look forward to seeing you in Lima, Peru at MICCAI 2020!

October 2019

Dinggang Shen
Tianming Liu
Terry M. Peters
Lawrence H. Staib
Caroline Essert
Sean Zhou
Pew-Thian Yap
Ali Khan

# Organization

## General Chairs

Dinggang Shen      The University of North Carolina at Chapel Hill, USA
Tianming Liu      The University of Georgia, USA

## Program Executive

Terry Peters      Robarts Research Institute, Western University, Canada
Lawrence H. Staib      Yale University, USA
Sean Zhou      United Imaging Intelligence (UII), China
Caroline Essert      University of Strasbourg, France
Pew-Thian Yap      The University of North Carolina at Chapel Hill, USA
Ali Khan      Robarts Research Institute, Western University, Canada

## Submissions Manager

Kitty Wong      Robarts Research Institute, Western University, Canada

## Workshops/Challenges/Tutorial Chairs

Kenji Suzuki      Illinois Institute of Technology, USA
Hayit Greenspan      Tel Aviv University, Israel
Bram van Ginneken      Radboud University Medical Center, The Netherlands
Qian Wang      Shanghai Jiao Tong University, China
Luping Zhou      The University of Sydney, Australia
Hongen Liao      Tsinghua University, China

## MICCAI Society, Board of Directors

Leo Joskowicz (President)      The Hebrew University of Jerusalem, Israel
Stephen Aylward      Kitware, Inc., NY, USA
  (Treasurer)
Josien Pluim (Secretary)      Eindhoven University of Technology, The Netherlands
Wiro Niessen      Erasmus Medical Centre, The Netherlands
  (Past President)
Marleen de Bruijne      Erasmus Medical Centre, The Netherlands
                 and University of Copenhagen, Denmark
Hervé Delinguette      Inria, Sophia Antipolis, France
Caroline Essert      University of Strasbourg, France
Alejandro Frangi      University of Leeds, UK
Lena Maier-Hein      German Cancer Research Center, Germany

| | |
|---|---|
| Shuo Li | Western University, London, Canada |
| Tianming Liu | University of Georgia, USA |
| Anne Martel | University of Toronto, Canada |
| Daniel Racoceanu | Pontifical Catholic University of Peru, Peru |
| Julia Schnabel | King's College, London, UK |
| Guoyan Zheng | Institute for Surgical Technology & Biomechanics, Switzerland |
| Kevin Zhou | Chinese Academy of Sciences, China |

## Industry Forum

| | |
|---|---|
| Xiaodong Tao | iFLYTEK Health, China |
| Yiqiang Zhan | United Imaging Intelligence (UII), China |

## Publication Committee

| | |
|---|---|
| Gang Li | The University of North Carolina at Chapel Hill, USA |
| Li Wang | The University of North Carolina at Chapel Hill, USA |

## Finance Committee

| | |
|---|---|
| Dong Ni | Shenzhen University, China |
| Janette Wallace | Robarts Research Institute, Western University, Canada |
| Stephen Aylward | Kitware, Inc., USA |

## Local Organization Chairs

| | |
|---|---|
| Dong Ni | Shenzhen University, China |
| Jing Qin | The Hong Kong Polytechnic University, SAR China |
| Qianjin Feng | Southern Medical University, China |
| Dong Liang | Shenzhen Institutes of Advanced Technology, Chinese Academy of Sciences, China |
| Xiaoying Tang | Southern University of Science and Technology, China |

## Sponsors and Publicity Liaison

| | |
|---|---|
| Kevin Zhou | Institute of Computing Technology, Chinese Academy of Sciences, China |
| Hongen Liao | Tsinghua University, China |
| Wenjian Qin | Shenzhen Institutes of Advanced Technology, Chinese Academy of Sciences, China |

# Keynote Lectures Chairs

Max Viergever          University Medical Center Utrecht, The Netherlands
Kensaku Mori           Nagoya University, Japan
Gözde Ünal             Istanbul Technical University, Turkey

# Student Travel Award Committee

Huiguang He            Institute of Automation, Chinese Academy of Sciences,
                         China
Jun Shi                Shanghai University, China
Xi Jiang               University of Electronic Science and Technology
                         of China, China

# Student Activities Liaison

Julia Schnabel         King's College London, UK
Caroline Essert        University of Strasbourg, France
Dimitris Metaxas       Rutgers University, USA
MICCAI Student Board Members

# Area Chairs

Purang Abolmaesumi     The University of British Columbia, Canada
Shadi Albarqouni       The Technical University of Munich (TUM), Germany
Elsa Angelini          Imperial College London, UK
Suyash Awate           Indian Institute of Technology (IIT) Bombay, India
Ulas Bagci             University of Central Florida (UCF), USA
Kayhan Batmanghelich   University of Pittsburgh, USA
Christian Baumgartner  Swiss Federal Institute of Technology Zurich,
                         Switzerland
Ismail Ben Ayed        Ecole de Technologie Superieure (ETS), Canada
Weidong Cai            The University of Sydney, Australia
Xiaohuan Cao           United Imaging Intelligence (UII), China
Elvis Chen             Robarts Research Institute, Western University, Canada
Xinjian Chen           Soochow University, China
Jian Cheng             Beihang University, China
Jun Cheng              Cixi Institute of Biomedical Engineering, Chinese
                         Academy of Sciences, China
Veronika Cheplygina    Eindhoven University of Technology, The Netherlands
Elena De Momi          Politecnico di Milano, Italy
Ayman El-Baz           University of Louisville, USA
Aaron Fenster          Robarts Research Institute, Western University, USA
Moti Freiman           Philips Healthcare, The Netherlands
Yue Gao                Tsinghua University, China

| Xiujuan Geng | Chinese University of Hong Kong, SAR China |
| Stamatia Giannarou | Imperial College London, UK |
| Orcun Goksel | Swiss Federal Institute of Technology Zurich, Switzerland |
| Xiao Han | AI Healthcare Center, Tencent Inc., China |
| Huiguang He | Institute of Automation, Chinese Academy of Sciences, China |
| Yi Hong | The University of Georgia, USA |
| Junzhou Huang | The University of Texas at Arlington, USA |
| Xiaolei Huang | The Pennsylvania State University, USA |
| Juan Eugenio Iglesias | University College London, UK |
| Pierre Jannin | The University of Rennes, France |
| Bernhard Kainz | Imperial College London, UK |
| Ali Kamen | Siemens Healthcare, USA |
| Jaeil Kim | Kyungpook National University, South Korea |
| Andrew King | King's College London, UK |
| Karim Lekadir | Universitat Pompeu Fabra, Spain |
| Cristian Linte | Rochester Institute of Technology, USA |
| Mingxia Liu | The University of North Carolina at Chapel Hill, USA |
| Klaus Maier-Hein | German Cancer Research Center, Germany |
| Anne Martel | Sunnybrook Research Institute, USA |
| Andrew Melbourne | University College London, UK |
| Anirban Mukhopadhyay | Technische Universität Darmstadt, Germany |
| Anqi Qiu | National University of Singapore, Singapore |
| Islem Rekik | Istanbul Technical University, Turkey |
| Hassan Rivaz | Concordia University, USA |
| Feng Shi | United Imaging Intelligence (UII), China |
| Amber Simpson | Memorial Sloan Kettering Cancer Center, USA |
| Marius Staring | Leiden University Medical Center, The Netherlands |
| Heung-Il Suk | Korea University, South Korea |
| Tanveer Syeda-Mahmood | University Medical Center Utrecht, The Netherlands |
| Xiaoying Tang | Southern University of Science and Technology, China |
| Pallavi Tiwari | Case Western Reserve University, USA |
| Emanuele Trucco | University of Dundee, UK |
| Martin Urschler | Graz University of Technology, Austria |
| Hien Van Nguyen | University of Houston, USA |
| Archana Venkataraman | Johns Hopkins University, USA |
| Christian Wachinger | Ludwig Maximilian University of Munich, Germany |
| Linwei Wang | Rochester Institute of Technology, USA |
| Yong Xia | Northwestern Polytechnical University, China |
| Yanwu Xu | Baidu Inc., China |
| Zhong Xue | United Imaging Intelligence (UII), China |
| Pingkun Yan | Rensselaer Polytechnic Institute, USA |
| Xin Yang | Huazhong University of Science and Technology, China |
| Yixuan Yuan | City University of Hong Kong, SAR China |

Daoqiang Zhang                Nanjing University of Aeronautics and Astronautics,
                              China
Miaomiao Zhang                Washington University in St. Louis, USA
Tuo Zhang                     Northwestern Polytechnical University, China
Guoyan Zheng                  Shanghai Jiao Tong University, China
S. Kevin Zhou                 Institute of Computing Technology, Chinese Academy
                              of Sciences, China
Dajiang Zhu                   The University of Texas at Arlington, USA

# Reviewers

Abdi, Amir                              Barbu, Adrian
Abduljabbar, Khalid                     Bardosi, Zoltan
Adeli, Ehsan                            Bateson, Mathilde
Aganj, Iman                             Bathula, Deepti
Aggarwal, Priya                         Batmanghelich, Kayhan
Agrawal, Praful                         Baumgartner, Christian
Ahmad, Ola                              Baur, Christoph
Ahmad, Sahar                            Baxter, John
Ahn, Euijoon                            Bayramoglu, Neslihan
Akbar, Shazia                           Becker, Benjamin
Akhondi-Asl, Alireza                    Behnami, Delaram
Akram, Saad                             Beig, Niha
Al-Kadi, Omar                           Belyaev, Mikhail
Alansary, Amir                          Benkarim, Oualid
Alghamdi, Hanan                         Bentaieb, Aicha
Ali, Sharib                             Bernal, Jose
Allan, Maximilian                       Beyeler, Michael
Amiri, Mina                             Bhatia, Parmeet
Anton, Esther                           Bhole, Chetan
Anwar, Syed                             Bhushan, Chitresh
Armin, Mohammad                         Bi, Lei
Audigier, Chloe                         Bian, Cheng
Aviles-Rivero, Angelica                 Bilinski, Piotr
Awan, Ruqayya                           Bise, Ryoma
Awate, Suyash                           Bnouni, Nesrine
Aydogan, Dogu                           Bo, Wang
Azizi, Shekoofeh                        Bodenstedt, Sebastian
Bai, Junjie                             Bogunovic, Hrvoje
Bai, Wenjia                             Bozorgtabar, Behzad
Balbastre, Yaël                         Bragman, Felix
Balsiger, Fabian                        Braman, Nathaniel
Banerjee, Abhirup                       Bridge, Christopher
Bano, Sophia                            Broaddus, Coleman

Bron, Esther
Brooks, Rupert
Bruijne, Marleen
Bühler, Katja
Bui, Duc
Burlutskiy, Nikolay
Burwinkel, Hendrik
Bustin, Aurelien
Cabeen, Ryan
Cai, Hongmin
Cai, Jinzheng
Cai, Yunliang
Camino, Acner
Cao, Jiezhang
Cao, Qing
Cao, Tian
Carapella, Valentina
Cardenes, Ruben
Cardoso, M.
Carolus, Heike
Castro, Daniel
Cattin, Philippe
Chabanas, Matthieu
Chaddad, Ahmad
Chaitanya, Krishna
Chakraborty, Jayasree
Chakraborty, Rudrasis
Chang, Ken
Chang, Violeta
Charaborty, Tapabrata
Chatelain, Pierre
Chatterjee, Sudhanya
Chen, Alvin
Chen, Antong
Chen, Cameron
Chen, Chao
Chen, Chen
Chen, Elvis
Chen, Fang
Chen, Fei
Chen, Geng
Chen, Hanbo
Chen, Hao
Chen, Jia-Wei
Chen, Jialei
Chen, Jianxu

Chen, Jie
Chen, Jingyun
Chen, Lei
Chen, Liang
Chen, Min
Chen, Pingjun
Chen, Qingchao
Chen, Xiao
Chen, Xiaoran
Chen, Xin
Chen, Xuejin
Chen, Yang
Chen, Yuanyuan
Chen, Yuncong
Chen, Zhiqiang
Chen, Zhixiang
Cheng, Jun
Cheng, Li
Cheng, Yuan
Cheng, Yupeng
Cheriet, Farida
Chong, Minqi
Choo, Jaegul
Christiaens, Daan
Christodoulidis, Argyrios
Christodoulidis, Stergios
Chung, Ai
Çiçek, Özgün
Cid, Yashin
Clarkson, Matthew
Clough, James
Collins, Toby
Commowick, Olivier
Conze, Pierre-Henri
Cootes, Timothy
Correia, Teresa
Coulon, Olivier
Coupé, Pierrick
Courtecuisse, Hadrien
Craley, Jeffrey
Crimi, Alessandro
Cury, Claire
D'souza, Niharika
Dai, Hang
Dalca, Adrian
Das, Abhijit

Das, Dhritiman
Deeba, Farah
Dekhil, Omar
Demiray, Beatrice
Deniz, Cem
Depeursinge, Adrien
Desrosiers, Christian
Dewey, Blake
Dey, Raunak
Dhamala, Jwala
Ding, Meng
Distergoft, Alexander
Dobrenkii, Anton
Dolz, Jose
Dong, Liang
Dong, Mengjin
Dong, Nanqing
Dong, Xiao
Dong, Yanni
Dou, Qi
Du, Changde
Du, Lei
Du, Shaoyi
Duan, Dingna
Duan, Lixin
Dubost, Florian
Duchateau, Nicolas
Duncan, James
Duong, Luc
Dvornek, Nicha
Dzyubachyk, Oleh
Eaton-Rosen, Zach
Ebner, Michael
Ebrahimi, Mehran
Edwards, Philip
Egger, Bernhard
Eguizabal, Alma
Einarsson, Gudmundur
Ekin, Ahmet
Elazab, Ahmed
Elhabian, Shireen
Elmogy, Mohammed
Eltanboly, Ahmed
Erdt, Marius
Ernst, Floris
Esposito, Marco

Esteban, Oscar
Fan, Jingfan
Fan, Xin
Fan, Yong
Fan, Yonghui
Fang, Xi
Farag, Aly
Farzi, Mohsen
Fauser, Johannes
Fawaz, Hassan
Fedorov, Andrey
Fehri, Hamid
Feng, Chiyu
Feng, Jun
Feng, Xinyang
Feng, Yuan
Fenster, Aaron
Ferrante, Enzo
Feydy, Jean
Fischer, Lukas
Fischer, Peter
Fishbaugh, James
Fletcher, Tom
Flores, Kevin
Forestier, Germain
Forkert, Nils
Fotouhi, Javad
Fountoukidou, Tatiana
Franz, Alfred
Frau-Pascual, Aina
Freysinger, Wolfgang
Fripp, Jurgen
Fu, Huazhu
Funka-Lea, Gareth
Funke, Isabel
Funke, Jan
Fürnstahl, Philipp
Furukawa, Ryo
Gahm, Jin
Galassi, Francesca
Galdran, Adrian
Gan, Yu
Gao, Fei
Gao, Mingchen
Gao, Siyuan
Gao, Zhifan

Gardezi, Syed
Ge, Bao
Gerber, Samuel
Gerig, Guido
Gessert, Nils
Gevaert, Olivier
Gharabaghi, Sara
Ghesu, Florin
Ghimire, Sandesh
Gholipour, Ali
Ghosal, Sayan
Giraud, Rémi
Glocker, Ben
Goceri, Evgin
Goetz, Michael
Gomez, Alberto
Gong, Kuang
Gong, Mingming
Gonzalez, German
Gopal, Sharath
Gopinath, Karthik
Gordon, Shiri
Gori, Pietro
Gou, Shuiping
Granados, Alejandro
Grau, Vicente
Green, Michael
Gritsenko, Andrey
Grupp, Robert
Gu, Lin
Gu, Yun
Gu, Zaiwang
Gueziri, Houssem-Eddine
Guo, Hengtao
Guo, Jixiang
Guo, Xiaoqing
Guo, Yanrong
Guo, Yong
Gupta, Kratika
Gupta, Vikash
Gutman, Boris
Gyawali, Prashnna
Hacihaliloglu, Ilker
Hadjidemetriou, Stathis
Haldar, Justin
Hamarneh, Ghassan

Hamze, Noura
Han, Hu
Han, Jungong
Han, Xiaoguang
Han, Xu
Han, Zhi
Hancox, Jonny
Hanson, Erik
Hao, Xiaoke
Haq, Rabia
Harders, Matthias
Harrison, Adam
Haskins, Grant
Hatamizadeh, Ali
Hatt, Charles
Hauptmann, Andreas
Havaei, Mohammad
He, Tiancheng
He, Yufan
Heimann, Tobias
Heldmann, Stefan
Heller, Nicholas
Hernandez-Matas, Carlos
Hernandez, Monica
Hett, Kilian
Higger, Matt
Hinkle, Jacob
Ho, Tsung-Ying
Hoffmann, Nico
Holden, Matthew
Hong, Song
Hong, Sungmin
Hou, Benjamin
Hsu, Li-Ming
Hu, Dan
Hu, Kai
Hu, Xiaowei
Hu, Xintao
Hu, Yan
Hu, Yipeng
Huang, Heng
Huang, Huifang
Huang, Jiashuang
Huang, Kevin
Huang, Ruobing
Huang, Shih-Gu

Huang, Weilin
Huang, Xiaolei
Huang, Yawen
Huang, Yixing
Huang, Yufang
Huang, Zhongwei
Huaulmé, Arnaud
Huisman, Henkjan
Huo, Xing
Huo, Yuankai
Husch, Andreas
Hussein, Sarfaraz
Hutter, Jana
Hwang, Seong
Icke, Ilknur
Igwe, Kay
Ingalhalikar, Madhura
Irmakci, Ismail
Ivashchenko, Oleksandra
Izadyyazdanabadi, Mohammadhassan
Jafari, Mohammad
Jäger, Paul
Jamaludin, Amir
Janatka, Mirek
Jaouen, Vincent
Jarayathne, Uditha
Javadi, Golara
Javer, Avelino
Jensen, Todd
Ji, Zexuan
Jia, Haozhe
Jiang, Jue
Jiang, Steve
Jiang, Tingting
Jiang, Weixiong
Jiang, Xi
Jiao, Jianbo
Jiao, Jieqing
Jiao, Zhicheng
Jie, Biao
Jin, Dakai
Jin, Taisong
Jin, Yueming
John, Rogers
Joshi, Anand
Joshi, Shantanu

Jud, Christoph
Jung, Kyu-Hwan
Jungo, Alain
Kadkhodamohammadi, Abdolrahim
Kakileti, Siva
Kamnitsas, Konstantinos
Kang, Eunsong
Kao, Po-Yu
Kapoor, Ankur
Karani, Neerav
Karayumak, Suheyla
Kazi, Anees
Kerrien, Erwan
Kervadec, Hoel
Khalifa, Fahmi
Khalili, Nadieh
Khallaghi, Siavash
Khalvati, Farzad
Khan, Hassan
Khanal, Bishesh
Khansari, Maziyar
Khosravan, Naji
Kia, Seyed
Kikinis, Ron
Kim, Geena
Kim, Hosung
Kim, Hyo-Eun
Kim, Jae-Hun
Kim, Jinman
Kim, Jinyoung
Kim, Minjeong
Kim, Namkug
Kim, Seong
Kim, Young-Ho
Kitasaka, Takayuki
Klein, Stefan
Klinder, Tobias
Kolli, Kranthi
Kong, Bin
Kong, Xiang-Zhen
Konukoglu, Ender
Koo, Bongjin
Koohbanani, Navid
Kopriva, Ivica
Kose, Kivanc
Koutsoumpa, Christina

Liu, Bin
Liu, Daochang
Liu, Dong
Liu, Dongnan
Liu, Fang
Liu, Feihong
Liu, Feng
Liu, Hong
Liu, Hui
Liu, Jianfei
Liu, Jiang
Liu, Jin
Liu, Jing
Liu, Jundong
Liu, Kefei
Liu, Li
Liu, Mingxia
Liu, Na
Liu, Peng
Liu, Shenghua
Liu, Siqi
Liu, Siyuan
Liu, Tianming
Liu, Tiffany
Liu, Xianglong
Liu, Yixun
Liu, Yong
Liu, Yue
Liu, Zhe
Loddo, Andrea
Lopes, Daniel
Lorenzi, Marco
Lou, Bin
Lu, Allen
Lu, Donghuan
Lu, Jiwen
Lu, Le
Lu, Weijia
Lu, Yao
Lu, Yueh-Hsun
Luo, Gongning
Luo, Jie
Lv, Jinglei
Lyu, Ilwoo
Lyu, Junyan
Ma, Benteng

Ma, Burton
Ma, Da
Ma, Kai
Ma, Xuelin
Mahapatra, Dwarikanath
Mahdavi, Sara
Mahmoud, Ali
Maicas, Gabriel
Maier-Hein, Klaus
Maier, Andreas
Makrogiannis, Sokratis
Malandain, Grégoire
Malik, Bilal
Malpani, Anand
Mancini, Matteo
Manhart, Michael
Manjon, Jose
Mansoor, Awais
Mao, Yunxiang
Martel, Anne
Martinez-Torteya, Antonio
Mathai, Tejas
Mato, David
Mcclelland, Jamie
Mcleod, Jonathan
Medrano-Gracia, Pau
Mehta, Ronak
Meier, Raphael
Melbourne, Andrew
Meng, Qingjie
Meng, Xianjing
Meng, Yu
Menze, Bjoern
Mi, Liang
Miao, Shun
Michielse, Stijn
Midya, Abhishek
Milchenko, Mikhail
Min, Zhe
Miyamoto, Tadashi
Mo, Yuanhan
Molina, Rafael
Montillo, Albert
Moradi, Mehdi
Moreno, Rodrigo
Mortazi, Aliasghar

Mozaffari, Mohammad
Muetzel, Ryan
Müller, Henning
Muñoz-Barrutia, Arrate
Munsell, Brent
Nadeem, Saad
Nahlawi, Layan
Nandakumar, Naresh
Nardi, Giacomo
Neila, Pablo
Ni, Dong
Nichols, Thomas
Nickisch, Hannes
Nie, Dong
Nie, Jingxin
Nie, Weizhi
Niethammer, Marc
Nigam, Aditya
Ning, Lipeng
Niu, Shuaicheng
Niu, Sijie
Noble, Jack
Noblet, Vincent
Novo, Jorge
O'donnell, Thomas
Obeid, Mohammad
Oda, Hirohisa
Oda, Masahiro
Odry, Benjamin
Oeltze-Jafra, Steffen
Oksuz, Ilkay
Oliveira, Marcelo
Oliver, Arnau
Oñativia, Jon
Onofrey, John
Orasanu, Eliza
Orihuela-Espina, Felipe
Orlando, Jose
Osmanlioglu, Yusuf
Otalora, Sebastian
Pace, Danielle
Pagador, J.
Pai, Akshay
Pan, Yongsheng
Pang, Shumao
Papiez, Bartlomiej

Parajuli, Nripesh
Park, Hyunjin
Park, Jongchan
Park, Sanghyun
Park, Seung-Jong
Paschali, Magdalini
Paul, Angshuman
Payer, Christian
Pei, Yuru
Peng, Jialin
Peng, Tingying
Pennec, Xavier
Perdomo, Oscar
Pereira, Sérgio
Pérez-Carrasco, Jose-Antonio
Pesteie, Mehran
Peter, Loic
Peters, Jorg
Petitjean, Caroline
Pezold, Simon
Pfeiffer, Micha
Phellan, Renzo
Phophalia, Ashish
Pisharady, Pramod
Playout, Clement
Pluim, Josien
Pohl, Kilian
Portenier, Tiziano
Pouch, Alison
Prasanna, Prateek
Prevost, Raphael
Ps, Viswanath
Pujades, Sergi
Qi, Xin
Qian, Zhen
Qiang, Yan
Qiao, Lishan
Qiao, Yuchuan
Qin, Chen
Qin, Wenjian
Qirong, Bu
Qiu, Wu
Qu, Liangqiong
Raamana, Pradeep
Rabbani, Hossein
Rackerseder, Julia

Rad, Reza
Rafii-Tari, Hedyeh
Rajpoot, Kashif
Ramachandram, Dhanesh
Ran, Lingyan
Raniga, Parnesh
Rashwan, Hatem
Rathore, Saima
Ratnarajah, Nagulan
Raval, Mehul
Ravikumar, Nishant
Raviprakash, Harish
Raza, Shan
Reaungamornrat, Surreerat
Rekik, Islem
Remeseiro, Beatriz
Rempfler, Markus
Ren, Jian
Ren, Xuhua
Ren, Yudan
Reyes-Aldasoro, Constantino
Reyes, Mauricio
Riedel, Brandalyn
Rieke, Nicola
Risser, Laurent
Rittner, Leticia
Rivera, Diego
Ro, Yong
Robinson, Emma
Robinson, Robert
Rodas, Nicolas
Rodrigues, Rafael
Rohr, Karl
Roohani, Yusuf
Roszkowiak, Lukasz
Roth, Holger
Rouco, José
Roy, Abhijit
Ruijters, Danny
Rusu, Mirabela
Rutter, Erica
S., Sharath
Sabuncu, Mert
Sachse, Frank
Safta, Wiem
Saha, Monjoy

Saha, Pramit
Sahu, Manish
Samani, Abbas
Samek, Wojciech
Sánchez-Margallo, Francisco
Sánchez-Margallo, Juan
Sankaran, Sethuraman
Sanroma, Gerard
Sao, Anil
Sarhan, Mhd
Sarikaya, Duygu
Sarker, Md.
Sato, Imari
Saut, Olivier
Savardi, Mattia
Savitha, Ramasamy
Scarpa, Fabio
Scheinost, Dustin
Scherf, Nico
Schirmer, Markus
Schlaefer, Alexander
Schmid, Jerome
Schnabel, Julia
Schultz, Thomas
Schwartz, Ernst
Sdika, Michael
Sedai, Suman
Sekou, Taibou
Sekuboyina, Anjany
Selvan, Raghavendra
Semedo, Carla
Senouf, Ortal
Seoud, Lama
Sermesant, Maxime
Serrano, Carmen
Sethi, Amit
Shaban, Muhammad
Shaffie, Ahmed
Shah, Meet
Shalaby, Ahmed
Shamir, Reuben
Shan, Hongming
Shao, Yeqin
Sharma, Harshita
Shehata, Mohamed
Shen, Haocheng

Shen, Li
Shen, Mali
Shen, Yiru
Sheng, Ke
Shi, Bibo
Shi, Jun
Shi, Kuangyu
Shi, Xiaoshuang
Shi, Yonggang
Shi, Yonghong
Shigwan, Saurabh
Shin, Hoo-Chang
Shin, Jitae
Shontz, Suzanne
Signoroni, Alberto
Siless, Viviana
Silva, Carlos
Silva, Wilson
Simonovsky, Martin
Simson, Walter
Sinclair, Matthew
Singh, Vivek
Soans, Rajath
Sohel, Ferdous
Sokooti, Hessam
Soliman, Ahmed
Sommen, Fons
Sommer, Stefan
Song, Ming
Song, Yang
Sotiras, Aristeidis
Sparks, Rachel
Spiclin, Ziga
St-Jean, Samuel
Steinbach, Peter
Stern, Darko
Stimpel, Bernhard
Strait, Justin
Studholme, Colin
Styner, Martin
Su, Hai
Su, Yun-Hsuan
Subramanian, Vaishnavi
Subsol, Gérard
Sudre, Carole
Suk, Heung-Il

Sun, Jian
Sun, Li
Sun, Tao
Sung, Kyunghyun
Suter, Yannick
Tajbakhsh, Nima
Tan, Chaowei
Tan, Jiaxing
Tan, Wenjun
Tang, Min
Tang, Sheng
Tang, Thomas
Tang, Xiaoying
Tang, Youbao
Tang, Yuxing
Tang, Zhenyu
Tanner, Christine
Tanno, Ryutaro
Tao, Qian
Tarroni, Giacomo
Tasdizen, Tolga
Thung, Kim
Tian, Jiang
Tian, Yun
Toews, Matthew
Tong, Yubing
Topsakal, Oguzhan
Torosdagli, Neslisah
Toussaint, Nicolas
Troccaz, Jocelyne
Trzcinski, Tomasz
Tulder, Gijs
Tustison, Nick
Tuysuzoglu, Ahmet
Ukwatta, Eranga
Unberath, Mathias
Ungi, Tamas
Upadhyay, Uddeshya
Urschler, Martin
Uslu, Fatmatulzehra
Uyanik, Ilyas
Vaillant, Régis
Vakalopoulou, Maria
Valindria, Vanya
Varela, Marta
Varsavsky, Thomas

Vedula, S.
Vedula, Sanketh
Veeraraghavan, Harini
Vega, Roberto
Veni, Gopalkrishna
Verma, Ujjwal
Vetter, Thomas
Vialard, Francois-Xavier
Villard, Pierre-Frederic
Villarini, Barbara
Virga, Salvatore
Vishnevskiy, Valery
Viswanath, Satish
Vlontzos, Athanasios
Vogl, Wolf-Dieter
Voigt, Ingmar
Vos, Bob
Vrtovec, Tomaz
Wang, Bo
Wang, Changmiao
Wang, Chengjia
Wang, Chunliang
Wang, Dadong
Wang, Guotai
Wang, Haifeng
Wang, Haoqian
Wang, Hongkai
Wang, Hongzhi
Wang, Hua
Wang, Huan
Wang, Jiazhuo
Wang, Jingwen
Wang, Jun
Wang, Junyan
Wang, Kuanquan
Wang, Kun
Wang, Lei
Wang, Li
Wang, Liansheng
Wang, Manning
Wang, Mingliang
Wang, Nizhuan
Wang, Pei
Wang, Puyang
Wang, Ruixuan
Wang, Shanshan

Wang, Sheng
Wang, Shuai
Wang, Wenzhe
Wang, Xiangxue
Wang, Xiaosong
Wang, Xuchu
Wang, Yalin
Wang, Yan
Wang, Yaping
Wang, Yuanjun
Wang, Ze
Wang, Zhe
Wang, Zhinuo
Wang, Zhiwei
Wang, Zilei
Weber, Jonathan
Wee, Chong-Yaw
Weese, Jürgen
Wei, Benzheng
Wei, Dong
Wei, Donglai
Wei, Dongming
Weigert, Martin
Wein, Wolfgang
Wels, Michael
Wemmert, Cédric
Werner, Rene
Wesierski, Daniel
Williams, Bryan
Williams, Jacqueline
Williams, Travis
Williamson, Tom
Wilms, Matthias
Wiskin, James
Wittek, Adam
Wollmann, Thomas
Wolterink, Jelmer
Wong, Ken
Woo, Jonghye
Wu, Guoqing
Wu, Ji
Wu, Jian
Wu, Jiong
Wu, Pengxiang
Wu, Xi
Wu, Ye

Wu, Yicheng
Wuerfl, Tobias
Xi, Xiaoming
Xia, Jing
Xia, Wenfeng
Xiao, Deqiang
Xiao, Yiming
Xie, Hai
Xie, Hongtao
Xie, Jianyang
Xie, Long
Xie, Weidi
Xie, Yiting
Xie, Yuanpu
Xie, Yutong
Xing, Fuyong
Xiong, Tao
Xu, Chenchu
Xu, Jiaofeng
Xu, Jun
Xu, Kele
Xu, Rui
Xu, Ting
Xu, Yan
Xu, Yongchao
Xu, Zheng
Xu, Zhenlin
Xu, Zhoubing
Xu, Ziyue
Xue, Jie
Xue, Wufeng
Xue, Yuan
Yahya, Faridah
Yan, Chenggang
Yan, Ke
Yan, Weizheng
Yan, Yu
Yan, Yuguang
Yan, Zhennan
Yang, Guang
Yang, Guanyu
Yang, Hao-Yu
Yang, Jie
Yang, Lin
Yang, Shan
Yang, Xiao

Yang, Xiaohui
Yang, Xin
Yao, Dongren
Yao, Jianhua
Yao, Jiawen
Ye, Chuyang
Ye, Jong
Ye, Menglong
Ye, Xujiong
Yi, Jingru
Yi, Xin
Ying, Shihui
Yoo, Youngjin
Yousefi, Bardia
Yousefi, Sahar
Yu, Jinhua
Yu, Kai
Yu, Lequan
Yu, Renping
Yu, Weichuan
Yushkevich, Paul
Zanjani, Farhad
Zenati, Marco
Zeng, Dong
Zeng, Guodong
Zettinig, Oliver
Zhan, Liang
Zhang, Baochang
Zhang, Chuncheng
Zhang, Dongqing
Zhang, Fan
Zhang, Haichong
Zhang, Han
Zhang, Haopeng
Zhang, Heye
Zhang, Jianpeng
Zhang, Jiong
Zhang, Jun
Zhang, Le
Zhang, Lichi
Zhang, Mingli
Zhang, Pengyue
Zhang, Pin
Zhang, Qiang
Zhang, Rongzhao
Zhang, Shengping

Zhang, Shu
Zhang, Songze
Zhang, Tianyang
Zhang, Tong
Zhang, Wei
Zhang, Wen
Zhang, Wenlu
Zhang, Xiang
Zhang, Xin
Zhang, Yi
Zhang, Yifan
Zhang, Yizhe
Zhang, Yong
Zhang, Yongqin
Zhang, You
Zhang, Yu
Zhang, Yue
Zhang, Yueyi
Zhang, Yungeng
Zhang, Yunyan
Zhang, Yuyao
Zhang, Zizhao
Zhao, Haifeng
Zhao, Jun
Zhao, Qingyu
Zhao, Rongchang
Zhao, Shijie
Zhao, Shiwan
Zhao, Tengda
Zhao, Wei
Zhao, Yitian
Zhao, Yiyuan

Zhao, Yu
Zhao, Zijian
Zheng, Shenhai
Zheng, Yalin
Zheng, Yinqiang
Zhong, Zichun
Zhou, Bo
Zhou, Jianlong
Zhou, Luping
Zhou, Niyun
Zhou, S.
Zhou, Shoujun
Zhou, Tao
Zhou, Wenjin
Zhou, Yuyin
Zhou, Zhiguo
Zhu, Hancan
Zhu, Junjie
Zhu, Qikui
Zhu, Weifang
Zhu, Wentao
Zhu, Xiaofeng
Zhu, Xinliang
Zhu, Yingying
Zhu, Yuemin
Zhu, Zhuotun
Zhuang, Xiahai
Zia, Aneeq
Zimmer, Veronika
Zolgharni, Massoud
Zou, Ju
Zuluaga, Maria

# Accepted MICCAI 2019 Papers

## By Region of First Author

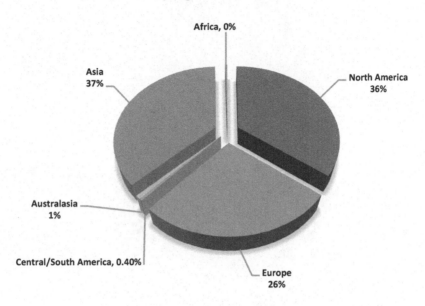

Africa, 0%

Asia
37%

North America
36%

Australasia
1%

Central/South America, 0.40%

Europe
26%

## By Technical Keyword

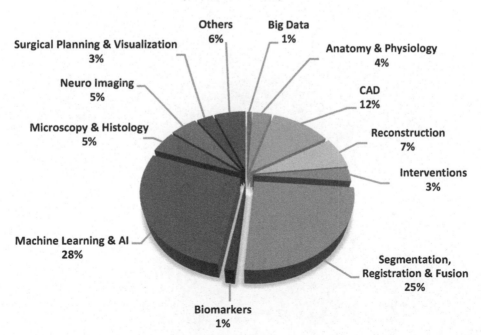

Others
6%

Big Data
1%

Surgical Planning & Visualization
3%

Anatomy & Physiology
4%

Neuro Imaging
5%

CAD
12%

Microscopy & Histology
5%

Reconstruction
7%

Interventions
3%

Machine Learning & AI
28%

Segmentation,
Registration & Fusion
25%

Biomarkers
1%

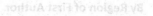

# Accepted MICCAI 2019 Papers

## By Region of First Author

Africa, 0%
North America 35%
Asia 37%
Australasia 1%
Central/South America 0.xx%
Europe 26%

## By Technical Keyword

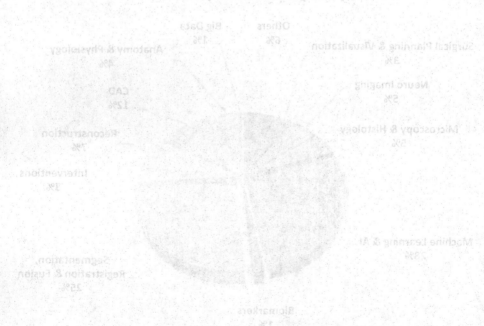

Big Data 1%
Others 6%
Anatomy & Physiology 4%
Surgical Planning & Visualization 3%
CAD 12%
Neuro Imaging 5%
Reconstruction 7%
Microscopy & Histology 5%
Interventions 1%
Machine Learning & AI 28%
Segmentation, Registration & Fusion 25%
Biomarkers 1%

# Awards Presented at MICCAI 2018, Granada, Spain

MICCAI Society Enduring Impact Award: The Enduring Impact Award is the highest award of the MICCAI Society. It is a career award for continued excellence in the MICCAI research field. The 2018 Enduring Impact Award was presented to Sandy Wells, Brigham and Women's Hospital/Harvard Medical School, USA.

MICCAI Society Fellowships: MICCAI Fellowships are bestowed annually on a small number of senior members of the society in recognition of substantial scientific contributions to the MICCAI research field and service to the MICCAI community. In 2018, fellowships were awarded to:

- Pierre Jannin (Université de Rennes, France)
- Anne Martel (University of Toronto, Canada)
- Julia Schnabel (King's College London, UK)

Medical Image Analysis Journal Award Sponsored by Elsevier: Jianyu Lin, for his paper entitled "Dual-modality Endoscopic Probe for Tissue Surface Shape Reconstruction and Hyperspectral Imaging Enabled by Deep Neural Networks," authored by Jianyu Lin, Neil T. Clancy, Ji Qi, Yang Hu, Taran Tatla, Danail Stoyanov, Lena Maier-Hein, and Daniel S. Elson.

Best Paper in *International Journal of Computer-Assisted Radiology and Surgery* (IJCARS) journal: Arash Pourtaherian for his paper entitled "Robust and Semantic Needle Detection in 3D Ultrasound Using Orthogonal-Plane Convolutional Neural Networks," authored by Arash Pourtaherian, Farhad Ghazvinian Zanjani, Svitlana Zinger, Nenad Mihajlovic, Gary C. Ng, Hendrikus H. M. Korsten, and Peter H. N. de With.

Young Scientist Publication Impact Award: MICCAI papers by a young scientist from the past 5 years were eligible for this award. It is made to a researcher whose work had an impact on the MICCAI field in terms of citations, secondary citations, subsequent publications, h-index. The 2018 Young Scientist Publication Impact Award was given to Holger R Roth: "A New 2.5D Representation for Lymph Node Detection Using Random Sets of Deep Convolutional Neural Network Observations" authored by Holger R. Roth, Le Lu, Ari Seff, Kevin M. Cherry, Joanne Hoffman, Shijun Wang, Jiamin Liu, Evrim Turkbey, and Ronald M. Summers.

MICCAI Young Scientist Awards: The Young Scientist Awards are stimulation prizes awarded for the best first authors of MICCAI contributions in distinct subject areas. The nominees had to be full-time students at a recognized university at, or within, two years prior to submission. The 2018 MICCAI Young Scientist Awards were given to:

- Erik J. Bekkers for the paper entitled: "Roto-Translation Covariant Convolutional Networks for Medical Image Analysis"
- Bastian Bier for the paper entitled: "X-ray-transform Invariant Anatomical Landmark Detection for Pelvic Trauma Surgery"

- Yuanhan Mo for his paper entitled: "The Deep Poincaré Map: A Novel Approach for Left Ventricle Segmentation"
- Tanya Nair for the paper entitled: "Exploring Uncertainty Measures in Deep Networks for Multiple Sclerosis Lesion Detection and Segmentation"
- Yue Zhang for the paper entitled: "Task-Driven Generative Modeling for Unsupervised Domain Adaptation: Application to X-ray Image Segmentation"

# Contents – Part I

# Optical Imaging

# Enhancing OCT Signal by Fusion of GANs: Improving Statistical Power of Glaucoma Clinical Trials

Georgios Lazaridis[1,3,4](✉), Marco Lorenzi[2], Sebastien Ourselin[3], and David Garway-Heath[4,5]

[1] Centre for Medical Image Computing, University College London, London, UK
G.Lazaridis@cs.ucl.ac.uk
[2] Université Côte d'Azur, Inria Sophia Antipolis, Epione Research Project,
Nice, France
[3] School of Biomedical Engineering and Imaging Sciences, King's College London,
London, UK
[4] NIHR Biomedical Research Centre at Moorfields Eye Hospital NHS Foundation
Trust, London, UK
[5] Institute of Ophthalmology, University College London, London, UK

**Abstract.** Accurately monitoring the efficacy of disease-modifying drugs in glaucoma therapy is of critical importance. Albeit high resolution spectral-domain optical coherence tomography (SDOCT) is now in widespread clinical use, past landmark glaucoma clinical trials have used time-domain optical coherence tomography (TDOCT), which leads, however, to poor statistical power due to low signal-to-noise characteristics. Here, we propose a probabilistic ensemble model for improving the statistical power of imaging-based clinical trials. TDOCT are converted to synthesized SDOCT images and segmented via Bayesian fusion of an ensemble of generative adversarial networks (GANs). The proposed model integrates super resolution (SR) and multi-atlas segmentation (MAS) in a principled way. Experiments on the UK Glaucoma Treatment Study (UKGTS) show that the model successfully combines the strengths of both techniques (improved image quality of SR and effective label propagation of MAS), and produces a significantly better separation between treatment arms than conventional segmentation of TDOCT.

## 1 Introduction

Glaucoma is the leading cause of irreversible blindness. Evaluating the progression rate of the pathology is crucial in order to assess the risk of functional impairment and to establish sound treatment strategies [1]. Clinically, optical coherence tomography (OCT) is used as a surrogate measure to evaluate retinal

**Electronic supplementary material** The online version of this chapter (https://doi.org/10.1007/978-3-030-32239-7_1) contains supplementary material, which is available to authorized users.

© Springer Nature Switzerland AG 2019
D. Shen et al. (Eds.): MICCAI 2019, LNCS 11764, pp. 3–11, 2019.
https://doi.org/10.1007/978-3-030-32239-7_1

ganglion cell loss by measuring retinal nerve fibre layer (RNFL) thickness around the optic nerve head (ONH), whereas standard automated perimetry (SAP) is employed to assess the status of the visual field (VF) [1].

Glaucoma research has produced several clinical trials, trying to monitor the disease progression and the efficacy of disease-modifying drugs. Up until the introduction of high-resolution spectral-domain OCT (SDOCT), trials relied on time-domain OCT (TDOCT), characterized by lower quality acquisitions and signal-to-noise (SNR) ratio. Thus, structural measurements in past studies provided low statistical power in detecting significant treatment effects. Such an example is the UK Glaucoma Treatment Study (UKGTS) [1]. The UKGTS is the only glaucoma study to assess the vision-preserving efficacy of one disease-modifying drug with both VF and OCT outcome. Nonetheless, TDOCT information could not be effectively combined with VF outcomes to improve detection of a treatment effect. Improving the quality of image-related anatomical measurements is therefore imperative for increasing statistical power in clinical trials.

While prospective studies seek to modify the statistical power determinants [2], retrospective analyses aim to maximize effect size in order to gain insight on the efficacy of disease-modifying drugs. For instance, optimal spatial image smoothing [3] prior to analysis can improve statistical power to detect group differences. In [4], it has been proposed to use reference images to guide statistical analysis of a new dataset through transfer learning, and to select only relevant voxels in novel studies. When image segmentation is required, multi-atlas segmentation (MAS) [5] is successful in leveraging diverse reference image information, by propagating atlas labels to novel image coordinates.

Meanwhile, various methods for super resolution (SR) using convolutional neural networks (CNNs), such as generative adversarial networks (GANs), have been proposed to transform image quality and appearance [6–10]. In medical imaging, GANs have been successfully employed to address the ill-posed nature of cross-modal synthesis. For example, in [6–8], GANs have been proposed to predict computed tomography (CT) and positron emission tomography (PET) images from magnetic resonance imaging (MRI). Concerning signal enhancement as well, in [9] and [10], synthesis was achieved at different resolution scales and by enforcing cycle-consistency, albeit not focusing on medical applications. These works may, however, present important limitations for SR in medical imaging. First, due to the restricted view of GANs spatial window, preservation of spatial smoothness and anatomical features in predictions is not always guaranteed. Second, single GAN predictions are characterized by spatial and intensity variability. Therefore, in order to extract robust anatomical quantifications from the output of GANs, principled schemes accounting for prediction uncertainty must be developed. This requires, for instance, probabilistic modeling of the uncertainty of the underlying signal distributions on distinct image parts, to preserve anatomical structures and account for spatial coherency.

This paper presents a novel method to improve the statistical power of clinical trials with low quality images. Our methodology leverages Bayesian fusion of GANs to infer morphological descriptors from low to high quality anatomical information. The transfer mapping is learned in an independent dataset and the proposed method is demonstrated on the UKGTS, enhancing the power of TDOCT via quality transfer from SDOCT. As a result, RNFL segmentations are improved and further refined via the effective label-propagation of MAS.

## 2 Materials and Methods

### 2.1 Data

We used two studies to validate and test our proposed methodology. For training and validation, we used the RAPID study: 82 glaucoma patients attended for up to 10 visits within a 3-month period, consisting of 4.902 TDOCT (StratusOCT, ZEISS) and 1.789 SDOCT (SpectralisOCT, Heidelberg Engineering) images. For testing, we used the UKGTS subset of participants with TDOCT imaging available [1]: 373 glaucoma patients, attended for up to 2 years. Eligible patients were assigned to treatment with Latanoprost 0.005% or placebo. The UGKTS consists solely of 78.415 TDOCT (StratusOCT, ZEISS) images.

### 2.2 Proposed Methodology

The definition of our framework requires to address a number of challenges. First, due to different acquisition protocols, the pairing between target SDOCT and predictor TDOCT training images is ill-defined. To solve this issue, we propose an automated method for target-predictor image pairing (Sect. 2.2.1). Second, OCT signal is characterized by diverse degrees of noise and spatial information, whereas RNFL segmentation is subject to variability due to the different attributes of the synthesized images. This problem is tackled in Sect. 2.2.2, where we present our method to obtain representations accounting for the different spatial coherence of OCT images. Finally, in Sect. 2.2.3 we identify a probabilistic consensus strategy for RNFL segmentations on the average synthesized image.

### 2.2.1 Training Pairs Generation

Although TDOCT and SDOCT images were acquired at each patient visit, there is not a correspondence between the two sets of predictor and target modalities. Our method finds a matching based on global and local image information represented by (i) the vessel profile given by the average retinal pigment epithelium (RPE) pixel intensity, (ii) the internal limiting membrane (ILM) contour and (iii) the average norm of the deformation fields between TDOCT and SDOCT images within a patient's longitudinal history. First, as the topography around the ONH undulates, we flatten all images using a pilot estimate of the hyper-reflective RPE layer. Hence, images are aligned according to a fixed vertical RPE offset. We further exploit the RPE identification to detect the vessels, as they appear as shaded bands in the RPE. We then segment the ILM contour (upper high-contrast boundary on the dark-to-bright gradient image) and smooth it by Gaussian Process interpolation. Iterative closest point was used to evaluate the matching between the sets of features in (i) and (ii), and mutual information to evaluate the image registration in (iii). We evaluate the robustness of our pairing method on a benchmark of synthetic images with spatial variability, achieving 100% sensitivity (see Supplementary material). We note that a patient with N TDOCT and M SDOCT can theoretically produce a maximum of N×M images. Application to the RAPID dataset lead to 24.792 TDOCT and SDOCT pairs.

### 2.2.2  Ensemble GANs

To account for the specific anatomical geometry and signal properties in OCT images, we propose an adaptation of standard cycle-consistent GANs (cycle-GANs) [10], to improve robustness and accuracy of the modality transfer. OCT images have a very specific geometry where the background, i.e. vitreous cavity, is clearly separated from the layers at the ILM. Thus, we used image stitching, exploiting the ILM identification, to separate background from layer signal. Moreover, cycleGANs require a fixed window on which spatial filters and mappings are learned. However, since OCT signal and noise properties are characterized by different spatial scales, a modality transfer method based on a fixed spatial window might not be able to capture all the necessary spatial information needed for synthesis. This reduces the chance for cross-modal distributions to share supports in latent space. To address this problem, we propose an ensemble of spatially coherent cycleGANs [10] to learn the TDOCT-to-SDOCT mapping and to translate a TDOCT into a synthesized SDOCT image. The scheme is the following. Each GAN is trained by employing a different spatial window size: $128 \times 128$, $256 \times 256$ and $512 \times 512$, learning a mapping from the observed TDOCT image $I_{TD}$ and random noise vector $z$, to the target SDOCT image $I_{SD}$, $G \colon \{I_{TD},\, z\} \to I_{SD}$. As a result, we train six GANs: three with background pairs and three with layer pairs. The synthesized backgrounds and layers are stitched back according to the window size, i.e. $I_{128 \times 128}$, $I_{256 \times 256}$, $I_{512 \times 512}$ and the average synthesized stitched image $\bar{I}$ is obtained. To preserve the morphological correlation between training pairs, cycleGANs were trained with windows centered at the same geometrical location in both pairs. Figure 1 shows the proposed framework for OCT synthesis via the ensemble of GANs.

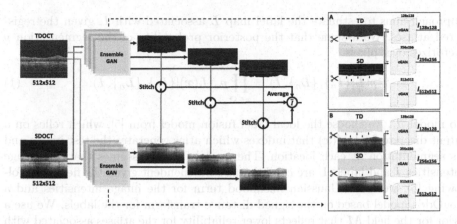

**Fig. 1.** SDOCT synthesis via ensemble of GANs. Three GANs are trained with backgrounds (box A) and three with layers (box B). Synthesized images are stitched back and the average synthesized stitched image is obtained. Separation of layers and background is illustrated with scissors.

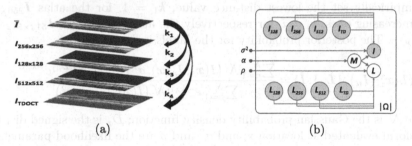

(a)                                   (b)

**Fig. 2.** (a) Stack of images, where $k_1, k_2, k_3, k_4$ are the distances between $\bar{I}$ and $I_{256\times256}$, $I_{128\times128}$, $I_{512\times512}$ and $I_{\text{TDOCT}}$. (b) Graphical model representing the relationship between the model variables in MAS. Replications are illustrated with plates. Shaded variables are observed.

## 2.2.3   Multi-atlas Segmentation

Once the average synthesized stitched image $\bar{I}$ is obtained, the problem consists in finding a robust RNFL segmentation accounting for the signal variability introduced by the synthesis. We treat images as being in a stack where $\bar{I}$ is used as test image, and, $I_{128\times128}$, $I_{256\times256}$, $I_{512\times512}$, and the original $I_{\text{TDOCT}}$ as atlases, here denoted by $\{I_n(\boldsymbol{x})\}_{n=1,\dots,4}$ (Fig. 2a). We want to propagate the atlas RNFL labels to the novel test image coordinates, where the segmentation of each pixel is decided through a label fusion approach. To account for the variability across atlases, we rely on a Bayesian model averaging technique, the graphical model of which is shown in Fig. 2b. Let $\{L_n(\boldsymbol{x})\}_{n=1,\dots,4}$ be segmentations corresponding to the atlases $\{I_n(\boldsymbol{x})\}$. We assume that these atlases are co-registered to the test image $\bar{I}(\boldsymbol{x})$, with unknown labels $L(\boldsymbol{x})$. A label fusion approach aims to estimate the label map $L$ associated with $\bar{I}$, given the registered atlases. We assume that the posterior probability of the segmentation $p$ factorizes over pixels:

$$p(L|\{I_n\},\{L_n\},\bar{I}) = \prod_{x \in \Omega} p_x(L(x)|\{I_n\},\{L_n\},\bar{I}) \tag{1}$$

To model $p_x$, we choose the local label fusion model from [5], which relies on a latent discrete field $M(x)$ that indexes which atlas generates the test image and its segmentation at each location. The model further assumes that the image intensities $\bar{I}$ and labels $L$ are conditionally independent given the field $M$. Following [5], we use a Gaussian likelihood term for the image intensities and a LogOdds model based on the signed distance transform for the labels. We use a prior for the field $M$ that reflects lower reliability for the atlases associated with lower registration accuracy [11]. For each 2D location $x$, the prior takes the form $p(M(x) = n) \propto \exp(-k_n\alpha)$, where the coefficients $k_n$, $n = 1, 2, 3, 4$, are the distances between the test image $\bar{I}$ and the atlases, while $\alpha$ is a parameter controlling the sharpness of the prior. Based on our experimental registration results, we empirically set the lowest distance value, $k_1 = 1$, for the atlas $I_{256 \times 256}$, and increasing ones, $k_i = i$, for respectively the atlases $I_{128 \times 128}$, $I_{512 \times 512}$ and $I_{\text{TDOCT}}$. The posterior probability for the labels is finally [5]:

$$p(L(x)|\{I_n\},\{L_n\},\bar{I}) = \frac{\sum_{n=1}^{N} \mathcal{N}\left(\bar{I}(x); I_n(x), \sigma^2\right) e^{\rho D_x[L(x); L_n]} e^{-k_n\alpha}}{\sum_{n=1}^{N} e^{-k_n\alpha} \mathcal{N}\left(\bar{I}(x); I_n(x), \sigma^2\right)} \tag{2}$$

where $\mathcal{N}$ is the Gaussian probability density function; $D_x$ is the signed distance transform evaluated at location x; and $\sigma^2$ and $\rho$ are the likelihood parameters.

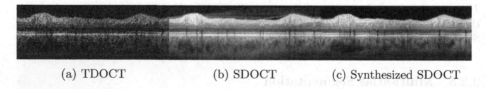

|  (a) TDOCT  |  (b) SDOCT  |  (c) Synthesized SDOCT  |

**Fig. 3.** OCT synthesis results via fusion of GANs. (a) and (b) illustrate a pair of TDOCT and SDOCT images. (c) Synthesized SDOCT from (a).

## 3   Experiments and Results

### 3.1   Experimental Setup

We compared our method with respect to the results obtained with each single GAN used in our pipeline (Fig. 1), to a label fusion strategy on the GANs output, and to the original images provided by the StratusOCT machine. Testing on UKGTS was instead performed by quantifying the statistical power relative to the measurements obtained with our method, as compared with those derived from the StratusOCT, following the same evaluation protocol from prior image-to-image translation studies [10]. To quantify the quality of the synthesized SDOCT images, we segmented their RNFL and compared the resulting average RNFL thickness with the original SDOCT average RNFL thickness. The intuition is that if we can produce realistic SDOCT images, an off-the-shelf segmentation model should output the same RNFL thickness obtained with the original data. We adopt the layer segmentation model of Mayer et al. [12]. For label fusion, as atlases, we used the segmented RNFL sections of the synthesized SDOCT and the original TDOCT RNFL segmentation. For the test image, we used the average synthesized stitched image in which we registered the retinal layers of the atlases. We used the method from [13] for non-rigid registration of OCT layers, and computed predictions for the final RNFL labels with Eq. 2. The parameters were kept constant for all experiments: $\sigma^2 = 625$, $\rho = 30\,\mu m^{-1}$, $\alpha = 1\,mm^{-1}$. Decaying weights were set depending on the agreement measured when evaluating GANs performance individually. We used 9-Block Resnet models as generators, and $70 \times 70$ PatchGANs as the two discriminators [10]. All experiments were performed on a NVIDIA Titan X (12 GB) GPU.

**Table 1.** Limits of agreement, mean difference, correlation of all methods versus ground truth, and mean SD of the first three visits difference for both eyes.

| Method | GAN | | | Label Fusion | | StratusOCT |
|---|---|---|---|---|---|---|
| | 128x128 | 256x256 | 512x512 | Direct | Proposed | |
| 95% LOA | [22.53, -18.7] | [16.9, -14.2] | [23.34, -19.35] | [11.72, -9.72] | **[8.11, -6.73]** | [26.64, -22.95] |
| Mean Diff. | 1.92 | 1.44 | 1.99 | 1.00 | **0.69** | 1.84 |
| Pearson r | 0.79 | 0.85 | 0.71 | 0.89 | **0.92** | 0.76 |
| Mean SD | 2.27 | 1.87 | 3.01 | 1.33 | **1.29** | 2.67 |

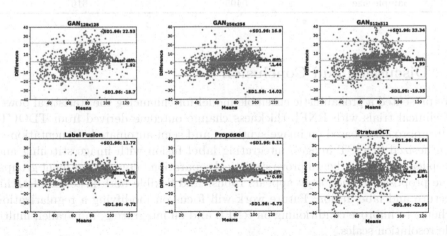

**Fig. 4.** Bland-Altman plots on the agreement between all methods versus ground truth on RAPID. The proposed method leads to significantly better agreement.

## 3.2  Results

Table 1 shows the 95% limits of agreement (LOA), mean difference, correlation and the mean standard deviation (SD) of the difference for three visits across all subjects of the RAPID study. $GAN_{256\times256}$ yields better scores compared to $GAN_{128\times128}$ and $GAN_{512\times512}$. Label fusion, without image stitching, on the average synthesized image outperforms the individual output of GANs, while a further improvement is obtained by integrating image stitching. These results suggest that combining the synthesized images of each GAN enables us to take advantage of the strengths of all architectures. Figure 4 illustrates the compatibility of the measurements with respect to the ground truth SDOCT segmentation in Bland-Altman plots. Our approach not only manages to produce a RNFL segmentation close to the ground truth, but also reduces the variability in the measurements. We applied our method to the TDOCT images available from the UKGTS and subsequently segmented the newly synthesized SDOCT images. Table 2 shows the results of our method compared to the original StratusOCT. We appreciate a statistically significant improvement in the separation between treatment and placebo groups ($p = 0.0017$), leading to sensibly lower sample size in power analysis.

**Table 2.** Comparison of rate of RNFL change between our method and Stratus OCT in the UKGTS. Significant difference between treatment and placebo progression rates ($p < 0.05$, Mann–Whitney U test) is indicated with (*). Sample size for 80% power with $p = 0.05$.

| Method | StratusOCT | | Proposed | |
|---|---|---|---|---|
| | Treatment | Placebo | Treatment | Placebo |
| Mean (SD) ($\mu$m/visit) | 0.0344 (1.964) | -0.0733 (2.066) | -0.0760 (1.5019) | -0.341 (1.8027) |
| Diff. in mean rate (95% CI) | 0.107 (-0.358 to 0.574) | | 0.265* (-0.118 to 0.648) | |
| Sample size | 5495 | | 616 | |

## 4  Discussion and Conclusion

We presented a probabilistic ensemble model for enhancing the statistical power of clinical trials with RNFL thickness change outcome derived from TDOCT. Our approach is based on image synthesis and semi-automated segmentation of synthesized SDOCT images, integrating label fusion with image stitching and deep learning to further improve statistical separation between treatment groups. The proposed methodology appears robust and flexible both in terms of architecture and label fusion. Future work will focus on modifying a regularization scheme to improve conditioning on RNFL and on integrating, in parallel, multiple resolution scales.

**Acknowledgements.** This work was supported by the EPSRC (CDT in Medical Imaging, EP/L016478/1) and Santen Pharmaceutical Co., Ltd.

# References

1. Garway-Heath, D.F., Crabb, D.P., et al.: Latanoprost for open-angle glaucoma (UKGTS): a randomised, multicentre, placebo-controlled trial. The Lancet **385**(9975), 1295–1304 (2015)
2. Button, K., Ioannidis, J., et al.: Power failure: why small sample size undermines the reliability of neuroscience. Nat. Rev. Neurosci. **14**, 365–376 (2013)
3. Zhang, T., Davatzikos, C.: Optimally-discriminative voxel-based analysis. In: Jiang, T., Navab, N., Pluim, J.P.W., Viergever, M.A. (eds.) MICCAI 2010. LNCS, vol. 6362, pp. 257–265. Springer, Heidelberg (2010). https://doi.org/10.1007/978-3-642-15745-5_32
4. Schwartz, Y., Varoquaux, G., Pallier, C., Pinel, P., Poline, J.-B., Thirion, B.: Improving accuracy and power with transfer learning using a meta-analytic database. In: Ayache, N., Delingette, H., Golland, P., Mori, K. (eds.) MICCAI 2012. LNCS, vol. 7512, pp. 248–255. Springer, Heidelberg (2012). https://doi.org/10.1007/978-3-642-33454-2_31
5. Sabuncu, M.R., Yeo, B.T.T., Van Leemput, K., Fischl, B., Golland, P.: A generative model for image segmentation based on label fusion. IEEE Trans. Med. Imaging **29**(10), 1714–1729 (2010)
6. Nie, D., et al.: Medical image synthesis with context-aware Generative Adversarial Networks. In: Descoteaux, M., Maier-Hein, L., Franz, A., Jannin, P., Collins, D.L., Duchesne, S. (eds.) MICCAI 2017. LNCS, vol. 10435, pp. 417–425. Springer, Cham (2017). https://doi.org/10.1007/978-3-319-66179-7_48
7. Wolterink, J.M., Dinkla, A.M., Savenije, M.H.F., Seevinck, P.R., van den Berg, C.A.T., Išgum, I.: Deep MR to CT synthesis using unpaired data. In: Tsaftaris, S.A., Gooya, A., Frangi, A.F., Prince, J.L. (eds.) SASHIMI 2017. LNCS, vol. 10557, pp. 14–23. Springer, Cham (2017). https://doi.org/10.1007/978-3-319-68127-6_2
8. Ben-Cohen, A., Klang, E., Raskin, S.P., Amitai, M.M., Greenspan, H.: Virtual PET images from CT data using deep convolutional networks: initial results. In: Tsaftaris, S.A., Gooya, A., Frangi, A.F., Prince, J.L. (eds.) SASHIMI 2017. LNCS, vol. 10557, pp. 49–57. Springer, Cham (2017). https://doi.org/10.1007/978-3-319-68127-6_6
9. Wang, T.C., Liu, M.Y., et al.: High-resolution image synthesis and semantic manipulation with conditional GANs. In: 2018 IEEE CVPR, pp. 8798–8807, June 2018
10. Zhu, J.Y., Park, T., Isola, P., Efros, A.A.: Unpaired image-to-image translation using cycle-consistent adversarial networks. In: IEEE ICCV, pp. 2242–2251 (2017). https://doi.org/10.1109/ICCV.2017.244
11. Atzeni, A., Jansen, M., Ourselin, S., Iglesias, J.E.: A probabilistic model combining deep learning and multi-atlas segmentation for semi-automated labelling of histology. In: Frangi, A.F., Schnabel, J.A., Davatzikos, C., Alberola-López, C., Fichtinger, G. (eds.) MICCAI 2018. LNCS, vol. 11071, pp. 219–227. Springer, Cham (2018). https://doi.org/10.1007/978-3-030-00934-2_25
12. Mayer, M.A., Hornegger, J., Mardin, C.Y., Tornow, R.P.: Retinal nerve fiber layer segmentation on FD-OCT scans of normal subjects and glaucoma patients. Biomed. Opt. Express **1**(5), 1358–1383 (2010). https://doi.org/10.1364/BOE.1.001358
13. Du, X., Gong, L., Shi, F., Chen, X., Yang, X., Zheng, J.: Non-rigid registration of retinal OCT images using conditional correlation ratio. In: Cardoso, M., et al. (eds.) FIFI/OMIA -2017. LNCS, vol. 10554, pp. 159–167. Springer, Cham (2017). https://doi.org/10.1007/978-3-319-67561-9_18

# A Deep Reinforcement Learning Framework for Frame-by-Frame Plaque Tracking on Intravascular Optical Coherence Tomography Image

Gongning Luo[1], Suyu Dong[1], Kuanquan Wang[1(✉)], Dong Zhang[2,3], Yue Gao[4], Xin Chen[5], Henggui Zhang[1], and Shuo Li[2,3]

[1] Harbin Institute of Technology, Harbin, China
wangkq@hit.edu.cn
[2] Department of Medical Imaging and Medical Biophysics, Western University, London, ON, Canada
[3] Digital Imaging Group of London, London, ON N6A 3K7, Canada
[4] Tsinghua University, Beijing, China
[5] Wuhan Asia Heart Hospital, Wuhan, China

**Abstract.** Intravascular Optical Coherence Tomography (IVOCT) is considered as the gold standard for the atherosclerotic plaque analysis in clinical application. A continuous and accurate plaque tracking algorithm is critical for coronary heart disease diagnosis and treatment. However, continuous and accurate plaque tracking frame-by-frame is very challenging because of some difficulties from IVOCT imaging conditions, such as speckle noise, complex and various intravascular morphology, and large numbers of IVOCT images in a pullback. To address such a challenging problem, for the first time we proposed a novel Reinforcement Learning (RL) based framework for accurate and continuous plaque tracking frame-by-frame on IVOCT images. In this framework, eight transformation actions are well-designed for IVOCT images to fit any possible changes of plaque's location and scale, and the spatio-temporal location correlation information of adjacent frames is modeled into state representation of RL to achieve continuous and accurate plaque detection, avoiding potential omissions. What's more, the proposed method has strong expansibility, because the fully-automated and semi-automated tracking patterns are both allowed to fit the clinical practice. Experiments on the large-scale IVOCT data show that the plaque-level accuracy of the proposed method can achieve 0.89 and 0.94 for the fully-automated tracking pattern and semi-automated tracking pattern respectively. This proves that our method has big application potential in future clinical practice. The code is open accessible: https://github.com/luogongning/PlaqueRL.

**Keywords:** Plaque tracking · Reinforcement Learning · Intravascular Optical Coherence Tomography Image · Spatio-temporal location correlation

© Springer Nature Switzerland AG 2019
D. Shen et al. (Eds.): MICCAI 2019, LNCS 11764, pp. 12–20, 2019.
https://doi.org/10.1007/978-3-030-32239-7_2

# 1    Introduction

Continuous and accurate atherosclerotic plaque detection and tracking is critical for coronary heart disease diagnosis and treatment [1]. Intravascular Optical Coherence Tomography (IVOCT) has higher resolution and feasibility than intravascular ultrasound, and is considered as the gold standard for the intravascular plaque analysis in clinical application [2]. Hence, plaque detection and tracking based on IVOCT is an important and valuable task in computer-aided coronary heart disease treatment field.

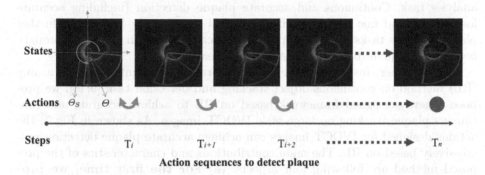

**Fig. 1.** A sequence of actions taken by the proposed framework to localize a plaque. The red sector is the ground truth region of a plaque. The blue sector is the detected region of the plaque after every action. The algorithm transforms sector region to achieve accurate detection based on RL. (Color figure online)

However, continuous and accurate plaque detection and tracking is very challenging because: (1) A lot of speckle noise on IVOCT images and the low contrast of plaque edges make it difficult to identify plaques without experts' guide. (2) Complex and various intravascular morphology makes it difficult to achieve continuous and accurate plaque detection frame-by-frame. (3) In a single pullback, hundreds of IVOCT images are gotten, analysing images one-by-one is impossible without an efficient analysis method during the clinical routine.

Some methods were proposed to address plaque analysis problem on IVOCT images. In [1], Gessert et al. used convolution neural networks (CNNs) to address automatic plaque detection problem on IVOCT images. In [3], Ughi et al. proposed an algorithm to achieve the automated characterization of plaque tissue based on textural features on IVOCT images. In [4], Wang et al. used a gradient based level-set model to achieve semi-automatic segmentation and quantification of calcified plaques. In [5], Soest et al. proposed a method to achieve automatic classification of plaque constituents based on the optical attenuation coefficient. In [6], Abdolmanafi et al. used the CNNs as feature extractor to achieve automated plaque tissue classification. In [7], He et al. used CNNs to achieve automatic plaque characterization for IVOCT images. In [8], Oliveira et al. used CNNs to address coronary calcification identification problem.

In summary, computer aided plaque analysis based on IVOCT images is an emerging research area and has big study potential. Recently, some works [1, 6, 7] have proven that CNNs have big application potential on computer aided plaque analysis problem. However, to our best knowledge, most of existing methods focus on addressing plaque classification or identification problems. Few methods can address region-level plaque localization and scale-level quantification problem simultaneously. What's more, no methods can achieve continuous plaque localization and scale quantification frame-by-frame (i.e., **plaque tracking**) with high accuracy (a plaque generally exists across consecutive frames). However, plaque tracking is a fundamental problem for computer aided plaque analysis task. Continuous and accurate plaque detection (including accurate localization and fine scale quantification) will significantly benefit the further plaque analysis tasks and has important clinical application value for coronary heart disease quantification, diagnosis, and treatment.

In this paper, inspired by the good performance of reinforcement learning (RL) method on continuous object tracking and detection task [9, 10], we propose a newly-designed framework based on RL to achieve accurate and continuous plaque tracking on large-scale IVOCT images. As shown in Fig. 1, the actions designed for IVOCT images can achieve accurate plaque detection progressively based on RL. The main contributions and characteristics of the proposed method are following four aspects: (a) **For the first time, we proposed an RL-based framework to achieve accurate plaque tracking on IVOCT images.** (b) **The proposed framework models the spatio-temporal information of adjacent frames to achieve continuous and accurate plaque detection frame-by-frame, avoiding potential omissions.** (c) **The proposed method has strong expansibility, because the fully-automated and semi-automated tracking styles are both allowed to fit the clinical practice.** (d) **On the collected large-scale IVOCT data, the proposed method achieves high tracking accuracy.**

## 2    Architecture of the Proposed Framework

The architecture of the proposed framework is illustrated in Fig. 2. The proposed framework includes three modules, i.e., the feature encoding module, the spatio-temporal correlation RL module (see Sect. 2.1), and the aided plaque localization and identification module (see Sect. 2.2). To achieve high computation efficiency, we design a simple CNNs structure as shown in Fig. 2 (Some new network structures, such as ResNet and DenseNet, can also be used, if computation power is sufficient). Specifically, in the feature encoding module, five convolution layers and one fully connected (FC) layer (i.e., FC1 layer) are used to achieve frame-by-frame feature encoding of IVOCT images. In an IVOCT image, the center coordinate is the localization of probe in physical space. Hence, we denote the detected plaque section as a sector with unified radius. The sector is represented as two-tuples $d = (\Theta_S, \Theta)$, where $\Theta$ denotes the **scale** (included angle) of the detected sector, $\Theta_S \in [0, 2\pi)$ denotes the **localization** (starting angle on the

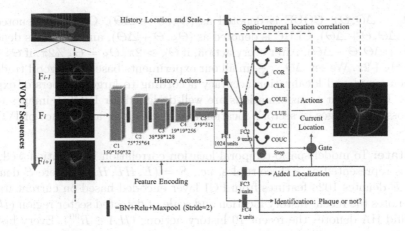

**Fig. 2.** Architecture of the proposed framework. The proposed deep reinforcement framework can utilize the spatio-temporal location correlation information to achieve continuous and accurate plaque tracking.

polar coordinate space) of the detected sector. In the following sections, we will introduce the details of the proposed framework.

## 2.1  Spatio-Temporal Correlation RL Module

To achieve continuous and accurate plaque tracking frame-by-frame without sampling or omissions, we formulate the plaque tracking task as an RL problem. This setting enables providing a continuous spatio-temporal location correlation to model an agent which makes a sequence of accurate actions to achieve accurate tracking. Our RL module is modeled based on FC2 layer (states are the input of FC2 layer and actions are the output of FC2 layer), and it considers a sequence of continuous IVOCT images as the **environment**, where the agent transforms a sector using a set of **actions** based on spatio-temporal location correlation information. The goal of the agent is to generate a tight sector in a plaque object to achieve precise location and scale quantification. The agent also has a **state** representation as the input of FC2 layer with spatio-temporal correlation information on the history localizations, scales, and actions, and receives positive and negative **rewards** for each action to learn a proper policy.

(1) **Actions:** The action set $A$ is composed of eight well-designed transformations that is used to transform the sector flexibly and one stop action to terminate the transformation process on current frame and start a series of new actions on next frames. Specifically, the eight transform actions are Bidirectional Expansion (BE), Bidirectional Contraction (BC), Contra Rotation (COR), Clockwise Rotation (CLR), Contra Unilateral Expansion (COUE), Clockwise Unilateral Expansion (CLUE), Clockwise Unilateral Contraction (CLUC), and Contra Unilateral Contraction (COUC). BE is denoted as $(\Theta_S - \Delta\Theta, \Theta + 2\Delta\Theta)$, BC is denoted as $(\Theta_S + \Delta\Theta, \Theta - 2\Delta\Theta)$, COR is denoted as $(\Theta_S + \Delta\Theta, \Theta)$, CLR is denoted

as $(\Theta_S - \Delta\Theta, \Theta)$, COUE is denoted as $(\Theta_S, \Theta + \Delta\Theta)$, CLUE is denoted as $(\Theta_S - \Delta\Theta, \Theta + \Delta\Theta)$, CLUC is denoted as $(\Theta_S, \Theta - \Delta\Theta)$, and COUC is denoted as $(\Theta_S + \Delta\Theta, \Theta - \Delta\Theta)$. After every action, if $\Theta_S > 2\pi$, $\Theta_S = \Theta_S \% 2\pi$, if $\Theta_S < 0$, $\Theta_S = \Theta_S + 2\pi$. We set $\Delta\Theta = \frac{\pi}{12}$ in all our experiments based on a good trade-off between speed and localization accuracy according to large numbers of experiments. These eight transformations are well-designed for IVOCT images to fit any possible changes of sector's location and scale along a sequence of IVOCT frames.

(2) **State:** To model spatio-temporal location correlation information well, the state is represented as a three-tuples, i.e., $S = (E, HL, HA)$, where $S$ denotes state, $E$ denotes 1024 features from FC1 layer encoded based on current frame, HL denotes the recent history location and scale of detected sector region ($HL \in R^2$), and HA denotes the recent 10 history actions ($HA \in R^{90}$). Every history action is represented by a 9-dimensional vector with one-hot form. **The spatio-temporal location correlation information is modeled into the $HL$ and $HA$ based on the fact that the past location, scale, and actions are always related to future actions whether intra frame or inter frames. In particular, the location and scale of a plaque across adjacent frames are spatially continuous.** Hence, based on such state representation $S$, the FC2 layer can learn a policy to generate proper actions to achieve accurate plaque detection in current frame, as well as accurate tracking in continuous IVOCT sequences.

(3) **Reward Function:** To achieve an accurate and timely feedback for every action, we design a reward function based on the change of intersection-over-union (IOU) index to quantify whether an action improves tracking or not. Specifically, the reward function is:

$$R = \begin{cases} 1, & IOU(d^a, g) - IOU(d, g) > 0 \\ -1, & IOU(d^a, g) - IOU(d, g) < 0 \\ 1, & IOU(d^a, g) - IOU(d, g) = 0 \& IOU(d^a, g) > 0.95 \\ -1, & IOU(d^a, g) - IOU(d, g) = 0 \& IOU(d^a, g) < 0.95 \end{cases} \tag{1}$$

where $g$ is the ground truth sector region from experts' label, $d$ denotes the current detected sector (CDS) region, and $d^a$ is the next detected sector (NDS) based on current selected action. $IOU(d^a, g) - IOU(d, g) = 0$ only happens when stop action is selected. 0.95 is set according to clinical application standard to define a proper stop condition, as well as avoid too many unnecessary actions.

## 2.2   Aided Plaque Localization and Identification Module

Aided localization and identification module not only can provide initial plaque location and scale for initial plaque frame (IPF), but also can avoid over-tracking on images without plaque through a well designed gate. In an IVOCT sequence, the plaque emerges in some continuous frames, and disappears also in some continuous frames. We denote the frame when plaque emerges firstly as IPF, and denote the frame when plaque disappears firstly as stop plaque frame (SPF) along IVOCT image sequences.

**(1) Localization and Identification:** We formulated the localization and identification into a multi-task framework. A multi-task loss is designed to guide the network generate an initial plaque location and scale for IPF (based on the output of FC3) and an identification for whether a plaque object exists in current frame (based on the output of FC4). The multi-task loss function is

$$L = \frac{1}{m} \sum_{i=1}^{m} L_r(d_i, g_i) + \frac{1}{m} \sum_{i=1}^{m} L_c(c_i, cg_i) \tag{2}$$

where $i$ is the index of a frame, $m$ denotes the size of batch size, $d_i$ is the predicted plaque sector on a frame (is denoted as two-dimensional vector $(\Theta_S, \Theta)$), $g_i$ denotes the ground truth plaque sector, $c_i$ is the predicted probability of a plaque existing on current frame, $cg_i$ is ground truth label of a plaque existing or not on current frame (is 1 if the plaque exists, is 0 if the plaque does not exist), $L_r$ is the L2 regularization loss, and $L_c$ is the two-class Softmax loss.

**2) Gate Design:** A gate is designed to improve the tracking accuracy avoiding over-tracking (avoid tracking on frames without plaque), and to transfer the spatio-temporal information to the current selected action. When spatio-temporal information transformation happens intra frame, $G = d_h$, where $G$ denotes the output of gate, and $d_h$ denotes the recent history location and scale of sector. When information transformation happens between adjacent frames, the output of gate is:

$$G = \begin{cases} d_h, & I_i = 1 \& I_{i-1} = 1 \\ d_i, & I_i = 1 \& I_{i-1} = 0, I_0 = 0, i \geq 1, \\ NULL, & I_i = 0 \end{cases} \tag{3}$$

where $d_h$ is used to transfer spatio-temporal information across adjacent frames, $d_i$ denotes the predicted sector from FC3 layer, $I_i$ denotes the identification of current frame, and $I_{i-1}$ denotes the identification of previous frame. When $I_i = 1 \& I_{i-1} = 0$, IPF appears, $d_i$ is used as the initial sector for the selected action to conduct transformation. When $G = NULL$, the tracking based RL is stopped in current frame to avoid over-tracking.

### 2.3 Implementation and Application Process

Implementation and application process includes two aspects, i.e., training and clinical application:

**Training and Optimization Process:** The parameters in all layers are initialized with Gaussian distribution. The proposed framework are trained using alternate pattern based on Tensorflow and Titan X GPU, and the learning rate was 0.0001. Specifically, we firstly fixed FC2 layer and trained other layers based on loss function in (2) using stochastic gradient descent with 10 epochs, and then trained FC2 layer (RL module) fixing other layers based on the action-reward function in (1) using strategy gradient [10] with 10 epochs. In this way, the proposed framework can achieve good compatibility of two training modes (i.e., traditional regression and RL).

**Clinical Application Strategy: Fully-automated tracking (FAT)** can be achieved based on the above description about the proposed framework. What's more, **the proposed framework is flexible and semi-automated tracking (SAT) is also allowed in the proposed framework.** To fit the clinical application based on the trade-off between accuracy and efficiency, a clinical physician can manually label the sector region in IPF, and specify the SPF. The proposed method can achieve automated tracking between IPF and SPF. Note that in the semi-automated tracking pattern, the gate's output is simplified as $G = d_h$ to only transfer the recent history location and scale to the selected action.

## 3 Experiment and Analysis

We selected IVOCT images by ILUMIEN OPTIS system from 120 patients with 132 pullbacks. 10000 continuous frames (including 154 plaques with experts' label on plaque location, scale and identification) are used to evaluate the proposed framework, in which the 2000 images are used for training and 8000 images are used for final testing. All images are converted into Cartesian and resized into unified size $150 * 150$. Data augmentation is conducted by randomly rotating images during training. According to the widely used measure metrics (i.e., accuracy, sensitivity, specificity) in [1], we evaluated the proposed framework's tracking performance in frame-level (i.e., accuracy on every independent frame) and plaque-level (i.e., accuracy on continuous frame sequence including a whole plaque, in which accuracy denotes plaque on all frames is detected accurately and continuously) respectively, and compared with state-of-the-art method [1] (To our best knowledge, [1] is the only plaque detection method before us). The accurate plaque detection on an IVOCT image is denoted as $IOU > 0.95$. However, $IOU > 0.95$ is not suitable for [1], because [1] only can achieve binary-level plaque detection. Hence, such a comparison is strict for the proposed framework.

Table 1 shows that the proposed framework (whether FAT or SAT) achieves better tracking performance on frame-level and plaque-level compared with the state-of-the-art method and ablation model (i.e., FAT-RL), which proves the superiority of the proposed framework. Specifically, FAT can achieve better performance than FAT-RL especially on plaque-level accuracy, which proves that the RL module can enhance the precision of plaque tracking with a strict standard ($IOU > 0.9$). Additionally, though FAT gets relatively lower accuracy than SAT, FAT achieves 10 times faster tracking (average 100 frames every second) than SAT. Hence, FAT and SAT both have superiority in clinical practice.

**Table 1.** Tracking performance comparison among the proposed method, state-of-the-art method, and ablation model. (FAT-RL denotes removing RL module from FAT, the output of FAT-RL directly comes from FC3 layer.)

| Level | Frame-level | | | Plaque-level | | |
|---|---|---|---|---|---|---|
| Metrics | Accuracy | Sensitivity | Specificity | Accuracy | Sensitivity | Specificity |
| SAT | **0.99** | **0.99** | **0.98** | **0.94** | **0.96** | **0.96** |
| FAT | **0.92** | **0.93** | **0.94** | **0.89** | **0.91** | **0.92** |
| [1] | 0.87 | 0.89 | 0.87 | N/A | N/A | N/A |
| FAT-RL | 0.86 | 0.85 | 0.89 | 0.82 | 0.81 | 0.83 |

# 4   Conclusion

For the first time, we proposed a novel RL-based framework for accurate and continuous plaque tracking frame-by-frame on IVOCT images. The proposed framework models the spatio-temporal information of adjacent frames to achieve continuous and accurate plaque detection, avoiding potential omissions. Besides, the proposed method has strong expansibility, because the fully-automated and semi-automated tracking styles are both allowed to fit the clinical practice. On large-scale IVOCT data, the high tracking accuracy of the proposed method has been proven. Hence the proposed method has big application potential in future.

**Acknowledgments.** This work was supported by the National Key R&D Program of China under Grant 2017YFC0113000.

# References

1. Gessert, N., et al.: Automatic plaque detection in IVOCT pullbacks using convolutional neural networks. IEEE Trans. Med. imaging **38**(2), 426–434 (2019)
2. Jang, I.K., et al.: Visualization of coronary atherosclerotic plaques in patients using optical coherence tomography: comparison with intravascular ultrasound. J. Am. Coll. Cardiol. **39**(4), 604–609 (2002)
3. Ughi, G.J., Adriaenssens, T., Sinnaeve, P., Desmet, W., D'hooge, J.: Automated tissue characterization of in vivo atherosclerotic plaques by intravascular optical coherence tomography images. Biomed. Opt. Express **4**(7), 1014–1030 (2013)
4. Wang, Z., et al.: Semiautomatic segmentation and quantification of calcified plaques in intracoronary optical coherence tomography images. J. Biomed. Opt. **15**(6), 061711 (2010)
5. Van Soest, G., et al.: Atherosclerotic tissue characterization in vivo by optical coherence tomography attenuation imaging. J. Biomed. Opt. **15**(1), 011105 (2010)
6. Abdolmanafi, A., Duong, L., Dahdah, N., Cheriet, F.: Deep feature learning for automatic tissue classification of coronary artery using optical coherence tomography. Biomed. Opt. Express **8**(2), 1203–1220 (2017)

7. He, S., et al.: Convolutional neural network based automatic plaque characterization for intracoronary optical coherence tomography images. In: Medical Imaging 2018: Image Processing, vol. 10574. International Society for Optics and Photonics (2018). 1057432
8. Oliveira, D.A., Macedo, M.M., Nicz, P., Campos, C., Lemos, P., Gutierrez, M.A.: Coronary calcification identification in optical coherence tomography using convolutional neural networks. In: Medical Imaging 2018: Biomedical Applications in Molecular, Structural, and Functional Imaging, vol. 10578. International Society for Optics and Photonics (2018). 105781Y
9. Caicedo, J.C., Lazebnik, S.: Active object localization with deep reinforcement learning. In: Proceedings of the IEEE International Conference on Computer Vision, pp. 2488–2496 (2015)
10. Yun, S., Choi, J., Yoo, Y., Yun, K., Young Choi, J.: Action-decision networks for visual tracking with deep reinforcement learning. In: Proceedings of the IEEE Conference on Computer Vision and Pattern Recognition, pp. 2711–2720 (2017)

# Multi-index Optic Disc Quantification via MultiTask Ensemble Learning

Rongchang Zhao[1,2] , Zailiang Chen[1,2], Xiyao Liu[1,2], Beiji Zou[1,2], and Shuo Li[3,4](✉)

[1] School of Computer Science and Engineering, Central South University, Changsha, China
[2] Hunan Engineering Research Center of Machine Vision and Intelligent Medicine, Changsha, China
byrons.zhao@gmail.com
[3] Department of Medical Imaging and Medical Biophysics, Western University, London, Canada
[4] Digital Imaging Group of London, London, ON, Canada
slishuo@gmail.com

**Abstract.** Accurate quantification of optic disc (OD) is clinically significant for the assessment and diagnosis of ophthalmic disease. Multi-index OD quantification, i.e., to simultaneously quantify a set of clinical indices including 2 vertical diameters (cup and disc), 2 whole areas (disc and rim), and 16 regional areas, is an untouched challenge due to its complexity of the multi-dimensional nonlinear mapping and various visual appearance across patients. In this paper, we propose a novel multitask ensemble learning framework (DMTFs) to automatically achieve accurate multi-types multi-index OD quantification. DMTFs creates an ensemble of multiple OD quantification tasks (OD segmentation and indices estimation) that are individually accurate and mutually complementary, and then learns the ensemble under a multi-task learning framework which is formed as a tree structure with a root network for shared feature representation, two branches for task-specific prediction, and a multitask ensemble module for aggregation of multi-index OD quantification. DMTFs models the consistency correlation between OD segmentation and indices estimation tasks to conform to the accurate multi-index OD quantification. Experiments on the ORIGA datasets show that the proposed method achieves impressive performance with the average mean absolute error on 20 indices of $0.99 \pm 0.20$, $0.73 \pm 0.14$ and $1.23 \pm 0.24$ for diameters, whole areas and regional area, respectively. Besides, the obtained quantitative indices achieve competitive performance (AUC $= 0.8623$) on glaucoma diagnosis. As the first multi-index OD quantification, the proposed DMTFs demonstrates great potential in clinical application.

## 1 Introduction

Accurate quantification of optic disc (OD) from fundus images is the most clinically important for the comprehensive assessment of ophthalmic disease. Accord-

D. Shen et al. (Eds.): MICCAI 2019, LNCS 11764, pp. 21–29, 2019.
https://doi.org/10.1007/978-3-030-32239-7_3

ing to [7], multi-index OD quantification is defined as simultaneously quantifying a set of clinical indices, i.e., 2 vertical diameters (cup and disc), 2 whole areas (disc and rim), and 16 regional areas (as shown in Fig. 1), to characterize the global and focal appearance of OD. Clinically, accurate quantification provides effective assessment tools and detailed information for diagnosis, treatment, and follow-up of many ophthalmic diseases, especially chronic glaucoma [8,12,14].

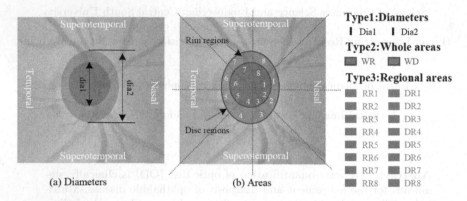

(a) Diameters        (b) Areas

**Fig. 1.** Multi-index OD quantification includes three type of indices: diameters, whole areas and regional areas. (a) diameters of optic disc and cup. (b) areas of optic disc and neuroretinal rim for the whole disc and for individual 45° regions followed as [7] to characterize the global and local appearance. RR: rim regions; DR: disc regions; WR: whole rim; WD: whole disc.

Existing methods address only single index OD quantification by either learning a nonlinear mapping between fundus image and quantitative index, such as CDR [16], or measuring on the segmented OD mask [2,4,9]. However, those methods are still open challenging to achieve multi-index OD quantification because the former approach (direct estimation) always implements a complex nonlinear regression which is hard to train individually [5,17]; the latter is a common segmentation-based approach, but the great variability of shape and inhomogeneity in OD appearance, especially the ambiguity optic cup borders, easily cause critical inconsistency of OD indices compared to actual ones.

No work has successfully achieved multi-index OD quantification due to three challenges: (1) estimating multiple indices from fundus image is complicated and difficult due to the complexity of nonlinear mapping from fundus image to multivariate vector. (2) Large variation of fundus appearance cross patients increases the difficulty of feature representation for comprehensive OD quantification. OD appearance changes in different ways with different pathology, e.g., cupping caused by thinning of rim and notch caused by focal enlargement of the cup [1]. (3) Combining OD segmentation and direct index estimation for accurate quantification is challenging due to the modeling difficulty of correlations between the two approaches.

Multi-task learning (MTL) [6,10,15,16] has great potential since it improves the performance of the individual task by joint learning of the two OD quantification approaches (OD segmentation and indices estimation). However, traditional MTL methods can not formulate the two approaches into an ensemble model to aggregate their quantitative indices effectively. Our work constructs a particular case of multi-task learning when OD quantification is divided into an ensemble of multiple correlated but diverse tasks by modeling the consistency correlation between those tasks. The multi-task learning structure is encoded as a tree, where the root indicates task-shared representation, and branches implement a set of decision trees which obtain the confident task-specific predictions that can be aggregated into a consistent OD quantification in multiple granularities [11].

In this paper, we propose a novel multitask ensemble learning framework (DMTFs) to automatically quantify optic disc (OD) by obtaining multi-type quantitative indices. DMTFs is capable of achieving accurate OD quantification by: (1) creatively formulating multi-index OD quantification as multitask ensemble learning to learn OD segmentation and indices estimation tasks jointly; (2) modeling consistency correlations between two quantification tasks based on the advantages integration of multi-task and ensemble learning frameworks; and (3) addressing the multitask ensemble learning with multi-objective optimization to find the effective solution. Benefit from the multitask ensemble learning, DMTFs enables high-efficiency solution on accurate multi-index OD quantification.

Our main contributions are three-folds: (1) For the first time, multi-index OD quantification is achieved to help the clinician to assess global and focal changes of optic disc for diagnosis, treatment, and follow-up of many ophthalmic diseases. (2) The proposed distribution regression forest provides an effective approach for task-specific feature selection and distribution regression to handle the task-specific prediction problem in each individual task. (3) Multitask ensemble learning framework (DMTFs) is innovatively proposed to create an ensemble of multiple OD quantification tasks (OD segmentation and indices estimation) to effectively achieve accurate multi-index OD quantification.

## 2 Deep Multi-task Forests (DMTFs)

DMTFs (Fig. 2) creates an ensemble of multiple OD quantification tasks (OD segmentation and indices estimation), and learns the ensemble under a multi-task learning framework by modeling the consistency correlations between the two quantification tasks. Taking advantages of multi-task learning and ensemble learning, DMTFs promotes performance improvement on each individual task and achieves accurate multi-index OD quantification by multitask ensemble.

### 2.1 Architectures of DMTFs

The proposed DMTFs consists of a root network for shared feature representation, followed with two branches for task-specific prediction (OD segmentation and indices estimation) by implementing a set of distribution regression forests,

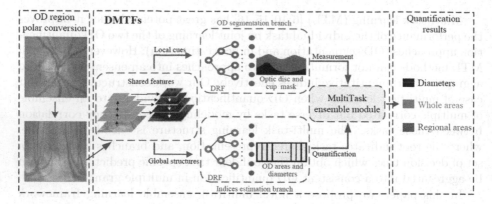

**Fig. 2.** Overview of DMTFs, which is a multitask ensemble learning framework consisting of a root CNN for task-shared feature representation, two task-specific branches for OD segmentation and indices estimation tasks, and a multitask ensemble module for joint optimization and final OD quantification. Each branch implements a distribution regression forest, randomly linked with the shared root network. The DMTFs is trained by the multi-objective optimization algorithm with the end-to-end manner.

and a multitask ensemble module for final OD quantification. The DMTFs allows for learning of the inter-task correlation by shared feature representation and consistency regularization, whilst simultaneously allows for modeling of task-specific correlation by task-specific feature selection and ensemble learning. To learn those correlations, the objective of DMTFs is formulated as

$$\underset{\mathbf{w},\mathbf{p}_{seg},\mathbf{p}_{est}}{\arg\min} ( \underbrace{\mathbf{L}_{seg}(\mathbf{w},\mathbf{p}_{seg})}_{segmentation\ task\ loss} , \underbrace{\mathbf{L}_{est}(\mathbf{w},\mathbf{p}_{est})}_{estimation\ task\ loss} , \underbrace{\mathbf{L}_{cons}(\mathbf{w},\mathbf{p}_{est},\mathbf{p}_{seg})}_{consistency\ loss})^{\intercal} \quad (1)$$

where $L_{seg}$ is the loss to ensure the precise of OD segmentation task, $L_{est}$ is the estimation loss to ensure the accuracy of the indices regression task, and $L_{cons}$ denotes the consistency regularization to impose a penalty for the consistent OD quantification from segmentation and estimation tasks. $\mathbf{w}$ is the parameters, $\mathbf{p}_{seg}, \mathbf{p}_{est}$ are predicted indices vectors by the segmentation and estimation tasks, respectively. Notes $\mathbf{p} = (Dia1, Dia2, WR, WD, RR1 : RR8, DR1 : DR8)$.

Multi-task learning often requires modeling of the trade-off between OD segmentation and indices estimation tasks, for example, the direct estimated area of the regional rim is conflicting with the segmented rim region. To find the solutions that are not dominated by any tasks, DMTFs is formulated as multi-objective optimization and the loss function is defined as a vector-valued loss as shown in Eq. 1 with the overall objective of finding a Pareto optimal solution.

## 2.2  Task-Specific Branches with Distribution Regression Forest

Task-specific branches employ distribution regression forests (DRF) to individually achieve OD segmentation and indices estimation tasks by constructing a multitude of differentiable decision trees [13] linked with the root network. Each task-specific branch extracts task-related features and obtains task-specific prediction based on the feature selection and distribution regression of DRF module.

Each DRF module is consisted of a set of split nodes $\mathcal{N}$ and leaf nodes $\mathcal{L}$. Split and leaf nodes construct a multitude of decision trees at training time and output the prediction of the individual branch. To enable the tree with task-related feature selection, a routing function $\mu_l(\mathbf{x}|\mathbf{w})$ is defined to provide the probability that input $\mathbf{x}$ will reach leaf node $l$ as

$$\mu_l(\mathbf{x}|\mathbf{w}) = \prod_{n \in \mathcal{N}} h_n(\mathbf{x}; \mathbf{w})^{\mathbb{1}(l \in \mathcal{N}_n^l)} (1 - h_n(\mathbf{x}; \mathbf{w}))^{\mathbb{1}(l \in \mathcal{N}_n^r)} \tag{2}$$

where $\mathbb{1}(\cdot)$ is an indicator function, $h_n(\mathbf{x}; \mathbf{w})$ indicates the probability that split node $n \in \mathcal{N}$ selects input feature $\mathbf{x}$ as its task-specific feature.

To enable the forest with the capability to be optimized end-to-end together with the shared root network, the differentiable split function is defined as $h_n(\mathbf{x}; \mathbf{w}) = \sigma(f_{\varphi(n)}(\mathbf{x}; \mathbf{w}))$, where $\sigma(\cdot)$ is the sigmoid function, $f_{\varphi(n)}(\mathbf{x}; \mathbf{w})$ is outputs of the root network, adopted as the shared feature extraction function to end-to-end learn the expressive representation of fundus image. $\varphi(\cdot)$ is an index function to assign the connection between the output of function $f(\mathbf{x}; \mathbf{w})$ and split node $n$. In this work, the index function $\varphi(\cdot)$ is a random function to link split nodes with the shared root network randomly.

**OD Segmentation Branch.** OD segmentation branch formulates OD segmentation task as the regression segmentation problem to learn the distribution of OD and OC (optic cup) region with DRF module. To improve the segmentation for OD quantification, we develop a novel distribution-aware segmentation loss to guide the DRF to capture the smoothness priors of the OD and OC region. The segmentation loss includes a dice coefficient loss $\mathbf{L}_{dice}$ measuring the overlap between the prediction and ground truth, and a distribution loss $\mathbf{L}_{dist}$ encouraging the predictive borders of OD and OC regions to be similar to the ground truth. Therefore, the distribution-aware segmentation loss is defined as

$$\mathbf{L}_{seg}(\mathbf{w}, \mathbf{p}_{seg}) = 1 - \underbrace{\frac{2 \sum_i p_i y_i}{\sum_i p_i^2 + \sum_i y_i^2}}_{\mathbf{L}_{dice}} + \underbrace{\sum_c d_c log(s_c)}_{\mathbf{L}_{dist}} \tag{3}$$

where $p$ and $y$ denote the predicted probability map and ground truth, respectively. $s$ and $d$ denote the predicted and ground truth distribution of border pixels, and $c$ is the length of the distribution.

**Indices Estimation Branch.** Indices estimation branch handles direct indices estimation task by learning a nonlinear mapping from shared feature to the OD quantitative indices with another DRF module. In this work, the discrete distribution concatenated with the normalized OD areas and diameters acts as the ground truth to train DMTFs together with OD segmentation labels. To enable the DRF module with the ability of nonlinear regression, the Kullback-Leibler

(K-L) divergence is adopted to measure the similarity between predicted distribution $\mathbf{p}_{est}$ and ground truth $\mathbf{d}$. Therefore, the learning procedure is minimizing the following cross-entropy loss as $\mathbf{L}_{est}(\mathbf{w}, \mathbf{p}_{est}) = -\frac{1}{N} \sum \mathbf{d} log(\mathbf{p}_{est})$.

### 2.3  MultiTask Ensemble Module for Multi-index OD Quantification

To learn the ensemble of two OD quantification tasks and model the consistency correlation between tasks, multitask ensemble module is developed, which contains a consistency loss function to impose the penalty for the consistent OD quantification between segmentation and estimation tasks, and a two-stage aggregation for final OD quantitative indices. Consistency loss is designed to minimize the prediction difference between two branches, i.e., OD segmentation and indices estimation tasks. Ideally, indices predicted by the two branches are the same. To ensure the indices from different branches as consistent as possible, the consistency loss is defined as the difference between the indices vectors $\mathbf{L}_{cons} = \frac{1}{2}(\mathbf{p}_{est} - \mathbf{p}_{seg})^2$, $\mathbf{p}_{est}$ and $\mathbf{p}_{seg}$ denote indices vectors coming from estimation branch and OD segmentation branch, respectively.

To integrate predictions from each leaf node of the two task branches, two-stage aggregation is adopted. (1) Inter-task aggregation: with the prediction on each leaf nodes of DRF, the task-specific quantitative indices are obtained by aggregating those leaf nodes predictions into a single coherent output followed ensemble learning as $\sum_{l \in \mathcal{L}} \mu_l(\mathbf{x}|\mathbf{w})\mathbf{p}^l$, where $\mu_l(\mathbf{x}|\mathbf{w})$ is the probability that feature $\mathbf{x}$ be selected by leaf node $l$ and defined in Eq. 2, $\mathbf{p}^l$ is the predicted indices vector on leaf node $l$. Note that $\mathbf{p}^l$ is measured based on the segmented mask when node $l$ belongs to OD segmentation branch, while directly regressed when belongs to indices estimation branch. (2) Intra-task aggregation: with the prediction of each task-specific branch, the final quantitative indices are build based on the simple yet effective adaptive weighting method. DMTFs learns to average task weighting by considering the loss for each task, and the task weighting for segmentation and estimation tasks are defined as:

$$\lambda_{seg} = \frac{\exp(\mathbf{L}_{seg}^t)}{\exp(\mathbf{L}_{seg}^t) + \exp(\mathbf{L}_{est}^t)}, \quad \lambda_{est} = \frac{\exp(\mathbf{L}_{est}^t)}{\exp(\mathbf{L}_{seg}^t) + \exp(\mathbf{L}_{est}^t)} \tag{4}$$

where $\mathbf{L}_{seg}^t$ and $\mathbf{L}_{est}^t$ are the average loss from segmentation and estimation task branches in the $t$-$th$ epoch over several iterations.

## 3  Experiments

The effectiveness of DMTFs is validated with the open accessible dataset ORIGA [3]. Experimental results show that DMTFs accurately quantifies optic disc with multiple types of 20 indices with average mean absolute error (MAE) of $0.99 \pm 0.20$, $0.73 \pm 0.14$, $1.23 \pm 0.24$ for diameters, whole areas and regional areas.

**Datasets and Configurations.** The ORIGA contains 650 images (168 glaucomatous and 482 normal eyes) with manual labeled optic disc mask, divided into

325 training and 325 testing images. To leverage the powerful representation for the circle-shaped OD appearance, the input fundus images are pixel-wisely converted into the polar coordinate system. Pixels in optic disc region are re-sampled along the angular and radius dimension, therefore resulting in the regions of OC, OD, and background in the ordered layout.

The pyramid integration structure [16] is adopted as the shared root network for shared feature representation. We apply the alternating optimization strategy to obtain the optimistic parameters and prediction on leaf nodes.

**Overall Performance.** Results (Table 1) demonstrate that DMTFs successfully delivers accurate multi-index OD quantification with average MAE of $0.99 \pm 0.20$, $0.73 \pm 0.14$, $1.23 \pm 0.24$ for diameters, whole areas and regional areas, respectively. Meanwhile, the results indicate DMTFs achieves more accurate multi-index OD quantification than other single-task-based approaches with the lowest average MAE $0.98 \pm 0.19$ over all the 20 quantitative indices. Experimental results on glaucoma diagnosis show that the quantitative indices provide more effective assessment tools (with 0.8623 AUC) for ophthalmic diseases diagnosis.

**Effectiveness of MultiTask Ensemble Learning.** Indices shown in the third and fourth columns are independently obtained with only one task branch (OD segmentation or estimation). The results clearly indicate that multitask ensemble improves average 3.3%, 2.2% of 20 indices compared with the single segmentation and estimation task branch, respectively. Compared with the single task, DMTFs obtains the smallest bias overall indices and lowest average MAE overall 20 indices. The average MAE and bias show multitask ensemble learning framework brings clearly improvements for all the indices quantification.

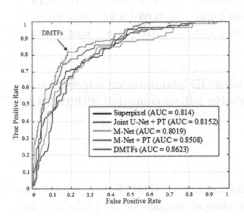

**Comparison.** Results, compared with measured indices on the state-of-the-art segmented mask [4], show that DMTFs achieves the average improvement of 2.15% on 20 indices. Comparing column 2 and 5 of Table 1, it clearly shows DMTFs obtains more accurate multi-index OD quantification than single segmentation-based approach, which demonstrates the remarkable advantages in more detailed OD quantification.

**Fig. 3.** The ROC curves with AUC scores for glaucoma diagnosis based on the quantitative multi-types indices for our DMTFs while only CDR for others. Source: Fu et al. [4] with our results added.

**Effectiveness of Glaucoma Diagnosis.** Figure 3 shows the success of the proposed DMTFs on glaucoma diagnosis based on the quantitative 20 indices. Evidenced by ROC curves and AUC value (0.8623), the glaucoma

**Table 1.** Performance of DMTFs under different configurations and state-of-the-art method for multi-index OD quantification. Average Mean Absolute Error (MAE) is used for the quantification evaluation criterion.

| Method | MNet [4] | DMTFs | | |
|---|---|---|---|---|
| | | Only segmentation | Only estimation | Ensemble |
| *Diameter* ($10^2$ pixel) | | | | |
| Dia1 | $0.97 \pm 0.23$ | $0.98 \pm 0.27$ | $0.97 \pm 0.29$ | $\mathbf{0.96 \pm 0.21}$ |
| Dia2 | $1.09 \pm 0.28$ | $1.08 \pm 0.21$ | $1.05 \pm 0.25$ | $\mathbf{1.05 \pm 0.19}$ |
| *Whole areas* ($10^4$ pixel) | | | | |
| WR | $\mathbf{0.32 \pm 0.09}$ | $0.34 \pm 0.18$ | $0.32 \pm 0.15$ | $0.32 \pm 0.12$ |
| WD | $1.67 \pm 0.16$ | $1.68 \pm 0.15$ | $1.65 \pm 0.20$ | $\mathbf{1.65 \pm 0.15}$ |
| *Regional areas* ($10^4$ pixel) | | | | |
| RR1 | $0.74 \pm 0.21$ | $0.74 \pm 0.25$ | $0.75 \pm 0.23$ | $\mathbf{0.73 \pm 0.21}$ |
| RR2 | $0.39 \pm 0.13$ | $0.35 \pm 0.12$ | $0.34 \pm 0.13$ | $\mathbf{0.34 \pm 0.10}$ |
| RR3 | $0.11 \pm 0.08$ | $0.12 \pm 0.12$ | $0.12 \pm 0.10$ | $\mathbf{0.11 \pm 0.09}$ |
| RR4 | $\mathbf{0.55 \pm 0.25}$ | $0.57 \pm 0.33$ | $0.55 \pm 0.32$ | $0.55 \pm 0.29$ |
| RR5 | $0.70 \pm 0.31$ | $\mathbf{0.68 \pm 0.32}$ | $0.68 \pm 0.34$ | $0.69 \pm 0.21$ |
| RR6 | $0.30 \pm 0.15$ | $0.30 \pm 0.23$ | $0.31 \pm 0.14$ | $\mathbf{0.30 \pm 0.13}$ |
| RR7 | $0.15 \pm 0.26$ | $0.14 \pm 0.32$ | $0.15 \pm 0.25$ | $\mathbf{0.13 \pm 0.24}$ |
| RR8 | $0.26 \pm 0.17$ | $0.27 \pm 0.31$ | $0.25 \pm 0.22$ | $\mathbf{0.25 \pm 0.18}$ |
| DR1 | $1.28 \pm 0.19$ | $1.29 \pm 0.14$ | $\mathbf{1.25 \pm 0.23}$ | $1.26 \pm 0.12$ |
| DR2 | $\mathbf{3.17 \pm 0.54}$ | $3.21 \pm 0.57$ | $3.29 \pm 0.53$ | $3.21 \pm 0.46$ |
| DR3 | $3.80 \pm 0.38$ | $3.79 \pm 0.42$ | $3.78 \pm 0.39$ | $\mathbf{3.78 \pm 0.29}$ |
| DR4 | $3.32 \pm 0.36$ | $3.30 \pm 0.24$ | $3.29 \pm 0.22$ | $\mathbf{3.30 \pm 0.20}$ |
| DR5 | $\mathbf{2.55 \pm 0.31}$ | $2.64 \pm 0.41$ | $2.57 \pm 0.23$ | $2.57 \pm 0.18$ |
| DR6 | $1.77 \pm 0.29$ | $1.76 \pm 0.27$ | $1.77 \pm 0.32$ | $\mathbf{1.76 \pm 0.18}$ |
| DR7 | $0.68 \pm 0.24$ | $0.66 \pm 0.23$ | $\mathbf{0.60 \pm 0.24}$ | $0.61 \pm 0.17$ |
| DR8 | $0.09 \pm 0.08$ | $0.08 \pm 0.19$ | $0.06 \pm 0.06$ | $\mathbf{0.06 \pm 0.05}$ |

diagnosis results indicate that our multi-index OD quantification achieves a competitive performance using the 20 quantitative indices compared with the other methods only using the CDR value.

## 4    Conclusion

In this paper, multitask ensemble learning framework (DMTFs) is proposed to achieve multi-index OD quantification for clinical assessment of ophthalmic disease. The DMTFs innovatively creates an ensemble of multiple OD quantification tasks (OD segmentation and indices estimation) and learns the ensemble with a multi-task learning framework by modeling the consistency correlation between the two tasks. Experimental results show that DMTFs is capable of achieving impressive performance for multi-index OD quantification. The proposed method has great potential in clinical ophthalmic disease diagnoses.

**Acknowledgment.** This work was supported in part by the National Natural Science Foundation of China (61702558, 61602527), the Hunan Natural Science Foundation (2017JJ3411), the Key Research and Development Projects in Hunan (2017WK2074), the National Key Research and Development Program of China (2017YFC0840104) and the China Scholarship Council (201806375006).

# References

1. Caprioli, J.: Clinical evaluation of the optic nerve in glaucoma. Trans. Am. Ophthalmol. Soc. **92**, 589 (1994)
2. Cheng, J., Yin, F., Wong, D.W.K., Tao, D., Liu, J.: Sparse dissimilarity-constrained coding for glaucoma screening. IEEE TBME **62**(5), 1395–1403 (2015)
3. Cheng, J., et al.: Similarity regularized sparse group lasso for cup to disc ratio computation. Biomed. Opt. Express **8**(8), 3763–3777 (2017)
4. Fu, H., Cheng, J., Xu, Y., Wong, D.W.K., Liu, J., Cao, X.: Joint optic disc and cup segmentation based on multi-label deep network and polar transformation. IEEE TMI **37**(7), 1597–1605 (2018)
5. Gao, Z., et al.: Motion tracking of the carotid artery wall from ultrasound image sequences: a nonlinear state-space approach. IEEE TMI **37**(1), 273–283 (2017)
6. Gao, Z., et al.: Robust estimation of carotid artery wall motion using the elasticity-based state-space approach. Med. Image Anal. **37**, 1–21 (2017)
7. Garway-Heath, D., Hitchings, R.: Quantitative evaluation of the optic nerve head in early glaucoma. Br. J. Ophthalmol. **82**(4), 352–361 (1998)
8. Harizman, N., et al.: The ISNT rule and differentiation of normal from glaucomatous eyes. Arch. Ophthalmol. **124**(11), 1579–1583 (2006)
9. Jiang, Y., et al.: Optic disc and cup segmentation with blood vessel removal from fundus images for glaucoma detection. In: IEEE EMBC, pp. 862–865. IEEE (2018)
10. Kendall, A., Gal, Y., Cipolla, R.: Multi-task learning using uncertainty to weigh losses for scene geometry and semantics. In: CVPR, pp. 7482–7491 (2018)
11. Kim, S., Xing, E.P.: Tree-guided group lasso for multi-task regression with structured sparsity. In: ICML, vol. 2, p. 1 (2010)
12. Maninis, K.K., Pont-Tuset, J., Arbeláez, P., Van Gool, L.: Deep retinal image understanding. In: Ourselin, S., Joskowicz, L., Sabuncu, M., Unal, G., Wells, W. (eds.) MICCAI 2014. LNCS, vol. 9901, pp. 140–148. Springer Cham (2016). https://doi.org/10.1007/978-3-319-46723-8-17
13. Shen, W., Zhao, K., Guo, Y., Yuille, A.L.: Label distribution learning forests. In: NIPS, pp. 834–843 (2017)
14. Xu, Y., et al.: Optic cup segmentation for glaucoma detection using low-rank superpixel representation. In: Golland, P., Hata, N., Barillot, C., Hornegger, J., Howe, R. (eds.) MICCAI 2014. LNCS, vol. 8673, pp. 788–795. Springer Cham (2014) https://doi.org/10.1007/978-3-319-10404-1-98
15. Zhang, Y., Yang, Q.: A survey on multi-task learning. arXiv preprint arXiv:1707.08114 (2017)
16. Zhao, R., Liao, W., Zou, B., Chen, Z., Li, S.: Weakly-supervised simultaneous evidence identification and segmentation for automated glaucoma diagnosis. In: AAAI (2019)
17. Zhao, S., et al.: Robust segmentation of intima-media borders with different morphologies and dynamics during the cardiac cycle. IEEE JBHI **22**(5), 1571–1582 (2017)

# Retinal Abnormalities Recognition Using Regional Multitask Learning

Xin Wang[1], Lie Ju[1], Xin Zhao[1], and Zongyuan Ge[1,2(✉)]

[1] Airdoc LLC, Beijing, China
{wangxin,julie,zhaoxin,gezongyuan}@airdoc.com
[2] Monash eResearch Center, Monash University, Clayton, Australia

**Abstract.** The number of people suffering from retinal diseases increases with population aging and the popularity of electronic screens. Previous studies on deep learning based automatic screening generally focused on specific types of retinal diseases, such as diabetic retinopathy and glaucoma. Since patients may suffer from various types of retinal diseases simultaneously, these solutions are not clinically practical. To address this issue, we propose a novel deep learning based method that can recognise 36 different retinal diseases with a single model. More specifically, the proposed method uses a region-specific multi-task recognition model by learning diseases affecting different regions of the retina with three sub-networks. The three sub-networks are semantically trained to recognise diseases affecting optic-disc, macula and entire retina. Our contribution is two-fold. First, we use multitask learning for retinal disease classification and achieve significant improvements for recognising three main groups of retinal diseases in general, macular and optic-disc regions. Second, we collect a multi-label retinal dataset to the community as standard benchmark and release it for further research opportunities.

## 1 Introduction

Many retinal diseases, such as glaucoma, age-related macular degeneration (AMD) and diabetic retinopathy (DR), lead to irreversible vision loss or even blindness [1]. Fundus photograph, where the microcirculation can be observed directly, is widely used to examine and screen eye diseases for early intervention in the asymptomatic stage. Deep learning has been used for computer-aided diagnosis of retinal diseases on fundus images [2–5]. For DR screening, [2,3] used convolutional neural networks (CNNs) to perform lesion detection and DR grading. Although the performance of those methods is impressive in controlled experimental settings, most of them are designed and tested for one specific retinal disease only. Real clinical scenarios where some patients suffer from various

---

**Electronic supplementary material** The online version of this chapter (https://doi.org/10.1007/978-3-030-32239-7_4) contains supplementary material, which is available to authorized users.

D. Shen et al. (Eds.): MICCAI 2019, LNCS 11764, pp. 30–38, 2019.
https://doi.org/10.1007/978-3-030-32239-7_4

and multiple retinal diseases are not considered in those models. For instance, people who suffer from DR may suffer from macular edema and optic-disc edema as well. Diseases such as hypertensive retinopathy, retinal detachment, epiretinal membrane, macular hole and macular edema may be co-occurrent with one another which leads to a challenging multi-label categorisation problem.

Moreover, global and local region information fusion has been used to improve the model performance. A novel Disc-aware ensemble network is proposed for glaucoma screening in [5], which integrates the deep hierarchical context of the entire retina and the local optic region. However, most existing methods use global and local network to target for diseases with the same distribution, region-based disease information is not explicitly used. Many researches show that the symptom from glaucoma is often associated with elevated intraocular pressure in optic-disc area. Various medical signs linked to some specific eye diseases including hemorrhage, blood vessel abnormalities (tortuosity, pulsation and new vessels) and pigmentation may tend to appear frequently in one region (e.g. macular or optic-disc region).

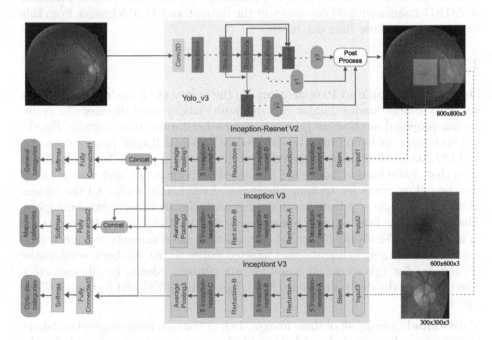

**Fig. 1.** The multi-label classification network has been split into three sub-networks and trained for three mutual exclusive tasks: a general task to detect diseases affect the whole retina (DR, CRVO/BRVO etc.), a **macular** sub-network to identify macular diseases (drusen, macular edema etc.) and a **optic-disc** network component to detect optic-disc related diseases (glaucoma, optic atrophy etc.). Because the features representing each of these region tasks are relevant, we design a hierarchical fusion strategy to combine late semantic representations.

In this paper, we propose a multi-task deep learning framework for identifying multi-label retinal diseases using fundus images. Our method is inspired by how ophthalmologists observe fundus images to make diagnoses and determine therapies. They firstly scan the whole fundus image to examine if there is any abnormality in color, texture or any dispersed lesion in general and then switch their attention to macular and optic-disc regions which are more vital to center vision. In order to simulate ophthalmologists' behaviour, we adopt the idea of multi-stream network [6] by using three separate sub-networks to extract features from **macula**, **optic-disc** and whole **fundus** regions separately. Additionally, we design the network in a multi-task manner by employing the prior clinical knowledge about label co-occurrence dependencies in each task (as shown in Fig. 1 from the Appendix). Our framework consists of two stages. The first stage contains a joint detector for detection of **optic-disc** and **macula** regions. The second stage is composed of a semantic multi-task network where each task is trained with exclusive region-related disease labels to output disease categories of whole fundus, optic-disc and macula concurrently, as shown in Fig. 1. To evaluate the performance of our proposed method, we collect and relabel a number of 200,817 images with 36 categories in the dataset and 17,385 images from this dataset contain more than one labels.

## 2   Datasets

**Data Annotation and Preparation.** To the best of our knowledge, there does not exist a large fundus dataset contains multi-label retinal diseases. To evaluate our proposed method, we present a multi-label dataset that contains 200,817 fundus images, including 18,614 re-labelled images from Kaggle contest dataset [1] and 182,203 de-identified samples collected from several private hospitals. Apart from that, 2,000 fundus images are annotated with optic-disc and macular location bounding boxes for training the region detection network. All the images from either Kaggle or private hospitals are re-labelled by three ophthalmologists. The labels of one fundus image preserve only if at least two ophthalmologists are in agreement. We choose 36 retinal diseases that are commonly examined during the screening including diseases affected entire retina (diabetic retinopathy etc.), optic-disc (glaucoma etc.) and macula (drusen, edema, membranes etc.). The dataset is divided for training (80%), validating (10%) and testing (10%) in this work.

**Multi-label.** Among all of these images, 183,432 images have single-class labels, 16,849 images have dual-class labels and 536 images have triple-class labels. The distribution of the categories and their co-occurrences are shown in Fig. 1 from the Appendix. To summarise, the most frequently co-occurrent labels are central or branch retinal vein occlusion (CRVO/BRVO) with macular edema (4,147 samples), and pathologic myopia with choroidal neovascularization (CNV) (2,467 samples). We will make the test dataset publicly available to the community for benchmark comparison and extenable future study.

---

[1] https://www.kaggle.com/c/diabetic-retinopathy-detection.

# 3  Methods

**Overview.** Our proposed method contains two parts: (1) macular and optic-disc region detection; (2) semantic multitask learning for retinal disease classification. We first train a joint CNN detector to localise optic disc and macula regions. The architecture extends the Yolov3 [7] with geometric constraints. The detected optic-disc and macular region bounding boxes along with whole fundus image are resized to $300 \times 300$, $600 \times 600$, $800 \times 800$ respectively and then fed into a three-stream multi-label disease classification network. The classification network uses the idea of semantic feature fusion to categorise regionally based diseases.

## 3.1  Macular and Optic-Disc Region Detection

Optic-disc and the macula are critical regions in the diagnosis of many diseases. To identify these regions, recent works such as [8] trained a Yolo detector and demonstrated accurate detection results. We extend Yolov3 [7]'s structure to infer and calibrate optic disc and macula regions. Yolov3 predicts candidate bounding boxes with 3 different scales (i.e. $y1$, $y2$ and $y3$ in Fig. 1) and perform postprocessing techniques such as non-maxima suppression [9] to select the most appropriate bounding boxes for each object. With prior knowledge of the centre distance between optic-disc and macula is approximately equivalent to two and half times as the diameter of the optic disc [10], it becomes reasonable to model and infer target regions from one another. Therefore, based on the bounding box annotations of macula and optic-disc, we add an auxiliary bounding box including those two regions as an extra cue for training and inference.

**Geometric Constraints.** Let $(x_0^{OD}, y_0^{OD}, x_1^{OD}, y_1^{OD})$ denote the locations (upper left and bottom right coordinates of optic-disc for the bounding box) and $(x_0^{MA}, y_0^{MA}, x_1^{MA}, y_1^{MA})$ as macular bounding box. The auxiliary bounding box is defined as,

$$x_0^{AUX} = \min(x_0^{OD}, x_0^{MA}), x_1^{AUX} = \max(x_1^{OD}, x_1^{MA})$$
$$y_0^{AUX} = \min(y_0^{OD}, y_0^{MA}), y_1^{AUX} = \max(y_1^{OD}, y_1^{MA})$$

as shown in Fig. 2(a). During training, the auxiliary bounding box is regressed to assists the model learning the implicit relations between the macula and optic-disc regions. While in inference process, the auxiliary bounding box could be used to deduce the optic disc or macula location in some circumstances where one of the two regions is failed to be detected. Because the individual region detectors are less than perfect, the candidate region window is not always correct or even missing occasionally, especially when macula or optic-disc region is at low quality or with occlusion. In such circumstances, when the proposed auxiliary bounding box can be used to deduce the optic disc or macula location explicitly, as shown in Fig. 2(b) and (c), the missing macula bounding box location is calculated as:

$$s = sgn(|x_1^{AUX} - x_1^{OD}| - |x_0^{AUX} - x_0^{OD}|), w^{AUX} = x_1^{AUX} - x_0^{AUX}$$

$$x_0^{MA} = \max\left(s\left(x_1^{AUX} - \frac{1}{3}w^{AUX}\right), x_0^{AUX}\right), x_1^{MA} = x_0^{MA} + \frac{1}{3}w^{AUX}$$

$$y_0^{MA} = y_0^{AUX}, y_1^{MA} = y_1^{AUX}$$

where, $sgn$ indicates signum function and $s$ indicates whether the detected optic-disc box is at the left of the auxiliary box; $w^{AUX}$ denotes the width of the auxiliary box. Based on the prior domain knowledge, we approximate the location of the macular box to be at either left or right (depends on which eye being scanned) one-third part of the auxiliary box, in which of in the opposite direction to the optic-disc box. To be complete, in the rare case where both macula and optic-disc boxes are missing even with the assistance of auxiliary box, the whole fundus image is adjusted and used as input to the macula and optic-disc stream.

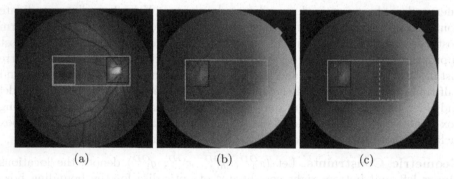

(a)                              (b)                              (c)

**Fig. 2.** Illustration of auxiliary bounding box $AUX$. (a) annotations of optic-disc bounding box $OD$ in red, macular box $MA$ in blue and the auxiliary bounding box $AUX$ of joint region in yellow; (b) the detection result with missing macula $MA$ because of low quality/blurry region; (c) localisation of macula $MA$ in dash blue from (b) through $AUX$ post-processing described in Sect. 3.1 (Color figure online)

### 3.2 Semantic Multitask Learning for Retinal Disease Classification

There are three main groups of retinal diseases, general retina diseases indicate diseases that influence the entire retina, such as DR, hypertensive retinopathy and CRVO/BRVO etc. Macular diseases include age-related macular degeneration (AMD), macular edema and macular hole, while optic-disc diseases contain glaucoma, optic-disc edema, optic atrophy etc. By analyzing medical signs of these diseases, many studies found that some diseases belong to different tasks share some common pathological features or have some medical signs correlations with each other. From those observations, we propose a collaborative multi-task learning framework with three streams. Each stream of the network represents learning process for one group of retinal diseases. One important concept of the proposed framework is that part of the model layer is shared across independent tasks. In this work, the layer sharing strategy is semantically designed with respect to the knowledge of regionally disease correlation.

**General task stream** is designed to be a task that determines the general retinal disease affecting the entire retina based on the features from optic-disc and macular regions as well as the whole fundus image. The motivation to design this branch is inspired by the fact that most general retinal diseases are diagnosed in consideration of lesions on the macula and optic disc. For instance, one of the vital medical signs to diagnose proliferative diabetic retinopathy (PDR) is whether there is neovascularisation on the optic-disc. As for diagnosing pathologic myopic, atrophy on macula can serve as a strong evidence. Therefore, it is reasonable to add region-specific features of macula and optic-disc as supporting information to determine the general retinal disease category. **Macular task stream** takes advantage of features from macular region and entire retina because some sub-type macular edema diseases are closely correlated to general retinal disease such as DR. To further improve the intra-class performance of this branch, we made macular edema into three sub-categories, macular edema caused by DR or hypertensive retinopathy, CRVO/BRVO and other diseases. The same operation is applied to pathologic myopia w/o CNV. **Optic-disc task stream** is a relatively independent task because its categories are self-contained and the regionally independent compared to other regions.

**Inference:** During inference process, each task stream outputs either healthy or diseased class which has the highest confidence score. A patient is diagnosed as healthy when all task streams (macular, optic-disc and whole fundus regions) indicate non-disease outcome.

**Implementation:** Inception-V3 is used as backbone for optic-disc and macular task streams, and Inception-Resnet-V2 is used for general retinal task[2]. Each task stream is initialised with ImageNet pre-trained parameters and trained separately before jointly trained together.

## 4    Experiments

### 4.1    Results on Optic-Disc and Macula Joint Detection

The joint detection YoloV3 network with joint constraint is trained and validated on 2,000 fundus images with annotated macular and optic-disc bounding boxes. All the 2,000 images are divided into training, validating and testing in the

---

[2] We experimented with all Inception-V3/Inception-Resnet-V2 settings and figured out a mixture of them gave the best performance of all. Network training used Adam with a learning rate of 1e-5 which decayed every three epochs with ratio of 0.9 for total 14 epochs. We used Keras distributed machine learning system with 8 replicas running each on a NVidia 1080Ti GPU. The input size of general stream is 800, while the input size of macular and optic-task stream is 600 and 300 respectively.

proportion of 8:1:1. Experiment on the testing dataset obtains 83.45% mAP with minimal IoU 0.5, with macula(90.03% AP) and optic disc (96.73% AP). We then run the trained detector on the whole fundus dataset with 200,817 images. After carefully checked by three ophthalmologists, only 4,824 (about 2.4% out of the whole dataset) macular or optic-disc regions are not correctly detected. Most of these cases are either blurry or with very serious lesions (see Appendix Fig. 2).

### 4.2 Quantitative Evaluation on Multitask Learning

Table 1 shows average precision and recall for task based classification. We evaluate the effectiveness of applying multi-stream on macular task and general task. For macular task, we first obtain the results of one-stream network which is trained on macular images (detected by YoloV3 detector) with 14 macular (MA) relevant retinal diseases (**MA-One-Stream (with single task)**), and compare it to **MA-Two-Stream (with single task)** which takes both the whole fundus image and macular image as inputs. We then conduct the same experiment on the general disease task (GC). In both experiments of MA and GC, our multi-stream method works better than single stream network baseline. We then extend the multi-stream experiments with extra multitask label learning, marginal performance improvements can be observed for **GC-Three-Stream (with multitask)**. More detailed confusion matrix of these frameworks for various tasks are shown in Figs. 3 and 4 in the Appendix.

**Table 1.** Results on task based classification

| Methods | Average recall | Average precision |
|---|---|---|
| MA-One-Stream (single task) | 68.8% | 61.3% |
| MA-Two-Stream (single task) | **73.6%** | 67.6% |
| MA-Two-Stream (multitask) | 73.1% | **68.6%** |
| GC-One-Stream (single task) | 65.2% | 60.8% |
| GC-Three-Stream (single task) | 67.5% | 61.5% |
| GC-Three-Stream (multitask) | **67.8%** | **62.2%** |

The second set of results in Table 2 focuses on fully 36 diseases trained multitask deep neural network performance for each disease group (macula, optic-disc and whole fundus). As Table 2 shows, in this setting our proposed multi-task method works much better than the baseline single stream model. The performance of all diseases has improvements in both precision and recall, while diseases relevant to macula and disc acquire greater improvement than diseases not relevant to these two regions compared with single stream.

**Table 2.** Results on 36 category classification on different disease regions

| Methods | Regions | Average recall | Average precision |
|---|---|---|---|
| One-Stream | Macula | 60.9% | 61.1% |
| Three-Stream | Macula | **62.6%** | **63.0%** |
| One-Stream | Disc | 57.5% | 69.7% |
| Three-Stream | Disc | **62.4%** | **70.0%** |
| One-Stream | General | 69.2% | 60.5% |
| Three-Stream | General | **70.6%** | **61.4%** |

## 4.3 Visualization

In order to gain a better understanding of the proposed model, we draw the class activation maps (CAM) [11] for each stream with respect to each task. As shown in Fig. 3, the case in Fig. 3 is a fundus image with PDR, macular edema and other optic-disc disease[3]. Our model gives three correct labels via the multitask architecture. From the CAM generated by the general task of individual regions, we can observe that when PDR, proliferative membranes and hemorrhage appear over the whole fundus image, neovascularisation grows around the optic-disc, and more activation of exudates from macular region are taken into consideration. Moreover, lesions from the entire fundus are also used to help distinguish diabetic macular edema (DME) from other macular diseases. The membrane and neovascularisation on the optic-disc are highlighted by its task stream to correctly give the label of other optic-disc disease.

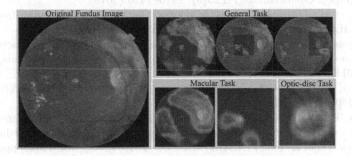

**Fig. 3.** Class activation maps (CAM) of a challenging multi-label sample, CAM generated for each task from a fundus image with PDR, macular edema and other optic-disc disease.

---

[3] We set a label named as other general, macular or optic-disc disease to indicate a gathering of rare diseases in each task. This label for optic-disc task represents disease such as morning glory syndrome, melanocytoma of optic disc, membrane tissue on the optic disc and etc.

From visualization of this case, we can see that the proposed model can mine the region-specific information with respective to various disease types and improve the performance of disease recognition through collaborative multi-label learning.

## 5    Conclusion

In this work, we demonstrate the effectiveness of multitask learning approach for recognising the general, macular and optic-disc diseases, as opposed to single task classification. The presented method and new benchmark open the possibility for large scale multi-label retinal abnormalities recognition.

## References

1. Tham, Y.-C., Li, X., Wong, T.Y., Quigley, H.A., Aung, T., Cheng, C.-Y.: Global prevalence of glaucoma and projections of glaucoma burden through 2040: a systematic review and meta-analysis. Ophthalmology **121**(11), 2081–2090 (2014)
2. Wang, P., et al.: Development and validation of a deep-learning algorithm for the detection of polyps during colonoscopy. Nat. Biomed. Eng. **2**(10), 741 (2018)
3. Playout, C., Duval, R., Cheriet, F.: A multitask learning architecture for simultaneous segmentation of bright and red lesions in fundus images. In: Frangi, A.F., Schnabel, J.A., Davatzikos, C., Alberola-López, C., Fichtinger, G. (eds.) MICCAI 2018. LNCS, vol. 11071, pp. 101–108. Springer, Cham (2018). https://doi.org/10. 1007/978-3-030-00934-2_12
4. Grassmann, F., et al.: A deep learning algorithm for prediction of age-related eye disease study severity scale for age-related macular degeneration from color fundus photography. Ophthalmology **125**(9), 1410–1420 (2018)
5. Fu, H., et al.: Disc-aware ensemble network for glaucoma screening from fundus image. IEEE Trans. Med. Imaging **37**(11), 2493–2501 (2018)
6. Simonyan, K., Zisserman, A.: Two-stream convolutional networks for action recognition in videos. In: Advances in Neural Information Processing Systems, pp. 568–576 (2014)
7. Redmon, J., Farhadi, A.: Yolov3: An incremental improvement. arXiv preprint arXiv:1804.02767 (2018)
8. Araújo, T., Aresta, G., Galdran, A., Costa, P., Mendonça, A.M., Campilho, A.: UOLO - automatic object detection and segmentation in biomedical images. In: Stoyanov, D., et al. (eds.) DLMIA/ML-CDS -2018. LNCS, vol. 11045, pp. 165–173. Springer, Cham (2018). https://doi.org/10.1007/978-3-030-00889-5_19
9. Bodla, N., Singh, B., Chellappa, R., Davis, L.S.: Soft-NMS-improving object detection with one line of code. In: Proceedings of the IEEE International Conference on Computer Vision, pp. 5561–5569 (2017)
10. Sinthanayothin, C., Boyce, J.F., Cook, H.L., Williamson, T.H.: Automated localisation of the optic disc, fovea, and retinal blood vessels from digital colour fundus images. Br. J. Ophthalmol. **83**(8), 902–910 (1999)
11. Zhou, B., Khosla, A., Lapedriza, A., Oliva, A., Torralba, A.: Learning deep features for discriminative localization. In: Proceedings of the IEEE Conference on Computer Vision and Pattern Recognition, pp. 2921–2929 (2016)

# Unifying Structure Analysis and Surrogate-Driven Function Regression for Glaucoma OCT Image Screening

Xi Wang[1], Hao Chen[2(✉)], Luyang Luo[1], An-ran Ran[3], Poemen P. Chan[3], Clement C. Tham[3], Carol Y. Cheung[3], and Pheng-Ann Heng[1,4]

[1] Department of Computer Science and Engineering,
The Chinese University of Hong Kong, Hong Kong, China
{xiwang,hchen}@cse.cuhk.edu.hk
[2] Imsight Medical Technology, Co., Ltd., Shenzhen, China
[3] Department of Ophthalmology and Visual Sciences, The Chinese University
of Hong Kong, Hong Kong, China
[4] Guangdong Provincial Key Laboratory of Computer Vision and Virtual Reality
Technology, Shenzhen Institutes of Advanced Technology,
Chinese Academy of Sciences, Shenzhen, China

**Abstract.** Optical Coherence Tomography (OCT) imaging plays an important role in glaucoma diagnosis in clinical practice. Early detection and timely treatment can prevent glaucoma patients from permanent vision loss. However, only a dearth of automated methods has been developed based on OCT images for glaucoma study. In this paper, we present a novel framework to effectively classify glaucoma OCT images from normal ones. A semi-supervised learning strategy with *smoothness assumption* is applied for surrogate assignment of missing function regression labels. Besides, the proposed multi-task learning network is capable of exploring the structure and function relationship from the OCT image and visual field measurement simultaneously, which contributes to classification performance boosting. Essentially, we are the first to unify the structure analysis and function regression for glaucoma screening. It is also worth noting that we build the largest glaucoma OCT image dataset involving 4877 volumes to develop and evaluate the proposed method. Extensive experiments demonstrate that our framework outperforms the baseline methods and two glaucoma experts by a large margin, achieving 93.2%, 93.2% and 97.8% on accuracy, F1 score and AUC, respectively.

## 1 Introduction

Glaucoma is the most frequent cause of irreversible blindness worldwide, which is a heterogeneous group of disease that damages the optic nerve and leads to vision loss [1]. It is featured by loss of retinal ganglion cells, thinning of retinal nerve fibre layer (RNFL), and cupping of the optic disc. Early detection and diagnosis

© Springer Nature Switzerland AG 2019
D. Shen et al. (Eds.): MICCAI 2019, LNCS 11764, pp. 39–47, 2019.
https://doi.org/10.1007/978-3-030-32239-7_5

are essential as they can facilitate immediate treatment and prevent the progression of the disease, especially for early-stage glaucoma patients. On clinical grounds, diagnosis of glaucoma usually requires a variety of tests, including functional measurement (e.g., visual field test) and structure assessment (e.g., optical coherence tomography). In general, visual field (VF) test provides three important global indices: visual field index (VFI), mean deviation (MD) and pattern standard deviation (PSD) to depict the functional changes. Optical coherence tomography (OCT) is a non-contact and non-invasive imaging modality that generates high-resolution, cross-sectional images (B-scans) of the retina. It can provide objective and quantitative assessment of various retinal structures. However, the examination of OCT imaging requires highly trained ophthalmologist, which is always partly subjective and time-consuming. Thus, automated glaucoma OCT image screening tool is of great needs in clinical practice. Moreover, evaluation of the relationship between structural and functional damage can provide valuable insight into how visual function works according to the degree of structural damage, which can help our understanding of glaucoma. This is quite significant in diagnosing, staging and monitoring glaucomatous patients.

Many researchers have devoted their efforts to solving the glaucoma OCT image screening problem and have achieved significant progress. Nevertheless, most of the previous works were based on machine learning methods and heavily relied on established features, such as the measurements on retinal nerve fiber layer thickness and ganglion cell layer thickness [2–4]. Differently, Ramzan et al. [5] proposed an approach that first segmented inner limiting membrane and retinal pigment epithelium layers in OCT images for cup-to-disc ratio calculation, and then differentiated glaucoma based on the calculated ratio. A pioneering work [6] recently proposed a 3D convolutional neural network (CNN) to directly classify the downsampled OCT volumes into glaucoma or normal, which considerably outperformed various feature-based machine learning algorithms. With respect to modelling the structure-function relationship [7,8], Leite et al. utilized locally weighted scatterplot smoothing and regression analysis to evaluate parapapillary RNFL thickness sectors and corresponding topographic standard automated perimetry locations [8]. However, there are still three main challenges that have not been fully investigated yet. First, heretofore there is a dearth of studies that explores the structure and function relationship based on the raw OCT image and visual field measurement for glaucoma screening. Second, owing to very limited images in current datasets, validation experiments of previous methods were not comprehensive, which indeed constrained the development of robust and reliable approaches. Third, building a large medical dataset is always confronted with many difficulties, e.g., it is inevitable to acquire incomplete clinical records due to some unexpected reasons, which is a common phenomenon in retrospective studies.

In this paper, we carried thorough investigation on all of the aforementioned challenges. To the best of our knowledge, we are the first to unify structure analysis and function regression for glaucoma screening based on OCT images. We develop a novel framework that explores the structure and function relationship between OCT image and visual field measurement via a semi-supervised multi-task learning network. Specifically, a semi-supervised learning method is first introduced to find the surrogates to fill the vacancy of missing visual field measurements. Afterwards, both class labels (glaucoma/normal) and visual field measurements (ground truth and pseudo labels) are utilized to jointly train a multi-task learning network. In particular, we concatenate the classification features with those learned from the regression module to identify glaucoma. It indicates that the structure and function relationship learned by our network indeed contributes to classification performance improvement. It is worthwhile to emphasize that to our best knowledge, the largest glaucoma OCT image dataset composed of 4877 volumes of the optic disc is constructed in this study for algorithm development and evaluation.

## 2  Method

Our main goal is to effectively classify glaucoma OCT images assisted by exploring the structure and function relationship of glaucoma. Figure 1 illustrates the overview of the proposed method, which consists of two parts. The first part uses a semi-supervised learning technique to solve the missing label problem for function regression. In particular, a B-scan-based CNN is trained under full supervision of class labels, aiming to extract the holistic representation for each OCT volume. Afterwards, pseudo labels are automatically generated by probing the nearest neighbour of OCT images without VF measurement among homogeneous groups with CNN-encoded features. In the second part, a multi-task learning network is trained to unify structure analysis and surrogate-driven function regression for more accurate glaucoma screening.

### 2.1  Surrogate-Driven Labelling with Semi-supervised Learning

In order to solve the problem of missing VF measurement labels, we borrow the spirit from semi-supervised learning and come up with an appropriate solution. In semi-supervised learning domain, the *smoothness assumption* points out that features close to each other are more likely to share the same label. This assumption is intimately linked to a definition of what it means for one feature to be near another feature, which can be embodied in a similarity function $S(\cdot, \cdot)$ on input space [9].

To project OCT volumes into the input space for similarity calculation, we adopted ResNet18 [10] as the feature representation model. Specifically, this CNN is first trained based on B-scans under full supervision of class labels. Then we apply the trained model to extract the embedded feature of each B-scan from the Global Average Pooling (GAP) layer. Finally following [11], the norm-3 pooling, $\mathcal{F} = (\sum_{i=1}^{n} f_i^3)^{\frac{1}{3}}$, is applied to aggregate B-scan features into a holistic representation $\mathcal{F}$ for each OCT volume. Here, $f$ is the feature representation of B-scan input, and $n$ is the number of B-scans from the same volume.

Based on the availability of class labels and the VF measurements, we group the training set into four clusters: (1) $G^l$: glaucoma images with VF measurement; (2) $G^u$: glaucoma images without VF measurement; (3) $N^l$: normal images

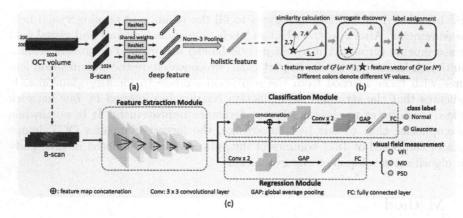

**Fig. 1.** An overview of the proposed method. (a) Initially, we train a CNN model with class labels (glaucoma/normal) to extract features of B-scans. Then the extracted features are aggregated to form a global representation of an OCT volume. (b) Next, we compute similarities between homogeneous groups to find the nearest neighbour of OCT images without VF measurement and enable its VF values for surrogate assignment. Here, $G^l$ and $G^u$ indicate glaucoma images with and without VF labels while $N^l$ and $N^u$ denote normal images with and without VF labels. (c) Lastly, class labels and VF labels (ground truth and pseudo labels) are unified to train a multi-task learning network.

with VF measurement and (4) $N^u$: normal images without VF measurement. Through the feature representation model, each OCT volume is represented by a feature vector, $\mathcal{F} \in \mathbb{R}^{512}$. The similarity between any pair of homogeneous OCT images, e.g., $\mathcal{F}^l \in G^l$ and $\mathcal{F}^u \in G^u$, is measured by *Euclidean distance*:

$$S(\mathcal{F}^l, \mathcal{F}^u) = \left[ \sum_{i=1}^{m} (\mathcal{F}_i^l - \mathcal{F}_i^u)^2 \right]^{\frac{1}{2}} \tag{1}$$

Inspired by the semi-supervised *smoothness assumption*, for each OCT image without VF measurement $\mathcal{F}_j^u \in G^u$ (or $\mathcal{F}_j^u \in N^u$), we find its nearest neighbour in the group of the same class that has VF measurement $\mathcal{F}_{i*}^l \in G^l$ (or $\mathcal{F}_{i*}^l \in N^l$), where $i^* = \arg\min_i S(\mathcal{F}_i^l, \mathcal{F}_j^u)$, and appoint the VF measurement of $\mathcal{F}_{i*}^l$ to $\mathcal{F}_j^u$. Consequently, we successfully find suitable surrogates for all missing VF measurements in this semi-supervised learning fashion.

## 2.2   Multi-task Learning for Structure and Function Analysis

We proposed an end-to-end multi-task learning CNN with a primary task to classify B-scan images into glaucomatous and normal, and an auxiliary task to investigate the relationship between structural and functional changes of glaucoma eyes. Particularly, this network is composed of three components, the shared feature extraction module, the classification module and the regression module.

As illustrated in Fig. 1(c), we employ ResNet18, initialized with ImageNet pre-trained weights, as the backbone in the feature extraction module whose weights are shared by both classification and regression tasks. The rest of the network is composed of two branches, one for glaucoma discrimination and the other for visual field measurement regression. These tasks are trained jointly.

**Visual Field Measurement Regression.** For each attribute of visual field measurement, i.e., VFI, MD and PSD, we formulate it as an individual regression task. Within the regression module, two convolutional layers with ReLU activation and batch-normalization are inserted before GAP. Fully connected layers with sigmoid activation are then used to regress these attributes. The regression tasks are driven by minimizing the mean square error:

$$\mathcal{L}_{reg} = \frac{1}{N} \sum_{i=1}^{N} \|y_i^r - \hat{y}_i^r(x_i; \theta_s, \theta_{reg})\|_2^2 \tag{2}$$

where $N$ denotes the number of training samples, $x_i$ is the input of three adjacent B-scan images, $y_i^r$ is the clinical measurement of visual field attribute and $\hat{y}_i^r$ is the corresponding prediction of the network. $\theta_s$ denotes shared weights in the feature extraction module and $\theta_{reg}$ denotes features in the regression module, respectively. In this paper, we use superscripts $r$ and $c$ for discrimination between regression and classification tasks.

**Glaucoma Classification.** The classification module performs the primary task for glaucoma screening. In routine clinical practice, visual field measurement is an important indicator of functional change for glaucoma diagnosis. Hence, it is reasonable to hypothesize that if the relationship between structure and function is appropriately discovered, the learned features in the regression module could exert a positive influence on the classification task. Based on this assumption, we concatenate the attribute regression feature maps with those originated from the feature extraction module, supposing that the features learned in the regression module could provide the classifier with helpful guidance. Here, the typical binary cross-entropy loss is utilized to train this classifier:

$$\mathcal{L}_{cls} = -\frac{1}{N} \sum_{i=1}^{N} y_i^c \log \hat{y}_i^c(x_i; \theta_s, \theta_{cls}) \tag{3}$$

where $y_i^c$ is the ground truth label while $\hat{y}_i^c$ is the likelihood predicted by the classifier. Similarly, $\theta_{cls}$ stands for weights in the classification module.

**Joint Training of Multi-task Learning Network.** Finally, the multi-task learning network is trained by minimizing the weighted combination of the mean square error losses and the binary cross-entropy loss.

$$\mathcal{L}_{total} = \mathcal{L}_{cls} + \sum_{j=1}^{3} \alpha_j \mathcal{L}_{reg}^j \tag{4}$$

where $\alpha_j$ is the hyper-parameter balancing $\mathcal{L}_{cls}$ and $\mathcal{L}_{reg}^j$ determined by cross validation. At the inference stage, we take the average of multiple B-scan-level probabilities as a single volume-level prediction.

## 3    Experiments and Results

**Dataset:** In this study, we constructed the largest scale cohort for evaluation. This dataset consists of 4877 volumetric OCT images (glaucoma: 2926; normal: 1951) from 930 subjects. It is worth noting that each investigated subject (one eye or both two eyes involved) might have several follow-ups, and also several OCT images may be taken during each follow-up, which eventually results in 3182 eye visits (glaucoma: 1901; normal: 1281) in total. Specially, we denote the eye-visit result as *case-level* result. A part of VF measurements for some follow-ups are unavailable in this study. Two glaucoma specialists worked individually to label all the OCT images into glaucoma and normal, taking VF tests and other clinical records as reference. A senior glaucoma expert was consulted in case of disagreement. Subsets of 2895, 1015 and 967 images are randomly selected for training, validation and testing, respectively. The random sampling is at patient level so as to prevent leakage and biased estimation of the testing performance. According to the accessibility of VF measurements in the training set, we re-configure the training set as follows: (i) *Part*: 1979 images whose VF measurements exist. (ii) *All*: all 2895 images.

**Quantitative Evaluation and Comparison:** The performance is measured via three criteria: classification accuracy, F1 score and Area Under ROC Curve (AUC). To obtain the *case-level* prediction, averaging method is used to aggregate the results of several images during each eye visit to a single one.

At present, there is only a dearth of studies on glaucoma OCT image classification. Hence, several baseline methods, including an existing method as well as three variants of the proposed method, were implemented for comparison: (i). 3D-CNN: the implementation of the approach proposed in [6] which is trained with downsampled 3D volumes. (ii). 3D-ResNet: A 3D implementation of ResNet18 [10] that takes raw volumes as input. (iii). 2D-ResNet: ResNet18 trained with B-scan images from OCT volumes. (iv). 2D-ResNet-MT: 2D-ResNet with Multi-Task learning network as shown in Fig. 1(c) without surrogate label assignment. Specifically, if the training sample is lack of visual field measurement, the regression loss is ignored. (v). 2D-ResNet-SEMT: The proposed SEmi-supervised Multi-Task learning network with surrogate label assignment.

The experimental results are listed in Table 1. At first, trained with the same set *All*, 2D-ResNet is superior to 3D-ResNet. There are two possible reasons. One is that training a 3D network with such high-dimensional input is extremely difficult. In fact, validation loss oscillates wildly during training, which makes it hard for selecting models. The other is that there is a deficiency of 3D pre-trained model available, thus training from scratch could readily result in local optima. By exploring the structure and function relationship in 2D-ResNet-MT, the classification performance is improved, which verifies our hypothesis that the extra information from the regression module is helpful. Inspiringly, the proposed framework achieves the best results among the aforementioned methods on all metrics. With surrogate label assignment for VF measurement, the classification module can receive more reliable information from the regression branch.

**Table 1.** Comparison with different methods and expert performance.

| Data | Methods | Accuracy | | F1 Score | | AUC | |
|---|---|---|---|---|---|---|---|
| | | Image-level | Case-level | Image-level | Case-level | Image-level | Case-level |
| *Part* | 2D-ResNet | 0.823 | 0.829 | 0.835 | 0.830 | 0.960 | 0.955 |
| | 2D-ResNet-MT | 0.878 | 0.882 | 0.890 | 0.887 | 0.971 | 0.968 |
| *All* | 3D-CNN [6] | 0.884 | 0.889 | 0.881 | 0.890 | 0.962 | 0.959 |
| | 3D-ResNet | 0.880 | 0.875 | 0.878 | 0.874 | 0.958 | 0.956 |
| | 2D-ResNet | 0.908 | 0.911 | 0.904 | 0.909 | 0.968 | 0.964 |
| | 2D-ResNet-MT | 0.915 | 0.912 | 0.923 | 0.917 | 0.975 | 0.971 |
| | 2D-ResNet-SEMT | **0.932** | **0.924** | **0.932** | **0.924** | **0.978** | **0.973** |
| | Expert 1 | 0.912 | 0.912 | 0.917 | 0.917 | 0.918 | 0.918 |
| | Expert 2 | 0.905 | 0.905 | 0.913 | 0.913 | 0.914 | 0.914 |

When compared to the pioneering work 3D-CNN [6], our method outperforms it by a large margin, with 4.8%, 5.1%, and 1.6% performance improvement on accuracy, F1 score and AUC at image level. By and large, 3D-CNN has two drawbacks. First, the input volumes are compressed intensively, which may lead to discriminative information loss. Second, its capability is quite limited due to the shallow network structure. To further explore the efficacy of our method, we invited another two glaucoma experts to identify glaucoma based on the printout of the OCT images in the format that ophthalmologists usually read in clinic. They reviewed the printouts individually masked from any other clinical notes to make the decision, either glaucoma or normal, for each testing image. Apparently, the proposed method exceeds expert performance significantly, particularly on AUC.

**Qualitative Evaluation.** Class Activation Maps (CAMs) [12] were computed to visualize the discriminative regions that played a vital role in class prediction. For each pair in Fig. 2, the upper one is the input, and the lower one is the corresponding CAM overlapped with the input. Clearly, the discriminative regions found by CNN for glaucoma and normal images are quite different. In normal B-scan images, there is barely any response within retinal areas while such regions contrarily have high responses in glaucoma images. It is corresponding with the clinical diagnosis of glaucoma.

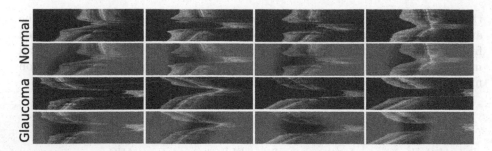

**Fig. 2.** Visualization of discriminative regions. The first two rows show the pairs of normal B-scan and corresponding CAM. The last two rows show the pairs of glaucomatous ones. (Best viewed in color)

## 4    Conclusion

In this study, we present a deep learning framework to screen glaucoma based on volumetric OCT images of the optic disc. We first use a semi-supervised learning method to address the problem of incomplete visual field measurement labels of training images. Then a multi-task learning network is built to explore the relationship between functional and structural changes of glaucoma, which is verified beneficial to classification improvement. Extensive experiments on our large-scale dataset manifested the effectiveness of the proposed approach, which outperforms the baseline methods by a large margin. In addition, the comparison with glaucoma specialists provides strong evidence that our proposed framework has promising potential for automated glaucoma screening in the near future.

**Acknowledgements.** This project is supported in part by the National Basic Program of China 973 Program under Grant 2015CB351706, grants from the National Natural Science Foundation of China with Project No. U1613219, Research Grants Council - General Research Fund, Hong Kong (Ref: 14102418) and Shenzhen Science and Technology Program (No. JCYJ20180507182410327).

## References

1. Jonas, J.B., Aung, T., Bourne, R.R., Bron, A.M., Ritch, R., Panda-Jonas, S.: Glaucoma. Lancet **390**, 2183–2193 (2017)
2. Huang, M.-L., Chen, H.-Y.: Development and comparison of automated classifiers for glaucoma diagnosis using stratus optical coherence tomography. Invest. Ophthalmol. Vis. Sci. **46**(11), 4121–4129 (2005)
3. Kim, H.J., Lee, S.-Y., Park, K.H., Kim, D.M., Jeoung, J.W.: Glaucoma diagnostic ability of layer-by-layer segmented ganglion cell complex by spectral-domain optical coherence tomography. Invest. Ophthalmol. Vis. Sci. **57**(11), 4799–4805 (2016)
4. Christopher, M., et al.: Retinal nerve fiber layer features identified by unsupervised machine learning on optical coherence tomography scans predict glaucoma progression. Invest. Ophthalmol. Vis. Sci. **59**(7), 2748–2756 (2018)

5. Ramzan, A., Akram, M.U., Shaukat, A., Khawaja, S.G., Yasin, U.U., Butt, W.H.: Automated glaucoma detection using retinal layers segmentation and optic cup-to-disc ratio in optical coherence tomography images. IET Image Processing **13**, 409–420 (2018)
6. Maetschke, S., Antony, B., Ishikawa, H., Garvani, R.: A feature agnostic approach for glaucoma detection in OCT volumes, arXiv preprint arXiv:1807.04855 (2018)
7. El Beltagi, T.A., et al.: Retinal nerve fiber layer thickness measured with optical coherence tomography is related to visual function in glaucomatous eyes. Ophthalmology **110**(11), 2185–2191 (2003)
8. Leite, M.T., Zangwill, L.M., Weinreb, R.N., Rao, H.L., Alencar, L.M., Medeiros, F.A.: Structure-function relationships using the Cirrus spectral domain optical coherence tomograph and standard automated perimetry. J. Glaucoma **21**(1), 49 (2012)
9. Chapelle, O., Scholkopf, B., Zien, A.: Semi-supervised learning (chapelle, o. et al., eds.; 2006)[book reviews]. IEEE Trans. Neural Netw. **20**(3), 542 (2009)
10. He, K., Zhang, X., Ren, S., Sun, J.: Deep residual learning for image recognition. In: Proceedings of the IEEE Conference on Computer Vision and Pattern Recognition, pp. 770–778 (2016)
11. Wang, X., et al.: Weakly supervised learning for whole slide lung cancer image classification. In: Medical Imaging with Deep Learning (2018)
12. Zhou, B., Khosla, A., Lapedriza, A., Oliva, A., Torralba, A.: Learning deep features for discriminative localization. In: Proceedings of the IEEE Conference on Computer Vision and Pattern Recognition, pp. 2921–2929 (2016)

# Evaluation of Retinal Image Quality Assessment Networks in Different Color-Spaces

Huazhu Fu[1], Boyang Wang[1], Jianbing Shen[1(✉)], Shanshan Cui[1], Yanwu Xu[3], Jiang Liu[2,3], and Ling Shao[1]

[1] Inception Institute of Artificial Intelligence, Abu Dhabi, UAE
jianbing.shen@inceptioniai.org
[2] Southern University of Science and Technology, Shenzhen, China
[3] Cixi Institute of Biomedical Engineering, CAS, Ningbo, China
https://github.com/hzfu/EyeQ

**Abstract.** Retinal image quality assessment (RIQA) is essential for controlling the quality of retinal imaging and guaranteeing the reliability of diagnoses by ophthalmologists or automated analysis systems. Existing RIQA methods focus on the RGB color-space and are developed based on small datasets with binary quality labels (i.e., 'Accept' and 'Reject'). In this paper, we first re-annotate an Eye-Quality (EyeQ) dataset with 28,792 retinal images from the EyePACS dataset, based on a three-level quality grading system (i.e., 'Good', 'Usable' and 'Reject') for evaluating RIQA methods. Our RIQA dataset is characterized by its large-scale size, multi-level grading, and multi-modality. Then, we analyze the influences on RIQA of different color-spaces, and propose a simple yet efficient deep network, named Multiple Color-space Fusion Network (MCF-Net), which integrates the different color-space representations at both a feature-level and prediction-level to predict image quality grades. Experiments on our EyeQ dataset show that our MCF-Net obtains a state-of-the-art performance, outperforming the other deep learning methods. Furthermore, we also evaluate diabetic retinopathy (DR) detection methods on images of different quality, and demonstrate that the performances of automated diagnostic systems are highly dependent on image quality.

**Keywords:** Retinal image · Quality assessment · Deep learning

## 1 Introduction

Retinal images are widely used for early screening and diagnosis of several eye diseases, including diabetic retinopathy (DR), glaucoma, and age-related macular degeneration (AMD). However, retinal images captured using different cameras, by people with various levels of experience, have a large variation in quality. A study based on UK BioBank showed that more than 25% of the retinal images

© Springer Nature Switzerland AG 2019
D. Shen et al. (Eds.): MICCAI 2019, LNCS 11764, pp. 48–56, 2019.
https://doi.org/10.1007/978-3-030-32239-7_6

are not of high enough quality to allow accurate diagnosis [8]. The quality degradation of retinal images, e.g., from inadequate illumination, noticeable blur and low contrast, may prevent a reliable medical diagnosis by ophthalmologists or automated analysis systems [1]. Thus, retinal image quality assessment (RIQA) is required for controlling the quality of retinal image. However, RIQA is a subjective task that depends on the experience of the ophthalmologists and the type of eye disease. Moreover, the traditional general quality assessment methods for natural images are not suitable for the RIQA task.

Recently, several methods for RIQA specifically have been proposed, which can be divided into two main categories: structure-based methods and feature-based methods. **Structure-based methods** employ segmented structures to determine the quality of retinal images. For example, an image structure clustering method was proposed to extract compact representations of retinal structures to determine image quality levels [10]. Blood vessel structures are also widely used for identifying the quality of retinal images [7,8,15]. However, structure-based methods rely heavily on the performance of structure segmentation, and cannot obtain latent visual features from images. **Feature-based methods**, on the other hand, directly extract feature representations from images, without structure segmentation. For example, features quantifying image color, focus, contrast and illumination can be calculated to represent the quality grade [12]. Wang et al. employed features based on the human visual system, with a support vector machine (SVM) or a decision tree to identify high-quality images [16]. A fundus image quality classifier that analyzes illumination, naturalness, and structure was also provided to assess quality [14]. Recently, deep learning techniques that integrate multi-level representations have been shown to obtain significant performances in a wide variety of medical imaging tasks. A combination of unsupervised features from saliency maps and supervised deep features from convolutional neural networks (CNNs) have been utilized to predict the quality level of retinal images [17]. For instance, Zago et al. adapted a deep neural network by using the pre-trained model from ImageNet to deal with the quality assessment task [18]. Although these deep methods have successfully overcome the limitations of hand-crafted features, they nevertheless have several of their own drawbacks. First, they focus on the RGB color-space, without considering other color-spaces that from part of the human visual system. Second, the existing RIQA datasets only contain binary labels (i.e., 'Accept' and 'Reject'), which is a coarse grading standard for complex clinical diagnosis. Third, the RIQA community lacks a large-scale dataset, which limits the development of RIQA related methods, especially for deep learning techniques, since these require large amounts of training data.

To address the above issues, in this paper, we discuss the influences on RIQA of different color-spaces in deep networks. We first re-annotate an **Eye-Quality (EyeQ) dataset** with 28,792 retinal images selected from the EyePACS dataset, using a three-level quality grading system (i.e., 'Good', 'Usable' and 'Reject'). Our EyeQ dataset considers the differences between ophthalmologists and automated systems, and can be used to evaluate other related works, including quality assessment methods, the influence of image quality on disease diagnosis, and retinal image enhancement. Second, we analyze the influences on RIQA of different color-spaces, and propose a general **Multiple Color-space Fusion Network (MCF-Net)** for retinal image quality classification. Our MCF-Net utilizes multiple base networks to jointly learn image representations from different color-spaces and fuses the outputs of all the base networks, at both a feature-level and prediction-level, to produce the final quality grade. Experiments demonstrate that our MCF-Net outperforms the other deep learning methods. In addition, we also apply the EyeQ dataset to evaluate the performances of DR detection methods for images of various qualities.

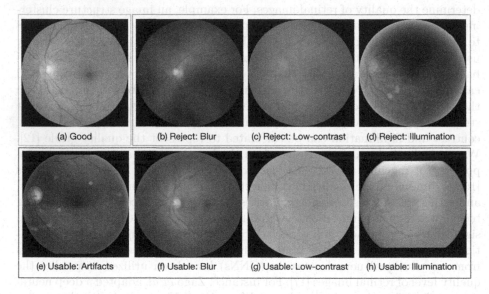

**Fig. 1.** Examples of different retinal image quality grades. The images of 'Good' quality (a) provide clear diagnostic information, while the images of 'Reject' quality (b–d) are insufficient for reliable diagnosis. However, some images are between 'Good' and 'Reject' (e–h), having some poor-quality indicators, but the main structures (e.g., disc and macular regions) and lesion are clear enough to be identified by ophthalmologists.

## 2    Eye-Quality Dataset

There are several publicly available RIQA datasets with manual quality annotations, such as HRF [7], DRIMDB [13], and DR2 [11]. However, they have various drawbacks. First, the image quality assessment of these datasets is based on binary labels, i.e., 'Accept' and 'Reject'. However, several images fall somewhere between these two categories. For example, some retinal images of poor-quality, e.g., containing a few artifacts (Fig. 1(e)), or slightly blurred (Fig. 1(f)), are still gradable by clinicians, so should not be labeled as 'Reject', but they may mislead automated medical analysis methods, so can also not be labeled as 'Accept'. Second, retinal images of the existing RIQA datasets are often captured by the same camera, which can not be used to evaluate the robustness of RIQA methods against various imaging modalities. Third, the existing datasets are limited in size, and there lacks a large-scale quality grade dataset for developing deep learning methods.

**Table 1.** Summary of our EyeQ dataset, where DR-i denotes the DR presence on grade i based on the labels in EyePACS dataset.

| | Training set | | | | | | Testing set | | | | | |
|---|---|---|---|---|---|---|---|---|---|---|---|---|
| | DR-0 | DR-1 | DR-2 | DR-3 | DR-4 | All | DR-0 | DR-1 | DR-2 | DR-3 | DR-4 | All |
| Good | 6,342 | 699 | 1,100 | 167 | 39 | 8,347 | 5,966 | 886 | 1,354 | 199 | 65 | 8,470 |
| Usable | 1,353 | 103 | 283 | 79 | 58 | 1,896 | 3,201 | 359 | 721 | 145 | 133 | 4,559 |
| Reject | 1,544 | 109 | 426 | 87 | 154 | 2,320 | 2,195 | 153 | 569 | 104 | 199 | 3,220 |
| Total | 9,239 | 911 | 1,809 | 333 | 251 | **12,543** | 1,1362 | 1,398 | 2,644 | 448 | 397 | **16,249** |

To address the above issues, in this paper, we re-annotate an Eye-Quality (EyeQ) dataset from the EyePACS dataset, which is a large retinal image dataset captured by different models and types of cameras, under a variety of imaging conditions. Our EyeQ dataset utilizes a three-level quality grading system by considering four common quality indicators, including blurring, uneven illumination, low-contrast, and artifacts. Our three quality grades are defined as:

- **'Good' grade**: the retinal image has no low-quality factors, and all retinopathy characteristics are clearly visible, as shown in Fig. 1(a).
- **'Usable' grade**: the retinal image has some slight low-quality indicators, which can not observe the whole image clearly (e.g., low-contrast and blur) or affect the automated medical analysis methods (e.g., artifacts), but the main structures (e.g., disc, macula regions) and lesion are clear enough to be identified by ophthalmologists, as shown in Fig. 1(e–h). For the uneven illumination case, the readable region of fundus image is larger than 80%.
- **'Reject' grade**: the retinal image has a serious quality issue and cannot be used to provide a full and reliable diagnosis, even by ophthalmologists, as shown in Fig. 1(b–d). Moreover, the fundus image with invisible disc or macula region is also be treated as 'Reject' grade.

To re-annotate the EyeQ dataset, we asked two experts to grade the quality of images in EyePACS. Then, the images with ambiguous labels were discarded, yielding a collection of 28,792 retinal images. A summary of this EyeQ dataset is given in Table 1. Note that some images with 'Reject' grades still have DR grade labels from the EyePACS dataset. The reason is that our quality standard is based on the diagnosability for general eye diseases, such as glaucoma,

AMD, etc., rather than only DR. Although some low-quality images have visible lesions for DR diagnosis, they are not of high enough quality for diagnosing other diseases, lacking, for example, clear views of optic disc and cup regions for glaucoma screening, or visible macula regions for AMD analysis.

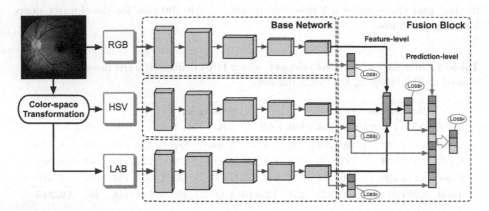

**Fig. 2.** The architecture of our MCF-Net, which contains multiple base networks for different color-spaces. A fusion block is employed to integrate the multiple outputs of these base networks on both feature-level and prediction-level.

## 3 Multiple Color-Space Fusion Network

Recently, deep learning techniques have been shown to obtain satisfactory performances in retinal image quality assessment [17,18]. However, these methods only focus on the RGB color-space, and ignore other color-spaces that included in the human visual system. A color-space identifies a particular combination of the color model and the mapping function. Different color-spaces represent different characteristics, and can be used to extract diverse visual features, which have been demonstrated to affect the performances of deep learning networks [9]. In this paper, we analyze the influences of different color-spaces on the RIQA task, and propose a general Multiple Color-space Fusion Network (MCF-Net) to integrate the representations of various color-spaces. Besides the original RGB color-space, we also consider HSV and LAB color-spaces, which are widely used in computer vision tasks and are obtained through nonlinear conversions from the RGB color-space.

Figure 2 illustrates the architecture of our MCF-Net. The original RGB image is first transferred to HSV and LAB color-spaces, and fed into the base networks. The base networks generate image features by employing multi-scale CNN layers. Then, a fusion block is used to combine the output of each base network at both a feature-level and prediction-level. First, the feature maps from the base networks are concatenated and input to a fully connected layer to generate a feature-level fusion prediction. Then, the predictions of all the base networks and feature-level fusion are concatenated and fed into a fully connected layer to produce the final prediction-level fusion result. Our two-level fusion block guarantees the full integration of the different color-spaces. On the other hand, our fusion block also maintains the independence and integrity of the base networks, which enables any deep network to be implemented as the base network. Different from existing deep fusion networks, which only use the loss function of the last layer to train the whole model, our MCF-Net retains all loss functions of the base networks, to improve their transparency for each color-space, and combines them with the fusion loss of the last layer, as:

$$Loss_{total} = \sum_{i=1}^{3} w_i Loss_i + w_F Loss_F + w_P Loss_P, \qquad (1)$$

where $Loss_i$, $Loss_F$ and $Loss_P$ denote the *multi-class cross-entropy* loss functions of the base networks and the two-level fusion layers, respectively. $w_i$, $w_F$ and $w_m$ are trade-off weights, which are set to $w_i = 0.1$, $w_F = 0.1$ and $w_m = 0.6$ to highlight the final prediction-level fusion layer.

## 4    Experiments

**Implementation Details:** For each input image, we first detect the retinal mask using the Hough Circle Transform, and then crop the mask region to reduce the influence of black background. Finally, the image is resized to 224 × 224 and normalized to $[-1, 1]$, before being fed to our MCF-Net. For data augmentation, we apply vertical and horizontal flipping, random drifting and rotation. The initial weights of the base networks are loaded from pre-trained models based on ImageNet, and the parameters of the final fully connected layer are randomly initialized. Our model is optimized using the SGD algorithm with a learning rate of 0.01. The framework is implemented on PyTorch.

**Experimental Settings:** Our EyeQ dataset is divided into a training set (12,543 images) and a testing set (16,249 images), following the EyePACS settings, as shown in Table 1. We evaluate our MCF-Net utilizing three state-of-the-art networks: ResNet18 [5], ResNet50 [5], and DenseNet121 [6]. For each base network, we compare our MCF-Net in terms of the network with individual color-space (i.e., RGB, HSV and LAB). We also report the average result (AVG) when combining the predictions of the three color-spaces directly, without the fusion block. For the non-deep learning baseline, we implement the RIQA method from [16], which is based on three visual characteristics (i.e., multi-channel sensation, just noticeable blur, and the contrast sensitivity function) and an SVM classifier with a radial based function. For evaluation metrics, we employ average accuracy, precision, recall, and F-measure ($\frac{2*precision*recall}{precision+recall}$).

**Results and Discussion:** The performances of different methods are reported in Table 2. We can make the following observations: (1) The performance of the non-deep learning baseline [16] is obviously lower than those of deep learning based methods. This is reasonable because deep learning can extract highly discriminative representations from the retinal images directly, using multiple CNN layers, which are superior to the hand-crafted features in [16] and lead to better performance. (2) For the different color-spaces, the networks in RGB and LAB color-spaces perform better than that in HSV color-space. One possible reason is that the RGB color-space is closer to the raw data captured from the camera, and thus a more natural way to represent image data. Another possible reason is that the model pre-trained on ImageNet are based on RGB color-space, which is more suitable for fine-tuning in the same color-space. The LAB color-space represents the lightness and color components of green–red and blue–yellow. The lightness channel directly reflects the illustration status of images, which is the main quality indicator for retinal images. (3) Combinations of different color-spaces, even the simple average fusion (AVG), perform better than those of individual color-space. (4) Our MCF-Net outperforms the models with an individual color-spaces and average fusion. This demonstrates that the multi-level fusion block can produce a stable improvement to benefit the quality assessment task. Moreover, for deep learning models, DenseNet121-MCF obtains the best performance, outperforming ResNet18-MCF and ResNet50-MCF.

**Table 2.** Performances of different methods on test set.

| | Accuracy | Precision | Recall | F-measure |
|---|---|---|---|---|
| Baseline [16] | 0.8372 | 0.7404 | 0.6945 | 0.6991 |
| ResNet18-RGB | 0.8914 | 0.8044 | 0.8166 | 0.8087 |
| ResNet18-HSV | 0.8859 | 0.8010 | 0.7972 | 0.7980 |
| ResNet18-LAB | 0.8912 | 0.8071 | 0.8138 | 0.8083 |
| ResNet18-AVG | 0.8966 | 0.8164 | 0.8226 | 0.8176 |
| ResNet18-MCS | 0.9029 | 0.8457 | 0.8189 | 0.8288 |
| ResNet50-RGB | 0.8921 | 0.8123 | 0.8078 | 0.8100 |
| ResNet50-HSV | 0.8709 | 0.7706 | 0.7778 | 0.7735 |
| ResNet50-LAB | 0.8925 | 0.8078 | 0.8146 | 0.8091 |
| ResNet50-AVG | 0.8957 | 0.8156 | 0.8183 | 0.8163 |
| ResNet50-MCS | 0.9004 | 0.8389 | 0.8126 | 0.8230 |
| DenseNet121-RGB | 0.8943 | 0.8194 | 0.8114 | 0.8152 |
| DenseNet121-HSV | 0.8786 | 0.7963 | 0.7695 | 0.7808 |
| DenseNet121-LAB | 0.8882 | 0.8130 | 0.7937 | 0.8010 |
| DenseNet121-AVG | 0.8952 | 0.8240 | 0.8065 | 0.8143 |
| DenseNet121-MCS | 0.9175 | 0.8645 | 0.8497 | 0.8551 |

**DR Detection in Different-Quality Images:** In this paper, we also apply our EyeQ dataset to evaluate the performances of DR detection methods for different-quality images. We train three deep learning networks, e.g., ResNet-18 [5], ResNet-50 [5] and DenseNet-121 [6], on the whole EyePACS training set, and evaluate their performances on images of different quality. Table 3 shows the accuracy scores of the DR detection models. As expected, the performances of the methods decrease along with the quality degradation of the images. The accuracy scores of ResNet-18 [5], ResNet-50 [5] and DenseNet-121 [6] decrease by 0.21%, 0.04%, and 0.23%, respectively, from 'Good' to 'Usable', and by 1.45%, 0.82%, and 1.31% from 'Usable' to 'Reject'. Note that since we train the DR detection methods on the whole EyePACS training set, which includes different quality images, the networks are somewhat robust to poor-quality images. However, poor-quality images still pose challenges for automated diagnosis systems, even for the images labeled as 'Usable', which could provide diagnosable information to ophthalmologists.

**Table 3.** Accuracy score of DR detection methods on different-quality images.

|  | 'Good' | 'Usable' | 'Reject' |
| --- | --- | --- | --- |
| ResNet18 | 0.9014 | 0.8993 | 0.8848 |
| ResNet50 | 0.9154 | 0.9150 | 0.9068 |
| DenseNet121 | 0.9174 | 0.9151 | 0.9020 |

## 5    Conclusion

In this paper, we have constructed an Eye-Quality (EyeQ) dataset from the Eye-PACS dataset, with a three-level quality grading system (i.e., 'Good', 'Usable' and 'Reject'). Our EyeQ dataset has the advantages of a large-scale size, multi-level grading, and multi-modality. Moreover, we have also proposed a general Multiple Color-space Fusion Network (MCF-Net) for retinal image quality classification, which integrates different color-spaces. Experiments have demonstrated that MCF-Net outperforms other methods. In addition, we have also shown that image quality affects the performances of automated DR detection methods. We hope our work can draw more interest from the community to work on the RIQA task, which plays a critical role in applications such as retinal image segmentation [3,4], and automated disease diagnosis [2].

## References

1. Cheng, J., et al.: Structure-preserving guided retinal image filtering and its application for optic disk analysis. IEEE Trans. Med. Imaging **37**(11), 2536–2546 (2018)
2. Fu, H., et al.: Disc-aware ensemble network for glaucoma screening from fundus image. IEEE Trans. Med. Imaging **37**(11), 2493–2501 (2018)

3. Fu, H., et al.: Joint optic disc and cup segmentation based on multi-label deep network and polar transformation. IEEE Trans. Med. Imaging **37**(7), 1597–1605 (2018)
4. Gu, Z., et al.: CE-Net: context encoder network for 2D medical image segmentation. IEEE TMI (2019, in press). https://doi.org/10.1109/TMI.2019.2903562
5. He, K., et al.: Deep residual learning for image recognition. In: CVPR, pp. 770–778 (2016)
6. Huang, G., et al.: Densely connected convolutional networks. In: CVPR, pp. 2261–2269 (2017)
7. Köhler, T., et al.: Automatic no-reference quality assessment for retinal fundus images using vessel segmentation. In: IEEE International Symposium on Computer-Based Medical Systems, pp. 95–100 (2013)
8. MacGillivray, T.J., et al.: Suitability of UK Biobank retinal images for automatic analysis of morphometric properties of the vasculature. PLoS One **10**(5), 1–10 (2015)
9. Mishkin, D., et al.: Systematic evaluation of convolution neural network advances on the imagenet. Comput. Vis. Image Underst. **161**, 11–19 (2017)
10. Niemeijer, M., et al.: Image structure clustering for image quality verification of color retina images in diabetic retinopathy screening. Med. Image Anal. **10**(6), 888–898 (2006)
11. Pires, R., et al.: Retinal image quality analysis for automatic diabetic retinopathy detection. In: SIBGRAPI Conference on Graphics, Patterns and Images, pp. 229–236 (2012)
12. Pires Dias, J.M., et al.: Retinal image quality assessment using generic image quality indicators. Inf. Fusion **19**, 73–90 (2014)
13. Sevik, U., et al.: Identification of suitable fundus images using automated quality assessment methods. J. Biomed. Opt. **19**(4), 1–11 (2014)
14. Shao, F., et al.: Automated quality assessment of fundus images via analysis of illumination, naturalness and structure. IEEE Access **6**, 806–817 (2017)
15. Tobin, K.W., et al.: Elliptical local vessel density: a fast and robust quality metric for retinal images. In: EMBC, pp. 3534–3537 (2008)
16. Wang, S., et al.: Human visual system-based fundus image quality assessment of portable fundus camera photographs. IEEE Trans. Med. Imaging **35**(4), 1046–1055 (2016)
17. Yu, F., et al.: Image quality classification for DR screening using deep learning. In: EMBC, pp. 664–667 (2017)
18. Zago, G.T., et al.: Retinal image quality assessment using deep learning. Comput. Biol. Med. **103**, 64–70 (2018)

# 3D Surface-Based Geometric and Topological Quantification of Retinal Microvasculature in OCT-Angiography via Reeb Analysis

Jiong Zhang[1,2], Amir H. Kashani[2], and Yonggang Shi[1(✉)]

[1] USC Stevens Neuroimaging and Informatics Institute,
University of Southern California (USC), Los Angeles, CA 90033, USA
yshi@loni.usc.edu
[2] USC Roski Eye Institute, Keck School of Medicine,
University of Southern California (USC), Los Angeles, CA 90033, USA

**Abstract.** 3D optical coherence tomography angiography (OCT-A) is a novel, non-invasive imaging modality for studying important retina-related diseases. Current works have been mainly focusing on the microvascular analysis of 2D enface OCT-A projections while direct 3D analysis using rich depth-resolved microvascular information is rarely considered. In this work, we aim to set up an innovative 3D microvascular modeling framework via Reeb analysis to explore rich geometric and topological information. We first use effective vessel extraction and surface reconstruction techniques to establish a complete 3D mesh representation of retinal OCT-A microvasculature. We propose to use geodesic distance as a feature function to build level contours with smooth transitions on mesh surface. Intrinsic Reeb graphs are thereby constructed through level contours to represent general OCT-A microvascular topology. Afterwards, specific geometric and topological analysis are performed on Reeb graphs to quantify critical microvascular characteristics. The proposed Reeb analysis framework is evaluated on a clinical DR dataset and shows great advantage in describing 3D microvascular changes. It is able to produce important surface-based microvascular biomarkers with high statistical power for disease studies.

**Keywords:** Optical coherence tomography angiography ·
Reeb graph · Diabetic retinopathy · Retinal microvasculature

## 1 Introduction

The recently developed 3D optical coherence tomography angiography (OCT-A) is an efficient and non-invasive imaging modality that is able to provide

Y. Shi—This work was supported in part by NIH grants UH3NS100614, R21EY027879, U01EY025864, K08EY027006, P41EB015922, P30EY029220, and Research to Prevent Blindness.

© Springer Nature Switzerland AG 2019
D. Shen et al. (Eds.): MICCAI 2019, LNCS 11764, pp. 57–65, 2019.
https://doi.org/10.1007/978-3-030-32239-7_7

rich micrometer-level axial resolution with rich depth-resolved 3D microvascular information. It has been widely applied to analyze microvascular diseases like diabetic retinopathy (DR) and age-related macular degeneration (AMD) [5]. The routine way for analyzing retinal microvasculature in OCT-A images is mostly based on the 2D *en face* projections, while direct 3D analysis including rich depth-resolved geometric and topological information is hardly considered due to the challenges of low image quality and high capillary complexity. A comprehensive overview including clinical applications using 2D *en face* images can be found in [5]. Most of the analysis [5,6] are performed on projected OCT-A images from different retinal layers to study the correlations between vessel biomarkers and disease progression. In comparison with other imaging modalities, OCT-A is proven to be a more useful tool for describing capillary loss between normal and non-proliferative diabetic retinopathy (NPDR) subjects based on the analysis of *en face* projections from different depth layers [3,5].

Despite the challenges of 3D OCT-A analysis, it is valuable to investigate and analyze 3D microvascular changes by considering the rich depth-resolved information instead of just performing 2D analysis. The demands for high-quality 3D OCT-A vessel visualization and processing motivate us to build a surface-based microvascular analysis framework. A unified Reeb analysis approach [10] was proposed to detect tissue outliers on smooth and triangulated cortical surface representation [9] of brain magnetic resonance images (MRI). In this work, we propose to design a similar routine by taking advantage of the analysis on Reeb graph which is built on a delicate feature function defined on 3D OCT-A vessel surface. Reeb analysis provides the possibility to analyze local geometric and topological changes based on the description of full vascular topology. A variety of functions [2,10] have been employed to set up Reeb graphs for removing surface outliers and identifying surface protrusions. In this work, we propose to employ the geodesic distance transform as a distinguishable feature function for precise Reeb graph construction on mesh surface.

Based on Reeb graph, we are able to extract potentially important biomarkers to perform 3D microvascular analysis on clinical data. To our knowledge, this is for the first time that a complete microvascular modeling framework is proposed to analyze geometric and topological biomarkers in 3D OCT-A images. The surface representation provides a high-quality 3D microvascular visualization to assist clinical practice. Meanwhile, the proposed Reeb analysis framework gives the possibility of analyzing 3D microvascular data in a new perspective.

## 2    Methodology

### 2.1    3D Surface Representation of OCT-A Microvasculature

To establish a high-quality 3D microvascular surface representation, we first design an effective enhancement and segmentation method to extract OCT-A vessel networks. Speckle noise reduction is achieved via 3D curvelet denoising on OCT-A volumes. Afterwards, we exploit the optimally oriented flux (OOF) filter [7] by considering its nice property of processing closely located curvi-linear structures to enhance the dense OCT-A microvasculature as shown in Fig. 1(b). The OOF is a quadratic function and defines a symmetric matrix $\mathcal{Q}(\mathbf{x}, r)$ which can be decomposed as $\mathcal{Q}(\mathbf{x}, r) = \sum_{i=1}^{3} \lambda_i(\mathbf{x}, r)\boldsymbol{v}_i(\mathbf{x}, r)\boldsymbol{v}_i(\mathbf{x}, r)^T$, where $\lambda_i(\mathbf{x}, r)$ and $\boldsymbol{v}_i(\mathbf{x}, r)$ denote eigenvalues and eigenvectors, respectively. One has $\lambda_1(\cdot) \leq \lambda_2(\cdot) \ll \lambda_3(\cdot) \approx 0$ inside vessels due to that the OCT-A vessel voxels have intensity values higher than background voxels. The final vesselness map for each voxel is defined by taking the largest magnitude: $\mathcal{P}(\mathbf{x}) := \max\{\max_{r}\{-\frac{1}{r^2}\lambda_1(\mathbf{x}, r)\}, 0\}$. The binarized vessel segmentations are obtained via a proper thresholding. We also extract the volume of interest (VOI) including superficial and deep layers from each corresponding OCT volume using OCTExplorer [1]. A continuous OCT-A vessel surface representation is constructed by defining triangular meshes on 3D segmented vessel boundary masks. See Fig. 1(c). Hence, a complete mesh surface $\mathcal{M}$ is represented by vertices and triangular faces, i.e. $\mathcal{M} = \{\mathcal{V}, \mathcal{T}\}$, where $\mathcal{V} = \{\mathcal{V}_i | i = 1, \cdots, N_{\mathcal{V}}\}$ and $\mathcal{T} = \{\mathcal{T}_j | j = 1, \cdots, N_{\mathcal{T}}\}$ denote the set of vertices and triangles, respectively.

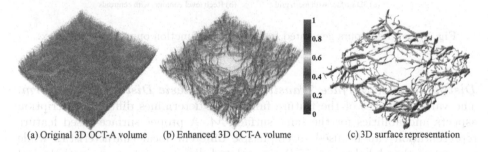

(a) Original 3D OCT-A volume    (b) Enhanced 3D OCT-A volume          (c) 3D surface representation

**Fig. 1.** 3D OCT-A microvascular enhancement surface reconstruction.

## 2.2    Intrinsic Reeb Graph Construction Using Geodesic Distance Transform on Vessel Mesh Surfaces

*Reeb Graph.* Based on the surface representation, we propose to analyze 3D OCT-A vessel geometry and topology in a new perspective via Reeb graph [8]. A Reeb graph $R(f)$ is intuitively a graph of level contours constructed by a Morse function $f$ [4] defined on manifold. The Reeb graph on vessel surface can reflect the intrinsic topological changes of retinal microvasculature since its level contours vary only at critical points of the Morse function. For a triangular mesh $\mathcal{M} = \{\mathcal{V}, \mathcal{T}\}$, the function $f$ is defined on each vertex in $\mathcal{V}$. The level sets of $f$ are sampled at a set of $K$ values $\xi_0 < \xi_1 < \cdots < \xi_k$ with the set of contours as $\mathcal{C} = \{\mathcal{C}_k^n, 0 \leq k \leq K - 1, 1 \leq n \leq N_k\}$, where $N_k$ is the number of contours at level $k$, and where $\mathcal{C}_k^n$ denotes the $n$-th contour at this level. In this work, we compute the Reeb graphs for 3D OCT-A microvascular surfaces by following the similar routine as in [10]. The edge $E_{k,k+1}$ between neighbouring level contours are established by connecting a contour $\mathcal{C}_k^{n_1}$ at level $\xi_k$ and a contour $\mathcal{C}_{k+1}^{n_2}$ at level $\xi_{k+1}$ if they belong to the same connected component in the vascular region $R_{k,k+1} = \{\mathcal{V}_i \in \mathcal{M} | \xi_k \leq f(\mathcal{V}_i) \leq \xi_{k+1}\}$. Finally, a complete Reeb graph on mesh surface $\mathcal{M}$ with undirected edge connection of level contours as nodes is constructed to represent the 3D microvascular networks. Figure 2 shows the neighboring contours generated from a feature function on each vertex. The centroid of each contour is visualized to intuitively represent the graph nodes.

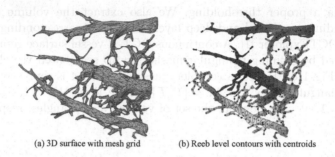

(a) 3D surface with mesh grid          (b) Reeb level contours with centroids

**Fig. 2.** Level contours generated from a feature function on each mesh vertex.

*Distinguishable Surface Transition via Geodesic Distance Transform.* The various choices of the feature function $f$ determines different description aspects and abilities for the same surface $\mathcal{M}$. A proper surface-based feature representation can be used to emphasize different local characteristics while preserving the global topology. Retina-related diseases often cause pathological variations that can gradually affect the microvascular geometry and topology during disease progression. It is of vital importance to investigate and quantify 3D microvascular changes at critical points such as bifurcations and small capillaries. Hence, we propose to integrate a novel feature, i.e. the mesh geodesic distances as the Morse function, into our Reeb analysis framework to represent the topological transitions on 3D OCT-A microvascular surface. See Fig. 3(a).

The length of the minimal geodesic from vertices $\mathcal{V}_i$ to $\mathcal{V}_j$ is called their geodesic distance on surface $\mathcal{M}$ and is represented by $d(\mathcal{V}_i, \mathcal{V}_j)$. Thus, the geodesic distance transform of a point $\mathcal{V}_p$ on the manifold $\mathcal{M}$ can be defined as $d_{\mathcal{V}_p}(\mathcal{V}_q) = d(\mathcal{V}_p, \mathcal{V}_q), \forall \mathcal{V}_q \in \mathcal{M}$. By calculating the geodesic distances between a given seed point $\mathcal{V}_p$ and the other vertices $\mathcal{V}_q$, we can conveniently obtain an intuitive representation of the microvascular topology on top of the complex linkages and hierarchical tree structures in OCT-A images. The seed point $\mathcal{V}_p$ in our framework is automatically defined by finding the closest vertex to the volume center. The geodesic distances can reflect vascular expansion and are distinguishable at different locations. In Fig. 3(b), we can see the level contours are nicely distributed in vessel perpendicular direction with smooth transitions based on the proposed feature function $f$. Then by following the routine defined in [10] we build a Reeb graph to precisely represent the partition of OCT-A vessel surfaces.

***Vessel Classification Based on Level-Set Contours.*** The OCT-A vessel topology can be easily affected by tailing artifact [12] which appears as connected "fake" blood flow signals and causes large vessel thickening below. This can result in unreliable microvascular measurements for further diseases study. Thus, we propose to analyze large vessels and small capillaries independently via a level-contour based classification step. A level contour is represented as a polyline composed of points intersecting edges of $\mathcal{M}$ at the level $\xi_k$. The proposed mesh geodesic distance function generates level contours that can fully represent the vessel cross-sectional boundaries as shown in Fig. 3(b). By considering the contour curve length $L(\mathcal{C}_k^n)$ obtained in the Reeb graph construction procedure, we can use it as a feature to categorize each level contour into large or small vessel groups. The original OCT-A vessel signal strengths can have large variations across healthy and pathological subjects, which cause differences in vessel geometry. Thus, we need define an automatic way to select suitable threshold values for different data. We first give a rough estimation of the large vessel contour size by taking the mean $\mu_L$ of the maximum 10% level contours. Then we empirically define the automatic thresholding levels $T_L$ at $0.5\mu_L$ for different subjects. In Fig. 3(c), we show a typical example of the segmented level contours on 3D microvascular surface. The level contours of large vessels and small capillaries are well separated into different classes.

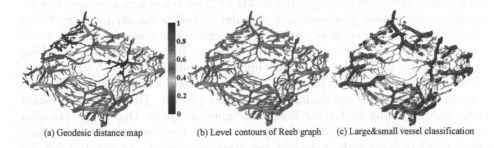

(a) Geodesic distance map    (b) Level contours of Reeb graph    (c) Large&small vessel classification

**Fig. 3.** Reeb graph construction and vessel classification on vessel surface.

## 2.3 Geometric and Topological Feature Extraction via Reeb Analysis

The Reeb graph provides the possibility and convenience to investigate 3D geometric and topological variations in OCT-A images. It is also interesting to see the great potential of using the 3D surface representation as a novel perspective for retinal microvascular analysis. To this end, we employ Reeb analysis to extract the following geometric and topological biomarkers on Reeb graph.

**Number of Bifurcations:** The bifurcation number indicates the complexity of the hierarchical retinal microvascular tree. By taking each level contour $\mathcal{C}_k^n$ as a node, we count the total number $B_k^n$ of its 1-ring connected nodes. If $B_k^n \geq 3$, we label it as 1 to indicate there exist a bifurcation point nearby. We label all its 1-ring connected nodes as 0 to avoid repeated counting in later iterations. The whole number of bifurcation points is obtained by summing the labels of all nodes, i.e. $B_{total} = \sum_{k=0}^{K-1} \sum_{n=1}^{N_k} B_k^n$. In Fig. 4(a), we highlight the closest level contour where a nearby bifurcation exist.

**Number of Ending Points:** The ending points can approximately represent the amount of 3D small capillary segments in the deepest microvascular level. We iteratively count each node which has only one connection in its 1-ring neighborhood and obtain the ending nodes summation as a biomarker. In Fig. 4(b), we highlight all the ending level contours.

**Number and Curve Length of Level Contours:** The contour curve length can represent the microvascular size at each level. Since the level contours are equally sampled for different volume images, the curve length summation of all level contours can be considered as a measure to roughly reflect the amount of 3D blood flow signals of the whole volume at each moment.

**Number of Microvascular Loops:** The complex linkages in retinal vessel circulation can easily form multiple closed capillary loop areas, as shown in the histology study [11] in deep retinal layers. One capillary can split out from the main vessel and again merge into the same structure. This motivates us to quantify the small loop quantity in 3D OCT-A vessel topology and find its relation with disease progression. A vascular "loop" is essentially a "cycle" in the graph since we may have multiple level contours as nodes in a single vessel segment. The cycle detection is achieved via an iterative dynamic searching process. A dynamic path is iteratively updated by addling nodes along the deep-first searching direction. One cycle path is detected when the starting node appears for the 2nd time during the searching process. Then it restarts again from the beginning by tracing another neighboring path. Due to the complex vessel connections, we restrict the loop counting process by considering only the *chordless* cycle without having any other edge inside. In Fig. 4(c), all the contours that belong to a loop are visualized and we can see that many loops appear below the main vessels.

## 3    Experimental Results

A clinical OCT-A dataset of diabetic retinopathy (OCTA-DR) has been established for analyzing the obtained Reeb-based biomarkers. There are in total 100 OCT-A volume images from 100 subjects including 40 normal controls (NC), 20 severe non-proliferative diabetic retinopathy (NPDR) and 40 proliferative diabetic retinopathy (PDR). Only one eye of each patient has been selected for analysis to ensure data independence.

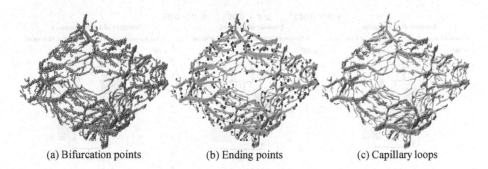

(a) Bifurcation points        (b) Ending points        (c) Capillary loops

**Fig. 4.** Visualization of the detected feature via Reeb analysis.

The proposed Reeb analysis framework is applied to extract geometric and topological biomarkers for each subject. We perform statistical analysis in a pair-wise way on all three groups based on Wilcoxon rank sum test with a significance level at 0.05. We calculate in total 11 biomarkers including the number of bifurcations, number of level contours, length of level contours for large, small and all vessels separately, as well as the number of ending points and loops.

The statistical analysis shows high significance (with $p < 0.05$) on 10 biomarkers except the bifurcation numbers on small capillaries in distinguishing normal and PDR groups. This could be caused by the fact that most of the detected bifurcations in OCT-A images are split from large vessels as shown in Fig. 4(a). We provide the box and whisker plot in Fig. 5(a) to present the significant difference between each group for the number of bifurcations in large vessels, which achieves a high significance with $p < 0.001$ between normal and PDR groups. Similarly, the number of ending points and the number of level contours in small capillaries also show strong differences (with $p < 0.001$) between this two groups as shown in Fig. 5(b)–(c). They also achieve significance (with $p < 0.05$) when their differences between normal and severe NPDR groups are compared. These indicate that there is a small capillary loss in severe NPDR groups compared with normal controls. However, the differences between severe NPDR and PDR groups are not so significant for both biomarkers. Some of the other biomarkers also show insignificant differences when the pair-wise analysis is performed against severe NPDR. These could be caused by the limited data usage and thus further analysis should be performed by collecting more data in the study.

In Fig. 5(d)–(e), we can observe that the length of overall level contours on large vessels and small capillaries present very significant differences between normal and severe NPDR groups, as well as normal and PDR groups with a $p$ value $< 0.001$. For the difference between severe NPDR and PDR groups, the length of level contours achieves a $p$ value $< 0.001$ on large vessels and a $p$ value $< 0.05$ on small capillaries. These findings indicate that the length of level contours can be considered as a potentially important feature for the discrimination of different disease stages. Although the proposed 3D microvascular segmenta-

64      J. Zhang et al.

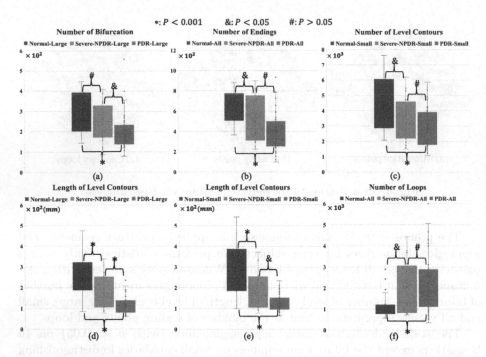

**Fig. 5.** Statistical analysis of Reeb graph based geometric and topological biomarkers for DR on large, small and all vessels separately.

tion method has extracted most of the small capillaries, but it is still restricted by the low OCT-A image quality and capillary visibility. More accurate statistical performance can be obtained by exploring precise vessel segmentations with better image quality. In Fig. 5(f), we present the statistical analysis based on the number of topological loops to describe the difference between DR stages. We can see that it shows strong significance in distinguishing normal with the other two groups severe NPDR and PDR with $p < 0.05$ and $p < 0.001$, respectively. There is an increasing tendency in the amount of loops along with disease progression. This may indicate that the topological changes in the later stages of DR cause more closed capillary areas. It shows the great value of exploring more potentially important topological features in further Reeb analysis.

## 4   Conclusion

In this work, we have proposed an innovative 3D OCT-A microvascular analysis method by designing a Reeb analysis framework on high-quality OCT-A vessel surface representations. Several important geometric and topological vessel biomarkers have been extracted from the Reeb graph built on geodesic distances. Significant statistical performance of microvascular biomarkers has been found on DR discrimination. The proposed Reeb analysis framework opens great promise for analyzing 3D retinal microvasculature in a new perspective.

# References

1. Antony, B., Abramoff, M.D., Tang, L., et al.: Automated 3-D method for the correction of axial artifacts in spectral-domain optical coherence tomography images. Biomed. Opt. Express **2**(8), 2403–2416 (2011)
2. Elad, A., Kimmel, R.: On bending invariant signatures for surfaces. IEEE Trans. Pattern Anal. Mach. Intell. **25**(10), 1285–1295 (2003)
3. Jia, Y., Bailey, S.T., Hwang, T.S., et al.: Quantitative optical coherence tomography angiography of vascular abnormalities in the living human eye. PNAS **112**(18), E2395–E2402 (2015)
4. Jost, J., Jost, J.: Riemannian Geometry and Geometric Analysis, vol. 42005. Springer, Heidelberg (2008)
5. Kashani, A.H., Chen, C.L., Gahm, J.K., et al.: Optical coherence tomography angiography: a comprehensive review of current methods and clinical applications. Prog. Retin. Eye Res. **60**, 66–100 (2017)
6. Kashani, A.H., Lee, S.Y., Moshfeghi, A., et al.: Optical coherence tomography angiography of retinal venous occlusion. Retina **35**(11), 2323–2331 (2015)
7. Law, M.W.K., Chung, A.C.S.: Three dimensional curvilinear structure detection using optimally oriented flux. In: Forsyth, D., Torr, P., Zisserman, A. (eds.) ECCV 2008. LNCS, vol. 5305, pp. 368–382. Springer, Heidelberg (2008). https://doi.org/10.1007/978-3-540-88693-8_27
8. Reeb, G.: Sur les points singuliers d'une forme de pfaff completement integrable ou d'une fonction numerique [on the singular points of a completely integrable pfaff form or of a numerical function]. Comptes Rendus Acad. Sci. Paris **222**, 847–849 (1946)
9. Shi, Y., Lai, R., Morra, J.H., et al.: Robust surface reconstruction via Laplace-Beltrami eigen-projection and boundary deformation. IEEE Trans. Med. Imag. **29**(12), 2009–2022 (2010)
10. Shi, Y., Lai, R., Toga, A.W.: Cortical surface reconstruction via unified reeb analysis of geometric and topological outliers in magnetic resonance images. IEEE Trans. Med. Imag. **32**(3), 511–530 (2013)
11. Tan, P.E.Z., Balaratnasingam, C., Xu, J., et al.: Quantitative comparison of retinal capillary images derived by speckle variance optical coherence tomography with histology. Invest. Ophthalmol. Vis. Sci. **56**(6), 3989–3996 (2015)
12. Zhang, A., Zhang, Q., Wang, R.K.: Minimizing projection artifacts for accurate presentation of choroidal neovascularization in OCT micro-angiography. Biomed. Opt. Express **6**(10), 4130–4143 (2015)

# Limited-Angle Diffuse Optical Tomography Image Reconstruction Using Deep Learning

Hanene Ben Yedder[1]([envelope]), Majid Shokoufi[2], Ben Cardoen[1], Farid Golnaraghi[2], and Ghassan Hamarneh[1]

[1] School of Computing Science, Simon Fraser University, Burnaby, Canada
{hbenyedd,bcardoen,hamarneh}@sfu.ca
[2] School of Mechatronic Systems Engineering, Simon Fraser University, Surrey, Canada
{mshokouf,mfgolnar}@sfu.ca

**Abstract.** Diffuse optical tomography (DOT) leverages near-infrared light propagation through in vivo tissue to assess its optical properties and identify abnormalities such as cancerous lesions. While this relatively new optical imaging modality is cost-effective and non-invasive, its inverse problem (i.e., recovering an image from raw signal measurements) is ill-posed, due to the highly diffusive nature of light propagation in biological tissues and limited boundary measurements. Solving the inverse problem becomes even more challenging in the case of limited-angle data acquisition given the restricted number of sources and sensors, the sparsity of the recovered information, and the presence of noise, representative of real world acquisition environments. Traditional optimization-based reconstruction methods are computationally intensive and thus too slow for real-time imaging applications. We propose a novel image reconstruction method for breast cancer DOT imaging. Our method is highlighted by two components: (i) a deep learning network with a novel hybrid loss, and (ii) a distribution transfer learning module. Our model is designed to focus on lesion specific information and small reconstruction details to reduce reconstruction loss and lesion localization errors. The transfer learning module alleviates the need for real training data by taking advantage of cross-domain learning. Both quantitative and qualitative results demonstrate that the proposed method's accuracy surpasses existing methods' in detecting tissue abnormalities.

**Keywords:** Diffuse optical tomography · Inverse problem · Reconstruction · Deep learning · Hybrid loss · Transfer learning · Fuzzy Jaccard

## 1 Introduction

Diffuse optical tomography has witnessed increased interest as an imaging modality and has recently demonstrated its clinical potential in probing

© Springer Nature Switzerland AG 2019
D. Shen et al. (Eds.): MICCAI 2019, LNCS 11764, pp. 66–74, 2019.
https://doi.org/10.1007/978-3-030-32239-7_8

tumors [1,2] for being an affordable, non-ionising alternative to X-ray mammography, the primary screening technique for breast cancer detection. Using near-infrared light in the spectral range of 600 to 950 nm, DOT enables measuring the distribution of the tissue's optical absorption and scattering parameters that can be used to quantitatively assess tissue malignancy. The main challenge then remains how to accurately recover these parameters given the ill-posedness of the DOT image reconstruction problem and the absence of exact analytic inverse.

Most image reconstruction methods are analytic and iterative approaches that often suffer from high computational complexity and are complicated by factors such as imaging geometry, source calibrations and sensor non-idealities [4]. While many deep learning based image reconstruction approaches were proposed recently [5] and showed increased reconstruction speed, resolution enhancement and artifact removal for a variety of imaging modalities, most methods focus on CT and MR image reconstruction [3,5–7] and only a few tackle ultrasound, photo-acoustic, multiple scattering, and DOT inverse problems [8–11].

Most DOT inverse problems consider a circular shape scanner with 16 or more point sources uniformly distributed along the field of view boundary to maximize the number of measurements thereby improving spatial resolution, especially in strongly scattering media. Most recently, a multi-layer perceptron network (MLP) was used to solve DOT image reconstruction problem using high source count [11]. However, increasing the number of sources and detectors adds complexity to the DOT scanner hardware and increases manufacturing cost and computational resources.

One common limitation of existing reconstruction methods is that they perform poorly on data with a very low number of point sources (limited projection data), limited-angle acquisition (e.g, acquisition from one view), or both [1].

Sun et al. [12,13] address the multiple scattering problem of microwaves in biological samples. They study the effect of decreasing the number of sources, to a limited extent (to a minimum of 20 sources), on deep learning based reconstruction methods for weak and strong scattering scenarios. While their proposed reconstruction model leverages the rich data representation collected from 20 up to 40 point sources, it relies on a computationally expensive analytic reconstruction step to provide a first estimate of the reconstructed image, prohibiting real time inference. Furthermore, their deep model is not optimized in an end-to-end manner.

Limited-angle and limited sources DOT image reconstruction in a strong scattering medium is a challenging task that has been considered in end-to-end fashion for a functional hand-held probe in a clinical trial by Ben Yedder et al. [14]. Yet, their results still suffer from noisy reconstruction and deviation of the reconstruction lesion compared to the ground truth location.

To address the aforementioned limitations, in this paper, we propose a deep learning DOT reconstruction method based on a novel loss function and transfer learning to solve the limited-angle and limited sources DOT image reconstruction problem in a strong scattering medium.

By adaptively focusing on important features and filtering irrelevant and noisy ones using the Fuzzy Jaccard loss, our network is able to reduce false positive reconstructed pixels and as a result reconstruct more accurate images.

Training machine learning based methods requires a high number of training samples, a challenging requirement in a medical setting, especially with relatively new imaging devices like DOT probes. Synthetic data simulators can provide an alternative source of training data. However, creating a realistic synthetic dataset is a challenging task as it requires careful modelling of the complex interplay of factors influencing real world acquisition environment. A potential remedy is to attempt to bridge the gap between real word acquisition and synthetic data simulation via transfer learning. To the best of our knowledge, this is the first work to employ a Jaccard based loss and transfer learning to the DOT reconstruction problem.

## 2 Methodology

### 2.1 Background

Given a set of raw acquired DOT measurements $y \in \mathbb{R}^{S \times D}$ from $S$ sources with $D$ sensors, our objective is to reconstruct an image $x \in \mathbb{R}^{W \times H}$, which represents the tissue's optical coefficients. This problem is commonly formulated as finding a reconstructed image $\hat{x}^*$ that minimizes the reconstruction error between the sensor-domain sampled data $y$ and the forward projection $\mathcal{F}(\cdot)$ from a possible reconstructed image $\hat{x}$:

$$\hat{x}^* = \underset{\hat{x}}{\operatorname{argmin}} \|\mathcal{F}(\hat{x}) - y\| + \lambda \mathcal{R}(\hat{x}) \tag{1}$$

where $\mathcal{F}(\cdot)$ is a known predefined forward projection that converts $\hat{x}$ to the sensor domain, $\mathcal{R}(\cdot)$ is a regularization term encoding the prior information about the data, and $\lambda$ is a hyper-parameter that controls the contribution of the regularization term. This objective function is traditionally minimized in an iterative manner until convergence. Alternatively we can learn the task of reconstructing the image from sensor-domain data by way of a deep neural network with a significant one-time, off-line training cost that is offset by a fast inference time.

### 2.2 Deep Learning Reconstruction

Given pairs of measurement vectors $y$ and their corresponding ground truth image $x$, our goal is to optimize the parameters $\theta$ of a fully convolutional neural network in an end-to-end manner to learn the mapping between the measurement vector $y$ and its reconstructed tomographic image $x$, which recovers the optical parameters of underlying imaged tissue. Therefore, we seek the inverse function $\mathcal{F}^{-1}(\cdot)$ that solves:

$$\theta^* = \underset{\theta}{\operatorname{argmin}} \mathcal{L} \left(\mathcal{F}^{-1}(y, \theta), x\right) + \lambda \mathcal{R}(\mathcal{F}^{-1}(y, \theta)) \tag{2}$$

where $\mathcal{L}$ is the loss function of the network that, broadly, penalizes the dissimilarity between the estimated reconstruction and the ground truth. We use an L2 regularization term ($\mathcal{R}$).

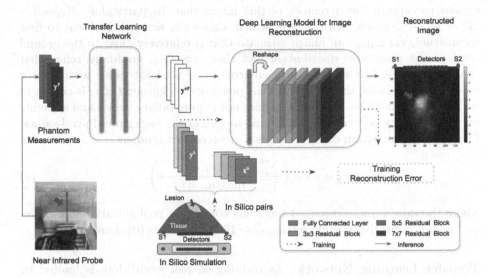

**Fig. 1.** The overall architecture of the proposed model. (lower left) The probe (in black) is positioned to image a phantom (white) with an embedded synthetic lesion (red arrow). The transfer learning (multilayer perceptron) network maps phantom measurements $y^p$ to the domain of in silico training measurements $y^s$. The mapped measurements are passed through the reconstruction network to produce the reconstructed image $\hat{x}^*$ (rightmost image) (Color figure online)

**Deep Network.** The proposed architecture, which extends Yedder et al.'s [14] FCNN architecture with a transfer learning and novel loss components, is a decoder-like network that consists of a fully connected layer followed by a set of residual layers. The fully connected layer maps the measurement vector to a two-dimensional array and provides a coarse image estimate, while the subsequent residual blocks refine the image estimate by passing it through a set of nonlinear transformations to produce the final reconstruction image. The architecture of our proposed model is shown in Fig. 1, where each residual block uses convolutions with batch normalization and ReLU.

**Novel Loss Function.** To address DOT image reconstruction from a limited information representation (one view with few sources), we propose a novel loss function, $\mathcal{L}$, that dynamically combines two loss terms:

$$\mathcal{L} = \mathcal{L}_{\text{MSE}} + \beta(epoch)\mathcal{L}_{\text{FJ}} \tag{3}$$

where $\mathcal{L}_{\mathrm{MSE}}$ is the mean squared error (MSE) loss, which focuses on pixel-wise similarity. $\mathcal{L}_{\mathrm{FJ}}$ is similarity coefficient based fuzzy Jaccard term designed to promote lesion location and appearance similarity while penalizing artifacts. $\beta$ is a hyper-parameter balancing the two terms and varies with the training epochs to capture the dynamics of this interaction. In particular, $\beta(epoch + \Delta) = \beta_0 + \gamma\beta(epoch)$ with $\gamma > 0$, which allows the network to learn to first reconstruct, via $\mathcal{L}_{\mathrm{MSE}}$, an image estimate that is relatively close to the ground truth image pixel wise distribution and then, via $\mathcal{L}_{\mathrm{FJ}}$, gradually refine that candidate image. In DOT image reconstruction of a breast tissue with zero or more isolated lesions, the majority of the pixels are background, $\mathcal{L}_{\mathrm{FJ}}$ is chosen to address this imbalance. Further, $\mathcal{L}_{\mathrm{FJ}}$ does not require binary values and accounts for the similarity between the foreground as well as the background pixel values. Finally, a log transform of $\mathcal{L}_{\mathrm{FJ}}$ ensures a steep convex gradient,

$$\mathcal{L}_{\mathrm{FJ}} = -\log\left(\frac{\sum_{i=1}^{n}\min(a_i, a_i')}{\sum_{i=1}^{n}\max(a_i, a_i')} + \epsilon\right) \tag{4}$$

where the $min(\cdot, \cdot)$ and $max(\cdot, \cdot)$ functions compute a probabilistic intersection and union, respectively while setting $\epsilon = 10^{-5}$ avoids $\log(0)$ domain errors.

**Transfer Learning Network.** As training on real world data is limited by availability of samples, we resort to generating artificial training data via a simulator. A transfer learning network, implemented as a multilayer perceptron, tackles the domain shift between the real data measurement $y^p$, as collected from the probe and used during inference, and the in silico data measurement $y^s$ used during training time (Fig. 1-upper left). By minimizing a loss $\mathcal{L}_{TL}$, the transfer learning network learns to translate the real world data distribution onto the in silico data distribution while avoiding overfitting on the in silico model. Finally, by retraining or fine-tuning this transfer learning network only, our proposed approach can be generalized to new DOT sensors and or source configurations.

Given the $i$-th phantom $x_i^p$ we simulate its $x_i^s$ tissue equivalent and derive the corresponding sensor measurements $y_i^s$, while we collect $y_i^p$ using a physical probe. By minimizing $\mathcal{L}_{TL}$ over $N_p$ phantom experiments, the transfer learning module learns the mapping $\phi(y_i^p) \approx y_i^s$ to ensure it is in the same domain as $y^s$,

$$\theta^* = \operatorname*{argmin}_{\theta} \mathcal{L}_{\mathrm{TL}}(\theta) \quad \text{where} \quad \mathcal{L}_{\mathrm{TL}}(\theta) = \sum_{i=1}^{N_p} ||\phi(y_i^p; \theta) - y_i^s|| \tag{5}$$

where a final test reconstructed image is computed as, $\hat{x}_i^* = \mathcal{F}^{-1}(\phi(y_i^p))$.

## 3 Experiments and Results

We compare our proposed approach to the state of the art FCNN architecture for limited angle data [14] and the aforementioned MLP approach [11], as well as the analytic reconstruction approach described by Shokoufi et al. [15]. In addition, we evaluate the individual contributions of the terms of our loss function and the transfer learning.

## 3.1 Dataset

To train our network $\mathcal{F}^{-1}(\cdot)$ we use in silico training data pairs $(x^s, y^s)$. It includes images $x^s$ of optical tissue properties, discretized into finite-element nodes, and their corresponding forward projection measurements $y^s$ from the Toast++ software suite [17] using realistic human breast tissue and lesion optical parameters distribution values [16]. Simulated lesions have varying sizes, locations, and optical coefficients. The forward model mimics the functional hand-held probe sources and detectors geometries [1]. It comprises 2 LED light sources that illuminate the tissue symmetrically and surrounds 128 detectors where both LED and all detectors are co-linear. The output of the forward model is a 1 × 256 vector $y^s$. A total of 21,590 samples data pairs are used.

The test-set is based on a tissue-equivalent solution where an intralipid solution is used to mimic background breast tissue due to its similarity in optical properties to breast tissue. A tube with 4 mm cross-sectional diameter was filled with an Indian-ink tumor-like liquid and was placed at different locations inside the solution container/solid phantom to mimics cancerous lesions. All phantom measurements $y^p$ are collected with the DOB-probe.

## 3.2 Implementation

The model was implemented in the Keras framework and trained for a total of 1,000 epochs on an Nvidia Titan X GPU using the Adam optimizer. By optimizing the model's performance on the validation set, we set all hyper-parameters as follows: Batch size to 64; learning rate to 0.001; AMS Grad optimizer set to true; and ($\Delta = 10$, $\beta_0 = 0.2$, $\gamma = 0.002$), which describe the update equation of the hyper-parameter $\beta$ in (3); We use a 80/10/10 training/validation/test split of the in silico data.

## 3.3 Qualitative Results

Our model is trained on the in silico data and tested on the phantom dataset. In Fig. 2, we visually compare our proposed reconstruction method to the competing methods' results on sample phantom cases. As mentioned earlier, the transfer learning module maps the real world distribution onto the learned in silico distribution. Without such mapping, unsurprisingly, we notice artifacts in the reconstructed image; note the extensive scattering of false positives with different scales and locations (Fig. 2 - FCNN (MSE)). Adopting transfer learning clearly reduces these artifacts (Fig. 2 - FCNN (MSE+TL)). Further, observe how incorporating both the new loss term $\mathcal{L}_{FJ}$ and transfer learning module significantly reduces the artifacts and improves lesion localization, which otherwise could compromise diagnosis (Fig. 2 - FCNN (MSE+TL+FJ)).

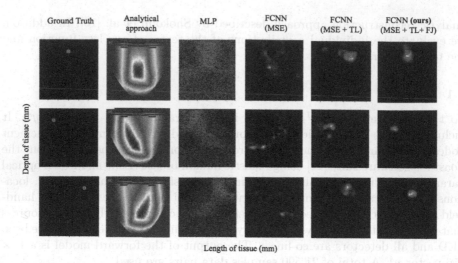

Length of tissue (mm)

**Fig. 2.** Qualitative reconstruction performance of our model compared to state of the art techniques on phantom samples with known lesion ground truth locations. The parabolic shape of the reconstruction produced by the analytical approach is due to the algorithm used.

While MLP showed good performance in the complete information case, namely a circular shape scanner with 16+ uniformly distributed point sources [11], it underperforms on the limited angle experiments (Fig. 2 - MLP). We hypothesize that this difference in performance is due to the convolution operators' ability to extract comprehensive contextual information and synthesize more complex robust features.

### 3.4 Quantitative Results

We measure the reconstruction quality via: (i) Lesion localization error, i.e. the distance between the centre of the lesions in the ground truth image versus the reconstructed image; (ii) peak signal to noise ratio (PSNR); (iii) structural similarity index (SSIM); and (iv) the Fuzzy Jaccard [18]. All reconstructed

**Table 1.** Quantitative results on 32 phantom experiments.

|  | Loc. Error (pixel) | PSNR (db) | SSIM | Fuzzy Jaccard | Time (ms) |
|---|---|---|---|---|---|
| Analytic approach [1] | 77.4 ± 32.2 | 15.0 ± 6.0 | 0.32 ± 0.26 | 0.17 ± 0.15 | 83.3 |
| MLP [11] | 42.0 ± 17.3 | 12.5 ± 1.5 | 0.05 ± 0.03 | 0.07 ± 0.05 | 1.2 |
| FCNN (MSE) [14] | 33.2 ± 23.4 | 20.1 ± 4.6 | 0.46 ± 0.28 | 0.32 ± 0.06 | 7.3 |
| FCNN (MSE+TL) | 16.6 ± 6.60 | 20.6 ± 0.4 | 0.61 ± 0.17 | 0.45 ± 0.08 | 11.5 |
| Proposed | **14.8 ± 7.40** | **21.7 ± 0.9** | **0.73 ± 0.03** | **0.64 ± 0.10** | 16.9 |

images were first normalized prior to calculating the performance metrics. Table 1 presents the results on the phantom dataset.

Using the transfer learning $\phi(\cdot)$ module, we observe ~10% improvement in Fuzzy Jaccard and ~16% in SSIM compared to state of the art FCNN with MSE only. Adding the new $\mathcal{L}_{FJ}$ loss term boosts the improvement in these two metrics further to ~34% and ~33%, respectively. The lesion localization error is also considerably reduced when using transfer learning and $\mathcal{L}_{FJ}$.

# 4   Conclusion

We proposed novel extensions to deep learning based diffuse optical tomography image reconstruction. We have shown empirically that our model, trained with the novel hybrid loss function, attains superior quantitative results on multiple evaluation metrics and, qualitatively, improves the reconstructed images, showing fewer artifacts that could compromise clinical diagnosis. The transfer learning module renders an in silico trained network applicable to real world data. More importantly our approach is decoupled from a change in real world measurements and can be generalized to new source configurations. Our next phase in this research is to improve further the lesion localization and validate our approach on real patient data to assess its diagnostic accuracy.

**Acknowledgments.** We thank NVIDIA Corporation for the donation of Titan X GPUs used in this research, Compute Canada for HPC resources, Michael Smith Foundation, BC Cancer Agency, and the Natural Sciences and Engineering Research Council of Canada (NSERC) and NSERC-CREATE-Bioinformatics for partial funding. The authors also thank Dr. Ramani Ramaseshan from the BC Cancer Agency for his suggestions.

# References

1. Shokoufi, M., Golnaraghi, F.: Handheld diffuse optical breast scanner probe for cross-sectional imaging of breast tissue. J. Innov. Opt. Health Sci. **12**(02), 1950008 (2019)
2. Flexman, M.L., Kim, H.K., Stoll, et al.: A wireless handheld probe with spectrally constrained evolution strategies for diffuse optical imaging of tissue. Rev. Sci. Instrum. **83**(3), 033108 (2012)
3. Jin, K.H., McCann, M.T., Froustey, E., Unser, M.: Deep convolutional neural network for inverse problems in imaging. IEEE Trans. Image Process. **26**(9), 4509–4522 (2017)
4. Wang, G.: A perspective on deep imaging. IEEE Access **4**, 8914–8924 (2016)
5. Wang, G., Ye, J.C., Mueller, et al.: Image reconstruction is a new frontier of machine learning. IEEE Trans. Med. Imaging **37**(6), 1289–1296 (2018)
6. Gupta, H., Jin, K.H., Nguyen, H.Q., et al.: CNN-based projected gradient descent for consistent CT image reconstruction. IEEE Trans. Med. Imaging **37**(6), 1440–1453 (2018)

7. Würfl, T., Hoffmann, M., Christlein, V., et al.: Deep learning computed tomography: learning projection-domain weights from image domain in limited angle problems. IEEE Trans. Med. Imaging **37**(6), 1454–1463 (2018)
8. Wu, S., Gao, Z., Liu, Z., Luo, J., Zhang, H., Li, S.: Direct reconstruction of ultrasound elastography using an end-to-end deep neural network. In: Frangi, A.F., Schnabel, J.A., Davatzikos, C., Alberola-López, C., Fichtinger, G. (eds.) MICCAI 2018. LNCS, vol. 11070, pp. 374–382. Springer, Cham (2018). https://doi.org/10.1007/978-3-030-00928-1_43
9. Yoon, Y.H., Khan, S., Huh, J., Ye, J.C.: Efficient b-mode ultrasound image reconstruction from sub-sampled data using deep learning. IEEE Trans. Med. Imaging **38**(2), 325–336 (2019)
10. Cai, C., Deng, K., Ma, C., Luo, J.: End-to-end deep neural network for optical inversion in quantitative photoacoustic imaging. Opt. Lett. **43**(12), 2752–2755 (2018)
11. Feng, J., Sun, Q., Li, Z., Sun, Z., Jia, K.: Back-propagation neural network-based reconstruction algorithm for diffuse optical tomography. J. Biomed. Opt. **24**(5), 051407 (2018)
12. Sun, Y., Xia, Z., Kamilov, U.S.: Efficient and accurate inversion of multiple scattering with deep learning. Opt. Express **26**(11), 14678–14688 (2018)
13. Sun, Y., Kamilov, U.S.: Stability of Scattering Decoder for Nonlinear Diffractive Imaging. arXiv preprint arXiv:1808015 (2018)
14. Ben Yedder, H., BenTaieb, A., Shokoufi, M., Zahiremami, A., Golnaraghi, F., Hamarneh, G.: Deep learning based image reconstruction for diffuse optical tomography. In: Knoll, F., Maier, A., Rueckert, D. (eds.) MLMIR 2018. LNCS, vol. 11074, pp. 112–119. Springer, Cham (2018). https://doi.org/10.1007/978-3-030-00129-2_13
15. Shokoufi, M.: Multi-modality breast cancer assessment tools using diffuse optical and electrical impedance spectroscopy. Ph.D. thesis (2016)
16. Ghosh, N., Mohanty, S.K., Majumder, S.K., et al.: Measurement of optical transport properties of normal and malignant human breast tissue. Appl. Opt. **40**(1), 176–184 (2001)
17. Schweiger, M., Arridge, S.R.: The Toast++ software suite for forward and inverse modeling in optical tomography. J. Biomed. Opt. **19**(4), 040801 (2014)
18. Crum, W.R., Camara, O., Hill, D.L.: Generalized overlap measures for evaluation and validation in medical image analysis. IEEE Trans. Med. Imaging **11**(25), 1451–1461 (2006)

# Data-Driven Enhancement of Blurry Retinal Images via Generative Adversarial Networks

He Zhao, Bingyu Yang, Lvchen Cao, and Huiqi Li[✉]

Beijing Institute of Technology, Beijing, China
huiqili@bit.edu.cn

**Abstract.** In this paper, we aim at improving the quality of blurry retinal images that are caused by ocular diseases. The blurry images could affect clinical diagnosis for both ophthalmologists and automatic aided system. Inspired by the great success of generative adversarial networks, a data-driven approach is proposed to enhance the blurry images in a weakly supervised manner. That is to say, instead of paired blurry and high-quality images, our approach can be trained with two sets of unpaired images. The advantage of unpaired training setting makes our approach easily applicable, since the annotated data are very limited in medical images. Compared with traditional methods, our model is an end-to-end approach without human designed adjustments or prior knowledge. However, it achieves a superior performance on blurry images. Besides, a dynamic retinal image feature constraint is proposed to guide the generator to improve the performance and avoid over-enhancing the extremely blurry region. Our approach can work on large image resolution which makes it widely beneficial to clinic images.

## 1 Introduction

Retinal imaging is widely used by ophthalmologists for early disease detection and diagnosis including glaucoma, diabetic retinopathy, hypertensive retinopathy. However, the unsatisfied quality of retinal images such as poor illuminance, low contrast and blurriness makes it hard to distinguish different diseases and also decrease the accuracy of diagnosis for doctors [9]. Meanwhile, the poor quality image leads to an unsatisfied result for automatic image processing (*e.g.* segmentation, tracking) which may further influence the analysis of diseases. Recent years, there are many researchers trying to enhance the retinal images with low quality. Most of the methods focus on improving illuminance and contrast of retinal image using normalization techniques, while little effort is putting on deblurriness.

In this paper, we propose a novel deep learning approach to enhance the blurry images. Different from other retinal image enhancement methods with sophisticated adjustments of parameters, our approach is very straightforward with an end-to-end framework. We propose a solution of using an image-to-image

© Springer Nature Switzerland AG 2019
D. Shen et al. (Eds.): MICCAI 2019, LNCS 11764, pp. 75–83, 2019.
https://doi.org/10.1007/978-3-030-32239-7_9

translation pipeline with a two-way GAN that is restricted by feature constraint. In addition, our approach only requires two sets of unpaired blurry/high-quality images as inputs, which is applicable in many cases where paired medical images are rare and not accessible. The contribution of our approach can be summarized as follows. (1) To the best of our knowledge, our approach is the first end-to-end deep generative model to enhance the blurry retinal images, which is not based on prior knowledge and designed adjustment. (2) Our model can learn the mapping by a weakly supervision manner (*i.e.* no paired blurry/high quality images are required), which is appropriate to the situation that paired data are limited in medical images. (3) The proposed dynamic feature descriptor provides a feature constraint that helps the model to produce more reliable enhancement containing the core information and fewer artifacts. (4) Besides, our enhanced images are helpful on improving the performance of automatic processing, such as vessel segmentation and tracking.

## 2   Related Work

***Retinal Image Enhancement.*** Image enhancement has been well studied in recent years, and various methods are proposed [3,8,10]. They have achieved a good performance on luminance and contrast enhancement. For medical images, image enhancement has been explored and methods are focusing on specific tasks. The histogram based method, contrast limited adaptive histogram equalization (CLAHE), is widely used and applied to improve the poor quality retinal images. A luminosity and contrast adjustment method is proposed in [13]. The luminance is enhanced by a luminance gain matrix from gamma correction and the contrast is enhanced by CLAHE in the Lab color space. This kind of methods is based on the knowledge of the neighborhood region. In [6], Fourier transformation is utilized to remove the opacity and CLAHE is used to enhance the contrast based on HIS color space. The blurriness of retinal images are modelled using scattering process in [11] and the images are enhanced with estimation of transmission map and background illuminance. Predefined parameters and prior knowledge such as enhancing details or region selected are required in the above models, and this may make their model sensitive.

***Generative Adversarial Model.*** The generative adversarial model that is designed as a two-player zero-sum game between a discriminator and a generator [2], has been developed rapidly in the past five years. The generator is trained to generate samples as similar as the real ones, while the discriminator is designed to distinguish the generated samples. The model is utilized to generate realistic images of both natural images [4,14] and medical images [7,12]. For example, Isola *et al.* [4] present a general translator to transform image from one domain to another, which requires the paired training data. Later, Zhu *et al.* [14] loose the constraint by introducing a backward mapping from output to input. Application based on Zhu *et al.* is also studied to enhance the photos in terms of color and sharpness with modified model structure and training scheme for stability [1]. In medical imaging, the adversarial learning is widely used in other tasks such as registration, reconstruction and segmentation and have achieved satisfied results, in which it is applied as an additional constraint.

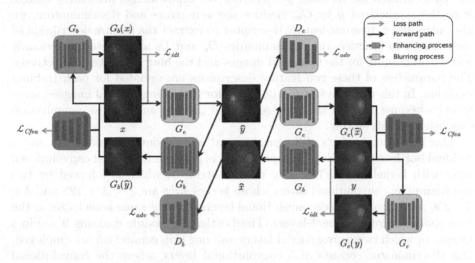

**Fig. 1.** Flowchart of our approach focusing on the low-quality to high-quality process. Blue boxes indicate the generator and discriminator for enhancing process, while green boxes are for blurring process. $G_e$ and $G_b$ represent enhanced generator and blurred generator respectively, while $D_e$ and $D_b$ indicate the corresponding discriminators. The yellow box refers to the dynamic feature descriptor for feature consistent constraint. $x$ indicates the blurry image, while $y$ refers to the high quality image. (Color figure online)

## 3   Method

In this section, we propose a retinal image enhancement model based on the generative adversarial networks with feature consistent constraint. Denote the training dataset as $\{x_i, y_i\}_{i=1}^{N}$, where $x \in \mathbb{R}^{W \times H \times 3}$ refers to the blurry images and $y \in \mathbb{R}^{W \times H \times 3}$ is the high quality images. Our goal is to enhance the blurry image $x$ and produce the enhanced image $\hat{y}$ to make it as clear as the normal retinal image $y$. In order to achieve this target, two generative models are employed $G_e : x \to y$ and $G_b : y \to x$. The first generator $G_e$ is used to enhance the image from low-quality to high-quality and $G_b$ is used for providing a training reference by converting the high-quality to low-quality. This mechanism forms a feedback of information and makes the model trainable using a weakly supervised manner, where the feature descriptor is proposed for a perceptual constraint.

### 3.1   Model Structure

The flowchart of our approach is displayed in Fig. 1. The two generators $G_e$ and $G_b$ share the same model structure but with different tasks, while the two discriminators $D_e$ and $D_b$ also have the same model structure. The $D_e$ aims to distinguish the enhanced images $\hat{y}$ from the real high quality images $y$, while the $D_b$ is utilized for checking out whether the input images are blurry images $x$ or the synthesized $\hat{y}$ by $G_b$. Besides the generators and discriminators, we also introduce a dynamic feature descriptor to extract the feature description of each image. In practice, the discriminators $D_e$ and $D_b$ are selected as dynamic feature descriptors for the enhanced images and the blurred images respectively. The parameters of these two feature descriptors are updated for each training iteration. In this way, the features designed for describing the real image characteristics become stronger and stronger during training and it's less computation expensive for this setting.

Our generator consists of 3 convolutional and deconvolutional layers and a residual bottleneck module. The input image is passed into the first convolutional layer with kernel size of $7 \times 7 \times 64$ and stride 1, which is followed by two downsampling convolutional layers whose kernel sizes are $3 \times 3 \times 128$ and $3 \times 3 \times 256$ respectively. The deconvolutional layers have the same kernel sizes as the corresponding convolutional layers. The bottleneck module contains 9 residual blocks, in which two convolutional layers and one skip connection are employed. Our discriminator consists of 5 convolutional layers, where the convolutional kernels with $3 \times 3$ and stride 2 are applied for 4 times downsampling. The Patch-GAN [4] is utilized here which classifies whether the image patches are real or fake instead of the whole image. This setting decreases the number of parameters and improves the ability of the discriminators.

## 3.2 Objective Function

The entire enhancement process can be described as $G_e(x) : x \rightarrow \hat{y}$, while a discriminator function is defined as $D_e : X \rightarrow d \in [0, 1]$. When the input $X$ is the real high quality image $y$, $d$ should be closed to 1 and when $X$ is the enhanced image $\hat{y}$, $d$ should be closed to 0. Different from the traditional GAN, another pair of generator $G_b$ and discriminator $D_b$ is employed here to train the model using a weakly supervised manner. We follow the GAN's idea and combine the two pairs of $G$ and $D$, and the optimization problem which needs to be solved is:

$$\min_{G_e, G_b} \max_{D_e, D_b} \mathcal{L} = \omega_{adv}\mathcal{L}_{adv} + \omega_{Cfea}\mathcal{L}_{Cfea} + +\omega_{idt}\mathcal{L}_{idt} \tag{1}$$

where the adversarial loss is $\mathcal{L}_{adv} = (D_e(y)-1)^2 + D_e(\hat{y})^2 + (D_b(x)-1)^2 + D_b(\hat{x})^2$, with $\mathcal{L}_{Cfea}$ and $\mathcal{L}_{idt}$ being the feature consistent constraint and identity loss respectively. Here, we use a least-squares loss [5] to obtain a more stable training process and better results. These three terms form our final loss function and will be introduced in the following.

*Feature Consistent Constraint.* In general, the generator $G_e$ can produce many "enhanced" outputs if the adversarial loss is the only restriction. In order to make $G_e$ enhance the blurry images in the direction we expect, the consistent mapping function is introduced. The intuition of this restriction is that one blurry image $\hat{x}$ generated by $G_b$ from $y$ should be converted back by the enhanced function $G_b$. Similarly, for each enhanced image $\hat{y}$ generated by $G_e$ should also satisfy the cycle consistency, where $G_b(\hat{y}) \rightarrow x$. So the consistent constraint can be defined as:

$$\mathcal{L}_C = \|G_b(\hat{y}) - x\|_1 + \|G_e(\hat{x}) - y\|_1 \tag{2}$$

where $\hat{y} = G_e(x)$ and $\hat{x} = G_b(y)$ indicate the outputs of enhanced and blurry result respectively. This consistent strategy creates a supervisory signal to train the enhanced generator $G_e$ and the blurred generator $G_b$, which somehow makes this unpaired training task into a "pair-wise" learning. However, due to the complex background and foreground of retinal images, image-level consistent constraint is not enough and leads to unsatisfactory artifacts on the enhanced images. A feature consistent constraint is further proposed to overcome this issue. In practice, we choose to measure the difference of feature maps coming from convolutional layers. For specific layer $l$ and the convolutional function $F$, the final feature consistent constraint is defined as:

$$\mathcal{L}_{Cfea} = \left\|F^l(G_b(\hat{y})) - F^l(x)\right\|_1 + \left\|F^l(G_e(\hat{x})) - F^l(y)\right\|_1 \tag{3}$$

*Identity Loss.* The identity loss is applied to regularize the generator $G_e$ to produce an identity mapping when a high-quality image $y$ is fed into $G_e$. The same operation is also applied to the output of another generator $G_b$. Then the final identity loss is defined as:

$$\mathcal{L}_{idt} = (\|G_e(y) - y\|_1 + \|G_b(x) - x\|_1) \tag{4}$$

Intuitively, the same image should be obtained when a high-quality image is fed into the enhanced generator. This additional loss is very helpful to preserve the color between the input and output by adding a restriction to the generator. Without the identity loss, the model is free to generate and the enhanced image $\hat{y}$ is corrupted with unsatisfied color appearance.

## 4   Experiment and Results

In practice, we set $\omega_{adv} = 1$, $\omega_{Cfea} = 10$, $\omega_{idt} = 10$ as the weights of each single loss. Empirically, all convolutional layers in discriminator are selected to computing $\mathcal{L}_{Cfea}$. The dataset used for training and testing are from hospitals. There are 550 blurry images and 550 high quality images used for training and 60 blurry images are used for testing. The blurry images are from cataract patients and the high quality are from normal people. There are two subsets of testing set. The first one contains only fifty blurry images, while the second one consists of ten images with ground-truths. Images of cataract patients are blurry due to the opacity of lens, and the images after surgery are regarded as ground-truth. To evaluate our retinal image enhancement performance, we carry out the following experiments including visual and quantitative evaluation.

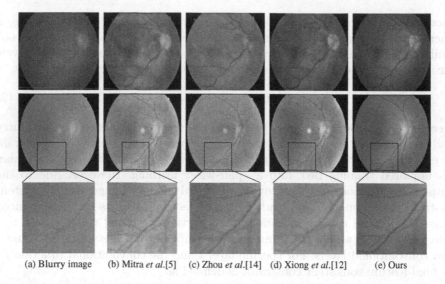

(a) Blurry image     (b) Mitra *et al.*[5]     (c) Zhou *et al.*[14]     (d) Xiong *et al.*[12]     (e) Ours

**Fig. 2.** Visual comparison between our approach and other methods. Two different image samples are shown in the first and the second rows, while the last row is the zoom-in views of selected regions.

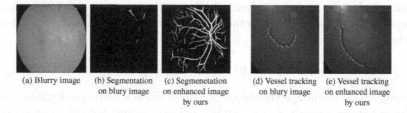

(a) Blurry image     (b) Segmentation on blury image     (c) Segmenetation on enhanced image by ours     (d) Vessel tracking on blury image     (e) Vessel tracking on enhanced image by ours

**Fig. 3.** Results of two retinal image processing tasks on blurry and enhanced images. (a–c) show the segmentation task, while (d–e) display the tracking task.

## 4.1 Enhancement Evaluation – Visual and Quantitative

In this section, two kinds of image quality assessment are adopted, full-reference and no-reference evaluation. For no-reference assessment, Blind/Referenceless Image Spatial Quality Evaluator (BRISQUE), Natural Image Quality Evaluator (NIQE) and Entropy are chosen to assess each enhanced image and its original blurry retinal image. Fifty blurry images are employed in the no-reference evaluation. All these no-reference quality metrics give us an absolute image quality but not the proximity to a reference. As to full-reference assessment, Signal-to-Noise Ratio (PSNR) and structural similarity index measure (SSIM) are utilized. SSIM and PSNR give the comparison between the enhanced image and the ground truth. For this assessment, images of ten cataract patients before and after cataract surgery are used for evaluation. The quantitative results are displayed in Table 1. The lower values of BRISQUE and NIQE indicate better

**Table 1.** Quantitative comparison between our approach and other methods, where full-reference and no-reference assessments are included. The lower the score of BRISQUE and NIQE, the better, while opposite for others.

| | No-reference | | | Full-reference | |
|---|---|---|---|---|---|
| | BRISQUE | NIQE | Entropy | PSNR | SSIM |
| Mitra *et al.* [6] | 45.16 | 3.32 | 6.69 | 16.38 | 0.78 |
| Zhou *et al.* [13] | 46.13 | 4.30 | 6.74 | 17.73 | 0.73 |
| Xiong *et al.* [11] | 43.61 | 3.87 | 6.67 | 17.26 | 0.87 |
| Ours w/o feature constraint | 41.39 | 2.78 | 6.67 | 19.03 | 0.88 |
| Ours | **40.62** | **2.74** | **6.89** | **19.24** | **0.89** |

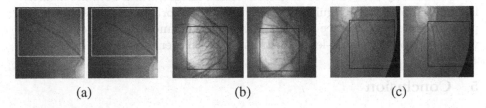

| (a) | (b) | (c) |
|---|---|---|

**Fig. 4.** Visual comparison between feature-level constraint and image-level constraint on enhanced retinal images. For each panel, images on the left are outputs from model with image-level constraint and images on the right are the outputs from model with feature constraint. (Color figure online)

image quality, while higher entropy scores refer to better quality. Our approach achieves the best BRISQUE, NIQE and entropy scores which are 40.62, 2.74 and 6.89 respectively. As to the full-reference assessment, our approach still obtains the highest value of PSNR with 19.24 and SSIM with 0.89. This superior performance can also be supported by the visual comparison of enhanced results shown in Fig. 2, in which three methods (Mitra *et al.* [6], Zhou *et al.* [13] and Xiong *et al.* [11]) are compared with ours. All these four methods can produce an overall good performance and enhance vessels more or less. But the results obtained by our approach are visually better. Our approach can generate a clean image with a similar appearance of raw image, while other methods may produce irregular color appearance. Besides, the boundaries of vessels are sharper than other methods and the background is cleaner without noises. The results obtained by the other methods contain more blurred vessels. This is more obvious in the zoomed-in views of the selected patches.

The enhanced images can benefit other retinal image processing, such as vessel segmentation or vessel tracking. To demonstrate the improvement, we conduct experiments on both blurry and enhanced images for different tasks. Figure 3 displays the results of vessel segmentation and tracking with the same model for each task. As we can see, more vessels can be segmented out on our enhanced image, while the wrong vessel tracking will be corrected.

## 4.2 Ablation Test on Feature Constraint

To evaluate the performance of our dynamic feature constraint compared with image-level constraint, we measure the results of these two models separately. The second last row of Table 1 displays the quantitative results of model without feature constraint. It's a bit worse than the final model of our approach both on no-reference and full-reference assessment. Figure 4 shows the visual comparison of these two models.

Overall, the results enhanced by image-level constraint are satisfied. However, the image-level model usually produces artifacts when the area is extremely unclear (shown with blue boxes in figure), and some parts are not well enhanced compared with our final model (shown with red boxes in figure). Retinal structures can hardly be seen on the extreme blurred images, which becomes a barrier for image-level model to guide the enhanced generator. On the other hand, the pattern in the feature space can still provide the guidance, this is also the reason why our proposed feature-level constraint works better than image-level one.

## 5 Conclusion

We propose a novel deep learning approach to enhance blurry retinal images in a data-driven fashion. It is trained in a weakly supervised manner without the requirement of paired data, which is extremely important for medical images where not much paired data are available. These two advantages (*i.e.* data-driven fashion and unpaired data) make our approach flexible and could be easily used. The proposed approach outperforms the state-of-art retinal image enhancement methods in both visual and quantitative evaluation. Furthermore, it can be used to improve the performance of image processing, including retinal vessel segmentation and tracking. The proposed method can be extend from retinal images to other medical images.

## References

1. Chen, Y.S., Wang, Y.C., Kao, M.H., Chuang, Y.Y.: Deep photo enhancer: unpaired learning for image enhancement from photographs with gans. In: IEEE Conference on Computer Vision and Pattern Recognition, pp. 6306–6314 (2018)
2. Goodfellow, I., et al.: Generative adversarial nets. In: Advances in Neural Information processing Systems, pp. 2672–2680 (2014)
3. He, K., Sun, J., Tang, X.: Single image haze removal using dark channel prior. IEEE Trans. Pattern Anal. Mach. Intell. **33**(12), 2341–2353 (2011)
4. Isola, P., Zhu, J.Y., Zhou, T., Efros, A.A.: Image-to-image translation with conditional adversarial networks. In: IEEE Conference on Computer Vision and Pattern Recognition, pp. 5967–5976. IEEE (2017)
5. Mao, X., Li, Q., Xie, H., Lau, R.Y., Wang, Z., Paul Smolley, S.: Least squares generative adversarial networks. In: Proceedings of the IEEE International Conference on Computer Vision, pp. 2794–2802 (2017)

6. Mitra, A., Roy, S., Roy, S., Setua, S.K.: Enhancement and restoration of non-uniform illuminated fundus image of retina obtained through thin layer of cataract. Comput. Methods Program. Biomed. **156**, 169–178 (2018)

7. Nie, D., et al.: Medical image synthesis with context-aware generative adversarial networks. In: Descoteaux, Maxime, Maier-Hein, Lena, Franz, Alfred, Jannin, Pierre, Collins, D.Louis, Duchesne, Simon (eds.) MICCAI 2017. LNCS, vol. 10435, pp. 417–425. Springer, Cham (2017). https://doi.org/10.1007/978-3-319-66179-7_48

8. Polesel, A., Ramponi, G., Mathews, V.J.: Image enhancement via adaptive unsharp masking. IEEE Trans. Image Process. **9**(3), 505–510 (2000)

9. Sevik, U., Kose, C., Berber, T., Erdol, H.: Identification of suitable fundus images using automated quality assessment methods. J. Biomed. Opt. **19**(4), 046006 (2014)

10. Starck, J.L., Murtagh, F., Candès, E.J., Donoho, D.L.: Gray and color image contrast enhancement by the curvelet transform. IEEE Trans. Image Process. **12**(6), 706–717 (2003)

11. Xiong, L., Li, H., Xu, L.: An enhancement method for color retinal images based on image formation model. Comput. Methods Program. Biomed. **143**, 137–150 (2017)

12. Zhao, H., Li, H., Maurer-Stroh, S., Cheng, L.: Synthesizing retinal and neuronal images with generative adversarial nets. Med. Image Anal. **49**, 14–26 (2018)

13. Zhou, M., Jin, K., Wang, S., Ye, J., Qian, D.: Color retinal image enhancement based on luminosity and contrast adjustment. IEEE Trans. Biomed. Eng. **65**(3), 521–527 (2018)

14. Zhu, J.Y., Park, T., Isola, P., Efros, A.A.: Unpaired image-to-image translation using cycle-consistent adversarial networks. In: International Conference on Computer Vision, pp. 2242–2251. IEEE (2017)

# Dual Encoding U-Net for Retinal Vessel Segmentation

Bo Wang[1,2], Shuang Qiu[2], and Huiguang He[1,2,3(✉)]

[1] School of Artifical Intelligence, University of Chinese Academy of Sciences,
Beijing 100049, People's Republic of China
[2] Research Center for Brain-inspired Intelligence and National Laboratory
of Pattern Recognition, Institute of Automation, Chinese Academy of Sciences,
Beijing 100190, People's Republic of China
huiguang.he@ia.ac.cn
[3] Center for Excellence in Brain Science and Intelligence Technology,
Chinese Academy of Sciences, Beijing 100190, People's Republic of China

**Abstract.** Retinal Vessel Segmentation is an essential step for the early diagnosis of eye-related diseases, such as diabetes and hypertension. Segmentation of blood vessels requires both sizeable receptive field and rich spatial information. In this paper, we propose a novel Dual Encoding U-Net (DEU-Net), which have two encoders: a spatial path with large kernel to preserve the spatial information and a context path with multiscale convolution block to capture more semantic information. On the top of the two paths, we introduce a feature fusion module to combine the different level of feature representation. Besides, we apply channel attention to select useful feature map in a skip connection. Furthermore, low-level and high-level prediction are combined in multiscale prediction module for a better accuracy. We evaluated this model on the digital retinal images for vessel extraction (DRIVE) dataset and the child heart and health study (CHASEDB1) dataset. Results show that the proposed DEU-Net model achieved the state-of-the-art retinal vessel segmentation accuracy on both datasets.

**Keywords:** Retinal vessel segmentation · Spatial path · Context path · Attention mechanism

## 1 Introduction

Segmentation of blood vessels plays an important role in the diagnosis of eye-related diseases such as diabetics, hypertension and retinopathy of prematurity [3]. However, manual annotation of retina blood vessels by ophthalmologist is time consuming task and requires training and skill. Therefore, automatic segmentation of retinal blood vessels from funds images is particularly significant.

Many automatic retinal vessel segmentation algorithms have been reported in the past decades and can be divided into two broad categories. The first

© Springer Nature Switzerland AG 2019
D. Shen et al. (Eds.): MICCAI 2019, LNCS 11764, pp. 84–92, 2019.
https://doi.org/10.1007/978-3-030-32239-7_10

category is image processing algorithms, including pre-processing, segmentation and postprocessing. For example, Bankhead et al. [2] developed wavelet transform approach to enhance the foreground and background for fast vessel detection. The other category is machine learning based algorithms, which utilizes extracted feature vectors to train a classifier to determine whether a pixel from retinal image belong to vessel or not. As a typical example, Lupascu et al. [5] constructed 41-D feature vector for each pixel, and an AdaBoost classifier was trained for classifying each pixel in retinal image.

Recently, deep learning method has shown its excellence in many computer version tasks. Since U-Net [8] has the encoder-decoder structure with skip connections which allows efficient information flow, it provides state-of-the-art performance in many medical image analysis. Wu et al. [11] proposed the multiscale network followed network (MS-NFN) model for retinal vessel segmentation and each submodel consists of two identical U-Net models. Zhuang et al. [12] reported a chain of multiple U-Nets (LadderNet), which has multiple pairs of encoder-decoder branches. However, in order to incorporate more spatial information of pixels into the pixel classification, all these variants just stack various U-Net, with low interpretability and high computational complexity.

This paper proposed a Dual Encoding U-Net (DEU-Net) model that greatly enhances deep neural networks' capability of segmenting vessels with an end-to-end and pixel-to-pixel manner. The main uniqueness of this model includes: (1) a spatial encoding path, which has a small stride and large kernel to preserve the spatial information; a context path, which has multiscale convolution modules to capture more semantic information; (2) channel attention mechanism is applied for skip connection to flow and select useful feature map. (3) low-level and high-level prediction are generated by decoding path and a multiscale predict module is introduced to fusion different scale feature for a better prediction. The proposed model has been evaluated on DRIVE and CHASEDB1 dataset. Results show that the proposed DEU-Net model achieved the state-of-the-art retinal vessel segmentation accuracy on both datasets.

## 2   Method

In this paper, we propose a Dual Encoding U-Net approach for retinal vessel segmentation. The proposed method for retinal vessel segmentation mainly consists of the following steps: (1) retinal image preprocessing, (2) patch extraction, (3) feeding each patch into Dual Encoding U-Net for segmentation, (4) segmentation result reconstruction. The overview of the retinal vessel segmentation framework is shown in Fig. 1.

### 2.1   Retinal Image Preprocessing and Patch Extraction

Retinal images usually comprise noise and uneven illumination, thus it is necessary to make an image enhancement before postprocessing. Firstly, we converted an RGB fundus image to a gray image, and the gray imaged was normalized.

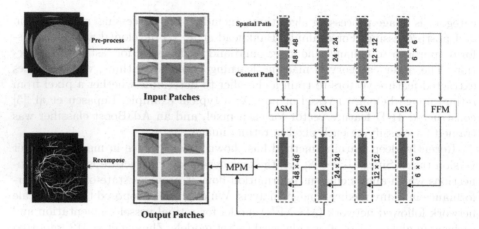

**Fig. 1.** Illustration of the Dual Encoding U-Net model-based retinal vessel segmentation. Components of the network architecture contains: Attention Skip Module(ASM), Feature Fusion Module (FFM) and Multiscale Predict Module (MPM).

Secondly, contrast limited adaptive histogram equalization and gamma adjustment was applied to improve the image contrast and the suppress noise. Finally, the intensity values are scaled range from 0 to 1. We randomly sampled 190,000 patches of size 48 × 48 from the DRIVE dataset and 760,000 patches from the CHASEDB1 dataset for training our model.

## 2.2 The Proposed Architecture

Inspired by U-Net [8], we proposed a Dual Encoding U-Net (DEU-Net) for retinal vessel segmentation. Figure 1 illustrates the network architecture. The proposed network has a U-shaped architecture with encoder and decoder. In encoder, a spatial path was designed to preserve the spatial information and a context path was used to capture more semantic information. Furthermore, channel attention mechanism was applied for skip connection to transfer information and select useful feature map. Finally, in decoder, low-level and high-level prediction were combined to predict a better accuracy.

**Spatial Path.** In semantic task, the spatial information and the receptive field are crucial to achieving high accuracy. However, it is hard to meet these two demands simultaneously. Refer to the Global Convolutional Network [7], we propose a spatial path with large kernels to encode the affluent spatial information from original input image. The spatial path contains four layers and each layer includes a convolution with stride = 7,12,9,6 in order, followed by batch normalization and ReLU. Since the input size of network is 48 × 48, these relatively large convolution kernels encode rich spatial information with large spatial size of feature maps.

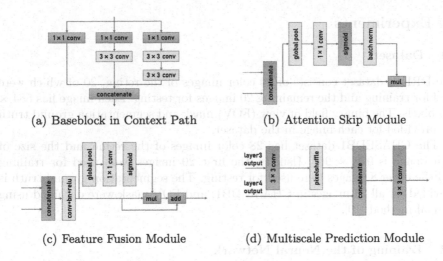

(a) Baseblock in Context Path        (b) Attention Skip Module

(c) Feature Fusion Module        (d) Multiscale Prediction Module

**Fig. 2.** Structure of components in Dual Encoding U-Net

**Context Path.** The spatial path is used to encode spatial information, also, we design a context path to provide sufficient semantic information. The context path also contains four layers. Each layer includes a baseblock with numbers of size convolution filters (see Fig. 2(a)), which can improve the expressive ability of the convolution layer and raise efficiency of the network parameters.

**Attention Skip Module.** In skip layers, we propose a specific channel attention mechanism to select necessary feature map. As shown in Fig. 2(b), attention skip module employs global average pooling on the combined output of spatial and context path, which computes an attention vector to guide the feature map learning. This module is a self-attention mechanism, which can increase the network's sensitivity to informative features which is important in decoder without any supervisory information. Efficient information of encoder can make a better prediction.

**Feature Fusion Module.** The features of the two paths are different in level of feature representation. The spatial information captured by the spatial path encodes mostly rich detail information, which is known as low level. Moreover, the output feature of the context path mainly encodes context information, which is known as high level. Therefore, we introduce a feature fusion module to fuse these features as shown in Fig. 2(c).

**Multiscale Predict Module.** Given the different level of the prediction, a multiscale predict module is introduced to fusion different scale feature. PixelShuffle [9] is applied to upsample low level prediction feature to high resolution, which can preserve spatial information. Finally, low-level and high-level predictions with the same size are combined and followed by a convolution process (see Fig. 2(d)).

# 3   Experiments

## 3.1   Datasets

The DRIVE dataset consists of 40 color images of the retina, 20 of which were used for training and the remaining 20 images for testing. Each image has 584 × 565 pixels. The binary field of view (FOV) mask and segmentation ground truth are provided for each image in the dataset.

The CHASEDB1 dataset has 28 color images of the retina and the size of each image is 999 × 960. Usually, the first 20 images were used for training and the other 8 images were used for testing. The segmentation ground truth is provided for all 28 images in CHASE DB1, and FOV mask were obtained using manual method [10].

## 3.2   Training of the Neural Network

We randomly sampled 190,000 patches of size 48 × 48 from the training images in DRIVE, and used 10% of the training samples as validation data. For the CHASEDB1 dataset, we sampled 760,000 patches of size 48 × 48 from the training images, and used 10% of the training samples as validation. Instead of only cross-entropy loss for segmentation, we use a hybrid loss function that is a weighted sum of two terms. The first is a binary-class cross-entropy term that encourages the segmentation model to predict the right class label at each pixel location independently, which is defined as:

$$Loss_{ce}(y, \hat{y}) = - \sum y_i \log \hat{y}_i + (1 - y_i) \log(1 - \hat{y}_i) \tag{1}$$

where both $y_i$ is ground truth and $\hat{y}_i$ is predicted vectors. The second loss term is based on Intersection over Union (Iou), named the jaccard loss, which is defined as:

$$Loss_{jaccard}(y, \hat{y}) = 1 - \frac{|y \cap \hat{y}|}{|y \cup \hat{y}|} \tag{2}$$

where $y$ is ground truth image and $\hat{y}$ is predicted image. The jaccard loss can detect and correct higher-order inconsistencies between ground truth segmentation maps and the ones produced by the segmentation net, nor measured by a per-pixel cross-entropy loss. Finally, the joint loss function is:

$$Loss = \lambda_1 Loss_{ce} + \lambda_2 Loss_{jaccard} \tag{3}$$

where $\lambda_1$ and $\lambda_2$ are the weight of two terms, satisfied with $\lambda_1 = 0.8$ and $\lambda_2 = 0.2$ in this paper. Adam optimizer with default parameters is applied to train the model and batch size is 256. Besides, we use "reduce learning rate on plateau" strategy, and set the learning rate as 0.01, 0.001, 0.0001 on epochs 0, 25 and 50 respectively, and set the total learning epochs as 200.

### 3.3 Evaluation Metrics

In retinal vessel segmentation, we divide the pixels in the vessel map into true positive (TP), false positive (FP), negative (FN) and true negative (TN) by comparing them with the corresponding ground truth labels. Then, accuracy (AC), sensitivity (SE), specificity (SP) and F1-score are used to evaluate the performance of DEU-Net. To further evaluate the performance of different neural networks, we also calculated the area under receiver operating characteristics curve (AUC).

## 4 Results

To evaluate the proposed Dual Encoding U-Net framework, we conduct experiments on the DRIVE and CHASEDB1 datasets. The retinal vessel segmentation results of DEU-Net are shown in Fig. 3, where in each column the input image, the ground truth, and the result of our segmentation method are shown from top to bottom. From Fig. 4, it can be observed that DEU-Net produces more distinct vessel segmentation results and preserve more details than Laddernet [12].

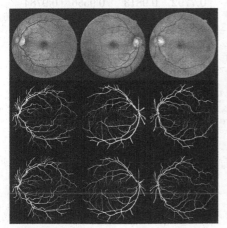 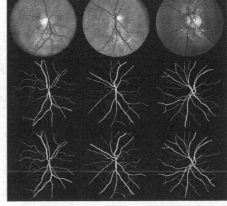

(a) Test results on DRIVE dataset.     (b) Test results on CHASE-DB1 dataset.

**Fig. 3.** Test results on DRIVE and CHASE DB1 dataset. From top to bottom: input image, ground truth and predictions.

A quantitative evaluation of the results obtained on our experiments is presented in Tables 1 and 2. The experimental result shows that the proposed method is competitive with other existing methods by achieving the highest F1-score, sensitivity, specificity and accuracy for both tasks. DEU-Net also generates high AUC on two tasks. So the proposed method is a robust tool for vessel segmentation and the comparison demonstrate that the proposed method is very competitive with the stage-of-the-art methods.

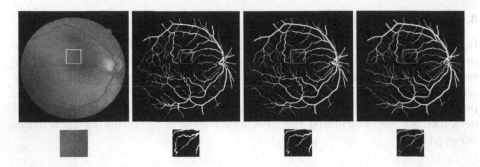

**Fig. 4.** A test image from the DRIVE dataset (1st column), ground truth (2th column), the segmentation results obtained by using our DEU-Net (3nd column) and Laddernet [12] (4rd column).

**Table 1.** Results of DEU-Net and other methods on DRIVE datasets.

| Methods | Year | F1-score | SE | SP | AC | AUC |
|---|---|---|---|---|---|---|
| Li et al. [4] | 2016 | N.A | 0.7569 | **0.9816** | 0.9527 | 0.9738 |
| Orlando et al. [6] | 2017 | 0.7857 | 0.7897 | 0.9684 | N.A | 0.9507 |
| R2U-Net [1] | 2018 | 0.8171 | 0.7792 | 0.9813 | 0.9556 | 0.9784 |
| Recurrent UNet [1] | 2018 | 0.8155 | 0.7751 | **0.9816** | 0.9556 | 0.9782 |
| LadderNet [12] | 2018 | 0.8202 | 0.7856 | 0.9810 | 0.9561 | **0.9793** |
| **Dual Encoding U-Net** | 2019 | **0.8270** | **0.7940** | **0.9816** | **0.9567** | 0.9772 |

**Table 2.** Results of DEU-Net and other methods on CHASE-DB1 datasets.

| Methods | Year | F1-score | SE | SP | AC | AUC |
|---|---|---|---|---|---|---|
| Li et al. [4] | 2016 | N.A | 0.7507 | 0.9793 | 0.9581 | 0.9716 |
| Orlando et al. [6] | 2017 | 0.7332 | 0.7277 | 0.9712 | N.A | 0.9524 |
| R2U-Net [1] | 2018 | 0.7928 | 0.7756 | 0.9712 | 0.9634 | 0.9815 |
| Residual U-Net [1] | 2018 | 0.7800 | 0.7726 | 0.9820 | 0.9553 | 0.9779 |
| LadderNet [12] | 2018 | 0.8031 | 0.7978 | 0.9818 | 0.9656 | **0.9839** |
| **Dual Encoding U-Net** | 2019 | **0.8037** | **0.8074** | **0.9821** | **0.9661** | 0.9812 |

We also analyzed the speed of our algorithm. It took more than 13 hours to train the DEU-Net on the DRIVE dataset and more than 20 hours on the CHASEDB1 dataset (Intel Xeon CPU E5-2650 v4 CPU, NVIDIA GTX 1080Ti GPU, 125 GB Memory, and pytorch 0.4.0). However, it only took 6.75 s to segment a 584 × 565 retinal image on DRIVE and 12.82 seconds to segment a 999 × 960 retinal image on CHASEDB1 dataset. The speed is faster than MS-NFN [11], thus, our proposed network has low computational complexity.

## 5 Conclusions

Dual Encoding U-Net is proposed in this paper to improve the accuracy of retinal vessel segmentation. Our proposed DEU-Net contains two encoders: a spatial path and a context path which is designed to preserve spatial information and capture semantic information, separately. Besides, channel attention mechanism is applied to select necessary feature map in skip connection. All the designs improve the interpretability of U-Net. Our results indicate that the proposed method has significantly outperforms the-state-of-the-art for retinal blood vessel segmentation on both datasest.

**Acknowledgements.** This work was supported in part by The National Key Research and Development Program of China (2017YFB1302704) and the Chinese Academy of Sciences (CAS) Scientific Equipment Development Project under Grant YJKYYQ20170050, the Beijing Municipal Science and Technology Commission under Grant Z181100008918010, Youth Innovation Promotion Association CAS and Strategic Priority Research Program of CAS.

## References

1. Alom, M.Z., Hasan, M., Yakopcic, C., Taha, T.M., Asari, V.K.: Recurrent residual convolutional neural network based on u-net (r2u-net) for medical image segmentation. arXiv preprint arXiv:1802.06955 (2018)
2. Bankhead, P., Scholfield, C.N., McGeown, J.G., Curtis, T.M.: Fast retinal vessel detection and measurement using wavelets and edge location refinement. PloS One **7**(3), e32435 (2012)
3. Kanski, J.J., Bowling, B.: Clinical Ophthalmology: a Systematic Approach. Elsevier, Amsterdam (2011)
4. Li, Q., Feng, B., Xie, L., Liang, P., Zhang, H., Wang, T.: A cross-modality learning approach for vessel segmentation in retinal images. IEEE Trans. Med. Imaging **35**(1), 109–118 (2016)
5. Lupascu, C.A., Tegolo, D., Trucco, E.: FABC: retinal vessel segmentation using adaboost. IEEE Trans. Inf. Technol. Biomed. **14**(5), 1267–1274 (2010)
6. Orlando, J.I., Prokofyeva, E., Blaschko, M.B.: A discriminatively trained fully connected conditional random field model for blood vessel segmentation in fundus images. IEEE Trans. Biomed. Eng. **64**(1), 16–27 (2017)
7. Peng, C., Zhang, X., Yu, G., Luo, G., Sun, J.: Large kernel matters-improve semantic segmentation by global convolutional network. In: Proceedings of the IEEE Conference on Computer Vision and Pattern Recognition, pp. 4353–4361 (2017)
8. Ronneberger, O., Fischer, P., Brox, T.: U-Net: convolutional networks for biomedical image segmentation. In: Navab, N., Hornegger, J., Wells, W.M., Frangi, A.F. (eds.) MICCAI 2015. LNCS, vol. 9351, pp. 234–241. Springer, Cham (2015). https://doi.org/10.1007/978-3-319-24574-4_28
9. Shi, W., et al.: Real-time single image and video super-resolution using an efficient sub-pixel convolutional neural network. In: Proceedings of the IEEE Conference on Computer Vision and Pattern Recognition, pp. 1874–1883 (2016)
10. Soares, J.V., Leandro, J.J., Cesar, R.M., Jelinek, H.F., Cree, M.J.: Retinal vessel segmentation using the 2-D gabor wavelet and supervised classification. IEEE Trans. Med. Imaging **25**(9), 1214–1222 (2006)

11. Wu, Y., Xia, Y., Song, Y., Zhang, Y., Cai, W.: Multiscale network followed network model for retinal vessel segmentation. In: Frangi, A.F., Schnabel, J.A., Davatzikos, C., Alberola-López, C., Fichtinger, G. (eds.) MICCAI 2018. LNCS, vol. 11071, pp. 119–126. Springer, Cham (2018). https://doi.org/10.1007/978-3-030-00934-2_14
12. Zhuang, J.: Laddernet: multi-path networks based on u-net for medical image segmentation. arXiv preprint arXiv:1810.07810 (2018)

# A Deep Learning Design for Improving Topology Coherence in Blood Vessel Segmentation

Ricardo J. Araújo[1,2($\boxtimes$)], Jaime S. Cardoso[1,3], and Hélder P. Oliveira[1,2]

[1] INESC TEC, Campus da Faculdade de Engenharia da Universidade do Porto,
Rua Dr. Roberto Frias, 4200-465 Porto, Portugal
ricardo.j.araujo@inesctec.pt
[2] Faculdade de Ciências da Universidade do Porto,
Rua do Campo Alegre, 4169-007 Porto, Portugal
[3] Faculdade de Engenharia da Universidade do Porto,
Rua Dr. Roberto Frias, 4200-465 Porto, Portugal

**Abstract.** The segmentation of blood vessels in medical images has been heavily studied, given its impact in several clinical practices. Deep Learning methods have been applied to supervised segmentation of blood vessels, mainly the retinal ones due to the availability of manual annotations. Despite their success, they typically minimize the Binary Cross Entropy loss, which does not penalize topological mistakes. These errors are relevant in graph-like structures such as blood vessel trees, as a missing segment or an inadequate merging or splitting of branches, may severely change the topology of the network and put at risk the extraction of vessel pathways and their characterization. In this paper, we propose an end-to-end network design comprising a cascade of a typical segmentation network and a Variational Auto-Encoder which, by learning a rich but compact latent space, is able to correct many topological incoherences. Our experiments in three of the most commonly used retinal databases, DRIVE, STARE, and CHASEDB1, show that the proposed model effectively learns representations inducing better segmentations in terms of topology, without hurting the usual pixel-wise metrics. The implementation is available at https://github.com/rjtaraujo/dvae-refiner.

**Keywords:** Blood vessel segmentation · Deep learning · Topology

## 1 Introduction

Blood vessel imaging plays a crucial role in several clinical domains, from diagnosis of diseases such as atherosclerosis and aneurysms, to surgery eligibility in organ transplantation, and even surgery planning and guiding. The high volume of data and the large effort required by clinicians to analyse these images led to the need of automatizing the process, such that computer vision methodologies

© Springer Nature Switzerland AG 2019
D. Shen et al. (Eds.): MICCAI 2019, LNCS 11764, pp. 93–101, 2019.
https://doi.org/10.1007/978-3-030-32239-7_11

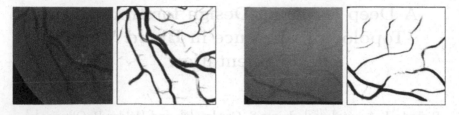

**Fig. 1.** Example images and corresponding segmentations obtained with the Unet model [8]. Topological errors are common in challenging cases.

started being developed in the end of the past century. Methods relying on strong but intuitive priors quickly advanced the state-of-the-art. With the disposal of labelled databases, essentially containing retinal images and expert delineation of blood vessels, a branch of methodologies using supervision emerged. Lately, with the advent of deep learning, supervised segmentation of blood vessels has reached new performance levels.

Nonetheless, these systems are far from being flawless, as small vessels are still occasionally missed, and the segmented trees often contain topological errors, such as broken vessel segments and sub-segmentation due to central reflex (see Fig. 1). These errors may put at risk applications that require vessel pathways extraction and/or characterization [1], as they may induce relevant differences in the overall blood vessel graph. The state-of-the-art methodologies are prone to commit these topological errors as they rely on minimizing the Binary Cross Entropy (BCE) loss (which only penalizes pixel-wise errors) and mostly use model designs that are not aware of topological incoherences.

Recently, there have been attempts of incorporating topological awareness in deep learning models targeting different applications. A loss encoding hierarchical relations between labels, such as containment and detachment, was designed to improve the multi-class segmentation of histology glands [2]. In [3], a process for consecutive refinement of a segmentation given the grayscale image and previous mask was proposed, guided by the differences between high-level features of the current segmentation and the ground truth. None of these works was applied to vessel segmentation. Bifurcation detection has been addressed in a parallel fashion [4], aiming to enhance the overall segmentation process of vascular networks, and consequently, the overall network topology. Nonetheless, topological errors do not arise in bifurcations only, appearing frequently in the middle of branches due to local loss of signal, as can be seen in Fig. 1.

In this work, we consider adding a refinement step after a typical segmentation network, looking for an end-to-end design that is capable of learning the true vascular topology from noisy and occasionally topological-incoherent observations. To achieve such end, we cascaded a Variational Auto-Encoder (VAE) [5] after a typical segmentation network. We let this VAE take segmentations produced by the latter and reconstruct the ground truth annotation, aiming to learn a latent space that is capable of avoiding topological incoherences when sufficient evidence is present, leading to topologically coherent segmentations in the end.

## 2 Methodology

In this section, we present an end-to-end deep neural network design for improving topological consistency in blood vessel segmentation. The methodology comprises a typical segmentation network followed by a refinement model which aims to enforce the learning of meaningful features from corrupted data. We discuss how such design can be used as a strategy to reduce topological mistakes. In what follows, $\mathbf{x}$ and $\mathbf{y}$ denote, respectively, the grayscale input and the ground truth vessel mask, and $\mathbf{y}'$ and $\mathbf{y}''$ represent the outputs of the segmentation network and the refinement model, respectively.

### 2.1 Auto-Encoding for Learning Local Topology

We can interpret errors committed by the segmentation network as a hidden noise process affecting the true vessel signal $\mathbf{y}$. Thus, we seek an encoding of $\mathbf{y}'$ that does not model this noise, allowing $\mathbf{y}''$ to better depict the topology of $\mathbf{y}$.

Usually, auto-encoding designs encode the entire image $\mathbf{x}$ into a vector $\mathbf{z} \in \mathbb{R}^D$, assuming that complex large scale spatial interactions may be learned. This is not the most adequate option for encoding images where recurring patterns exist, as is the case of blood vessels. In this type of data, for inference purposes, it is better to follow [6], where we have latent variables $\mathbf{z}$ as a 3D tensor (stack of feature maps) instead, for explicitly capturing spatial information.

Let us consider for now the generation process of ground truth vessel masks $\mathbf{y}$. It consists of sampling latent variables from a prior distribution $p_{\theta^*}(\mathbf{z})$ and generating masks according to a conditional distribution $p_{\theta^*}(\mathbf{y}|\mathbf{z})$. We assume these distributions belong to parametric families of distributions $p_\theta(\mathbf{z})$ and $p_\theta(\mathbf{y}|\mathbf{z})$. Given observations $\mathbf{y}$, we want to perform inference in this model, $p_\theta(\mathbf{z}|\mathbf{y}) = (p_\theta(\mathbf{y}|\mathbf{z})p_\theta(\mathbf{z}))/p_\theta(\mathbf{y})$, to obtain distributions over the latent space explaining the different observations.

The described approach leads to an intractable problem because evaluating the marginal likelihood of the data, $p_\theta(\mathbf{y})$, requires integrating over the entire latent space. This limitation can be circumvented using variational inference by approximating the posterior probability with a family of distributions $q_\lambda(\mathbf{z})$. The optimal parameters $\lambda^*$ are the ones minimizing the Kullback-Leibler divergence between the two distributions:

$$\mathbb{D}_{\mathrm{KL}}(q_\lambda(\mathbf{z})\|p_\theta(\mathbf{z}|\mathbf{y})) = \mathbb{E}_{q_\lambda(\mathbf{z})}\left[\log\left(\frac{q_\lambda(\mathbf{z})}{p_\theta(\mathbf{z}|\mathbf{y})}\right)\right]$$

$$= \mathbb{E}_{q_\lambda(\mathbf{z})}\left[\log q_\lambda(\mathbf{z}) - \log p_\theta(\mathbf{z},\mathbf{y})\right] + \log p_\theta(\mathbf{y}) \tag{1}$$

However this optimization problem also requires computing the marginal likelihood, thus being once again intractable. By noting that $\mathbb{D}_{\mathrm{KL}}$ is a non-negative quantity and rearranging (1):

$$\log p_\theta(\mathbf{y}) = \mathbb{D}_{\mathrm{KL}}(q_\lambda(\mathbf{z})||p_\theta(\mathbf{z}|\mathbf{y})) + \mathbb{E}_{q_\lambda(\mathbf{z})}\left[\log p_\theta(\mathbf{z}, \mathbf{y}) - \log q_\lambda(\mathbf{z})\right]$$
$$\geq \mathbb{E}_{q_\lambda(\mathbf{z})}\left[\log p_\theta(\mathbf{y}|\mathbf{z})\right] - \mathbb{D}_{\mathrm{KL}}\left(q_\lambda(\mathbf{z})||p_\theta(\mathbf{z})\right) \tag{2}$$

we obtain the Evidence Lower BOund (ELBO), which can equivalently be maximized, allowing us to do approximate posterior inference.

The Variational Auto-Encoder (VAE) [5] conditions the approximate posterior on the data. This distribution, $q_\phi(\mathbf{z}|\mathbf{y})$, and the data likelihood one, $p_\theta(\mathbf{y}|\mathbf{z})$, are both parameterized by neural networks, which are commonly designated as recognition and generative models, respectively. The weights of both networks are jointly learned using the Stochastic Gradient Variational Bayes estimator introduced in the same work. Since parameters $\phi$ are shared among all observations, this model performs amortized inference.

Until now, we considered the case of auto-encoding the vessel masks $\mathbf{y}$. However, the aim of this work is to use the VAE as a segmentation refiner. Therefore, our recognition model is conditioned by the segmentation output $\mathbf{y}'$, while the generative model produces masks $\mathbf{y}''$ closer to the ground truth $\mathbf{y}$. As we shall discuss next, this formulation is a particular case of a Denoising VAE [7].

## 2.2   Refinement Model as a Denoising VAE

The Denoising VAE (DVAE) [7] is trained on noisy observations, where the noise is modeled by a distribution conditioned on the data, $p_\gamma(\mathbf{y}'|\mathbf{y})$. In our use case, the outcome of the segmentation network, $\mathbf{y}'$, is interpreted as a corrupted version of the true vessel signal, $\mathbf{y}$. In a DVAE, the recognition model is given by:

$$\tilde{q}_\phi(\mathbf{z}|\mathbf{y}) = \int q_\phi(\mathbf{z}|\mathbf{y}')p_\gamma(\mathbf{y}'|\mathbf{y})d\mathbf{y}' \tag{3}$$

The modified ELBO of the DVAE comes as:

$$\mathbb{E}_{\tilde{q}_\phi(\mathbf{z}|\mathbf{y})}\left[\log\left(\frac{p_\theta(\mathbf{z}, \mathbf{y})}{\mathbb{E}_{p_\gamma(\mathbf{y}'|\mathbf{y})}\left[q_\phi(\mathbf{z}|\mathbf{y}')\right]}\right)\right] \tag{4}$$

but a more practical lower bound was proven to be eligible for optimization by the authors [7]:

$$\mathbb{E}_{\tilde{q}_\phi(\mathbf{z}|\mathbf{y})}\left[\log\left(\frac{p_\theta(\mathbf{z}, \mathbf{y})}{q_\phi(\mathbf{z}|\mathbf{y}')}\right)\right] \tag{5}$$

which is equivalent to training a regular VAE on corrupted examples. From (5) follows the conclusion that the recognition model in the DVAE is trying to learn meaningful features from the noisy observations, in order to obtain latent representations that allow the generative model to produce a result that is close to the noiseless data. Our proposed refinement model can be seen as a particular case of a DVAE, when the noise model is not known and is encoded in the observations $\mathbf{y}'$. In Fig. 2, we present the proposed design for obtaining segmentation masks that are topologically more coherent.

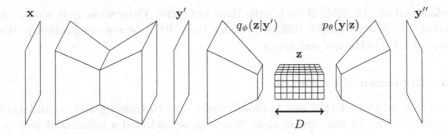

**Fig. 2.** Design of the proposed model for blood vessel segmentation.

## 3    Experiments and Discussion

The Unet model [8] is very popular for segmenting biomedical images, given its capability of accounting for both low and high-level features of the images. In this work, the Unet was used as the segmentation network. Our proposed method (*prop*) was compared against two baselines: (i) a single Unet which produces the vessel masks (*unet*), and (ii) a cascade of two Unet models which performs segmentation and refinement tasks (*dunet*). The losses of these models are, respectively, $\mathcal{L}_{prop} = \alpha\mathcal{L}_1(\mathbf{y}',\mathbf{y}) + (1-\alpha)\left(\mathcal{L}_2(\mathbf{y}'',\mathbf{y}) + \mathbb{D}_{KL}(q_\phi(\mathbf{z}|\mathbf{y}')\|p_\theta(\mathbf{z}))\right)$, $\mathcal{L}_{unet} = \mathcal{L}_1(\mathbf{y}',\mathbf{y})$ and $\mathcal{L}_{dunet} = \alpha\mathcal{L}_1(\mathbf{y}',\mathbf{y}) + (1-\alpha)\mathcal{L}_2(\mathbf{y}'',\mathbf{y})$, with $p_\theta(\mathbf{z})$ being the standard Gaussian. We tested the impact of using losses $\mathcal{L}_1$ and $\mathcal{L}_2$ other than BCE to train the models: the class-weighted BCE (BCEw), which penalizes more false negatives than false positives (weights of 0.7 and 0.3 were found appropriate for vessel and non-vessel classes); and the focal loss (FL) [9], which is an extension of BCE focusing more on the misclassified examples.

### 3.1    Datasets

We performed experiments in three of the most used benchmarks for retinal vessel segmentation, DRIVE [10], STARE [11], and CHASEDB1 [12] databases. DRIVE contains some images showing signs of early diabetic retinopathy, half of the images from STARE are pathological, and CHASEDB1 comprises data where central vessel reflex is abundant. Only DRIVE splits by default the images into train and test sets, each with 20 images. In this work, we set apart the last 10 images of STARE and CHASEDB1 for testing purposes, and used the remaining for training the models.

### 3.2    Metrics

To compare the performance of the models, we considered usual pixel-wise metrics such as: the area under the ROC curve (AUC), sensitivity, and specificity. To evaluate the topological coherence of the masks, we followed a similar approach to [13]. A connected path is randomly chosen from the ground truth and the equivalent path in the binarized prediction mask is analysed. The prediction is classified as infeasible if such path does not exist. Otherwise, it is wrong or correct whether its length differs by more than 10%, or not, respectively. We sampled 1000 paths per test image.

## 3.3   Implementation Details

The train data of DRIVE was randomly split into 15 training and 5 validation images, in order to tune the models. When these included a refinement step, $\alpha$ was set to 1 and decreased 5e-3 each epoch until 0.3, and $\mathcal{L}_1 = \mathcal{L}_2$. For stability purposes, when using the focal loss, we set $\mathcal{L}_1 = \text{BCE}$ and $\mathcal{L}_2 = \text{FL}$. The training procedure lasted for 150 epochs where, in each, 300 batches of 16 patches of size $64 \times 64$ were used. Patches were taken from the green channel of images and augmented via random transformations including horizontal and vertical flips, rotations in the range $\left[-\frac{\pi}{2}, +\frac{\pi}{2}\right]$, and addition of an intensity bias.

The original Unet model comprises 4 condensing and expanding levels, however we concluded that 2 were ideal in this scenario, when considering the AUC metric. Afterwards, we tuned the refiners in the Double Unet and proposed models, considering the number of correct paths. Both pipelines ended having around 4M parameters. The best performing Double Unet model was a cascade of two Unets as described above. Our proposed recognition model was constituted by 4 convolutional layers ($3 \times 3$ kernels and padding of 1) producing, respectively, 64, 64, 256, and 256 feature maps. Each of the first 3 is followed by a max pooling layer (kernel size of 2). Then, convolutional layers ($1 \times 1$ kernels, no padding) learning $D$ feature maps, parameterize the diagonal Gaussian over the latent space. D was tuned to 100. Regarding the generative model, it includes 3 transposed convolutional layers ($4 \times 4$ kernels, padding and stride of 2) producing, respectively, 256, 256, and 64 feature maps, followed by 2 convolutional layers ($3 \times 3$ kernels and padding of 1), where the first learns 64 kernels and the last outputs the parameters of a Bernoulli distribution. ReLUs were used in the intermediate layers of the proposed VAE, and a Sigmoid activation function in the last one. The modulating constant of $\mathbb{D}_{\text{KL}}$ was tuned to 1e-3.

Having tuned the structure and hyperparameters of the models, they were trained as before, but this time using all the train data. Note that we perform patch-based training, but the design of the models allows single-pass prediction.

## 3.4   Results and Discussion

The average performance of the models on 5 different runs is shown in Table 1. The focal loss slightly increased the AUC of the models, meaning that they became better at separating both classes. However, that did not necessarily translate into better topological masks in the end. This is not surprising, as giving more focus to hard cases does not guarantee we are giving more weight to the pixels that generate topological mistakes. Instead, using BCEw, thus giving more weight to the vessel class, allowed to improve the sensitivity and the topology, as was expected. Proceeding to model design comparison, the proposed method was able to significantly decrease the number of infeasible paths, essentially

**Table 1.** Performance of the models, in percentage, averaged over 5 runs. *AUC*, *sen*, *spe*, *inf*, and *cor* stand for, respectively, area under the roc curve, sensitivity, specificity, infeasible, and correct paths. Note that lower *inf* values are better.

| | | BCE | | | BCEw | | | FL | | |
|---|---|---|---|---|---|---|---|---|---|---|
| | | unet | dunet | prop | unet | dunet | prop | unet | dunet | prop |
| DRIVE | *AUC* | 97.7 | 97.8 | 97.8 | 97.9 | 97.9 | 97.9 | **98.0** | **98.0** | 97.9 |
| | *sen* | 79.2 | 79.6 | 85.1 | 87.4 | 87.8 | 89.7 | 78.4 | 79.0 | 82.3 |
| | *spe* | 98.1 | 98.0 | 96.7 | 96.2 | 96.1 | 95.3 | 98.1 | 98.1 | 97.4 |
| | *inf* | 47.0 | 45.0 | 34.1 | 34.8 | 31.8 | **29.1** | 48.6 | 44.8 | 40.4 |
| | *cor* | 45.5 | 47.3 | 56.7 | 56.7 | 59.2 | **61.2** | 43.8 | 48.3 | 51.4 |
| STARE | *AUC* | 98.0 | 98.2 | 98.3 | 98.1 | 98.4 | 98.6 | 98.7 | **98.8** | **98.8** |
| | *sen* | 80.5 | 82.7 | 87.3 | 87.7 | 89.1 | 90.1 | 81.1 | 82.7 | 85.2 |
| | *spe* | 98.5 | 98.4 | 97.3 | 97.3 | 97.2 | 96.8 | 98.5 | 98.4 | 97.9 |
| | *inf* | 53.4 | 43.2 | 27.9 | 38.9 | 29.2 | **23.1** | 49.7 | 38.4 | 34.9 |
| | *cor* | 40.8 | 51.8 | 61.9 | 55.3 | 64.3 | **69.2** | 43.6 | 54.4 | 58.1 |
| CHASE | *AUC* | 97.6 | 97.7 | 97.9 | 97.8 | 98.0 | 98.0 | 97.9 | **98.2** | **98.2** |
| | *sen* | 80.7 | 80.5 | 82.8 | 87.8 | 88.4 | 89.8 | 80.6 | 80.9 | 84.2 |
| | *spe* | 97.6 | 97.6 | 97.4 | 95.9 | 95.9 | 95.6 | 97.5 | 97.7 | 97.2 |
| | *inf* | 74.9 | 74.0 | 64.7 | 60.5 | 54.6 | **48.0** | 73.7 | 71.4 | 62.2 |
| | *cor* | 20.9 | 22.8 | 29.8 | 32.4 | 38.1 | **45.6** | 21.6 | 24.5 | 31.8 |

due to finding the correct topology, as demonstrated by the increase of correct paths. This was achieved without hurting pixel-wise metrics, as may be seen by analysing the AUC. In fact, this metric was even improved in some cases. Note that there is a compromise between the sensitivity and specificity of the

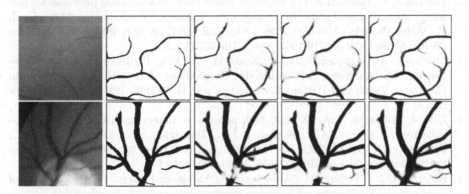

**Fig. 3.** Example masks obtained by using the BCEw loss. From left to right: original images, ground truth, and predictions from Unet, Double Unet, and proposed method.

models, such that using them for direct comparison of models is often not trivial. By comparing against the Double Unet results, which is also a model with more capacity, we conclude that our proposed design effectively learned better features for ensuring topological coherence. Figure 3 shows some visual results of the three models trained with BCEw.

## 4   Conclusion

We proposed a design where a VAE is cascaded after a segmentation network, with the purpose of improving the topological coherence of the predicted blood vessel masks. The experiments showed that our methodology achieves that objective by predicting more correct paths and less infeasible paths, without negatively affecting pixel-wise metrics. The results of comparing the proposed method with a cascade of two Unet models sustain that the improvement comes from the model design and not from the increased complexity of the pipeline. Future works will include investigating a differentiable loss that is aware of the topology. Besides, we believe the design here proposed may be useful for semi-supervised segmentation of blood vessels.

**Acknowledgements.** This work was financed by National Funds through the Portuguese funding agency, FCT - Fundação para a Ciência e a Tecnologia within PhD grant number SFRH/BD/126224/2016 and within project UID/EEA/50014/2019.

## References

1. Zhao, Y., et al.: Retinal artery and vein classification via dominant sets clustering-based vascular topology estimation. In: Frangi, A.F., Schnabel, J.A., Davatzikos, C., Alberola-López, C., Fichtinger, G. (eds.) MICCAI 2018. LNCS, vol. 11071, pp. 56–64. Springer, Cham (2018). https://doi.org/10.1007/978-3-030-00934-2_7
2. BenTaieb, A., Hamarneh, G.: Topology aware fully convolutional networks for histology gland segmentation. In: Ourselin, S., Joskowicz, L., Sabuncu, M.R., Unal, G., Wells, W. (eds.) MICCAI 2016. LNCS, vol. 9901, pp. 460–468. Springer, Cham (2016). https://doi.org/10.1007/978-3-319-46723-8_53
3. Mosinska, A., Marquez-Neila, P., Koziński, M., Fua, P.: Beyond the pixel-wise loss for topology-aware delineation. In: Proceedings of the IEEE Conference on Computer Vision and Pattern Recognition, pp. 3136–3145. IEEE, Salt Lake City (2018)
4. Uslu, F., Bharath, A.A.: A multi-task network to detect junctions in retinal vasculature. In: Frangi, A.F., Schnabel, J.A., Davatzikos, C., Alberola-López, C., Fichtinger, G. (eds.) MICCAI 2018. LNCS, vol. 11071, pp. 92–100. Springer, Cham (2018). https://doi.org/10.1007/978-3-030-00934-2_11
5. Kingma, D.P., Welling, M.: Auto-encoding variational bayes. In: Proceedings of International Conference on Learning Representations 2014, Banff (2014)
6. Kingma, D.P., Salimans, T., Jozefowicz, R., Chen, X., Sutskever, I., Welling, M.: Improved variational inference with inverse autoregressive flow. In: Advances in Neural Information Processing Systems, vol. 29, pp. 4743–4751. Curran Associates Inc., Barcelona (2016)

7. Im, D.I.J., Ahn, S., Memisevic, R., Bengio, Y.: Denoising criterion for variational auto-encoding framework. In: Thirty-First AAAI Conference on Artificial Intelligence. AAAI Press, San Francisco (2017)
8. Ronneberger, O., Fischer, P., Brox, T.: U-Net: convolutional networks for biomedical image segmentation. In: Navab, N., Hornegger, J., Wells, W.M., Frangi, A.F. (eds.) MICCAI 2015. LNCS, vol. 9351, pp. 234–241. Springer, Cham (2015). https://doi.org/10.1007/978-3-319-24574-4_28
9. Lin, T.Y., Goyal, P., Girshick, R., He, K., Dollár, P.: Focal loss for dense object detection. In: Proceedings of the IEEE International Conference on Computer Vision, pp. 2980–2988. IEEE, Venice (2017)
10. Staal, J., Abrámoff, M.D., Niemeijer, M., Viergever, M.A., van Ginneken, B.: Ridge-based vessel segmentation in color images of the retina. IEEE Trans. Med. Imaging 23(4), 501–509 (2004)
11. Hoover, A., Kouznetsova, V., Goldbaum, M.: Locating blood vessels in retinal images by piecewise threshold probing of a matched filter response. IEEE Trans. Med. Imaging 19(3), 203–210 (2000)
12. Owen, C.G., et al.: Measuring retinal vessel tortuosity in 10-year-old children: validation of the computer-assisted image analysis of the retina (caiar) program. Investig. Ophthalmol. Vis. Sci. 50(5), 2004–2010 (2009)
13. Wegner, J.D., Montoya-Zegarra, J.A., Schindler, K.: A higher-order CRF model for road network extraction. In: Proceedings of the IEEE Conference on Computer Vision and Pattern Recognition, pp. 1698–1705. IEEE, Portland (2013)

# Boundary and Entropy-Driven Adversarial Learning for Fundus Image Segmentation

Shujun Wang[1(✉)], Lequan Yu[1], Kang Li[1], Xin Yang[1], Chi-Wing Fu[1,2], and Pheng-Ann Heng[1,2]

[1] Department of Computer Science and Engineering,
The Chinese University of Hong Kong, Sha Tin, Hong Kong SAR, China
`sjwang@cse.cuhk.edu.hk`
[2] Guangdong Provincial Key Laboratory of Computer Vision and Virtual Reality
Technology, Shenzhen Institutes of Advanced Technology,
Chinese Academy of Sciences, Shenzhen, China

**Abstract.** Accurate segmentation of the optic disc (OD) and cup (OC) in fundus images from different datasets is critical for glaucoma disease screening. The cross-domain discrepancy (domain shift) hinders the generalization of deep neural networks to work on different domain datasets. In this work, we present an unsupervised domain adaptation framework, called *Boundary and Entropy-driven Adversarial Learning (BEAL)*, to improve the OD and OC segmentation performance, especially on the ambiguous boundary regions. In particular, our proposed BEAL framework utilizes the adversarial learning to encourage the boundary prediction and mask probability entropy map (uncertainty map) of the target domain to be similar to the source ones, generating more accurate boundaries and suppressing the high uncertainty predictions of OD and OC segmentation. We evaluate the proposed BEAL framework on two public retinal fundus image datasets (Drishti-GS and RIM-ONE-r3), and the experiment results demonstrate that our method outperforms the state-of-the-art unsupervised domain adaptation methods. Our code is available at https://github.com/EmmaW8/BEAL.

**Keywords:** Unsupervised domain adaptation · Optic disc and cup segmentation · Fundus images · Adversarial learning

## 1 Introduction

Automated segmentation of the optic disc (OD) and cup (OC) from fundus images is beneficial to glaucoma screening and diagnosis [4]. Deep convolutional neural networks (CNNs) have brought significant improvement for automated OD and OC segmentation under the supervised learning setting, but fail to generate satisfactory predictions on new datasets due to cross-domain discrepancy

---

S. Wang and L. Yu—Equal contribution.

© Springer Nature Switzerland AG 2019
D. Shen et al. (Eds.): MICCAI 2019, LNCS 11764, pp. 102–110, 2019.
https://doi.org/10.1007/978-3-030-32239-7_12

(domain shift) [8]. For instance, the M-Net [4] achieves the state-of-the-art performance on the ORIGA testing dataset, but has poor generalization ability to work on other testing datasets [12].

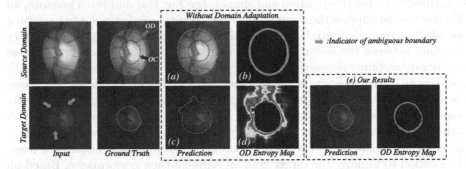

**Fig. 1.** Comparison of the OD and OC predictions and the entropy maps of OD. The middle two columns show results on source and target domain images of the model trained without domain adaptation. The right most two columns show the results of our method on the same target domain image. Red color in the entropy maps ((b) and (d)) indicates high entropy values. (Color figure online)

Very recently, unsupervised domain adaptation methods have been explored to deal with the performance degradation caused by the domain shift in medical imaging community, since acquiring extra annotations on the target domain is time- and money-consuming. Some of the previous unsupervised domain adaptation methods improved the performance of network on a target domain by transferring the input images from the target domain to the source domain, and then applying the network trained on the source domain to transferred images [1,13]. Without any paired images, Cycle-GAN [14] and its variants were the popular methods to transfer image appearance. Besides, high-level feature alignment was used to explore the shared hidden feature space between different domain datasets and aimed to generate similar predictions for both datasets [3,8]. Recently, output space alignment was exploited to incorporate the spatial and geometry structures information of predictions [10,12]. For example, Wang *et al.* [12] presented a novel patch-based output space adversarial learning framework to jointly segment the OD and OC from different fundus image datasets. However, most previous methods fail to produce reliable predictions on soft boundary regions of the target domain images, *i.e.*, the areas among different structures without clear boundary, due to the large appearance difference between the source and target domain images and the low intensity contrast between different structures. Therefore, developing an effective domain adaptation method to improve the prediction performance on soft boundary regions of the target domain images is still a challenging problem.

In this work, we present a novel unsupervised domain adaptation framework, called *Boundary and Entropy-driven Adversarial Learning (BEAL)*, to improve the accuracy to segment the OD and OC over different fundus image datasets. Our method is based on two main observations. First, deep networks trained on the source domain tend to generate ambiguous and inaccurate boundaries for target domain images, while the boundary prediction of source domain is more structured (*i.e.*, relative position and shape); see Fig. 1(a) and (c). Therefore, an effective way to improve the accuracy of target domain predictions is to perform a boundary-driven adversarial learning, which enforces domain-invariant boundary structure between the source and target domains. Second, the network is prone to generate certainty (low-entropy) predictions on the source domain images [11], resulting in a clear prediction entropy map with high entropy values only along the object boundaries, as shown in Fig. 1(b). While the predictions of target domain are uncertain, and the entropy map of mask prediction is noisy with high entropy outputs; see the OD entropy map in Fig. 1(d). Accordingly, enforcing certainty predictions (low-entropy) on the target domain becomes a feasible solution to improve the target domain segmentation performance. Based on these observations, we develop a boundary and entropy-driven adversarial learning method to segment the OD and OC from the target domain fundus images by generating accurate boundaries and suppressing the high uncertainty regions; see our results in Fig. 1(e). Specifically, we exploit the adversarial learning technique to simultaneously encourage the boundary and entropy map predictions to be domain-invariant simultaneously. The proposed method was extensively evaluated on two public fundus image datasets, *i.e.*, RIM-ONE-r3 [5] and Drishti-GS [9], demonstrating state-of-the-art results. We also conducted an ablation study to show the effectiveness of each component in our method.

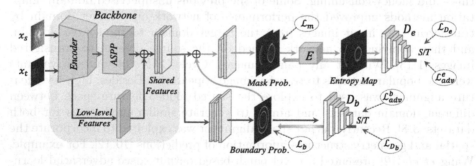

**Fig. 2.** Overview of our BEAL framework for unsupervised domain adaptation. The backbone is based on the DeepLabv3+ [2] architecture with Atrous Spatial Pyramid Pooling (ASPP) component followed by boundary and mask branches. We then apply Shannon Entropy ($E$) to obtain the entropy maps. Finally, we add two discriminators to apply adversarial learning on the boundary and entropy maps.

# 2   Methodology

Figure 2 overviews our proposed BEAL framework for segmenting OD and OC in fundus images from different domains to segment OD and OC in fundus images from different domains. The key technical contribution in our method is a boundary and entropy-driven adversarial learning framework for accurate and confident predictions on the target domain.

## 2.1   Boundary-Driven Adversarial Learning (BAL)

For target domain images, the segmentation network optimized by source domain supervision tends to generate ambiguous and unstructured predictions. To mitigate this problem, we formulate a boundary-driven adversarial learning model to enforce the predicted boundary structure in the target domain to be similar to that in the source domain. Specifically, we adopt a boundary prediction branch to regress the boundary and a mask prediction branch for the OD and OC segmentation by changing the decoder of the segmentation network (Network details will be presented later). Then, we introduce an adversarial learning model by taking the regressed boundary as input.

Formally, we consider a source domain image set $\mathcal{I}_S \subset \mathbb{R}^{H \times W \times 3}$ along with ground truth segmentation maps $\mathcal{Y}_S \subset \mathbb{R}^{H \times W}$, and another target domain image set $\mathcal{I}_T \subset \mathbb{R}^{H \times W \times 3}$ without any ground truth. For each source domain input image $x_s \in \mathcal{I}_S$, our network produces the boundary prediction $p_{x_s}^b$ and mask probability prediction $p_{x_s}^m$. Similarly, our network also generates the boundary prediction $p_{x_t}^b$ and mask prediction $p_{x_t}^m$ for each target domain input image $x_t \in \mathcal{I}_T$. To use the boundary to drive the adversarial learning model, we utilize a boundary discriminator $D_b$ to align the distributions of the boundary predictions $(p_{x_s}^b, p_{x_t}^b)$. The discriminator network $D_b$ aims to figure out whether the boundary is from the source or from the target domain. So, the training objective for the boundary discriminator is formulated as

$$\mathcal{L}_{D_b} = \frac{1}{N} \sum_{x_s \in \mathcal{I}_S} \mathcal{L}_D(p_{x_s}^b, 1) + \frac{1}{M} \sum_{x_t \in \mathcal{I}_T} \mathcal{L}_D(p_{x_t}^b, 0), \tag{1}$$

where $\mathcal{L}_D$ is the binary cross-entropy loss, and $N$ and $M$ are the total number of source and target domain images, respectively. To further align the boundary structure distribution, we utilize the adversarial learning to optimize the segmentation network with the boundary adversarial objective

$$\mathcal{L}_{adv}^b = \frac{1}{M} \sum_{x_t \in \mathcal{I}_T} \mathcal{L}_D(p_{x_t}^b, 1). \tag{2}$$

## 2.2   Entropy-Driven Adversarial Learning (EAL)

With the boundary-driven adversarial learning model, the predictions on the target domain are still prone to be *high-entropy* (under-confident) on the soft boundary regions. To suppress uncertain predictions, we further adopt an entropy-driven adversarial learning model to narrow down the performance gap between the source and target domains by enforcing the entropy maps of the target domain predictions to be similar to the source ones. In detail, given the pixel-wise mask probability prediction $p_x^m$ of input image $x$, we use the Shannon Entropy to calculate the entropy map in pixel level [11] following

$$E(x) = p_x^m \cdot \log(p_x^m). \tag{3}$$

To conduct the entropy-driven adversarial learning, we construct an entropy discriminator network $D_e$ to align the distributions of entropy maps $E(x_s)$ and $E(x_t)$. Similar to boundary-driven adversarial learning, we train the entropy discriminator to figure out whether the entropy map is from the source or the target domain. Specifically, the objective function of $D_e$ is

$$\mathcal{L}_{D_e} = \frac{1}{N} \sum_{x_s \in \mathcal{I}_S} \mathcal{L}_D(E(x_s), 1) + \frac{1}{M} \sum_{x_t \in \mathcal{I}_T} \mathcal{L}_D(E(x_t), 0). \tag{4}$$

At the same time, we optimize the segmentation network to fool the discriminator using the following adversarial loss

$$\mathcal{L}_{adv}^e = \frac{1}{M} \sum_{x_t \in \mathcal{I}_T} \mathcal{L}_D(E(x_t), 1), \tag{5}$$

which encourages the segmentation network to generate prediction entropy on the target domain images similar to the source domain ones.

### 2.3   Network Architecture and Training Procedure

We use an adapted DeepLabv3+ [2] as the segmentation backbone of our BEAL framework. Specifically, we replace the Xception with a lightweight and handy MobileNetV2 to reduce the number of parameters and accelerate the computation, and add the boundary and mask prediction branches after the high-level and low-level feature concatenation. The boundary branch consists of three convolutional layers with output channel of {256, 256, 1} followed by ReLU and batch normalization, except the last one with Sigmoid activation. The mask branch has one convolutional layer with taking the concatenation of boundary predictions and shared features as input. The final prediction are obtained after bilinear interpolation to the same size of the input image. The discriminators consist of five convolutional layers following the previous work [12].

We optimize the segmentation network and the discriminators in an alternate way. To optimize the boundary and entropy discriminators, we minimize the objective function in Eqs. (1) and (4), respectively. To optimize the segment network, we calculate the mask prediction loss $\mathcal{L}_m$ and the boundary regression loss $\mathcal{L}_b$ on the source domain images, and the adversarial loss $\mathcal{L}_{adv}^b$ and $\mathcal{L}_{adv}^e$ on the target domain images. The overall objective of segmentation network is

$$\mathcal{L} = \mathcal{L}_m + \mathcal{L}_b + \lambda(\mathcal{L}_{adv}^b + \mathcal{L}_{adv}^e),$$

$$\mathcal{L}_b = \frac{1}{N} \sum_{x_s \in \mathcal{I}_S} (y_{x_s}^b - p_{x_s}^b)^2,$$

$$\text{and } \mathcal{L}_m = -\frac{1}{N} \sum_{x_s \in \mathcal{I}_S} [y_{x_s}^m \cdot log(p_{x_s}^m) + (1 - y_{x_s}^m) \cdot log(1 - p_{x_s}^m)], \quad (6)$$

where $y^m$ and $y^b$ are the ground truth of the mask and boundary, respectively, and $\lambda$ is a balance coefficient. We formulate the mask prediction as a multi-label learning [12] and generate the probability maps of OD and OC simultaneously. We take the entropy map of OD and OC together as the discriminator input. To acquire the boundary ground truth, we apply the Sobel operation and Gaussian filter to the ground truth masks.

**Table 1.** Statistics of the datasets used in evaluating our method.

| Domain | Dataset | Number of samples |
|---|---|---|
| Source | REFUGE[a] (Train) | 400 |
| Target | RIM-ONE-r3 [5] (Train + Test) | 99 + 60 |
| Target | Drishti-GS [9] (Train + Test) | 50 + 51 |

[a]https://refuge.grand-challenge.org/

**Table 2.** Comparison with other methods on the target domain datasets.

| Method | RIM-ONE-r3 [5] | | Drishti-GS [9] | |
|---|---|---|---|---|
| | $DI_{cup}$ | $DI_{disc}$ | $DI_{cup}$ | $DI_{disc}$ |
| w/o DA | 0.744 | 0.779 | 0.836 | 0.944 |
| Upper bound | 0.856 | 0.968 | 0.901 | 0.974 |
| TD-GAN [13] | 0.728 | 0.853 | 0.747 | 0.924 |
| Hoffman et al. [6] | 0.755 | 0.852 | 0.851 | 0.959 |
| Javanmardi et al. [7] | 0.779 | 0.853 | 0.849 | 0.961 |
| OSAL-pixel [12] | 0.778 | 0.854 | 0.851 | 0.962 |
| pOSAL [12] | 0.787 | 0.865 | 0.858 | **0.965** |
| **BEAL** (ours) | **0.810** | **0.898** | **0.862** | 0.961 |

## 3  Experiments and Results

**Dataset.** To evaluate our method, we utilize the training part of the REFUGE challenge dataset as the source domain, and the public Drishti-GS [9], and the RIM-ONE-r3 [5] dataset as the target domains including both the training and testing parts. The detailed statistics of the datasets are shown in Table 1.

**Implementation Details.** Our framework was implemented with the PyTorch library. We trained the whole framework directly without the warm-up phase of supervised learning in a minibatch of size 8. The discriminator $D_e$ and $D_b$ were optimized with the SGD algorithm, while the Adam optimizer was utilized for optimizing the segmentation network. We set the initial learning rate of SGD as $1e-3$ and divided it by 0.2 every 100 epochs for a total of 200 epochs. The learning rate of discriminator training was set as $2.5e-5$. We cropped $512 \times 512$ ROIs centering at OD as the network input following the previous work [12] by utilizing a simple U-Net architecture. We used the standard data augmentation, including random rotation, flipping, elastic transformation, contrast adjustment, adding Gaussian noise, and random erasing [12].

**Quantitative Analysis.** We use the dice coefficients ($DI$) of OD and OC to quantitatively evaluate the results produced from our method. The segmentation results of our approach and others on RIM-ONE-r3 and Drishti-GS are presented in Table 2. We compare our framework with the baseline (w/o DA), the supervised method (*Upper bound*), and other unsupervised domain adaptation methods, including TD-GAN [13], high-level feature alignment [6] and output space-based adaptation [7,12]. The results of other methods are inherited from the previous work [12]. Compared with the state-of-the-art unsupervised domain adaptation method $p$OSAL, our BEAL framework achieves 2.3% and 3.3% DI improvement for the OC and OD segmentation on the RIM-ONE-r3 dataset, demonstrating the effectiveness of the boundary and entropy-driven domain adaption method. Since the domain distribution gap between the REFUGE and Drishti-GS data is smaller than the difference between REFUGE and RIM-ONE-r3 data [12], the absolute DI values of optic cup and disc on Drishti-GS is higher than that on RIM-ONE-r3. Therefore, the room for improvement on the Drishti-GS dataset is limited, as the current performance is approaching the upper bound. Nevertheless, our method still outperforms the state-of-the-arts for the cup segmentation, and achieves comparable results with $p$OSAL for the disc segmentation on the Drishti-GS dataset, demonstrating the effectiveness of our method to handle with varying degrees of domain shifts.

**Qualitative Analysis.** We show some visual results of the OD and OC segmentation, prediction entropy map, and predicted boundary on the RIM-ONE-r3 dataset in Fig. 3. It shows that the $p$OSAL hardly predicts accurate boundary on the ambiguous regions and generates high entropy values. By leveraging the proposed boundary and entropy-driven adversarial learning, our method produces more accurate boundaries and clean entropy maps of the mask predictions.

**Ablation Study.** We conducted a set of ablation experiments to evaluate the effectiveness of each component: (i) DeepLabv3+ network (Baseline w/o boundary), (ii) DeepLabv3+ network equipped with a boundary branch (Baseline), (iii) boundary-driven adversarial learning (Baseline+BAL), (iv) entropy-driven

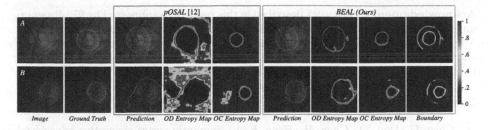

Fig. 3. Qualitative results of pOSAL [12] and our method on the RIM-ONE-r3 dataset [5]. Our method can improve the segmentation results with accurate boundary, and generate clear prediction entropy maps. Green and blue lines represent the disc and cup contours, respectively. The entropy values are rescaled to [0,1] for better visualization. (Color figure online)

**Table 3.** Ablation study on different components.

| Method | RIM-ONE-r3 [5] | | Drishti-GS [9] | |
|---|---|---|---|---|
| | $DI_{cup}$ | $DI_{disc}$ | $DI_{cup}$ | $DI_{disc}$ |
| Baseline w/o boundary | 0.744 | 0.779 | 0.836 | 0.944 |
| Baseline | 0.779 | 0.885 | 0.841 | 0.951 |
| Baseline+BAL | 0.781 | 0.893 | 0.847 | 0.958 |
| Baseline+EAL | 0.800 | **0.898** | 0.851 | 0.960 |
| **BEAL (ours)** | **0.810** | **0.898** | **0.862** | **0.961** |

adversarial learning (Baseline+EAL); and (v) our proposed method (BEAL). The results are shown in Table 3. With extra constraint information from the boundary prediction, the Baseline improves performance for both two datasets compared with Baseline w/o boundary. With additional adversarial learning model, the results show that both BAL and EAL improve the OD and OC segmentations on the two datasets. By combining the two adversarial learning methods, we observe a further improvement in the performance, confirming that the effectiveness of our combined adversarial learning model.

## 4    Conclusion

We proposed a novel boundary and entropy-driven adversarial learning method for the OC and OD segmentation in fundus images from different domains. To address the domain shift challenge, our method encourages the boundary and the entropy map of prediction simultaneously to be domain-invariant, generating more accurate boundaries and suppressing uncertain predictions of OD and OC. Our method outperforms the state-of-the-art methods, as clearly demonstrated on the two public fundus segmentation datasets. It is effective and could be generalized to other unsupervised domain adaptation problems.

110     S. Wang et al.

**Acknowledgments.** The work described in this paper was supported by 973 Program under Project No. 2015CB351706, and Research Grants Council of Hong Kong Special Administrative Region under Project No. CUHK14225616, and Hong Kong Innovation and Technology Fund under Project No. ITS/426/17FP, and National Natural Science Foundation of China under Project No. U1613219.

# References

1. Chen, C., Dou, Q., Chen, H., Heng, P.-A.: Semantic-aware generative adversarial nets for unsupervised domain adaptation in chest x-ray segmentation. In: Shi, Y., Suk, H.-I., Liu, M. (eds.) MLMI 2018. LNCS, vol. 11046, pp. 143–151. Springer, Cham (2018). https://doi.org/10.1007/978-3-030-00919-9_17
2. Chen, L.-C., Zhu, Y., Papandreou, G., Schroff, F., Adam, H.: Encoder-decoder with atrous separable convolution for semantic image segmentation. In: Ferrari, V., Hebert, M., Sminchisescu, C., Weiss, Y. (eds.) ECCV 2018. LNCS, vol. 11211, pp. 833–851. Springer, Cham (2018). https://doi.org/10.1007/978-3-030-01234-2_49
3. Dou, Q., Ouyang, C., Chen, C., Chen, H., Heng, P.A.: Unsupervised cross-modality domain adaptation of convnets for biomedical image segmentations with adversarial loss. In: IJCAI, pp. 691–697 (2018)
4. Fu, H., Cheng, J., Xu, Y., et al.: Joint optic disc and cup segmentation based on multi-label deep network and polar transformation. IEEE TMI **37**(7), 1597–1605 (2018)
5. Fumero, F., Alayón, S., Sanchez, J.L., Sigut, J., Gonzalez-Hernandez, M.: RIM-ONE: an open retinal image database for optic nerve evaluation. In: 24th International Symposium on Computer-Based Medical Systems (CBMS), pp. 1–6 (2011)
6. Hoffman, J., Wang, D., Yu, F., Darrell, T.: FCNs in the wild: pixel-level adversarial and constraint-based adaptation. arXiv preprint arXiv:1612.02649 (2016)
7. Javanmardi, M., Tasdizen, T.: Domain adaptation for biomedical image segmentation using adversarial training. In: ISBI, pp. 554–558. IEEE (2018)
8. Kamnitsas, K., Baumgartner, C., et al.: Unsupervised domain adaptation in brain lesion segmentation with adversarial networks. In: Niethammer, M., et al. (eds.) IPMI 2017. LNCS, vol. 10265, pp. 597–609. Springer, Cham (2017). https://doi.org/10.1007/978-3-319-59050-9_47
9. Sivaswamy, J., Krishnadas, S., Chakravarty, A., et al.: A comprehensive retinal image dataset for the assessment of glaucoma from the optic nerve head analysis. JSM Biomed. Imaging Data Pap. **2**(1), 1004 (2015)
10. Tsai, Y.H., Hung, W.C., Schulter, S., et al.: Learning to adapt structured output space for semantic segmentation. In: CVPR, pp. 7472–7481 (2018)
11. Vu, T.H., Jain, H., Bucher, M., Cord, M., Pérez, P.: ADVENT: adversarial entropy minimization for domain adaptation in semantic segmentation. In: CVPR, pp. 2517–2526 (2019)
12. Wang, S., Yu, L., Yang, X., Fu, C.W., Heng, P.A.: Patch-based output space adversarial learning for joint optic disc and cup segmentation. IEEE TMI (2019, to appear)
13. Zhang, Y., Miao, S., Mansi, T., Liao, R.: Task driven generative modeling for unsupervised domain adaptation: application to x-ray image segmentation. In: Frangi, A.F., Schnabel, J.A., Davatzikos, C., Alberola-López, C., Fichtinger, G. (eds.) MICCAI 2018. LNCS, vol. 11071, pp. 599–607. Springer, Cham (2018). https://doi.org/10.1007/978-3-030-00934-2_67
14. Zhu, J.Y., Park, T., Isola, P., Efros, A.A.: Unpaired image-to-image translation using cycle-consistent adversarial networks. In: ICCV, pp. 2223–2232 (2017)

# Unsupervised Ensemble Strategy
# for Retinal Vessel Segmentation

Bo Liu[1,4], Lin Gu[2], and Feng Lu[1,3,4(✉)]

[1] State Key Laboratory of VR Technology and Systems,
School of Computer Science and Engineering, Beihang University, Beijing, China
lufeng@buaa.edu.cn
[2] National Institute of Informatics, Tokyo, Japan
[3] Peng Cheng Laboratory, Shenzhen, China
[4] Beijing Advanced Innovation Center for Big Data-Based Precision Medicine,
Beihang University, Beijing, China

**Abstract.** Retinal vessel segmentation is a fundamental step in diagnosis for retinal image analysis. Though many segmentation methods are proposed, little research considers how to ensemble their results to fully exploit the advantages of each method. In this work, we propose a novel unsupervised ensemble strategy to automatically combine multiple segmentation results for an accurate result. There is a no-reference network that could assess the vessel segmentation quality without knowing the ground truth. We then optimize the weight of individual result to maximize this segmentation quality score to enhance the final result. Through extensive experiments, our method has shown superior performance over the state-of-the-art on the DRIVE, STARE, CHASE_DB1 datasets.

**Keywords:** Vessel segmentation · Ensemble strategy

## 1 Introduction

Retinal vessels are commonly examined in the diagnosis of diverse ophthalmological diseases, such as diabetic retinopathy (DR), age-related macular degeneration (AMD), glaucoma and hypertension. Thus, retinal vessel segmentation plays a crucial role in the diagnosis task of retinopathy [17].

A broad variety of unsupervised and supervised methods have been proposed to segment retinal vessels automatically. For instance, Frangi *et al.* [3] proposed a representative handcrafted feature which exams the second-order local structure of an image (Hessian) to develop a vessel enhancement filter. Nguyen *et al.* [16] proposed an unsupervised algorithm based on multi-scale line operators. Orlando *et al.* [18] segmented the vessels with the fully-connected conditional random field. Gu *et al.* [6] proposed an iterative two-step learning-based approach to boost the performance of segmentation.

The past recent years have witnessed the rapid development and successful application of deep learning, especially in the field of computer vision.

© Springer Nature Switzerland AG 2019
D. Shen et al. (Eds.): MICCAI 2019, LNCS 11764, pp. 111–119, 2019.
https://doi.org/10.1007/978-3-030-32239-7_13

Ronneberger *et al.* [19] proposed U-Net, a fully convolutional network developed for biomedical segmentation that utilizes features on multiple levels. Recently, many deep learning architectures inspired by U-Net, such as Laibacher *et al.* (M2UNet) [10] and Zhuang *et al.* (LadderNet) [23], achieved quite nice performance on vessel segmentation task. Each method has its pros and cons in certain conditions. However, few research ensembles these different segmentation results to fully exploit the advantages of each method.

As shown in Fig. 1, we propose a novel but simple strategy to ensemble the predictions from multiple methods for accurate retinal vessel segmentation. Galdran *et al.* [5] proposed a network that is able to blindly evaluate the quality of segmentation without knowing ground truth. As shown in Fig. 1, we use this no-reference evaluation network (orange color) to determine the weight $w$ of individual method's prediction when fusing the final result. Specifically, we formulate it into maximizing the quality score of the no-reference network [5] with respect to the weight $w$ of the individual base method. As shown in Fig. 2, our method manages to gradually increase the quality score $q$ while the segmentation quality is also consistently improved.

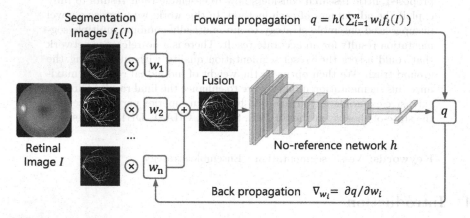

**Fig. 1.** Structure of our proposed ensemble method. Given an input image, we can obtain $n$ segmentation estimations by various base algorithms. Each estimation $y_i$ is multiplied by a weight $w_i$ and then added to a fused estimation. Fused result is then forwarded to the pre-trained no-reference evaluation network with fixed parameters to generate a quality score $q$. We then iteratively optimize the weights $w_1, w_2, ..., w_n$ through loss back propagation to maximize estimation score $q$. (Color figure online)

Our paper makes the following contributions: (1) We propose a novel strategy to ensemble multiple retinal vessel segmentation results. This is achieved by optimizing the ensemble weight of individual method to maximize the no-reference segmentation quality of final segmentation. (2) Our method has significantly improved the performance over base algorithms. Extensive experiments shows our superior performance over state-of-the-art on DRIVE [20], STARE [7] and CHASE_DB1 [4].

## 2    Methodology

### 2.1    No-Reference Segmentation Evaluation

Galdran *et al.* [5] proposed a no-reference network for retinal vessel segmentation quality assessment in the absence of a referenced ground truth. We name it the no-reference network in this paper. This method at first artificially simulates segmentation of diverse quality levels from the expert annotation. Then the no-reference network, a convolutional neural network (CNN), is trained to regress the similarity between degraded vessel tree and the manually segmented via Normalized Mutual Information (NMI). The similarity could be interpreted as a visually meaningful quality score that predicts the segmentation quality.

Given ground truth $v$ and degraded binary vessel tree $\deg(v)$, the normalized mutual information $\mathcal{NMI}$ is formulated as follows:

$$\mathcal{NMI}(v, \deg(v)) = 2 \cdot [1 - \frac{\mathcal{H}(v, \deg(v)}{\mathcal{H}(v) + \mathcal{H}(\deg(v))}], \tag{1}$$

where $\mathcal{H}(v)$ and $\mathcal{H}(\deg(v))$ is the marginal entropy of $v$ and $deg(v)$ respectively, and $\mathcal{H}(v, \deg(v))$ is the entropy of their joint probability distribution. $\mathcal{NMI}(v, \deg(v))$ ranges from 0 to 1, representing the segmentation quality from bad to good.

As shown in Fig. 1 (orange), the no-reference network containing 10 convolution layers are grouped into pairs with down-sampling between each group. A Group Average Pooling (GAP) layer is used to reduce the total number of parameters and lift restrictions on the input size. Finally, two fully connected layers with Sigmoid activation produce a score in $[0, 1]$. We use the $L_1$ loss by $\sum_{i=0}^{n} |y_i - \hat{y_i}|$ computed through the actual $\mathcal{NMI}$ score $y_i$ and the predicted one $\hat{y_i}$. Though this method is originally designed to evaluate binary segmentation, in Sect. 3.2, we demonstrate this network is also able to access the grayscale segmentation estimation ranging from $[0, 1]$. In this paper, we independently train the no-reference network and then fix the parameters for our ensemble system.

### 2.2    Our Method

Given the input retinal image $I$, we have several base segmentation algorithms $f_i : f_1, f_2, f_3, ... f_n$ that predict the pixel-wise probability of vessel: $f_i(I) \in [0, 1]$. Thus, our final ensemble prediction would be $y(I) = \sum_{i=1}^{n} w_i f_i(I)$, where $w_i \geq 0$. In our system, we would the clip $y(I)$ to $[0, 1]$.

As discussed above, no-reference network is able to blindly evaluate the segmentation $f(I)$ and produces a quality score $q = h(y(I)) = h(\sum_i^n w_i f_i(I))$. Therefore, for individual retinal image $I$, seeking optimized $w_i^*$ for an accurate fused segmentation could be formulated as maximizing the quality score $q$ with respect to $w_1$ to $w_n$:

$$w_i^*(I) = \underset{w_i}{\operatorname{argmax}} h(\sum_i^n w_i f_i(I)), \tag{2}$$

We adopt Adam algorithm [9] to optimize this equation. The loss function is defined as $(1 - q)^2$. Specifically, we update the weight $w_i$ according to the back-propagated gradient as shown in Fig. 1. The gradient is given as:

$$\nabla_{w_i} loss = \frac{\partial (1 - h(\sum_i^n w_i f_i(I)))^2}{\partial h} \frac{\partial h}{\partial w_i}. \tag{3}$$

When optimizing Eq. (2), the parameters of the no-reference network are fixed during forwarding propagation and backpropagation. We set the initial learning rate 1e − 3. We use early stopping when the no-reference score doesn't improve for 20 epochs. Typically, our method searches about 200 iterations in less than 5 s for one sample. The final segmentation is the sum of segmentation images multiplied by corresponding weights.

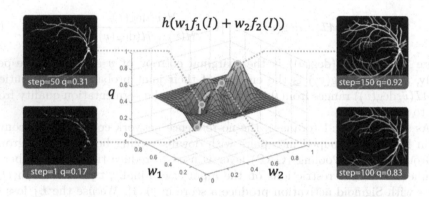

**Fig. 2.** Illustration of optimization of $w$ and corresponding ensemble results.

As illustrated in Fig. 2, taking two-segmentation ensemble as an example, the weight of each base segmentation result is repeatedly updated according to Eq. (3). The quality score increases with the steps while the segmentation result also consistently improves.

## 3    Experiments

In the experiments, we will first introduce the involved datasets. Then we describe the implementation details of the no-reference method [5] and individual base methods. Finally, We will show our results.

### 3.1    Datasets

To evaluate our method, we experiment on three public datasets: DRIVE [20], STARE [7] and CHASE_DB1 [4]. Manual segmentations by two expert annotators are included for each dataset. We use the segmentations of the first annotator

as the gold standard to train and test, and regard the ones from the second annotator as human performance. The DRIVE dataset has 40 images with binary filed
of view (FOV) masks. We use standard train/test split: 20 images for training
and 20 images for testing. The STARE dataset consists of 20 images, and we
split the data into 10 images for training and 10 images for testing, following [21].
For CHASE_DB1, the first 20 are chosen as the training set and remaining 8 as
the testing set, a setting also used in [22,23]. Binary FOV masks of STARE and
CHASE_DB1 are obtained by manual thresholding.

### 3.2   Implementation Details

**Training of No-Reference Network:** Following [5], we train the no-reference
network on DRIVE [20] dataset. We take more degradation situations into consideration compared with [5] shown in Fig. 3(c)–(d). The learning rate is set
to $5e^{-5}$. Figure 3(e)–(f) demonstrate that the no-reference network can also be
applied on gray scale vessel estimation and give appropriate quality scores.

**Base Methods:** We implement several segmentation algorithms and choose
three methods to fuse: M2UNet [10], LadderNet [23] and VesselNet [2]. Experiments show that more inputs does not necessarily lead to better results. Evaluated on DRIVE [20], their vessel estimation map generates the consistent no-
reference score as the binary segmentation.

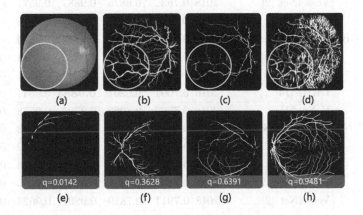

**Fig. 3.** Segmentation degradation and assessment of no-reference network. (a) Retinal
image from DRIVE dataset; (b) Ground truth; (c)–(d) Degradation of under segmentation and over segmentation based on ground truth; (e)–(h) Four U-net [19] segmentation estimation score selected from kaggle dataset [8], with quality scores evaluated
by the no-reference network.

**Table 1.** Performance comparison on three datasets

| Datasets | Methods | Year | F1score | Se | Sp | Acc | AUC |
|---|---|---|---|---|---|---|---|
| DRIVE | 2nd Observer | – | 0.7881 | 0.7760 | 0.9725 | 0.9473 | – |
| | M2UNet [10] | 2015 | 0.8025 | 0.7863 | 0.9755 | 0.9511 | 0.9544 |
| | Qiaoliang Li [12] | 2016 | – | 0.7569 | 0.9816 | 0.9527 | 0.9738 |
| | DRIU [14] | 2016 | 0.7361 | 0.6480 | 0.9844 | 0.9413 | 0.9486 |
| | U-Net [1] | 2018 | 0.8142 | 0.7537 | 0.9820 | 0.9531 | 0.9755 |
| | Residual UNet [1] | 2018 | 0.8149 | 0.7726 | 0.9820 | 0.9553 | 0.9779 |
| | Recurrent UNet [1] | 2018 | 0.8155 | 0.7751 | 0.9816 | 0.9556 | 0.9782 |
| | R2U-Net [1] | 2018 | 0.8171 | 0.7792 | 0.9813 | 0.9556 | **0.9784** |
| | LadderNet [23] | 2018 | 0.8205 | **0.8081** | 0.9770 | 0.9553 | 0.9767 |
| | VesselNet [2] | 2018 | 0.8125 | 0.7626 | **0.9839** | 0.9555 | 0.9772 |
| | Ours | 2019 | **0.8225** | 0.8072 | 0.9780 | **0.9559** | 0.9779 |
| STARE | 2nd Observer | – | 0.7401 | **0.8951** | 0.9386 | 0.9350 | – |
| | M2UNet [10] | 2015 | 0.7725 | 0.7056 | 0.9883 | 0.9581 | 0.9754 |
| | Liskowski et al. [13] | 2016 | – | 0.8554 | 0.9862 | **0.9729** | **0.9928** |
| | DRIU [14] | 2016 | 0.7139 | 0.5949 | **0.9938** | 0.9534 | 0.9240 |
| | Mo et al. [15] | 2017 | – | 0.8147 | 0.9844 | 0.9674 | 0.9885 |
| | Leopold et al. [11] | 2017 | – | 0.6433 | 0.9472 | 0.9045 | 0.7952 |
| | LadderNet [23] | 2018 | 0.7319 | 0.6321 | 0.9898 | 0.9535 | 0.9609 |
| | VesselNet [2] | 2018 | 0.7632 | 0.6875 | 0.9887 | 0.9577 | 0.9427 |
| | Ours | 2019 | **0.8036** | 0.7771 | 0.9843 | 0.9623 | 0.9793 |
| CHASE_DB1 | 2nd Observer | – | 0.7978 | 0.8328 | 0.9744 | 0.9614 | – |
| | M2UNet [10] | 2015 | 0.7725 | 0.7056 | 0.9883 | 0.9581 | 0.9754 |
| | Qiaoliang Li [12] | 2016 | – | 0.7507 | 0.9743 | 0.9581 | 0.9793 |
| | DRIU [14] | 2016 | 0.7091 | 0.6207 | **0.9884** | 0.9547 | 0.8962 |
| | U-Net [1] | 2018 | 0.7783 | 0.8288 | 0.9701 | 0.9578 | 0.9772 |
| | Residual UNet [1] | 2018 | 0.7800 | 0.7726 | 0.9820 | 0.9553 | 0.9779 |
| | Recurrent UNet [1] | 2018 | 0.7810 | 0.7459 | 0.9836 | 0.9622 | 0.9803 |
| | R2U-Net [1] | 2018 | 0.7928 | 0.7756 | 0.9820 | 0.9634 | 0.9815 |
| | LadderNet [23] | 2018 | 0.7895 | 0.7856 | 0.9799 | 0.9620 | 0.9772 |
| | VesselNet [2] | 2018 | 0.7911 | 0.7819 | 0.9807 | 0.9624 | 0.9758 |
| | Ours | 2019 | **0.8598** | **0.8769** | 0.9843 | 0.9742 | **0.9905** |

## 3.3    Results

Here, we conduct extensive comparison with existing methods on three datasets: DRIVE [20], STARE [7] and CHASE_DB1 [4]. At first, we report their precision-recall curves in Fig. 4. Our method has achieved superior performance over other methods except for M2UNet on CHASE_DB1. However, it is noted that our segmentation is more precise before recall reaching 0.78 than M2UNet. This area covers most of the practical scenarios.

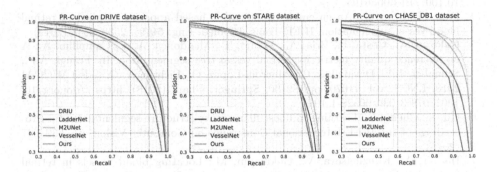

**Fig. 4.** PR-curve on three datasets.

We also provide Table 1, which demonstrates the quantitative results of different methods with F1-score, sensitivity, specificity, accuracy, and area under the ROC curve (AUC). It shows that our method achieves state-of-the-art performance on three datasets with the highest F1-score and almost highest scores on other metrics.

## 4 Conclusion

In this paper, we propose a novel but simple ensemble method to fuse the result of different retinal vessel segmentation methods. Noted that no-reference network could blindly evaluate the segmentation and generate a quality score. We are able to determine the weight of each base method by maximizing the quality score of the ensemble result with respect to the weights. We evaluate our method on DRIVE, STARE, and CHASE_DB1. Experimental results demonstrate that our method achieves, to our knowledge, the state-of-the-art performance on the three datasets. Looking forward, we believe this strategy could also be extended to more applications.

**Acknowledgments.** This work was supported by the National Natural Science Foundation of China (NSFC) under Grant 61602020.

## References

1. Alom, M.Z., Hasan, M., Yakopcic, C., Taha, T.M., Asari, V.K.: Recurrent residual convolutional neural network based on u-net (r2u-net) for medical image segmentation. arXiv preprint arXiv:1802.06955 (2018)
2. ChenCong, X.: Retina-vesselnet: a denseblock-unet for retinal blood vessel segmentation. https://github.com/DeepTrial/Retina-VesselNet. Accessed 3 Mar 2019

3. Frangi, A.F., Niessen, W.J., Vincken, K.L., Viergever, M.A.: Multiscale vessel enhancement filtering. In: Wells, W.M., Colchester, A., Delp, S. (eds.) MICCAI 1998. LNCS, vol. 1496, pp. 130–137. Springer, Heidelberg (1998). https://doi.org/10.1007/BFb0056195

4. Fraz, M.M., et al.: An ensemble classification-based approach applied to retinal blood vessel segmentation. IEEE Trans. Biomed. Eng. **59**(9), 2538–2548 (2012)

5. Galdran, A., Costa, P., Bria, A., Araújo, T., Mendonça, A.M., Campilho, A.: A no-reference quality metric for retinal vessel tree segmentation. In: Frangi, A.F., Schnabel, J.A., Davatzikos, C., Alberola-López, C., Fichtinger, G. (eds.) MICCAI 2018. LNCS, vol. 11070, pp. 82–90. Springer, Cham (2018). https://doi.org/10.1007/978-3-030-00928-1_10

6. Gu, L., Cheng, L.: Learning to boost filamentary structure segmentation. In: Proceedings of the IEEE International Conference on Computer Vision, pp. 639–647 (2015)

7. Hoover, A., Kouznetsova, V., Goldbaum, M.: Locating blood vessels in retinal images by piece-wise threshold probing of a matched filter response. In: Proceedings of the AMIA Symposium, p. 931. American Medical Informatics Association (1998)

8. Kaggle: diabetic retinopathy detection. https://www.kaggle.com/c/diabetic-retinopathy-detection. Accessed 3 Mar 2019

9. Kingma, D.P., Ba, J.: Adam: a method for stochastic optimization. arXiv preprint arXiv:1412.6980 (2014)

10. Laibacher, T., Weyde, T., Jalali, S.: M2u-net: effective and efficient retinal vessel segmentation for resource-constrained environments. arXiv preprint arXiv:1811.07738 (2018)

11. Leopold, H.A., Orchard, J., Zelek, J.S., Lakshminarayanan, V.: Pixelbnn: augmenting the pixelcnn with batch normalization and the presentation of a fast architecture for retinal vessel segmentation. J. Imaging **5**(2), 26 (2019)

12. Li, Q., Feng, B., Xie, L., Liang, P., Zhang, H., Wang, T.: A cross-modality learning approach for vessel segmentation in retinal images. IEEE Trans. Med. Imaging **35**(1), 109–118 (2016)

13. Liskowski, P., Krawiec, K.: Segmenting retinal blood vessels with deep neural networks. IEEE Trans. Med. Imaging **35**(11), 2369–2380 (2016)

14. Maninis, K.-K., Pont-Tuset, J., Arbeláez, P., Van Gool, L.: Deep retinal image understanding. In: Ourselin, S., Joskowicz, L., Sabuncu, M.R., Unal, G., Wells, W. (eds.) MICCAI 2016. LNCS, vol. 9901, pp. 140–148. Springer, Cham (2016). https://doi.org/10.1007/978-3-319-46723-8_17

15. Mo, J., Zhang, L.: Multi-level deep supervised networks for retinal vessel segmentation. Int. J. Comput. Assist. Radiol. Surg. **12**(12), 2181–2193 (2017)

16. Nguyen, U.T., Bhuiyan, A., Park, L.A., Ramamohanarao, K.: An effective retinal blood vessel segmentation method using multi-scale line detection. Pattern Recognit. **46**(3), 703–715 (2013)

17. Niu, Y., et al.: Pathological evidence exploration in deep retinal image diagnosis. arXiv preprint arXiv:1812.02640 (2018)

18. Orlando, J.I., Blaschko, M.: Learning fully-connected CRFs for blood vessel segmentation in retinal images. In: Golland, P., Hata, N., Barillot, C., Hornegger, J., Howe, R. (eds.) MICCAI 2014. LNCS, vol. 8673, pp. 634–641. Springer, Cham (2014). https://doi.org/10.1007/978-3-319-10404-1_79

19. Ronneberger, O., Fischer, P., Brox, T.: U-Net: convolutional networks for biomedical image segmentation. In: Navab, N., Hornegger, J., Wells, W.M., Frangi, A.F. (eds.) MICCAI 2015. LNCS, vol. 9351, pp. 234–241. Springer, Cham (2015). https://doi.org/10.1007/978-3-319-24574-4_28

20. Staal, J., Abramoff, M., Niemeijer, M., Viergever, M., van Ginneken, B.: Ridge based vessel segmentation in color images of the retina. IEEE Trans. Med. Imaging **23**(4), 501–509 (2004)
21. Tetteh, G., Rempfler, M., Zimmer, C., Menze, B.H.: Deep-FExt: deep feature extraction for vessel segmentation and centerline prediction. In: Wang, Q., Shi, Y., Suk, H.-I., Suzuki, K. (eds.) MLMI 2017. LNCS, vol. 10541, pp. 344–352. Springer, Cham (2017). https://doi.org/10.1007/978-3-319-67389-9_40
22. Wu, Y., Xia, Y., Song, Y., Zhang, Y., Cai, W.: Multiscale network followed network model for retinal vessel segmentation. In: Frangi, A.F., Schnabel, J.A., Davatzikos, C., Alberola-López, C., Fichtinger, G. (eds.) MICCAI 2018. LNCS, vol. 11071, pp. 119–126. Springer, Cham (2018). https://doi.org/10.1007/978-3-030-00934-2_14
23. Zhuang, J.: Laddernet: multi-path networks based on U-Net for medical image segmentation. arXiv preprint arXiv:1810.07810 (2018)

# Fully Convolutional Boundary Regression for Retina OCT Segmentation

Yufan He[1($\boxtimes$)], Aaron Carass[1,2], Yihao Liu[1], Bruno M. Jedynak[3],
Sharon D. Solomon[4], Shiv Saidha[5], Peter A. Calabresi[5], and Jerry L. Prince[1,2]

[1] Department of Electrical and Computer Engineering,
The Johns Hopkins University, Baltimore, MD 21218, USA
yhe35@jhu.edu
[2] Department of Computer Science, The Johns Hopkins University,
Baltimore, MD 21218, USA
[3] Department of Mathematics and Statistics, Portland State University,
Portland, OR 97201, USA
[4] Wilmer Eye Institute, The Johns Hopkins University School of Medicine,
Baltimore, MD 21287, USA
[5] Department of Neurology, The Johns Hopkins University School of Medicine,
Baltimore, MD 21287, USA

**Abstract.** A major goal of analyzing retinal optical coherence tomography (OCT) images is retinal layer segmentation. Accurate automated algorithms for segmenting smooth continuous layer surfaces, with correct hierarchy (topology) are desired for monitoring disease progression. State-of-the-art methods use a trained classifier to label each pixel into background, layer, or surface pixels. The final step of extracting the desired smooth surfaces with correct topology are mostly performed by graph methods (e.g. shortest path, graph cut). However, manually building a graph with varying constraints by retinal region and pathology and solving the minimization with specialized algorithms will degrade the flexibility and time efficiency of the whole framework. In this paper, we directly model the distribution of surface positions using a deep network with a fully differentiable soft argmax to obtain smooth, continuous surfaces in a single feed forward operation. A special topology module is used in the deep network both in the training and testing stages to guarantee the surface topology. An extra deep network output branch is also used for predicting lesion and layers in a pixel-wise labeling scheme. The proposed method was evaluated on two publicly available data sets of healthy controls, subjects with multiple sclerosis, and diabetic macular edema; it achieves state-of-the art sub-pixel results.

**Keywords:** Retina OCT · Deep learning segmentation · Surface segmentation

## 1 Introduction

Optical coherence tomography (OCT), which uses light waves to rapidly obtain 3D retina images, is widely used in the clinic. Retinal layer thicknesses change

© Springer Nature Switzerland AG 2019
D. Shen et al. (Eds.): MICCAI 2019, LNCS 11764, pp. 120–128, 2019.
https://doi.org/10.1007/978-3-030-32239-7_14

with certain diseases [15] and the analysis of OCT images improves disease monitoring. Manually segmenting the images and measuring the thickness is time consuming, and fast automated retinal layer segmentation tools are routinely used for this purpose.

The goal of layer segmentation is to obtain smooth, continuous retina layer surfaces with the correct anatomical ordering; these results can then be used for thickness analysis or registration [14]. State-of-the-art methods use a trained classifier (e.g, random forest (RF) [13] or deep network [5]) for coarse pixel-wise labeling and then level set [2] or graph methods [3,5,6,13] for surface estimation. Deep networks, which can learn features automatically, have been used in retina layer segmentation. ReLayNet [18] uses a fully convolutional network (FCN) to segment eight layers and edema by classify each pixel into layer or background classes. The main problem with this pixel-wise labeling scheme is that the layer topology is not guaranteed and final continuous and smooth surfaces are not always obtained. Ben-Cohen et al. [1] extract the boundaries from the layer maps using a Sobel filter and then use a shortest path algorithm to extract the surfaces. Other work focuses on classifying the pixels into surface pixels or background. Fang et al. [5] use a convolutional neural network (CNN) and Kugelman et al. [12] use a recurrent neural network (RNN) to classify the center pixel of a patch into boundary pixel or background; then a graph method is used to extract the final surfaces. In order to build a topologically correct graph [6,13], surface distances and smoothness constraints, which are spatially varying, must be experimentally assigned and an energy minimization must be solved outside the deep learning framework. A simpler shortest path graph method [3] was used by [5,12]; however, the shortest path extracts each surface separately, thus the hierarchy is not guaranteed compared to [6,13], especially at the fovea where surface distances can be zero.

The aforementioned graph method cannot be integrated into a deep network, and it needs special parameter settings, which make the method harder to optimize. He et al. [7,9] use a second network to replace the graph method to obtain the smooth, topology-guaranteed surfaces, but this requires much more computation.

In this paper, we propose a new method for obtaining smooth, continuous layer surfaces with the correct topology in an end-to-end deep learning scheme. We use a fully convolutional network to model the position distribution of the surfaces and use a soft-argmax method to infer the final surface positions. The proposed fully convolutional regression method can obtain sub-pixel surface positions in a single feed forward propagation without any fully-connected layer (thus requiring many fewer parameters). Our network has the benefit of being trained end-to-end, with improved accuracy against the state-of-the-art, and it is also light-weight because it does not use a fully-connected layer for regression.

## 2   Method

Our framework is shown in Fig. 1, we provide a description below for each step. The network has two output branches: the first branch outputs a pixel-wise labeling segmentation of layers and lesions and the second branch models the distribution of surface positions and outputs the positions of each surface at each column. These two branches share the same feature extractor, a residual U-Net [17]. The input to the network is a three-channel image. One channel is the original flattened OCT image [13], and the other two images are the spatial $x$ and $y$ positions (normalized to the interval $[0, 1]$) of each pixel to provide additional spatial information.

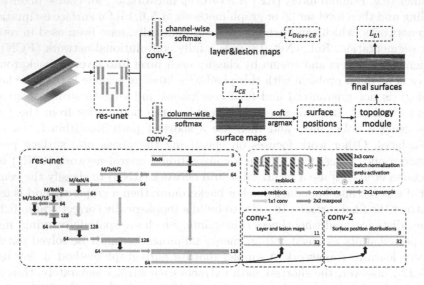

**Fig. 1.** A schematic of the proposed method (top) and network structure (bottom).

**Preprocessing.** To reduce memory usage, we flatten a retinal B-scan image to the estimated Bruch's membrane (BM) using an intensity gradient method [13] and crop the retina out.

**Surface Position Modeling.** Given an image $I$ and a ground truth surface represented by row indexes $x_1^g, \ldots, x_N^g$ across $N$ columns (correspondingly $N$ A-scans), a conventional pixel-wise labeling scheme builds a surface probability map $H$, where $H(x_j^g, j) = 1$ ($j = 1, \ldots, N$) and zero else where. A U-Net [17] takes $I$ as input and learns to generate $H$. Ideally, the surface should be continuous across the image and intersect each column only once. However, the generated probability map may produce zero or multiple positions with high prediction probability in a single column, thus breaking the continuity. Extreme class imbalance between the one-pixel-wide boundary and non-boundary pixels may also cause problems.

In contrast to the pixel-wise labeling scheme, we want to model the surface position distribution $p = p(x_1, \cdots, x_N, I)$ by approximating it with $q = \Pi_{i=1}^{N} q_i(x_i | I; \boldsymbol{\theta}) p(I)$. For an input image I, the network generates N independent surface position distributions $q_i(x_i | I; \boldsymbol{\theta}), i = 1, \cdots, N$ at each column. $\boldsymbol{\theta}$ are the network parameters to be trained by minimizing the K-L divergence between the data distribution $p$ and $q$. This idea has similarities with Variational Bayesian methods. The direct inference of each $x_i$ from the joint distribution $p$ is hard but it is easier given the simpler independent $q_i$'s. To train the network by minimizing the K-L divergence using the input image $I$ and ground truth $x_i^g$'s, we have

$$\operatorname*{argmin}_{\theta} KL(p||q) = \operatorname*{argmin}_{\theta} \iint_{\vec{x},I} p(x_1,\cdots,x_N,I) \log \frac{p(x_1,\cdots,x_N,I)}{\Pi_{i=1}^{N} q_i(x_i|I;\theta)p(I)}, \quad (1)$$

$$= -\operatorname*{argmin}_{\theta} \iint_{\vec{x},I} p(x_1,\cdots,x_N,I) \sum_{i=1}^{N} \log q_i(x_i|I,\theta), \quad (2)$$

$$= -\operatorname*{argmin}_{\theta} \operatorname*{E}_{\vec{x},I \sim p} \left( \sum_{i=1}^{N} \log q_i(x_i|I,\theta) \right). \quad (3)$$

The $\vec{x}$ is a vector of surface positions at N columns and is sampled from data distribution $p$. In a stochastic gradient descent training scheme, the expectation in Eq. (3) can be removed with a training sample $(I, x_1^g, \cdots, x_N^g)$ and the position $x_i^g$ of the $i^{\text{th}}$ column is on the image grid which can only be an integer from 1 to the image row number $R$. So the loss becomes,

$$\mathcal{L}_{\text{CE}} = -\sum_{i=1}^{N} \sum_{j=1}^{R} \mathbb{1}(x_i^g = j) \log q_i(x_i^g|I,\theta). \quad (4)$$

$\mathbb{1}(x_i^g = j)$ is the indicator function where $\mathbb{1}(x_i^g = j) = 1$ if $x_i^g = j$ and zero elsewhere. Equation (4) is the cross entropy loss for a single surface. In multiple surfaces segmentation, we use the network to output M feature maps (each map has the same size as the input image) for M surfaces. A column-wise softmax is performed independently on these M feature maps to generate surface position probabilities $q_i(x_i|I;\theta)$, $i = 1,\ldots,N$ for each column and each surface. An intuitive explanation of the proposed formulation is: instead of classifying each pixel into surfaces or backgrounds, we are selecting a row index at each column for each surface.

**Soft-argmax.** The deep network outputs marginal conditional distributions $q_i(x_i|i,\theta)$ for each column $i$, so the exact inference of the boundary position at column $i$ from $q_i$ can be performed independently. The differentiable soft-argmax operation (5) used in keypoint localization [10] is used to estimate the final surface position $x_i^{sa}$ at each column $i$. Thus, we directly obtain the surface positions from the network with soft-argmax,

$$x_i^{sa} = \sum_{r=1}^{R} r q_i(r|I,\theta)). \quad (5)$$

We further regularize $q_i$ by directly encouraging the soft-argmax of $q_i$ to be the ground truth, $x_i^g$, with a smooth $L1$ loss,

$$\mathcal{L}_{L1} = \sum_{i=1}^{N} 0.5 d_i^2 \, \mathbb{1}(|d_i| < 1) + (|d_i| - 0.5) \, \mathbb{1}(|d_i| \geq 1), \quad d_i = x_i^{sa} - x_i^g. \quad (6)$$

**Topology Guarantee Module.** The layer boundaries within the retina have a strict anatomical ordering. For M surfaces $s_1, \cdots, s_M$ from inner to outer retina, the anatomy requires $s_1(i) \leq s_2(i) \cdots \leq s_M(i), i = 1, \ldots, N$ where $s_j(i)$ is the position of the $j^{\text{th}}$ surface at the $i^{\text{th}}$ column. The soft-argmax operation produces exact surfaces $s_1, \ldots, s_M$ but may not satisfy the ordering constraint. We update each $s_j(i)$ as $s_j(i)^{new} = s_{j-1}(i) + \text{ReLU}(s_j(i) - s_{j-1}(i))$ iteratively to guarantee the ordering. We implement this as the deep network output layer to guarantee the topology both in the training and testing stages.

**Layer and Lesion Pixel-Wise Labeling.** Our multi-task network has two output branches. The first branch described above outputs the correctly ordered surfaces whereas the second branch outputs pixel-wise labelings for both layers and lesions. A combined Dice and cross entropy loss [18] is used for the output of this branch. $C$ is the total number of classes, $g_c(x)$ and $p_c(x)$ are the ground truth and predicted probability that pixel $x$ belongs to class $c$, and $\Omega_c$ is the number of pixels in class $c$ and our combined loss is,

$$\mathcal{L}_{\text{Dice+CE}} = \sum_{c=1}^{C} \sum_{x \in \Omega_c} w_c(x) g_c(x) \log(p_c(x)) - \frac{1}{C} \sum_{c=1}^{C} \frac{\epsilon + \sum_{x \in \Omega_i} 2 g_c(x) p_c(x)}{\epsilon + \sum_{x \in \Omega_c} g_c(x)^2 + p_c(x)^2}.$$

Here, $\epsilon = 0.001$ is a smoothing constant and $w_c(x)$ is a weighting function for each pixel [18]. The final network training loss is $\mathcal{L} = \mathcal{L}_{\text{Dice+CE}} + \mathcal{L}_{\text{CE}} + \mathcal{L}_{L1}$.

## 3 Experiments

The proposed method was validated on two publicly available data sets. The first data set [8] contains 35 (14 healthy controls (HC) and 21 subjects with multiple sclerosis (MS)) macula Spectralis OCT scans, of which nine surfaces are manually delineated. Each scan has 49 B-scans of size $496 \times 1024$. We train on the last 6 HC and last 9 MS subjects and test on the other 20 subjects. The second data set [4] contains 110 B-scans ($496 \times 768$) from 10 diabetic macular edema patients (each with 11 Bscans). Eight retina surfaces and macular edema have been manually delineated. We train on the last 55 B-scans and test on the challenging first 55 B-scans with large lesions. The network is implemented with Pytorch and trained with an Adam optimizer with an initial learning rate of $10^{-4}$, weight decay of $10^{-4}$, and a minibatch size of 2 until convergence. The training image is augmented with horizontal flipping and vertical scaling both with probability 0.5.

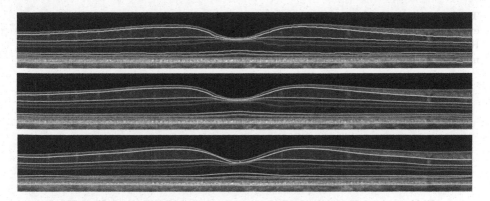

**Fig. 2.** Visualization of shortest path (top), our result (middle), and manual segmentation (bottom) from a healthy subject.

**HC and MS Data Set.** We compare our proposed method with several baselines. The AURA tool [13] is a graph based method and it is the state-of-the-art compared to other publicly available tools as shown in [19]. The RNet [9] is a regression deep network that can obtain smooth surfaces from layer segmentation maps. ReLayNet [18] is a variation of U-Net and only outputs layer maps; we obtain the final surface positions by summing up the output layer maps in each column. The shortest path (SP) algorithm [3,5,12] is also compared. We extract the final surfaces using SP on our predicted $q_i$'s (the surface map as shown in Fig. 1). All the baseline methods are retrained on the same data as our proposed method. The mean absolute distances (MADs) for each method are shown in Table 1 (Fig. 2).

**DME Data Set.** We compare our results with three graph based methods (for final surface extraction): Chiu et al. [4], Rathke et al. [16], and Karri et al. [11]. Since ReLayNet layer surfaces cannot be obtained by simply summing up layer maps (due to lesions), we compare the lesion Dice scores with it. We ignore the positions where Chiu et al. [4]'s result or manual delineation are NaN. The boundary MAD is shown in Table 2. Our network has an extra branch for lesion prediction; however, Rathke's and Karri's method can only output layer surfaces. The Dice score of diabetic macular edema for Chiu's method [4], ReLayNet [18] and ours are 0.56, 0.7, 0.7 respectively. Qualitative results are shown in Fig. 3.

**Table 1.** Mean absolute distance (MAD) and standard deviation (Std. Dev.) in $\mu$m evaluated on 20 manually delineated scans of 9 surfaces, comparing AURA toolkit [13], R-Net [9], ReLayNet [18], SP (shortest path on our surface map), and our proposed method. Depth resolution is 3.9 $\mu$m. Numbers in bold are the best in that row.

| Boundary | MAD (Std. Dev.) | | | | |
| --- | --- | --- | --- | --- | --- |
| | AURA | R-Net | ReLayNet | SP | Our's |
| ILM | **2.37** (0.36) | 2.38 (0.36) | 3.17 (0.61) | 2.70 (0.39) | 2.41 (0.40) |
| RNFL-GCL | 3.09 (0.64) | 3.10 (0.55) | 3.75 (0.84) | 3.38 (0.68) | **2.96** (0.71) |
| IPL-INL | 3.43 (0.53) | 2.89 (0.42) | 3.42 (0.45) | 3.11 (0.34) | **2.87** (0.46) |
| INL-OPL | 3.25 (0.48) | **3.15** (0.56) | 3.65 (0.34) | 3.58 (0.32) | 3.19 (0.53) |
| OPL-ONL | 2.96 (0.55) | 2.76 (0.59) | 3.28 (0.63) | 3.07 (0.53) | **2.72** (0.61) |
| ELM | 2.69 (0.44) | **2.65** (0.66) | 3.04 (0.43) | 2.86 (0.41) | **2.65** (0.73) |
| IS-OS | 2.07 (0.81) | 2.10 (0.75) | 2.73 (0.45) | 2.45 (0.31) | **2.01** (0.57) |
| OS-RPE | 3.77 (0.94) | 3.81 (1.17) | 4.22 (1.48) | 4.10 (1.42) | **3.55** (1.02) |
| BM | **2.89** (2.18) | 3.71 (2.27) | 3.09 (1.35) | 3.23 (1.36) | 3.10 (2.02) |
| Overall | 2.95 (1.04) | 2.95 (1.10) | 3.37 (0.92) | 3.16 (0.88) | **2.83** (0.99) |

**Table 2.** Mean absolute distance (MAD) in $\mu$m for eight surfaces (and the mean of those eight surfaces) evaluated on 55 manually delineated scans comparing Chiu et al. [4], Karri et al. [11], Rathke et al. [16], and our proposed method. Numbers in bold are the best in that column.

| | Mean | #1 | #2 | #3 | #4 | #5 | #6 | #7 | #8 |
| --- | --- | --- | --- | --- | --- | --- | --- | --- | --- |
| Chiu | 7.82 | 6.59 | 8.38 | 9.04 | 11.02 | 11.01 | 4.84 | 5.74 | 5.91 |
| Karri | 9.54 | **4.47** | 11.77 | 11.12 | 17.54 | 16.74 | 4.99 | 5.35 | **4.30** |
| Rathke | 7.71 | 4.66 | 6.78 | 8.87 | 11.02 | 13.60 | 4.61 | 7.06 | 5.11 |
| Ours | **6.70** | 4.51 | **6.71** | **8.29** | **10.71** | **9.88** | **4.41** | **4.52** | 4.61 |

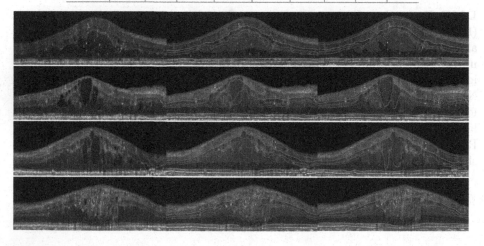

**Fig. 3.** Visualization of original image (left), our results (middle), manual segmentation (right) of four B-scans from diabetic macular edema subjects.

# 4 Discussion and Conclusion

In this paper, we proposed a new way for retina OCT layer surface and lesion segmentation without using handcrafted graph based methods. The direct modeling of surface position and the fully differentiable soft-argmax operation generates sub-pixel surface positions in a single feed forward propagation. The generated sub-pixel accuracy surface is smooth and continuous and guarantees correct layer ordering, thus overcoming conventional pixel-wise labeling problems. The topology module affects the network training and thus is not simply a post-processing step. Currently the algorithm works on each B-scan individually, and future work will consider context among different B-scans.

**Acknowledgments.** This work was supported by the NIH/NEI under grant R01-EY024655.

# References

1. Ben-Cohen, A., et al.: Retinal layers segmentation using fully convolutional network in OCT images. In: RSIP Vision (2017)
2. Carass, A., et al.: Multiple-object geometric deformable model for segmentation of macular OCT. Biomed. Opt. Express **5**(4), 1062–1074 (2014)
3. Chiu, S.J., et al.: Automatic segmentation of seven retinal layers in SDOCT images congruent with expert manual segmentation. Opt. Express **18**(18), 19413–19428 (2010)
4. Chiu, S.J., et al.: Kernel regression based segmentation of optical coherence tomography images with diabetic macular edema. Biomed. Opt. Express **6**(4), 1172–1194 (2015)
5. Fang, L., et al.: Automatic segmentation of nine retinal layer boundaries in OCT images of non-exudative AMD patients using deep learning and graph search. Biomed. Opt. Express **8**(5), 2732–2744 (2017)
6. Garvin, M.K., et al.: Automated 3-D intraretinal layer segmentation of macular spectral-domain optical coherence tomography images. IEEE Trans. Med. Imag. **28**(9), 1436–1447 (2009)
7. He, Y., et al.: Towards topological correct segmentation of macular OCT from cascaded FCNs. In: Cardoso, M.J., et al. (eds.) FIFI/OMIA -2017. LNCS, vol. 10554, pp. 202–209. Springer, Cham (2017). https://doi.org/10.1007/978-3-319-67561-9_23
8. He, Y., et al.: Retinal layer parcellation of optical coherence tomography images: data resource for multiple sclerosis and healthy controls. Data Brief **22**, 601–604 (2018)
9. He, Y., et al.: Topology guaranteed segmentation of the human retina from OCT using convolutional neural networks. arXiv preprint arXiv:1803.05120 (2018)
10. Honari, S., et al.: Improving landmark localization with semi-supervised learning. In: The IEEE Conference on Computer Vision and Pattern Recognition (2018)
11. Karri, S., et al.: Learning layer-specific edges for segmenting retinal layers with large deformations. Biomed. Opt. Express **7**(7), 2888–2901 (2016)
12. Kugelman, J., et al.: Automatic segmentation of oct retinal boundaries using recurrent neural networks and graph search. Biomed. Opt. Express **9**(11), 5759–5777 (2018)

128 Y. He et al.

13. Lang, A., et al.: Retinal layer segmentation of macular OCT images using boundary classification. Biomed. Opt. Express **4**(7), 1133–1152 (2013)
14. Lee, S., et al.: Atlas-based shape analysis and classification of retinal optical coherence tomography images using the functional shape (fshape) framework. Med. Image Anal. **35**, 570–581 (2017)
15. Medeiros, F.A., et al.: Detection of glaucoma progression with stratus OCT retinal nerve fiber layer, optic nerve head, and macular thickness measurements. Invest. Ophthalmol. Vis. Sci. **50**(12), 5741–5748 (2009)
16. Rathke, F., Desana, M., Schnörr, C.: Locally adaptive probabilistic models for global segmentation of pathological OCT scans. In: Descoteaux, M., Maier-Hein, L., Franz, A., Jannin, P., Collins, D.L., Duchesne, S. (eds.) MICCAI 2017. LNCS, vol. 10433, pp. 177–184. Springer, Cham (2017). https://doi.org/10.1007/978-3-319-66182-7_21
17. Ronneberger, O., Fischer, P., Brox, T.: U-Net: convolutional networks for biomedical image segmentation. In: Navab, N., Hornegger, J., Wells, W.M., Frangi, A.F. (eds.) MICCAI 2015. LNCS, vol. 9351, pp. 234–241. Springer, Cham (2015). https://doi.org/10.1007/978-3-319-24574-4_28
18. Roy, A.G., et al.: Relaynet: retinal layer and fluid segmentation of macular optical coherence tomography using fully convolutional networks. Biomed. Opt. Express **8**(8), 3627–3642 (2017)
19. Tian, J., et al.: Performance evaluation of automated segmentation software on optical coherence tomography volume data. J. Biophotonics **9**(5), 478–489 (2016)

# PM-Net: Pyramid Multi-label Network for Joint Optic Disc and Cup Segmentation

Pengshuai Yin[1], Qingyao Wu[1], Yanwu Xu[4($\boxtimes$)], Huaqing Min[1], Ming Yang[2], Yubing Zhang[2], and Mingkui Tan[1,3($\boxtimes$)]

[1] South China University of Technology, Guangzhou, China
mingkuitan@scut.edu.cn
[2] Guangzhou Shiyuan Electronic Technology Company Limited, Guangzhou, China
[3] Peng Cheng Laboratory, Shenzhen, China
[4] Cixi Institute of Biomedical Engineering, Ningbo Institute of Materials Technology and Engineering, Chinese Academy of Sciences, Ningbo, China
ywxu@ieee.org

**Abstract.** Accurate segmentation of optic disc (OD) and optic cup (OC) is a fundamental task for fundus image analysis. Most existing methods focus on segmenting OD and OC inside the optic nerve head (ONH) area but paying little attention to accurate ONH localization. In this paper, we propose a Mask-RCNN based paradigm to localize ONH and jointly segment OD and OC in a whole fundus image. However, directly using Mask-RCNN faces some critical issues: First, for some glaucoma cases, the highly overlapping of OD and OC may lead to the missing of OC proposals. Second, some proposals may not fully surround the object, and thus the segmentation can be incomplete. Last, the instance head in Mask-RCNN cannot well incorporate the prior such as the OC is inside the OD. To address these issues, we first propose a segmentation based region proposal network (RPN) to improve the accuracy of proposals and then propose a pyramid RoIAlign module to aggregate the multi-level information to get a better feature representation. Furthermore, we employ a multi-label head strategy to incorporate the prior for better performance. Extensive experiments verify our method.

**Keywords:** Medical image process · Fundus image · Optic disc · Segmentation

## 1 Introduction

Fundus images assist doctors to diagnose many eye diseases such as glaucoma, which is one of the leading causes of blindness. The early detection and treatment for glaucoma often protect the eyes against serious vision loss. Clinically, the

---

P. Yin and Q. Wu—Equally contribution to this work.

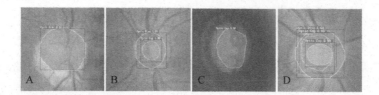

**Fig. 1.** Issues when adopting Mask-RCNN framework for OD and OC segmentation. (A): No proposals for OC and the proposal does not fully surround the OD. (B): The proposal does not fully surround the OD but the objectness score of this proposal is 1. (C): No proposals for OD. (D): Multiple instances of OC.

vertical cup to disc ratio (CDR) is a popular optic nerve head (ONH) assessment that is widely adopted by trained glaucoma specialists to screen glaucoma. The CDR is the comparison of the diameter of the cup to disc [11]. A larger CDR may indicate glaucoma or other diseases such as neuro-ophthalmic diseases. Accurate optic disc and cup segmentation are essential for CDR measurement. However, manual CDR assessment is time-consuming and costly, so an automatic glaucoma screening method is necessary.

OD and OC segmentation is a fundamental task in fundus image analysis [1]. Initially, many methods are based on hand-craft features, such as template based methods [2,5], deformable based methods [10,15,21], pixel classification based methods [16,20], label transfer based methods [18] and superpixel based methods [6,7,19]. However, these methods are limited in performance and can be easily affected by pathological regions. Recently, deep learning based methods show promising performance on OD and OC segmentation [3,4,8,9,23]. Most methods employ a two-step paradigm: first locate ONH area, and then segment OD and OC within the ONH area to avoid the influence from other fundus regions. In practice, accurate ONH localization is essential for accurate OD and OC segmentation. However, most methods focus on the second step and pay little attention to the accurate ONH localization.

In this paper, we propose a Mask-RCNN based method to jointly localize ONH and segment OD and OC in a whole fundus image. Unfortunately, directly using Mask-RCNN for OD and OC segmentation [14] may suffer from several issues, as shown in Fig. 1. Essentially, the performance of Mask-RCNN highly depends on the accuracy and compactness of bounding boxes. However, the proposals generated from the region proposal network may not completely enclose the object. More critically, in some glaucoma cases, the highly overlapping of OD and OC leads to the missing of OC proposals. Moreover, the instance segmentation may produce multiple instances of OC, but each fundus image in fact has only one OD and OC. Last but not least, the instance head is hard to model the prior that the OD contains the OC.

To solve these issues, we improve Mask-RCNN framework in three aspects. First, we introduce a segmentation branch on the region proposal network (RPN) to segment the ONH area from the whole image. Second, we propose a pyramid

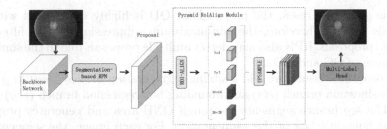

**Fig. 2.** The flowchart of our proposed network. The whole network can be trained end-to-end. A fundus image is fed into a convolutional neural network to extract features for segmentation based region proposal network to localize the ONH area. The pyramid RoIAlign module is developed to aggregate multi-level context information in proposals. Last, a multi-label segmentation head is used to jointly segment OD and OC.

RoIAlign module to aggregate multi-level information. The pyramid RoIAlign module helps to incorporate global features and learn stronger feature representations. Last, we employ a multi-label segmentation head instead of the instance segmentation head to better incorporate the prior that the OD is inside the OC.

The main contributions of this paper are listed as follows:

- We propose a segmentation-based RPN to generate more accurate and complete proposals for localizing ONH area.
- We propose a pyramid RoIAlign module to aggregate multi-level context information within proposals, which makes the final prediction more reliable.
- We propose a multi-label head to segment OD and OC jointly by better modeling the relation of OD and OC.

## 2  Proposed Method

The flowchart of our pyramid multi-label network (PM-Net) is shown in Fig. 2. A fundus image is first fed into a backbone network to extract features. Here, to increase the accuracy of proposals, we propose a **segmentation-based RPN** to segment the ONH area and produce proposals from the segmentation. Which helps to avoid proposal missing and accurately localize the ONH area based on the extracted features. We then propose a pyramid RoIAlign module to aggregate multi-level information in proposals to learn stronger representations. Last, we employ a multi-label head to jointly segment OD and OC by considering the relations between OD and OC. The whole network can be trained end-to-end.

### 2.1  Segmentation-Based Region Proposal Network

The RPN takes an image as input and produces rectangle proposals for OC and OD, each with an objectness score [12]. Unfortunately, as shown in Fig. 1, the rectangle proposals commonly do not fully surround the object. More seriously, the anchor based method may miss the proposals for OD or OC. Especially for some glaucoma cases, the proposals of OD is highly overlapped with the proposals of OC. Therefore, the non-maximum suppression (NMS) filters out some OC proposals. RPN also may detect multiple proposals due to the similarity appearance of OC and OD.

To solve these issues, we add a sibling segmentation branch ($seg$) in parallel with classification branch ($cls$) and bounding box regression branch ($reg$) in the RPN. The $seg$ branch segments the rough ONH area and generates proposals from the bounding box of the segmentation. For each image, the segmentation branch generates only one proposal for the ONH area and does not generate proposals for OC. Therefore, our segmentation-based RPN avoids generating multiple instances of an object and we enlarge the proposal by 20 pixels in order to let the proposal completely enclose the ONH area.

Our RPN is implemented with a $3 \times 3$ convolution followed by three sibling $1 \times 1$ convolution layers (for $cls$, $reg$ and $seg$ respectively). The $seg$ branch segments the ONH area from the whole image and it is trained simultaneously with $cls$ and $reg$ branches. The segmentation-based region proposal network is trained by minimizing the objective function following the multi-task loss defined in [12]:

$$Loss_{segrpn} = Loss(\{p_i\}, \{t_i\}) + Loss_{seg}. \tag{1}$$

$$Loss(\{p_i\}, \{t_i\}) = \frac{1}{N_{cls}} \sum_i L_{cls}(p_i, p_i^*) + \lambda \frac{1}{N_{reg}} \sum_i p_i^* L_{reg}(t_i, t_i^*). \tag{2}$$

$$Loss_{seg} = g_i log c_i + (1 - g_i) log(1 - c_i). \tag{3}$$

Here, $i$ is the index of an anchor, $L_{cls}(p_i, p_i^*)$ is the log loss between the predicted probability $p_i$ of anchor $i$ and the corresponding ground-truth label $p_i^*$. $L_{reg}(t_i, t_i^*) = R(t_i - t_i^*)$ where $R$ is the smooth $L_1$ loss, $t_i$ is a vector representing the 4 parameterized coordinates of the predicted bounding box and $t_i^*$ is the corresponding ground-truth bounding box. $loss_{seg}$ is a binary cross-entropy loss between ground-truth class $g_i$ at pixel $i$ and the corresponding prediction $c_i$.

During the training, we use both anchor and segmentation based proposals to train the mask branch. In the testing phase, we use only segmentation based proposals.

## 2.2   Pyramid RoIAlign Module

The network tends to misclassify OC and OD due to the similar appearance of these objects. Motivated by [22], we solve this issue by incorporating suitable global features. We extend the RoIAlign layer to pyramid RoIAlign module. RoIAlign layer converts the feature inside any valid region into a feature map with a fixed spatial content of $H \times W$ by using bilinear interpolation to avoid quantization. Different output spatial sizes of the RoIAlign layer represent different level of context information. Small output spatial sizes represent the global context. Our pyramid RoIAlign module is a five-level RoiAlign layer with output spatial sizes of $\{1 \times 1\}$, $\{3 \times 3\}$, $\{7 \times 7\}$, $\{14 \times 14\}$ and $\{28 \times 28\}$ respectively. These output features are upsampled to $\{28 \times 28\}$ and concatenated together to form the final feature representation, which carries different level context information. The local and global context together make the final prediction more reliable. The representation is sent to multi-label head to predict the final segmentation.

## 2.3   Multi-label Head for Joint OD and OC Segmentation

Note that the OD contains OC so the pixels within OC has the same labels to OD. The instance head assigns one label to each class and predicts a binary mask. Instead, multi-label head learns an independent binary classifier for each class and assigns each pixel to multiple binary labels. The multi-label head can better use the relative relation of OD and OC. Moreover, for some glaucoma cases, the OC occupy the most area of OD. Using instance head leads to imbalance pixel number for OD and OC. The multi-label head solves the imbalance problem since the classifier is independent for OD and OC. For the above reasons, we treat the OD and OC segmentation problem as a multi-label problem. Our multi-label head divide this multi-label problem into two binary classification problem with single label: {OD,¬OD}, {OC,¬OC} (¬ represents negative examples), our multi-label loss is defined as:

$$Loss_m = -\frac{1}{N} \sum_{n=1}^{N} [g_{n,i} log p_{n,i} + (1 - g_{n,i}) log(1 - p_{n,i})]. \tag{4}$$

Here, $N$ is the class number. $p_{n,i}$ represents the predicted probability when assign pixel $i$ to class $n$. $g_{n,i}$ represents the ground truth label for pixel $i$.

## 3   Experiments

We compare our method with several state-of-the-art methods, including R-Bend [10], ASM [21], LRR [17], U-Net [13], Superpixel [7], M-Net [8] and Faster-RCNN based method [14].

**Datasets.** We test our method on two datasets: ORIGA and REFUGE. ORIGA has 650 images with 168 glaucomatous eyes and 482 normal eyes. Following [8], we use 325 images for training (including 73 glaucoma cases) and 325 images for testing (including 95 glaucoma cases). For REFUGE, we use 400 images for training and 400 images for validation.

**Implementation Details.** We train our model with 15000 iterations using the initial learning rate 0.002. Then, we decay the learning rate to 0.0002 and fine-tune the model with another 15000 iterations. For architecture, we adopt the ResNet-50 with feature pyramid network (FPN) as the backbone and pretrain the model on MS COCO dataset to avoid overfitting.

**Evaluation Metrics.** We adopt the overlapping error $(E)$ and balanced accuracy $(A)$ as the evaluation metrix for OD, OC and rim regions:

$$OE = 1 - \frac{Area(S \bigcap G)}{Area(S \bigcup G)}, A = \frac{1}{2}(Sen + Spe), \tag{5}$$

with $Sen = \frac{TP}{TP+FN}$, and $Spe = \frac{TN}{TN+FP}$. Here, $S$ and $G$ denote the predicted mask and corresponding ground-truth. TP and FP denote true and false positives, respectivel. TN and FN denote true and false negatives, respectively. Moreover, we also calculate CDR and adopt absolute CDR error $\delta_E$ as an evaluation metric: $\delta_E = |CDR_S - CDR_G|$, where $CDR_G$ is the ground-truth CDR from trained clinician and $CDR_S$ is calculated on segmentation result.

**Table 1.** Performance evaluation on ORIGA dataset.

| Method | $E_{disc}$ | $E_{cup}$ | $E_{rim}$ | $\delta_E$ | $A_{disc}$ | $A_{cup}$ | $A_{rim}$ |
|---|---|---|---|---|---|---|---|
| R-Bend [10] | 0.129 | 0.395 | - | 0.154 | - | - | - |
| ASM [21] | 0.148 | 0.313 | - | 0.107 | - | - | - |
| LRR [17] | - | 0.244 | - | 0.078 | - | - | - |
| U-Net [13] | 0.115 | 0.287 | 0.303 | 0.102 | 0.959 | 0.901 | 0.921 |
| Superpixel [7] | 0.102 | 0.264 | 0.299 | 0.077 | 0.964 | 0.918 | 0.905 |
| M-Net [8] | 0.083 | 0.256 | 0.265 | 0.078 | 0.972 | 0.914 | 0.921 |
| M-Net+PT [8] | 0.071 | 0.230 | 0.233 | 0.071 | 0.983 | 0.930 | 0.941 |
| Sun's [14] | 0.069 | 0.213 | - | 0.067 | - | - | - |
| Mask-RCNN(Baseline) | 0.074 | 0.231 | 0.260 | 0.079 | 0.985 | 0.941 | 0.929 |
| PM-Net(Ours) | **0.066** | **0.208** | **0.224** | **0.065** | **0.986** | **0.942** | **0.949** |

## 3.1   Comparison with State-of-the-arts

We compare our method with several baselines on ORIGA dataset and record results in Table 1. Our method does not rely on post-processing such as ellipse fitting. From Table 1, our PM-Net method outperforms all other methods. There are several reasons accounting for this. First, our segmentation based region proposal network produces more accurate proposals for the ONH area. Conversely, faster-RCNN based methods [14] may miss OC proposals or generate proposals that do not fully surround the ONH area. Second, the multi-label head considers the relation of OD and OC for joint segmentation while the instance head segment OD and OC separately. For M-Net, it is performed on the ONH area; While our method is performed on the whole image. Although the background accounts for a large content of the image compared to the OD, our method is still better than M-Net. One possible reason is that our proposed pyramid RoIAlign module helps to learn stronger representations than M-Net.

**Table 2.** Segmentation results on REFUGE validation set.

| Method | $E_{disc}$ | $E_{cup}$ | $E_{rim}$ | $\delta_E$ | $A_{disc}$ | $A_{cup}$ | $A_{rim}$ |
|---|---|---|---|---|---|---|---|
| Mask-RCNN | 0.092 | 0.228 | 0.211 | 0.055 | 0.973 | 0.976 | 0.923 |
| PM-Net | **0.088** | **0.223** | **0.204** | **0.048** | **0.979** | **0.980** | **0.936** |

We have the same observations on the experiments on REFUGE validation set in Table 2, which further verifies our method. We also show example segmentation results and discussions in Fig. 3.

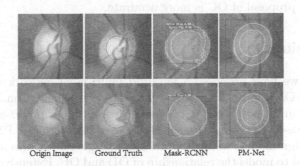

Origin Image        Ground Truth        Mask-RCNN        PM-Net

**Fig. 3.** Example segmentation results. The first row is a normal eye while the second row is a glaucoma eye. Our method achieve more accurate and reliable results.

**Table 3.** Effect of the pyramid RoIAlign module on ORIGA dataset.

| Method | $E_{disc}$ | $E_{cup}$ | $E_{rim}$ | $\delta_E$ | $A_{disc}$ | $A_{cup}$ | $A_{rim}$ |
|---|---|---|---|---|---|---|---|
| Baseline | 0.074 | 0.231 | 0.260 | 0.079 | 0.985 | 0.941 | 0.929 |
| Max-pooling | 0.073 | 0.210 | 0.234 | **0.067** | 0.982 | 0.938 | 0.944 |
| Sum-average | **0.069** | 0.211 | 0.237 | 0.068 | **0.987** | **0.942** | 0.942 |
| Concatenation | 0.070 | **0.207** | **0.228** | 0.069 | 0.986 | 0.936 | **0.950** |

## 3.2   Ablative Studies

In this part, we conduct ablative studies on ORIGA dataset. First, we evaluate the different feature map fusion strategy for the pyramid RoIAlign module. Then, we evaluate each module of our proposed method. Table 3 shows the performance

**Table 4.** Effect of different components of our method on ORIGA dataset. ML is for multi-label head. SegRPN is for segmentation based region proposal network.

| Method | $E_{disc}$ | $E_{cup}$ | $E_{rim}$ | $\delta_E$ | $A_{disc}$ | $A_{cup}$ | $A_{rim}$ |
|---|---|---|---|---|---|---|---|
| Mask-RCNN(Baseline) | 0.074 | 0.231 | 0.260 | 0.079 | 0.985 | 0.941 | 0.929 |
| ML | 0.071 | 0.217 | 0.232 | 0.071 | 0.984 | 0.940 | 0.947 |
| RoIAlign | 0.069 | 0.211 | 0.237 | 0.068 | **0.987** | **0.942** | 0.942 |
| ML + RoiAlign | 0.068 | 0.217 | 0.237 | 0.073 | 0.986 | **0.942** | 0.941 |
| ML + SegRPN | 0.069 | 0.219 | 0.230 | 0.070 | 0.986 | 0.933 | **0.950** |
| ML + RoiAlign + SegRPN | **0.066** | **0.208** | **0.224** | **0.065** | 0.986 | **0.942** | 0.949 |

using different feature fusion strategy for pyramid RoIAlign module. All three strategies improve $E_{cup}$ and $\delta_E$ significantly. Table 4 shows the effect of different components on our PM-Net. The multi-label head and pyramid RoiAlign module improve $A_{cup}$ significantly. Moreover, the segmentation based RPN improve $A_{disc}$ since the proposal of OC is more accurate.

## 4 Conclusions

In this paper, we have proposed a pyramid multi-label network (PM-Net) for simultaneously ONH localization and joint OD/OC segmentation. PM-Net produces more accurate proposals and avoids missing object proposals by using a segmentation-based RPN to locate the ONH area. Furthermore, PM-Net adopts pyramid RoIAlign module to incorporate suitable global features and employs a multi-label head to model the relationship of OD and OC. Extensive experiments verify the effectiveness of our method.

**Acknowledgement.** This work was supported by National Natural Science Foundation of China (NSFC) 61602185, 61876208, Guangdong Introducing Innovative and Entrepreneurial Teams 2017ZT07X183, Guangdong Provincial Scientific and Technological Fund 2018B010107001, 2017B090901008, 2018B010108002, Pearl River S&T Nova Program of Guangzhou 201806010081, CCF-Tencent Open Research Fund RAGR20190103.

## References

1. Almazroa, A., Burman, R., et al.: Optic disc and optic cup segmentation methodologies for glaucoma image detection: a survey. J. Ophthalmol. (2015)
2. Aquino, A., Gegúndez-Arias, M.E., et al.: Detecting the optic disc boundary in digital fundus images using morphological, edge detection, and feature extraction techniques. IEEE TMI **29**(11), 1860–1869 (2010)
3. Chen, X., Xu, Y., Yan, S., Wong, D.W.K., Wong, T.Y., Liu, J.: Automatic feature learning for glaucoma detection based on deep learning. In: Navab, N., Hornegger, J., Wells, W.M., Frangi, A.F. (eds.) MICCAI 2015. LNCS, vol. 9351, pp. 669–677. Springer, Cham (2015). https://doi.org/10.1007/978-3-319-24574-4_80
4. Chen, X., Xu, Y., et al.: Glaucoma detection based on deep convolutional neural network. In: EMBC, pp. 715–718. IEEE (2015)
5. Cheng, J., Liu, J., et al.: Automatic optic disc segmentation with peripapillary atrophy elimination. In: EMBC, pp. 6224–6227. IEEE (2011)
6. Cheng, J., Liu, J., et al.: Superpixel classification for initialization in model based optic disc segmentation. In: EMBC, pp. 1450–1453. IEEE (2012)
7. Cheng, J., Liu, J., et al.: Superpixel classification based optic disc and optic cup segmentation for glaucoma screening. IEEE TMI **32**(6), 1019–1032 (2013)
8. Fu, H., Cheng, J., et al.: Joint optic disc and cup segmentation based on multi-label deep network and polar transformation. IEEE TMI **37**, 1597–1605 (2018)
9. Fu, H., Cheng, J., et al.: Disc-aware ensemble network for glaucoma screening from fundus image. IEEE TMI **30**, 2493–2501 (2018)

10. Joshi, G.D., Sivaswamy, J., et al.: Optic disk and cup segmentation from monocular color retinal images for glaucoma assessment. IEEE TMI **30**(6), 1192–1205 (2011)
11. Kaufman, P.L., Levin, L.A., Adler, F.H., Alm, A.: Adler's Physiology of the Eye. Elsevier Health Sciences (2011)
12. Ren, S., He, K., et al.: Faster R-CNN: towards real-time object detection with region proposal networks. In: NeurIPS, pp. 91–99 (2015)
13. Ronneberger, O., Fischer, P., Brox, T.: U-Net: convolutional networks for biomedical image segmentation. In: Navab, N., Hornegger, J., Wells, W.M., Frangi, A.F. (eds.) MICCAI 2015. LNCS, vol. 9351, pp. 234–241. Springer, Cham (2015). https://doi.org/10.1007/978-3-319-24574-4_28
14. Sun, X., Xu, Y., et al.: Optic disc segmentation from retinal fundus images via deep object detection networks. In: EMBC, pp. 5954–5957, July 2018
15. Tang, L., Garvin, M.K., et al.: Segmentation of optic nerve head rim in color fundus photographs by probability based active shape model. IOVS **53**(14), 2144 (2012)
16. Wong, D.W.K., Liu, J., et al.: Learning-based approach for the automatic detection of the optic disc in digital retinal fundus photographs. In: EMBC. IEEE (2010)
17. Xu, Y., Duan, L., Lin, S., Chen, X., Wong, D.W.K., Wong, T.Y., Liu, J.: Optic cup segmentation for glaucoma detection using low-rank superpixel representation. In: Golland, P., Hata, N., Barillot, C., Hornegger, J., Howe, R. (eds.) MICCAI 2014. LNCS, vol. 8673, pp. 788–795. Springer, Cham (2014). https://doi.org/10.1007/978-3-319-10404-1_98
18. Xu, Y., Lin, S., Wong, D.W.K., Liu, J., Xu, D.: Efficient reconstruction-based optic cup localization for glaucoma screening. In: Mori, K., Sakuma, I., Sato, Y., Barillot, C., Navab, N. (eds.) MICCAI 2013. LNCS, vol. 8151, pp. 445–452. Springer, Heidelberg (2013). https://doi.org/10.1007/978-3-642-40760-4_56
19. Xu, Y., et al.: Efficient optic cup detection from intra-image learning with retinal structure priors. In: Ayache, N., Delingette, H., Golland, P., Mori, K. (eds.) MICCAI 2012. LNCS, vol. 7510, pp. 58–65. Springer, Heidelberg (2012). https://doi.org/10.1007/978-3-642-33415-3_8
20. Xu, Y., et al.: Sliding window and regression based cup detection in digital fundus images for glaucoma diagnosis. In: Fichtinger, G., Martel, A., Peters, T. (eds.) MICCAI 2011. LNCS, vol. 6893, pp. 1–8. Springer, Heidelberg (2011). https://doi.org/10.1007/978-3-642-23626-6_1
21. Yin, F., Liu, J., et al.: Model-based optic nerve head segmentation on retinal fundus images. In: EMBC, pp. 2626–2629. IEEE (2011)
22. Zhao, H., Shi, J., et al.: Pyramid scene parsing network. In: CVPR (2017)
23. Zilly, J., Buhmann, J.M., et al.: Glaucoma detection using entropy sampling and ensemble learning for automatic optic cup and disc segmentation. Comput. Med. Imaging Graph. **55**, 28–41 (2017)

# Biological Age Estimated from Retinal Imaging: A Novel Biomarker of Aging

Chi Liu[1,2], Wei Wang[1], Zhixi Li[1], Yu Jiang[1], Xiaotong Han[1], Jason Ha[3], Wei Meng[4], and Mingguang He[1,5,6(✉)]

[1] State Key Laboratory of Ophthalmology, Zhongshan Ophthalmic Center, Sun Yat-sen University, Guangzhou, China
mingguang_he@yahoo.com
[2] Department of Computer Science, University of Technology Sydney, Sydney, Australia
[3] Faculty of Medicine, Nursing and Health Sciences, Monash University, Clayton, Australia
[4] Guangzhou Healgoo Interactive Medical Technology Co. Ltd., Guangzhou, China
[5] Ophthalmology, Department of Surgery, University of Melbourne, Melbourne, Australia
[6] Centre for Eye Research Australia, Melbourne, Australia

**Abstract.** Biological age (BA) is widely introduced as a biomarker of aging, which can indicate the individual difference underlying the aging progress objectively. Recently, a new type of BA - 'brain age' predicted from brain neuroimaging has been proved to be a novel effective biomarker of aging. The retina is considered to share anatomical and physiological similarities with the brain, and rich information related with aging can be visualized non-invasively from retinal imaging. However, there are very few studies exploring BA estimation from retinal imaging. In this paper, we conducted a pilot study to explore the potential of using fundus images to estimate BA. Modeling the BA estimation as a multi-classification problem, we developed a convolutional neural network (CNN)-based classifier using 12,000 fundus images from healthy subjects. An image detail enhancement method was introduced for global anatomical and physiological features enhancement. A joint loss function with label distribution and error tolerance was proposed to improve the model performance in learning the time-continuous nature of aging within an acceptable range of ambiguity. The proposed methods were evaluated in healthy subjects from a clinical dataset based on the VGG-19 network. The optimal model achieved a mean absolute error of 3.73 years, outperforming existing 'brain age' models. An additional individual-based validation was conducted in another real-world dataset, which showed an increasing BA difference between healthy subjects and unhealthy subjects with aging. Results of our study indicate that retinal imaging–based BA could be potentially used as a novel candidate biomarker of aging.

© Springer Nature Switzerland AG 2019
D. Shen et al. (Eds.): MICCAI 2019, LNCS 11764, pp. 138–146, 2019.
https://doi.org/10.1007/978-3-030-32239-7_16

# 1 Introduction

Aging is a common risk factor for many common diseases, however, no universal biomarker for aging exists in current clinical practice [1]. The biological age (BA) of individual organs is now widely applied as an aging biomarker, which can help quantify the individual differences in senescence of a specific system or organ [2]. Recently, the rapid development of machine learning (ML)-based medical image understanding has heralded a novel type of BA – the BA of brain or 'brain age'. This type of BA was estimated principally from machine learning frameworks applied to magnetic resonance imaging (MRI) brain scans, and has been proved to be an effective biomarker for common age-related brain diseases [3, 4]. However, the utility of this BA is limited by the difficulty and cost associated with obtaining this MRI data.

The retina is considered to share anatomical and physiological similarities with the brain generally, arising from its development from the diencephalon during the embryonic period. Previous studies have found substantial correlations between retinal neuronal/vascular changes and age-related brain diseases such as dementia and stroke [5, 6]. These correlations make the 'retinal age' a plausible surrogate measure of BA. In addition, anatomical and physiological features of the retina can be visualized non-invasively using retinal imaging (e.g. fundus photography by the ocular fundus camera), which is more accessible and cost-effective compared with MRI. Therefore, it is worth exploring the effect of ML-based fundus image understanding for BA estimation.

However, despite the increasing promise of ML in fundus image-based eye disease classification [7], to the best of our knowledge, few studies have directly investigated BA estimation using fundus imaging. Poplin et al. [8] developed a deep convolutional neural network (CNN) to predict age from fundus images. But a considerable part of their training data was collected from unhealthy population (e.g., diabetes patients), thereby the predicted age could not be regarded as the gold standard of BA [2]. Generally speaking, three major challenges exist in fundus imaging-derived BA estimation: (1) The lack of specific features which could indicate aging on fundus images. Unlike eye diseases which can be characterized by pathological fundus lesions, the non-specific global anatomical and physiological features in fundus images are all relevant to aging, as suggested in the previous studies [5, 6]. (2) Compared with traditional disease classification models that divide the progression of disease into multiple discrete stages, aging is a gradual, time-continuous process which cannot be easily classified into isolated age stages. Each age stage is supposed to be associated with neighboring age stages. (3) With consideration to the progressive nature of aging, the age representation of a ML model should be 'ambiguous'. A model capable of tolerating a small margin of error is relatively more robust and practical. For example, the model is expected to describe an instance aged 50 years old as 'about 48 to 52' rather than 'exactly equaling to 50'.

To address the above challenges, in this paper, we conduct a pilot study of fundus image-based BA estimation using CNN. Specifically, we introduce an image detail manipulation method for global feature enhancement on fundus images. We also propose a joint loss function to deal with the difficulties of representing the progressive nature of aging and tolerating minor error in CNN modeling. Moreover, the proposed method are evaluated within the VGG-19 network [9] in an independent validation. The optimal model is further applied for an individual-based real-world validation in a clinical dataset. Our results show the effectiveness of 'retinal age' used as a potential biomarker for aging.

## 2　Method

In this study, the age estimation is formulated as a multi-class classification problem. Let $\chi = \{(X_i, y_i)\}_{i=1}^N, y_i \in \{1, \ldots, K\}$ be the training dataset, where $X_i$, $y_i$ denote the $i$-th fundus image and its corresponding age label; $K$, $N$ denote the total number of different age labels and images. For the $i$-th image $X_i$, the output of the model can be denoted as a $K$-dimensional vector $P_i = \{p_i^k\}_{k=1}^K$, where $p_i^k$ is the predicted probability of the class $k$.

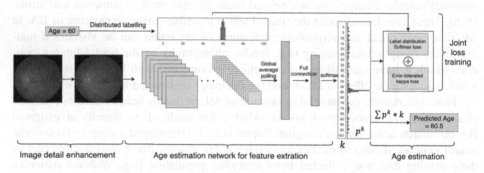

**Fig. 1.** The overview of the biological age estimation workflow

The overview of our approach is shown in Fig. 1. Firstly, the global feature representation of each image is improved by imposing the detail enhancement method, with the corresponding age label encoded by distributed labelling. A CNN is then constructed for high-dimensional feature extraction and outputs a $K$-dimensional probability vector through a softmax classifier. The proposed joint loss is embedded into the network to enable the model to be trained with label ambiguity and error-tolerance. The final BA of the $i$-th image is obtained by calculating the expected value over the softmax-normalized output probabilities as $BA_i = \sum_{k=1}^K p_i^k \cdot k$.

### 2.1　Image Detail Enhancement

Previous studies have suggested that the non-specific global anatomical and physiological features on fundus images are all relevant to aging plausibly [5, 6]. Therefore, the global detail enhancement of these features is important for model performance improvement. Hence, we introduce a detail manipulation method based on domain transform filtering [10] for global detail enhancement. Firstly, the source RGB image is converted into CIE Lab color space, in which the first channel $L$ represents the image lightness. Secondly, the domain transform filter is performed on $L$ iteratively to produce three progressively smoother versions, denoted as $\tilde{L}_0, \tilde{L}_1, \tilde{L}_2$, where $\tilde{L}_0 = L$. We follow the parameter setting of domain transform filter suggested in [10]. Thirdly, the manipulated lightness channel $L_{man}$ is obtained by

$$L_{man} = \tilde{L}_2 + S(\tilde{L}_1 - \tilde{L}_2) + S(\tilde{L}_0 - \tilde{L}_1), \tag{1}$$

where $S(\cdot)$ is the sigmoid function used for detail manipulation, and the inside subtraction results in the detail layer between two adjacent smooth versions of $L$. Lastly, $L_{man}$ is merged into the source image by replacing the original channel $L$, and the CIE Lab color space is then converted back to RGB.

The effectiveness of the detail enhancement method can be seen in Fig. 2 intuitively. As expected, there is considerable improvement in the quality of anatomical and physiological features such as blood vessels (even the barely visible microvessels in the source image) on the example fundus image.

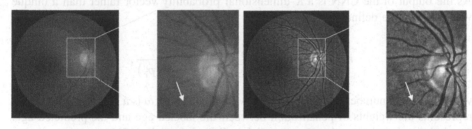

**Fig. 2.** A fundus image before/after detail enhancement, with a zoom-in region. The features have been well improved, even the micro ends of microvessels (green arrow). (Color figure online)

## 2.2   Joint Loss Function

The BA estimation model is expected to be capable of reflecting the time-continuous nature of aging with label ambiguity to some extent, as discussed in Sect. 1. In this section, we propose a joint loss function to address this particular need.

**Label Distribution Softmax Loss.** The softmax loss is a widely-used loss function for image classification. In most cases, the softmax loss is computed based on the one-hot encoding labelling, which encodes the source label into a sparse 0-1 vector of the dimension corresponding to the number of classes, where the target class is encoded as 1, otherwise 0. The one-hot encoding emphasizes the independence of different classes while ignoring the continuity of neighboring labels, which is crucial for representing the continuous and progressive nature of aging. Therefore, we propose a label distribution learning method inspired by [11]. The principle idea is to transform the one-hot values into a Gaussian distribution centered at the target age. Additionally, a double-boundary is imposed on the distribution to restrict the model attention to a limited age range. Consequently, the label distribution softmax loss is denoted as

$$\mathcal{L}_s(\chi) = -\frac{1}{N}\sum_{i=1}^{N}\sum_{k=1}^{K} d_i^k \log p_i^k, \tag{2}$$

where $d_i^k$ is the $k$-th dimension of the corresponding Gaussian label distribution for the age label $y_i$, defined as

$$d_i^k = \begin{cases} \frac{1}{\sigma\sqrt{2\pi Z}}\exp\left(-\frac{(k-y_i)^2}{2\sigma^2}\right), k \in [y_i - b, y_i + b] \\ 0, k \in [1, y_i - b) \cup (y_i + b, K] \end{cases}, \tag{3}$$

where $\sigma$ is the standard deviation of the distribution, $Z$ is a normalization factor to ensure $\sum_{k=1}^{K} d_i^k = 1$; $b$ is the age boundary around $y_i$, which is set as 2 in this study.

**Error-Tolerated Weighted Kappa Loss.** This loss function is derived from Cohen's Weighted Kappa $\kappa_\omega$, which is a measurement of the disagreement between two raters. As the output of the CNN is a $K$-dimensional probability vector rather than a unique value, $\kappa_\omega$ can be defined as

$$\kappa_\omega = 1 - \frac{\sum_{i=1}^{N}\sum_{k=1}^{K} \omega_{y_i,k} p_i^k}{\sum_{m=1}^{K}\frac{N_m}{N}\sum_{n=1}^{K}\left(\omega_{m,n}\sum_{i=1}^{N} p_i^n\right)}, \tag{4}$$

where $N_m$ is the number of image samples with age label $m$. $\omega$ is a $K \times K$ matrix which represents the weights of penalization between the labeled age and the predicted age. The index pair indicates the corresponding cell in the matrix [12].

This loss function aims to improve the robustness of the model in a real-world setting by tolerating errors within an acceptable range. Moreover, during the training stage, the penalization of misclassification should be increased with higher error levels, rather than staying constant. For instance, the penalization of misclassifying an age of 60 years as 65 years should be larger than when misclassified as 62 years. Therefore, we propose a novel weight matrix with $\varepsilon$-level error tolerance, denoted as

$$\omega_{m,n} = \begin{cases} \frac{(m-n)^2}{K^2}, |m - n| > \varepsilon \\ 0, |m - n| \le \varepsilon \end{cases}, \tag{5}$$

which means that no penalization is imposed when the classification error is less than $\varepsilon$, otherwise the penalization increases with the error degree. In this study, $\varepsilon$ is set as 2.

As a larger $\kappa_\omega$ represents greater accuracy of the BA estimation, the optimization of $\kappa_\omega$ is a typical maximization problem, while the loss function optimization is generally modeled as a minimization problem. Thus, the loss function is rewritten as

$$\mathcal{L}_\kappa(\chi) = \log(1 - \kappa_\omega), \tag{6}$$

Note that the logarithm transformation is involved to enhance the penalization.

**Joint Loss Function.** Consequently, based on the label distribution softmax loss and the error tolerated weighted Kappa loss, the overall joint loss is given as follows,

$$\mathcal{L}_{overall}(\chi) = \lambda\mathcal{L}_s(\chi) + (1 - \lambda)\mathcal{L}_\kappa(\chi), \tag{7}$$

where $\lambda$ is the trade-off factor between $\mathcal{L}_s(\chi)$ and $\mathcal{L}_\kappa(\chi)$, and is set as 0.9 in this study.

## 3   Experiment Setup and Results

### 3.1   Data and Implementation Detail

Two datasets from two independent eye studies in China: the Yangxi Eye Study [13] and the Shenzhen Eye Study, which enrolled 5825 and 2911 adults aged 50 years or older in Yangxi and Shenzhen, Guangdong respectively, were included in our experiment, and named as Yangxi Dataset and Shenzhen Dataset. At least one 45-degree fundus image was obtained from each eye of the study subjects using multiple types of fundus cameras. As the appropriateness of BA is normally assessed in reference to the chronological age of healthy people [2], the models were trained on 12000 random selected images of healthy subjects from the Yangxi Dataset (healthy was defined as the absence of common systemic diseases, as substantiated by clinical examination records and questionnaires), using a six-fold cross validation protocol. The cross validation was performed at the patient level guided by individual ID to ensure that all images from the same patient were allocate to at most one subset per cross. Two independent validations were conducted. One was performed in healthy subjects solely in the Yangxi Dataset for models comparison, while the other one was performed in both healthy and unhealthy subjects in the Shenzhen Dataset as a clinical validation for real-world BA estimation. Details of the datasets are shown in Table 1.

**Table 1.** Details of the two datasets.

| Dataset | Allocation | Health condition | Images | Subjects | Age range (yrs.) | Age mean (±SD, yrs.) |
|---------|-----------|------------------|--------|----------|------------------|----------------------|
| Yangxi dataset | Training | Healthy | 12000 | – | 50–94 | 65.06 (±9.78) |
|  | validation | Healthy | 2016 | – | 50–94 | 64.81 (±9.81) |
| Shenzhen dataset | Clinical | Healthy | 1692 | 1132 (38.88%) | 50–73 | 53.63 (±4.08) |
|  | validation | Unhealthy | 4373 | 1779 (61.11%) | 50–93 | 59.55 (±8.49) |

One of the state-of-the-art CNN architectures - VGG-19 [9] was involved for network construction, initialized with the weights pre-trained in the ImageNet dataset. All input images were cropped with retaining the main color area of retinal fundus, then resized to 299 × 299 after image detail enhancement. The batch size, learning rate, weight decay and momentums were set as 64, 0.001, 0.008 and 0.9 respectively for weights optimization using mini-batch gradient descent algorithm. To avoid overfitting, the final model was achieved when the training performance stopped improving for consecutive 30 epochs during each training period. The models were implemented by Keras v2.2.4 and trained within two NVIDIA GeForce Titan X 12 GB processors. Mean Absolute Error (MAE) and Cumulative Score (CS) were used for model performance evaluation, denoted as

$$MAE = \frac{1}{N} \sum_{i=1}^{N} |y_i - BA_i|, \tag{8}$$

$$CS(t) = \frac{1}{N} \sum_{i=1}^{N} [|y_i - BA_i| \le t], \tag{9}$$

In Eq. (9), $t$ is the threshold of error level between the predicted BA and the age label. $[\cdot]$ is the truth-test operator equalling 1 if the inner condition is true, otherwise 0.

## 3.2    Validations Results

We firstly analyzed the effectiveness of our proposed methods in the Yangxi Dataset by a four-step ablation experiment, including the original network, the network with image detail enhancement, the network with image detail enhancement and Gaussian label distribution loss, as well as the network with image detail enhancement and joint loss. The results are shown in Table 2. An increasing trend in model performance was observed with the successive addition of different methods to the network. The final network with image detail enhancement and joint loss achieved a MAE of 3.73 years and a CS ($t = 2$) of 0.396, which is significantly superior to the original network, as well as the recently proposed MRI-derived 'brain ages' in terms of MAE [3, 4]. Compared with the single label distribution loss, the joint loss model performed much better in terms of CS, but similarly or even worse in terms of MAE. That is likely because the error-tolerated Kappa loss in the joint loss is able to improve the model robustness by accepting minor errors, which may compromise the overall MAE performance to some extent. The effect of different methods in the ablation experiment can be seen more directly in the CS curves, as show in Fig. 3(a). The network with image detail enhancement and joint loss outperformed the other methods at all error levels. Note that the biggest difference occurred at the error level of 2 years, which was due to the pre-set error tolerance $\varepsilon$ of 2 in the joint loss.

**Table 2.**  Results of different methods in the Yangxi Dataset (Network = VGG-19 network).

| Methods | Age range (yrs.) | MAE (yrs.) | CS ($t = 2$) |
|---|---|---|---|
| Brain age 1 [3] | 18–90 | 5.02 | – |
| Brain age 2 [4] | 18–90 | 4.16–5.14 | – |
| Network | 50–94 | 4.13 | 0.319 |
| Network + DE | 50–94 | 3.85 | 0.353 |
| Network + DE + GL | 50–94 | **3.67** | 0.353 |
| Network + DE + JL | 50–94 | 3.73 | **0.396** |

In order to evaluate the effectiveness of introducing retinal imaging-based BA as a biomarker of aging, we applied the final BA model (VGG-19 with image detail enhancement and joint loss) in the Shenzhen Dataset for real-world validation. Subjects were divided into the healthy and unhealthy groups, and the BA model was performed in the two groups independently. Given that at least one image was obtained from each eye, the final individual BA was calculated as the mean of BAs predicted from all included images from the same subject. The MAE was 3.39 years and 4.21 years in the healthy group and unhealthy group respectively, showing a statistically significant difference (the p-value was less than 0.001 in hypothesis test). For an intuitive representation of the result, we provided the scatterplots with best-fit lines computed by linear regression for the predicted BA in each group, as show in Fig. 3(b). An increasing difference between two groups with aging can be observed.

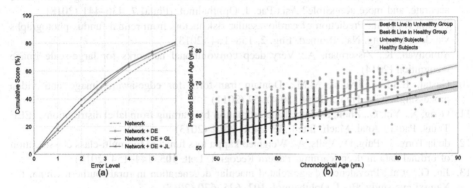

**Fig. 3.** (a) Cumulative score curves of different methods in the Yangxi Dataset. Network = VGG-19 network. DE = image detail enhancement. GL = Gaussian label distribution loss. JL = joint loss. (b) Scatterplots of the predicted biological age (BA) of healthy and unhealthy groups in the real-world clinical validation experiment in the Shenzhen Dataset. The regression lines show the increasing BA difference with aging.

## 4   Conclusion

We proposed a CNN framework for BA estimation from retinal imaging, in which image detail enhancement was introduced for global feature improvement, and a joint loss function was proposed to improve the model robustness in reflecting the time-continuous nature of aging. Our model demonstrated effectiveness in two independent datasets and could further demonstrate statistically significant BA difference between healthy and unhealthy subjects in real-world validation. The overall MAE of the proposed retinal imaging-derived BA was lower than the recently reported 'brain age'. Results of our study indicate that retinal imaging–derived BA could be used as a novel effective biomarker of aging.

# References

1. Wagner, K.H., Cameron-Smith, D., Wessner, B., Franzke, B.: Biomarkers of aging: from function to molecular biology. Nutrients **8**, 338 (2016)
2. Jia, L., Zhang, W., Chen, X.: Common methods of biological age estimation. Clin. Interv. Aging **12**, 759–772 (2017)
3. Cole, J.H., et al.: Brain age predicts mortality. Mol. Psychiatry **23**, 1385–1392 (2018)
4. Cole, J.H., et al.: Predicting brain age with deep learning from raw imaging data results in a reliable and heritable biomarker. NeuroImage **163**, 115–124 (2017)
5. London, A., Benhar, I., Schwartz, M.: The retina as a window to the brain—from eye research to CNS disorders. Nat. Rev. Neurol. **9**, 44 (2012)
6. Cheung, C.Y., Ikram, M.K., Chen, C., Wong, T.Y.: Imaging retina to study dementia and stroke. Prog. Retin. Eye Res. **57**, 89–107 (2017)
7. Li, Z., Keel, S., Liu, C., Hc, M.: Can artificial intelligence make screening faster, more accurate, and more accessible? Asia Pac. J. Ophthalmol. (Phila) **7**, 436–441 (2018)
8. Poplin, R., et al.: Prediction of cardiovascular risk factors from retinal fundus photographs via deep learning. Nat. Biomed. Eng. **2**, 158–164 (2018)
9. Simonyan, K., Zisserman, A.: Very deep convolutional networks for large-scale image recognition (2014)
10. Gastal, E.S.L., Oliveira, M.M.: Domain transform for edge-aware image and video processing. ACM Trans. Graph. **30**(4), 69 (2011)
11. Geng, X., Yin, C., Zhou, Z.: Facial age estimation by learning from label distributions. IEEE Trans. Pattern Anal. Mach. Intell. **35**, 2401–2412 (2013)
12. de la Torre, J., Puig, D., Valls, A.: Weighted kappa loss function for multi-class classification of ordinal data in deep learning. Pattern Recognit. Lett. **105**, 144–154 (2018)
13. Jin, G., et al.: Prevalence of age-related macular degeneration in rural southern China: the Yangxi eye study. Br. J. Ophthalmol. **102**, 625–630 (2018)

# Task Adaptive Metric Space for Medium-Shot Medical Image Classification

Xiang Jiang[1,2](✉) [iD], Liqiang Ding[2] [iD], Mohammad Havaei[2] [iD],
Andrew Jesson[2] [iD], and Stan Matwin[1] [iD]

[1] Dalhousie University, Halifax, Canada
{xiang.jiang,stan}@dal.ca
[2] Imagia Inc., Montreal, Canada
{liqiang.ding,mohammad,andrew.jesson}@imagia.com

**Abstract.** In the medical domain, one challenge of deep learning is to
build sample-efficient models from a small number of labeled data. In
recent years, meta-learning has become an important approach to few-
shot image classification. However, current research on meta-learning
focuses on learning from a few examples; we propose to extend few-
shot learning to medium-shot to evaluate medical classification tasks
in a more realistic setup. We build a baseline evaluation procedure by
analyzing two representative meta-learning methods through the lens of
bias-variance tradeoff, and propose to fuse the two techniques for better
bias-variance equilibrium. The proposed method, Task Adaptive Metric
Space (TAMS), fine-tunes parameters of a metric space to represent medical data in a more semantically meaningful way. Our empirical studies
suggest that TAMS outperforms other baselines. Visualizations on the
metric space show TAMS leads to better-separated clusters. Our baselines and evaluation procedure of the proposed TAMS opens the door to
more research on medium-shot medical image classification.

**Keywords:** Meta-learning · Image classification · Medium-shot
learning

## 1 Introduction

Learning new concepts from a small number of examples is an essential ability of
human cognition. While deep learning models typically require a large number
of labeled examples, datasets in the medical imaging domain tend to have a limited number of training examples. Efforts towards more sample-efficient training

---

X. Jiang, L. Ding—Equal contribution.

---

**Electronic supplementary material** The online version of this chapter (https://
doi.org/10.1007/978-3-030-32239-7_17) contains supplementary material, which is
available to authorized users.

© Springer Nature Switzerland AG 2019
D. Shen et al. (Eds.): MICCAI 2019, LNCS 11764, pp. 147–155, 2019.
https://doi.org/10.1007/978-3-030-32239-7_17

procedures address this data hindrance, thereby enabling the wider use of deep learning techniques for medical applications.

Meta-learning [1,8,10,13], or "learning to learn", is an important approach to few-shot classification. The meta-learner is trained across many tasks to acquire meta-knowledge with the goal of learning a new task with few labeled examples. Despite the recent popularity of meta-learning, we find two main limitations in applying meta-learning to medical image classification tasks.

The first limitation is the discrepancy of the number of training examples between few-shot tasks and medical datasets. While in the literature meta-learning mostly deals with tasks with only a few training examples, i.e., five or fewer, datasets in the medical domain tend to have tens to a few hundred labeled examples. This discrepancy necessitates the extension from few-shot learning to *medium-shot* for more realistic evaluations on the medical domain.

The second limitation is the lack of meta-learning evaluation procedures on medical datasets. We propose to evaluate representative meta-learning methods under different amounts of data per class, to better understand their generalization properties. We choose key advances in meta-learning—*gradient-based* [2] and *metric-based* [12] methods—to establish the baseline performances.

We empirically evaluate and analyze the baseline meta-learning methods through the lens of bias-variance tradeoff. Our analysis suggests gradient-based methods tend to overfit few-shot datasets while metric-based methods tend to underfit medium-shot datasets. To get the best of both worlds for bias-variance equilibrium, we propose Task Adaptive Metric Space (TAMS) that uses gradient-based fine-tuning to adjust parameters of the metric space so that distances between examples in the medical dataset can better reflect their semantics. We show that our proposed model outperforms gradient-based and metric-based meta-learning models on a medical image classification task. We report visualizations on the metric space that validates the impacts of metric adaptation.

Our main contributions are three-fold: (1) We propose *medium-shot learning* that aligns meta-learning with realistic situations of medical image classification. (2) We establish baseline evaluation procedures to evaluate meta-learners on various situations to better understand their generalization properties. (3) Through bias-variance analysis, we propose a new meta-learning method—Task Adaptive Metric Space—that takes advantage of both gradient-based and metric-based methods. We show that TAMS outperforms the meta-learning baselines.

## 2   Background and Motivation

*Medium-Shot Learning for Medical Data.* Medical datasets raise many practical challenges especially because they tend to have tens to a few hundred labeled examples [6]. The size of medical datasets does not align with the prevalent approaches in few-shot learning that only focus on five or fewer training examples per class. For this reason, we propose *medium-shot* learning with the intention of more realistic assessments in the medical domain. We define "medium-shot" as classification tasks with tens to a few hundred labeled examples each class.

*Overview of Meta-learning.* The goal of meta-learning is to acquire meta-knowledge from many tasks to help better learn a new task. In recent years, meta-learning has become an important approach for few-shot learning [14]. A meta-learning system first aims to *meta-train* the meta-learner from $\mathcal{D}_{\text{meta}-\text{train}}$, which is composed of many classification tasks $\mathcal{D}_i \in \mathcal{D}_{\text{meta}-\text{train}}$ and each task can be further split into a training and test set $(\mathcal{D}_{\text{train}}, \mathcal{D}_{\text{test}}) \in \mathcal{D}$. Once the meta-learner is trained, we *meta-test* a new task $\mathcal{D}_{\text{meta}-\text{test}}$ using the meta-learned inductive bias in the form of weight initializations or a metric space. We discuss two representative meta-learning methods through the lens of bias-variance tradeoff [3].

*Gradient-Based Meta-learning.* Gradient-based methods, such as Model-Agnostic Meta-Learning (MAML) [2], aim to optimize representations for fast adaptation across many tasks. The meta-learned knowledge is encoded through parameter initializations to support fast adaptation when fine-tuned on $\mathcal{D}_{\text{meta}-\text{test}}$. In the medical domain, MAML has been explored in breast screening classification to meta-learn initializations with curriculum learning [7]. Gradient-based methods tend to have a low bias and high variance. They can take advantage of more data to better adapt model representations towards a new task. However, gradient-based methods are more complex and may overfit because the fine-tuning procedure updates all parameters to adapt to $\mathcal{D}_{\text{meta}-\text{test}}$.

*Metric-Based Meta-learning.* Metric-based methods, such as Prototypical Networks [12], learn a metric space across many tasks such that distances between examples are semantically meaningful. The metric space is parameterized with a neural network meta-trained on $\mathcal{D}_{\text{meta}-\text{train}}$. At meta-test time, each class is represented by a prototype in the metric space, and classification labels are assigned with distance-based inference. Metric-based methods tend to have high bias and low variance. An advantage of metric-based methods is their non-parametric classification procedure that prevents overfitting on a few examples, but their static metric space may result in underfitting when more data is available.

*The Best of Both Worlds.* The bias-variance tradeoff [3] tells us that the gradient-based and metric-based methods complement each other with different amounts of training data. In TAMS, we fuse these methods and demonstrate the improved generalization under several setups, which is congruent with out intuition.

# 3  Task Adaptive Metric Space for Improved Medium-Shot Generalization

We propose Task Adaptive Metric Space (TAMS) to exploit the inherent expressiveness of gradient-based methods and the non-parametric property of metric-based methods. We note that TAMS is built upon a metric space that is meta-trained using Prototypical Networks [12] on $\mathcal{D}_{\text{meta}-\text{train}}$, and we focus

on how to adapt the meta-learned metric space to better fit the medical classi-
fication task $(\mathcal{D}_{\text{train}}, \mathcal{D}_{\text{test}}) \in \mathcal{D}_{\text{meta-test}}$. The metric space $f_\phi$ is initialized with
meta-learned parameters from $\mathcal{D}_{\text{meta-train}}$ prior to task adaptive fine-tuning
on $\mathcal{D}_{\text{meta-test}}$.

*Partition the Training Set* $\mathcal{D}_{\text{train}}$. Prototypical networks use all training data
to construct prototypes and the training examples are never evaluated against
their labels, hence *cannot* provide a loss function to estimate the quality of the
metric space. However, for metric fine-tuning, we need to quantify the extent to
which the metric space fits $\mathcal{D}_{\text{train}}$ to penalize errors and to improve the metric
space. To address this, we propose to randomly partition the training examples
into disjoint sets: $\mathcal{D}_{\text{train}}^{\text{prototype}}$ for computing a prototype for each class and $\mathcal{D}_{\text{train}}^{\text{predict}}$
for assessing the quality of the prototypes. This provides an evaluation measure
that estimates how suitable the metric is for the training data, which further
allows us to fine-tune the metric space to better represent the medical dataset.

*Construct Prototypes from* $\mathcal{D}_{\text{train}}^{\text{prototype}}$. Prototypical networks reduce the training
data into points $\mathbf{c}_t$ on the metric space as prototypical representations of class
$t$. We only use $\mathcal{D}_{\text{train}}^{\text{prototype}}$ to construct $\mathbf{c}_t = \frac{1}{K} \sum_{(\mathbf{x}_i, y_i) \in \mathcal{D}_{\text{train}}^{\text{prototype}}} \mathbb{1}_{\{y_i=t\}} f_\phi(\mathbf{x}_i)$,
where $K$ denotes the number of examples for class $t$, $\mathbb{1}_{\{y_i=t\}}$ denotes an indicator
function of $y_i$ which takes value 1 when $y_i = t$ and 0 otherwise. The metric space
is parameterized by $\phi$ in the form of a convolutional or a residual network.

*Make Predictions on* $\mathcal{D}_{\text{train}}^{\text{predict}}$. We evaluate the prototypes $\mathbf{c}_t$ on $\mathcal{D}_{\text{train}}^{\text{predict}}$ to
estimate the quality of the metric space for the medical image classification
task. To obtain the prediction labels, each example $\mathbf{x} \in \mathcal{D}_{\text{train}}^{\text{predict}}$ is first mapped
to $f_\phi(\mathbf{x})$ on the metric space, then being classified based on its relative distances
with each prototype $\mathbf{c}_t$, according to the distance function $d$:

$$p(y = t|\mathbf{x}) = \frac{\exp(-d(f_\phi(\mathbf{x}), \mathbf{c}_t))}{\sum_{t'} \exp(-d(f_\phi(\mathbf{x}), \mathbf{c}_{t'}))}. \tag{1}$$

*Loss for Metric Fine-Tuning.* We use the cross-entropy loss to evaluate the
predictions on the medical dataset $\mathcal{D}_{\text{train}}^{\text{predict}}$. The loss can be reinterpreted as a
maximum-likelihood objective that aims at minimizing the distance between an
example and its corresponding class centroid while maximizing its distance to
other class centroids [12].

*Make Predictions on* $\mathcal{D}_{\text{test}}$. With the task-adapted metric space on $\mathcal{D}_{\text{train}}$, we
can make predictions on the testing data $\mathcal{D}_{\text{test}}$. Unlike the metric fine-tuning
step that constructs prototypes from $\mathcal{D}_{\text{train}}^{\text{prototype}}$, in this prediction step, we use
all training examples in $\mathcal{D}_{\text{train}}$ to represent the prototypes. We use the same
distance-based classifier as Eq. (1) on $\mathcal{D}_{\text{test}}$ as final predictions on the test data.

To summarize, TAMS adapts a meta-learned metric space to better represent medical data. This improves medium-shot generalization in spite of domain
difference between $\mathcal{D}_{\text{meta-train}}$ and $\mathcal{D}_{\text{meta-test}}$ which would otherwise be challenging for current meta-learning methods. TAMS constitutes a natural bridge

between gradient-based and metric-based methods. In few-shot situations, the non-parametric classification procedure prevents our model from overfitting. In medium-shot situations, fine-tuning the metric space exploits the expressive richness of gradient-based methods to fit the target medical classification task better.

## 4    Empirical Results

### 4.1    Data and Evaluation Setup

The experiments first pre-train a model with meta-learning or transfer learning on $\mathcal{D}_{meta-train}$, then evaluate the generalization properties on the target meta-test dataset $\mathcal{D}_{meta-test}$, i.e., the target medical classification task.

*Meta-train Dataset.* We use *mini*ImageNet [9,14]—a standard meta-learning dataset—as $\mathcal{D}_{meta-train}$. Because the goal of this paper is to propose TAMS and evaluate it against other meta-learning baselines in unseen domains, we do not incorporate other medical datasets in meta-training.

**Table 1.** OCT test accuracy with "conv4" architecture (%)

| Shots | Proto | 16 gradient steps | | | | 32 gradient steps | | | |
|---|---|---|---|---|---|---|---|---|---|
| | | Scratch | Transfer | MAML | TAMS | Scratch | Transfer | MAML | TAMS |
| 1 | **28.18** | 25.72 | 26.97 | 27.80 | — | 25.88 | 26.93 | 27.84 | — |
| 2 | 33.14 | 27.58 | 28.93 | 33.63 | 32.13 | 27.78 | 29.05 | **34.04** | 32.02 |
| 4 | 35.51 | 26.84 | 30.31 | 33.12 | 37.34 | 27.62 | 31.20 | 33.93 | **37.80** |
| 8 | 40.93 | 29.37 | 34.52 | 38.00 | **42.73** | 30.11 | 36.27 | 38.50 | 42.49 |
| 16 | 41.53 | 32.83 | 40.27 | 42.29 | 47.55 | 34.75 | 41.98 | 44.27 | **48.07** |
| 32 | 46.38 | 35.72 | 41.97 | 43.23 | 53.71 | 38.25 | 45.32 | 45.45 | **53.74** |
| 64 | 48.20 | 38.84 | 44.49 | 44.91 | 56.30 | 42.45 | 48.48 | 48.59 | **57.51** |
| 128 | 49.17 | 43.45 | 47.95 | 48.68 | 57.53 | 48.62 | 52.84 | 54.35 | **60.55** |
| 250 | 49.80 | 46.89 | 50.28 | 50.00 | 60.83 | 53.72 | 57.34 | 57.65 | **63.57** |

*Meta-test Dataset.* We use Optical Coherence Tomography (OCT) [4] as $\mathcal{D}_{meta-test}$. OCT aims to classify each image into one of the four classes: NORMAL, CNV, DME, DRUSEN. We created our train-test split that consists of up to 250 examples per class as $\mathcal{D}_{train}$, and 250 examples per class as $\mathcal{D}_{test}$. We include more details about data statistics and preprocessing in the supplementary material.

*Evaluation Setup.* To examine the impact of training data on model performance, we vary the number of training examples and use 1 to 250 examples per class as training data $\mathcal{D}_{train}$. All experiments are repeated ten times with controlled random seeds. In terms of model architectures, we first evaluate different methods with a standard meta-learning architecture: "conv4"—a 4-layer convolutional network. We then experiment with "resnet12", a 12-layer residual network, to assess the impact of added model capacity.

*Baselines.* We use the following transfer learning and meta-learning baselines:

1. "Scratch": a basic model that trains $\mathcal{D}_{train}$ from random initialization.
2. "Transfer": a transfer learning baseline where the model is pre-trained on $mini$ImageNet, and then fine-tuned on $\mathcal{D}_{train}$.
3. "MAML": a gradient-based meta-learning baseline that meta-trains MAML parameters on $mini$ImageNet, and fine-tunes on $\mathcal{D}_{train}$.
4. "Proto": a metric-based prototypical network meta-trained on $mini$ImageNet.

## 4.2   Results and Discussions

Table 1 summarizes the test accuracies on OCT with various shots per class. All models use "conv4" architecture, and the accuracy is averaged over ten runs.

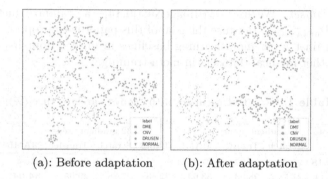

(a): Before adaptation          (b): After adaptation

**Fig. 1.** t-SNE visualization of sampled test data on "resnet12" metric space.

*Transfer Learning and Gradient-Based Meta-learning.* We first investigate the impact of transfer learning and gradient-based meta-learning by comparing "Scratch" with "Transfer" and "MAML". The three methods only differ in parameter initialization: "Scratch" is randomly initialized, "Transfer" is initialized from a pre-trained classifier, and "MAML" is initialized from meta-learned parameters. In Table 1, under the same number of gradient steps, we find "Transfer" and "MAML" perform better than "Scratch" because of better parameter initializations. We also find "MAML" works better than "Scratch" and "Transfer" when shots are less than 32 because "MAML" is optimized for few-shot learning.

*The Bias-Variance Tradeoff.* As a critical motivation to TAMS, we highlight the bias-variance tradeoff by comparing "MAML" with "Transfer" and "Proto". In few-shot scenarios, as shown in Table 1, "Proto" outperforms "Transfer" and "MAML" under 1, 4 and 8 shots, even after "Transfer" and "MAML" are fine-tuned with more gradient steps. This suggests gradient-based methods tend to overfit in few-shot. However, as we increase the number of training examples, we find that "MAML" with 32 gradient steps outperforms "Proto" at 16, 64, 128 and 250 shots, suggesting metric-based methods tend to underfit in medium-shot.

*The Effect of Metric Adaptation.* To validate the effectiveness of our proposed method, we compare TAMS with all baseline methods under the same number of gradient steps. Table 1 shows that TAMS achieves the best test accuracy in most cases. Take 128-shot classification as an example, under 32 gradient steps, TAMS outperforms MAML by 6% and outperforms Proto by 10%. This suggests TAMS achieves better bias-variance equilibrium, alleviating the overfitting of gradient-based methods while preventing underfitting of metric-based methods. Figure 1 shows testing examples projected on the metric space before and after metric adaptation. While examples from different classes are mixed before metric adaptation, TAMS results in well-separated clusters that reflect their labels. This confirms that TAMS is capable of adjusting parameters of the metric space to better represent examples in semantically meaningful ways. Furthermore, TAMS is efficient to train as it requires a small number of gradient steps.

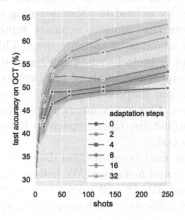

Fig. 2. Metric adaptation steps.

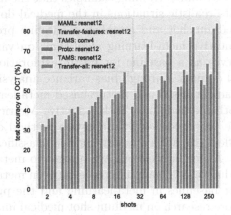

Fig. 3. Impact of model architecture.

*The Impact of Metric Adaptation Steps.* Figure 2 shows the impact of metric adaptation steps on the test accuracy. We find that a few adaptations steps are sufficient in few-shot, but more adaptations steps are needed in medium-shot.

*The Impact of Model Capacity.* As an ablation study, we investigate the impact of model capacity on different meta-learners. We have the following findings from Fig. 3: (i) With respect to metric adaptation, TAMS improves dramatically as the model capacity increases from "conv4" to "resnet12". We also highlight the improved performance over "Proto" and "MAML" brought by our proposed TAMS. (ii) Concerning different transfer learning approaches, we find transfer learning without updating the features on the new task—"Transfer-features"— does not work well. This difference can be attributed to the domain difference between $\mathcal{D}_{meta-train}$ and $\mathcal{D}_{meta-test}$ and the need for the model to adjust its feature representations to better fit $\mathcal{D}_{meta-test}$. (iii) We find the transfer learning method "Transfer-all", that fine-tunes both feature representations and the classifier, performs best with "resnet12". We find the transfer learning method "Transfer-all", that fine-tunes both feature representations and the classifier, performs best with "resnet12". Despite this, we highlight that the proposed TAMS greatly outperforms other meta-learning methods indicating the exciting potential of metric-adaptive meta-learning. We believe better metric loss functions, such as contrastive loss [5] and triplet loss [11], could further improve the performance of TAMS for better medium-shot medical image classification.

Due to page limits, we include more empirical results in supplementary materials.

## 5    Conclusions and Future Work

With this paper, we hope to draw the attention of the medical imaging community to the rich field of meta-learning, which offers feasible solutions to situations of the limited training examples that the field is often faced with. To better evaluate realistic situations in the medical domain, we extend few-shot learning to medium-shot and establish a baseline procedure that aims to evaluate representative meta-learning algorithms on various amounts of training data. This serves as a baseline for future explorations using meta-learning in the medical domain. Through bias-variance analysis, we identify complementary roles of gradient-based and metric-based meta-learning and propose to fuse the best of both methods into Task Adaptive Metric Space. Our experiments reveal that the proposed metric adaptation method can adjust the metric space to better reflect examples of a new medical classification task.

As for future work, we suggest to meta-train models on medical datasets to reduce the domain difference between meta-train and meta-test. We believe that our baselines in meta-learning and the proposed TAMS will open the door to more research on medium-shot medical image classification, to better unlock the potential of deep learning.

**Acknowledgement.** The authors thank Tanya Nair, Martine Bertrand and the Imagia team for their support. XJ acknowledges the support of NVIDIA Corporation with the donation of the Titan X GPU used for this research.

## References

1. Bengio, S., Bengio, Y., Cloutier, J., Gecsei, J.: On the optimization of a synaptic learning rule. In: Preprints Conference on Optimality in Artificial and Biological Neural Networks, pp. 6–8. University of Texas (1992)
2. Finn, C., Abbeel, P., Levine, S.: Model-agnostic meta-learning for fast adaptation of deep networks. In: International Conference on Machine Learning, pp. 1126–1135 (2017)
3. Friedman, J., Hastie, T., Tibshirani, R.: The Elements of Statistical Learning. Springer Series in Statistics, vol. 1. Springer, New York (2001). https://doi.org/10.1007/978-0-387-21606-5
4. Kermany, D.S., et al.: Identifying medical diagnoses and treatable diseases by image-based deep learning. Cell **172**(5), 1122–1131 (2018)

5. Koch, G., Zemel, R., Salakhutdinov, R.: Siamese neural networks for one-shot image recognition. In: ICML Deep Learning Workshop, vol. 2 (2015)
6. Litjens, G., et al.: A survey on deep learning in medical image analysis. Med. Image Anal. **42**, 60–88 (2017)
7. Maicas, G., Bradley, A.P., Nascimento, J.C., Reid, I., Carneiro, G.: Training medical image analysis systems like radiologists. In: Frangi, A.F., Schnabel, J.A., Davatzikos, C., Alberola-López, C., Fichtinger, G. (eds.) MICCAI 2018. LNCS, vol. 11070, pp. 546–554. Springer, Cham (2018). https://doi.org/10.1007/978-3-030-00928-1_62
8. Mitchell, T.M., Thrun, S.B.: Explanation-based neural network learning for robot control. In: Advances in Neural Information Processing Systems, pp. 287–294 (1993)
9. Ravi, S., Larochelle, H.: Optimization as a model for few-shot learning (2016)
10. Schmidhuber, J.: Evolutionary principles in self-referential learning. On learning now to learn: the meta-meta-meta...-hook. Diploma thesis, Technische Universitat Munchen, Germany, 14 May 1987. http://www.idsia.ch/~juergen/diploma.html
11. Schroff, F., Kalenichenko, D., Philbin, J.: FaceNet: a unified embedding for face recognition and clustering. In: Proceedings of the IEEE Conference on Computer Vision and Pattern Recognition, pp. 815–823 (2015)
12. Snell, J., Swersky, K., Zemel, R.S.: Prototypical networks for few-shot learning. CoRR abs/1703.05175 (2017). arXiv:1703.05175
13. Vilalta, R., Drissi, Y.: A perspective view and survey of meta-learning. Artif. Intell. Rev. **18**(2), 77–95 (2002)
14. Vinyals, O., Blundell, C., Lillicrap, T., Wierstra, D., et al.: Matching networks for one shot learning. In: Advances in Neural Information Processing Systems, pp. 3630–3638 (2016)

# Two-Stream CNN with Loose Pair Training for Multi-modal AMD Categorization

Weisen Wang[1,2,3], Zhiyan Xu[4,5], Weihong Yu[4,5], Jianchun Zhao[3],
Jingyuan Yang[4,5], Feng He[4,5], Zhikun Yang[4,5], Di Chen[4,5], Dayong Ding[3],
Youxin Chen[4,5], and Xirong Li[1,2,3(✉)]

[1] MOE Key Lab of DEKE, Renmin University of China, Beijing, China
xirong@ruc.edu.cn
[2] AI & Media Computing Lab, School of Information,
Renmin University of China, Beijing, China
[3] Vistel AI Lab, Visionary Intelligence Ltd., Beijing, China
[4] Key Lab of Ocular Fundus Disease, Chinese Academy of Medical Sciences,
Beijing, China
[5] Department of Ophthalmology, Peking Union Medical College Hospital,
Beijing, China

**Abstract.** This paper studies automated categorization of age-related macular degeneration (AMD) given a multi-modal input, which consists of a color fundus image and an optical coherence tomography (OCT) image from a specific eye. Previous work uses a traditional method, comprised of feature extraction and classifier training that cannot be optimized jointly. By contrast, we propose a two-stream convolutional neural network (CNN) that is end-to-end. The CNN's fusion layer is tailored to the need of fusing information from the fundus and OCT streams. For generating more multi-modal training instances, we introduce Loose Pair training, where a fundus image and an OCT image are paired based on class labels rather than eyes. Moreover, for a visual interpretation of how the individual modalities make contributions, we extend the class activation mapping technique to the multi-modal scenario. Experiments on a real-world dataset collected from an outpatient clinic justify the viability of our proposal for multi-modal AMD categorization.

**Keywords:** AMD categorization · Multi-modal · Fundus · OCT · Two-stream CNN

W. Wang, Z. Xu and W. Yu—Equal Contribution.

**Electronic supplementary material** The online version of this chapter (https://doi.org/10.1007/978-3-030-32239-7_18) contains supplementary material, which is available to authorized users.

D. Shen et al. (Eds.): MICCAI 2019, LNCS 11764, pp. 156–164, 2019.
https://doi.org/10.1007/978-3-030-32239-7_18

# 1    Introduction

This paper targets at automated categorization of age-related macular degeneration (AMD). As a common macular disease among people over 50, AMD may cause blurred vision or even blindness if not treated in time [15]. Depending on whether the retina contains choroidal neovascularization, AMD is classified into two subcategories, *i.e.*, *dry AMD* (non-neovascular) and *wet AMD* (neovascular) [5]. Due to different treatments, such a fine-grained classification is crucial. In the clinical practice, color fundus photography and optical coherence tomography (OCT) are used by an ophthalmologist to assess the condition of an eye. Not surprisingly, the lack of experienced ophthalmologists has driven the research towards automated AMD categorization based on either fundus images, OCT images or both.

The majority of previous works are based on a single modality, let it be color fundus images capturing the posterior pole [1–3,6] or OCT images [9,10,12–14]. In [1], for instance, Burlina *et al.* employ a deep convolutional neural network (CNN) pretrained on ImageNet to extract visual features from fundus images and then train a linear SVM classifier. As for OCT-based methods, Lee *et al.* [12] train a VGG16 model to classify OCT images either as *normal* or as *AMD*. Since fundus images capture the state of the retinal plane, while OCT images reflect the longitudinal section of the retina, they describe distinct aspects of the retina and can thus be complementary to each other. While jointly exploiting the two modalities seems to be natural, this direction is largely unexplored. To the best of our knowledge, Yoo *et al.* [16] make an initial attempt towards multi-modal AMD categorization. Given a pair of fundus and OCT images from a specific eye, the authors employ a VGG19 model pretrained on ImageNet to extract visual features from both images. The features are concatenated and used as input of a random forest classifier. Despite their encouraging result that the multi-modal method is better than its single-modal counterpart, some crucial questions remain open.

Note that both the VGG19 features and the classifier, *i.e.*, random forest, used in [16] are suboptimal in the context of deep learning based visual categorization. The following questions arise. First, when the single-modal baseline is re-implemented using a state-of-the-art CNN, say ResNet [7], in an end-to-end manner, is the multi-modal method by [16] still better? If the answer is negative, a follow-up question is can multi-modal AMD categorization be performed end-to-end as well? Training a deep network with multi-modal input is nontrivial because by definition, the number of paired multi-modal training instances is less than the number of single-modal training instances. Moreover, the method by [16] lacks the capability of interpreting how the individual modalities contribute to the final prediction.

Towards answering the above questions, we make contributions as follows.

– We propose a two-stream CNN specifically designed for multi-modal AMD categorization, see Fig. 1. Two-stream CNNs have been actively investigated in the context of video action recognition [4]. However, the fusion layer needs

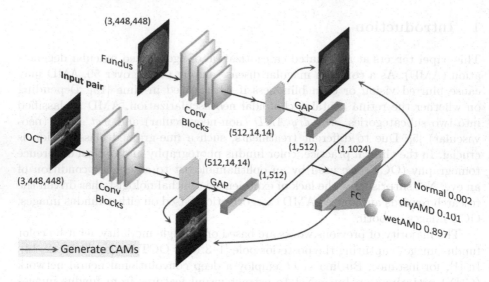

**Fig. 1.** A conceptual diagram of the proposed two-stream CNN for multi-modal AMD categorization. The network consists of two symmetric branches, one for processing fundus images while the other for processing OCT images. Given a pair of fundus and OCT images taken from a specific eye, the proposed network makes a three-class prediction concerning the probability of the eye being *normal*, *dryAMD* and *wetAMD*, respectively. Moreover, we adopt class activation mapping (CAM) [17] to visually interpret how the multi-modal input contributes to the prediction.

to be re-considered for the new task, not only for effectively combining the information from fundus and OCT images but also for visually interpreting their contributions.

- To attack the inadequacy of multi-modal training instances, we introduce Loose Pair Training, a simple sampling strategy that effectively increases the number of training instances.
- Experiments on real-world data collected from an outpatient clinic show the viability of the proposed method. The new method outperforms the state-of-the-art [16] with a large margin, *i.e.*, 0.971 *versus* 0.826 in terms of overall accuracy, for multi-modal AMD categorization.

## 2    Our Method

Given a color fundus image $I_f$ and an OCT image $I_o$ taken from a specific eye, we aim to build a multi-modal CNN (MM-CNN) that takes the paired input and categorizes the eye's condition to a specific class $c$:

$$c \leftarrow \text{MM-CNN}(\{I_f, I_o\}), \tag{1}$$

with $c \in \{normal, dryAMD, wetAMD\}$.

## 2.1 Multi-modal CNN

**Network Architecture.** To handle the multi-modal input, we design a two-stream network as illustrated in Fig. 1. It consists of two symmetric branches, one for processing the fundus image $I_f$ and the other for processing the OCT image $I_o$. Note that such an architecture resembles to some extent the two-stream network widely used for video action recognition [4]. The major difference is at which layer multi-modal fusion is performed. Feature maps generated by intermediate layers of a CNN preserves, to some extent, the spatial information of an input image. As different streams of video data are spatially correlated, the state-of-the-art for video action recognition performs fusion by combining feature maps from the individual streams [4]. By contrast, as $I_f$ and $I_o$ are not spatially correlated, we opt to perform the fusion after the global average pooling (GAP) layer, which removes the spatial information by averaging each feature map into a single value.

For each branch, we use convolutional blocks of ResNet-18 [7]. In principle, any other state-of-the-art CNN can be used here. We choose ResNet-18 as it has fewer parameters and thus requires less training data. Also, this CNN is shown to be effective for other fundus image analysis tasks [11]. For an OCT image, we convert each of its pixels from grayscale to RGB by duplicating the intensity for each RGB component. As such, the same architecture and initialization are applied to both branches.

Let $\mathbf{F}_f = \{F_{f,1}, \ldots, F_{f,512}\}$ be an array of $m \times m$ feature maps generated by the ResNet-18 module in the fundus branch. The value of $m$ depends on the size of the input, which is 14 for an input size of $448 \times 448$. Given a specific feature map $F_{f,i}$, the value of a specific position $(x, y)$ is acquired as $F_{f,i}(x, y)$. In a similar vein, we define the feature maps for the OCT branch as $\mathbf{F}_o = \{F_{o,1}, \ldots, F_{o,512}\}$.

Our fusion layer is implemented by first feeding separately $\mathbf{F}_f$ and $\mathbf{F}_o$ into a GAP layer to obtain two $1 \times 512$ vectors, denoted as $(\bar{F}_{f,1}, \ldots, \bar{F}_{f,512})$ and $(\bar{F}_{o,1}, \ldots, \bar{F}_{o,512})$, respectively. The two vectors are then concatenated to form a $1 \times 1024$ vector which contains information from the two modalities. For classification, the combined vector is fed into a fully connected (FC) layer to produce a score for a specific class $c$, denoted as $s^c$,

$$s^c = \sum_{i=1}^{512} w_{f,i}^c \cdot \bar{F}_{f,i} + \sum_{i=1}^{512} w_{o,i}^c \cdot \bar{F}_{o,i}, \tag{2}$$

where $\{w_{f,1}^c, \ldots, w_{f,512}^c\}$ and $\{w_{o,1}^c, \ldots, w_{o,512}^c\}$ are class-dependent weights parameterizing the FC layer. Classification as expressed in Eq. 1 is achieved by selecting the class with the maximum score.

**Multi-modal Class Activation Mapping for Visual Interpretation.** As Eq. 2 shows, the classification score $s^c$ for a given class $c$ is additively contributed by both modalities. For a more intuitive interpretation, we leverage class activation mapping (CAM) [17], which reveals the (implicit) attention of a CNN on an input image. We compute the multi-modal version of CAMs as

$$\begin{cases} CAM_f^c(x,y) = \sum_{i=1}^{512} w_{f,i}^c \cdot F_{f,i}(x,y), \\ \\ CAM_o^c(x,y) = \sum_{i=1}^{512} w_{o,i}^c \cdot F_{o,i}(x,y). \end{cases} \tag{3}$$

Note that $\bar{F}_{f,i} = \sum_{x,y} F_{f,i}(x,y)$ and $\bar{F}_{f,o} = \sum_{x,y} F_{f,o}(x,y)$. Putting Eqs. 2 and 3 together, $s^c$ can be rewritten as

$$s^c = \sum_{x,y} CAM_f^c(x,y) + \sum_{x,y} CAM_o^c(x,y). \tag{4}$$

According to Eq. 4, $CAM_f^c(x,y)$ and $CAM_o^c(x,y)$ indicate the contribution of a specific position of the fundus and OCT images, respectively. Consequently, the contribution of each modality can be visualized by overlaying with the corresponding up-sampled CAM, see Fig. 2.

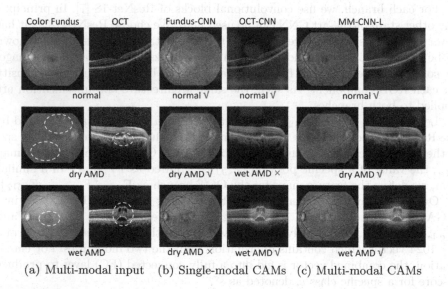

(a) Multi-modal input    (b) Single-modal CAMs    (c) Multi-modal CAMs

**Fig. 2.** CAM-based visualization of single-modal/multi-modal CNNs. White ellipses in (a) indicate regions related to a specific AMD class. Brighter areas in (b) and (c) indicate higher activations. MM-CNN-L is the proposed multi-modal CNN with loose pair training. Note that the color fundus images are shown in gray for better visualizing the heat maps. Best viewed in digital format.

## 2.2   Network Training

A conventional way to construct a multi-modal training instance is to strictly select a fundus image and an OCT image from the same eye, which we term strict pairing. By contrast, we construct instances based on labels instead of eyes. That is, a fundus image is allowed to be paired with an OCT image if their labels are identical. We coin this sampling strategy *Loose Pairing*. Such a strategy expands the size of the training set quadratically. Note that loose pairing is applied only on the training data.

All fundus and OCT images are resized to 448 × 448. As the input of the pretrained ResNet-18 model is 224 × 224, we adjust the kernel size of the GAP layer from 7 × 7 to 14 × 14. Following [8], we enhance fundus images by contrast-limited adaptive histogram equalization. Meanwhile, median filtering is applied on OCT images for noise reduction. For image-level data augmentation, random rotation, crop, flip and random changes in brightness, saturation and contrast are performed on training images.

**Table 1.** Dataset used in our experiments. Data split is made based on eyes. In parentheses are number of eyes per class in each split.

| Class | Training images | | Validation images | | Test images | |
|---|---|---|---|---|---|---|
| | *Fundus* | *OCT* | *Fundus* | *OCT* | *Fundus* | *OCT* |
| *normal* | 155 (155) | 156 (155) | 20 (20) | 20 (20) | 20 (20) | 20 (20) |
| *dryAMD* | 67 (67) | 33 (22) | 20 (20) | 35 (20) | 20 (20) | 38 (20) |
| *wetAMD* | 717 (717) | 821 (484) | 20 (20) | 42 (20) | 20 (20) | 46 (20) |

Our deep models are implemented in the PyTorch (version 1.0.0) framework. ResNet-18 was pretrained on ImageNet. We use cross-entropy, a common loss function for multi-class classification. SGD with momentum of 0.9 and weight decay of 1e−4 is used as the optimizer. Each convolution layer is followed by batch normalization. No dropout is used. The model that obtaining the best validation performance is selected.

## 3 Evaluations

### 3.1 Experimental Setup

**Dataset for Multi-modal AMD Categorization.** We collect 1,059 color fundus images from 1,059 distinct eyes at the outpatient clinic of the Department of Ophthalmology, Peking Union Medical College Hospital. That is, one fundus image per eye. For 781 eyes, they are associated with one to five OCT images, which are central B-scans manually selected by technicians. The fundus images were acquired from a Topcon fundus camera, while OCT images came from a Topcon OCT camera and a Heidelberg OCT camera. For each eye, two ophthalmologists jointly classify its condition as *normal*, *dryAMD* or *wetAMD*, by examining the corresponding fundus image plus OCT, fluorescein angiography (FA) or indocyanine green angiography (ICGA) images, if applicable. Fundus and OCT images associated with a specific eye are assigned with the same class.

In order to build a multi-modal test set, per class we select 20 eyes at random from the eyes that have both fundus and OCT images available. Such a setting

**Table 2.** Performance of different models on the test set. MM-CNN-L, which is the proposed multi-modal CNN with loose pair training, performs the best.

| Model | Normal | | | dryAMD | | | wetAMD | | | Overall | |
|---|---|---|---|---|---|---|---|---|---|---|---|
| | Sen. | Spe. | F1 | Sen. | Spe. | F1 | Sen. | Spe. | F1 | F1 | Accuracy |
| **Single-modal:** | | | | | | | | | | | |
| Fundus-CNN | 1.000 | 0.975 | 0.975 | 0.700 | 0.975 | 0.800 | 0.950 | 0.875 | 0.863 | 0.879 | 0.883 |
| OCT-CNN | 1.000 | 1.000 | **1.000** | 0.815 | 1.000 | 0.898 | 1.000 | 0.879 | 0.929 | 0.942 | 0.932 |
| **Multi-modal:** | | | | | | | | | | | |
| Yoo et al. [16] | 1.000 | 0.976 | 0.952 | 0.552 | 1.000 | 0.711 | 0.978 | 0.724 | 0.841 | 0.835 | 0.826 |
| Yoo et al.-L | 1.000 | 0.988 | 0.975 | 0.763 | 0.954 | 0.828 | 0.913 | 0.844 | 0.866 | 0.890 | 0.875 |
| MM-CNN-S | 1.000 | 1.000 | **1.000** | 0.842 | 0.984 | 0.901 | 0.978 | 0.896 | 0.927 | 0.943 | 0.932 |
| MM-CNN-L | 1.000 | 1.000 | **1.000** | 0.921 | 1.000 | **0.958** | 1.000 | 0.948 | **0.968** | **0.975** | **0.971** |

allows us to justify the effectiveness of multi-modal input against its single-modal counterpart. Moreover, it enables a head-to-head comparison between the two single modalities, *i.e.*, fundus versus OCT. In a similar vein, we construct a multi-modal validation set from the remaining data for model selection. All the rest is used for training. Table 1 shows data statistics.

**Performance Metrics.** Per class we report three metrics, *i.e.*, sensitivity, specificity and F1 score defined as the harmonic mean between sensitivity and specificity. For an overall comparison, the average F1 score over the three classes is used. In addition, we report accuracy, computed as the ratio of correctly classified instances (which are fundus or OCT images for single-modal CNNs and fundus-OCT pairs for MM-CNNs).

### 3.2   Experiment 1. Multi-modal *versus* Single-modal

**Single-modal Baselines.** For single-modal models, we train two ResNet-18 on the fundus images and the OCT images, respectively. For the ease of reference we term the two models Fundus-CNN and OCT-CNN.

**Results.** As Table 2 shows, OCT-CNN is on par with MM-CNN-S, which is trained on the strict pairs. The result suggests that training an effective multi-modal model requires more training data. The proposed loose pair training strategy is effective, resulting in MM-CNN-L that presenting the best performance.

Comparing the two single-modal models, OCT-CNN is better than Fundus-CNN (0.942 versus 0.879 in terms of the overall F1). Confusion matrices are provided in the supplementary material. While the two single-modal CNNs recognize the normal class with ease, they tend to misclassify dryAMD as wetAMD. Such mistakes are reduced by MM-CNN-L. The above results justify the advantage of multi-modal models for AMD categorization.

### 3.3   Experiments 2. Comparison with the State-of-the-Art

**Multi-modal Baselines.** As aforementioned, the only existing work on multi-modal AMD categorization is by Yoo *et al.* [16], where the authors employ a

VGGNet pretrained on ImageNet to extract visual features from fundus and OCT images and then train a random forest classifier on strictly matched pairs. We therefore consider that work as our multi-modal baseline. As their data is not fully available, we replicate their method and evaluate on our test set. For a fair comparison, we substitute ResNet-18 for VGGNet. Moreover, we investigate if the proposed loose pair strategy is also beneficial for the baseline. So we train another random forest with loose pairs. We term this variant Yoo *et al.*-L.

**Results.** As Table 2 shows, MM-CNN-L outperforms the baseline with a large margin (0.975 *versus* 0.835 in terms of overall F1). The two single-modal baselines outperform Yoo *et al.* [16]. These results justify the necessity of end-to-end learning. The loose pair training strategy is found to be useful for the baseline also, improving its overall F1 from 0.835 to 0.890.

## 4  Conclusions

Multi-modal AMD categorization experiments on a clinical dataset allow us to answer the questions asked in Sect. 1 as follows. When end-to-end trained, a single-modal CNN, in particular OCT-CNN, is a nontrivial baseline to beat. Multi-modal CNN recognizes dry AMD and wet AMD at a higher accuracy. This advantage is obtained by the proposed two-stream CNN with loose pair training.

**Acknowledgments.** This work was supported by NSFC (No. 61672523), the Fundamental Research Funds for the Central Universities and the Research Funds of Renmin University of China (No. 18XNLG19), and CAMS Initiative for Innovative Medicine (No. 2018-I2M-AI-001).

## References

1. Burlina, P., Freund, D.E., Joshi, N., Wolfson, Y., Bressler, N.M.: Detection of age-related macular degeneration via deep learning. In: ISBI (2016)
2. Burlina, P.M., Joshi, N., Pekala, M., Pacheco, K.D., Freund, D.E., Bressler, N.M.: Automated grading of age-related macular degeneration from color fundus images using deep convolutional neural networks. JAMA Ophthalmol. **135**(11), 1170–1176 (2017)
3. Burlina, P., Pacheco, K.D., Joshi, N., Freund, D.E., Bressler, N.M.: Comparing humans and deep learning performance for grading AMD: a study in using universal deep features and transfer learning for automated AMD analysis. Comput. Biol. Med. **82**, 80–86 (2017)
4. Feichtenhofer, C., Pinz, A., Zisserman, A.: Convolutional two-stream network fusion for video action recognition. In: CVPR (2016)
5. Ferris, F.L., et al.: Clinical classification of age-related macular degeneration. Ophthalmology **120**(4), 844–851 (2013)
6. Grassmann, F., et al.: A deep learning algorithm for prediction of age-related eye disease study severity scale for age-related macular degeneration from color fundus photography. Ophthalmology **125**(9), 1410–1420 (2018)

7. He, K., Zhang, X., Ren, S., Jian, S.: Deep residual learning for image recognition. In: CVPR (2016)
8. Jintasuttisak, T., Intajag, S.: Color retinal image enhancement by Rayleigh contrast-limited adaptive histogram equalization. In: ICCAS (2014)
9. Karri, S.P.K., Chakraborty, D., Chatterjee, J.: Transfer learning based classification of optical coherence tomography images with diabetic macular edema and dry age-related macular degeneration. Biomed. Opt. Express **8**(2), 579–592 (2017)
10. Kermany, D.S., et al.: Identifying medical diagnoses and treatable diseases by image-based deep learning. Cell **172**(5), 1122–1131.e9 (2018)
11. Lai, X., Li, X., Qian, R., Ding, D., Wu, J., Xu, J.: Four models for automatic recognition of left and right eye in fundus images. In: Kompatsiaris, I., Huet, B., Mezaris, V., Gurrin, C., Cheng, W.-H., Vrochidis, S. (eds.) MMM 2019. LNCS, vol. 11295, pp. 507–517. Springer, Cham (2019). https://doi.org/10.1007/978-3-030-05710-7_42
12. Lee, C.S., Baughman, D.M., Lee, A.Y.: Deep learning is effective for classifying normal versus age-related macular degeneration OCT images. Ophthalmol. Retina **1**(4), 322–327 (2017)
13. Russakoff, D.B., Lamin, A., Oakley, J.D., Dubis, A.M., Sivaprasad, S.: Deep learning for prediction of AMD progression: a pilot study. Investig. Ophthalmol. Vis. Sci. **60**(2), 712–722 (2019)
14. Treder, M., Lauermann, J.L., Eter, N.: Automated detection of exudative age-related macular degeneration in spectral domain optical coherence tomography using deep learning. Graefe's Arch. Clin. Exp. Ophthalmol. **256**(2), 259–265 (2018)
15. Wong, W.L., et al.: Global prevalence of age-related macular degeneration and disease burden projection for 2020 and 2040: a systematic review and meta-analysis. Lancet Glob. Health **2**(2), e106–e116 (2014)
16. Yoo, T.K., Choi, J.Y., Seo, J.G., Ramasubramanian, B., Selvaperumal, S., Kim, D.W.: The possibility of the combination of OCT and fundus images for improving the diagnostic accuracy of deep learning for age-related macular degeneration: a preliminary experiment. Med. Biol. Eng. Comput. **57**(3), 677–687 (2019)
17. Zhou, B., Khosla, A., Lapedriza, A., Oliva, A., Torralba, A.: Learning deep features for discriminative localization. In: CVPR (2016)

# Deep Multi-label Classification
# in Affine Subspaces

Thomas Kurmann[1]([✉]), Pablo Márquez-Neila[1], Sebastian Wolf[2],
and Raphael Sznitman[1]

[1] University of Bern, Bern, Switzerland
thomas.kurmann@artorg.unibe.ch
[2] University Hospital of Bern, Bern, Switzerland

**Abstract.** Multi-label classification (MLC) problems are becoming increasingly popular in the context of medical imaging. This has in part been driven by the fact that acquiring annotations for MLC is far less burdensome than for semantic segmentation and yet provides more expressiveness than multi-class classification. However, to train MLCs, most methods have resorted to similar objective functions as with traditional multi-class classification settings. We show in this work that such approaches are not optimal and instead propose a novel deep MLC classification method in affine subspace. At its core, the method attempts to pull features of class-labels towards different affine subspaces while maximizing the distance between them. We evaluate the method using two MLC medical imaging datasets and show a large performance increase compared to previous multi-label frameworks. This method can be seen as a plug-in replacement loss function and is trainable in an end-to-end fashion.

## 1 Introduction

In recent years, multi-label classification (MLC) tasks have gained important relevance in medical imaging. In essence, MLC is focused on training prediction functions that can tag image data with multiple labels that are not necessarily mutually exclusive [1]. With the advent of Deep Learning, impressive performance in the area of chest X-ray tagging [2], identification of disease comorbidity [3] and retinal image characterization [4] have already been shown.

Yet, at its core, MLC is challenging because of the large number of possible label combinations a method needs to be able to predict and that some output configurations may be extremely rare even though they are important. For instance, for a MLC task with 11 binary labels as depicted in Fig. 1, the number of possible prediction configuration outcomes is $2^{11}$. Given that generating groundtruth annotations for large dataset is often both time consuming and expensive, it is thus common for MLC training sets to not have any examples for many label combinations.

To overcome this, MLC problems were initially treated as direct extensions of binary classification tasks, whereby multiple binary classifiers were trained

© Springer Nature Switzerland AG 2019
D. Shen et al. (Eds.): MICCAI 2019, LNCS 11764, pp. 165–173, 2019.
https://doi.org/10.1007/978-3-030-32239-7_19

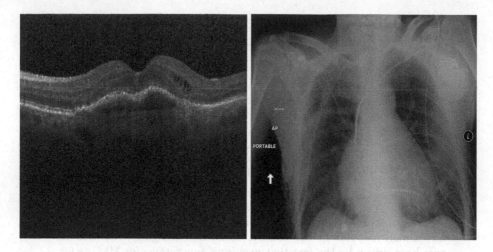

**Fig. 1.** Left: Retinal Optical Coherence Tomography scan containing 11 possible biomarkers. In this example Intraretinal Cysts and Fibrovascular PED are present. Right: Chest X-Ray scan [2] with Cardiomegaly and Emphysema present.

independently to predict each label [5]. In an effort to leverage common image features, recent approaches have looked to share information across different labeling tasks using deep neural networks [2]. In particular, while feature sharing is achieved via network weights, classification boundaries are optimized using traditional binary multi-class objectives. An alternative is to consider that features associated to specific labels should be similar to each other, so to group these together in a subspace and be modeled by density approximators such as k-Nearest Neighbor (kNN) [6]. Similarly, ranking loss functions have been used to disentangle labels in the feature space [7]. Recently, methods performing MLC in latent embedding spaces have been proposed for low dimensional input spaces which are not trainable end-to-end [8] or require multiple networks [9].

To overcome these shortcomings, we present a novel framework for MLC. Unlike most traditional approaches that attempt to discriminate training samples via decision boundaries that separate different labels, our approach is to enforce that samples with the same label values lie on a dedicated subspace. To do this, we introduce a novel loss function that on one hand enforces that samples with the same label value are close to the same subspace, and on the other, that different subspaces are far apart from each other. As such, when training a neural network (NN) with our approach, samples are pulled towards the learned subspaces and can easily be classified by means of a density estimation approach. To show this, we validated our approach on two MLC tasks (i.e., OCT biomarker classification and chest X-ray tagging) using common NN architectures. We show that our approach provides superior performances to a number of state-of-the-art methods for the same task.

## 2   Method

In a MLC, each input image $\mathbf{x} \in \mathbb{R}^{h \times w \times c}$ has $n$ different binary labels $\mathbf{y} = (y_0, \ldots, y_n)$ with $y_i \in \{0, 1\}$. The goal is finding a deep network $f : \mathbb{R}^{h \times w \times c} \to [0, 1]^n$ such that $f(\mathbf{x})_i$ is the estimated probability that label $y_i$ is 1 for the input image $\mathbf{x}$. For convenience, we express our deep network as the composition of two functions $f = g \circ h$: the *feature extraction* function $h : \mathbb{R}^{h \times w \times c} \to \mathbb{R}^d$ builds a $d$-dimensional descriptor vector for the given image $\mathbf{x}$, and $g : \mathbb{R}^d \to [0, 1]^n$ is a multi-output binary classifier. Typically, the choice for $g$ is the standard multi-output logistic regression,

$$g(\mathbf{z}) = \sigma(\mathbf{V}\mathbf{z} + \mathbf{v}), \tag{1}$$

where $\mathbf{V} \in \mathbb{R}^{n \times d}$ and $\mathbf{v} \in \mathbb{R}^n$ define an affine transformation mapping from the feature space to $\mathbb{R}^n$, and $\sigma$ is the element-wise logistic function that provides final probabilities. In this case, the logistic regression splits the feature space using $n$ different $(d-1)$-dimensional hyperplanes, one for each label, and pushes each sample towards one side of each hyperplane depending on its labels. That is, it defines $2^n$ disjoint regions in the feature space (assuming that $d \geq n$), one for each possible combination of labels, and moves samples to their corresponding regions as shown in Fig. 2(left). We claim that this procedure is not well suited in MLC for two fundamental reasons: (1) regions defined by a collection of splitting hyperplanes are highly irregular with some regions unbounded and others with small volumes. This leads to some combinations of labels being easier to represent than others in the feature space. (2) Logistic regression does not promote feature vectors to be similar for samples that share the same label. Instead it only enforces that samples fall on the correct side of the hyperplanes.

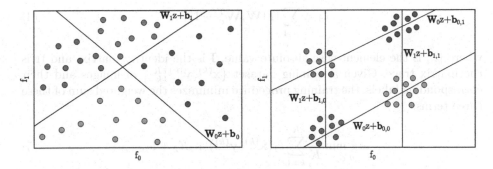

**Fig. 2.** Illustration of MLC (left) and our proposed **AS-MLC** method (right). This synthetic example the feature space is of size $d = 2$ with $n = 2$ labels: Red points = (00), Green = (01), Pink = (10) and Blue = (11). Note how the joint distribution of labels is clustered at the intersections of the hyperplanes. (Color figure online)

To address these issues, we introduce a new Affine Subspace multi-label classifier (**AS-MLC**). Instead of pushing points toward different regions, our method pulls points towards different affine subspaces. This simple idea solves the two aforementioned problems. First, all affine subspaces are homogenenous in dimension such that no combination of labels is easier to represent than others. Second, pulling points towards affine subspaces makes them share similarities in the feature space, that is, the distance to the subspace.

Formally, for each label $i$, we define two parallel $(d-e)$-dimensional affine subspaces $(\mathbf{W}_i, \mathbf{b}_{i0})$ and $(\mathbf{W}_i, \mathbf{b}_{i1})$, determined by the intersection of $e$ hyperplanes, where $\mathbf{W}_i \in \mathbb{R}^{e \times d}$ are the shared hyperplane normals and $\mathbf{b}_{i0}, \mathbf{b}_{i1} \in \mathbb{R}^e$ are the bias terms of both subspaces. For a given label $i$, points with $y_i = 0$ will be pulled towards $(\mathbf{W}_i, \mathbf{b}_{i0})$ and points with $y_i = 1$ will be pulled towards $(\mathbf{W}_i, \mathbf{b}_{i1})$.

**Training:** To train our method, we first minimize the distances of samples to their corresponding subspaces, using the following loss function term,

$$\ell_1(\mathbf{x}, \mathbf{y}) = \sum_{i=1}^{n} \alpha_{i,y_i} \left\| \mathbf{W}_i \mathbf{z} + \mathbf{b}_{i,y_i} \right\|_2^2, \tag{2}$$

where $\mathbf{z} = h(\mathbf{x})$ and $\alpha$ is a class-label specific weight. At the same time, we also want subspaces corresponding to the same label to be as far apart as possible from each other. This can be formalized with the additional loss term,

$$\ell_2 = \sum_{i=1}^{n} \frac{1}{\left\| \mathbf{b}_{i0} - \mathbf{b}_{i1} \right\|_2^2 + \epsilon}, \tag{3}$$

that maximizes the distance between the parallel subspaces. Finally, to avoid that the loss terms are minimized by scaling down the magnitude of the weights, we add a regularization term to enforce that normals have unit magnitude,

$$\ell_3 = \sum_{i=1}^{n} \operatorname{tr} \left| \mathbf{W}_i \mathbf{W}_i^T - \mathbf{I} \right|, \tag{4}$$

where $| \cdot |$ is the element-wise absolute value, $\mathbf{I}$ is the identity matrix, and tr is the matrix trace. Given a training dataset $\{\mathbf{x}^{(k)}, \mathbf{y}^{(k)}\}_{k=1}^{K}$ of images and their corresponding labels, the training procedure minimizes the weighted sum of these three terms:

$$\arg\min_{\theta,\phi} \frac{1}{K} \sum_{k=1}^{K} \ell_1(\mathbf{x}^{(k)}, \mathbf{y}^{(k)}) + \beta \ell_2 + \ell_3, \tag{5}$$

where $\theta$ are the parameters of the feature extractor $h$, $\beta$ is a distance weighting hyperparameter and $\phi = \{(\mathbf{W}_i, \mathbf{b}_{i0}, \mathbf{b}_{i1})\}_{i=1}^{n}$ are the weights and bias terms of our **AS-MLC**. This loss function is trainable in an end-to-end manner. After training, the intersections of the $2n$ learned subspaces define $2^n$ $(d - n \cdot e)$-dimensional affine subspaces, one for each combination of labels. See Fig. 2(right) for an example where $n = d = 2$ and $e = 1$. In this case, the final subspaces are 0-dimensional, namely, points.

**Inference:** At test time, one could use the ratio of distances to each subspace as our criterion for assigning the probability of every label (we denote this method as **AS-MLC-Distance**). However, we found that a data-driven approach reaches better performance in practice. For each label $i$ and class $j$, we thus build a kernel density estimation of the likelihood using the projected training data,

$$p(\mathbf{W}_i \mathbf{z} \mid \mathbf{y}_i = j) = \frac{1}{K} \sum_{k=1}^{K} G_\delta \left( \mathbf{W}_i (\mathbf{z} - \mathbf{z}^{(k)}) \right), \tag{6}$$

where $G_\delta$ is the Gaussian kernel with bandwidth $\delta$, $\mathbf{z}^{(k)} = h(\mathbf{x}^{(k)})$ is the descriptor vector of the $k$-th element of the training data, and $\mathbf{z} = h(\mathbf{x})$ is the descriptor vector of the input image. Note that bias terms are not required to define the density, as they are implicitly encoded in the set of descriptor vectors $\{\mathbf{z}^{(k)}\}_{k=1}^{K}$. We define the posterior (assuming uniform priors)

$$g(\mathbf{z})_i \equiv P(\mathbf{y}_i = 1 \mid \mathbf{W}_i \mathbf{z}) = \frac{p(\mathbf{W}_i \mathbf{z} \mid \mathbf{y}_i = 1)}{\sum_{j \in \{0,1\}} p(\mathbf{W}_i \mathbf{z} \mid \mathbf{y}_i = j)}, \tag{7}$$

which is the $i$-th output of our multi-label binary classifier $g$.

## 3   Experiments

To evaluate the performance of our proposed method, we perform experiments on two medical MLC image datasets.

**Dataset 1 – OCT Biomarker Identification**
This dataset consists of volumetric Optical Coherence Tomography (OCT) scans of the retina with 11 pathological biomarker labels annotated. The data is split into 23'030 and 1'029 images for the training and testing sets, respectively, with no patient images in both splits. The image labels include: Healthy, Sub Retinal Fluid, Intraretinal Fluid, Intraretinal Cysts, Hyperreflective Foci, Drusen, Reticular Pseudodrusen, Epirential Membrane, Geographic Atrophy, Outer Retinal Atrophy and Fibrovascular PED. Figure 1 (Left) shows a training example with two biomarkers being present.

To compare our approach to existing methods, we evaluated a number of baselines using two different NN architectures: a pre-trained DRND-54 [10] and a ResNet-50 [11]. All methods are trained using the Adam optimizer [12] with a base learning rate of $10^{-3}$. We apply the same data augmentation scheme (flipping, rotation, translation, gamma and brightness) for all experiments. Results are reported with 5-fold cross validation where the training data was split into training 80% and validation 20%. Baselines include:

- **Softmax:** Two class outputs per label that are normalized using the softmax operator and the binary cross-entropy loss is optimized.

**Table 1.** Experimental results comparing our proposed method to other approaches. Testing is performed by taking the weights at the epoch where the maximum macro mAP was achieved on the validation set. (*) indicates test time augmentation.

| | Loss | Macro mAP | Micro mAP | Macro mAP* | Micro mAP* |
|---|---|---|---|---|---|
| ResNet-50 | Softmax | $0.790 \pm 0.015$ | $0.805 \pm 0.035$ | $0.797 \pm 0.011$ | $0.815 \pm 0.031$ |
| | Ranking | $0.747 \pm 0.043$ | $0.759 \pm 0.052$ | $0.764 \pm 0.040$ | $0.752 \pm 0.050$ |
| | Ml-kNN | $0.770 \pm 0.004$ | $0.799 \pm 0.005$ | $0.781 \pm 0.005$ | $0.806 \pm 0.005$ |
| | AS-MLC-Distance | $0.762 \pm 0.015$ | $0.778 \pm 0.022$ | $0.773 \pm 0.017$ | $0.789 \pm 0.022$ |
| | AS-MLC | $\mathbf{0.800 \pm 0.004}$ | $\mathbf{0.814 \pm 0.021}$ | $\mathbf{0.810 \pm 0.002}$ | $\mathbf{0.822 \pm 0.015}$ |
| DRND-54 | Softmax | $0.806 \pm 0.011$ | $0.801 \pm 0.026$ | $0.813 \pm 0.014$ | $0.830 \pm 0.006$ |
| | Ranking | $0.770 \pm 0.012$ | $0.782 \pm 0.022$ | $0.781 \pm 0.011$ | $0.789 \pm 0.021$ |
| | Ml-kNN | $0.790 \pm 0.008$ | $0.817 \pm 0.009$ | $0.805 \pm 0.006$ | $0.828 \pm 0.07$ |
| | AS-MLC-Distance | $0.824 \pm 0.017$ | $0.814 \pm 0.012$ | $0.823 \pm 0.017$ | $0.834 \pm 0.011$ |
| | AS-MLC | $\mathbf{0.831 \pm 0.013}$ | $\mathbf{0.848 \pm 0.016}$ | $\mathbf{0.840 \pm 0.009}$ | $\mathbf{0.8567 \pm 0.013}$ |

- **Ranking:** We use the ranking loss as described by Li et al. [7]. As ranking losses are typically thresholded, we omit this threshold and scale outputs between 0 and 1 during training and testing. We acknowledge that this is a disadvantage for the ranking method, but include it for the sake of comparision.
- **Ml-kNN:** We apply a distance weighted kNN ($n = 50$) to $z$ extracted from the **Softmax** method as in [6].
- **AS-MLC:** We set $\beta = 5, \alpha = 1$ and $e = 32$. The Gaussian kernel density estimation bandwidth is set to $\delta = 0.1$ and uses the features of the training images and their horizontally flipped versions. We also compare to the distance function method **AS-MLC-Distance**.

Mean Average Precision (mAP) results are presented in Table 1 and show that our proposed method outperforms the commonly used loss functions for all metrics and both networks. We show both the micro and macro averaged results, when using and not using test time data augmentation (original image + left/right flip). We see a performance increase of up to 5.7% using our method over the softmax cross-entropy loss. In Fig. 3 (Left), we show the influence of the bandwidth $\delta$ value when using a 10-fold cross-validations. Here we see that unless the bandwidth value is chosen to be too small, the performance remains stable for a wide range of values. Similarly, we also analyse the effects of the size of the feature space $e$, which we consider to be an additional hyperparameter. From Fig. 3 (Right) we can conclude that extremely small feature space sizes are not sufficient for our method but for values greater than 5, performances are consistently high.

### Dataset 2 – ChestX-ray14
The dataset contains 112'120 X-ray scans associated to 14 different labels [2]. The data is split according to the original patient-level data splits which results in 70% training, 10% validation and 20% test sets. We resize images to $512 \times 512$ pixels and optimize the network using the Adam optimizer [12]. In this case, we compare the weighted cross-entropy loss and add the weighting term $\alpha$ to the

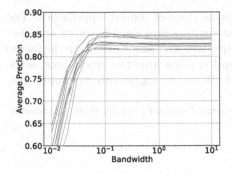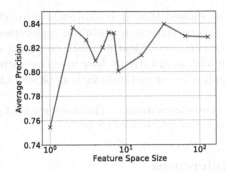

**Fig. 3.** Left: 10 fold cross validation of bandwith size using a fixed feature size $e = 32$. Right: Impact analysis for the feature dimension size $e$ at a fixed bandwidth $\delta = 0.1$.

**Table 2.** Area under the curve values for ROC results on the ChestX-ray14 dataset.

| Method | Atelectasis | Cardiomegaly | Effusion | Infiltration | Mass |
|---|---|---|---|---|---|
| Original [2] | 0.7003 | 0.8100 | 0.7585 | 0.6614 | 0.6933 |
| Softmax | 0.7290 | **0.8514** | 0.7893 | **0.6692** | 0.7853 |
| AS-MLC | **0.7471** | 0.8481 | **0.8203** | 0.6647 | **0.7957** |

| Method | Nodule | Pneumonia | Pneumothorax | Consolidation | Edema |
|---|---|---|---|---|---|
| Original [2] | 0.6687 | 0.658 | 0.7993 | 0.7032 | 0.8052 |
| Softmax | 0.7217 | **0.700** | 0.8371 | 0.7134 | 0.8291 |
| AS-MLC | **0.7759** | 0.6997 | **0.8663** | **0.7294** | **0.8306** |

| Method | Emphysema | Fibrosis | PT | Hernia | Average |
|---|---|---|---|---|---|
| Original [2] | 0.833 | 0.7859 | 0.6835 | 0.8717 | 0.7451 |
| Softmax | 0.9051 | 0.8042 | 0.7283 | 0.8560 | 0.7800 |
| AS-MLC | **0.9200** | **0.8222** | **0.7626** | **0.9288** | **0.8008** |

class labels due to the significant class imbalances in the data (i. e., weights are equal to the inverse class occurrence). For all experiments we use a DRND-54 [10] CNN as the base architecture. We fix the hyperparameters $\beta = 5$ and find the best bandwidth using cross-validation ($\delta = 1.0$).

Results of our **AS-MLC** method are given in Table 2 and yield a 0.8008 mean AUC. Our method thus outperforms the softmax cross entropy loss by nearly 3% in mean ROC values. These results using a standard network are in range of previously published state-of-the-art results that used large amounts of additional training data [13] (0.806), attention based models [14,15] (0.8027 and 0.816) and significantly outperform the original publication [2].

## 4   Conclusion

We presented **AS-MLC**, a novel MLC method which attempts to overcome the short-comings of classical MLC methods by classifying in affine subspaces. To do so, we propose a novel loss function which pulls class-labels towards affine subspaces and maximizes their distance. We evaluated our method on two datasets and showed that it consistently outperforms state-of-the-art approaches. The proposed method is a plug-in replacement for standard deep learning architectures and can be learnt end-to-end using standard backpropagation. In the future we wish to investigate how to extract attention maps from the predictions as the application of methods such as GradCAM [16] are no longer directly applicable.

**Acknowledgements.** This work received partial financial support from the Innosuisse Grant #6362.1 PFLS-LS.

# References

1. Gibaja, E., Ventura, S.: Multi-label learning: a review of the state of the art and ongoing research. Wiley Interdiscip. Rev.: Data Min. Knowl. Discov. **4**(6), 411–444 (2014)
2. Wang, X., Peng, Y., Lu, L., Lu, Z., Bagheri, M., Summers, R.M.: ChestX-ray8: hospital-scale chest X-ray database and benchmarks on weakly-supervised classification and localization of common thorax diseases. In: CVPR (2017)
3. Adeli, E., Kwon, D., Pohl, K.M.: Multi-label transduction for identifying disease comorbidity patterns. In: Frangi, A.F., Schnabel, J.A., Davatzikos, C., Alberola-López, C., Fichtinger, G. (eds.) MICCAI 2018. LNCS, vol. 11072, pp. 575–583. Springer, Cham (2018). https://doi.org/10.1007/978-3-030-00931-1_66
4. Fauw, D., et al.: Clinically applicable deep learning for diagnosis and referral in retinal disease. Nat. Med. **24**(9), 1342–1350 (2018)
5. Read, J., Pfahringer, B., Holmes, G., Frank, E.: Classifier chains for multi-label classification. Mach. Learn. **85**(3), 333 (2011)
6. Zhang, M.L., Zhou, Z.H.: ML-KNN: a lazy learning approach to multi-label learning. Pattern Recognit. **40**(7), 2038–2048 (2007)
7. Li, Y., Song, Y., Luo, J.: Improving pairwise ranking for multi-label image classification. In: Proceedings of the IEEE Conference on Computer Vision and Pattern Recognition, pp. 3617–3625 (2017)
8. Li, X., Guo, Y.: Multi-label classification with feature-aware non-linear label space transformation. In: Twenty-Fourth International Joint Conference on Artificial Intelligence (2015)
9. Yeh, C.K., Wu, W.C., Ko, W.J., Wang, Y.C.F.: Learning deep latent spaces for multi-label classification (2017)
10. Yu, F., Koltun, V., Funkhouser, T.: Dilated residual networks. In: CVPR (2017)
11. He, K., Zhang, X., Ren, S., Sun, J.: Deep residual learning for image recognition. In: CVPR, pp. 770–778 (2016)
12. Kingma, D.P., Ba, J.: Adam: a method for stochastic optimization. arXiv preprint arXiv:1412.6980 (2014)
13. Guendel, S., Grbic, S., Georgescu, B., Zhou, K., Ritschl, L., Meier, A., Comaniciu, D.: Learning to recognize abnormalities in chest X-rays with location-aware dense networks (2018)
14. Tang, Y., Wang, X., Harrison, A.P., Lu, L., Xiao, J., Summers, R.M.: Attention-guided curriculum learning for weakly supervised classification and localization of thoracic diseases on chest radiographs. In: Shi, Y., Suk, H.-I., Liu, M. (eds.) MLMI 2018. LNCS, vol. 11046, pp. 249–258. Springer, Cham (2018). https://doi.org/10.1007/978-3-030-00919-9_29

15. Guan, Q., Huang, Y.: Multi-label chest X-ray image classification via category-wise residual attention learning. Pattern Recognit. Lett. (2018)
16. Selvaraju, R.R., Cogswell, M., Das, A., Vedantam, R., Parikh, D., Batra, D.: Grad-CAM: visual explanations from deep networks via gradient-based localization (2016)

# Multi-scale Microaneurysms Segmentation Using Embedding Triplet Loss

Mhd Hasan Sarhan[1,2]([✉]) [iD], Shadi Albarqouni[1] [iD], Mehmet Yigitsoy[2] [iD],
Nassir Navab[1,3], and Abouzar Eslami[2] [iD]

[1] Computer Aided Medical Procedures,
Technical University of Munich, Munich, Germany
hasan.sarhan@tum.de
[2] Carl Zeiss Meditec AG, Munich, Germany
mhd-hasan.sarhan@zeiss.com
[3] Computer Aided Medical Procedures, Johns Hopkins University, Baltimore, USA

**Abstract.** Deep learning techniques are recently being used in fundus image analysis and diabetic retinopathy detection. Microaneurysms are an important indicator of diabetic retinopathy progression. We introduce a two-stage deep learning approach for microaneurysms segmentation using multiple scales of the input with selective sampling and embedding triplet loss. The model first segments on two scales and then the segmentations are refined with a classification model. To enhance the discriminative power of the classification model, we incorporate triplet embedding loss with a selective sampling routine. The model is evaluated quantitatively to assess the segmentation performance and qualitatively to analyze the model predictions. This approach introduces a 30.29% relative improvement over the fully convolutional neural network.

**Keywords:** Deep learning · Segmentation · Ophthalmology

## 1 Introduction

Diabetic retinopathy (DR) is the leading cause of vision impairment and blindness for middle-aged groups [11]. DR early detection is important for the treatment planning. Severity of DR falls into one of five levels (none, mild, moderate, severe, or proliferative) [1]. Microaneurysms are considered as the first signs for detecting early stages of DR. Hence, detecting these lesions is important for Computer Aided Diagnosis systems. Microaneurysms are abnormalities in the microvascular structure and appear as small red dots in color fundus images. Screening programs use colored fundus images of the retina for their rich information and ease of access. Detecting microaneurysms in colored fundus images

**Electronic supplementary material** The online version of this chapter (https://doi.org/10.1007/978-3-030-32239-7_20) contains supplementary material, which is available to authorized users.

is a challenging task due to the small size of the lesion which makes up less than 1% of the entire image [3], and the low contrast between microaneurysms and background.

Microaneurysms are the strongest determinant for DR since they are the first lesion that appears during the early stages. Various approaches for microaneurysms detection using deep learning are proposed [7,10,14]. These methods are patch-wise approaches and use deep architectures to extract representative features. These features could be added to a set of hand-crafted features [14] and passed to a classification model or used solely in an end-to-end network [7,10]. Deep learning techniques in the literature of microaneurysms detection use random patches selection, hence, they are prone to be biased towards the oversampled class. Moreover, no work in the microaneurysms segmentation context has leveraged the embedding space of the input patches to impose an additional constraint on the learning process.

*Contributions:* In this work, a multi-scale patch-wise approach for segmenting microaneurysms in retinal fundus images is proposed. The main contributions of this work are (1) fusing segmentation on multiple scales for microaneurysms detection, and (2) using embedding triplet loss [16] with selective sampling [6] to increase the descriptiveness of the feature representation while focusing the training on informative examples. The model is agnostic to other lesions (i.e. the model differentiates between healthy and microaneurysm patches regardless of information about other lesions). Being agnostic to other lesions is important in such cases as it may be difficult to obtain an annotated dataset with all DR lesions annotated.

## 2   Methodology

Our proposed microaneurysms segmentation framework, depicted in Fig. 1, consists of two stages; the *hypothesis generation network* (**HGN**), where multi-scale fully convolutional networks (FCNs) are employed to propose a region of interest (ROI), and *patch-wise refinement network* (**PRN**), where extracted patches around ROIs are passed to the classifier. In the next sections we introduce the details of the applied method. First, we go through the fully convolutional hypothesis generation networks, the reasoning behind having multiple scales, and the details of the loss function used for optimization. The second section is dedicated for the PRN. In which, the motive behind this network is explained and the details of triplet loss and selective sampling are presented.

*Hypothesis Generation Network (HGN):*  High-resolution fundus images where a microaneurysm covers a very small part of the image are examined to segment microaneurysm. Using a zoomed-in patch would allow for high spatial accuracy on account of losing semantic information, whilst a zoomed-out patch would have a richer semantic representation on the account of losing spatial resolution [4]. As a trade-off, we use equally sized patches on two scales of the image to build two HGNs, one for each scale.

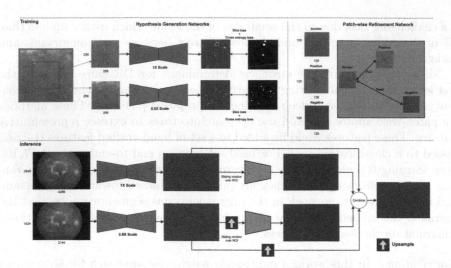

**Fig. 1.** Pipeline for the multi-scale microaneurysms segmentation framework. Top part shows the pipeline in the training mode where each model is trained separately. Bottom part shows the pipeline at inference time where the image is used rather than patches for the hypothesis generation networks.

HGN is a fully convolutional neural network trained on patches of size 256 × 256 extracted from the fundus images. Two HGNs are trained for two different scales of the fundus image (1x, 0.5x). This allows the extraction of scale-related features while at the same time preserve full resolution image information. The architecture used is the full resolution residual network type A [15] for its good results in segmentation.

To select the training patches, we define images that contain no signs of DR as healthy (negative) images and images with microaneurysms as lesion (positive) images. Healthy pixels are extracted only from healthy patients' scans and lesion pixels are extracted from DR patients at the microaneurysms locations. As a loss function, weighted cross entropy loss is used to compensate for the imbalance negative and positive patches. Moreover, dice loss is optimized to enhance the spatial overlap between a segmentation map output and the gold standard segmentation. We use a differentiable approximation of the dice loss as in [12].

*Patch-Wise Refinement Network:* PRN is a classification network that is used as on top of the HGN. The input of the network is an image patch and the output is the probability of the patch center pixel being a microaneurysm or healthy. The segmentation maps of the HGN are used as regions of interest for the PRN. The architecture of classification networks allows for receptive fields larger than fully convolutional networks that consume more memory because of the decoder part and skip connections. The larger receptive field allows for feature maps that incorporate more spatial information about the image which enriches the extracted features. The architecture employed for this network is an adopted version of the Resnet-50 [8]. One downsampling step is omitted from the original architecture because the input image size in our case is smaller than what is expected in the Resnet-50 scenario. In the training phase, patches are extracted from images in the same manner of extracting 1x resolution patches for HGN. The only difference is the size of PRN patches is $129 \times 129$.

To extract discriminative features in PRN we propose the utilization of triplet loss [16]. Triplet loss is applied on the embedding of a patch around pixel $x$ into a $d$-dimensional feature space. The aim of triplet loss is to make similar patches closer to each other in the embedding space while pushing dissimilar patches away from each other in the embedding space using a predefined distance measure. We found the feature representation of the last convolution layer after the global average pooling (GAP) as a good representation in the embedding space due to its high descriptive power while having a compact representation. The optimization of triplet loss requires three input patches namely the anchor patch $x^a$, the positive patch $x^p$ and the negative patch $x^n$. The goal is to make the embedding of the positive patch closer to the anchor patch than the embedding of the negative patch. Patches with microaneurysms at the center pixels are used as anchor and positive patches, while healthy patches are used as negative patches. The loss is defined as

$$\mathcal{L}_{triplet} = \sum_i^N \left[ d(f(x_i^a), f(x_i^p)) - d(f(x_i^a), f(x_i^n)) + a \right]_+ \tag{1}$$

where $a$ is a margin to enforce a distance between positive and negative pairs, $d(.,.) \in \mathbb{R}^1$ is the distance measure in the embedding space, and $N$ is the number of all possible triplets. As a distance measure, angular cosine distance is utilized as it shows better performance on high dimensional representations when training deep networks [13]. In addition to triplet loss, cross entropy loss for patches is optimized.

Generating all triplets, in this case, would be computationally prohibitive. Moreover, the imbalance in the dataset is high. To counter these problems, we use selective sampling [6]. This approach of training proved to enhance the results in training scenarios where data from different classes are not balanced. In our use case, the healthy class is over-represented. In selective sampling, patches with higher loss have a higher probability of being picked for the next epoch as they are considered representative samples.

## 3   Experiments

### 3.1   Experimental Setup

*Dataset:* For our evaluations of the segmentation pipeline, we use the IDRiD[1] publicly available dataset. All images are captured with the same device that has 50-degree field of view and have size of $4288 \times 2848$ pixels. Before patch

---

[1] https://idrid.grand-challenge.org/.

**Table 1.** IDRiD dataset splits

|  | Healthy | | Microaneurysms | |
|---|---|---|---|---|
|  | Images | Patches | Images | Patches |
| Train set | 80 | 6M | 44 | ˜500K |
| Validation set | 9 | ˜6M | 10 | ˜132K |
| Test set | 27 | - | 45 | - |

extraction, the published train dataset is split into two parts: training, and validation sets. The validation set is used for monitoring the training. Table 1 shows the dataset splits.

*Implementation Details:* We employ contrast enhancement following the formula $I_{pre}(x,y) = 4I(x,y) - 4G_\sigma * I(x,y) + 1024/30$. To train HGN, we define a mini-batch of size 10 and consider each epoch to be 1000 mini-patches. The learning rate for the full-scale network is $1e-6$ and for the half-scale network is $1e-5$.

PRN is trained with mini-batches of triplets. The size of a mini-batch is $90 \times 3$ patches. We sample $90 \times 2$ patches from the pool of lesion patches randomly with uniform distribution, and $90 \times 1$ samples from the healthy patches pool with selective sampling. This neural network has a Siamese structure [2], this means that each part of the triplet's three parts is run through identical versions of the network and the gradients are combined at the output to update the weights of the network. In addition to triplet loss, cross entropy loss for pairs is optimized. To this end, we optimize the cross-entropy loss between the anchor and the negative pair. Every 1000 mini-batches is considered as an epoch. We run selective sampling routine every 10 epoch, this is because of the big number of training patches. Which takes a significant amount of time to evaluate. Learning rate is set to $1e-5$ and decreased by a factor of 10 after 20 epochs. The optimization of the losses is done using Adam optimizer [9].

## 3.2  Multi-scale Effect

In this evaluation, we study the effect of using multiple scalse. To this end, two HGNs are trained, one for the full resolution image and one for the downsampled image by a factor of two. The evaluation is done on the publicly published test set images. We compare results from each scale with the results of combining the two scales in two different ways. First the output of the half scale is upsampled using linear interpolation, then the prediction maps of the two scales are combined either with pixelwise arithmetic or geometric averaging. The results of this evaluation are presented in Table 2. FCN 1x, FCN 0.5x represent the evaluation on the prediction map of the full scale and half scale HGNs, respectively. FCN geometric and FCN arithmetic refer to the results of combining the two scales with geometric and arithmetic averaging, respectively. The results show that combining the two scales gives better performance either way. We notice a higher recall from the half scale network but lowest precision, this reflects that the model is very sensitive to microaneurysms and generates a high number of false positives that drops down the overall performance.

### 3.3    Patch-Wise Refinement and Triplet Loss Effect

We evaluate the effect of (1) using a classification network to refine the classifications of HGNs and (2) using triplet loss in the classification network to refine HGNs results (i.e PRN). To evaluate the classification network, we utilize patches from the image in a sliding window fashion and use the classification probability of each point to obtain segmentation maps. It is worth noting that sliding window does not go over all the image, but only the parts higher than a preset probability threshold (0.5 in our case) from HGN. Two segmentation maps will be obtained by sliding over the image masked with two HGNs outputs. Two prediction maps from two HGNs and two prediction maps from refining HGNs results with the classification networks combined as shown in Fig. 1.

We first demonstrate the effect of incorporating a classification network to refine the results of HGNs. To this end, we use an edited version of PRN that uses only cross entropy loss without the triplet embedding optimization. This network is denoted as *cls*. Using the classification network on top of the fully convolutional networks enhances the results of the overall segmentation. The larger receptive field allows for more descriptive representations which in turn could suppress false positives that are triggered by HGNs. The effect of utilizing triplet embedding loss is then evaluated by training a PRN using triplets from the training set. We set the margin value $a$ from Eq. 1 to 0.5. At test time, this network is utilized in a sliding window fashion similar to *cls*.

Using triplet loss in a multi-scale approach with geometric averaging has an overall 30.29% PR AUC improvement over the baseline fully convolutional neural network trained with weighted cross entropy. The improvement when incorporating triplet loss could be attributed to the quality of the learned representations where lesion patches are forced to be close to each other with a certain margin of difference from healthy ones.

Our results come in 4th place in the IDRiD challenge outdated leaderboard based on the metric used on the released test set. The challenge submission is currently closed. iFLYTEK-MIG used Mask-RCNN to segment 3 lesions at the same time. VRT used a U-net to segment four lesions all together. PATech used a patch-wise approach with false positives bootstrapping on lesions simultaneously. We notice that in all these models, information about lesions other than microaneurysms is utilized. This makes the disambiguation between lesion types (**e.g.** hemorrhages and microaneurysms) learned inherently in the model but has the drawback of requiring full annotation of multiple lesion types. The proposed model does not require information from other lesions to be trained.

**Table 2.** Ablation test for emphasizing each part of the pipeline

|                    | AUC PR | F1-score | Precision | Recall |
|--------------------|--------|----------|-----------|--------|
| HGN 1x - baseline  | 0.3374 | 0.3618   | 0.2970    | **0.4626** |
| HGN 0.5x           | 0.3411 | 0.4001   | 0.4380    | 0.3682 |
| HGN geometric      | 0.3622 | 0.3866   | 0.5115    | 0.3108 |
| HGN arithmetic     | 0.3701 | 0.4156   | 0.4741    | 0.3701 |
| *cls* geometric    | 0.3895 | 0.4153   | **0.5402** | 0.3374 |
| *cls* arithmetic   | **0.3905** | **0.4368** | 0.4973 | 0.3895 |
| PRN arithmetic     | 0.3978 | **0.4323** | 0.54051 | 0.3602 |
| PRN geometric      | **0.4196** | 0.38477 | **0.61128** | 0.2807 |
| IDRiD iFLYTEK-MIG  | **0.5017** | –      | –         | –      |
| IDRiD VRT          | 0.4951 | –        | –         | –      |
| IDRiD PATech       | 0.4740 | –        | –         | –      |

## 3.4   Visual Evaluation

We study the misclassifications of the model by visually examining samples of the results. In Fig. 2 an example of a segmentation is presented. From the example, we notice that false positives mostly lay in the area around hemorrhages or on top of a blood vessel where a higher intensity occur. False negatives are more difficult to be detected because they sometimes appear very close to hemorrhage and

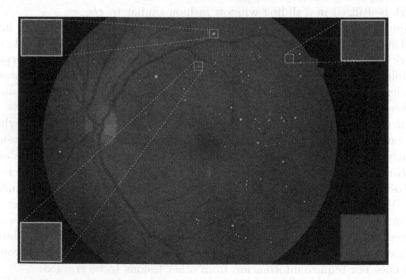

**Fig. 2.** An example of a segmented microaneurysms in a fundus image. Green is for true positives, red is for false positives, and cyan is for false negatives. (Color figure online)

blend in or the contrast in the image is low enough to lose the microaneurysm. In the top left example, we see a false negative example where the microaneurysm is misclassified because of very light edges and irregular shape that leans towards hemorrhage. In the other false negative examples (in cyan), the cases are very difficult to be distinguished and variability between raters may occur in such cases. The bottom right example shows a false positive example where a darker area around the bright exudates appears similar to microaneurysm. The variability in illumination parameters of the capturing device has also a significant effect on the training and may lead to a bias towards a certain image appearance. It is important to note that images in the IDRiD dataset are compressed with a lossy compression which leads to big jumps in intensity values next to each other. For more examples please refer to supplementary material.

## 4 Discussion and Conclusion

We hypothesize that using multiple fully convolutional networks for multiple scales of the inputs enhances the segmentation of small objects similar to microaneurysms because it gives a better trade-off between semantic and spatial accuracy. Embedding loss is employed mainly in learning image descriptors [17]. We use the triplet embedding loss in our model to treat deeper layers of the classification network as a local descriptor of the keypoint represented by the healthy or microaneurysm patch. The classification performance increases by adding this additional constraint on the features created by the network.

The segmentation results could be used in report generation for the doctors or in future studies to do big data analysis of populations. Microaneurysms turnover is also an important factor in the progression analysis of DR [5] and could be studied better with reliable models for microaneurysms segmentation.

## References

1. American Academy of Ophthalmology. International clinical diabetic retinopathy disease severity scale detailed table. http://www.icoph.org/downloads/Diabetic-Retinopathy-Detail.pdf. Accessed 10 Sept 2018
2. Bromley, J., Guyon, I., LeCun, Y., Säckinger, E., Shah, R.: Signature verification using a "siamese" time delay neural network. In: Advances in Neural Information Processing Systems, pp. 737–744 (1994)
3. Gargeya, R., Leng, T.: Automated identification of diabetic retinopathy using deep learning. Ophthalmology **124**(7), 962–969 (2017)
4. Ghiasi, G., Fowlkes, C.C.: Laplacian pyramid reconstruction and refinement for semantic segmentation. In: Leibe, B., Matas, J., Sebe, N., Welling, M. (eds.) ECCV 2016. LNCS, vol. 9907, pp. 519–534. Springer, Cham (2016). https://doi.org/10.1007/978-3-319-46487-9_32
5. Goatman, K.A., Cree, M.J., Olson, J.A., Forrester, J.V., Sharp, P.F.: Automated measurement of microaneurysm turnover. Investig. Ophthalmol. Vis. Sci. **44**(12), 5335–5341 (2003)

6. van Grinsven, M.J., van Ginneken, B., Hoyng, C.B., Theelen, T., Sánchez, C.I.: Fast convolutional neural network training using selective data sampling: application to hemorrhage detection in color fundus images. IEEE Trans. Med. Imaging **35**(5), 1273–1284 (2016)
7. Haloi, M.: Improved microaneurysm detection using deep neural networks. arXiv preprint arXiv:1505.04424 (2015)
8. He, K., Zhang, X., Ren, S., Sun, J.: Deep residual learning for image recognition. In: Proceedings of the IEEE Conference on Computer Vision and Pattern Recognition, pp. 770–778 (2016)
9. Kingma, D.P., Ba, J.: Adam: a method for stochastic optimization. arXiv preprint arXiv:1412.6980 (2014)
10. Lam, C., Yu, C., Huang, L., Rubin, D.: Retinal lesion detection with deep learning using image patches. Investig. Ophthalmol. Vis. Sci. **59**(1), 590–596 (2018)
11. Lee, R., Wong, T.Y., Sabanayagam, C.: Epidemiology of diabetic retinopathy, diabetic macular edema and related vision loss. Eye Vis. **2**(1), 17 (2015)
12. Milletari, F., Navab, N., Ahmadi, S.A.: V-net: fully convolutional neural networks for volumetric medical image segmentation. In: 2016 Fourth International Conference on 3D Vision (3DV), pp. 565–571. IEEE (2016)
13. Nair, V., Hinton, G.E.: Rectified linear units improve restricted Boltzmann machines. In: Proceedings of the 27th International Conference on Machine Learning (ICML 2010), pp. 807–814 (2010)
14. Orlando, J.I., Prokofyeva, E., del Fresno, M., Blaschko, M.B.: Learning to detect red lesions in fundus photographs: an ensemble approach based on deep learning. arXiv preprint arXiv:1706.03008 (2017)
15. Pohlen, T., Hermans, A., Mathias, M., Leibe, B.: Full-resolution residual networks for semantic segmentation in street scenes. arXiv preprint (2017)
16. Schroff, F., Kalenichenko, D., Philbin, J.: FaceNet: a unified embedding for face recognition and clustering. In: Proceedings of the IEEE Conference on Computer Vision and Pattern Recognition, pp. 815–823 (2015)
17. Wohlhart, P., Lepetit, V.: Learning descriptors for object recognition and 3D pose estimation. In: Proceedings of the IEEE Conference on Computer Vision and Pattern Recognition, pp. 3109–3118 (2015)

# A Divide-and-Conquer Approach Towards Understanding Deep Networks

Weilin Fu[1]([✉]), Katharina Breininger[1], Roman Schaffert[1], Nishant Ravikumar[1], and Andreas Maier[1,2]

[1] Pattern Recognition Lab, Friedrich-Alexander University Erlangen-Nürnberg, 91058 Erlangen, Germany
weilin.fu@fau.de
[2] Erlangen Graduate School in Advanced Optical Technologies (SAOT), 91058 Erlangen, Germany

**Abstract.** Deep neural networks have achieved tremendous success in various fields including medical image segmentation. However, they have long been criticized for being a black-box, in that interpretation, understanding and correcting architectures is difficult as there is no general theory for deep neural network design. Previously, precision learning was proposed to fuse deep architectures and traditional approaches. Deep networks constructed in this way benefit from the original known operator, have fewer parameters, and improved interpretability. However, they do not yield state-of-the-art performance in all applications. In this paper, we propose to analyze deep networks using known operators, by adopting a divide-and-conquer strategy to replace network components, whilst retaining networks performance. The task of retinal vessel segmentation is investigated for this purpose. We start with a high-performance U-Net and show by step-by-step conversion that we are able to divide the network into modules of known operators. The results indicate that a combination of a trainable guided filter and a trainable version of the Frangi filter yields a performance at the level of U-Net (AUC 0.974 vs. 0.972) with a tremendous reduction in parameters ($111,536$ vs. $9,575$). In addition, the trained layers can be mapped back into their original algorithmic interpretation and analyzed using standard tools of signal processing.

**Keywords:** Precision learning · Debugging · CNN

## 1 Introduction

Deep learning (DL) technology [6] has been successfully applied in various fields including medical image segmentation, which provides substantial support for diagnosis, therapy planning and treatment procedures. Despite their outstanding achievements, DL-based algorithms have long been criticized for being a black-box and many design choices in Convolutional Neural Network (CNN) topologies are driven rather by experimental improvements than theoretical founda-

© Springer Nature Switzerland AG 2019
D. Shen et al. (Eds.): MICCAI 2019, LNCS 11764, pp. 183–191, 2019.
https://doi.org/10.1007/978-3-030-32239-7_21

tion. Accordingly, understanding the actual working principle of the architectures is difficult. One option to gain interpretability is to constrain the network with known operators. Precision learning [8,9], which integrates known operators [3,13] into DL models, can provide a suitable mechanism to design CNN architectures. This strategy integrates prior knowledge into the deep learning pipeline, thereby improving interpretability, providing guarantees and quality control in certain settings. However, the quantitative performance of these approaches often falls short compared to completely data-driven approaches.

In this work, we propose an approach to debug and identify the limitation/bottleneck of a known operator workflow. Frangi-Net [3], which is the deep learning counterpart of the Frangi filter [2] is utilized as an exemplary network. The performance of different methods is evaluated on the retinal vessel segmentation task, using data from the Digital Retinal Images for Vessel Extraction (DRIVE) database [11]. Experiments are designed under the assumption that if the replacement of one step leads to a performance boost, then this step is the probable bottleneck of the overall workflow. In our case, we debug the Frangi-Net by replacing the preprocessing step with the powerful U-Net [10]. With the output from the U-Net as input, Frangi-Net approaches state-of-the-art performance. Thereby, we conclude that the preprocessing method is the weakness of the Frangi-Net segmentation pipeline. In other words, given a proper preprocessing algorithm, Frangi-Net may be capable of accomplishing the retinal vessel segmentation task. To verify this hypothesis, we further utilize the guided filter layer [12], which is a deep learning module designed for image quality enhancement. Experimental results confirm our hypothesis: the additional guided filter layer indeed brings about a substantial improvement in performance. Due to the modular design, analysis of the trained filter block is possible which reveals slightly unexpected behaviour. Our work has two main contributions: Firstly, we propose a feasible way to identify the bottleneck of a precision learning-based workflow. Secondly, the debugging procedure yields a network pipeline with well-defined explainable steps for retinal vessel segmentation, i.e., guided filter layer for preprocessing, and Frangi-Net for vesselness computation.

## 2    Methods

### 2.1    Frangi-Net

In this work, Frangi-Net, which is the deep learning counterpart of the Frangi filter [2], is utilized as the segmentation network in different pipelines. The Frangi filter is a widely used multi-scale tube segmentation method, which calculates vesselness response $V_0$ of dark tubes at scale $\sigma$ with Hessian eigenvalues ($|\lambda_1| \leq |\lambda_2|$) using:

$$V_0(\sigma) = \begin{cases} 0, & \text{if } \lambda_2 < 0, \\ \exp(-\frac{R_B^2}{2\beta^2})(1 - \exp(-\frac{S^2}{2c^2})), & \text{otherwise,} \end{cases} \quad (1)$$

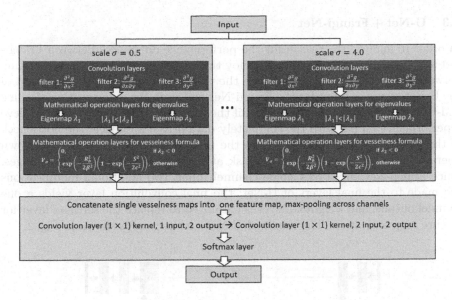

**Fig. 1.** Architecture of the 8-scale Frangi-Net.

where $S = \sqrt{\lambda_1^2 + \lambda_2^2}$ is the second-order structureness, $R_B = \frac{\|\lambda_1\|}{\|\lambda_2\|}$ is the blobness measure, and $\beta, c$ are image-dependent parameters for blobness and structureness terms. Frangi-Net is constructed by representing each step in the multi-scale Frangi filter as a layer. Here, we employ a Frangi-Net with 8 different Gaussian scales ranging from 0.5 to 4.0. The convolution kernels are initialized as the second-order partial derivatives of the Gaussian kernel at the corresponding scales. We employ two additional $1 \times 1$ convolution layers before the final softmax output layer, to regulate the data range. The hyper-parameters $\beta, c$ in Eq. 1 of all scales are initialized to 0.5 and 1.0, respectively. The network has 6,525 weights, and the overall architecture is shown in Fig. 1.

## 2.2   U-Net

In this work, a U-Net [10] is directly applied to retinal vessel segmentation, and forms the baseline method for all comparisons. U-Net is a successful encoder-decoder CNN architecture, popularized in the field of medical image segmentation. It combines location information in the contracting encoder path, with contextual information in the expanding decoder path via skip connections. Here, we adapt a three-level U-Net with 16 initial features with two main modifications. Firstly, batch normalization layers are added after convolution layers to stabilize the training process. Secondly, deconvolution layers are replaced with upsampling layers followed by a $1 \times 1$ convolution layer. The overall architecture contains 111,536 trainable weights.

### 2.3   U-Net + Frangi-Net

In order to analyze the reason for the performance differences between Frangi-Net and the U-Net, we propose to employ the latter as a "wildcard preprocessing network". To this end, we concatenate the two networks such that the output of the U-Net serves as input for the Frangi-Net and train the segmentation pipeline end-to-end. The intuition here is that, if the combined network is able to achieve a performance on par with the completely data driven approach, the bottleneck of the known-operator network lies in the preprocessing. Otherwise, the known operator is inadequate to solve the task at hand, even with optimized images. Since Frangi-Net only takes single channel input, two additional modifications are made to the final layers of U-Net: the final convolution layer yields a one channel output, and a sigmoid layer is employed to replace the softmax layer for feature map activation. The modified U-Net architecture is shown in Fig. 2.

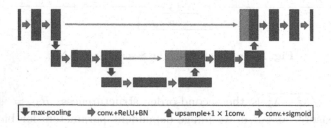

**Fig. 2.** U-Net architecture adapted for preprocessing.

### 2.4   Guided Filter Layer + Frangi-Net

Preliminary experiments conducted using U-Net and U-Net + Frangi-Net indicated that the preprocessing step was indeed the bottleneck in the vessel segmentation pipeline. Consequently, we propose to replace the "wildcard" U-Net with a guided filter layer. The guided filter layer was proposed as differentiable neural network counterpart of the guided filter [4], which can be utilized as an edge-preserving, denoising approach. The guided filter takes one image $p$ and one guidance image $I$ as input to produce one output image $q$. This translation-variant filtering process can be simplified and described in Eq. 2:

$$q_i = \sum_j W_{ij}(I)p_j, \tag{2}$$

where $i, j$ are pixel indices, and $W_{ij}$ is the kernel which is a function of the guidance image $I$ and is independent of $p$.

A guided filter layer with two trainable components is used as the preprocessing block. First, the guidance map $I$ is generated with a CNN, using image $p$ as input. Here, the CNN is configured as a five-layer Context Aggregation Network (CAN) [1]. Subsequently, a small feature extractor is applied to image $p$ before being passed to the guided filter layer. This feature extractor is composed of two $3 \times 3$ convolution layers with five intermediate channels, and one final output feature map. The guided filter block contains $3,050$ parameters. The architecture is shown in Fig. 3.

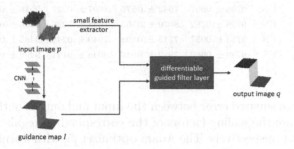

**Fig. 3.** Architecture of guided filter layer adapted for preprocessing.

# 3    Experiments and Results

## 3.1    Data

The DRIVE database is employed to evaluate different pipelines in this study. The database contains 40 RGB fundus photographs of size $565 \times 584$ pixels, which are evenly divided into a training and a testing set. A validation set of four images is further separated from the training set to monitor the training process and avoid overfitting. The green channels, which have the best contrast between vessels and the background, are extracted and processed using Contrast Limited Adaptive Histogram Equalization (CLAHE) [14] to balance inhomogeneous illuminations. Manual labels and Field Of View (FOV) masks are provided for all images. For each image of the training set, a weighting map $w$ which emphasizes thin vessels is generated on the basis of the manual label using the equation $w = \frac{1}{\alpha \times d}$, where $d$ denotes the vessel diameter in the ground truth, and $\alpha$ is a factor manually set to 0.18. In order to have a meaningful and fair comparison between different methods, all FOV masks are eroded inward by four pixels to remove potential border effects. Performance evaluation is conducted inside the FOV masks.

## 3.2    Network Training

The objective functions for all learning-based methods in this work are constructed with three parts as: $L_{total} = w \cdot L_{focal} + \lambda_w \cdot R_w + \lambda_s \cdot R_s$, where $w$ is the weighting map which emphasizes small vessels; $L_{focal}$ is the class balanced focal loss [7], with a focusing factor of 2.0; $R_w$ denotes an $\ell_2$-norm regularizer on the network weights to prevent overfitting; $R_s$ represents a similarity regularizer

**Table 1.** Performance evaluation on DRIVE testing set. *prep.*, *reg.*, *seg.* denote *preprocessing net, regularizer,* and *segmentation method,* respectively.

| Prep. | Reg. | Seg. | Specificity | Sensitivity | F1 score | Accuracy | AUC |
|-------|------|------|-------------|-------------|----------|----------|-----|
| - | - | FF | .9616 ± .0150 | .7528 ± .0612 | .7477 ± .0323 | .9341 ± .0089 | .9401 |
| - | - | FN | .9633 ± .0125 | .8008 ± .0590 | .7812 ± .0256 | .9419 ± .0070 | .9610 |
| - | $R_w$ | UN | .9756 ± .0057 | .7942 ± .0576 | .8097 ± .0227 | .9516 ± .0056 | .9743 |
| UP | $R_w$ | FN | .9726 ± .0082 | .8070 ± .0565 | .8088 ± .0236 | .9506 ± .0054 | .9743 |
| UP | $R_w, R_s$ | FN | .9753 ± .0057 | .7715 ± .0598 | .7949 ± .0248 | .9485 ± .0060 | .9703 |
| GF | - | FN | .9729 ± .0060 | .7982 ± .0546 | .8048 ± .0191 | .9498 ± .0048 | .9719 |

which is the mean squared error between the input and output of the preprocessing net. $\lambda_w, \lambda_s$ are the scaling factors of the corresponding regularizers, and are set to 0.2 and 0.1, respectively. The Adam optimizer [5] with learning rate decay is utilized to minimize the objective function. The initial learning rate is $5 \times 10^{-4}$ for U-Net, and $5 \times 10^{-5}$ for all other pipelines. All networks are trained with a batch size of 50, and with $168 \times 168$ image patches. Data augmentation in form of rotation, shearing, additive Gaussian noise, and intensity shifting is employed. All methods are implemented in Python 3.5.2 using TensorFlow 1.10.0.

### 3.3   Evaluation and Results

The evaluation performance of six different segmentation workflows is evaluated on the DRIVE testing set, and is summarized in Table 1. Binarization of the output probability maps from the network pipelines is performed with a single threshold which maximizes the F1 score on the validation set. The input, intermediate outputs of the preprocessing nets and the corresponding probability map results from the Frangi-Net for an representative region of interest (ROI) of an image from the testing set are presented in Fig. 4.

From Table 1, we observe that the Frangi-Net without additional preprocessing (FN) performs better than the original Frangi filter (FF), but worse than the completely data-driven U-Net (UN). Using the U-Net as a preprocessing network (UP + FN), we observe a performance boost, achieving results on-par with UN, with respect to all evaluation metrics and reaching an AUC score of 0.975. With an additional regularizer $R_s$ that enforces the similarity between the input and output of the preprocessing network, the performance is only modestly impaired. When looking at the intermediate outputs of the preprocessing nets (see Fig. 4(b) and (c)), we observe that the UP substantially enhances the contrast for small vessels and reduces noise compared to the input image (a). Low frequency information, e.g., the illumination in the bright optic disc and the dark macula region, is removed when no additional $R_s$ is applied. This provides further confirmation of the hypothesis that the main bottleneck of the proposed known-operator pipeline lies in the preprocessing, and can be combated by an appropriate adaption of this step. This is supported by the results achieved using the guided filter layer for preprocessing (GF + FN).

The guided filter layer, however, does not simply learn an edge-preserving denoising filtering as the intermediate output reveals (see Fig. 4(d)). It performs a substantial enhancement of small vessels and removal of the low-frequency background comparable to UP (see Fig. 4(b)). In this case, the performance of the pipeline is only marginally inferior to that of the U-Net, approaching an AUC score of 0.972.

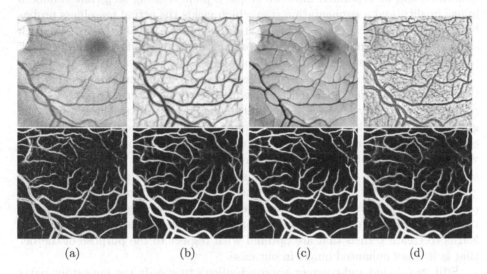

(a)                    (b)                    (c)                    (d)

**Fig. 4.** The input (a) and output (b–d) of preprocessing networks for a representative ROI are shown in the upper row, the corresponding probability map results after Frangi-Net are presented in the lower row for: (a) no preprocessing network, (b) UP, (c) UP with $R_s$, (d) GF.

## 4   Discussion and Conclusion

We proposed a method to analyze and interpret a DL-based algorithm, via step-by-step conversion of a fully-data driven approach, to construct a pipeline using well-defined known operators. The approach helps to identify and combat bottlenecks in a known-operator pipeline, by localizing the components responsible for drops in performance. Additionally, it provides a mechanism to interpret deep network architectures in a divide-and-conquer pattern, by replacing each step in the network pipeline with a well-defined operator.

The potential of the proposed framework to improve our understanding of deep neural networks and enable intelligent network design was demonstrated for the exemplary task of retinal vessel segmentation. The previously proposed known-operator network Frangi-Net enables easy interpretation, but performs worse than a fully data-driven approach such as the U-Net. Conversely, an interpretation of the fully data-driven approach remains vague despite satisfactory performance. By using the U-Net as a debugging tool, we confirm that with appropriate preprocessing, the Frangi-Net is capable of achieving on-par performance. This performance boost also indicates that the preprocessing is the bottleneck of the Frangi-Net workflow. Subsequently, we identify the guided filter layer as a suitable known operator that can serve as a replacement for the U-Net in terms of preprocessing, while retaining performance.

The quantitative results support our hypothesis that the task of vessel segmentation can be separated into two steps: a preprocessing step that enhances image quality, and a segmentation step which yields the actual vesselness probability map. By replacing these elements step-by-step, we are able to preserve high segmentation performance while incorporating interpretability into the network pipeline with well-defined, understandable steps.

While the results of the U-Net preprocessing with similarity regularization demonstrate that there exists an edge-preserving filtering approach that results in an equally effective segmentation based on the vesselness filter, the guided filter layer does not fulfill the expected filtering behavior. Instead of edge-preserving filtering, the guided filter layer learns a domain transfer to a vessel-enhancing representation that removes low frequency information at the same time. Looking at Eq. 2 this seems surprising, as the guided filter uses the guidance image only for design of the filter kernel in a shift-variant filtering process. Yet, this design does not guarantee an edge-preserving filtering per se as the guidance image may also result in band-pass kernels. As a result, the filter learns to create kernels that are optimal with respect to the purpose of the net that is a vessel enhanced image in our case.

Still, our divide-and-conquer approach allows to specify the important parts of a network. This is achieved by showing that a known operator network which is restricted in what it can learn with $9,575$ vs. $111,536$ parameters, performs comparably to a completely data-driven network with an AUC score of $0.972$ vs. $0.974$. The use of a powerful network, i.e., U-Net in this case, supplements the performance and addresses the shortcomings of the known operators, and thus helps to improve understanding of the network for a specific task. Future work will look into exploiting the divide-and-conquer approach to aid network interpretation and performance improvement for other tasks, based on known operator modules. It provides a systematic framework to design interpretable network pipelines with minimal loss in performance, relative to completely data-driven approaches, which is compelling for the intelligent design of networks in the future.

# References

1. Chen, Q., Xu, J., Koltun, V.: Fast image processing with fully-convolutional networks. In: Proceedings of the IEEE International Conference on Computer Vision, pp. 2497–2506 (2017)
2. Frangi, A.F., Niessen, W.J., Vincken, K.L., Viergever, M.A.: Multiscale vessel enhancement filtering. In: Wells, W.M., Colchester, A., Delp, S. (eds.) MICCAI 1998. LNCS, vol. 1496, pp. 130–137. Springer, Heidelberg (1998). https://doi.org/10.1007/BFb0056195

3. Fu, W., et al.: Frangi-Net. In: Maier, A., Deserno, T., Handels, H., Maier-Hein, K., Palm, C., Tolxdorff, T. (eds.) Bildverarbeitung für die Medizin 2018. INFOR-MAT, pp. 341–346. Springer, Heidelberg (2018). https://doi.org/10.1007/978-3-662-56537-7_87
4. He, K., Sun, J., Tang, X.: Guided image filtering. IEEE Trans. Pattern Anal. Mach. Intell. **35**(6), 1397–1409 (2013)
5. Kingma, D.P., Ba, J.: Adam: a method for stochastic optimization. arXiv preprint arXiv:1412.6980 (2014)
6. LeCun, Y., Bengio, Y., Hinton, G.: Deep learning. Nature **521**(7553), 436 (2015)
7. Lin, T.Y., Goyal, P., Girshick, R., He, K., Dollár, P.: Focal loss for dense object detection. In: Proceedings of the IEEE International Conference on Computer Vision, pp. 2980–2988 (2017)
8. Maier, A., et al.: Precision learning: towards use of known operators in neural networks. In: ICPR, pp. 183–188. IEEE (2018)
9. Maier, A.K., et al.: Learning with known operators reduces maximum training error bounds. arXiv preprint arXiv:1907.01992 (2019)
10. Ronneberger, O., Fischer, P., Brox, T.: U-Net: convolutional networks for biomedical image segmentation. In: Navab, N., Hornegger, J., Wells, W.M., Frangi, A.F. (eds.) MICCAI 2015. LNCS, vol. 9351, pp. 234–241. Springer, Cham (2015). https://doi.org/10.1007/978-3-319-24574-4_28
11. Staal, J., Abràmoff, M.D., Niemeijer, M., Viergever, M.A., Van Ginneken, B.: Ridge-based vessel segmentation in color images of the retina. IEEE Trans. Med. Imaging **23**(4), 501–509 (2004)
12. Wu, H., Zheng, S., Zhang, J., Huang, K.: Fast end-to-end trainable guided filter. In: CVPR, pp. 1838–1847 (2018)
13. Würfl, T., Ghesu, F.C., Christlein, V., Maier, A.: Deep learning computed tomography. In: Ourselin, S., Joskowicz, L., Sabuncu, M.R., Unal, G., Wells, W. (eds.) MICCAI 2016. LNCS, vol. 9902, pp. 432–440. Springer, Cham (2016). https://doi.org/10.1007/978-3-319-46726-9_50
14. Zuiderveld, K.: Contrast limited adaptive histogram equalization. In: Graphics Gems IV, pp. 474–485. Academic Press Professional, Inc. (1994)

# Multiclass Segmentation as Multitask Learning for Drusen Segmentation in Retinal Optical Coherence Tomography

Rhona Asgari[✉], José Ignacio Orlando, Sebastian Waldstein, Ferdinand Schlanitz, Magdalena Baratsits, Ursula Schmidt-Erfurth, and Hrvoje Bogunović

Christian Doppler Laboratory for Ophthalmic Image Analysis, Department of Ophthalmology, Medical University of Vienna, Vienna, Austria
fatemeh.asgari@meduniwien.ac.at

**Abstract.** Automated drusen segmentation in retinal optical coherence tomography (OCT) scans is relevant for understanding age-related macular degeneration (AMD) risk and progression. This task is usually performed by segmenting the top/bottom anatomical interfaces that define drusen, the outer boundary of the retinal pigment epithelium (OBRPE) and the Bruch's membrane (BM), respectively. In this paper we propose a novel multi-decoder architecture that tackles drusen segmentation as a multitask problem. Instead of training a multiclass model for OBRPE/BM segmentation, we use one decoder per target class and an extra one aiming for the area between the layers. We also introduce connections between each class-specific branch and the additional decoder to increase the regularization effect of this surrogate task. We validated our approach on private/public data sets with 166 early/intermediate AMD Spectralis, and 200 AMD and control Bioptigen OCT volumes, respectively. Our method consistently outperformed several baselines in both layer and drusen segmentation evaluations.

## 1 Introduction

Age-related macular degeneration (AMD) is one of the leading causes of blindness in elderly population in the developed world [1]. One of the first clinical hallmarks of AMD is the presence of drusen, waste material accumulations in the area delimited by the outer boundary of the retinal pigment epithelium (OBRPE) and the Bruch's membrane (BM). Optical coherence tomography (OCT) is the state-of-the-art imaging modality to assess AMD patients, as it allows to visualize the retinal layers and study pathological changes due to AMD, including drusen. Segmenting drusen in OCT is relevant for quantifying disease progression [2], although doing it manually is costly, tedious and time consuming. Current methods for automated drusen segmentation are based on identifying the OBRPE and BM interfaces, as every non-overlapped area in between those surfaces is considered drusen [3,4]. Deep learning techniques based on convolutional neural network (CNNs) have been recently explored for this task [3–6]. In

© Springer Nature Switzerland AG 2019
D. Shen et al. (Eds.): MICCAI 2019, LNCS 11764, pp. 192–200, 2019.
https://doi.org/10.1007/978-3-030-32239-7_22

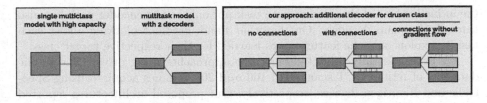

**Fig. 1.** Different multiclass segmentation approaches. From left to right: single multi-class model with high capacity, multitask model with 2 decoders [7] and our approaches with an additional decoder for drusen class: no connections and surrogate decoder, with connections and gradient flow, and with connections but no gradient flow. Box sizes indicate the capacity of the module.

[4], a patch-based CNN is applied for feature extraction, combined with graph search strategies and standard classifiers. In [5], an image-level classification CNN is applied to predict the vertical coordinates of each surface. A similar idea is followed in [6] to predict surface positions using a 2D-to-1D approach.

Segmenting the OBRPE and the BM is a multiclass segmentation problem that can be tackled in different ways (Fig. 1). The common solution [3] is to use a multiclass model with high capacity (e.g. encoder/decoder architectures such as the U-Net [8]) and a multiclass loss function (e.g. cross-entropy). This model learns how to discriminate between classes and which features are needed to identify them. This interaction cannot be explicitly controlled, and it is not possible to assign portions of capacity to specific classes (although it can be approached by weighting classes in the loss function, e.g. under class imbalance).

An alternative is to pose the multiclass segmentation task as a multitask learning problem. Instead of having a single encoder and a single decoder, both shared among the $K$ target classes, the architecture is split into $K$ decoders. Each decoder is focused on a binary segmentation task, providing class-specific capacities that are exclusively dedicated to the target problem. Simultaneously, a single encoder is shared among them to characterize common features. This architecture can be trained using a linear combination of $K$ binary loss functions, and benefits from the inductive bias of each task by updating the encoder parameters. This approach has been previously explored in [7] for red/bright lesion segmentation in fundus images, with promising results.

In this paper we bring the multitask approach in [7] one step further. In particular, we exploit the fact that our drusen segmentation task comprises the segmentation of the OBRPE and the BM to capture the area between them. Hence, instead of having one decoder for each layer class, we introduce a third one aiming to segment the region between both layers (Fig. 2). Our assumption is that this additional branch will aid the encoder to characterize the appearance of both drusen and non-pathological regions where OBRPE and BM are overlapped. We also explore the influence resulting from introducing additional connections between each of the layer decoders and this intermediate one, with and without gradient flow. Allowing gradient flow is expected to further transfer the inductive bias of the intermediate task not only to the encoder path but also through the main decoders. On the other hand, gradient blocking allows each task to exploit only the feature maps learned for their respective target class.

We experimentally validated our three approaches using private and public data sets of retinal OCT scans with 166 and 200 volumes acquired using Spectralis and Bioptigen devices, respectively. Our proposed architectures reported the best performance for drusen segmentation compared to several baselines.

## 2   Methods

### 2.1   Multiclass Segmentation as Multitask Learning

Given an input image $\mathbf{x} \in \mathcal{X}$, our goal is to produce a label $y$ for each pixel $x$, in the label space $\mathcal{L} = \{0, 1, ..., K\}$, with 0 being background and $K$ the total number of classes of interest. This task is usually performed using a supervised deep learning model, $f_\theta(\mathcal{X}) \rightarrow \mathcal{Y}$, where $\mathcal{X}$ and $\mathcal{Y}$ are the set of B-scans and labelings, respectively. The parameters $\theta$ are learned using a training set $S = \{(\mathbf{x}^{(i)}, \mathbf{y}^{(i)}), 0 < i < N\}$, with $N$ the total number of pairs $(\mathbf{x}^{(i)}, \mathbf{y}^{(i)})$ of training images and their labels, respectively. This is done by minimizing a loss function $J(\mathbf{y}, \hat{\mathbf{y}})$, where $\mathbf{y}$ and $\hat{\mathbf{y}}$ are the manual and predicted multiclass segmentations.

Network parameters can be decomposed as the union of the weights of the encoder $\theta_E$ and the decoder $\theta_D$, $\theta = \theta_E \cup \theta_D$. In a typical multiclass setting, all the parameters are shared among classes and it is not possible to assign part of them to each class. In [7], the authors proposed to replace the unique decoder by two decoders, one per target. Formally, this is equivalent to model $\theta_D = \bigcup_{k=1}^{K} \theta_D^k$, where each $\theta_D^k$ is the set of parameters of the decoder for the $k$-th class. This model is trained by means of a multitask loss function, which is defined as a linear combination of binary segmentation losses $J(\mathbf{y}, \hat{\mathbf{y}}) = \sum_{k=1}^{K} \lambda_k J_k(\mathbf{y}_k, \hat{\mathbf{y}}_k)$. $\lambda_k$ denotes a weight for the $k$-th loss function, while $\mathbf{y}_k$ and $\hat{\mathbf{y}}_k$ are binary predictions for each class $k$ vs. every other, including the background class.

### 2.2   Drusen Segmentation in OCT as Multitask Learning

A retinal OCT scan is a 3D volume composed of consecutive 2D images or B-scans, captured by means of low-coherence interferometry. We seek the model $f$ to produce a labeling for each input B-scan $\mathbf{x}$. The classical strategy to do so is to aim for the OBRPE and the BM interfaces: a multiclass segmentation problem with background vs. $K = 2$ classes [3,5]. In healthy cases, both classes are overlapped and there is no region in between them. In early/intermediate AMD cases, however, a third class $k = 3$, is implicit in the non-overlapped areas of these layers. Instead of considering this class as background, we propose to learn its properties by considering $K = 3$ during training. This is done by: (i) adding an extra decoder for this class, and (ii) incorporating another binary segmentation term to the loss function that penalizes errors in the segmentation of this region. Our hypothesis is that the existing decoders will benefit from the inductive bias

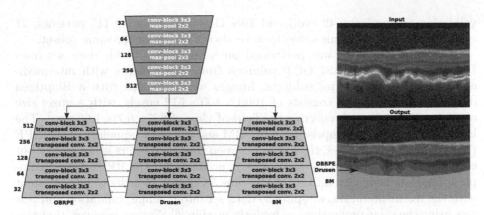

**Fig. 2.** Our multitask segmentation network for layer/drusen segmentation in OCT. Skip connections between each parallel encoder/decoder block were omitted for clarity. The number of output filters of each block are denoted on their left side. (Color figure online)

of this new task through the gradient updates in the encoder, better characterizing the non-overlapped cases. To further increase the regularization effect of this extra task, we also propose to incorporate inbound/outbound connections between each $\theta_D^k$ and $\theta_D^3$, with $k \neq 3$, both with and without gradient flow.

Figure 2 depicts our U-shaped architecture. Skip connections between each parallel encoder/decoder convolutional/deconvolutional blocks were omitted for clarity. Each convolutional block comprises two convolutional layers with $3 \times 3$ pixels convolutions. The Generalized Dice loss function was applied for each $J_k(\mathbf{y}_k, \hat{\mathbf{y}}_k)$ [9], and the predicted labels were binary masks for each target class, as depicted in Fig. 2. These outputs were combined to produce the final segmentation. Any segmented component with an area smaller than expected size for BM region (yellow in Fig. 2) or for RPE region (red in Fig. 2), in the output mask was treated as noise and removed from the mask. To retrieve the surfaces of the BM/OBRPE layers, a postprocessing strategy was applied: for each vertical column in the B-scan (or A-scan), the first/last row of activated pixels was taken as the surface boundary, respectively.

## 3    Experimental Setup

Our private data set consisted of 560 fovea-centered Spectralis OCT volumes of patients with early/intermediate AMD. In total, there are $51K$ B-scans acquired from 48 patients and 63 eyes. Each scan comprises $1024 \times 97 \times 496$ voxels, with a voxel size of $5.7 \times 60.5 \times 3.87 \,\mu m^3$, covering the field of view of $6 \times 6 \times 2 \, mm^3$. A manual labelling was produced for each B-scan on every volume. The Iowa Reference Algorithms [10] were used to generate a first raw segmentation, which was subsequently manually corrected by an expert clinician. To train and evaluate the networks, we split the data into 41K B-scans for training and validation (33 patients, 42 eyes) and 10K B-scans for testing (15 patients, 21 eyes). Scans from the same subjects were always placed in the same subset.

A second evaluation was performed on a publicly available data set from Duke [11], comprising 384 OCT volumes from 269 patients with intermediate AMD and 115 control subjects. Images were acquired with a Bioptigen device, where each scan consists of $1000 \times 100 \times 512$ voxels, with a voxel size of $6.54 \times 67 \times 3.23\,\mu m^3$, covering the field of view of $6.7 \times 6.7 \times 1.66\,mm^3$. The labels in this data set comprise both the BM and the inner boundary of the RPE (IBRPE). In healthy cases, the region between these two layers is not empty but covers the RPE, while in diseased cases it accounts for the RPE+drusen complex. The data is divided into 165 AMD plus 5 Control, In order to be consistent with the recent literature, we split the data set into training, validation and test sets using the same proportions as recently used in [6]. Notice, however, that this does not ensure that the same images are used for comparison. We performed the evaluation both in control and AMD diseased cases.

*Training Setup.* Our method and the baselines were trained with a batch size of 16 for at least 50 epochs, using Adam optimization with an initial learning rate of $\eta = 10^{-5}$, decreased by a factor of $10^{-7}$ after every epoch. Training was halted if no improvement in loss function(dice coefficient) was observed in 4 consecutive epochs. Each input B-scan was resized to $256 \times 256$ pixels and normalized to zero mean and unit variance. Data augmentation was applied in the form of flipping and translation. An equal weighting $\lambda_k = 1$ was used for each loss function $J_k$.

# 4    Results

We evaluated our method in terms of drusen and layer segmentation performance. For drusen segmentation, we used classical binary evaluation metrics such as Dice index, precision and recall (sensitivity). For layer segmentation, we used mean absolute error. Since our data set includes multiple scans for the same eye of different patients, the evaluation metrics were first computed at an eye level and then averaged by the number of visits. This ensures to have independent samples for subsequent statistical analysis. The significance of the results was evaluated using a paired Wilcoxon signed-rank test with $\alpha = 0.05$.

Three baselines were quantitatively compared with respect to our three proposed models using our private data set of early/intermediate AMD subjects: a binary U-Net trained for background vs. drusen segmentation [3]; a multiclass U-Net trained for segmenting OBRPE and BM [3]; and a multidecoder alternative such as the one in [7], with two decoders for segmenting OBRPE and BM, without connections between them. Enough capacity was given to these baselines to match the one of our models. These quantitative results for drusen segmentation are summarized in Table 1. Figure 3 depicts boxplots representing the mean absolute error in BM and OBRPE segmentation. Our method performed better than the baselines in any of its forms. Inbound/outbound connections with the drusen decoder were observed to significantly increase performance when no

**Table 1.** Quantitative evaluation of drusen segmentation results in our private data set. Values are reported across averaged eye-level performance.

| Method | Dice | Precision | Recall |
|---|---|---|---|
| Binary U-Net [3] (Drusen) | 0.66 ± 0.14 | 0.79 ± 0.09 | 0.58 ± 0.17 |
| Multiclass U-Net [3] (OBRPE/BM) | 0.68 ± 0.13 | 0.79 ± 0.12 | 0.59 ± 0.18 |
| Multitask [7] (OBRPE/BM decoders) | 0.69 ± 0.18 | 0.79 ± 0.16 | 0.62 ± 0.2 |
| Ours (disconnected decoders) | 0.71 ± 0.13 | 0.83 ± 0.07 | 0.64 ± 0.17 |
| Ours (connected with gradient flow) | 0.72 ± 0.12 | 0.83 ± 0.08 | 0.65 ± 0.16 |
| Ours (connected w/o gradient flow) | **0.73 ± 0.12** | **0.84 ± 0.07** | **0.67 ± 0.1** |

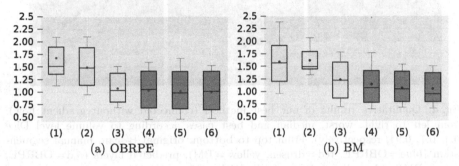

**Fig. 3.** Mean absolute error of OBRPE and BM surface segmentation in pixels on our private data set. (1) Multiclass U-Net with OBRPE/BM targets, (2) Multiclass U-Net with OBRPE/BM/drusen targets, (3) Multitask approach with 2 decoders, (4–6) Our model with (4) disconnected decoders, (5) connected decoders and gradient flow and (6) connected decoders and without gradient flow.

gradient flow is allowed through them (with vs. without gradients, $p < 0.05$). Exemplary results on the central B-scan of volumes with the highest, median and lowest volume level dice are depicted in Fig. 4. Our approach is able to consistently detect drusen of any size. The median case (second column) presents small material accumulations that are slightly undersegmented by our method. A similar behavior is observed in the worst case (first column) for the large drusen in the center of the image. Nevertheless, both cases present visual ambiguities that are difficult to address even for human readers.

Finally, Table 2 presents an evaluation of our best model in the public data set. To match the available annotations, our approach was trained for ILM, IBRPE and BM segmentation, with one branch per target surface. Our model clearly outperformed two recently proposed methods [5,6] that reported their performance on the same dataset.

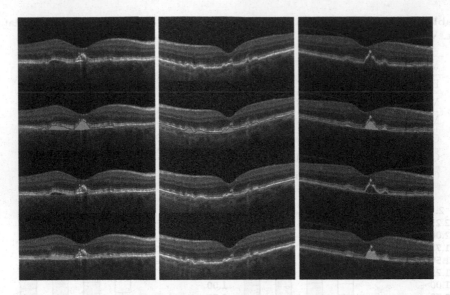

**Fig. 4.** Qualitative results of our best method (connected without gradient flow). From left to right: worst, median and best cases according to volume level Dice (0.4, 0.7, 0.94, respectively). From top to bottom: original B-scan, manual segmentation (blue = OBRPE, red = drusen, yellow = BM), predicted layers (red = OBRPE, green = BM) and predicted drusen (red). (Color figure online)

**Table 2.** Quantitative evaluation of BM, IBRPE and ILM segmentation in terms of absolute surface differences in pixels on Duke data sets [11]. This evaluation is done on AMD and control subjects for 100 AMD cases and 100 healthy cases.

| Method | ILM | IBRPE | BM |
|---|---|---|---|
| *AMD set* | | | |
| Shah *et al.* [5] | $1.15 \pm 0.25$ | $1.88 \pm 0.57$ | $1.81 \pm 0.56$ |
| Liefers *et al.* [6] | 1.055 | 1.568 | 1.858 |
| Ours (connected w/o gradients) | **$0.88 \pm 0.09$** | **$1.23 \pm 0.11$** | **$1.15 \pm 0.1$** |
| *Control (healthy) set* | | | |
| Shah *et al.* [5] | $1.04 \pm 0.07$ | $1.19 \pm 0.18$ | $1.54 \pm 0.31$ |
| Liefers *et al.* [6] | 0.84 | 1.28 | 1.227 |
| Ours (connected w/o gradients) | **$0.65 \pm 0.06$** | **$1.06 \pm 0.12$** | **$0.9 \pm 0.08$** |

## 5    Discussion

We introduced a novel multitask approach for multiclass segmentation in retinal OCT images. In particular, we showed that our multi-decoder architecture is able to outperform standard baselines by incorporating an intermediate decoder that targets the area between two stacked interfaces. This improvement, for example, is observed in drusen segmentation, with an increment of 3% in Dice index with respect to the multitask approach presented in [7]. Introducing connections between decoders also allowed for further improvement on Dice for drusen segmentation, while also improving performance for OBRPE and BM segmentation. Surprisingly, the best results were observed when no gradient flow was allowed between the connected decoders. This implies that, at least on our data set, local information provided by neighbouring classes can improve results. Finally, we also include an evaluation for layer segmentation in OCT images using the Duke public available data set, to further compare our method with the state-of-the-art. We used the same portion size of data as this work, clearly reported the lowest error for all the evaluated surfaces. This promising empirical evidence leads us to envision further applications that might benefit from our approach, such as layer segmentation in retinal diseased cases with fluid, where an extra decoder can be added targeting only those lesions.

**Acknowledgements.** This work was funded by the Christian Doppler Research Association, the Austrian Federal Ministry for Digital and Economic Affairs and the National Foundation for Research, Technology and Development. We thank the NVIDIA corporation for a GPU donation. JIO is funded by WWTF AugUniWien/FA7464A0249 (Medical University of Vienna); VRG12-009 (University of Vienna).

# References

1. Wong, W.L., et al.: Global prevalence of age-related macular degeneration and disease burden projection for 2020 and 2040: a systematic review and meta-analysis. Lancet **2**(2), e106–e116 (2014)
2. Schlanitz, F.G., et al.: Drusen volume development over time and its relevance to the course of age-related macular degeneration. BJO **101**(2), 198–203 (2017)
3. Gorgi Zadeh, S., et al.: CNNs enable accurate and fast segmentation of drusen in optical coherence tomography. In: Cardoso, M., et al. (eds.) DLMIA/ML-CDS-2017. LNCS, vol. 10553, pp. 65–73. Springer, Cham (2017). https://doi.org/10.1007/978-3-319-67558-9_8
4. Fang, L., et al.: Automatic segmentation of nine retinal layer boundaries in OCT images of non-exudative AMD patients using deep learning and graph search. Biomed. Opt. Express **8**(5), 2732–2744 (2017)
5. Shah, A., et al.: Multiple surface segmentation using convolution neural nets: application to retinal layer segmentation in OCT images. Biomed. Opt. Express **9**(9), 4509–4526 (2018)
6. Liefers, B., et al.: Dense segmentation in selected dimensions: application to retinal optical coherence tomography. In: MIDL (2019)
7. Playout, C., Duval, R., Cheriet, F.: A multitask learning architecture for simultaneous segmentation of bright and red lesions in fundus images. In: Frangi, A.F., Schnabel, J.A., Davatzikos, C., Alberola-López, C., Fichtinger, G. (eds.) MICCAI 2018. LNCS, vol. 11071, pp. 101–108. Springer, Cham (2018). https://doi.org/10.1007/978-3-030-00934-2_12
8. Ronneberger, O., Fischer, P., Brox, T.: U-Net: convolutional networks for biomedical image segmentation. In: Navab, N., Hornegger, J., Wells, W.M., Frangi, A.F. (eds.) MICCAI 2015. LNCS, vol. 9351, pp. 234–241. Springer, Cham (2015). https://doi.org/10.1007/978-3-319-24574-4_28

9. Crum, W.R., Camara, O., Hill, D.L.G.: Generalized overlap measures for evaluation and validation in medical image analysis. IEEE-TMI **25**(11), 1451–1461 (2006)
10. Chen, X., Niemeijer, M., Zhang, L., Lee, K., Abràmoff, M.D., Sonka, M.: Three-dimensional segmentation of fluid-associated abnormalities in retinal OCT: probability constrained graph-search-graph-cut. IEEE-TMI **31**(8), 1521–1531 (2012)
11. Farsiu, S., et al.: Quantitative classification of eyes with and without intermediate age-related macular degeneration using optical coherence tomography. Ophthalmology **121**(1), 162–172 (2014)

# Active Appearance Model Induced Generative Adversarial Network for Controlled Data Augmentation

Jianfei Liu, Christine Shen, Tao Liu, Nancy Aguilera, and Johnny Tam[✉]

National Eye Institute, National Institutes of Health, Bethesda, MD, USA
johnny@nih.gov

**Abstract.** Data augmentation is an important strategy for enlarging training datasets in deep learning-based medical image analysis. This is because large, annotated medical datasets are not only difficult and costly to generate, but also quickly become obsolete due to rapid advances in imaging technology. Image-to-image conditional generative adversarial networks (C-GAN) provide a potential solution for data augmentation. However, annotations used as inputs to C-GAN are typically based only on shape information, which can result in undesirable intensity distributions in the resulting artificially-created images. In this paper, we introduce an active cell appearance model (ACAM) that can measure statistical distributions of shape and intensity and use this ACAM model to guide C-GAN to generate more realistic images, which we call A-GAN. A-GAN provides an effective means for conveying anisotropic intensity information to C-GAN. A-GAN incorporates a statistical model (ACAM) to determine how transformations are applied for data augmentation. Traditional approaches for data augmentation that are based on arbitrary transformations might lead to unrealistic shape variations in an augmented dataset that are not representative of real data. A-GAN is designed to ameliorate this. To validate the effectiveness of using A-GAN for data augmentation, we assessed its performance on cell analysis in adaptive optics retinal imaging, which is a rapidly-changing medical imaging modality. Compared to C-GAN, A-GAN achieved stability in fewer iterations. The cell detection and segmentation accuracy when assisted by A-GAN augmentation was higher than that achieved with C-GAN. These findings demonstrate the potential for A-GAN to substantially improve existing data augmentation methods in medical image analysis.

**Keywords:** Generative adversarial network · Active appearance model · Data augmentation · Cell segmentation · Cell detection · Adaptive optics retinal imaging

D. Shen et al. (Eds.): MICCAI 2019, LNCS 11764, pp. 201–208, 2019.
https://doi.org/10.1007/978-3-030-32239-7_23

# 1   Introduction

Deep learning has fundamentally changed the field of medical image analysis. Central to many deep learning-based applications is data augmentation [7,16], an important step because annotated medical imaging datasets are not only difficult and costly to generate, but also because they quickly become obsolete as imaging technology improves. Existing methods for data augmentation are based on operations such as image rotation, shearing, translation, flipping, and Gaussian blurring [7]. Image retrieval has also been suggested for augmenting medical data through the selection of unlabeled medical images that are similar to labeled ones [16]. However, it is rare that these data augmentation strategies alone can lead to large improvements in results.

Recently, generative adversarial networks (GAN) [5], which combine generative and discriminative networks to generate data similar to real data, have shown great promise for data augmentation in medical imaging analysis [8], as in the case of spine segmentation [6] or liver lesion classification [4]. Among GAN techniques, image-to-image conditional GAN (C-GAN) [9] is of particular interest because it can generate artificial medical images from input annotations, which can substantially reduce the need for a large database of human annotations. For example, C-GAN has been adapted to transfer annotations between cardiovascular CT and MRI images and to align segmentations between two modalities [17], as well as to pair PET/CT and MRI/CT images [1]. Artificial lesions have also been created through C-GAN to balance training samples when there were insufficient numbers of pathological cases [10,15].

However, these existing data augmentation approaches are based primarily on shape information, which can result in unrealistic intensity distributions when there are anisotropic intensity distributions (e.g. adaptive optics retinal imaging [13,14], a rapidly-advancing technology for visualizing photoreceptor cells, shown in Fig. 1A). Images of photoreceptor cells exhibit low image contrast at boundaries (white arrows, Fig. 2), which is a common feature of many medical imaging modalities, including MRI and CT images. Whereas data augmentation often utilizes arbitrary data transformations that could easily give rise to datasets that are not representative of real data (e.g. different shape distributions that do not fall within the expected characteristics of real data), we propose that a more realistic approach would be to generate a population of images that captures the natural variations observed within real data. An additional challenge is that it is difficult for C-GAN to capture strong anisotropic intensity distributions because this information is not contained within binary cell contour input annotations. To overcome these challenges, we propose the use of an active cell appearance model (ACAM) [3] to statistically model the shape and intensity distributions of cells. We integrate ACAM with C-GAN, which we call A-GAN.

The contributions of A-GAN are as follows. A-GAN can utilize both shape information as well as intensity distributions for input annotations, a key step for generating more realistic images. This intensity information is useful not only for forcing the generative network to produce objects with similar intensities, but also for helping to stabilize the generative process. Augmented data from A-GAN is more representative of the original population of images because the transformation is applied locally to each cell in a manner that is consistent with the statistical distributions contained in ACAM, as opposed to arbitrary transformations that are applied globally. Evaluation of A-GAN for cell detection and segmentation from medical imaging data showed a clear improvement in performance using A-GAN-based data augmentation compared to existing methods.

## 2    Methods

An overview of A-GAN is shown in Fig. 1. The two main elements are (1) ACAM to compute the statistical distributions of cell contour shapes and intensities and (2) an improved C-GAN to generate realistic cell images by importing cell contours with their respective intensity information.

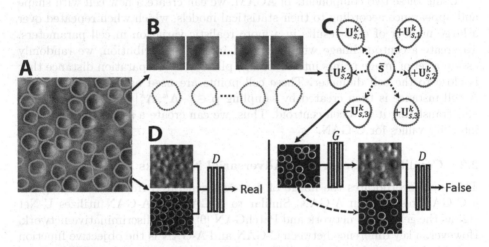

**Fig. 1.** Overview of A-GAN, which augments medical imaging data. (A) Cells (cone photoreceptors) imaged in a patient using an adaptive optics ophthalmoscope [13, 14]. (B) Cells and their contours are extracted. (C) Active cell appearance model (ACAM). (D) Sampling the intensity distributions from ACAM generates cell contours with representative intensity information, which are used to guide an image-to-image conditional GAN (C-GAN).

### 2.1    Active Cell Appearance Model

The goal of this step is to create ACAM in order to compute statistical distributions of cell shapes and intensities in medical imaging data. A set of cell contours and corresponding image patches are extracted from annotated medical images (Figs. 1A and B). Along each contour, $N$ evenly-spaced landmarks (circles, bottom row of Fig. 1B) are defined as a one-dimensional vector $\mathbf{s} = (\mathbf{x}_1, \cdots, \mathbf{x}_N)$. Given $M$ training contours, $\mathcal{S} = \{\mathbf{s}_1, \cdots, \mathbf{s}_M\}$, we can derive a linear contour shape model $\{\bar{\mathbf{s}}, \mathbf{U}_s^k\}$, where $\bar{\mathbf{s}}$ is the mean shape vector of $\mathcal{S}$ and $\mathbf{U}_s^k$ is an orthonormal basis of the first $k$ eigenvectors using principal component analysis (PCA). The corresponding $k$ eigenvalues are in the matrix $\mathbf{\Lambda}_s^k$. A new cell shape instance can be generated as $\mathbf{s}(\mathbf{p}) = \bar{\mathbf{s}} + \mathbf{U}_s^k \cdot \mathbf{p}$, where $\mathbf{p} = (p_1, \cdots, p_k)$ is a shape parameter vector (Fig. 1C).

In addition to shape, anisotropic intensity information at cell contours needs to be embedded into ACAM. We follow a similar procedure as was done for shape. For a set of image patches from $\mathcal{S}$ defined as $\mathcal{I} = \{I_1, \cdots, I_M\}$, we again sample a set of sub-image patches $\mathcal{L}_i = \{L_{i,1}, \cdots, L_{i,N}\}$ of $I_i$ around all contour points of $\mathbf{s}_i$ and align all $\mathcal{L}$ because we are concerned with the intensity distribution near cell contours. Vectoring $\mathcal{L}_i$ as $\mathbf{a}_i$ and applying the PCA results $\{\bar{\mathbf{a}}, \mathbf{U}_a^k\}$, where $\bar{\mathbf{a}}$ is the mean appearance vector and $\mathbf{U}_a^k$ is the orthonormal basis of the first $k$ eigenvectors, we obtain a second eigenvalue matrix $\mathbf{\Lambda}_a^k$. A new appearance instance can be created as $\mathbf{a}(\mathbf{t}) = \bar{\mathbf{a}} + \mathbf{U}_a^k \cdot \mathbf{t}$, where $\mathbf{t} = (t_1, \cdots, t_k)$ is an appearance parameter.

Using these two components of ACAM, we can create a new cell with shape and appearance according to their statistical models, which when repeated over a large number of cells results in a more realistic variation in cell parameters. To create a contour image with a defined intensity distribution, we randomly assign a set of image points into the image plane with a separation distance that is close to the cell diameter. These cell points are used as the cell centroids. A cell instance is then created by sampling $\mathbf{p} \in [-\mathbf{\Lambda}_s^k, \mathbf{\Lambda}_s^k]$ and $t \in [-\mathbf{\Lambda}_a^k, \mathbf{\Lambda}_a^k]$, and translating it to a cell centroid. Thus, we can create a set of contours with intensity values for C-GAN.

## 2.2    Conditional Generative Adversarial Networks

This step incorporates the image of contours generated from ACAM to guide a C-GAN resulting in A-GAN. Similar to C-GAN [9], A-GAN utilizes U-Net [12] as the generative network and PatchGAN [9] as the discriminative network. However, a key difference between C-GAN and A-GAN is the objective function to optimize networks which is different because the input of A-GAN carries partial intensity information for the image to be generated.

During training, a contour image $C$ (bottom image, left panel of Fig. 1D) is created by assigning intensity values from real images to contour positions while all other positions are assigned with the background value (0 in this case). The main purpose of A-GAN is thus to learn a mapping from $C$ and a random noise vector $\mathbf{n}$ to a real image of cells, $I$; i.e., $G : \{C, \mathbf{n}\} \rightarrow I$. The generative network $G$ attempts to produce realistic medical images $I$ that are indistinguishable from the adversely discriminative network $D$, while $D$ tries to improve its ability to flag fake medical images from $G$ during the adversarial process. We define the first component of the objective of A-GAN as

$$F_{GAN}(G, D) = \mathbb{E}_{C,I}[\log D(C, I)] + \mathbb{E}_{C,\mathbf{n}}[\log(1 - D(C, G(C, \mathbf{n})))] \qquad (1)$$

where $G$ attempts to minimize Eq. 1 while $D$ tries to maximize it. Next, A-GAN also incorporates an L1 distance to encourage less blurring (similar to C-GAN),

$$F_{L1}(G) = \mathbb{E}_{C,I,\mathbf{n}}[\|I - G(C, \mathbf{n})\|_1] \qquad (2)$$

Finally, since $C$ contains the partial intensity information of $I$ at cell boundaries, it is also used as an additional term for the objective function of A-GAN,

$$F_C(G) = \mathbb{E}_{C,\mathbf{n}}[\|C - G(C, \mathbf{n})\|_1], \text{ where } C \neq 0 \tag{3}$$

Here, $C \neq 0$ means Eq. 3 only considers the image points that do not belong to the background. Combining Eqs. 1–3 leads to the objective function for A-GAN:

$$F(G, D) = F_{GAN}(G, D) + \lambda_1 F_{L1}(G) + \lambda_2 F_C(G) \tag{4}$$

where $\lambda_1$ and $\lambda_2$ are two constants to balance the terms in Eq. 4. The expected $G$ is $G^* = \arg\min_G \max_D F(G, D)$.

During testing, the contour image created by ACAM is used as the input for A-GAN to produce realistic images (right panel, Fig. 1D). Importantly, the contour image from ACAM contains intensity information, which is a key feature of our approach.

## 2.3 Experiments and Validation Methods

Medical imaging data obtained using an adaptive optics ophthalmoscope [13,14] from 20 human subjects (age: $24.8 \pm 5.1$ years) was used to validate A-GAN. We created four groups of training datasets with $32, 64, 128$, and $256$ medical images ($150 \times 150$ pixels), as well as one separate group of test data with 256 images. The purpose of using a small number of training images was to facilitate the observation of data augmentation effects. All images were randomly selected from these subjects and then cells were annotated by experienced graders.

To evaluate the robustness of A-GAN, we generated four different models of ACAM from the four training groups. ACAM models were used to generate $32, 64, 128$, and $256$ contour images with and without intensity values. Paired image sets with and without intensity values were used in A-GAN and C-GAN, respectively. In this manner, we obtained four pairs of results from C-GAN and A-GAN. We visually evaluated the robustness of these GANs using the generated images.

We assessed whether A-GAN-based data augmentation improved cell detection and cell segmentation results. Here, we used U-Net to perform cell detection by computing the centroid of each cell from the annotated contour images and creating centroid images as the labeled training data. Similarly, cell segmentation was performed using the contour image as the labeled training data. The test dataset was used to evaluate detection and segmentation accuracy. For each training dataset, we also compared three different types of U-Net trained with real medical images incorporating conventional data augmentation, doubled medical images from C-GAN, and doubled medical images from A-GAN. Recall and precision were used to evaluate detection accuracy and Dice coefficient and area difference for segmentation accuracy.

## 3    Experimental Results

### 3.1    Robustness Evaluation

Across the four training groups, A-GAN quickly achieved stability and generated a realistic medical image with only 20 iterations, while C-GAN resulted in many unrealistic cells even after 400 iterations (Fig. 2). These results clearly demonstrate that intensity information from ACAM is a key factor for stabilizing the generative network and improving the accuracy of generated images.

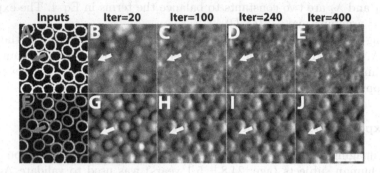

**Fig. 2.** Comparison of generated medical images from C-GAN (top row) and A-GAN (bottom row) following different numbers of iterations using a set of contours with the same shapes, but with intensity information used by A-GAN (no intensity information used by C-GAN). A-GAN quickly achieved stability after only 20 iterations while C-GAN yielded unrealistic cells (white arrows) even after 400 iterations. The scale bar is 20 μm.

### 3.2    Cell Detection

Improvements in detection accuracy through data augmentation of medical images was most readily achieved through A-GAN when compared to both conventional and C-GAN-based data augmentation (Table 1). For conventional data augmentation we applied random rotations, translations, scaling, and shearing to the images. The highest recall and precision values were achieved through A-GAN-based data augmentation.

### 3.3    Cell Segmentation

A-GAN-based data augmentation also resulted in the highest segmentation accuracy (Table 2). Despite the extremely low number of images used for training (as few as 32), A-GAN-based data augmentation was able to outperform existing methods that utilized 8 times more training data (256 images), which demonstrates the effectiveness of our approach. Similar to above, conventional data augmentation was also based on applying random rotations, translations, scaling, and shearing.

**Table 1.** Comparison of cell detection accuracy across the four training datasets based on conventional, C-GAN, and A-GAN-based data augmentation (mean ± SD).

| Training images | Conventional | | C-GAN | | A-GAN | |
|---|---|---|---|---|---|---|
| | Recall (%) | Precision (%) | Recall (%) | Precision (%) | Recall (%) | Precision (%) |
| 32 | 39.8 ± 41.8 | 38.4 ± 40.7 | 71.7 ± 38.9 | 68.3 ± 35.9 | **71.9 ± 31.9** | **77.4 ± 30.6** |
| 64 | 41.6 ± 41.8 | 38.8 ± 39.6 | 71.7 ± 39.6 | 66.2 ± 38.0 | **73.6 ± 34.1** | **78.0 ± 33.7** |
| 128 | 41.8 ± 38.8 | 41.5 ± 39.2 | 72.5 ± 39.3 | 65.9 ± 37.6 | **75.0 ± 34.3** | **77.8 ± 33.5** |
| 256 | 65.6 ± 41.4 | 62.1 ± 39.5 | 72.3 ± 39.3 | 67.0 ± 38.0 | **79.5 ± 33.4** | **79.0 ± 32.1** |

**Table 2.** Comparison of cell segmentation accuracy using Dice coefficient (DC) and area difference (AD) across the four training datasets based on conventional, C-GAN and A-GAN-based data augmentation (mean ± SD).

| Training images | Conventional | | C-GAN | | A-GAN | |
|---|---|---|---|---|---|---|
| | DC (%) | AD (%) | DC (%) | AD (%) | DC (%) | AD (%) |
| 32 | 52.1 ± 12.7 | 46.0 ± 22.7 | 64.3 ± 17.5 | 41.7 ± 48.9 | **75.5 ± 10.5** | **27.9 ± 38.5** |
| 64 | 64.4 ± 17.8 | 48.8 ± 45.5 | 65.6 ± 17.4 | 41.8 ± 34.8 | **80.3 ± 9.9** | **25.5 ± 23.5** |
| 128 | 63.8 ± 17.3 | 38.0 ± 48.3 | 66.2 ± 18.3 | 40.0 ± 37.8 | **85.3 ± 9.2** | **20.1 ± 34.7** |
| 256 | 75.2 ± 12.3 | 21.9 ± 27.9 | 65.7 ± 19.4 | 35.9 ± 40.7 | **86.4 ± 9.8** | **20.2 ± 29.7** |

## 4 Conclusion and Future Work

This work introduces A-GAN, an improved GAN method to augment medical images in a controlled manner that converges to realistic images faster than existing methods and that generates images with characteristics that are statistically representative of real data. This is achieved by using an active cell appearance model (ACAM) to constrain cell shapes and appearances in a statistical space. Unlike arbitrary global data transformation by conventional data augmentation, cell operations based on ACAM are performed locally with variances that are necessarily representative of real data. The intensity values of contours from ACAM are a key factor in defining the object of A-GAN as well as in stabilizing the image generation process. The improvement in cell detection and segmentation accuracy from data augmentation (A-GAN) is substantially greater than that from conventional data augmentation and C-GAN. The proposed methods may be useful for other applications, including fluorescent cell analysis [11], spine segmentation [6], or melanoma segmentation [2], in which anisotropic intensity distributions can be modeled using active appearance models [3]. These results demonstrate that A-GAN is an improved, efficient strategy for augmenting medical imaging data in situations where pixel intensity information is critical in addition to shape information.

**Acknowledgments.** This work was supported by the Intramural Research Program of the National Institutes of Health, National Eye Institute.

# References

1. Armanious, K., Yang, C., Fischer, M., et al.: MedGAN: medical image translation using GANs. CoRR abs/1806.06397 (2018)
2. Chi, Y., Bi, L., Kim, J., Feng, D., Kumar, A.: Controlled synthesis of dermoscopic images via a new color labeled generative style transfer network to enhance melanoma segmentation. In: Proceedings of the IEEE Conference on Engineering in Medicine and Biology Society, pp. 2591–2594 (2018)
3. Cootes, T., Edwards, G., Taylor, C.: Active appearance models. IEEE Trans. Pattern Anal. Mach. Intell. **23**(6), 681–685 (2001)
4. Frid-Adar, M., Diamant, J., Klang, E., et al.: GAN-based synthetic medical image augmentation for increased CNN performance in liver lesion classification. Neurocomputing **321**, 321–331 (2018)
5. Goodfellow, I., Pouget-Abadie, J., Mirae, M., et al.: Generative adversarial networks. In: NIPS, pp. 2672–2680 (2014)
6. Han, Z., Wei, B., Mercado, A., et al.: Spine-GAN: semantic segmentation of multiple spinal structures. Med. Image Anal. **50**, 23–35 (2018)
7. Hussain, Z., Gimenez, F., Yi, D., Rubin, D.: Differential data augmentation techniques for medical imaging classification tasks. In: AMIA Annual Symposium Proceedings, pp. 979–984 (2017)
8. Iqbal, T., Ali, H.: Generative adversarial network for medical images (MI-GAN). J. Med. Syst. **42**(11), 1–11 (2018)
9. Isola, P., Zhu, J., Zhou, T., Efros, A.: Image-to-image translation with conditional adversarial networks. In: IEEE CVPR (2017)
10. Liu, S., Gibson, E., Grbic, S., et al.: Decompose to manipulate: manipulable object synthesis in 3D medical images with structured image decomposition. CoRR abs/1812.01737 (2018)
11. Ramesh, N., Tasdizen, T.: Cell segmentation using a similarity interface with a multi-task convolutional neural network. IEEE J. Biomed. Health Inform. **23**(4), 1457–1468 (2019)
12. Ronneberger, O., Fischer, P., Brox, T.: U-Net: convolutional networks for biomedical image segmentation. In: Navab, N., Hornegger, J., Wells, W.M., Frangi, A.F. (eds.) MICCAI 2015. LNCS, vol. 9351, pp. 234–241. Springer, Cham (2015). https://doi.org/10.1007/978-3-319-24574-4_28
13. Roorda, A., Duncan, J.: Adaptive optics ophthalmoscopy. Ann. Rev. Vis. Sci. **1**, 19–50 (2015)
14. Scoles, D., Sulai, Y., Langlo, C., et al.: In vivo imaging of human cone photoreceptor inner segments. Invest. Ophthalmol. Vis. Sci. **55**(7), 4244–4251 (2014)
15. Wu, E., Wu, K., Cox, D., Lotter, W.: Conditional infilling GANs for data augmentation in mammogram classification. In: Stoyanov, D., et al. (eds.) RAMBO/BIA/TIA-2018. LNCS, vol. 11040, pp. 98–106. Springer, Cham (2018). https://doi.org/10.1007/978-3-030-00946-5_11
16. Zhang, C., Tavanapong, W., Wong, J., de Groen, P.C., Oh, J.H.: Real data augmentation for medical image classification. In: Cardoso, M.J., et al. (eds.) LABELS/CVII/STENT-2017. LNCS, vol. 10552, pp. 67–76. Springer, Cham (2017). https://doi.org/10.1007/978-3-319-67534-3_8
17. Zhang, Z., Yang, L., Zheng, Y.: Translating and segmenting multimodal medical volumes with cycle- and shape-consistency generative adversarial network. In: IEEE CVPR (2018)

# Biomarker Localization by Combining CNN Classifier and Generative Adversarial Network

Rong Zhang[1,2], Shuhan Tan[1], Ruixuan Wang[1,2(✉)], Siyamalan Manivannan[3],
Jingjing Chen[4], Haotian Lin[4], and Wei-Shi Zheng[1,2]

[1] School of Data and Computer Science, Sun Yat-sen University, Guangzhou, China
wangruix5@mail.sysu.edu.cn
[2] Key Laboratory of Machine Intelligence and Advanced Computing,
MOE, Guangzhou, China
[3] Department of Computer Science, University of Jaffna, Jaffna, Sri Lanka
[4] Zhongshan Ophthalmic Center, Sun Yat-sen University, Guangzhou, China

**Abstract.** This paper proposes a novel deep neural network architecture to effectively localize potential biomarkers in medical images, when only the image-level labels are available during model training. The proposed architecture combines a CNN classifier and a generative adversarial network (GAN) in a novel way, such that the CNN classifier and the discriminator in the GAN can effectively help the encoder-decoder in the GAN to remove biomarkers. Biomarkers in abnormal images can then be easily localized and segmented by subtracting the output of the encoder-decoder from its original input. The proposed approach was evaluated on diabetic retinopathy images with real biomarkers and on skin images with simulated biomarkers, showing state-of-the-art performance in localizing biomarkers even if biomarkers are irregularly scattered and are of various sizes in images.

**Keywords:** Biomarker localization · Encoder-decoder · Generative adversarial networks

## 1 Introduction

Visual biomarkers in medical images are important indicators for radiologists to investigate the risks, categories, and status of particular diseases. Therefore, automatic localization and segmentation of existing or potentially novel biomarkers from various medical images would be a key step for intelligent diagnosis and treatment of diseases. While it is relatively easier for human experts to roughly locate biomarkers (e.g., with bounding boxes surrounding biomarker regions), it is challenging, if not impossible, for humans to precisely localize and

**Electronic supplementary material** The online version of this chapter (https://doi.org/10.1007/978-3-030-32239-7_24) contains supplementary material, which is available to authorized users.

© Springer Nature Switzerland AG 2019
D. Shen et al. (Eds.): MICCAI 2019, LNCS 11764, pp. 209–217, 2019.
https://doi.org/10.1007/978-3-030-32239-7_24

segment biomarkers particularly when they are irregularly scattered in images. As a result, it is highly desirable to precisely localize biomarkers only based on weak annotations, e.g., image-level labels representing whether images contain diseases (labelled 'abnormal') or not (labelled 'normal').

Multiple approaches have been proposed to alleviate the great challenge of biomarker localization only based on image-level annotations. One traditional approach is multiple instance learning [7], a weakly supervised technique which can train a classifier not only predicting the labels of images, but also roughly localizing the discriminative regions (possible biomarkers) in abnormal images. Such technique has been applied to solve various medical imaging problems, such as segmenting retinal nerve fibers from retinal fundus images [6] and cancer detection in digital pathology images [5]. Another group of approaches, proposed in the computer vision community, is through visualizing image regions on which convolutional neural network (CNN) classifiers focus when predicting classes of images. Among them, perturbation methods occlude or mask each possible local region and check the changes in classifier outputs, with larger drops in output indicating higher importance in predicting image classes [14]. In comparison, feature activation methods locate important local regions based on activated regions in feature maps of certain convolutional layer's output, e.g., the popular class activation mapping (CAM) [13] and its variants Grad-CAM [10] etc. Recently, the CAM-based methods have been widely applied in medical image analyses, e.g., for pneumonia detection on chest X-ray images [8], bladder cancer prediction in digital pathology images [12] and Alzheimer diagnosis in MRI images [11]. However, all the above methods can only roughly locate biomarker or lesion regions, leaving the precise localization of biomarkers as an open problem.

In this paper, to precisely localize biomarkers, we propose a deep neural network architecture by combining a CNN classifier, a generator and a discriminator. The generator aims to output a normal version of each abnormal input image by removing potential biomarkers from the input image, such that the biomarkers in abnormal images can be easily localized and segmented by subtracting the output of the generator from its input. To help achieve this goal, a CNN classifier is added to encourage biomarker removal by classifying the subtraction (of the output of the generator from its input) as normal or abnormal. On the other hand, to make the output of the generator realistically normal, a discriminator is added and trained adversarially to discriminate real and generated normal images. Note that the generator and discriminator naturally form a generative adversarial network (GAN) [4]. Qualitative and quantitative evaluations on diabetic retinopathy images with real biomarkers and on skin images with simulated biomarkers showed superior performance of the proposed architecture to that of the CAM-based methods in precisely localizing biomarkers.

## 2    Method

The purpose is to precisely localize potential biomarkers or lesion regions in abnormal images when only the image-level labels are available. Different from the visualization methods (e.g., CAM or Grad-CAM) which can only approximately localize potential biomarkers at low resolution in images after training a classifier, the motivation of our idea is to design a new architecture which can learn to directly find precise locations of potential biomarkers. With this motivation, we proposed a novel deep neural network by combining two different learning architectures (Fig. 1): a supervised CNN classifier and a GAN (composed of an encoder-decoder and a discriminator).

In the proposed architecture, the encoder-decoder network tries to remove any potential biomarkers from the input image, generating a fake normal image for abnormal input image, or keeping the output image the same as the input if the input is normal. By subtracting the output of the encoder-decoder from its input, any biomarkers can be easily localized and segmented. While it is possible to train such an encoder-decoder just with normal images, this does not make use of the existing abnormal images, therefore not directly learning biomarker features for localization. Instead, to more effectively achieve the goal of the encoder-decoder, a CNN classifier is added on top of the encoder-decoder, with input being the subtraction of the encoder-decoder's output from its input, and expected output being the label of the original input image to the auto-encoder. In order to accurately classify images, the CNN classifier together with the encoder-decoder would have to differentiate abnormal images from normal ones. Ideally, if the input to the classifier contains only biomarkers for abnormal original images and contains nothing (zero values everywhere) for normal images, the classifier would more easily and accurately predict the category of the original images. In other words, training a more accurate classifier could help the encoder-decoder's output keep the normal regions and remove biormakers from the original image, such that the input to the classifier only contains biomarker signals.

However, the classifier may help localize just part of biomarkers from the original images. This is because localizing part of biomarker signals from original abnormal images (and localizing little signal from normal images) is enough for the classifier to easily differentiate between normal and abnormal images. In this case, the encoder-decoder output would still contain some biomarkers.

To further help the encoder-decoder remove potential biomarkers from original (abnormal) images, a discriminator is added to judge whether the output of the encoder-decoder looks like a real normal image or not. By forcing the encoder-decoder's outputs to look more like normal images, the discriminator helps the encoder-decoder remove as much biomarker signals as possible from original images.

It is clear that the encoder-decoder and the discriminator together form a generative adversarial network (GAN). One may consider that the GAN itself, without the classifier component in the architecture, may be enough to help the encoder-decoder remove potential biomarkers from images. However, GAN itself could help too much such that, although the encoder-decoder generates quite normal images, the normal regions of the encoder-decoder's output may also be changed compared to the input. In this case, the subtraction of the

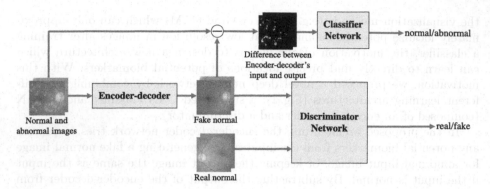

**Fig. 1.** The proposed architecture for biomarker localization. The classifier and the discriminator together can help the encoder-decoder more effectively remove biomarkers from input images. Biomarkers can then be localized by subtracting the encoder-decoder's output from its input.

encoder-decoder's output from its input, i.e., the input to the classifier, would contain both normal and biomarker signals, which in turn makes it relatively more difficult for the classifier to differentiate abnormal images from normal ones. That means, the classifier and the discriminator should work together to help the encoder-decoder remove potential biomarkers, i.e., the discriminator helps the encoder-decoder output normal images and the classifier helps the encoder-decoder only change biomarker regions to generate normal outputs. This has been experimentally confirmed (see Sect. 3.2).

In the proposed architecture, let us denote the encoder-decoder by $G$, the discriminator by $D$, and the classifier by $C$, then the problem of biomarker localization can be formulated as optimizing the deep neural network model by

$$\min_{G,C} \max_{D} \; L_{GAN}(D,G) + \lambda_1 L_{CE}(C,G) + \lambda_2 L_{ED}(G), \quad (1)$$

where $L_{GAN}(D,G)$ is the objective function of the GAN (here we used WGAN; [1]), $L_{CE}(C,G)$ is the cross-entropy loss for the classifier $C$, and $L_{ED}(G)$ is the encoder-decoder loss (here we used $L1$ loss) emphasizing the similarity between its output and input. $\lambda_1$ and $\lambda_2$ are coefficients balancing the three different parts.

During model training, an alternating strategy is adopted by updating different parts of the model iteratively, i.e.,

$$\min_{G,C} \; L_1 = \lambda_1 L_{CE}(C,G) + \lambda_2 L_{ED}(G), \quad (2)$$

$$\min_{G} \max_{D} \; L_2 = L_{GAN}(D,G) + \lambda_2 L_{ED}(G). \quad (3)$$

# 3   Experimental Evaluation

## 3.1   Experimental Settings

Two datasets were used to evaluate the proposed model. One was derived from the Kaggle Diabetic Retinopathy (DR) dataset[1], from which 2,101 abnormal images containing clear diabetic biomarkers and 2,101 normal images were selected. Uninformative dark regions in each image were removed before inputting to the neural network. Since it is highly costly for humans to precisely locate and segment the biomarkers in all abnormal images, here 40 abnormal images were randomly selected and then annotated at pixel level by two practising ophthalmologists. Note that the pixel-level annotations were not for model training but only for quantitative evaluation of the proposed model on the DR dataset.

The second dataset consists of skin images with artificial biomarkers. To generate this dataset, 2,920 normal images (actually image patches) of size $128 \times 128$ were firstly extracted from a dermoscopy image dataset [2]. To simulate varying number, size, and location of biomarkers in real skin images, the values of these parameters were randomly generated in a certain range for each simulated skin image. More specifically, for each image of the half dataset, one to three images were randomly selected from the ImageNet [3] and resized to either $4 \times 4$, $8 \times 8$ or $16 \times 16$ pixels. The thumbnail images were embedded into the skin image and then locally smoothed as artificial biomarkers. Pixel-level annotations were available for all artificial biomarkers.

In the proposed architecture, a modified UNet [9] was selected for the encoder-decoder network, with Tanh activation function added at last layer to constrain the pixel values of the UNet's output within the same range ($[-1, 1]$) as that of the UNet's input. The UNet is pre-trained with all images for each dataset. A Resnet-18 was used for the classifier network and a seven-layer CNN for the discriminator network. Gradient penalty coefficient $\eta$ in the WGAN loss was set to 10. Adam was used for model training, with default learning rate $= 0.0002$, batch size $= 32$. For all tests, $\lambda_1 = 0.4$ and $\lambda_2 = 10.0$. We use PR curves for quantitative evaluation, which were generated by comparing the pixel-level localization results with ground truth annotations. The heat maps of localization results were normalized to $[0, 1]$ before PR generation. Please note that ROC curves are not suitable for evaluating the biomarker localization performance, as the proportions of positive and negative pixels in each dataset are highly imbalanced (1:56 for DR dataset, 1:88 for skin dataset). Therefore, we only included the ROC curves for each experiment in the supplementary material.

Please note that our goal is to search for and localize visual (pixel-level) biomarkers from images with the help of image-level labels, rather than training a model to find biomarkers from new images. Therefore, for each dataset, all the images were used to train our model, and the model was then evaluated

---

[1]   https://www.kaggle.com/c/diabetic-retinopathy-detection/data.

qualitatively and quantitatively. Thus we trained and evaluated our model on the same dataset.

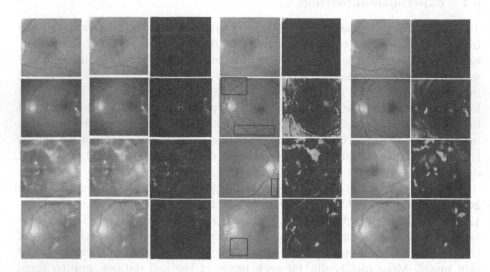

**Fig. 2.** Localization of biomarkers in retinal images. From left to right: original images, encoder-decoder output without the discriminator, the difference between first and second column, encoder-decoder output without the classifier, the difference between first and fourth column, encoder-decoder output with both classifier and discriminator included, the difference between first and sixth column. (Color figure online)

### 3.2  Roles of Architecture Components

This section evaluates the role of the classifier network and the discriminator network in the proposed architecture in localizing biomarkers from retinal images. We first compared the qualitative results. Figure 2 shows that, without the discriminator, the classifier helped localize only part of the biomarkers ($3^{rd}$ column), leaving most of biomarkers remained in the output of the encoder-decoder ($2^{nd}$ column). On the other hand, without the classifier, the discriminator localized most (if not all) biomarker regions ($5^{th}$ column). However, some normal regions were also altered (red boxes in $4^{th}$ column), causing some false biomarkers including some regions along vessels (see localized vessel curves in $5^{th}$ column). In comparison, the combination of the classifier and the discriminator in the proposed approach resulted in the precise localization of most biomarkers, with much fewer false biomarkers ($7^{th}$ column) and biomarkers removed in the output of the encoder-decoder ($6^{th}$ column). These results suggest that the classifier and the discriminator networks together help localize biomarkers as discussed in Sect. 2. This is further confirmed by quantitative evaluation of different model components, which shows that the proposed architecture (green 'G-D-C' curve in Fig. 3) performs better than that without the classifier (blue 'G-D' curve) or without the discriminator (red 'G-C' curve).

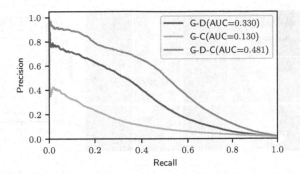

**Fig. 3.** Effect of model components. G-D represents encoder-decoder with only the discriminator, G-C represents encoder-decoder with only the classifier, and G-D-C represents our full model. The performance of the only encoder-decoder model was also evaluated, with AUC = 0.083 only (not shown in figure). The PR curves were generated as described in Sect. 3.1. (Color figure online)

### 3.3   Comparison with Visualization Methods for Localization

In this section we compare the localization ability of the proposed approach with the widely used visualization techniques CAM and Grad-CAM. ResNet-18 and VGG-19 binary classifiers were trained for CAM and Grad-CAM respectively. As can be seen from Fig. 4 (Left), while CAM found most biomarker regions, it also considered surrounding areas as part of biomarkers. This is largely due to the upsampling of the output of the last convolutional layer ($4 \times 4$) to the image size ($128 \times 128$). CAM also failed to detect most of the abnormal areas in the first image($3^{rd}$ column, $1^{st}$ row). As an extension of CAM, Grad-CAM allows us to generate visual explanations from multiple layers, e.g., the intermediate

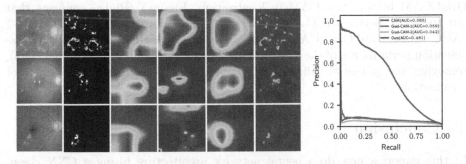

**Fig. 4.** Comparisons with visualization methods on real diabetic retinopathy dataset. Left-half: localization results by CAM ($3^{rd}$ column), Grad-CAM-1 ($4^{th}$ column), Grad-CAM-2 ($5^{th}$ column) and our approach ($6^{th}$ column) on exemplar retinal images ($1^{st}$ column). Red regions in the heatmaps indicate higher probabilities to be biomarkers and blue for normal regions. The binary ground truth annotations are shown in the $2^{nd}$ column. Right half: the PR curve for each method. (Color figure online)

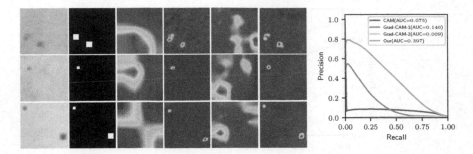

**Fig. 5.** Comparisons with visualization methods on skin image data. Left half: exemplar skin images ($1^{st}$ column), binary ground truth segmentation ($2^{nd}$ column), localization results by CAM ($3^{rd}$ column), Grad-CAM-1 ($4^{th}$ column), Grad-CAM-2 ($5^{th}$ column), and our approach ($6^{th}$ column). Right half: the PR curve for each method.

convolutional layer ($4^{th}$ column, denoted as Grad-CAM-1) and the last convolutional layer ($5^{th}$ column, denoted as Grad-CAM-2). Although relatively accurate localization of biomarkers is attained in the $4^{th}$ column by Grad-CAM, the results are still either not precise ($1^{st}$ row) or not accurate ($2^{nd}$ and $3^{rd}$ row) enough. In comparison, the proposed approach gave much more precise localization of biomarkers with irregular shapes and scattered distributions, proving its superior performance to that of CAM and Grad-CAM. This is confirmed by quantitative evaluation of each method (Fig. 4, Right), with the area under the PR curve (AUC) being 0.481 for the proposed model, 0.065 for CAM, and 0.061, 0.042 for different layers of Grad-CAM.

The superior performance of the proposed model was further confirmed on the skin images with artificial biomarkers. Figure 5 (Left half) shows that the proposed approach can almost perfectly and precisely localize the artificial biomarkers, while CAM and Grad-CAM again demonstrated inferior performance, with Grad-CAM better than CAM in localization. Figure 5 (Right) confirms that our model is better (AUC = 0.397) than CAM (AUC = 0.075), Grad-CAM-1 (AUC = 0.146) and Grad-CAM-2 (AUC = 0.009). Note that in all tests, the classification performance of the classifiers are similar (above 97% on both datasets), removing the potential influence of classification performance on biomarker localization.

## 4  Conclusion

In this paper, a new deep neural network architecture fusing a CNN classifier and GAN together was introduced to effectively localize biomarkers from medical images. Compared with widely used localization methods, the proposed model can more precisely localize potential biomarkers even if they are irregularly scattered and of various forms and sizes. This provides a new way to detect potentially novel biomarkers for various diseases, which will be investigated as future work.

**Acknowledgement.** This work is supported in part by the National Key Research and Development Program (grant No. 2018YFC1315402, No. 2018YFC0116500), the Guangdong Key Research and Development Program (grant No. 2019B020228001), and the National Natural Science Foundation of China (grant No. 81770967, No. 91846109).

# References

1. Arjovsky, M., Chintala, S., Bottou, L.: Wasserstein GAN. arXiv preprint arXiv:1701.07875 (2017)
2. Codella, N.C., Gutman, D., et al.: Skin lesion analysis toward melanoma detection: a challenge at the 2017 international symposium on biomedical imaging (ISBI), hosted by the international skin imaging collaboration (ISIC). In: ISBI (2018)
3. Deng, J., Dong, W., Socher, R., Li, L.J., Li, K., Fei-Fei, L.: ImageNet: a large-scale hierarchical image database. In: CVPR (2009)
4. Goodfellow, I., et al.: Generative adversarial nets. In: NIPS (2014)
5. Kandemir, M., Zhang, C., Hamprecht, F.A.: Empowering multiple instance histopathology cancer diagnosis by cell graphs. In: Golland, P., Hata, N., Barillot, C., Hornegger, J., Howe, R. (eds.) MICCAI 2014. LNCS, vol. 8674, pp. 228–235. Springer, Cham (2014). https://doi.org/10.1007/978-3-319-10470-6_29
6. Manivannan, S., Cobb, C., Burgess, S., Trucco, E.: Subcategory classifiers for multiple-instance learning and its application to retinal nerve fiber layer visibility classification. IEEE TMI **36**(5), 1140–1150 (2017)
7. Maron, O., Lozano-Pérez, T.: A framework for multiple-instance learning. In: NIPS (1998)
8. Rajpurkar, P., Irvin, J., Zhu, K., et al.: CheXNet: radiologist-level pneumonia detection on chest X-rays with deep learning. arXiv preprint arXiv:1711.05225 (2017)
9. Ronneberger, O., Fischer, P., Brox, T.: U-Net: convolutional networks for biomedical image segmentation. In: Navab, N., Hornegger, J., Wells, W.M., Frangi, A.F. (eds.) MICCAI 2015. LNCS, vol. 9351, pp. 234–241. Springer, Cham (2015). https://doi.org/10.1007/978-3-319-24574-4_28
10. Selvaraju, R.R., Cogswell, M., Das, A., Vedantam, R., Parikh, D., Batra, D., et al.: Grad-CAM: visual explanations from deep networks via gradient-based localization. In: ICCV (2017)
11. Yang, C., Rangarajan, A., Ranka, S.: Visual explanations from deep 3D convolutional neural networks for Alzheimer's disease classification. arXiv preprint arXiv:1803.02544 (2018)
12. Zhang, Z., Xie, Y., Xing, F., McGough, M., Yang, L.: MDNet: a semantically and visually interpretable medical image diagnosis network. In: CVPR (2017)
13. Zhou, B., Khosla, A., Lapedriza, A., Oliva, A., Torralba, A.: Learning deep features for discriminative localization. In: CVPR (2016)
14. Zintgraf, L.M., Cohen, T.S., Adel, T., Welling, M.: Visualizing deep neural network decisions: prediction difference analysis. arXiv preprint arXiv:1702.04595 (2017)

# Probabilistic Atlases to Enforce Topological Constraints

Udaranga Wickramasinghe[1]([⊠]), Graham Knott[2], and Pascal Fua[1]

[1] Computer Vision Laboratory, École Polytechnique Fédérale de Lausanne,
Lausanne, Switzerland
udaranga.wickramasinghe@epfl.ch
[2] BioEM Laboratory, École Polytechnique Fédérale de Lausanne,
Lausanne, Switzerland

**Abstract.** Probabilistic atlases (PAs) have long been used in standard segmentation approaches and, more recently, in conjunction with Convolutional Neural Networks (CNNs). However, their use has been restricted to relatively standardized structures such as the brain or heart which have limited or predictable range of deformations. Here we propose an encoding-decoding CNN architecture that can exploit rough atlases that encode only the topology of the target structures that can appear in any pose and have arbitrarily complex shapes to improve the segmentation results. It relies on the output of the encoder to compute both the pose parameters used to deform the atlas and the segmentation mask itself, which makes it effective and end-to-end trainable.

## 1 Introduction

Probabilistic atlases (PAs) are widely used for multi-atlas based segmentation [8]. With the advent of deep learning, there has been a push to incorporate them with Convolutional Neural Networks (CNNs) as well [1,7,14,15]. The published techniques relying on deep learning share a number of features: They work best for structures featuring relatively small variations in shape and position; the atlases are often created by fusing multiple manually annotated images; the atlases must also be pre-registered to the target images to align them with the structures of interest.

Thus, the PAs have been mostly used to segment structures such as the brain or heart for which the above requirements can be met. In this paper, we propose an approach to design and handle PAs that makes them usable in complex situations where the shape and position can vary dramatically, such as those shown in Fig. 1. Our PAs are coarse and only encode the relative position and topology of the structures we expect to find. To register them, we rely on affine transforms whose parameters are estimated at the same time as the segmentations

**Electronic supplementary material** The online version of this chapter (https://doi.org/10.1007/978-3-030-32239-7_25) contains supplementary material, which is available to authorized users.

D. Shen et al. (Eds.): MICCAI 2019, LNCS 11764, pp. 218–226, 2019.
https://doi.org/10.1007/978-3-030-32239-7_25

themselves using the end-to-end trainable encoder-decoder architecture depicted by Fig. 2, which we will refer to as **PA-Net**. The affine transforms are used to warp the atlases and feed the features of the warped atlases to the decoder. This differs significantly from earlier approaches [14,15] that rely on pre-registered atlases.

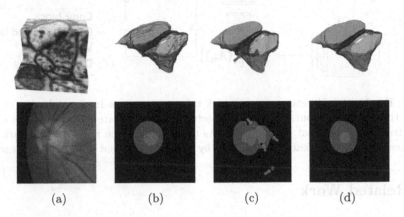

(a)                    (b)                    (c)                    (d)

**Fig. 1.** Eliminating topological mistakes. (a) A small FIBSEM image stack featuring a synaptic junction and a retinal fundus image. (b) Ground-truth segmentations. The pre-synaptic, synaptic-cleft, and post-synaptic regions shown in green, red, and blue respectively. Similarly, the optic disk and cup shown in green and red, respectively. (c) U-Net segmentations with orange arrows pointing to topological mistakes. (d) Our error-free result. (Color figure online)

We validate our approach on segmentation of synaptic junctions in Electron Microscopy (EM) images and optic nerve head segmentation in retinal fundus images. A synaptic junction has an arbitrary shape but always features a synaptic cleft sandwiched between a pre-synaptic bouton belonging to the axon of one neuron and a post-synaptic dendritic spine belonging to another. In this case, the shape complexity and unpredictability precludes the use of standard PAs. Optic nerve head consists of an optic disk and optic cup. Even though their shape does not vary significantly, there are significant variations in the size of the optic cup and the position of the optic nerve head.

We will show that **PA-Net** eliminates most of the topological mistakes its unaided V-Net [11] or U-Net [13] backbone makes on the EM and retinal images, while being generic and potentially applicable to other segmentation tasks. Our contribution is therefore a novel approach that makes it possible to use probabilistic atlases even in situations where shape variability is too great for existing approaches and methods to integrate the atlas registration process directly into the network. The code is publicly available[1].

---

[1] https://github.com/cvlab-epfl/PA-net.git.

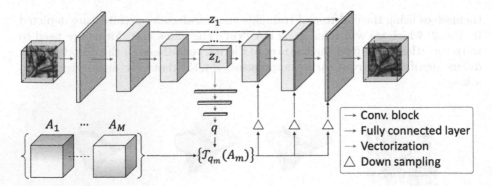

**Fig. 2. PA-Net** architecture. The network takes as input an image and a list of PAs. Given the decoder output, the fully connected layers estimate the parameters of the affine transformation that registers the PAs to the input. The registered PAs are then concatenated with the features computed by the convolutional decoder at each scale.

## 2    Related Work

PAs are commonly used in standard atlas-based segmentation approaches. In their piplines, CNNs are indirectly used to perform segmentation. These include using a CNN to infer deformation maps to register target images to atlas images [2] and using it to implicitly infer the segmentation masks [4,6]; using CNNs to improve the selection of best atlases from a library [10]. As this is not the focus of this paper, we will not discuss them further and will concentrate on methods that directly use the PAs to assist a CNN that perform segmentation.

A PA can provide localization priors to help a network find the target of interest. Such PAs are often referred to as seed layers. They come in two flavors, Gaussian priors [3,16] or binary seed layers [9]. Another popular way to focus the attention of the network is to provide an attention mask [5], which then serves the same purpose as a PA. However, the attention masks are derived from the input data itself and does not act as an external knowledge source.

PAs built by fusing multiple manually annotated images can be used to introduce even more prior knowledge about shape and topology of structures. In [14,15], this is done to improve segmentations of human brain by having the CNN take pre-registered PAs as input. In our work, we extend the idea by demonstrating that PAs can be used to introduce topological knowledge even when the structure of interest exhibits large shape variations and without pre-registration that the whole system is end-to-end trainable.

## 3    Approach

### 3.1    Network Architecture

The architecture of the proposed **PA-Net** is depicted in Fig. 2. Its backbone is an encoder-decoder architecture similar to the one used in popular networks such as U-Net [13] or V-Net [11]. These networks are designed to learn to approximate the distribution $p(\mathbf{Y}|\mathbf{X})$, where $\mathbf{X}$ is the input image and $\mathbf{Y}$ is the output segmentation. We extend the idea by learning the joint distribution $p(\mathbf{Y}, T_{\mathbf{q}}(\mathcal{A})|\mathbf{X}, \mathcal{A})$. The function $T_{\mathbf{q}}(\cdot)$ applies affine transformations to the set of PAs $\mathcal{A}$ given the pose vectors $\mathbf{q}$. We factorize this joint distribution as

$$p(\mathbf{Y}, T_{\mathbf{q}}(\mathcal{A})|\mathbf{X}, \mathcal{A}) = p(\mathbf{Y}|\mathbf{X}, T_{\mathbf{q}}(\mathcal{A}))p(\mathbf{q}|\mathbf{X}, \mathcal{A}) \tag{1}$$

**PA-Net** models it using a primary stream, the encoder-decoder backbone at the top of Fig. 2, and a secondary stream, the fully connected layers at the bottom of Fig. 2. The secondary stream $\mathcal{F}(\cdot, \theta_f)$ originates from the latent vector produced by the final stage of the encoder $\mathcal{E}(\cdot, \theta_e)$, estimates the affine parameter vector $\mathbf{q}$, uses it to warp the atlases, and feed them to the various layers of the decoder $\mathcal{D}(\cdot; \theta_d)$ after rescaling them to the resolution of feature vectors at each stage. Here $\theta_e, \theta_d$ and $\theta_f$ are the learned weights that control the behavior of $\mathcal{E}, \mathcal{D}$ and $\mathcal{F}$. Given the encoder output, $\mathcal{F}$ and $\mathcal{D}$ model $p(\mathbf{Y}|\mathbf{X}, T_{\mathbf{q}}(A))$ and $p(\mathbf{q}|\mathbf{X}, A)$, respectively. This guarantees that these two distributions are learned from the same features. Training the encoder to produce features that are effective for both tasks yield improved performance.

### 3.2 Atlas Design

Figure 3 depicts the topological atlases we use to segment synaptic junctions and optic disks and cups. In the first case, they are cubes and in the second, ordinary 2D arrays. They encode the probability of any pixel of voxel to belong to one of the possible classes—pre-synaptic, cleft, or post-synaptic for synapses and optic disk or cup for retinas—given its pose.

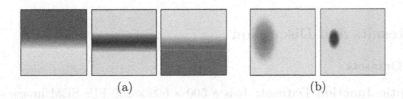

(a)                                          (b)

**Fig. 3.** Probabilistic atlases. (a) For synaptic junction segmentation, they are cubes and we show a single face. (b) For optic optic disk and cup segmentation, they are regular 2D arrays. The color hues denote the same areas as those in Fig. 1. The color saturation is proportional to the probability at a given location. (Color figure online)

### 3.3 Atlas Registration

Parameters necessary for PA registration is computed by estimating the pose vector $q$. When working with image cubes such as the one shown at the top of

Fig. 1, we take the pose vector to be $\mathbf{q} = [t_x, t_y, t_z, s_x, s_y, s_z, r_x, r_y, r_z]$, where $t_{\{x,y,z\}}$ represent translations and $s_{\{x,y,z\}}$ scalings in the $x, y$, and $z$ directions, respectively. We represent the orientation using the angle-axis vector $[r_x, r_y, r_z]$, whose direction is the axis of rotation. When working with 2D images, we drop $t_z$, $s_z$, and $r_z$ from $\mathbf{q}$.

**Table 1.** Comparative results for synaptic junction segmentation.

| | Jaccard index (%) | | | | TER |
|---|---|---|---|---|---|
| | Pre-synaptic | Synaptic junction | Post-synaptic | Mean | |
| V-Net | **63.0** | 56.0 | 80.6 | 66.5 | 5/15 |
| PA-VNet | 59.5 | **57.8** | **83.1** | **66.8** | 1/15 |
| U-Net | **73.6** | 59.7 | 79.1 | 70.7 | 7/15 |
| Naive PA-UNet | 73.4 | 58.0 | 78.4 | 69.9 | 7/15 |
| PA-UNet | 72.6 | **62.8** | **87.0** | **74.1** | 3/15 |

### 3.4 Loss Functions

Following standard practice, we formulate the loss terms as the negative log likelihood of the joint distribution $p(\mathbf{Y}, T_\mathbf{q}(A)|\mathbf{X}, \mathcal{A})$ of Eq. 1. This yields the composite loss

$$\mathcal{L} = \mathcal{L}_{seg} + \mathcal{L}_{pose}. \tag{2}$$

$\mathcal{L}_{seg}$ is the standard cross entropy loss that evaluates segmentation performance and take $\mathcal{L}_{pose}$ is the least square error in estimating the pose $\mathbf{q}$.

## 4    Results and Discussion

### 4.1    Datasets

**Synaptic Junction Dataset:** It is a $500 \times 500 \times 200$ FIB-SEM image stack of a mouse cortex. We used 50 xy slices for training, 50 for validation, and 100 for testing. From each set, we cropped $96 \times 96 \times 96$ image volumes containing a synaptic junction such as the one shown in the top row of Fig. 1(a) and they are zero-padded as necessary. This gave us 13, 10 and 15 volumes for training, validation and testing, respectively. The synapse is not necessarily perfectly centered and the task is to segment pre-synaptic region, post-synaptic region, and synaptic cleft.

**Retinal Fundus Image Dataset:** It comprises 400 $2124 \times 2056$ retinal fundus images acquired using a Zeiss Visucam 500 camera [12], which we resize and pad to be $512 \times 512$. We use 100 for training, 100 for validation, and 200 for testing.

**Table 2.** Comparative results for fetinal fundus image segmentation.

| | Jaccard index (%) | | | TER |
|---|---|---|---|---|
| | Optic disk | Optic cup | Mean | |
| V-Net | 78.4 | 72.5 | 75.5 | 7/200 |
| PA-VNet | **79.0** | **73.0** | **76.0** | 3/200 |
| U-Net | 81.3 | 73.8 | 77.6 | 18/200 |
| Naive PA-UNet | 80.8 | 74.1 | 77.3 | 16/200 |
| PA-UNet | **81.6** | **74.6** | **78.1** | **5/200** |

## 4.2   Quantitative and Qualitative Results

We evaluate segmentation performance in terms of the standard Jaccard Index and of an additional metric we dub the *Topological Error Ratio* (TER). We define TER as the ratio of segmentations containing topological errors to the total number of test images. A segmentation is considered to contain a topological error if it violates the expected topology of the target structure, that is, it features semantic labels appearing where they should not given the topological constraints. We compute this value by finding the connected components of the final segmentation and then finding instances that violate the topology.

We tested two versions of **PA-Net**, one based on the U-Net [13] architecture and the other based on the more recent V-Net [11]. We compare the results against those of the standard U-Net and V-Net. We report our comparative results on our two datasets in Tables 1 and 2. Figures 4 depict them qualitatively (see supplementary materials for further results). Using the atlas consistently improves over baseline performance. The gains are most visible in TER terms because our **PA-Net**s truly come into their own when the standard U-Net and V-Net fail, which is only a fraction of the time, as would be expected of architectures that are as popular as they are. Even when it fails to eliminate topological errors, it reduces the size of the errors as shown in the second row of Fig. 4. The one exception is the pre-synaptic region, for which the Jaccard numbers decrease. A closer inspection of the results show that the atlas sometimes encourages the segmentation to leak from weak boundary regions in few instances. We plan to address this issue by introducing an additional stream that specifically focus on predicting object boundaries and combining its results with **PA-Net**.

To demonstrate the importance of using the same features to compute the segmentation *and* the pose parameters, we implemented a naive version of our approach that uses two *separate* streams to compute the pose and the segmentation features, which we denote as Naive PA-Unet in Tables 1 and 2. The naive version fails to resolve the topological mistakes in the datasets. In the synaptic junction dataset, this occurs because the naive version has a mean orientation estimation error of $80.6°$ in contrast to the **PA-Net**'s error of $10.4°$. In the retinal fundus image dataset, the naive version has a mean localization error of 26.5 pixels compared to a 3.9 pixel error for **PA-Net**. As a result, in both instances, network fails to properly register PAs.

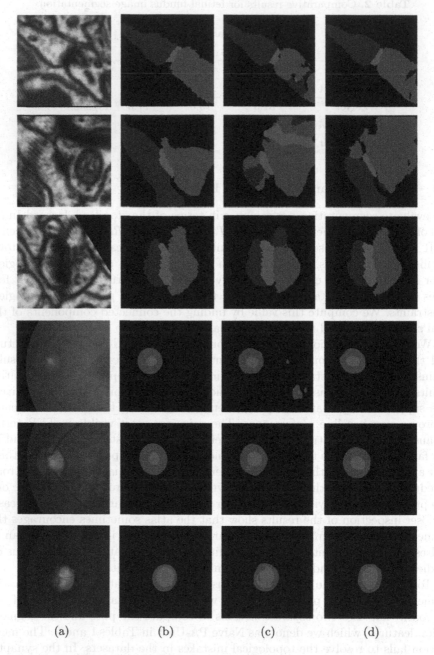

(a)          (b)          (c)          (d)

**Fig. 4.** U-Net vs **PA-Net**. Top three rows depict results from synaptic junction segmentation. The bottom three rows depict results from retinal fundus image segmentation. (a) Input images, (b) Ground-truth, (c) U-Net results (d) **PA-Net** results. The color hues denote the same areas as those in Fig. 1. (Color figure online)

# 5   Conclusion

We have proposed an encoding-decoding architecture that can exploit rough atlases that encode the topology of structures that can appear in any pose and have arbitrarily complex shapes to improve the segmentation results. One of its crucial components is that it relies on the output of the encoder to compute both the pose parameters used to deform the atlas and the segmentation mask itself, which makes it effective and end-to-end trainable. As future work, we plan to extend **PA-Net** by introducing an additional stream to produce edge maps and using it to address the minor loss in accaracy that occur when the structures have weak boundaries.

**Acknowledgments.** This work was supported in part by a Swiss National Science Foundation grant.

# References

1. Atzeni, A., Jansen, M., Ourselin, S., Iglesias, J.E.: A probabilistic model combining deep learning and multi-atlas segmentation for semi-automated labelling of histology. In: Frangi, A.F., Schnabel, J.A., Davatzikos, C., Alberola-López, C., Fichtinger, G. (eds.) MICCAI 2018. LNCS, vol. 11071, pp. 219–227. Springer, Cham (2018). https://doi.org/10.1007/978-3-030-00934-2_25
2. Balakrishnan, G., Zhao, A., Dalca, A., Durand, F., Guttag, J.: Synthesizing images of humans in unseen poses. In: CVPR (2018)
3. Bertasius, G., Park, H.S., Yu, S.X., Shi, J.: Unsupervised learning of important objects from first-person videos. In: ICCV (2017)
4. Dong, S., et al.: VoxelAtlasGAN: 3D left ventricle segmentation on echocardiography with atlas guided generation and voxel-to-voxel discrimination. In: Frangi, A.F., Schnabel, J.A., Davatzikos, C., Alberola-López, C., Fichtinger, G. (eds.) MICCAI 2018. LNCS, vol. 11073, pp. 622–629. Springer, Cham (2018). https://doi.org/10.1007/978-3-030-00937-3_71
5. Fei, W., et al.: Residual attention network for image classification. In: CVPR (2017)
6. Hering, A., Kuckertz, S., Heldmann, S., Heinrich, M.P.: Enhancing label-driven deep deformable image registration with local distance metrics for state-of-the-art cardiac motion tracking. In: Bildverarbeitung für die Medizin (2019)
7. Huo, Y., et al.: Spatially localized atlas network tiles enables 3D whole brain segmentation from limited data. In: Frangi, A.F., Schnabel, J.A., Davatzikos, C., Alberola-López, C., Fichtinger, G. (eds.) MICCAI 2018. LNCS, vol. 11072, pp. 698–705. Springer, Cham (2018). https://doi.org/10.1007/978-3-030-00931-1_80
8. Iglesias, J.E., Sabuncu, M.R.: Multi-atlas segmentation of biomedical images: a survey. Med. Image Anal. **24**, 205–219 (2015)
9. Januszewski, M., et al.: High-precision automated reconstruction of neurons with flood-filling networks. Nat. Methods **15**, 605 (2018)
10. Katouzian, A., et al.: Hashing-based atlas ranking and selection for multiple-atlas segmentation. In: Frangi, A.F., Schnabel, J.A., Davatzikos, C., Alberola-López, C., Fichtinger, G. (eds.) MICCAI 2018. LNCS, vol. 11073, pp. 543–551. Springer, Cham (2018). https://doi.org/10.1007/978-3-030-00937-3_62

11. Milletari, F., Navab, N., Ahmadi, S.: V-Net: fully convolutional neural networks for volumetric medical image segmentation. In: 3DV, pp. 565–571, October 2016
12. Retinal fundus glaucoma challenge (2018). http://refuge.grand-challenge.org. Accessed 24 Jun 2019
13. Ronneberger, O., Fischer, P., Brox, T.: U-Net: convolutional networks for biomedical image segmentation. In: Navab, N., Hornegger, J., Wells, W.M., Frangi, A.F. (eds.) MICCAI 2015. LNCS, vol. 9351, pp. 234–241. Springer, Cham (2015). https://doi.org/10.1007/978-3-319-24574-4_28
14. Spitzer, H., Amunts, K., Harmeling, S., Dickscheid, T.: Parcellation of visual cortex on high-resolution histological brain sections using convolutional neural networks. In: ISBI, pp. 920–923 (2017)
15. Spitzer, H., Kiwitz, K., Amunts, K., Harmeling, S., Dickscheid, T.: Improving cytoarchitectonic segmentation of human brain areas with self-supervised siamese networks. In: Frangi, A.F., Schnabel, J.A., Davatzikos, C., Alberola-López, C., Fichtinger, G. (eds.) MICCAI 2018. LNCS, vol. 11072, pp. 663–671. Springer, Cham (2018). https://doi.org/10.1007/978-3-030-00931-1_76
16. Yang, L., Wang, Y., Xiong, X., Yang, J., Katsaggelos, A.K.: Efficient video object segmentation via network modulation. In: CVPR (2018)

# Synapse-Aware Skeleton Generation for Neural Circuits

Brian Matejek[1]($\boxtimes$), Donglai Wei[1], Xueying Wang[2], Jinglin Zhao[2],
Kálmán Palágyi[3], and Hanspeter Pfister[1]

[1] John A. Paulson School of Engineering and Applied Sciences,
Harvard University, Cambridge, MA, USA
bmatejek@seas.harvard.edu
[2] Center for Brain Science, Department of Molecular and Cellular Biology,
Harvard University, Cambridge, MA, USA
[3] Department of Image Processing and Computer Graphics,
University of Szeged, Szeged, Hungary

**Abstract.** Reconstructed terabyte and petabyte electron microscopy image volumes contain fully-segmented neurons at resolutions fine enough to identify every synaptic connection. After manual or automatic reconstruction, neuroscientists want to extract wiring diagrams and connectivity information to analyze the data at a higher level. Despite significant advances in image acquisition, neuron segmentation, and synapse detection techniques, the extracted wiring diagrams are still quite coarse, and often do not take into account the wealth of information in the densely reconstructed volumes. We propose a synapse-aware skeleton generation strategy to transform the reconstructed volumes into an information-rich yet abstract format on which neuroscientists can perform biological analysis and run simulations. Our method extends existing topological thinning strategies and guarantees a one-to-one correspondence between skeleton endpoints and synapses while simultaneously generating vital geometric statistics on the neuronal processes. We demonstrate our results on three large-scale connectomic datasets and compare against current state-of-the-art skeletonization algorithms.

**Keywords:** Neural circuits · Connectomics · Skeleton generation

## 1 Introduction

Acquisition techniques [17], automatic segmentation methods [5], and synapse detection strategies [3] in connectomics have all progressed rapidly in the last decade, yielding densely reconstructed volumes at nanometer resolution. These terabyte and petabyte volumes contain hundreds of thousands of interconnected

**Electronic supplementary material** The online version of this chapter (https://doi.org/10.1007/978-3-030-32239-7_26) contains supplementary material, which is available to authorized users.

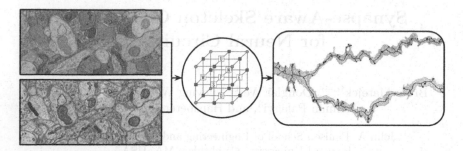

**Fig. 1.** Our method takes as input a segmentation dataset with cell body information and synapse locations (left). We generate a synapse-aware skeleton using a topological thinning strategy that relies only on local context (center) to produce accurate center-lines connecting all synapses to the cell body (right).

neurons and millions of synaptic connections. Despite the rich detail in the reconstructed 3D volumes, most analysis of this data occurs at a very coarse level [4].

Little research has focused on generating accurate wiring diagrams from the raw reconstructions. Current approaches [5] directly use an off-the-shelf skeletonization method to reduce these volumes into a series of nodes (neurons) and weighted edges (synapses). Unfortunately, such simplification eliminates valuable information needed for accurate biological analysis, such as geodesic distance from synapse to cell body and width of the neuron along the path. Concurrently, theoretical neuroscientists create biophysics-based simulations of simple neuronal circuits by numerically solving a series of differential equations that estimate the voltage change in a dynamic system [6]. These simulations often model neurites as a series of cylinders each with capacitance and resistances given a lack of accurate fine-resolution data, such as neurite width, length, and the accurate enumeration of connecting synapses. In addition, accurate skeleton representations of neuronal processes are increasingly important in the field of connectomics for biologically-constrained reconstruction [11], error correction [2], evaluation [5], and visualization [12].

The most commonly used skeletonization methods in the connectomic literature are the Tree-structure Extraction Algorithm for Accurate and Robust Skeletons (TEASER) [16] and its variants [19]. Alternative skeletonization approaches in the volume processing and graphics communities extract the medial axis from 3D volumes through the gradual erosion of their surfaces [9,13]. These methods rely only on local context to eliminate voxels while simultaneously preserving the topology of the original volume [13], but they do not maintain biologically relevant details. We present a novel synapse-aware skeleton generation strategy to transform volumetric connectomic data into a format for detailed analysis of the wiring diagram, accurate simulations, and improved reconstructions.

Our method builds on the class of topological thinning algorithms [9,10,13] and simplifies the input volume while still maintaining essential geometric attributes (Fig. 1). Our thinning based approach produces a center-line for the

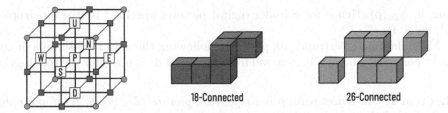

18-Connected                    26-Connected

**Fig. 2.** Following existing work, we use only the local neighborhood around a point $p$ to determine deletion (left). $N_6(p)$ contains the point $p$ and the six points labeled U, D, N, S, E, and W. $N_{18}(p)$ includes the points in $N_6(p)$ and the twelve ■ points. $N_{26}(p)$ is the set of $N_{18}(p)$ and the eight points marked by ●. Two points $x_0$ and $x_n$ are 18- (center) and 26-connected (right) if each point $x_i$ along the path is in $N_j(x_{i-1})$.

neuron with accompanying estimated neurite widths along the skeleton. We guarantee that the skeleton connects all detected synapses along the neuron. We further refine the skeleton to enforce specific topological properties based on the underlying biology and efficiently calculate the geodesic distance from each synapse to the cell body, i.e., the soma. Our parameterless algorithm requires no training data. We evaluate our method on three large-scale connectomic datasets from three different species and compare our results to state-of-the-art skeletonization algorithms. Our algorithm generalizes to other medical image domains such as skeleton generation of the cardiovascular or peripheral nervous system where the endpoints correspond to capillaries or nerve endings, respectively.

## 2   Methodology

Our synapse-aware skeleton generation approach adapts previous topological thinning algorithms [9,13] to guarantee a one-to-one correspondence between endpoints and synapses. We efficiently estimate the width of the neuronal processes during the thinning process. Subsequently, we calculate the geodesic distances from synapses to soma and refine the skeleton to enforce certain biological constraints—namely that neurons are acyclic.

**Notation.** Our method takes two inputs: a point cloud representing a neuronal process and a list of synapse locations. Here we use the following notations: $\mathbb{Z}^3$ is the set of points, $B$ is the set of object points, and $\mathbb{Z}^3 \setminus B$ is the set of background points.

We define three local neighborhoods of different scope around a pixel $p$ which we call $N_6(p)$, $N_{18}(p)$, and $N_{26}(p)$ (Fig. 2, left). Two points $x_0$ and $x_n$ are $j$-connected (for $j = 6, 18, 26$) if there exists a path $< x_0, x_1, ..., x_n >$ where each $x_i$ is in $N_j(x_{i-1})$ for $i = 1, ..., n$ (Fig. 2, center, right). An object is a maximally 26-connected set of object points. Conversely, a background component is a maximally 6-connected set of background points. An *endpoint* has only one object point in $N_{26}(p)$. Hence we consider digital pictures specified by the quadruple $(\mathbb{Z}^3, 26, 6, B)$ [7].

Malandain and Bertrand [10] prove the following theorem to determine if an object point $p$ is simple (i.e., removal from the set $B$ does not alter the topology):

**Theorem 1.** *An object point $p$ is simple in a picture $(\mathbb{Z}^3, 26, 6, B)$ if and only if all of the following conditions hold:*

1. *The set $N_{26}(p) \cap (B \setminus p)$ contains exactly one 26-component.*
2. *The set $N_6(p) \setminus B$ is not empty.*
3. *Any two points in $N_6(p) \setminus B$ are 6-connected in the set $N_{18}(p) \setminus B$.*

All simple points are surface points by Condition 2 of Theorem 1.

**Topological Thinning.** Every endpoint is a simple point by Theorem 1. Therefore to generate skeletons, specific points are preserved to avoid a complete reduction to a single point in the case of an acyclic input. Some strategies include preserving endpoints [1] or defining a second class of geometric constraints as non-simple isthmuses [13]. We differ from previous approaches by designating synapse locations as always non-simple and thus non-deletable. Any other point in the volume can be removed if it adheres to the requirements of Theorem 1. This synapse-aware endpoint strategy produces skeletons that are better suited for higher-level analysis.

We employ a sequential thinning procedure to erode the surface uniformly in all directions [13]. Each iteration consists of six sub-iterations where we consider surface points whose corresponding neighbor at location **U**, **N**, **E**, **S**, **W**, and **D** is a background point (Fig. 2, left). For each of these six sub-iterations, we identify the simple points that are potentially deletable. After collecting all the simple points, we reiterate through the list and delete any that are still simple. This dual-pass approach is necessary since a point may lose its simple designation based on neighboring deletions. After deletion, we add any neighboring points that are now on the surface to the list of surface voxels.

**Width Estimation.** For each object point, we store an estimate for the distance from the point to the surface. We initialize these estimates to 0 for all surface voxels and to $\infty$ for all internal voxels. When a surface point $p$ is deleted during a thinning iteration, we look at the neighborhood $N_{26}(p)$. We update the distance-to-surface estimate for a neighboring voxel only if its distance to $p$ plus the distance estimate at $p$ is less than its current value. As the surface erodes, our internal distance estimates better approximate the actual distance to the original surface. The distance estimates at the skeleton points correspond to half of the width of the neuronal process at that cross-section.

**Geodesic Distance Calculation.** Neuronal processes are acyclic, i.e., the genus of the cell membrane surface is zero. However, errors in the input volumes can produce bubbles and tunnels in the segmentation which our topological thinning strategy would preserve (Fig. 3). Furthermore, although we can quickly generate the neuron width at a given location with limited overhead, we have not yet determined the geodesic distance from each synapse to the cell body. We simultaneously enforce the acyclic constraint and produce geodesic distances with the following procedure. First, we run Dijkstra's shortest path algorithm on the skeleton with the soma as the source. We only keep skeleton points that belong on the shortest path from a synapse to the soma. This process removes any loops in the skeleton since any shortest path cannot contain loops. This additional step produces the geodesic distance from every skeleton point (including synapses) to the cell body and enforces the acyclic property of neurons on the skeleton.

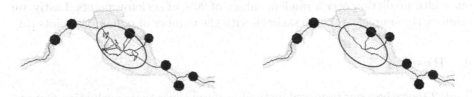

**Fig. 3.** *Loop Removal.* Since the thinning step preserves topology, any holes in the input segmentation cause loops in the skeleton. On the left, we see an example skeleton after thinning with several loops (the black spheres represent synapses). After refinement, these loops disappear, leaving a cleaner skeleton (right).

## 3   Experiments

We evaluate our methods on three large-scale connectomic datasets from three different species: rat, fruit fly, and zebra finch. JWR (rat) contains six fully-reconstructed neurons with manual segmentation and synapse identification. For FIB-25 (fruit fly), human proofreaders refined an initial segmentation produced by a context-aware two-stage agglomeration framework [14]. Synapses underwent a similar process of automatic detection and human refinement. Fully automatic techniques segmented neurons [5] and identified synapses [3] for the J0126 (zebra finch) dataset. The JWR, FIB-25, and J0126 datasets have resolutions of $32 \times 32 \times 30 \, \text{nm}^3$, $10 \times 10 \times 10 \, \text{nm}^3$, and $18 \times 18 \times 20 \, \text{nm}^3$, respectively (Table 1).

We compare our proposed method against two baselines: TEASER [16] and an isthmus-based topological thinning approach [13]. Both baselines are particularly susceptible to surface noise, which creates many spurious endpoints.

**Table 1.** We evaluate our method on three connectomic datasets from three different animal species. The FIB-25 and J0126 datasets contain many neuron fragments.

| Name | Species | Volume | No. neurons | No. synapses |
|------|---------|--------|-------------|--------------|
| JWR | Rat | $106 \times 106 \times 93 \, \mu\text{m}^3$ | 6 | 10,203 |
| FIB-25 [18] | Fruit Fly | $36 \times 29 \times 69 \, \mu\text{m}^3$ | 491 | 63,258 |
| J0126 [8] | Zebra Finch | $96 \times 98 \times 114 \, \mu\text{m}^3$ | 371 | 84,098 |

Additionally, the TEASER strategy requires a significant amount of memory per voxel. Therefore, we downsample the volumes for both of these datasets to a resolution of $100 \times 100 \times 100 \, \text{nm}^3$. Our proposed method is robust to surface noise since endpoints only occur at designated synapse locations.

We evaluate our results using three heuristics. The Neural Reconstruction Integrity (NRI) score indicates how well a given segmentation (or skeleton) maintains the underlying wiring diagram of the brain [15]. An NRI score near 1.0 indicates that most of the intracellular pathways between pairs of synapses are preserved. For our baselines, we link synapses to endpoints that fall within 800 nanometers of each other. Second, we calculate the mean absolute error of our width prediction over a random subset of 20% of skeleton points. Lastly, we evaluate the simplicity of each skeleton with the number of remaining points [13].

## 4    Results

Table 2 shows how our proposed method performs over three evaluation metrics.

**Table 2.** We evaluate the proposed method versus two baselines approaches on three metrics: NRI score, estimated neurite width error, and the number of points in the skeleton. The TEASER algorithm calculates the distance transform on the downsampled data, so the width given is the expected difference with upsampling.

| Method | JWR | | | FIB-25 | | | J0126 | |
| --- | --- | --- | --- | --- | --- | --- | --- | --- |
| | NRI ↑ | Width ↓ | Points ↓ | NRI ↑ | Width ↓ | Points ↓ | Width ↓ | Points ↓ |
| Proposed | 1.000 | 25.26 nm | 43,088 | 1.000 | 13.16 nm | 14,529 | 23.54 nm | 24,533 |
| TEASER | 0.265 | 20 nm* | 45,890 | 0.387 | 25 nm* | 13,577 | 24 nm* | 45,946 |
| Isthmus Thinning | 0.216 | N/A | 607,583 | 0.427 | N/A | 35,604 | N/A | 673,256 |

**NRI.** Our method guarantees a one-to-one correspondence between endpoints and synapses, we produce a perfect NRI score of 1.0 on the JWR and FIB-25 datasets. We cannot evaluate the NRI score on the J0126 dataset since there is no ground truth. With the addition of *merge* and *split* errors in the segmentation, our NRI score would continue to match that of the input data. Both the TEASER and the isthmus thinning strategies have significantly lower NRI scores ranging from 0.216 to 0.427.

**Width Estimation.** Our method achieves a mean absolute error of 25.26 nm, 13.16 nm, and 23.54 nm on the JWR, FIB-25, and J0126 datasets, respectively. The TEASER algorithm calculates the distance transform on the segmentation data as its first step. The mean absolute error for the TEASER skeleton generation strategy would be zero if the algorithm ran on the high-resolution data. However, since we need to downsample the data, the widths vary from the exact distances. We show the expected absolute error for any point between the downsampled distance transform and the correct surface distance.

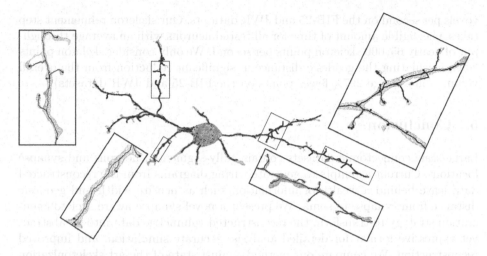

**Fig. 4.** Our synapse-aware skeleton generation strategy accurately produces center-lines on several neurons over three large-scale representative datasets. We zoom into four locations on one neuron from J0126 dataset. The black spheres indicate synapses.

**Skeleton Simplicity.** Our skeletons have the fewest total points on average on the JWR and J0126 datasets and are within 8% of the number of points of the TEASER skeletons on the Fib-25 dataset. The J0126 segmentation has numerous holes, particularly in the cell bodies. The isthmus thinning strategy preserves topology, which leads to a large number of skeleton points surrounding each hole. A refinement step would significantly reduce the number of skeleton points for this method.

**Geodesic Distance Calculation.** Using geodesic distances provides a much more accurate measurement of the path from a synapse to the soma than the frequently used Euclidean distance. The geodesic distance between each synapse and the soma is 47% ($12\,\mu m$) farther on average over the three datasets. Two of the JWR neurons share a synaptic connection. The geodesic distance from the soma to the presynaptic terminals and from the postsynaptic density to the neighboring soma is 145% farther than the corresponding Euclidean distance. These distances need to be accurate for neuron simulation.

**Qualitative Results.** Figure 4 shows the generated skeleton for a complete neuron from the J0126 dataset. The black spheres indicate synapse locations. Our skeleton refinement process removes self-loops caused by errors in the input segmentation enforcing the constraint that neurons are acyclic (Fig. 3). This refinement process reduces the number of skeleton points by a factor of $3.48\times$ on average on the FIB-25 dataset.

**Computational Efficiency.** For each point in the neuron, we require 8 bytes for a linear index, 1 byte for the status (surface, inside, or synapse), and 4 bytes for the distance to the surface estimation. We average throughput of over $100,000$

voxels per second on the FIB-25 and JWR datasets. Our skeleton refinement step takes a negligible amount of time for all tested neurons with an average throughput of nearly $65,000$ skeleton points per second. We only consider skeleton points when calculating the geodesic distance, a significant reduction from the overall volume (on average $297\times$ fewer points on the FIB-25 and JWR datasets).

## 5  Conclusion

Large-scale connectomic datasets contain fully-segmented neurons and synapse locations. Current attempts to generate wiring diagrams from the reconstructed data leave behind a wealth of information such as neurite width and geodesic distance from synapse to soma. We present a novel synapse-aware skeleton generation strategy to transform the reconstructed volumetric data into an abstract yet expressive format for detailed analysis, accurate simulation, and improved reconstruction. We compare our method against state-of-the-art skeletonization methods on 868 neurons and neuron fragments over three different datasets. Our code is freely available at https://www.rhoana.org/synapseaware.

**Acknowledgements.** H. Pfister is supported in part by NSF grant IIS-1607800. We thank Joergen Kornfeld and Winfried Denk's group for the J0126 data and synapses, and the Connectomics Group at Google led by Viren Jain for the segmentation. For the JWR dataset, we thank Jeff Lichtman's group at Harvard University for image acquisition, alignment, and ground truth labeling.

## References

1. Bertrand, G., Aktouf, Z.: Three-dimensional thinning algorithm using subfields. In: Vision Geometry III, vol. 2356, pp. 113–125. International Society for Optics and Photonics (1995)
2. Dmitriev, K., Parag, T., Matejek, B., Kaufman, A., Pfister, H.: Efficient correction for EM connectomics with skeletal representation. In: BMVC (2018)
3. Dorkenwald, S., et al.: Automated synaptic connectivity inference for volume electron microscopy. Nat. Methods **14**(4), 435 (2017)
4. Fornito, A., Zalesky, A., Breakspear, M.: Graph analysis of the human connectome: promise, progress, and pitfalls. Neuroimage **80**, 426–444 (2013)
5. Januszewski, M., et al.: High-precision automated reconstruction of neurons with flood-filling networks. Nat. Methods **15**(8), 605 (2018)
6. Koch, C.: Biophysics of Computation: Information Processing in Single Neurons. Oxford University Press, Oxford (2004)
7. Kong, T.Y., Rosenfeld, A.: Digital topology: introduction and survey. Comput. Vis. Graph. Image Process. **48**(3), 357–393 (1989)
8. Kornfeld, J., et al.: Em connectomics reveals axonal target variation in a sequence-generating network. Elife **6**, e24364 (2017)
9. Lee, T.C., Kashyap, R.L., Chu, C.N.: Building skeleton models via 3-D medial surface axis thinning algorithms. CVGIP: Graph. Models Image Process. **56**(6), 462–478 (1994)

10. Malandain, G., Bertrand, G.: Fast characterization of 3D simple points. In: 11th IAPR International Conference on Pattern Recognition, Conference C: Image, Speech and Signal Analysis, Proceedings, vol. III, pp. 232–235. IEEE (1992)

11. Matejek, B., Haehn, D., Zhu, H., Wei, D., Parag, T., Pfister, H.: Biologically-constrained graphs for global connectomics reconstruction. In: The IEEE Conference on Computer Vision and Pattern Recognition (CVPR), June 2019

12. Mohammed, H., et al.: Abstractocyte: a visual tool for exploring nanoscale astroglial cells. IEEE Trans. Vis. Comput. Graph. 24(1), 853–861 (2018)

13. Palágyi, K.: A sequential 3D curve-thinning algorithm based on isthmuses. In: Bebis, G., et al. (eds.) ISVC 2014. LNCS, vol. 8888, pp. 406–415. Springer, Cham (2014). https://doi.org/10.1007/978-3-319-14364-4_39

14. Parag, T., Chakraborty, A., Plaza, S., Scheffer, L.: A context-aware delayed agglomeration framework for electron microscopy segmentation. PloS One 10(5), e0125825 (2015)

15. Reilly, E.P., et al.: Neural reconstruction integrity: a metric for assessing the connectivity accuracy of reconstructed neural networks. Front. Neuroinform. 12, 74 (2018)

16. Sato, M., Bitter, I., Bender, M.A., Kaufman, A.E., Nakajima, M.: TEASAR: tree-structure extraction algorithm for accurate and robust skeletons. In: Proceedings of the Eighth Pacific Conference on Computer Graphics and Applications, pp. 281–449. IEEE (2000)

17. Suissa-Peleg, A., et al.: Automatic neural reconstruction from petavoxel of electron microscopy data. Microsc. Microanal. 22(S3), 536–537 (2016)

18. Takemura, S., et al.: Synaptic circuits and their variations within different columns in the visual system of drosophila. Proc. Natl. Acad. Sci. 112(44), 13711–13716 (2015)

19. Zhao, T., Olbris, D.J., Yu, Y., Plaza, S.M.: Neutu: software for collaborative, large-scale, segmentation-based connectome reconstruction. Front. Neural Circuits 12 (2018)

# Seeing Under the Cover: A Physics Guided Learning Approach for In-bed Pose Estimation

Shuangjun Liu[ID] and Sarah Ostadabbas[✉][ID]

Augmented Cognition Lab (ACLab), Northeastern University, Boston, USA
{shuliu,ostadabbas}@ece.neu.edu,
https://web.northeastern.edu/ostadabbas/

**Abstract.** Human in-bed pose estimation has huge practical values in medical and healthcare applications yet still mainly relies on expensive pressure mapping (PM) solutions. In this paper, we introduce our novel physics inspired vision-based approach that addresses the challenging issues associated with the in-bed pose estimation problem including monitoring a fully covered person in complete darkness. We reformulated this problem using our proposed Under the Cover Imaging via Thermal Diffusion (UCITD) method to capture the high resolution pose information of the body even when it is fully covered by using a long wavelength IR technique. We proposed a physical hyperparameter concept through which we achieved high quality groundtruth pose labels in different modalities. A fully annotated in-bed pose dataset called Simultaneously-collected multimodal Lying Pose (SLP) is also formed/released with the same order of magnitude as most existing large-scale human pose datasets to support complex models' training and evaluation. A network trained from scratch on it and tested on two diverse settings, one in a living room and the other in a hospital room showed pose estimation performance of 98.0% and 96.0% in PCK0.2 standard, respectively. Moreover, in a multi-factor comparison with a state-of-the art in-bed pose monitoring solution based on PM, our solution showed significant superiority in all practical aspects by being 60 times cheaper, 300 times smaller, while having higher pose recognition granularity and accuracy.

## 1 Introduction

The poses that we take while sleeping carry important information about our physical and mental health evident in growing research in the sleep monitoring

Supported by the NSF Award #1755695. Source code and SLP dataset available at: https://web.northeastern.edu/ostadabbas/2019/06/27/multimodal-in-bed-pose-estimation/.

**Electronic supplementary material** The online version of this chapter (https://doi.org/10.1007/978-3-030-32239-7_27) contains supplementary material, which is available to authorized users.

© Springer Nature Switzerland AG 2019
D. Shen et al. (Eds.): MICCAI 2019, LNCS 11764, pp. 236–245, 2019.
https://doi.org/10.1007/978-3-030-32239-7_27

field. These studies reveal that lying poses affect the symptoms of many complications such as sleep apnea [5], pressure ulcers [12], and even carpal tunnel syndrome [9]. Moreover, patients in hospitals are usually required to maintain specific poses after certain surgeries to get a better recovery result. Therefor, long-term monitoring and automatically detecting in-bed poses are of critical interest in healthcare [13].

Currently, besides self-reports obtained from the patients and/or visual inspection by the caregivers, in-bed pose estimation methods mainly rely on the use of pressure mapping (PM) systems. Although PM-based methods are effective at localizing areas of increased pressure and even automatically classifying overall postures [11], the pressure sensing mats are expensive and require frequent maintenance, which have prevented PM pose monitoring solutions from achieving large-scale popularity.

By contrast, camera-based methods for human pose estimation show great advantages including their low cost and ease of maintenance, yet are hindered by the natural sleeping conditions including being fully covered in full darkness. To employ computer vision for in-bed activity monitoring, some groups exclusively focus on detection of particularly sparse actions such as leaving or getting into a bed [3]. Depth modal is also extensively employed for this application [8], yet is limited to simple activity recognition or recognizing very few body parts such as head and torso. A patient motion capture (MoCap) system was proposed in [1] for 3D human pose estimation, however their experimental setup was never verified in a real setting for covered cases. Near infrared (IR) modality has also been employed [7] for long-term monitoring in full darkness, however it does not address the covered cases. Additionally, in the area of human in-bed pose estimation, there is no publicly-available dataset to train complex recognition models with acceptable generalizability, neither to fairly evaluate their performance.

In this paper, in contrast to the common RGB- or depth-based pose estimation methods, we propose a novel in-bed pose estimation technique based on a physics inspired imaging approach, which can effectively preserve human pose information in the imaging process, in complete darkness and even when the person is fully covered under a blanket. Our contributions in this paper can be summarized as follows: (1) reformulating the imaging process and proposing a passive thermal imaging method called Under the Cover Imaging via Thermal Diffusion (UCITD) based on a long wavelength IR (LWIR) technology; (2) proposing a physical hyperparameter concept that leads to quality multimodal groundtruth pose label generation; (3) building/publicly releasing the *first-ever* fully annotated in-bed human pose dataset, called Simultaneously-collected multimodal Lying Pose (SLP) (reads as Sleep dataset) under different cover conditions, with the size equivalent to the existing large-scale human pose datasets to facilitate complex models' training and evaluation; (4) training a state-of-the-art pose estimation model from scratch using our SLP dataset, which showed high estimation performance comparable to the recent successful RGB-based human pose estimation models; and (5) comparing with the existing methods with equivalent capabilities, our solution demonstrates higher pose estimation accuracy and granularity, with only a fraction of cost and size.

238    S. Liu and S. Ostadabbas

## 2  In-bed Pose Estimation

### 2.1  Problem Formulation

The major challenges that hinder the use of computer vision techniques for the in-bed pose estimation problem are monitoring in full darkness and potential cover conditions. To discover a proper imaging process capable of addressing these challenges, we reformulated the imaging process as follows. Let's assume the majority of the physical entities in the world (e.g. human body) can be modeled as articulated rigid bodies by ignoring their non-rigid deformation. The physical world composed of $N$ rigid bodies then can be described by a world state model [6], such that $W_s = \{\alpha_i, \beta_i, \phi(i,j)|i,j \in N\}$, where $\alpha_i$ and $\beta_i$ stand for the appearance and the pose of rigid body $i$, and $\phi(i,j)$ stands for the relationship between rigid bodies $i$ and $j$. For example, a human has $N$ (depending on the granularity of the template that we choose) articulated limbs in which each limb can be considered a rigid body and the joints between the limbs follow the biomechanical constraints of the body. Assuming light source $S$ as the source of illumination, image $I$ can then be modeled as a function $I = I(W_s, S)$. Based on these assumptions, we argue a necessary condition to recognized covered object using Lemma 1.

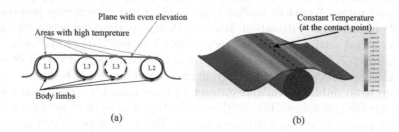

**Fig. 1.** (a) Multiple limbs under a cover, (b) Temperature simulation of a covered cylinder with constant temperature.

**Lemma 1.** *A physical object is recognizable after being covered by another physical entity, only if image of the world state after the cover being applied $W_{s \to c}$ is conditioned on the characteristics of the target object. or equivalently, $I = I(W_{s \to c}, S|\alpha_t, \beta_t) \neq I(W_{s \to c}, S)$ where, $\alpha_t, \beta_t$ stand for the target object's appearance and pose term.*

In RGB domain, we have $I(W_{s \to c}, S_{RGB}) = I(W_{s \to c}, S_{RGB}|\alpha_t, \beta_t)$. This means the resultant RGB image will be independent of the target object's shape and pose when fully covered. In comparison, the depth image of covered object is actually partially conditioned on the target object's pose and satisfies Lemma 1, hence it shows promising results for under cover conditions [1]. Yet, ambiguity exists as shown in Fig. 1(a), where human limbs are represented by cylinders. If the cover is tightly stretched over L1 and L2, the depth map will be independent of the exact location of L3.

## 2.2    Under the Cover Imaging via Thermal Diffusion (UCITD)

Although most imaging process is based on reflected light radiation, classical physics proves that all physical objects have their own radiation which can be approximated by their blackbody characteristics as Planck's radiation law. This law demonstrates two important characteristics: (1) blackbody has a specific spectrum and intensity that depends only on the body's temperature, and (2) at specific wavelength, object with higher temperature emits stronger radiation. The Planck's radiation law provides insights to solve our specific in-bed pose estimation problem, in which even though there is a lack of illumination from limbs under the cover, there will always be temperature differences between human body and the surrounding environment. The temperature of the skin of a healthy human is around 33 °C, while clothing reduces the surface temperature to about 28 °C, when the ambient temperature is 20 °C. Planck's law shows that in this range of temperature, the corresponding radiation energy concentrates in long wavelength infrared (LWIR) spectrum which is around 8–15 μm. Although blanket are not transparent to the LWIR radiation, in our specific context, the contact between cover and body parts while lying in bed introduces another physical phenomenon called heat transfer, which dramatically alters the temperature distribution around the contacted areas. This phenomenon can be described by the diffusion equation $\nabla^2 T = \frac{1}{a}\frac{\partial T}{\partial t}$, where $T = T(x, y, z, t)$ is the temperature as a function of coordinates $(x, y, z)$ and time $t$, $a$ is the thermal diffusivity, and $\nabla^2$ is a Laplacian operator.

Exact modeling of covered human body is beyond the scope of this paper, so we simulate such contact by simplifying each human limb as a cylinder with diameter 50 mm which is covered by a thin physical layer with a thickness of 2 mm in Solidworks (see Fig. 1(b)). To set boundary conditions, we assume the contact point of the cover will turn into a constant temperature similar to the human clothes temperature (≈28 °C) after sufficient time. Heat will diffuse into environment which has constant temperature around 20 °C. Such simplified model reveals that the contact point of a cover has the peak temperature. Furthermore, when a limb is covered with a sheet or a blanket, the location of the contact point directly depends on the shape and the location of the limb. In other words, the heat map will highly depend on the $\alpha$ and $\beta$ of the covered limbs, which satisfy the condition proposed in Lemma 1 and endorses the feasibility of LWIR for under the cover human pose estimation: $I = I(W_{s \to c}, S_{LWIR}|\alpha_t, \beta_t) \neq I(W_{s \to c}, S_{LWIR})$. Admittedly, real case is much more complicated than our simplified model. There could be multiple peaks in contacting area due to the wrinkles in the cover. Nearby limbs will also result in more complex temperature profile due to the overlapped heating effect. But the dependency of the heat map over the limb's $\alpha$ and $\beta$ will still hold. As we can see, human like profiles in the Fig. 2 via thermal imaging (second row) is well recognizable even when it is fully covered with a thick blanket. Figure 1(a) also shows the advantage of LWIR over depth as the heated area of $L3$ will depend on its location as long as it is contacted by the cover. We call this imaging approach that satisfies Lemma 1 under the cover imaging via thermal diffusion (UCITD).

## 3   UCITD Groundtruth Labeling

Although human profile under the cover is visible via UCITD, the pose details
are not always clearly recognizable by only looking at the LWIR images. Human
annotators are likely to assign wrong pose labels when labelling LWIR images,
which introduces noisy labels challenge to this problem. To address this issue,
we cast the imaging process as a function that maps the physical entity and
its cover into the image plane as $I = I(\alpha_t, \beta_t, \alpha_c, \beta_c)$, where $\alpha_t$, $\beta_t$, $\alpha_c$ and
$\beta_c$ stand for the target's and cover's appearance and pose, respectively. In this
formulation, $I$ could be the result of any of the feasible imaging modalities such
as $I \in \{I_{RGB}, I_{Depth}, I_{LWIR}, \dots\}$.

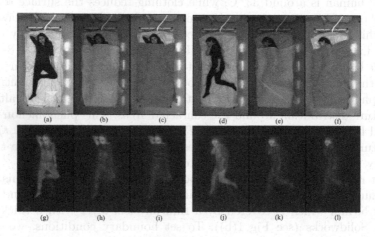

**Fig. 2.** Samples from in-bed supine and side postures: (a–f) show images captured using
RGB webcam, and (g–l) show images captured using LWIR camera. These images are
taken from subject without cover and with two different types (one thin and one thick)
of covers.

A labeling process then can be defined as a function $L$ that maps the
$I$ back to the target pose state $\beta_t$, such that the estimation target pose is
$\hat{\beta}_t = L\left(I(\alpha_t, \beta_t, \alpha_c, \beta_c)\right)$. Error $E(\hat{\beta}_t, \beta_t; \alpha_t, \alpha_c, \beta_c)$ depends on not only the pose
terms but also the appearance terms. As all these parameters (i.e. $\{\alpha_t, \alpha_c, \beta_c\}$)
can be decoupled from $\beta_t$ [6], they can be deemed as the hyperparameters of func-
tion $L$ and we can formulate the problems as an optimization: $\min\limits_{\alpha_t, \alpha_c, \beta_c} E$. Unlike
commonly referred hyperparameters in mathematical modeling, these variables
are directly related to the physical properties of the object, so we call them
*physical hyperparameters*. Due to the physical constraints, we can not adjust
them freely like other hyperparameters, yet we showed that in our application,
physical hyperparameters can also be altered effectively to optimize target $L$ performance. Based on this formulation, we propose the following three guidelines to

achieve a robust LWIR image groundtruth labeling. A labeling tool implemented following these guidelines will be released together with the paper.

_Guideline I:_ Perform labeling under settings with same $\beta_t$ but no cover to yield best pose labeling performance.

_Guideline II:_ Employ $I_{RGB}$ counterpart as a guide to prune out false poses in $I_{LWIR}$.

_Guideline III:_ When finding exact joint locations are intractable in one domain, employ labels from other domain with bounded bias via homography mapping.

## 4    Under the Cover Pose Estimation Evaluation

### 4.1    SLP Dataset Description

We setup two evaluation environments for our experiments, one in a lab setting turned into a regular living room and one in a simulated hospital room at Northeastern University Health Science Department. In each room, we mounted one RGB camera (a regular webcam) and one LWIR camera (a FLIR thermal imaging system) on the ceiling, where both were vertically aligned and adjacent to each other to keep small distance (detailed setup in the supplementary material). Using an IRB-approved protocol, we collected pose data from 102 subjects in the living room (called "Room" setting) and 7 volunteers in the hospital room (called "Hosp" setting), while lying in a bed and randomly changing their poses under three main categories of supine, left side, and right side. For each category, 15 poses are collected. For each pose, we altered the physical hyperparameters of the setting via manual intervention. We collected the images from both RGB and LWIR camera simultaneously to alter the function $I$. Moreover, we changed the cover condition from uncover, to cover one (a thin sheet with $\approx 1$ mm thickness), and then to cover two (a thick blanket with $\approx 3$ mm thickness) to alter $\alpha_c$ and $\beta_c$. In each cover condition, we waited around 10–20 s to mimic a stabilized pose during a real-life monitoring scenario. We follow pose definition of LSP [4] with 14 joints. Data collection in the living room and hospital room allowed us to form our Simultaneously-collected multimodal Lying Pose (SLP) dataset which will be public released with the paper. SLP dataset is collected under two different settings with 13,770 samples for "Room" and 945 for "Hosp", among which first 90 subjects with 12150 samples of "Room" set are for training and rest 12 subjects with 1620 samples are for testing. "Hosp" set is used for test purpose only to show its field performance under a simulated real application scenario. It is worth to mention that our SLP in-bed pose dataset has equivalent magnitude to most large-scale human pose dataset such as MPII [2] and LSP [4], which allows complex models' training from scratch.

### 4.2    In-bed Human Pose Estimation Performance

To evaluate the pose estimation performance of the proposed pipeline, we trained a state-of-the-art 2D human pose estimation model from scratch, the stacked hourglass (hg) network [10] which is one of top performance model for single human pose, using the LWIR images from 90 subjects training set in "Room" dataset with 8000 iterations, 30 epochs, and learning rate of 2.5e−4 as original settings for RGB domain. To investigate the effect of different cover conditions on model performance, we use probability of correct keypoint (PCK) as our metric which is extensively employed for human pose estimation [2,4]. In PCK metric, the distance between the estimated joint position and the ground-truth position is compared against a threshold defined as fraction of the person's torso length to form a joint level detection rate. Estimation results from each cover condition is reported. Due to the lack of public benchmark in this specific application, it is hard to provide a strict quantitative comparison. To launch a fair comparison, we fed pre-trained hg model with RGB samples without cover which suppose to have not only exact same uncover RGB domain as pre-trained model but also have similar "pose hardness" as test samples on UCITD. According to the evaluation shown in Fig. 3(a), our model demonstrated a 98.0% accuracy at PCK0.2 which is marginally higher than pre-trained hg in RGB domain. Please note that this cross-domain comparison is between our UCITD under darkness and covered condition against a well-illuminated RGB condition for the other models. Test result also shows that when subjects are covered tremendous impact is imposed on RGB hg but has only slight adverse effect on UCITD. Failure cases usually come when limbs are cuddled together that limbs will be misaligned to nearby body area due to the similar temperature of human profile or at transient moment caused by heat residue on bed.

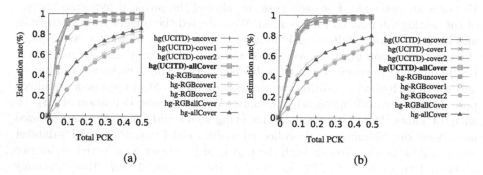

(a)                                    (b)

**Fig. 3.** PCK evaluation of in-bed human pose estimation models tested on data from (a) living room setting, and (b) hospital room setting, with different cover conditions. For test samples, we use RGB to specify the RGB modality otherwise it will be the LWIR modality. hg(UCITD) stands for the hourglass model trained via UCITD on SLP-LWIR set followed by different cover conditions. hg-allCover stands for applying pre-trained stacked hourglass (hg) model directly on SLP-LWIR test set with all cover conditions. hg-RGBallCover stands for applying pre-trained hg model directly on our SLP-RGB test set with all cover conditions.

### 4.3  Domain Adaptation Evaluation

Many datasets for healthcare applications are collected in extremely controlled environments, which limit their learning transferability to the real-life settings due to the gap between simulated and real-world data distributions (i.e. domain shift). With this consideration, to reveal the true performance of our technique in a practical application, we simulated a new deployment scenario by re-setting up the whole system in a hospital room, called "Hosp" setting. We intentionally altered all of the environment hyperparameters from the training set: (1) using a common hospital bed and mattress in "Hosp" setting, as supposed to a twin size metal bed-frame with middle firmness spring mattress used in "Room" setting; (2) repurchasing all covers to alter the cover appearance $\alpha_c$; (3) collecting data from new subjects to introduce a new $\alpha_t$; and (4) having different bed and room height which introduced a varied target distance from camera. We believe these are the most possibly changed parameters that can be seen in a real-world application. With a test dataset collected under the "Hosp" setting, our hg-trans model still showed 96.0% pose estimation performance over PCK0.2 as shown in Fig. 3b, which is also marginally higher than its pre-trained RGB counterpart.

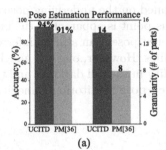 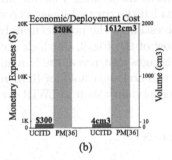

(a)     (b)

**Fig. 4.** Comparison between our UCITD and the PM-based pose estimation model presented in [11]: (a) Pose estimation performance in terms of pose detection accuracy and granularity, (b) Economic/deployment cost based on the monitory expense and the volume of each system.

### 4.4  Comparison with PM-Based Pose Estimation

Due to the lack of public benchmark and varying capabilities of different in-bed human pose estimation methods, we can hardly run an extensive comparison study. For a fair comparison, we believe the candidates should have following characteristics: (1) similar capabilities and pose granularity, and (2) concrete evaluation over real data instead of synthetic ones to reflect its practical value. Accordingly, candidate methods should be able to recognize multiple body parts simultaneously in darkness and varying cover conditions. As far as we know, none of the existing method can perfectly address all aforementioned standards except PM-based method in which the best one turns out to be the work by

[11] with comparable granularity. With close accuracy performance as shown in Fig. 4(a), our method shows higher granularity recognition ability with more joints being detected (14 vs. 8). Furthermore, authors in [11] evaluated accuracy via visual inspection for overlapping area, while UCITD employs widely acknowledged PCK0.2 metric for human pose estimation study.

Besides pose estimation performance, we further evaluated the cost-efficiency of UCITD against PM-based methods. We used a FLIR camera with 120 × 160 resolution. For equivalent resolution, we employed Tekscan® full body PM system with 192 × 84 sensor resolution. The price and space cost comparison is shown in Fig. 4(b). Our UCITD approach achieves tremendous cost efficiency, by being 60 times cheaper (a rough cost estimation is around $400) and 300 times smaller compared to the most advanced PM-based approach. Furthermore, by using unidentifiable heat map, UCITD is both privacy-reserving and radiation-free. As a contact-less method it requires much less maintenance compared to the PM-base approaches, which are prone to failure due to pressure sensors drift over time. Due to the small form-factor of the UCITD technology, it can be mounted unobtrusively in any indoor environment to be used in long-term in-bed pose monitoring applications.

It is worth mentioning that for other modalities (e.g. RGB), according to the Lemma 1 if the covered image is conditioned on the underlying pose $\alpha_c$, it is possible to estimate the pose accurately. This point is apparent in the images in the first row of the Fig. 2, in which the covered poses can still be inferred from the RGB images that reveal the human profiles. However, one can imagine such condition will no longer hold for RGB modality in the full darkness and the need for another modality such as LWIR for in-bed pose monitoring is inevitable.

# References

1. Achilles, F., Ichim, A.-E., Coskun, H., Tombari, F., Noachtar, S., Navab, N.: Patient MoCap: human pose estimation under blanket occlusion for hospital monitoring applications. In: Ourselin, S., Joskowicz, L., Sabuncu, M.R., Unal, G., Wells, W. (eds.) MICCAI 2016. LNCS, vol. 9900, pp. 491–499. Springer, Cham (2016). https://doi.org/10.1007/978-3-319-46720-7_57
2. Andriluka, M., Pishchulin, L., Gehler, P., Schiele, B.: 2D human pose estimation: new benchmark and state of the art analysis. In: CVPR, pp. 3686–3693, June 2014
3. Ding, J.R.: Bed status detection for elder-care center. In: 16th International Conference on Systems, Signals and Image Processing, pp. 1–4 (2009)
4. Johnson, S., Everingham, M.: Clustered pose and nonlinear appearance models for human pose estimation. In: BMVC, vol. 2, p. 5 (2010)
5. Lee, C.H., Kim, D.K., Kim, S.Y., Rhee, C.S., Won, T.B.: Changes in site of obstruction in obstructive sleep apnea patients according to sleep position: a dise study. Laryngoscope 125(1), 248–254 (2015)
6. Liu, S., Ostadabbas, S.: Inner space preserving generative pose machine. In: Ferrari, V., Hebert, M., Sminchisescu, C., Weiss, Y. (eds.) ECCV 2018. LNCS, vol. 11205, pp. 740–759. Springer, Cham (2018). https://doi.org/10.1007/978-3-030-01246-5_44

7. Liu, S., Yin, Y., Ostadabbas, S.: In-bed pose estimation: deep learning with shallow dataset. IEEE J. Transl. Eng. Health Med. **7**, 1–12 (2019)

8. Martinez, M., Schauerte, B., Stiefelhagen, R.: "BAM!" depth-based body analysis in critical care. In: Wilson, R., Hancock, E., Bors, A., Smith, W. (eds.) CAIP 2013. LNCS, vol. 8047, pp. 465–472. Springer, Heidelberg (2013). https://doi.org/10.1007/978-3-642-40261-6_56

9. McCabe, S.J., Gupta, A., Tate, D.E., Myers, J.: Preferred sleep position on the side is associated with carpal tunnel syndrome. Hand **6**(2), 132–137 (2011)

10. Newell, A., Yang, K., Deng, J.: Stacked hourglass networks for human pose estimation. In: Leibe, B., Matas, J., Sebe, N., Welling, M. (eds.) ECCV 2016. LNCS, vol. 9912, pp. 483–499. Springer, Cham (2016). https://doi.org/10.1007/978-3-319-46484-8_29

11. Ostadabbas, S., Pouyan, M., Nourani, M., Kehtarnavaz, N.: In-bed posture classification and limb identification. In: BioCAS, pp. 133–136 (2014)

12. Ostadabbas, S., Yousefi, R., Nourani, M., Faezipour, M., Tamil, L., Pompeo, M.: A posture scheduling algorithm using constrained shortest path to prevent pressure ulcers. In: BIBM, pp. 327–332 (2011)

13. Ostadabbas, S., Yousefi, R., Nourani, M., Faezipour, M., Tamil, L., Pompeo, M.Q.: A resource-efficient planning for pressure ulcer prevention. IEEE Trans. Inf. Technol. Biomed. **16**(6), 1265–1273 (2012)

# EDA-Net: Dense Aggregation of Deep and Shallow Information Achieves Quantitative Photoacoustic Blood Oxygenation Imaging Deep in Human Breast

Changchun Yang and Fei Gao[✉]

School of Information Science and Technology, ShanghaiTech University,
Shanghai, China
gaofei@shanghaitech.edu.cn

**Abstract.** Accurately and quantitatively imaging blood oxygen saturation ($sO_2$) is a very meaningful application of photoacoustic tomography (PAT), which is an important indicator for measuring physiological diseases and assisting cancer diagnostic and treatment. Yet, due to the complex optical properties of heterogeneous biological tissues, the diffusely scattered light in the tissue faces the unknown wavelength-dependent optical attenuation and causes the uncertain distribution of the fluence, which fundamentally limits the quantification accuracy of PAT for imaging $sO_2$. To tackle this problem, we propose an architecture, named EDA-Net, with Encoder, Decoder and Aggregator, which can aggregate features for a richer representation. We argue that the dense aggregated information helps to extract the comprehensive context information from the multi-wavelength PA images, then accurately infer the quantitative distribution of $sO_2$. The numerical experiment is performed by using PA images, which are obtained by Monte Carlo optical preprocessing and k-Wave acoustic preprocessing based on clinically-obtained female breast phantom. We also explore the effect of the combination of different wavelengths on the accuracy of estimating $sO_2$ to guide the design of PA imaging systems for meeting clinical needs. The experimental results demonstrate the efficacy and robustness of our proposed method, and also compare it with other methods to further prove the reliability of our quantitative $sO_2$ results.

**Keywords:** Quantitative photoacoustic imaging · $sO_2$ · Deep and shallow information · Dense aggregation

## 1 Introduction

Combining the advantages of optical imaging and ultrasound imaging, photoacoustic imaging (PAI), which meets both high optical contrast and high ultrasound penetration depth, has become an emerging imaging method [1]. PAI has the distinct advantage of being able to perform spectral analysis, and measurements based on multiple optical

---

**Electronic supplementary material** The online version of this chapter (https://doi.org/10.1007/978-3-030-32239-7_28) contains supplementary material, which is available to authorized users.

D. Shen et al. (Eds.): MICCAI 2019, LNCS 11764, pp. 246–254, 2019.
https://doi.org/10.1007/978-3-030-32239-7_28

wavelengths can be used to provide functional information about the molecular composition [2]. The goal of quantitative photoacoustic imaging (QPAI) is to convert multi-wavelength PA images into quantitative images of chromophore concentration (e.g. oxy/deoxy hemoglobin) and further ensure oxygen saturation estimation *in vivo*. However, the problem of light fluence correction has not yet been resolved, hence optical parameters are difficult to estimate (as a nonlinear ill-posed inverse problem), which results in inaccurate estimates of $sO_2$. Therefore, by neglecting the effects of the actual fluence distribution, the traditional method of QPAI [3] ignores its wavelength dependence and uses linear unmixing to estimate oxygen saturation, which introduces substantial errors. The accuracy of quantitative results can be improved by deep tissue correction, but relies on some assumptions such as prior knowledge of scattering coefficients, piecewise constancy of optical properties and uniform or known optical background, which however is too ideal and impractical. When the number of pixels in the image rises, these methods [1, 3] consume too many computing resources.

In recent years, machine learning, especially deep learning, has shown superior performance over traditional models in various fields. Based on the inspiration of emerging models, recently there have been reported a few developments on QPAI. A new principle underlying light fluence deep in tissues is proposed, named Eigenspectra Multispectral Optoacoustic Tomography [4], which models the wavelength dependence of light fluence as an affine function of several reference base spectra, and improves accuracy. However, it limits the scale invariance and the application scenarios. A machine learning method based on random forest regression factor, local context coding is proposed in [5]. It can analyze the characteristics of hidden quantitative information in PA images. It only relies on PA signals measured by local neighborhoods, while ignoring other measured signals containing relevant information. The ResU-net based on convolutional neural network is proposed to solve the optical inversion of QPAI with a good quantitative result, but the phantom is relatively simple [6]. From these prior works, we see that deep neural networks can be used to interpret key features and map inversion problems, indicating that it is a potential method to solve QPAI problems.

In this paper, we propose a novel deep learning architecture with three paths, the descending (Encoder) path and rising (Decoder) path with the dense block, and the horizontal (Aggregator) path with the aggregation block, which can concurrently use the deep and shallow information, to break the limitations of the independent layer. This network with encoder, decoder, and aggregator, named as EDA-Net, is used to quantify the concentration of $sO_2$ on clinically-obtained human breast dataset. The images of initial pressure distribution obtained from multi-wavelength PAT experiment, Monte Carlo optical simulation and k-Wave acoustic simulation, are used as inputs in EDA-Net, which can make the most of all measured signals and extract quantitative information from the spatial distribution of absorption. Quantitative $sO_2$ maps of the female breast are the outputs of the network. More excitingly, we also explore the effect of different wavelengths on the accuracy of estimating $sO_2$, hoping to have a guiding significance for the design of clinical QPAI systems.

# 2  Methods

## 2.1  Encoder, Decoder, Aggregator

The U-Net structure with Encoder and Decoder is originally proposed for medical image segmentation [7]. The method of skip connections helps the network to recover the full resolution of the medical image for output, and extracts the comprehensive information of the image, which is suitable for semantic segmentation. This idea later inspires many following works, and improves the network structure. Zhou *et al.* proposed U-Net++ with re-designed skip pathways and used deep supervision to connect subnets [8], which bring an interesting result, that is, pruning. Yu *et al.* proposed the concept of deep layer aggregation (DLA) [9], which is different from the existing linear aggregation of the shallowest layer. DLA uses a step-by-step aggregation approach to deepening representations. They believe that shallow features are propagated through different stages of aggregation and will be refined.

Motivated by the latest research of deep learning in medical imaging, we argue that dense aggregation of representations from different span levels and scales helps to extract the quantitative information from the multi-wavelength PA images, solve the problem of optical inversion, estimate absorption spectrum and finally perform accurate linear unmixing to get an accurate estimate of the concentration of $sO_2$.

## 2.2  Proposed Network: EDA-Net

In Fig. 1, we show the high-level description of the proposed architecture. In the encoder path, images shrink and extraction of local and global synthesis information from input images is achieved. The decoder path accepts feature images of different

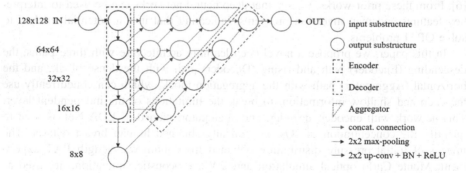

**Fig. 1.** The overall architecture of the EDA-Net, each circle node represents a layer substructure. The input substructure and output substructure change the number of channels. The image dimensions of each row are constant. The encoding and decoding nodes of the *i-th* row have the same dense block with a growth rate of $ki$ for learning the feature-maps of $f_i$. The residual structure is used in aggregation nodes to ensure better feature representation.

size from the aggregation nodes and performs up-sampling to increase the image size. The node $x_{i,j}$ in the $i$-th row and the $j$-th column can be formulated as

$$x_{i,j} = \begin{cases} \mathsf{E}\big(\mathsf{M}(x_{i-1,j})\big) & encoding \\ \mathsf{D}\big(x_{i,j-1}, \mathsf{U}(x_{i+1,j-1})\big) & decoding, \\ \mathsf{A}\big(x_{i,j-1}, \mathsf{U}(x_{i+1,j-1})\big) & aggregation \end{cases} \quad (1)$$

where subscripts are not out of bounds and do not include input and output sub-structures. For example, the encoding node $x_{0,0}$ accepts the output from the input node instead of the max-pooling output from the previous row. Function $\mathsf{M}(\bullet)$ is a max-pooling operation and $\mathsf{U}(\bullet)$ denotes the up-sampling layer. $\mathsf{E}(\bullet)$, $\mathsf{D}(\bullet)$ and $\mathsf{A}(\bullet)$ represent the encoding, decoding, and aggregation operation respectively.

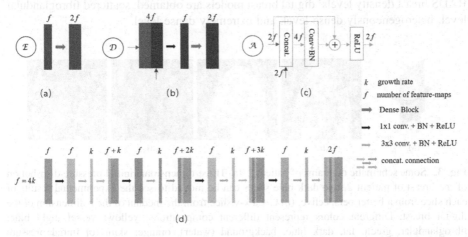

**Fig. 2.** The details of the EDA-Net. Each node is taken from the same row, so the scale factor of the corresponding feature-maps is specified in the figure, now we assumed the 0-$th$ row: $f_0 = 32, k_0 = 8$. (a) Encoding node with a dense-block, changing the feature-maps from $f_0$ to $2f_0$. (b) Decoding node ($[2f_0, 2f_0] \rightarrow 2f_0$) concatenates the result of the left node and the lower left node and operates via the convolution and dense block. (c) Aggregation node with residual structure. (d) Dense block: after four growths, feature-maps grow from $f_0$ to $2f_0$ (The concatenation result of the last growth is used the next time, and some of the arrows are omitted.).

The details of the encapsulated nodes are shown in Fig. 2. Since the dimension of the input images is the number of wavelengths used in QPAI, the number of channels is firstly changed from the wavelength number to 32 in the input substructure, and the output substructure finally changes it to 1. Dense block is used in encoding node (Fig. 2a) and decoding node (Fig. 2b) to match the number of feature-maps. All dense blocks (Fig. 2d) have undergone four growths, so they have the same number of convolutional layers, which means that each row's node uses different growth rate. The hyperparameter $k$ for different rows in our problem is 8, 16, 32, 64, 128. Since the residual connections are very important when the network is deeply assembled, it is also used in the aggregation node. $1 \times 1$ convolution can be used to increase computational efficiency before each $3 \times 3$ convolution, and the decoder nodes (Fig. 2b) also use the $1 \times 1$ convolution to reduce the number of feature-maps from the concatenated $4f$ to $f$.

## 3   Experiments and Results

**Datasets.** To make sure that quantitative imaging is realistic, and the measures of the $sO_2$ map can be utilized to guide the design of the QPAI system, our experiment is based on Optical and Acoustic Breast database (OA-Breast) [10], which is from three patients' clinical magnetic resonance (MR) data. After contrast enhancement and generation of optical and acoustic parameters, anatomically realistic three different BI-RADS breast density levels' digital breast models are obtained: scattered fibroglandular level, heterogeneously dense level, and extremely dense level.

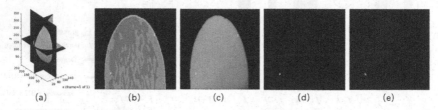

(a)                    (b)                    (c)                    (d)                    (e)

**Fig. 3.**  Some schematic diagrams of patient 2. (a) Three-dimensional initial pressure distribution of the breast of patient 2, two dark blue slices can be moved to see the experimental results of each slice from a better perspective. (b) Get a x-y slice from the median of the z dimension of the digital breast. Different colors represent different compositions: yellow: vessel, light blue: fibroglandular, green: fat, dark blue: background (water), orange: skin. (c) Initial pressure distribution of the slice in (b). Please note: both (a) and (c) use the log10 operation to enhance contrast. (d) Original initial pressure distribution of the slice in (b) (no enhanced contrast). (e) Reconstructed image with artifacts by k-Wave, homogeneous acoustic properties are used for acoustic preprocessing. (Color figure online)

**Optical Preprocessing.** Since the patient's breast is three-dimensional, for convenience, we use the GPU-accelerated Monte Carlo (MC) method [11] for 3-D simulation (number of photons we set: 5e8). The light surrounds the entire breast through four slit-shape sources, and the absorbed energy density map $H(r)$ can be obtained by Eq. (2):

$$H(r) = \mu_a(r)\Phi(r), \mathsf{p}_0(r) = \mathsf{T}H(r) \tag{2}$$

where $\mu_a(r)$ represents the optical absorption coefficient, $\Phi(r)$ represents optical fluence, which can be accumulated by the MC method in the fourth dimension (time dimension). Then the PA initial pressure $\mathsf{p}_0(r)$ can be obtained by calculating the product of the energy density and the Grüneisen parameter ($\mathsf{T}$, assumed to be a constant). Some results with patient 2 as an example are shown in Fig. 3. Due to page limitations, results of patient 1 and 3, and other details such as formulas or ablation study results, can be found in supplemental materials. Figure 3a is the three-dimensional light absorption induced initial pressure distribution after contrast enhancement, and we also show one slice of the result (Fig. 3c) and its original digital slice (Fig. 3b).

**Acoustic Preprocessing.** Light is scattered at the top and bottom of the breast, resulting in inaccurate energy deposition at those locations, so we remove a small number of the most edged slices from the 3-D volume optical preprocessing results, but still retain some edge slices, which is important for the robustness of the algorithm. Then select each 2-D slice after removal, perform acoustic preprocessing by k-Wave [12], where linear transducers (include 128 equally spaced transducer elements) are placed above the slice. Then we can obtain the pressure field of each transducer, given by propagating the initial pressure distribution forward, and the final result of iterative reconstruction is shown in Fig. 3e, which has some artifacts compared to the original value (Fig. 3d). And CNN can effectively reduce artifacts generated in PAT reconstruction, which has been proved in reference [13]. Our network also can be free from interference from these artifacts in dense aggregation to achieve a satisfactory quantitative $sO_2$ result.

**Experimental Setup.** 2880, 1444, and 3008 samples ($128 \times 128$) are generated using 3-D breast of patient 1, patient 2, and patient 3 respectively. Wavelengths in the range of 700–800 nm are used (wavelength in this range may produce more accurate oxygenation values) in step of 5 nm, which means that the initial pressure distribution induced by 21 wavelengths is obtained. Among the 5888 samples generated by Patient 1 and Patient 3, 4888 is used as the training set, and the remaining 1000 is used as the validation set. Test set uses all samples generated by patient 2.

The mean square error is used as a loss function, and the training time is almost 6 and a half hours in one 24 GB Tesla p40 GPU with 61,100 iterations, and batch size is 16 for each iteration. Then, the model based on training only takes an average of 21.3 ms to quantify the distribution of $sO_2$. We first select 9 of the 21 wavelengths for training.

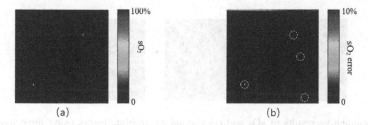

**Fig. 4.** $sO_2$ reconstruction results (a) using the slice of Fig. 3, and the corresponding absolute error (b) of the estimate result compared to the ground truth. It can be found that when the blood vessel is located deeper in the breast (the depth of the vessel in the lower left corner is greater than 6 mm), the error will be larger (but less than 7%).

**Results.** Estimated $sO_2$ result of the slice in Fig. 3 and the corresponding absolute error are shown in Fig. 4a and b. We also give our quantitative comparison results in

Table 1. We not only compare with the traditional linear unmixing method, but also ResU-net and UNet++, which shows that our proposed EDA-Net obviously outperforms the conventional methods ($\sim 10$ times less errors) and existing neural network models ($\sim 30\%$ less errors) for quantifying the $sO_2$ in PAT. Linear unmixing method, which is commonly used method for estimating $sO_2$, is significantly limited by the depth of the blood vessels *in vivo*, introducing large errors due to unknown optical fluence. Even if the measurement method is ideal, the blood vessel depth in the tissue is to at most 3 mm [14]. However, our proposed model greatly reduces the impact of the depth of tissue for estimating $sO_2$, see Fig. 4b.

**Table 1.** Quantitative results using 9 wavelengths compared to our proposed EDA-Net.

| Method | Linear unmixing | ResU-net [6] | UNet++ $L^4$ [8] | EDA-Net |
|---|---|---|---|---|
| Mean | 41.32% | 6.52% | 6.19% | **4.78%** |
| Standard deviation | 2.16% | 0.84% | 0.87% | **0.53%** |

In order to show the contrast more clearly and to illustrate the performance of our model, the estimation results of half test set (Patient 2, $722 \times 128 \times 128$) are reconstructed to a 3-D volume ($128 \times 256 \times 361$), then some blood vessels in it are projected to a plane, shown in Fig. 5. It can be seen that EDA-Net shows anti-interference ability to deep blood vessels, resulting in better reconstruction of $sO_2$ results.

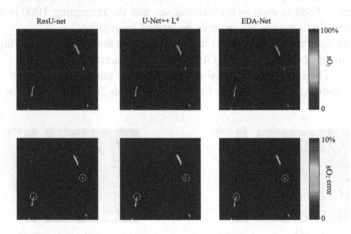

**Fig. 5.** Quantitative results of $sO_2$ and corresponding absolute errors using three models. The deeper blood vessels marked by dotted circles contribute most to the mean error and standard deviation of the estimation results. Each row shares the same color-bar. (Color figure online)

**Wavelength Effect.** More excitingly, we also explore the effect of the number of wavelengths on quantitative results. Table 2 shows that with more wavelengths, the mean error tends to decrease. However, when the wavelength is increased to a certain extent (greater than 9), mean error does not decrease significantly, but standard deviation still improves. We argue that more wavelengths can help to more effectively estimate the unknown fluence parameters, which improves the quantitative accuracy of deep blood vessels, and the result will be more robust with less deviation.

Table 2. The effect of the choice of the number of wavelengths on the estimation results.

| Number of wavelengths | 3 | 5 | 9 | 13 | 21 |
|---|---|---|---|---|---|
| Mean | 4.92% | 4.89% | 4.78% | 4.74% | 4.72% |
| Standard deviation | 1.24% | 0.93% | 0.53% | 0.46% | 0.41% |

## 4 Conclusion

We propose a novel deep learning architecture, named EDA-Net, with encoder, decoder, and aggregator, specifically for QPAI to achieve accurate quantitative $sO_2$ results. Our proposed model establishes a mapping between PA data and the quantitative concentration of $sO_2$, and $sO_2$ deep in breast can be accurately reconstructed in our experiments, achieving $\sim 10$ times less error compared with conventional linear mixing method, and $\sim 30\%$ less errors compared with other existing deep neural network models. We also study the effect of the number of wavelengths on the estimation results, which will be further investigated on the optimum combination of wavelengths in our future work. With further development of QPAI imaging system and optimization of EDA-Net algorithm towards clinical scenarios, we will validate our approach using larger data sets, even *in vivo* measured data in near future. We expect that QPAI will improve accuracy and specificity of breast cancer diagnostics, avoid unnecessary biopsy, and increase survival rate of patients.

## References

1. Cox, B.T., Laufer, J.G., Beard, P.C., Arridge, S.R.: Quantitative spectroscopic photoacoustic imaging: a review. J. Biomed. Opt. SPIE **17**, 061202 (2012)
2. Liu, Y., et al.: Photoacoustic molecular imaging: from multiscale biomedical applications towards early-stage theranostics. Trends Biotechnol. **34**, 420–433 (2016)
3. Brochu, F.M., Brunker, J., Joseph, J., Tomaszewski, M.R., Morscher, S., Bohndiek, S.E.: Towards quantitative evaluation of tissue absorption coefficients using light fluence correction in optoacoustic tomography. IEEE Trans. Med. Imaging **36**, 322–331 (2017)
4. Tzoumas, S., et al.: Eigenspectra optoacoustic tomography achieves quantitative blood oxygenation imaging deep in tissues. Nat. Commun. **7**, 12121 (2016)
5. Kirchner, T., Gröhl, J., Maier-Hein, L.: Context encoding enables machine learning-based quantitative photoacoustics. J. Biomed. Opt. SPIE **23**, 056008 (2018)
6. Cai, C., Deng, K., Ma, C., Luo, J.: End-to-end deep neural network for optical inversion in quantitative photoacoustic imaging. Opt. Lett. **43**, 2752–2755 (2018)
7. Ronneberger, O., Fischer, P., Brox, T.: U-net: convolutional networks for biomedical image segmentation. In: Navab, N., Hornegger, J., Wells, W.M., Frangi, A.F. (eds.) MICCAI 2015. LNCS, vol. 9351, pp. 234–241. Springer, Cham (2015). https://doi.org/10.1007/978-3-319-24574-4_28

8. Zhou, Z., Rahman Siddiquee, M.M., Tajbakhsh, N., Liang, J.: UNet++: a nested u-net architecture for medical image segmentation. In: Stoyanov, D., et al. (eds.) DLMIA/ML-CDS -2018. LNCS, vol. 11045, pp. 3–11. Springer, Cham (2018). https://doi.org/10.1007/978-3-030-00889-5_1

9. Yu, F., Wang, D., Shelhamer, E., Darrell, T.: Deep layer aggregation. In Proceedings of the IEEE Conference on Computer Vision and Pattern Recognition, pp. 2403–2412 (2018)

10. Lou, Y., Zhou, W., Matthews, T.P., Appleton, C.M., Anastasio, M.A.: Generation of anatomically realistic numerical phantoms for photoacoustic and ultrasonic breast imaging. J. Biomed. Opt. SPIE **24**, 041015 (2017)

11. Fang, Q., Boas, D.A.: Monte Carlo simulation of photon migration in 3D turbid media accelerated by graphics processing units. Opt. Express **17**, 20178–20190 (2009)

12. Treeby, B.E., Cox, B.T.: k-Wave: MATLAB toolbox for the simulation and reconstruction of photoacoustic wave fields. J. Biomed. Opt. **15**, 1–12 (2010)

13. Hauptmann, A., et al.: Model-based learning for accelerated, limited-view 3-D photoacoustic tomography. IEEE Trans. Med. Imaging **37**, 1382–1393 (2018)

14. Hochuli, R., Beard, P.C., Cox, B.: Effect of wavelength selection on the accuracy of blood oxygen saturation estimates obtained from photoacoustic images. In: Photons Plus Ultrasound: Imaging and Sensing, vol. 9323. International Society for Optics and Photonics (2015)

# Fused Detection of Retinal Biomarkers in OCT Volumes

Thomas Kurmann[1](✉), Pablo Márquez-Neila[1], Siqing Yu[2], Marion Munk[2],
Sebastian Wolf[2], and Raphael Sznitman[1]

[1] University of Bern, Bern, Switzerland
thomas.kurmann@artorg.unibe.ch
[2] University Hospital of Bern, Bern, Switzerland

**Abstract.** Optical Coherence Tomography (OCT) is the primary imaging modality for detecting pathological biomarkers associated to retinal diseases such as Age-Related Macular Degeneration. In practice, clinical diagnosis and treatment strategies are closely linked to biomarkers visible in OCT volumes and the ability to identify these plays an important role in the development of ophthalmic pharmaceutical products. In this context, we present a method that automatically predicts the presence of biomarkers in OCT cross-sections by incorporating information from the entire volume. We do so by adding a bidirectional LSTM to fuse the outputs of a Convolutional Neural Network that predicts individual biomarkers. We thus avoid the need to use pixel-wise annotations to train our method and instead provide fine-grained biomarker information regardless. On a dataset of 416 volumes, we show that our approach imposes coherence between biomarker predictions across volume slices and our predictions are superior to several existing approaches.

## 1 Introduction

Age-Related Macular Degeneration (AMD) and Diabetic Macular Edema (DME) are chronic sight-threatening conditions that affect over 250 million people world wide [1]. To diagnose and manage these diseases, Optical Coherence Tomography (OCT) is the standard of care to image the retina safely and quickly (see Fig. 1). However, with a growing global patient population and over 30 million volumetric OCT scans acquired each year, the resources needed to assess these has already surpassed the capacity of knowledgeable experts to do so [1].

For ophthalmologists, identifying biological markers of the retina, or *biomarkers*, plays a critical role in both clinical routine and research. Biomarkers can include the presence of different types of fluid buildups in the retina, retinal shape and thickness characteristics, the presence of cysts, atrophy or scar tissue. Beyond this, biomarkers are paramount to assess disease severity in clinical routine and have a major role in the development of new pharmaceutical therapeutics. With over a dozen clinical and research biomarkers, their identification is both challenging and time consuming due to their number, size, shape and extent.

© Springer Nature Switzerland AG 2019
D. Shen et al. (Eds.): MICCAI 2019, LNCS 11764, pp. 255–263, 2019.
https://doi.org/10.1007/978-3-030-32239-7_29

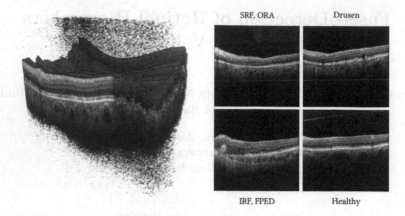

**Fig. 1.** (left) Example of an OCT volume of a patient with AMD. Slices are misaligned, even after post-processing registration. (right) four slices extracted from the volume, each containing a different set of biomarkers indicated for each image.

To support clinicians with OCT-based diagnosis, numerous automated methods have attempted to segment and identify specific biomarkers from OCT scans. For instance, retinal layer [2–4] and fluid [4] segmentation, as well as drusen detection [5] have previously been proposed. While these methods perform well, they are limited in the number of biomarkers they consider at a time and often use pixel-wise annotations to train supervised machine learning frameworks. Given the enormous annotation task involved in manually segmenting volumes, they are often trained and evaluated on relatively small amounts of data (20 to 100 volumes) [2,4,6].

Instead, we present a novel strategy that automatically identifies the presence of a wide range of biomarkers throughout an OCT volume. Our method does not require biomarker segmentation annotations, but rather biomarker tags as to which are present on a given OCT slice. Using a large dataset of OCT slices and annotated tags, our approach then estimates all biomarkers on each slice of a new volume separately. We do this first seperately, without considering adjacent slices, as these are typically highly anisotropic and not aligned within the volume. We then treat these predictions as sufficient statistics for each slice and impose biomarker coherence across slices using a bidirectional Long short-term memory (LSTM) neural network [7]. By doing so, we force our network to learn the wanted biomarker co-dependencies within the volume from slice predictions only, so as to avoid dealing with anisotropic and non-registered slices common in OCT volumes. We show in our experiments that this leads to superior performances over a number of existing methods.

## 2   Method

We describe here our approach for predicting biomarkers across all slices in an OCT volume. Formally, we wish to predict the presence of $B$ different biomarkers in a volume using a deep network, $f : [0,1]^{S \times W \times H} \rightarrow [0,1]^{S \times B}$, that maps from a volume of $S$ slices, $\mathbf{X} \in [0,1]^{S \times W \times H}$, to a set of predicted probabilities $\hat{\mathbf{Y}} \in [0,1]^{S \times B}$. We denote $\hat{\mathbf{Y}}_{sb}$ as the estimated probability that biomarker $b$ occurs in slice $s$.

While there are many possible network architectures for $f$, one simple approach would be to express $f$ as $S$ copies of the same CNN, $f' : [0,1]^{W \times H} \rightarrow [0,1]^B$, whereby each slice in the volume is individually predicted. However, such an architecture ignores the fact that biomarkers are deeply correlated across an entire volume. The other extreme would be to define $f$ as a single 3D CNN. Doing so however would be difficult because (1) 3D CNNs assume spatial coherence in their convolutional layers and (2) the output of $f$ would be of dimension $[0,1]^{S \times B}$. While (1) strongly violates OCT volume structure because there are they typically display non-rigid transformations between consecutive OCT slices, (2) would imply training with an enormous amount of training data.

For these reasons, we take an intermediate approach between the above mentioned extremes and express our network as a composition $f = f_{\mathcal{V}} \circ f_{\mathcal{S}}$, where $f_{\mathcal{S}} : [0,1]^{S \times W \times H} \rightarrow \mathbb{R}^{S \times D}$ processes slices individually and produces a $D$-dimensional descriptor for each slice. Then, $f_{\mathcal{V}} : \mathbb{R}^{S \times D} \rightarrow [0,1]^{S \times B}$ fuses all $S$ slice descriptors and predicts the biomarker probabilities for each slice, whereby taking into account the information of the entire volume. Figure 2 depicts our framework and we detail each of its components in the subsequent sections.

### 2.1   Slice Network $f_{\mathcal{S}}$

When presented with a volume $\mathbf{X}$, $f_{\mathcal{S}}$ processes each slice independently using the same *slice convolutional network*, $f'_{\mathcal{S}} : [0,1]^{W \times H} \rightarrow \mathbb{R}^D$ that maps from a single slice to a $D$-dimensional descriptor. The output of $f_{\mathcal{S}}$ is then the concatenation of the individual descriptors,

$$f_{\mathcal{S}}(\mathbf{X}) = [f'_{\mathcal{S}}(\mathbf{X}_1), \ldots, f'_{\mathcal{S}}(\mathbf{X}_S)]. \tag{1}$$

In our experiments, we implemented $f'_{\mathcal{S}}$ as the convolutional part of a Dilated Residual Network [8] up to the global pooling layer.

### 2.2   Volume Fusion Network $f_{\mathcal{V}}$

Let $\mathbf{D} = f_{\mathcal{S}}(\mathbf{X}) \in \mathbb{R}^{S \times D}$ be the set of descriptors of a volume $\mathbf{X}$ computed by $f_{\mathcal{S}}$. The fusion network $f_{\mathcal{V}}$ takes $\mathbf{D}$ and produces a final probability prediction $\hat{\mathbf{Y}}$.

The most straightforward architecture for $f_{\mathcal{V}}$ would be a multilayer perception (MLP), which is typical after convolutional layers. However, MLPs make no assumptions about the underlying nature of the data. Consequently, MLPs are hard to train, requiring either huge amounts of training data or resort to aggressive data augmentation techniques, particularly when the dimensionality of the input space is large as in this case. More importantly, a MLP would ignore two important aspects about $\mathbf{D}$: (1) the rows of $\mathbf{D}$ belong to the same feature space that share a common distribution; (2) volumes have spatial structure with respect to the biomarkers within them and slices that are nearby to one another have similar descriptors.

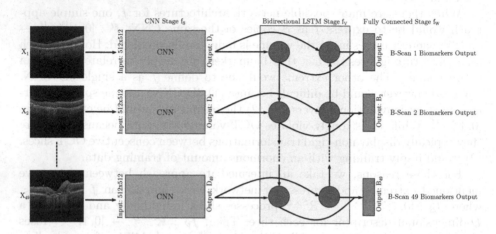

**Fig. 2.** Overview diagram of our approach including the CNN, $f_S$, the bidirectional LSTM, $f_V$, and the output of the fully connected stage. OCT volumes consist of 49 slices.

To account for this, we use an LSTM to process slices in a sequential way and implicitly leverage spatial dependencies, while performing the same operations on every input (i.e., implicitly assuming a common distribution in the input space). Formally, our LSTM is a network $f_\ell : \mathbb{R}^D \times \mathbb{R}^H \to \mathbb{R}^H$ that receives a descriptor and the previous $H$-dimensional LSTM state, to produce a new state. We use the LSTM to iteratively process the descriptors $\mathbf{D}$ generating a sequence of LSTM states,

$$\mathbf{h}_i = f_\ell(\mathbf{D}_s, \mathbf{h}_{s-1}), \quad s = 1, \ldots, S, \tag{2}$$

where $\mathbf{D}_s$ is the descriptor on slice $s$. Additionally, since the underlying distribution of OCT volumes is symmetric[1], we use the same LSTM to process the descriptors backwards,

$$\mathbf{h}'_i = f_\ell(\mathbf{D}_s, \mathbf{h}'_{s+1}), \quad s = S, \ldots, 1, \tag{3}$$

generating a second sequence of LSTM states. Initial states are $\mathbf{h}_0$ and $\mathbf{h}'_{S+1}$, respectively.

---

[1] Flipping the slice order in a volume produces another statistically correct volume.

Note that at each position $s$, $\mathbf{h}_s$ and $\mathbf{h}'_s$ combine the information from the current descriptor $\mathbf{D}_s$ with additional information coming from neighboring slices. We then concatenate both states in a single vector and feed it to a final fully connected layer $f_\omega : \mathbb{R}^{2H} \to \mathbb{R}^B$ that computes the estimated probabilities. The complete volume fusion network $f_\mathcal{V}$ is the concatenation of the outputs of $f_\omega$ for all the slices:

$$f_\mathcal{V}(\mathbf{D}) = [f_\omega([\mathbf{h}_1, \mathbf{h}'_1]), \ldots, f_\omega([\mathbf{h}_S, \mathbf{h}'_S])] \,. \tag{4}$$

### 2.3 Training

Training $f$ requires a dataset of $M$ annotated volumes, $\mathcal{D} = \{(\mathbf{X}^{(m)}, \mathbf{Y}^{(m)})\}_{m=1}^M$ where for each volume $\mathbf{X}^{(m)}$ a set of binary labels $\mathbf{Y}^{(m)}$ is provided. $\mathbf{Y}^{(m)}_{sb}$ is 1 if biomarker $b$ is present in slice $\mathbf{X}^{(m)}_s$. We then use the standard binary cross entropy as our loss function,

$$\ell(\mathbf{Y}, \hat{\mathbf{Y}}) = -\sum_s \sum_b (1 - \mathbf{Y}_{sb}) \log(1 - \hat{\mathbf{Y}}_{sb}) + \mathbf{Y}_{sb} \log \hat{\mathbf{Y}}_{sb}, \tag{5}$$

where $\hat{\mathbf{Y}} = f(\mathbf{X})$ is the estimation of our network for a given volume. The goal during training is then to minimize the expected value of the loss $\ell$ over the training dataset $\mathcal{D}$.

While we could perform this minimization with a gradient-based method in an end-to-end fashion from scratch, we found that a two-stage training procedure helped boost performances at test time. In the first stage, we train the *slice network* $f'_\mathcal{S}$ alone to predict the biomarkers of individual slices. More specifically, we append a temporary fully connected layer $f_t : \mathbb{R}^D \to [0, 1]^B$ at the end of $f'_\mathcal{S}$, and then minimize a cross entropy loss while presenting to the network randomly sampled slices from $\mathcal{D}$. In the second stage, we fix the weights of $f'_\mathcal{S}$ and minimize the loss of Eq. (5) for the whole architecture $f$ updating only the weights of the volume fusion network $f_\mathcal{V}$.

## 3 Experiments

### 3.1 Data

Our dataset consists of 416 volumes (originating from 327 individuals with Age-Related Macula Degeneration and Diabetic Retinopathy) whereby each volume scan consists of $S = 49$ slices for a total of 20'384 slices. Volumes were obtained using the Heidelberg Spectralis OCT and each OCT slice has a resolution of $496 \times 512$ pixels. Trained annotators provided slice level annotations for 11 common biomarkers: Subretinal Fluid (SRF), Interetinal Fluid (IRF), Hyperreflective Foci (HF), Drusen, Reticular Pseudodrusen (RPD), Epiretinal Membrane (ERM), Geographyic Atrophy (GA), Outer Retinal Atrophy (ORA), Intraretinal Cysts (IRC), Fibrovascular PED (FPED) and Healthy. The dataset was randomly split 90%/10% for training and testing purposes, making sure that no volume from the same individual was present in both the training and test sets. These sets contained a total of 18'179 and 2'205 slices, respectively. The distribution of biomarkers in the training and test sets are reported in Table 1. For all our experiments, we performed 10-fold cross validation, where the training set was split into a training (90%) and validation (10%) set.

## 3.2   Parameters and Baselines

For our approach, we set $D = 512$ for the size of the $f_S$ descriptors and $H = 512$ for the size of the LSTM hidden state. We train the fusion stage using a batch size of 4 volumes, while training using SGD with momentum of 0.9 and a base learning rate of $10^{-2}$ which we decrease after 10 epochs of no improvement in the validation score.

To demonstrate the performance of our approach, we compare it to the following baselines:

- **Base:** the output of $f_S$ (e.g. no slice fusion).
- **MLP:** output of size $49 \times 11$ using the $49 \times 512$ sized feature matrix from the **Base** classifier.
- **Conv-BLSTM:** fuses the last convolutional channels of $f_S$ with a size of $(49, 64, 64, 256)$ and a hidden state of $H = 256$ channels. This is then followed by a global pooling and a fully connected layer.
- **Conditional Random Field (CRF):** trained to learn co-occurrence of biomarkers within each slice and to smooth the predictions for each biomarker along different slices of the volume. Logit outputs of the **Base** classifier are used as unary terms, and learned pairwise weights are constrained to be positive to enforce submodularity of the CRF energy. We use the method from [9] for training and standard graph-cuts for inference at test time.

For all methods we use the same **Base** classifier and train it as a multi-label classification task using a learning rate of $10^{-2}$, a batch size of 32 with SGD and a momentum of 0.9. Rotational and flipping data augmentation was applied during training. We retain the best model for evaluation and do not perform test time augmentation or cropping. The network was pre-trained on ImageNet [10].

Our primary evaluation metric are the micro and macro mean Average Precision (mAP). In addition, we also report the Exact Match Ratio (EMR) which is equal to the percentage of slices predicted without failing to detect any biomarker in it. The mAP of the CRF baseline is not directly comparable as the CRF output is binary, hence allowing only a single precision-recall point to be evaluated. We therefore also state the maximum F1 scores for each method.

## 3.3   Results

Table 1 reports the performances of all methods. Using the proposed method we see an increase in mAP across all biomarkers except for GA and ORA. Both biomarkers have a very low sample size in the test set. The proposed method outperforms all other fusion methods in terms of mAP and F1 score and considerably improves over the unfused baseline, which confirms our hypothesis that inter-slice dependencies can be used to increase the per slice performance. The poor performance of the Convolutional BLSTM can be explained due to the misalignment of adjacent slices.

**Table 1.** Experimental results comparing our proposed method to other approaches. The per-biomaker scores are shown as mean Average Precision (mAP). The training and test label occurrence is stated beside the biomarker name (training/test). (*) threshold taken at the max F1 score.

| Biomarker | Base | MLP | Conv-BLSTM | CRF | Proposed |
|---|---|---|---|---|---|
| Healthy (5310/494) | 0.797 ± 0.023 | 0.730 ± 0.025 | 0.795 ± 0.013 | - | **0.800 ± 0.022** |
| SRF (942/103) | 0.847 ± 0.024 | 0.796 ± 0.043 | 0.877 ± 0.030 | - | **0.905 ± 0.017** |
| IRF (2019/339) | 0.691 ± 0.044 | 0.705 ± 0.039 | 0.701 ± 0.052 | - | **0.761 ± 0.047** |
| HF (4261/684) | 0.877 ± 0.008 | 0.839 ± 0.010 | 0.863 ± 0.018 | - | **0.896 ± 0.007** |
| Drusen (3990/399) | 0.762 ±0.024 | 0.731 ± 0.024 | 0.766 ± 0.029 | - | **0.775 ± 0.038** |
| RPD (1620/146) | 0.291 ± 0.044 | 0.302 ± 0.036 | 0.288 ± 0.069 | - | **0.335 ± 0.077** |
| ERM (4338/670) | 0.885 ± 0.009 | 0.849 ± 0.014 | 0.850 ± 0.022 | - | **0.903 ± 0.010** |
| GA (897/67) | **0.557 ± 0.063** | 0.234 ± 0.047 | 0.330 ± 0.049 | - | 0.556 ± 0.057 |
| ORA (1999/84) | **0.151 ± 0.018** | 0.105 ± 0.008 | 0.143 ± 0.025 | - | 0.131 ± 0.019 |
| IRC (3097/553) | 0.932 ± 0.006 | 0.880 ± 0.011 | 0.928 ± 0.012 | - | **0.940 ± 0.006** |
| FPED (3654/387) | 0.931 ± 0.007 | 0.920 ±0.008 | 0.936 ± 0.009 | - | **0.949 ± 0.006** |
| mAP (micro) | 0.814 ± 0.006 | 0.768 ± 0.012 | 0.794 ± 0.010 | 0.599 ± 0.003 | **0.834 ± 0.012** |
| mAP (macro) | 0.702 ± 0.008 | 0.645 ± 0.009 | 0.680 ± 0.012 | 0.523 ± 0.006 | **0.723 ± 0.014** |
| EMR* | 0.423 ± 0.015 | 0.164 ± 0.048 | 0.413 ± 0.019 | **0.440 ± 0.003** | 0.438 ± 0.011 |
| F1* | 0.676 ± 0.006 | 0.502 ± 0.024 | 0.676 ± 0.011 | 0.649 ± 0.013 | **0.694 ± 0.009** |

In Fig. 3, we show a typical example illustrating the performance improving ability of our proposed method. In particular, we show here the prediction of our approach on each slice for each biomarker and highlight three consecutive slices of the tested volume (right). For comparison, we also show the corresponding ground-truth (top left) and the outcome from the **Base** classifier (middle left). Here we see that our approach is capable of inferring more accurately the set of biomarkers across the different slices.

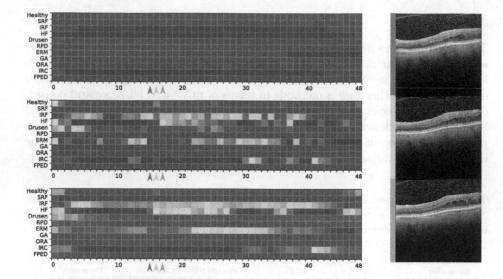

**Fig. 3.** Volume classification example, where (top left) depicts the ground truth, (middle left) the **Base** classification and (bottom left) our proposed method. Warm colors indicate higher likelihood of presence. (Right) Three consecutives slices where the **Base** classifier incorrectly misses biomarker IRF in the center slice (yellow). Our proposed method manages to fuse information from adjacent slices (pink and orange) to infer the proper prediction. (Color figure online)

## 4  Conclusion

We have presented a novel method to identify pathological biomarkers in OCT slices. Our approach involves detecting biomarkers first slice by slice in the OCT volume and then using a bidirectional LSTM to coherently adjust predictions. As far as we are aware, we are the first to demonstrate that such fine-grained biomarker detection can be achieved in the context of retinal diseases. We have shown that our approach performs well on a substantial patient dataset outperforming other common fusion methods. Future efforts will be focused on extending these results to infer pixel-wise segmentations of found biomarkers relying solely on the per-image labels.

**Acknowledgements.** This work received partial financial support from the Innosuisse Grant #6362.1 PFLS-LS.

## References

1. Bourne, R., et al.: Magnitude, temporal trends, and projections of the global prevalence of blindness and distance and near vision impairment: a systematic review and meta-analysis. Lancet Glob. Health **5**, e888–e897 (2017)

2. Apostolopoulos, S., De Zanet, S., Ciller, C., Wolf, S., Sznitman, R.: Pathological OCT retinal layer segmentation using branch residual U-shape networks. In: Descoteaux, M., Maier-Hein, L., Franz, A., Jannin, P., Collins, D.L., Duchesne, S. (eds.) MICCAI 2017. LNCS, vol. 10435, pp. 294–301. Springer, Cham (2017). https://doi.org/10.1007/978-3-319-66179-7_34
3. Hussain, M.A., et al.: Automatic identification of pathology-distorted retinal layer boundaries using SD-OCT imaging. IEEE Trans. Biomed. Eng. **64**(7), 1638–1649 (2017)
4. Roy, A.G., et al.: ReLayNet: retinal layer and fluid segmentation of macular optical coherence tomography using fully convolutional networks. Biomed. Opt. Express **8**(8) (2017)
5. Zhao, R., et al.: Automated drusen detection in dry age-related macular degeneration by multiple-depth, en faceoptical coherence tomography. Biomed. Opt. Express **8**(11), 5049–5064 (2017)
6. Bogunovic, H., et al.: RETOUCH - the retinal OCT fluid detection and segmentation benchmark and challenge. IEEE Trans. Med. Imaging **38**(8), 1858–1874 (2019)
7. Graves, A., Fernández, S., Schmidhuber, J.: Bidirectional LSTM networks for improved phoneme classification and recognition. In: Duch, W., Kacprzyk, J., Oja, E., Zadrożny, S. (eds.) ICANN 2005. LNCS, vol. 3697, pp. 799–804. Springer, Heidelberg (2005). https://doi.org/10.1007/11550907_126
8. Yu, F., Koltun, V., Funkhouser, T.: Dilated residual networks, May 2017
9. Szummer, M., Kohli, P., Hoiem, D.: Learning CRFs using graph cuts. In: Forsyth, D., Torr, P., Zisserman, A. (eds.) ECCV 2008. LNCS, vol. 5303, pp. 582–595. Springer, Heidelberg (2008). https://doi.org/10.1007/978-3-540-88688-4_43
10. Russakovsky, O., et al.: ImageNet large scale visual recognition challenge. Int. J. Comput. Vis. **115**(3), 211–252 (2015)

# Vessel-Net: Retinal Vessel Segmentation Under Multi-path Supervision

Yicheng Wu[1], Yong Xia[1(✉)], Yang Song[3], Donghao Zhang[2], Dongnan Liu[2],
Chaoyi Zhang[2], and Weidong Cai[2]

[1] National Engineering Laboratory for Integrated Aero-Space-Ground-Ocean Big
Data Application Technology, School of Computer Science and Engineering,
Northwestern Polytechnical University, Xi'an 710072, China
yxia@nwpu.edu.cn
[2] School of Computer Science, University of Sydney, Sydney, NSW 2006, Australia
[3] School of Computer Science and Engineering, University of New South Wales,
Sydney, NSW 2052, Australia

**Abstract.** Due to the complex morphology of fine vessels, it remains
challenging for most of existing models to accurately segment them, particularly the capillaries in color fundus retinal images. In this paper, we
propose a novel and lightweight deep learning model called Vessel-Net
for retinal vessel segmentation. First, we design an efficient inception-
residual convolutional block to combine the advantages of the Inception
model and residual module for improved feature representation. Next,
we embed the inception-residual blocks inside a U-like encoder-decoder
architecture for vessel segmentation. Then, we introduce four supervision
paths, including the traditional supervision path, a richer feature supervision path, and two multi-scale supervision paths to preserve the rich
and multi-scale deep features during model optimization. We evaluated
our Vessel-Net against several recent methods on two benchmark retinal
databases and achieved the new state-of-the-art performance (i.e. AUC of
98.21%/98.60% on the DRIVE and CHASE databases, respectively). Our
ablation studies also demonstrate that the proposed inception-residual
block and the multi-path supervision both can produce impressive performance gains for retinal vessel segmentation.

**Keywords:** Retinal vessel segmentation · Vessel-Net ·
Inception-residual block · Multi-path supervision

## 1 Introduction

Retinal vessel segmentation in color fundus images has been widely used for
quantitative analysis of ophthalmologic diseases including diabetic retinopathy
(DR) and glaucoma [1]. However, it remains challenging to achieve accurate segmentation of retinal vessels, especially the capillaries and other fine structures,
largely due to the complex vessel morphology (e.g. the thin and curved vessel).

© Springer Nature Switzerland AG 2019
D. Shen et al. (Eds.): MICCAI 2019, LNCS 11764, pp. 264–272, 2019.
https://doi.org/10.1007/978-3-030-32239-7_30

Traditionally, retinal vessel segmentation has been conducted by designing filter-based features to capture the unique morphological characteristics of vessels. For instance, various types of filters were used to extract the 41-dimensional visual features to describe retinal vessels [2], and a combination of shifted filter responses (COSFIRE) [3] was designed to segment the retinal vessels in fundus images. Recently, deep learning (DL) has been adopted to perform vessel segmentation with promising results. Several data augmentation algorithms were introduced to augment limited training data [4]. In addition, an unsupervised model with image matting was proposed to segment retinal vessels [5]. The additional labels of thick and thin vessels were introduced explicitly and an edge-based mechanism was incorporated into U-Net to achieve a better result [6]. Furthermore, the conditional random field (CRF) method was used for post-processing [7]. A cascaded architecture with multi-scale refinement was also proposed to further improve the segmentation performance [8]. While these DL-based methods have reported encouraging results, we hypothesize that the vessel segmentation performance can be further improved by more effective modeling the multi-scale visual information associated with vessels with varying thickness.

In this paper, we propose a novel and highly effective deep learning model called Vessel-Net for retinal vessel segmentation in color fundus images. The Vessel-Net contains five inception-residual (IR) blocks for better feature representation, and each IR block contains three parallel paths including one residual convolutional layer and two enhancement paths. To the best of our knowledge, we are the first to combine the advantages of Inception and residual methods for retinal vessel segmentation, without introducing too many additional parameters. Furthermore, we design four supervision paths called multi-path supervision to train the proposed Vessel-Net, in which the richer feature supervision combines all feature maps of our Vessel-Net and multi-scale supervision further preserves multi-scale features. With this multi-path supervision, multi-scale complementary information can be better preserved, which is critical to the segmentation of fine structures.

We evaluated our Vessel-Net against several recent retinal vessel segmentation algorithms on two benchmark databases: the digital retinal images for vessel extraction (DRIVE) database [9] and the child heart and health study (CHASE) database [10]. Our results show that the proposed Vessel-Net, even without adjusting any hyper-parameters for each experiment, achieves the area under the ROC curve (AUC) of 98.21% on DRIVE and 98.60% on CHASE and sets the new state of the art.

## 2   Method

The proposed Vessel-Net has a U-like encoder-decoder architecture, which contains five IR blocks, $2 \times 2$ convolutional layers, up-sampling layers, and four supervision paths (see Fig. 1). The convolutional layers with $2 \times 2$ kernels and a stride of 2 are designed to contract the feature maps, whereas the corresponding $2 \times 2$ up-sampling layers are used to expand the feature maps. Hence, the Vessel-Net takes $48 \times 48$ patches extracted from pre-processed retinal images as input and produces the vessel probability maps with the same size. We now delve into the details of the IR block and multi-path supervision.

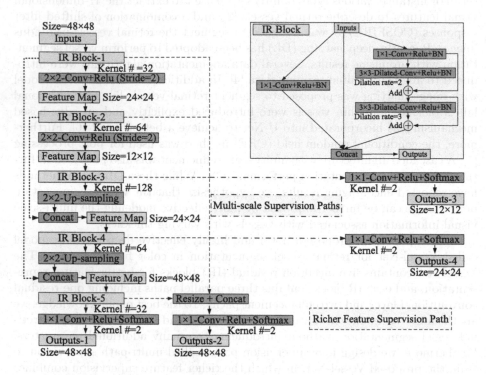

**Fig. 1.** Diagram of the proposed Vessel-Net.

## 2.1 Inception-Residual Block

The U-Net and its variants, such as the recurrent residual U-Net (R2U-Net) [11], are popular semantic segmentation tools, which have shown promising performance in many biomedical image applications [12]. The convolutional block in U-Net contains, sequentially, a $3 \times 3$ convolutional layer, a dropout layer, and another $3 \times 3$ convolutional layer (see Fig. 2). Nevertheless, convolutional block in R2U-Net consists of a $1 \times 1$ convolutional layer and two $3 \times 3$ convolutional layers, and replaces the dropout layer with skip connections and backward connections to achieve the recurrent learning (see Fig. 2).

To widen the model while avoiding superabundant parameters, we design the IR block (see Fig. 2) to replace the convolutional blocks in U-like networks for a higher feature representation capability. Specifically, we remove backward connections in the convolutional block of R2U-Net, then introduce two parallel enhancement paths (one includes a $1 \times 1$ convolutional layer, and the other is a skip connection from the input to output), and finally use a concatenation layer to combine the outputs of three parallel paths. Another difference between the IR block and the convolutional blocks in U-Net and R2U-Net is that we use dilated convolutions with a dilation rate of 2 and 3 in two 3 × 3 adjacent convolutional layers, respectively, to realize a large field of view. Compared to Inception block [13], the lightweight IR block does not leverage the convolutional layer of large kernels to extract features since it would cause over-fitting when the training data of retinal vessels is highly limited. Note that, each convolutional layer, with a stride of 1, is followed by the ReLU activation and a batch normalization layer to reduce over-fitting as much as possible.

As shown in Fig. 1, the channels of five IR blocks in our Vessel-Net are 32, 64, 128, 64 and 32 from top to bottom.

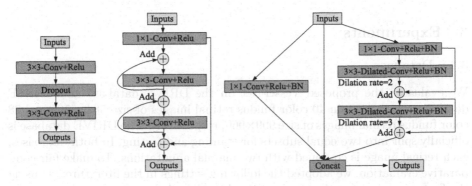

**Fig. 2.** U-Net block (left), R2U block (middle) and the proposed IR block (right).

## 2.2   Multi-path Supervision

It has been acknowledged that all feature maps contain essential image details and well deserve to be preserved [14,15]. This is especially true for vessel images, which contain complex structures at different scales. Therefore, we resize the feature maps produced by all IR blocks to 48 × 48 using the corresponding up-sampling layers, concatenate them, and thus feed them to a 1 × 1 convolutional layer followed by the ReLU activation and a Softmax layer to generate an auxiliary output $rP$ (see Fig. 1). This output path enables the feature maps obtained at different depths to be preserved and further processed to provide the richer feature supervision to model training. In addition, we feed the outputs of the 3rd and 4th IR block to a 1 × 1 convolutional layer followed by the ReLU activation and a Softmax layer, respectively, resulting in a 12 × 12 output $msP_3$ and a 24 × 24 output $msP_4$. These two paths enable the feature maps at two scales to provide the multi-scale supervision to model training. Therefore, Vessel-Net has four outputs, and hence the total loss can be defined as follows:

$$Loss = CE(P, GT) + \lambda_2 \times CE(rP, GT) + \sum_{i=3}^{4} \lambda_i \times CE(msP_i, msGT_i) \quad (1)$$

where $CE$ represents the categorical cross-entropy function, $P$ is the vessel probability map generated by the decoder, $GT$ is the ground truth, $msGT_3$ and $msGT_4$ denote the ground truth of size $12 \times 12$ and $24 \times 24$, respectively, and the weight parameters $\lambda_2 \sim \lambda_4$ represent the balance among four outputs. The $msGT_3$ and $msGT_4$ were obtained by down-sampling $GT$ via $2 \times 2$ and $4 \times 4$ max-pooling, respectively.

Consequently, the proposed Vessel-Net is trained under the main supervision provided by the decoder, the richer feature supervision, and two types of multiscale supervision. Thus, the complementary information acquired by five IR blocks can be combined to explore the effective representations of vessels of variable scales/thicknesses.

## 3    Experiments

### 3.1    Database

We evaluated the proposed Vessel-Net on the DRIVE database and CHASE database, which contain 40 color fundus retinal images of size $584 \times 565$ and 28 color fundus retinal images of size $999 \times 960$, respectively. The DRIVE database is officially split into two equal subsets for training and testing. In both databases, each retinal image is equipped with two manual annotations. To make fair comparative evaluation, we adopted the following settings in the literature: (1) using the first manual annotation as the ground truth and the second one as a human observer's segmentation [9]; (2) splitting the CHASE database into a training set of 20 images and a testing set of 8 images [8,16]; and (3) generating manually the field of view (FOV) mask for each image in the CHASE database [8,16,17].

### 3.2    Implementation Details

Fundus images were pre-processed by using the CLAHE [18], gamma adjusting and database normalization algorithms to reduce noise and improve contrast. In the training stage, we first randomly extracted 24.5K partly overlapped $48 \times 48$ patches in each pre-processed fundus image, resulting in a training set of 490K patches on each database. Then, we adopted the mini-batch stochastic gradient descent (mini-batch SGD) with a batch size of 32 as the optimizer, and set empirically the weight parameters $\lambda_2 \sim \lambda_4$ to 1, 1/3 and 2/3, respectively, the learning rate to 0.01, and the maximum epoch number to 150. Note that we used the same settings of hyper-parameters on both databases to demonstrate the robustness of our proposed Vessel-Net.

In the testing stage, we extracted $48 \times 48$ patches with a stride of 5 along both horizontal and vertical directions, and then fed each of them to the trained Vessel-Net. To recompose the entire images, we averaged the obtained probability maps of partly overlapped patches. Finally, we applied the threshold of 0.5 to the recomposed vessel probability map to generate the binary segmentation result.

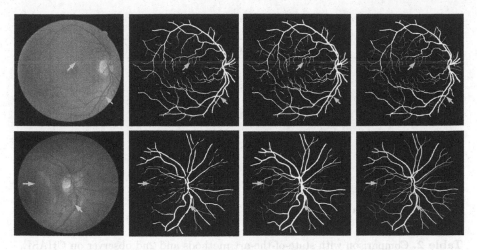

**Fig. 3.** Two examples of retinal images (1st column) from the DRIVE (top row) and CHASE (bottom row) databases, the segmentation results of U-Net (2nd column) and the proposed Vessel-Net (3rd column), and the ground truth (4th column). The samples of thin and thick vessels are pointed by blue and yellow arrows, respectively. (Color figure online)

## 4    Results

Figure 3 shows two retinal image examples from the DRIVE and CHASE databases, respectively, the corresponding segmentation results obtained by U-Net and the proposed Vessel-Net, and the ground truth. It reveals that Vessel-Net is able to delineate most thin and thick vessels and preserve more spatial structures of retinal vessels than U-Net (pointed by blue and yellow arrows). Such ability is essential for further topology estimation and reconstructions.

The retinal vessel segmentation results can be evaluated quantitatively by accuracy (ACC), specificity (SP), sensitivity (SE), and AUC. Tables 1 and 2 give the performance of the second human observer, several state-of-the-art methods, and the proposed Vessel-Net on the DRIVE and CHASE databases. Inter-observer variation is also included by assessing the second observer's annotations against the ground truth (first observer). It shows that our Vessel-Net achieves the highest AUC (i.e. 0.14%/0.35% higher than the second best), the highest accuracy (0.11%/0.24% higher than the second best), top-two sensitivity, and comparable specificity on both databases. It also shows that, compared to the inter-observer variation, our Vessel-Net produces a lower variation from the ground truth. This implies that our method can be used to provide more standardized segmentation of vessel images than manual processing. Furthermore, we suggest that, for potential clinical applications, our Vessel-Net can be combined with other post-processing operators [7,8] to further improve the segmentation of fine structures.

**Table 1.** Comparison with state-of-the-art methods and 2nd observer on DRIVE.

| Method | AUC (%) | Accuracy (%) | Specificity (%) | Sensitivity (%) |
|---|---|---|---|---|
| 2nd observer | N.A | 94.72 | 97.24 | 77.60 |
| Fu et al. [7] | N.A | 95.23 | N.A | 76.03 |
| Liskowski et al. [4] | 97.90 | 95.35 | 98.07 | 78.11 |
| Li et al. [16] | 97.38 | 95.27 | 98.16 | 75.69 |
| Orlando et al. [19] | 95.07 | N.A | 96.84 | 78.97 |
| Yan et al. [20] | 97.52 | 95.42 | 98.18 | 76.53 |
| Zhang et al. [6] | 97.99 | 95.04 | 96.18 | **87.23** |
| Wu et al. [8] | 98.07 | 95.67 | **98.19** | 78.44 |
| **Vessel-Net (ours)** | *98.21* | *95.78* | *98.02* | *80.38* |

**Table 2.** Comparison with state-of-the-art methods and 2nd observer on CHASE.

| Method | AUC (%) | Accuracy (%) | Specificity (%) | Sensitivity (%) |
|---|---|---|---|---|
| 2nd observer | N.A | 95.45 | 97.11 | 81.05 |
| Li et al. [16] | 97.16 | 95.81 | 97.93 | 75.07 |
| Orlando et al. [19] | 95.24 | N.A | 97.12 | 72.77 |
| Yan et al. [20] | 97.81 | 96.10 | 98.09 | 76.33 |
| Wu et al. [8] | 98.25 | 96.37 | **98.47** | 75.38 |
| **Vessel-Net (ours)** | *98.60* | *96.61* | *98.14* | *81.32* |

The ablation experiments were conducted on both databases to demonstrate the performance gain caused by each component of the proposed Vessel-Net. Table 3 shows, from top to bottom, the performance of baseline U-Net, R2U-Net, the U-Net with traditional Inception block, the Vessel-Net without using multi-path supervision (i.e. w/o MP), the Vessel-Net without IR blocks (w/o IR), and

**Table 3.** Ablation studies using the same experiment settings on both databases. (*The results of U-Net are obtained from [11])

| Database | DRIVE(%) | | | | CHASE(%) | | | |
|---|---|---|---|---|---|---|---|---|
| Indicator | AUC | ACC | SP | SE | AUC | ACC | SP | SE |
| U-Net [12]* | 97.55 | 95.31 | 98.20 | 75.37 | 97.72 | 95.78 | 97.01 | **82.88** |
| R2U-Net [11] | 97.84 | 95.56 | 98.13 | 77.92 | 98.15 | 96.34 | **98.20** | 77.56 |
| U-Net with Inception | 97.76 | 95.50 | 97.94 | 78.73 | 98.14 | 96.23 | 97.87 | 79.82 |
| Vessel-Net w/o MP | 98.15 | 95.74 | 98.24 | 78.65 | 98.52 | 96.55 | 98.20 | 80.09 |
| Vessel-Net w/o IR | 98.18 | 95.74 | **98.37** | 77.73 | 98.49 | 96.51 | 98.13 | 80.32 |
| Vessel-Net (ours) | **98.21** | **95.78** | 98.02 | **80.38** | **98.60** | **96.61** | 98.14 | 81.32 |

the proposed Vessel-Net. It reveals that, on both databases, (1) using both IR blocks and multi-path supervision results in an AUC gain of 0.66% and 0.88%; (2) using IR blocks to replace inception blocks results in an AUC gain of 0.39% and 0.38%; (3) using multi-path supervision (IR blocks are available) further results in an AUC gain of 0.06% and 0.08%; and (4) using IR blocks (multi-path supervision is available) further results in an AUC gain of 0.03% and 0.11%.

## 5  Conclusion

In this paper, we present the Vessel-Net, a novel U-like deep convolutional neural network, for retinal vessel segmentation in color fundus images. The newly designed IR blocks and multi-path supervision are highly effective in capturing rich multi-scale information. Our results on the DRIVE and CHASE databases suggest that the proposed Vessel-Net achieved the new state-of-the-art performance.

**Acknowledgements.** This work was supported in part by the National Natural Science Foundation of China under Grants 61771397, in part by the Science and Technology Innovation Committee of Shenzhen Municipality, China, under Grants JCYJ20180306171334997, in part by the Seed Foundation of Innovation and Creation for Graduate Students in NPU under Grants ZZ2019029, and in part by the Project for Graduate Innovation team of NPU.

## References

1. Fraz, M.M., et al.: Blood vessel segmentation methodologies in retinal images - a survey. Comput. Methods Progr. Biomed. **108**(1), 407–433 (2012)
2. Lupascu, C.A., Tegolo, D., Trucco, E.: FABC: retinal vessel segmentation using AdaBoost. IEEE Trans. Inf Technol. Biomed. **14**(5), 1267–1274 (2010)
3. Azzopardi, G., Strisciuglio, N., Vento, M., Petkov, N.: Trainable COSFIRE filters for vessel delineation with application to retinal images. Med. Image Anal. **19**(1), 46–57 (2015)
4. Liskowski, P., Krawiec, K.: Segmenting retinal blood vessels with deep neural networks. IEEE Trans. Med. Imaging **35**(11), 2369–2380 (2016)
5. Fan, Z., et al.: A hierarchical image matting model for blood vessel segmentation in fundus images. IEEE Trans. Image Process. **28**(5), 2367–2377 (2019)
6. Zhang, Y., Chung, A.C.S.: Deep supervision with additional labels for retinal vessel segmentation task. In: Frangi, A.F., Schnabel, J.A., Davatzikos, C., Alberola-López, C., Fichtinger, G. (eds.) MICCAI 2018. LNCS, vol. 11071, pp. 83–91. Springer, Cham (2018). https://doi.org/10.1007/978-3-030-00934-2_10
7. Fu, H., Xu, Y., Lin, S., Kee Wong, D.W., Liu, J.: DeepVessel: retinal vessel segmentation via deep learning and conditional random field. In: Ourselin, S., Joskowicz, L., Sabuncu, M.R., Unal, G., Wells, W. (eds.) MICCAI 2016. LNCS, vol. 9901, pp. 132–139. Springer, Cham (2016). https://doi.org/10.1007/978-3-319-46723-8_16
8. Wu, Y., Xia, Y., Song, Y., Zhang, Y., Cai, W.: Multiscale network followed network model for retinal vessel segmentation. In: Frangi, A.F., Schnabel, J.A., Davatzikos, C., Alberola-López, C., Fichtinger, G. (eds.) MICCAI 2018. LNCS, vol. 11071, pp. 119–126. Springer, Cham (2018). https://doi.org/10.1007/978-3-030-00934-2_14

9. Staal, J., Abr'amoff, M.D., Niemeijer, M., Viergever, M.A., Van Ginneken, B.: Ridge-based vessel segmentation in color images of the retina. IEEE Trans. Med. Imaging **23**(4), 501–509 (2004)
10. Fraz, M.M., et al.: An ensemble classification-based approach applied to retinal blood vessel segmentation. IEEE Trans. Biomed. Eng. **59**(9), 2538–2548 (2012)
11. Alom, M.Z., Hasan, M., Yakopcic, C., Taha, T.M., Asari, V.K.: Recurrent residual convolutional neural network based on U-Net (R2U-Net) for medical image segmentation. arXiv preprint arXiv:1802.06955 (2018)
12. Ronneberger, O., Fischer, P., Brox, T.: U-net: convolutional networks for biomedical image segmentation. In: Navab, N., Hornegger, J., Wells, W.M., Frangi, A.F. (eds.) MICCAI 2015. LNCS, vol. 9351, pp. 234–241. Springer, Cham (2015). https://doi.org/10.1007/978-3-319-24574-4_28
13. Szegedy, C., et al.: Going deeper with convolutions. In: CVPR 2015, pp. 1–9 (2015)
14. Liu, Y., Cheng, M.M., Hu, X., Wang, K., Bai, X.: Richer convolutional features for edge detection. In: CVPR 2017, pp. 3000–3009 (2017)
15. Zhang, J., Tao, D.: FAMED-Net: a fast and accurate multi-scale end-to-end dehazing network. arXiv preprint arXiv:1906.04334 (2019)
16. Li, Q., et al.: A cross-modality learning approach for vessel segmentation in retinal images. IEEE Trans. Med. Imaging **35**(1), 109–118 (2016)
17. Soares, J.V.B., Leandro, J.J.G., Cesar, R.M., Jelinek, H.F., Cree, M.J.: Retinal vessel segmentation using the 2-D Gabor wavelet and supervised classification. IEEE Trans. Med. Imaging **25**(9), 1214–1222 (2006)
18. Setiawan, A.W., Mengko, T.R., Santoso, O.S., Suksmono, A.B.: Color retinal image enhancement using CLAHE. In: ICISS, pp. 1–3 (2013)
19. Orlando, J., Prokofyeva, E., Blaschko, M.: A discriminatively trained fully connected conditional random field model for blood vessel segmentation in fundus images. IEEE Trans. Biomed. Eng. **64**(1), 16–27 (2017)
20. Yan, Z., Yang, X., Cheng, K.T.: Joint segment-Level and pixel-Wise losses for deep learning based retinal vessel segmentation. IEEE Trans. Biomed. Eng. **65**(9), 1912–1923 (2018)

# Ki-GAN: Knowledge Infusion Generative Adversarial Network for Photoacoustic Image Reconstruction *In Vivo*

Hengrong Lan[1], Kang Zhou[1,2], Changchun Yang[1], Jun Cheng[2],
Jiang Liu[2,3], Shenghua Gao[1(✉)], and Fei Gao[1(✉)]

[1] School of Information Science and Technology, ShanghaiTech University,
Shanghai 201210, China
{gaoshh,gaofei}@shanghaitech.edu.cn
[2] Cixi Institute of Biomedical Engineering, Chinese Academy of Sciences,
Ningbo 315201, China
[3] Department of Computer Science and Engineering,
Southern University of Science and Technology, Guangdong 518055, China

**Abstract.** Photoacoustic computed tomography (PACT) breaks through the depth restriction in optical imaging, and the contrast restriction in ultrasound imaging, which is achieved by receiving thermoelastically induced ultrasound signal triggered by an ultrashort laser pulse. The photoacoustic (PA) images reconstructed from the raw PA signals usually utilize conventional reconstruction algorithms, e.g. filtered back-projection. However, the performance of conventional reconstruction algorithms is usually limited by complex and uncertain physical parameters due to heterogeneous tissue structure. In recent years, deep learning has emerged to show great potential in the reconstruction problem. In this work, for the first time to our best knowledge, we propose to infuse the classical signal processing and certified knowledge into the deep learning for PA imaging reconstruction. Specifically, we make these contributions to propose a novel Knowledge Infusion Generative Adversarial Network (Ki-GAN) architecture that combines conventional delay-and-sum algorithm to reconstruct PA image. We train the network on a public clinical database. Our method shows better image reconstruction performance in cases of both full-sampled data and sparse-sampled data compared with state-of-the-art methods. Lastly, our proposed approach also shows high potential for other imaging modalities beyond PACT.

**Keywords:** Photoacoustic computed tomography · Generative adversarial network · Reconstruction · Knowledge infusion

---

Hengrong Lan and Kang Zhou contributed equally to this work.

---

**Electronic supplementary material** The online version of this chapter (https://doi.org/10.1007/978-3-030-32239-7_31) contains supplementary material, which is available to authorized users.

D. Shen et al. (Eds.): MICCAI 2019, LNCS 11764, pp. 273–281, 2019.
https://doi.org/10.1007/978-3-030-32239-7_31

# 1    Introduction

Photoacoustic imaging (PAI) is a hybrid imaging technique based on the photoacoustic (PA) effect that is excited by a laser pulse. The applications of PAI have covered many interesting biomedical imaging areas, such as imaging of oxyhemoglobin saturation, melanoma or chromophore for both cancer diagnostics and treatment monitoring [1, 2]. More specifically, photoacoustic computed tomography (PACT) acquires PA signals using multi-element ultrasound array, and rebuilds the image from PA signals using the reconstruction algorithm. Conventional reconstruction methods, e.g. back-projection and time reversal are widely applied in PA image reconstruction, which however suffers from artifacts and information loss.

Recently, deep learning based approach has been developed to resolve the inverse problem, which basically includes two schemes: training a model that map the raw signals to final image, or ameliorating the result of the conventional reconstruction algorithm (i.e. post-processing) [3, 4]. The input of the former scheme contains all of the physical informations about the target, but there is a huge gap between raw signals and final PA image, which lacks textural information to provide direct physical relationship. On the other hand, the input of the latter scheme reserves the direct physical relationship by conventional reconstruction method, which however only approximates the ground-truth and loses some detailed information. Furthermore, these methods rely on the brute force of big data.

To go beyond brute force and utilize the merits of both schemes, in this paper, we propose Knowledge Infusion Generative Adversarial Network (Ki-GAN) to boost reconstruction performance. The knowledge comes from two sources: (1) Traditional signal processing inspiration (e.g. raw PA signals); (2) Traditional certified reconstruction algorithm (e.g. PA images reconstructed from back-projection). We attempt to introduce signal processing knowledge for framework design and embedding certified knowledge into image feature for PA imaging reconstruction. We enlighten an innovative and effective convolutional kernel to bridge the gap between raw signals and image, and propose a novel Ki-GAN to reconstruct the PA image, which merges the conventional reconstruction algorithms (e.g. delay-and-sum) as a part of the architecture and is fed with the raw PA data as input. To infuse the knowledge, our primary contribution is to suggest a novel framework to infuse the signal processing knowledge and conventional reconstruction knowledge, and achieve better results compared with prior work. Hemoglobin is the main contrast of biological tissue in PAI, and we premise the vessel is the prime target for reconstruction. A set of vessels data is used for training and validating the architecture, which utilizes MATLAB to load the treated segmented blood vessels from the public clinical database [5]. To ensure the performance in different conditions, a set of sparse data is used to test our approach. Furthermore, the *in vivo* PA imaging experiments have also been performed to validate our approach further. The code is available at https://github.com/chenyilan/MICCAI19-Ki-GAN.

## 2   Methods

In this work, we mainly focus on how to infuse more knowledge into the deep learning based imaging framework in Fig. 1. In the following, we will introduce our proposed solution to bridge the gap between PA signals and image by designing a new Auto-Encoder (AE) with signal processing knowledge and embedding a certified algorithm into image feature.

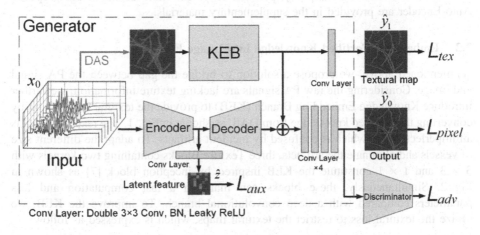

**Fig. 1.** The overall architecture of Ki-GAN; KEB is convolutional layers; DAS is a conventional reconstruction algorithm. KEB: knowledge embedding branch; DAS: delay-and-sum.

### 2.1   Introducing Signal Processing Knowledge for Auto-Encoder Design

As a backbone of our proposed Ki-GAN, our designed AE consists of two parts: (1) to adapt the AE to the physical PA signals, we propose the Auto-Encoder with PA Signal Sampling Inspired Kernel; (2) to further constrain the latent feature between PA signal and image, we introduce the Auto-Encoder with Image Feature Supervision.

**PA Signal Sampling Inspired Kernel.** As aforementioned, since the skip connection of U-Net for raw data is harmful to the decoder, we propose to adapt Auto-Encoder as our cornerstone rather than U-Net [6]. The input raw data has two dimensions: the transducer channel and the signal temporal distribution, where the dimension of signal temporal distribution is much larger than the transducer channel dimension. The large local receptive field is needed to identify the signal with larger length. Therefore, we apply convolutional kernel with $20 \times 3$ size to replace $3 \times 3$ size in the bottom layer of the encoder and kernel with $5 \times 3$ size to replace $3 \times 3$ size in other layers of the encoder, which is called PA Signal Sampling Inspired Kernel (PSSIK). We apply commonly-used MSE (mean square error) loss as our pixel loss, which is expressed as follow:

$$L_{pixel} = \|y - \hat{y}_0\|_F^2 \tag{1}$$

where $y$, $\hat{y}_0$ denote ground-truth and output image respectively.

**Image Feature Supervision.** To improve low-level features of the raw PA signal in the encoder, we assign auxiliary supervisions directly to the output of the encoder network (i.e. $\hat{z}$ in Fig. 1). The auxiliary loss is computed as follow:

$$L_{aux} = \|z - \hat{z}\|_F^2 = \|f(y) - \hat{z}\|_F^2 \tag{2}$$

where $\hat{z}$ denotes latent feature, and $z = f(y)$ denotes latent feature of ground-truth image $y$, where $f$ denotes down-sampling operation on $y$. The more details of our proposed Auto-Encoder are provided in the supplementary materials.

## 2.2 Embedding Certified Knowledge into Image Feature

As mentioned above, we propose a solution to bridge the gap between the PA signal and image. Considering the raw PA signals are lacking texture information, we further introduce Knowledge Embedding Branch (KEB) to provide the textural information by converting the certified knowledge from DAS, as shown in Fig. 1. The result of DAS is an imperfect image which is confused by incident artifacts. To adapt the different size of vessels and eliminate the artifacts, three Texture Blocks containing two kernels with $3 \times 3$ and $1 \times 1$ constitute the KEB inspired by inception block [7] as shown in Fig. 2. Simultaneously, these blocks can maintain a fast computation and less parameters compared with a deep convolutional branch. To improve the KEB, we utilize the textural loss to restrict the textural maps, which is expressed as follow:

$$L_{tex} = \|y - \hat{y}_1\|_F^2 \tag{3}$$

where $\hat{y}_1$ denotes the textural maps.

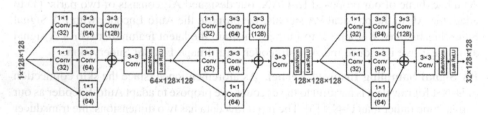

**Fig. 2.** Three Texture Blocks constitute the Knowledge Embedding Branch.

## 2.3 Ki-GAN: Knowledge Infusion GAN

As shown in Fig. 1, by integrating above two methods, we further propose to make use of adversarial learning [8] to improve the ineffectiveness of convolutional neural networks in modeling correlation between the PA signals and the detailed vessel reconstruction. On the other hand, pixel loss is an average operation, that is to say, the pixel loss will result in image smooth and blurring. Therefore, the generative adversarial network is needed. The generator outputs the reconstructed image $\hat{y}_0$, and is also restricted by adversarial loss, which is calculated as follow:

$$L_{advG} = \|D(y) - D(\hat{y}_0)\|_F^2 \tag{4}$$

where $D$ is a function that outputs an intermediate layer of the discriminator. Our discriminator is inspired by *Patch*GAN [9] to penalize the texture at the scale of patches (see Fig. S2 in supplementary materials), and the adversarial loss can be expressed as:

$$L_{advD} = -\mathbb{E}_{x_0,y}[\log D(x_0, y)] - \mathbb{E}_{x_0,\hat{y}_0}[\log(1 - D(x_0, \hat{y}_0))] \tag{5}$$

Finally, the generator network is trained by minimizing the total loss:

$$L_{total} = \lambda_{adv}L_{advG} + \lambda_{pix}L_{pixel} + \lambda_{aux}L_{aux} + \lambda_{tex}L_{tex} \tag{6}$$

where $\lambda_{adv}$, $\lambda_{pix}$, $\lambda_{aux}$ and $\lambda_{tex}$ are hyper-parameters.

## 3 Experiments and Results

### 3.1 Datasets and Evaluation

The proposed approach requires a large amount of data for training the model, which is difficult to obtain since the current PAI equipment is still in the stage translating from preclinical to clinical application, and not available in the clinic. Therefore, we convert the publicly available datasets of fundus oculi [5] as the photoacoustic initial pressure distribution. The toolbox of k-wave [10] in MATLAB reads the initial pressure to generate the raw PA signals for training.

The vessels are surrounded by 120 channels' transducers with 18 mm radius. For each PA signal, the total recorded points are 2560 with 150 MHz sampling rate. The pixel size of the initial pressure map is 128 × 128, and the output of the network is 128 × 128 as well. The center frequency of the ultrasound transducer is set as 5 MHz with 80% bandwidth, and the propagation velocity of ultrasound is 1500 m/s.

As the original dataset is small, we adopt some preprocessing to expand the data volume. Firstly, the complete blood vessel of fundus oculi is segmented into four equal parts; and then randomly transform (e.g. rotations and transpositions) and superpose two segmented blood vessels. After a series of treatment, we can acquire excessive initial pressure for PA imaging and generate sufficient training data.

The whole dataset is composed of 4300 training samples and 500 test samples. Simultaneously a set of sparse data are also utilized to evaluate the proposed approach, which compresses the signal channels from 120 to 40. In addition, we also explored rat thigh experimental data for the purpose of verifying the validity of the proposed approach in animal imaging *in vivo*.

### 3.2    Training Details

The framework is implemented in PyTorch. The network is fed the $2560 \times 120$ raw data as input with setting batch size as 32. The generator can be trained by Eq. (6), the $\lambda_{aux}$ and $\lambda_{tex}$ are set as 0.5 for both, which are optimum choices compared with different values (we also list the performance of different parameters values in supplementary materials). The $\lambda_{adv}$ and $\lambda_{pix}$ are set as 0.04 and 1 respectively. The discriminator can be trained by Eq. (5). In our evaluation, the simple delay-and-sum (DAS) algorithm is chosen as the image textural knowledge infused into Ki-GAN.

The computing platform we used is a high-speed graphics computing workstation consisting of Intel Xeon E5-2690 (2.6 GHz) $\times$ 2 central processing unit (CPU) and NVIDIA GTX 1080ti $\times$ 4 graphics processing units (GPU). The time consumption of every batch is 0.795 s in training stage.

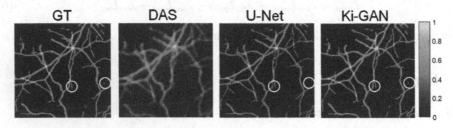

**Fig. 3.** Example of quantitative comparison using full-sampled data. From left to right: ground-truth, delay-and-sum, U-Net and Ki-GAN. The white circles indicate the local details.

### 3.3    Experimental Results

**Full-Sampled Data.** Figure 3 has shown a sample of results generated by different models, which comprise DAS, post-processing model (U-Net) and Ki-GAN. The images of DAS cannot avoid the artifacts albeit they preserve the vessel's sketch indistinctly. The images from our proposed Ki-GAN are closer to ground-truth than U-Net. To further compare the performance of different approaches, we compare the results of the test set using three indexes of quantitative metrics: (1) structural similarity index (SSIM); (2) peak signal-to-noise ratio (PSNR); (3) signal-to-noise ratio (SNR). We also list the ablation studies beyond the methods shown in Fig. 3, including Auto-Encoder (AE#1), AE#1 with PSSIK (AE#2), AE#2 with Image Feature Supervision (AE#3), AE#3 with Embedded Certified Knowledge (AE#4), and U-Net inputting the raw data (U-Net[1]). The quantitative comparison results are shown in Table 1, which indicate that our proposed Ki-GAN gets the upper hand compared with other models. Meanwhile, the ablation studies' results also validate the effectiveness of different modules of our proposed method. More results of ablation studies and comparative experiments are provided in the supplementary materials (Fig. S4–5).

**Table 1.** Evaluation results of different models for the test sets (full-sampled data). U-Net[1]: input the signals and resize to concatenation, U-Net[2]: input the result of DAS, AE#1: Auto-Encoder, AE#2: AE#1 with PSSIK, AE#3: AE#2 with Image Feature Supervision, AE#4: AE#3 with Embedded Certified Knowledge.

|      | DAS | U-Net[1] | U-Net[2] | AE#1 | AE#2 | AE#3 | AE#4 | Ki-GAN |
|------|-----|----------|----------|------|------|------|------|--------|
| SSIM | 0.2159 | 0.6453 | 0.8749 | 0.6519 | 0.6818 | 0.6931 | 0.9123 | **0.9285** |
| PSNR | 15.6176 | 18.4519 | 24.0175 | 18.7033 | 19.1193 | 19.1529 | 24.8951 | **25.5115** |
| SNR | 1.6386 | 4.3237 | 10.1285 | 4.7243 | 5.1403 | 5.1739 | 10.6161 | **11.5324** |

**Sparse-Sampled Data.** We further compare the performance of U-Net (post-processing) and Ki-GAN using the sparse data, which include only 40 channels' raw data to reconstruct the vessel image. It is noteworthy that we fill the zero data to keep the number of channel in 120 due to the fixed size of the input data. The qualitative comparison is shown in Fig. 4, which indicates that the performance of the proposed method is better than U-Net. The white circles marked three details in Fig. 4, showing that the result of Ki-GAN identifies with ground-truth image more closely compared with U-Net. The quantitative evaluation results also agree well with Fig. 4 as Table 2 showed.

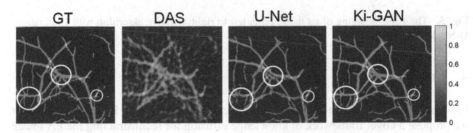

**Fig. 4.** Example of quantitative comparison using sparse-sampled data. From left to right: ground-truth, delay-and-sum, U-Net and Ki-GAN. The white circles indicate the local details.

**Table 2.** Evaluation results of different models for the test sets (sparse-sampled data).

|      | DAS | U-Net | Ki-GAN |
|------|-----|-------|--------|
| SSIM | 0.1842 | 0.8174 | **0.8617** |
| PSNR | 15.5123 | 21.348 | **22.7398** |
| SNR | 1.5333 | 7.4689 | **8.7607** |

**In Vivo Data.** Last but not least, the *in vivo* PA imaging experiments of a rat thigh have also been performed to validate our approach. Three methods including conventional iteration-based reconstruction, U-Net and Ki-GAN, are performed to illustrate the results in Fig. 5. It shows that our proposed model possesses a stronger contrast and fewer artifacts compared with other two methods in an insufficient training data set. The U-Net has a poor generalization performance compared with Ki-GAN in *in vivo* data, and suffers inevitable artifacts.

The time consumption of the iterative reconstruction algorithm with 10 iterations, U-Net and Ki-GAN are 331.51 s, 0.01 s and 0.025 s. The iterative algorithm depends on the repetitive calculation of the forward and backward models in the loop cycle. The image quality and time consumption show inevitable compromise in the iterative algorithm. U-Net shows the fastest mapping from image to image that consumes least time in three methods. The proposed Ki-GAN infuses the conventional reconstruction and raw-data based feature map. Meanwhile, the 0.025 s time consumption still sufficiently satisfies the requirement of real-time imaging for most clinical demands.

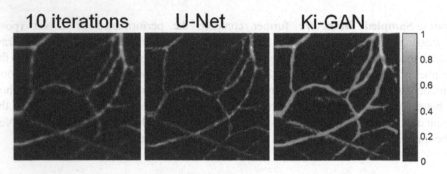

**Fig. 5.** The vessel imaging of rat thigh. From left to right: iterative algorithm with 10 iterations, U-Net and Ki-GAN.

## 4 Conclusion

Fast and accurate image reconstruction is a significant problem in PACT. In this paper, we propose a novel framework of knowledge infusion for reconstructing the PA image, which merges the conventional reconstruction with burgeoning deep learning. A novel Ki-GAN is proposed to rebuild the initial PA pressure of vessels. Ablation studies and comparative experiments show that the proposed model can perform very well in full-sampled data, sparse-sampled data, and *in vivo* experimental data. In the future work, we will try to exploit the real-time imaging system based on this method and extend the imaging dimension from 2D to 3D.

## References

1. Wang, L.V., Hu, S.: Photoacoustic tomography: in vivo imaging from organelles to organs. Science **335**, 1458–1462 (2012)
2. Lan, H., Duan, T., Zhong, H., Zhou, M., Gao, F.: Photoacoustic classification of tumor model morphology based on support vector machine: a simulation and phantom study. IEEE J. Sel. Top. Quantum Electron. **25**, 1–9 (2019)
3. Cai, C., Deng, K., Ma, C., Luo, J.: End-to-end deep neural network for optical inversion in quantitative photoacoustic imaging. Opt. Lett. **43**, 2752–2755 (2018)
4. Jin, K.H., McCann, M.T., Froustey, E., Unser, M.: Deep convolutional neural network for inverse problems in imaging. IEEE Trans. Image Process. **26**, 4509–4522 (2017)

5. Staal, J., Abramoff, M.D., Niemeijer, M., Viergever, M.A., van Ginneken, B.: Ridge-based vessel segmentation in color images of the retina. IEEE Trans. Med. Imaging **23**, 501–509 (2004)
6. Ronneberger, O., Fischer, P., Brox, T.: U-net: convolutional networks for biomedical image segmentation. In: Navab, N., Hornegger, J., Wells, W.M., Frangi, A.F. (eds.) MICCAI 2015. LNCS, vol. 9351, pp. 234–241. Springer, Cham (2015). https://doi.org/10.1007/978-3-319-24574-4_28
7. Szegedy, C., Ioffe, S., Vanhoucke, V., Alemi, A.A.: Inception-v4, inception-resnet and the impact of residual connections on learning. In: Thirty-First AAAI Conference on Artificial Intelligence (2017)
8. Goodfellow, I., et al.: Generative adversarial nets. In: Advances in Neural Information Processing Systems, pp. 2672–2680 (2014)
9. Isola, P., Zhu, J.-Y., Zhou, T., Efros, A.A.: Image-to-image translation with conditional adversarial networks. In: Proceedings of the IEEE Conference on Computer Vision and Pattern Recognition, pp. 1125–1134 (2017)
10. Treeby, B.E., Cox, B.T.: k-Wave: MATLAB toolbox for the simulation and reconstruction of photoacoustic wave fields. J. Biomed. Opt. **15**, 021314 (2010)

# Uncertainty Guided Semi-supervised Segmentation of Retinal Layers in OCT Images

Suman Sedai[1]($\boxtimes$), Bhavna Antony[1], Ravneet Rai[2], Katie Jones[2], Hiroshi Ishikawa[2], Joel Schuman[2], Wollstein Gadi[2], and Rahil Garnavi[1]

[1] IBM Research - Australia, Melbourne, VIC, Australia
ssedai@au1.ibm.com

[2] NYU Langone Eye Center, NYU School of Medicine, New York, NY, USA

**Abstract.** Deep convolutional neural networks have shown outstanding performance in medical image segmentation tasks. The usual problem when training supervised deep learning methods is the lack of labeled data which is time-consuming and costly to obtain. In this paper, we propose a novel uncertainty guided semi-supervised learning based on student-teacher approach for training the segmentation network using limited labeled samples and large number of unlabeled images. First, a teacher segmentation model is trained from the labeled samples using Bayesian deep learning. The trained model is used to generate soft segmentation labels and uncertainty map for the unlabeled set. The student model is then updated using the softly segmented samples and the corresponding pixel-wise confidence of the segmentation quality estimated from the uncertainty of the teacher model using a newly designed loss function. Experimental results on a retinal layer segmentation task show that the proposed method improves the segmentation performance in comparison to the fully supervised approach and is on par with the expert annotator. The proposed semi-supervised segmentation framework is a key contribution and applicable for biomedical image segmentation across various imaging modalities where access to annotated medical images is challenging.

**Keywords:** OCT retinal imaging · Semi-supervised segmentation · Bayesian deep learning

## 1 Introduction

Segmentation of anatomical regions in biomedical images such as optical coherence tomography (OCT) retinal scans is of great clinical significance especially for disease diagnosis, progression analysis and treatment planning. For example, the progressive thinning of circumpapillary retinal nerve fiber layer (cpRNFL)

© Springer Nature Switzerland AG 2019
D. Shen et al. (Eds.): MICCAI 2019, LNCS 11764, pp. 282–290, 2019.
https://doi.org/10.1007/978-3-030-32239-7_32

thickness measured by OCT can be used to predict the visual functional loss in patient with glaucoma [6].

In the past few years, Convolutional Neural Networks (CNNs) based methods such as Unet [9] and Dense-Unet [4,7] have achieved remarkable performance gain in medical image and natural image segmentation. The networks are trained end-to-end, pixels-to-pixels on semantic segmentation exceeded the most state-of-the-art methods without further machinery. For example, such network have been used for retinal structure segmentation in fundus [8] and OCT [10,11] images. Such fully supervised segmentation algorithms requires large number of annotated images to achieve reasonable robustness and accuracy. However, acquiring pixel-wise ground truth annotations can be time-consuming and costly in medical imaging domain where only experts can provide reliable annotations. The under-supply of the labeled data motivates the need for effective machine learning methods that require limited supervision, such as semi-supervised learning.

Semi-supervised learning tackle this problem by leveraging large number of readily available unlabeled data along with the limited labeled data to improve the performance. For example, semi-supervised approaches have been applied to different medical imaging tasks such as MRI segmentation [1], lung nodule detection and retinal vessel segmentation [14]. In another approaches, [2] uses auxiliary manifold learning in the latent space for MS lesion segmentation task and [12] uses the feature embedding obtained from unlabeled images to segment optic cup in retinal fundus images.

In this paper, we propose a novel semi-supervised approach to leverage unlabeled images to segment the retinal layers in OCT images. The proposed method consists of two components: (a) student segmentation network which is responsible for learning suitable data representation and learning the main segmentation task and (b) teacher segmentation network which controls the learning of the student network by modeling the unreliability in segmentation prediction. First, the teacher model is trained on the labeled set using Bayesian deep learning to capture the uncertainty map and is used to generate *soft segmentation labels* for the unlabeled samples. The uncertainty map indicates pixel-wise unreliability of the *soft labels*. Based on the uncertainty map, we further propose a novel loss function to guide the student model by adaptively weighting regions with unreliable *soft labels* to improve final segmentation performance. Our proposed algorithm has been applied to the task of retinal layer segmentation in OCT images from the optic nerve head. Experimental results indicate that our proposed algorithm can improve the segmentation accuracy compared to the state-of-the-art fully supervised OCT segmentation methods and is in par with the human expert.

## 2    Proposed Semi-supervised Segmentation Method

In this section, we describe our proposed uncertainty guided semi-supervised learning. We assume that we are given a large set of unlabeled images $D_u = (\mathbf{x}_i)$ and a small set of high quality labeled images $D_l = \{(\mathbf{x}_i, \mathbf{y}_i)\}$ where $\mathbf{x}_i$ is image and $\mathbf{y}_i$ is the segmentation annotation. As shown in Fig. 1(a), our proposed approach involves two kind of deep neural networks called the teacher segmentation network $F_T(\mathbf{x})$ and student segmentation network $F_S(\mathbf{x})$. The teacher network is trained using labeled dataset based on Bayesian deep learning to output both segmentation map as well as uncertainty map. The teacher network is then applied to each image in the unlabeled set to obtain the segmentation label and associated uncertainty map to generate the *softly labeled* samples. The uncertainty map captures the pixel-wise confidence values indicating the reliability of the segmentation output from the teacher network and it is used to guide the training of the student network learning which we describe in Sect. 2.2.

We use DenseUNet architecture [4,7] as our base model for both teacher and student networks. As shown in Fig. 1(b) the model consists of three dense blocks in encoder and decoder and a bottleneck dense block with Unet like skip connections between the output of the encoder dense blocks and input of the decoder dense blocks. Each dense block contains four convolution units each comprising of 8 (3 × 3) convolution, batch normalization (BN) and ReLU layer where the output of each unit is fed to the subsequent ones. Therefore each dense block produces 32 feature maps. The final prediction layer is a convolution layer with channel number equivalent to number of classes $C$ followed by a *softmax* activation function. We use *SpatialDropout* [13] layer before every convolution layer with *dropout rate* of 0.2.

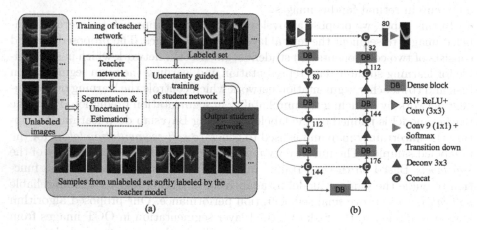

(a)　　　　　　　　　　　　　　　(b)

**Fig. 1.** (a) Proposed semi-supervised segmentation method based on Bayesian student-teacher learning. (b) Overview of the Dense-Unet architecture used by the teacher and the student models.

## 2.1　Teacher Segmentation Network as a Bayesian Model

We model the teacher segmentation network $F_T(\mathbf{x})$ using Bayesian deep learning to capture the segmentation uncertainties for the student model, estimated with respect to the labeled data. We adopt the approach introduced by [3] based

---

**Algorithm 1.** Training of the proposed semi-supervised learning method.

1. Given an unlabeled data $D_u = \{\mathbf{x}_1\}_{i=1}^{N_u}$ and the labeled set $D_l = \{(\mathbf{x}_i, \mathbf{y}_i)\}_{i=1}^{N_l}$
2. Train $F_T(\mathbf{x})$ using $D_l$ as described in Section 2.1.
3. For each iteration, until the validation loss converges:
   (a) Sample a minibatch $\hat{x}_u$ from $D_u$ and $\hat{x}_l$ from $D_l$.
   (b) Compute the *soft labels* $\mathbf{z}$ and uncertainty $\mathbf{u}$ for $\hat{x}_u$ using Equation 1 and 2.
   (c) Compute the confidence map from the uncertainty map using Equation 3.
   (d) Compute the labeled and unlabeled loss using Equation 6.
   (e) Update the parameter of the student model $F_S$ using back-propagation.

---

on the *dropout variational inference* to compute the segmentation uncertainty. First we train the $F_T(\mathbf{x})$ from the labeled sample set $D_l$ using the class weighted categorical cross entropy loss. For segmentation and uncertainty quantification, we enable the *dropout* in test phase and the output predictive distribution is obtained by performing $K$ stochastic forward passes through the network, i.e., $\mathbf{y}^k = F_T^k(x), k = 1, \cdots, K$ where $F_T^k$ is an effective network after the *spatial dropout* operation. In each forward pass, the fraction of convolution feature-maps (denoted by *dropout rate*) are disabled and the segmentation score is computed using only the remaining feature-maps. The segmentation score vector $\bar{\mathbf{y}}$ is obtained by averaging the $K$ samples, via *monte carlo integration*:

$$\bar{\mathbf{y}} = \frac{1}{K} \sum_{k=1}^{K} \mathbf{y}^k \tag{1}$$

The average score vector contains the probability score for each class, ie $\bar{\mathbf{y}} = [\bar{y}_1, \cdots, \bar{y}_C]$. The overall segmentation uncertainty for each pixel can be obtained by computing the entropy of the average probability vector:

$$U(\bar{\mathbf{y}}) = - \sum_{c=1}^{C} \bar{y}_c \log \bar{y}_c. \tag{2}$$

Higher segmentation uncertainty is obtained when the network assigns higher probabilities to different classes for different forward passes. Conversely, for the confident predictions, network assigns higher probability to the true class for any forward passes, resulting in lower uncertainty value.

## 2.2   Uncertainty Guided Learning of Student Network

Here, we describe the process of learning the student segmentation network $F_s(\mathbf{x})$ from both unlabeled and labeled data with the guidance from teacher segmentation network $F_T(\mathbf{x})$. We first apply $F_T(\mathbf{x})$ to the unlabeled images $\mathbf{x}_u \in U$ to obtain the soft segmentation map $\mathbf{z}$ using Eq. 1 and the associated segmentation uncertainty map $\mathbf{u}$ using Eq. 2. The higher values in the uncertainty map denotes the regions where generated *soft labels* are likely to be incorrect and needs to be down-weighted while updating $F_s(\mathbf{x})$. We convert the uncertainty map $\mathbf{u}$ to obtain the normalized confidence map as:

$$\omega = \exp\left[-\alpha\mathbf{u}\right] \tag{3}$$

where $\alpha$ is a positive scalar hyper-parameter and the confidence map $\omega \in [0, 1]$ provides the pixel-wise quality of the *soft labels* produced by $F_T(\mathbf{x})$ such that higher uncertainty values produces low quality score and vice versa. The unlabeled loss is then formulated as the confidence weighted cross entropy as:

$$L_{unlab} = \sum_{c=1}^{C} \zeta_c \sum_{\forall Z_c} \omega_t \log z_c^t \tag{4}$$

where

$$\zeta_c = \begin{cases} 1/\sum_{\forall Z_c} \omega_t, & \text{if } \sum_{\forall Z_c} \omega_t, > P \\ 0 & \text{otherwise,} \end{cases} \tag{5}$$

such that $\zeta_c$ weights the contribution of each class to mitigate the effect of class imbalance in *soft labels* due to its confidence weights; $Z_c$ denotes the pixels region of the $c^{th}$ class in the *soft label* $\mathbf{z}$ and $z_c^t$ is the *softmax* output from $F_s(\mathbf{x})$ for the $t^{th}$ pixel and $c^{th}$ class. The Eq. 5 sets $\zeta_c = 0$, when the effective number of pixels per class $\sum_{\forall Z_c} \omega_t \leq P$ to improve the stability of unlabeled loss which can happen when majority of pixels of $Z_c$ are uncertain. We empirically set $P = 50$ for our retinal segmentation task. Finally, semi-supervised loss is a sum of both labeled and unlabeled loss:

$$L_{semi\_sup} = L_{lab} + L_{unlab} \tag{6}$$

where $L_{lab}$ is a *categorical crossentropy* computed from the labeled mini-batch samples. The training steps of our method is shown in Algorithm 1.

The proposed semi-supervised loss function encourages the network to discard the pixels with inaccurate *soft labels* generated by $F_T(\mathbf{x})$. The hyper-parameter $\alpha$ in Eq. 3 controls the information flow from $F_T(\mathbf{x})$ to $F_s(\mathbf{x})$. Intuitively small $\alpha$ allows the student to blindly follow teacher, whereas the bigger $\alpha$ controls the learning by giving emphasis on the teacher's uncertainty. For example, setting $\alpha = 0$ is equivalent to using all the *soft labels* whereas setting $\alpha > 0$ allows probabilistic selection the *soft labels* that are more certain. We empirically set the value of $\alpha$ using validation which we describe in Sect. 3.

We train the student network for 40000 iterations or until the validation loss converges using mini-batch gradient descent and the Adam optimizer with momentum and a batch size of 1 for each labeled and unlabeled component. The learning rate is set to $10^{-5}$ which is decreased by one tenth after 10000 iterations of the training. We augment the training images and corresponding label map masks through a mirror-image reflection and random rotation within the range of $[-15, 15]$ degrees.

**Table 1.** Retinal segmentation performance in terms of dice coefficient of the proposed semi-supervised (U-SLS) method compared with the fully supervised (FS-DU) and Plain-SLS for different labeled training sizes.

| Method | U-SLS (Proposed) | | FS-DU | | Plain-SLS | |
|---|---|---|---|---|---|---|
| #Images | RNFL | Average | RNFL | Average | RNFL | Average |
| 490 | $0.90 \pm 0.04$ | $0.82 \pm 0.09$ | $0.88 \pm 0.08$ | $0.80 \pm 0.07$ | $0.87 \pm 0.08$ | $0.79 \pm 0.07$ |
| 240 | $0.87 \pm 0.07$ | $0.80 \pm 0.09$ | $0.85 \pm 0.07$ | $0.78 \pm 0.12$ | $0.83 \pm 0.11$ | $0.76 \pm 0.11$ |
| 120 | $0.84 \pm 0.09$ | $0.76 \pm 0.12$ | $0.81 \pm 0.09$ | $0.74 \pm 0.17$ | $0.77 \pm 0.12$ | $0.69 \pm 0.17$ |

## 3    Experiments

The dataset consists of 570 spectral-domain optical coherence tomography (OCT) optic nerve volumes acquired using commercial OCT device (Cirrus HD-OCT; Zeiss). Each OCT volume consists of 200 BScans of size $1024 \times 200$. We take 700 BScans sampled from 70 OCT volumes to create a labeled set where the ground truth has been obtained by manual annotation of the nine boundaries from eight retinal layers [5]. We convert the layer boundaries to the probability map for the eight layers regions and the background region. Therefore, the number of classes is $C = 9$.

Out of 700 labeled images, we select 490 images from 49 volumes to create a labeled training set, 70 images from 7 volumes for validation set and 140 images from 14 volume as a test set. Beside the annotation of expert E1 on the 700 labeled set, we also obtained a second set of annotation for the test from the second expert E2 to compare with E1. We then use 10000 BScans sampled from the remaining 500 volumes as an unlabeled set.

We compare our proposed uncertainty guided semi-supervised layer segmentation (U-SLS) method with the baseline fully supervised Dense-Unet (FS-DU) [4] that does not take unlabeled images into account and the plain semi-supervised learning (Plain-SL) method that blindly follows the teacher model without taking uncertainty into account, i.e., for the case where $\alpha = 0$ in Eq. 3. Figure 2(b)–(d) shows the examples of *soft labels* and uncertainty maps produced by the teacher model $F_T(\mathbf{x})$ on an unlabeled image. It can be seen that the teacher model trained on less number of labeled data produces less accurate

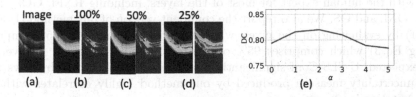

**Fig. 2.** (a)–(d) Examples of *soft labels* and corresponding uncertainty map produced by the teacher models trained using different number of labeled images. (e) The effect of different values of $\alpha$ on the performance of the student model.

*soft labels* and the corresponding uncertainty map correlates with the inaccuracies in the generated *soft labels*. For our method U-SLS, we set the optimal value of $\alpha = 2$ using validation set as shown in Fig. 2(e).

**Table 2.** Performance of our proposed method compared with the expert E2

| Layer | Dice Coefficient | | |
|---|---|---|---|
| | U-SLS (Proposed) | E2 vs E1 | U-SLS-Conf |
| RNFL | $0.90 \pm 0.04$ | $0.90 \pm 0.07$ | $0.95 \pm 0.03$ |
| GCL+IPL | $0.83 \pm 0.06$ | $0.84 \pm 0.11$ | $0.91 \pm 0.06$ |
| INL | $0.78 \pm 0.07$ | $0.78 \pm 0.14$ | $0.90 \pm 0.05$ |
| OPL | $0.68 \pm 0.09$ | $0.74 \pm 0.14$ | $0.79 \pm 0.01$ |
| ONL | $0.92 \pm 0.03$ | $0.91 \pm 0.06$ | $0.97 \pm 0.01$ |
| IS | $0.74 \pm 0.09$ | $0.77 \pm 0.14$ | $0.81 \pm 0.10$ |
| OS | $0.82 \pm 0.06$ | $0.83 \pm 0.10$ | $0.90 \pm 0.04$ |
| RPE | $0.82 \pm 0.06$ | $0.85 \pm 0.08$ | $0.89 \pm 0.001$ |
| Average | $0.82 \pm 0.07$ | $0.84 \pm 0.12$ | $0.91 \pm 0.08$ |

Table 1 compares the average Dice coefficient (DC) between the ground truth and generated segmentations by the proposed U-SLS, the plain-SLS methods and the fully supervised Dense-Unet method. The proposed method U-SLS resulted in average DC of 0.90 for RNFL layer and 0.82 across all eight layers when trained on the full labeled training set and the unlabeled set improving over both FS-DU and PLain-SLS. However, when we reduce the number of labeled training samples, the improvement of the proposed method was more significant than both FS-DU and Plain-SLS. This demonstrates that the proposed approach improves the segmentation performance when the number of labeled images are limited. Moreover, the lower performance of Plain-SLS shows that student model is corrupted by the soft labels when uncertainty is not taken into account. On the other hand U-SLS improves the performance by uncertainty guided learning from the unlabeled samples.

Table 2 compares the performance of our method with the performance of the human annotator E2. It can be observed that performance of our method is on par with the human expert for most of the layers, including RNFl, GCL+IPL, INL, ONL and OS. We also report the confident version of our method (U-SLS-Conf) by evaluating on the pixels whose confidence score $\omega > 0.5$ (computed using Eq. 3) which comprises 95% of the total number of pixels on average. As expected, U-SLS-Conf significantly improves over U-SLS which shows that the uncertainty measure produced by our method highly correlates with the segmentation inaccuracies.

Figure 3 (left) shows the examples of the retinal layers segmentation and the generated uncertainty map. Figure 3 (right) shows the precision recall curve for RNFL layer comparing our method with the human annotator. This shows that performance U-SLS is comparable with the human expert, whereas the confident version, U-SLS-Conf exceeded the human expert.

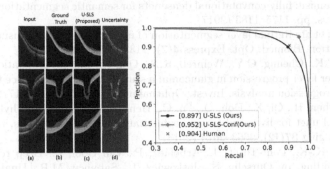

**Fig. 3.** Example of retinal layer segmentation and uncertainty quantification using proposed U-SLS method. Left: (a) test images, (b) ground truth, (c) predicted segmentation map from U-SLS (d) uncertainty map (warmer color denotes regions with higher uncertainty). Right: Precision recall curve comparing the proposed U-SLS method with the human expert for RNFL layer segmentation. (Color figure online)

## 4 Conclusion

In this paper, we presented a novel and effective semi-supervised method, based on student-teacher framework, for segmentation of OCT images of retina. The proposed method is able to leverage large volume of unlabeled noisy data and incorporate uncertainty for improved segmentation of retina structures, compared to the state-of-the-art fully and semi-supervised segmentation methods. We have demonstrated that the proposed uncertainty guided method can effectively transfer knowledge from the teacher to the student model for the segmentation task and is able to generate expert-level segmentation using limited number of labeled samples. Therefore, our approach is useful in clinical applications where access to large volume of annotated images (which is needed for state-of-the-art fully supervised approaches) is challenging. Although, we have applied our approach in retinal image segmentation, we believe that our method is equally applicable to other modalities.

## References

1. Bai, W., et al.: Semi-supervised learning for network-based cardiac MR image segmentation. In: Descoteaux, M., Maier-Hein, L., Franz, A., Jannin, P., Collins, D.L., Duchesne, S. (eds.) MICCAI 2017. LNCS, vol. 10434, pp. 253–260. Springer, Cham (2017). https://doi.org/10.1007/978-3-319-66185-8_29
2. Baur, C., Albarqouni, S., Navab, N.: Semi-supervised deep learning for fully convolutional networks. In: Descoteaux, M., Maier-Hein, L., Franz, A., Jannin, P., Collins, D.L., Duchesne, S. (eds.) MICCAI 2017. LNCS, vol. 10435, pp. 311–319. Springer, Cham (2017). https://doi.org/10.1007/978-3-319-66179-7_36

3. Gal, Y., Ghahramani, Z.: Dropout as a Bayesian approximation: representing model uncertainty in deep learning. In: ICML, pp. 1050–1059 (2016)
4. Jégou, S., Drozdzal, M., Vázquez, D., Romero, A., Bengio, Y.: The one hundred layers tiramisu: fully convolutional densenets for semantic segmentation. In: CVPR Workshops, pp. 1175–1183 (2017)
5. Lang, A., et al.: Retinal layer segmentation of macular OCT images using boundary classification. Biomed. Opt. Express 4(7), 1133–1152 (2013)
6. Leung, C.K., Cheung, C.Y., Weinreb, R.N., Qiu, K., Liu, S.: Evaluation of retinal nerve fiber layer progression in glaucoma: a study on optical coherence tomography guided progression analysis. Invest. Ophthalmol. Vis. Sci. 51(1), 217–222 (2010)
7. Li, X., Chen, H., Qi, X., Dou, Q., Fu, C., Heng, P.: H-DenseUNet: hybrid densely connected unet for liver and tumor segmentation from CT volumes. IEEE Trans. Med. Imaging 37(12), 2663–2674 (2018)
8. Maninis, K.-K., Pont-Tuset, J., Arbeláez, P., Van Gool, L.: Deep retinal image understanding. In: Ourselin, S., Joskowicz, L., Sabuncu, M.R., Unal, G., Wells, W. (eds.) MICCAI 2016. LNCS, vol. 9901, pp. 140–148. Springer, Cham (2016). https://doi.org/10.1007/978-3-319-46723-8_17
9. Ronneberger, O., Fischer, P., Brox, T.: U-net: convolutional networks for biomedical image segmentation. In: Navab, N., Hornegger, J., Wells, W.M., Frangi, A.F. (eds.) MICCAI 2015. LNCS, vol. 9351, pp. 234–241. Springer, Cham (2015). https://doi.org/10.1007/978-3-319-24574-4_28
10. Roy, A.G., et al.: ReLayNet: retinal layer and fluid segmentation of macular optical coherence tomography using fully convolutional networks. Biomed. Opt. Express 8(8), 3627–3642 (2017)
11. Sedai, S., Antony, B., Mahapatra, D., Garnavi, R.: Joint segmentation and uncertainty visualization of retinal layers in optical coherence tomography images using Bayesian deep learning. In: Stoyanov, D., et al. (eds.) OMIA/COMPAY -2018. LNCS, vol. 11039, pp. 219–227. Springer, Cham (2018). https://doi.org/10.1007/978-3-030-00949-6_26
12. Sedai, S., Mahapatra, D., Hewavitharanage, S., Maetschke, S., Garnavi, R.: Semi-supervised segmentation of optic cup in retinal fundus images using variational autoencoder. In: Descoteaux, M., Maier-Hein, L., Franz, A., Jannin, P., Collins, D.L., Duchesne, S. (eds.) MICCAI 2017. LNCS, vol. 10434, pp. 75–82. Springer, Cham (2017). https://doi.org/10.1007/978-3-319-66185-8_9
13. Tompson, J., Goroshin, R., Jain, A., LeCun, Y., Bregler, C.: Efficient object localization using convolutional networks. In: CVPR, pp. 648–656 (2015)
14. You, X., Peng, Q., Yuan, Y., Cheung, Y., Lei, J.: Segmentation of retinal blood vessels using the radial projection and semi-supervised approach. Pattern Recogn. 44(10–11), 2314–2324 (2011)

# Endoscopy

# Triple ANet: Adaptive Abnormal-aware Attention Network for WCE Image Classification

Xiaoqing Guo[iD] and Yixuan Yuan[✉][iD]

Department of Electrical Engineering,
City University of Hong Kong, Kowloon, Hong Kong, China
xiaoqiguo2-c@my.cityu.edu.hk, yxyuan.ee@cityu.edu.hk

**Abstract.** Accurate detection of abnormal regions in Wireless Capsule Endoscopy (WCE) images is crucial for early intestine cancer diagnosis and treatment, while it still remains challenging due to the relatively low contrasts and ambiguous boundaries between abnormalities and normal regions. Additionally, the huge intra-class variances, alone with the high degree of visual similarities shared by inter-class abnormalities prevent the network from robust classification. To tackle these dilemmas, we propose an Adaptive Abnormal-aware Attention Network (Triple ANet) with Adaptive Dense Block (ADB) and Abnormal-aware Attention Module (AAM) for automatic WCE image analysis. ADB is designed to assign one attention score for each dense connection in dense blocks and to enhance useful features, while AAM aims to adaptively adjust the respective field according to the abnormal regions and help pay attention to abnormalities. Moreover, we propose a novel Angular Contrastive loss (AC Loss) to reduce the intra-class variances and enlarge the inter-class differences effectively. Our methods achieved 89.41% overall accuracy and showed better performance compared with state-of-the-art WCE image classification methods. The source code is available at https://github.com/Guo-Xiaoqing/Triple-ANet.

## 1 Introduction

Wireless capsule endoscopy (WCE) is a noninvasive, wireless imaging tool that allows direct visualization of the entire gastrointestinal (GI) tract without discomfort to patients. Despite their prevalent and good application, the collected WCE videos are manually reviewed, which is time-consuming and extremely laborious for clinicians. Moreover, the GI diseases usually demonstrate various characteristics of shape, texture, and size. Even well trained clinicians may produce different diagnostic results. Therefore it is highly desirable to develop a computer-aided detection (CAD) method to automatic diagnose diseases with satisfying accuracy.

Common GI diseases includes inflammatory, vascular lesion and polyp. Effectively recognizing the abnormalities is a very challenging task due to intra-class

© Springer Nature Switzerland AG 2019
D. Shen et al. (Eds.): MICCAI 2019, LNCS 11764, pp. 293–301, 2019.
https://doi.org/10.1007/978-3-030-32239-7_33

variances, inter-class similarities and existence of artifacts. Numbers of scholars have been dedicated to solving these issues and proposing automatic algorithms for abnormality recognition in WCE images [3,5,7,9]. Fan et al. [3] directly utilized AlexNet to automatically recognize ulcer and erosion in WCE images. Jia et al. [5] extracted WCE image features with AlexNet and conducted automatic bleeding detection strategy based on support vector machine. Seguí et al. [7] proposed an early fusion approach, in which the Laplacian and Hessian streams were integrated with original WCE images as input of a VGG-based neural network for abnormality classification. In our previous work [9], we proposed a rotation-invariant and image similarity constrained neural network for polyp recognition by dealing with object rotation problems of the collected WCE images.

Despite the relatively good performance, deep learning based methods [3,5,7,9] could not localize abnormalities accurately and extract sufficiently distinguishable features with only image-level labels. Moreover, the performance of existing multi-class WCE classification task is not satisfactory. The challenges associated with these methods may lie in the following three parts. Firstly, the latest research [9] performed WCE image classification by utilizing the Densely Connected Convolutional Network (DenseNet) [4], in which every layer are concatenated to each other layer to aggregate information and learn features. However, this model treats every feature layer equally and ignores the importance variation of different connections. Second, existing works for WCE image classification extracted features directly from the whole image and assumed that different image parts contribute equally to the feature learning [3,5,7,9]. However, the background and noisy parts in the image may introduce redundant information for the network and lead to bad performance while some abnormal informative parts are the important cues for doctors to make diagnostic decisions. While the recent self-attention module [8] generated attention map by calculating the correlation matrix of the feature map to highlight the important regions in images, it has not been applied in the WCE image analysis filed. Moreover, this attention module only considers the pixel-to-pixel relationship, overlooking the context information. Thirdly, softmax loss was commonly utilized to learn WCE image features [3,7,9]. Thus, the calculated deep features could not support feature correlations across the entire data space. In reality, images within the same class should share similar feature information while the image features from different classes should be distinctly different.

To address the aforementioned challenges, we propose an Adaptively Abnormal Aware Network (Triple ANet) for WCE image classification. Our contributions lie in the following four points. (1) An Adaptive Dense Block (ADB) is developed to adaptively assign one attention score for each dense connected layer in dense blocks, and the score reveals importance of feature maps in different depth. In this way, ADB can selectively aggregate the most useful information of the images. (2) We propose an Abnormal-aware Attention Module (AAM) that can gradually adjust the respective field according to the abnormal regions. This AAM is aimed to combine local information with context and help network pay attention to the abnormal region. (3) A novel angular contrastive loss

(AC Loss) is proposed to reduce the intra-class variances and enlarge the inter-class differences effectively. Therefore, Triple ANet can better characterize and distinguish features of different diseases rendered in WCE images. (4) We validate the robustness of our proposed Triple ANet by conducting comprehensive experiments, and our method achieves the state-of-the-art WCE classification performance compared with existing methods.

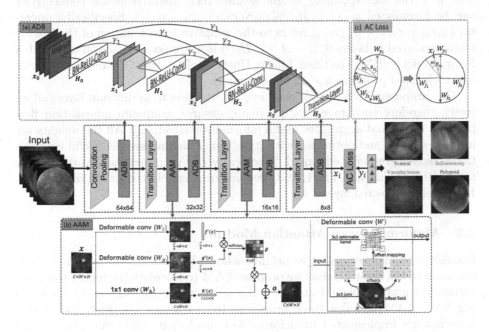

**Fig. 1.** Illustration of the proposed Triple ANet.

## 2   Method

In this paper, we propose the Triple ANet model to automatically differentiate inflammatory, vascular lesion and polyp from normal WCE images. The overall framework of our method is illustrated in Fig. 1. Given a WCE image, the deep features are extracted by alternate-cascaded ADBs, AAMs and transition layers. The size of feature maps in the four ADBs are $64 \times 64$, $32 \times 32$, $16 \times 16$, and $8 \times 8$, which makes network adaptively aggregate useful information at different scales. Before the first ADB, a $3 \times 3$ convolution with 24 output channels is performed on the input images. We use $1 \times 1$ convolution followed by $2 \times 2$ average pooling as transition layers following ADBs to reduce the number and dimension of feature maps. Two AAMs are inserted at $32 \times 32$ and $16 \times 16$ scales for capturing long range dependency information. At the end of the last ADB, a global average pooling is performed to squeeze feature maps into vectors for further classification. AC Loss is proposed to optimize the whole network and converge to learn discriminative features.

## 2.1  Adaptive Dense Block

To effectively train the deep neural network and aggregate information, we propose an ADB module in our classification network to introduce direct and suitable connections from any layer to all subsequent layers. The architecture of an ADB module is displayed in Fig. 1(a). Let $x_l$ denote the output of $l$th layer and $\gamma_l$ is the corresponding weight scalar, then adaptive dense connectivity can be formulated as $x_l = H_l([\gamma_0 x_0, \gamma_1 x_1, \cdots, \gamma_{l-1} x_{l-1}])$. Specifically, operator $[\gamma_0 x_0, \gamma_1 x_1, \cdots, \gamma_{l-1} x_{l-1}]$ refers to the adaptive concatenation of the feature maps produced in layers $0, 1, \cdots, l-1$. $H_l(\cdot)$ is a composite function with Batch Normalization (BN), Rectified Linear Units (ReLU) and Convolution (Conv), and each $H_l(\cdot)$ produces $k = 12$ feature maps.

Our proposed ADB module combines information from different layers adaptively, therefore encourages feature reuse, ensures maximum information flow between layers and aggregates useful information effectively. All the weights are initialized as $1s$ and optimized with iteration, which makes the useful convolutional signals gradually enhanced. Specifically, our proposed framework includes four ADBs as shown in Fig. 1, and they are respectively comprised of 6, 12, 24, 16 densely connected layers.

## 2.2  Abnormal-aware Attention Module

Considering that features in the neighbourhood of abnormalities also make contribution to the identification, we propose AAM to calculate the region-to-region correlation and highlight features in the most important region. As shown in Fig. 1(b), AAM includes three branches. In particular, the first and second branches are implemented by deformable convolution, while the third branch is implemented by $1 \times 1$ convolution. The deformable convolution adds an additional convolutional layer to learn offsets from preceding feature maps, and the offsets include offsets in horizontal and vertical direction. The weight in this additional layer is initialized to $N(0, \sigma^2)$ with $\sigma \ll 1$, and the bias is initialized to zeros. Through offset mapping, deformable convolution adds the learned offsets to the regular grid sampling locations in the standard convolution kernel, which enables the receptive fields to gradually expand around the abnormalities. Through these branches, the input features $x \in \mathbb{R}^{C \times W \times H}$ are gathered into three feature spaces $f$, $g$ and $h$. The channels of feature maps $f(x)$ and $g(x)$ are reduced to $\frac{C}{4}$, while channels of $h(x)$ remains to be $C$. Then the gathering feature maps are arranged into sequences $f'(x), g'(x) \in \mathbb{R}^{\frac{C}{4} \times N}$ and $h'(x) \in \mathbb{R}^{C \times N}$, and the response at a position in a sequence can be represented by a cross correlation matrix with $\alpha_{i,j} = f'(x)^\top \times g'(x)$. After that, the obtained cross correlation matrix is spatially normalized to be $\beta_{j,i} \in \mathbb{R}^{N \times N}$, representing the correlativity between regions in feature map respect to the other regions. Note that $\sum_i \beta_{i,j} = 1$. Then the spatial attention maps are computed by $\sum_{i=1}^{N} h(x)\beta_{j,i}$, which indicates the region-to-region correlation in a spatial feature map. The final attention maps is obtained by

$$O = x + \sum_{i=1}^{N} h(x)\beta_{j,i}. \tag{1}$$

With this formula, local information is combined with context information, and we could highlight the abnormality itself as well as the features around the boundaries of abnormalities. Compared with self-attention [8], our AMM could adaptively strengthen the response of abnormalities and suppress noise in normal regions with the expanded receptive fields. Additionally, the proposed AAM could be flexibly inserted to any deep neural networks for capturing long-range dependencies.

## 2.3 Angular Contrastive Loss

The softmax cross entropy loss is widely used to evaluate the classification loss and it can be formulated as $L_{softmax} = -\frac{1}{N} \sum_{i=1}^{N} \log \frac{e^{W_{y_i}^T x_i + b_{y_i}}}{\sum_{j=1}^{n} e^{W_j^T x_i + b_j}}$, where $x_i$ denotes the extracted features of the $i^{th}$ samples, and $y_i$ is the ground truth. $W_j$ is the weight for $j^{th}$ class in the fully connection (FC) layer, and $b_j$ is the bias. $N$ and $n$ represents batch size and number of classes respectively. However, softmax loss function does not explicitly optimize the feature to ensure higher differences for inter-class features and similarity for intra-class features.

To address the issue mentioned above, we propose AC Loss. For simplicity, we discard bias term as in [1] and rewrite the formula of FC layer as $F(W_j, x_i) = ||W_j|| \cdot ||x_i|| \cos \theta_j$, where $\theta_j$ is the angle between the features $x_i$ and the weight $W_j$. Then $x_i$ and $W_j$ are respectively normalized to $||x_i|| = 1$ and $||W_j|| = 1$ by $L_2$ normalization. A hyper parameter $s$ is introduced to rescale the length of $x_i$ to $s$, which could control the magnitude of loss value. This normalization method makes the predictions only relied on angle between the features and weights. Our proposed AC Loss takes the general form of $F(W_j, x_i) = s||W_j|| \cdot ||x_i|| \cdot A(\theta_j)$, where $A(\cdot)$ is a angular activation function. Obviously, appropriate angular activation function may lead better classification performance. In this paper, we define the angular activation function as:

$$A(\theta_j) = \frac{1 + e^{(-\frac{\pi}{2k})}}{1 - e^{(-\frac{\pi}{2k})}} \cdot \frac{1 - e^{(\frac{\theta_j}{k} - \frac{\pi}{2k})}}{1 + e^{(\frac{\theta_j}{k} - \frac{\pi}{2k})}}, \tag{2}$$

where $k$ is a hyper parameter to control the gradient of angular activation function and the performance of loss function directly. This characteristic makes our angular activation function more general compared with original cosine function [1]. In this paper, we choose $k = 0.3$. With $k = 0.3$, the loss function is more smooth when the loss value is large, which reduces the contribution of outliers and increases the robust of training. In the meanwhile, the loss function is more steep when the loss value is not large, to accelerate convergence of the network.

In order to further reduce the intra-class variances and inter-class similarities, we introduce an angle margin penalty $m$ and a regularization term to enhance the discrepancy of weights in FC layer for different classes. Therefore, the proposed AC loss function for Triple ANet training can be formulated as

$$L_{AC} = -\frac{1}{N} \sum_{i=1}^{N} \log \frac{e^{sA(\theta_{y_i}+m)}}{e^{sA(\theta_{y_i}+m)} + \sum_{j \neq y_i}^{n} e^{sA(\theta_j)}} + \frac{1}{n} \cdot \frac{1}{n-1} \sum_{y_i=1}^{n} \sum_{j \neq y_i}^{n} W_{y_i}^{\top} W_j. \quad (3)$$

Within a certain range, larger $m$ leads to more similar and compact intra-class features. As shown is Fig. 1(c), converged $L_{AC}$ maximizes the separability of inter-class features and enables intra-class features to cluster toward the weight of their corresponding class.

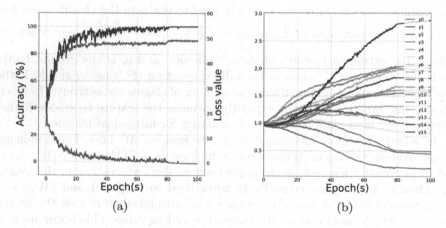

(a)                                    (b)

Fig. 2. (a) Accuracy and loss values for different epochs. The blue and red color curves respectively represent the train and test accuracy, while the green color one shows the training loss. (b) $\gamma$ values in the fourth ADB for different epochs. (Color figure online)

## 3   Experiments and Results

We evaluated Tripe ANet model on a combined WCE dataset from CAD-CAP [2], KID [6] and our collected polyp dataset. It consists of 2846 WCE images, including 771 normal frames, 728 inflammatory ones, 762 vascular lesion ones and 585 polyps. Considering different image resolution and quality, we resized the WCE images to $128 \times 128$ and applied a uniform circle mask to the dataset. Flip and rotation were implemented to augment the training data.

We implemented our model using TensorFlow. NVIDIA TITAN XP GPU and CUDA 8.0 are used for the training acceleration. Adam is chosen for optimization with $\beta_1 = 0.5$ and $\beta_2 = 0.999$. All training steps used batch size of 16. The initialized learning rate is set to 0.001, and is dropped by 0.1 at 80 epochs. Hyper parameters of $s, m, k$ are set as 64, 0.5, 0.3, respectively. Fourfold cross validation was adopted to evaluate our methods. The performance of classification was evaluated by per-class accuracy, overall accuracy (OA) and Cohen's Kappa score.

We first analyzed the learning process of Triple ANet. Figure 2(a) shows the train accuracy, test accuracy and train loss value. Our method rapidly reduces the loss values and reaches a relatively steady state after 80 epochs, which indicates that the network is successfully optimized and verifies the effectiveness of Triple ANet for WCE image classification.

Then we analyzed the influence of ADB module. Figure 2(b) shows the change of $\gamma$ values in the $4^{th}$ ADB with 16 connected layers, and $\gamma_i$ indicates the learned attention score for the $i^{th}$ layer. The assigned attention values for different layers vary significantly. It can be seen that the deeper the layer is, the higher the value of $\gamma$ is, indicating the deep feature will make more contributions for the WCE image classification. Actually, the deeper features usually contain more context and spatial structure information, while the shallow features contain more color and texture information. Thus we can make a conclusion that structure information plays more important role in classification.

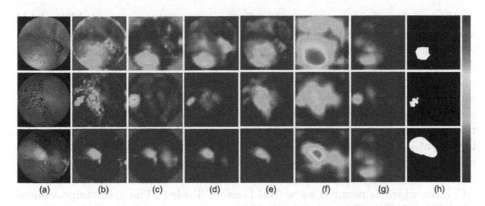

(a)        (b)        (c)        (d)        (e)        (f)        (g)        (h)

**Fig. 3.** From top to bottom, they are respectively inflammatory, vascular lesion and polyp samples. (a) Original image. (b)(c) show attention maps of the 1st and 2nd AAM. (d)(e) show offset fields in the 1st branch and 2nd branch of the 1st AMM while (f)(g) show offset fields in the 1st branch and 2nd branch of the 2st AMM. (h) Ground truth of mask

We further showed extracted attention maps and learned offset fields in Fig. 3. Figure 3(b–c) show the feature maps extracted from the two AAMs, and we could find that AAMs make feature maps highlight the abnormal regions successfully. Figure 3(d–g) show the offset fields obtained in these AAMs, and red regions indicate the large receptive fields. It can be seen that the respective fields are tend to be larger at abnormalities compared with normal regions. Therefore, context information of abnormalities are incorporated with local information to lead better classification performance.

**Table 1.** Comparison results for WCE image classification. w/ADB, w/AAM and w/AC Loss denote DenseNet with ADB (instead of original dense block), DenseNet with AAM and DenseNet minimized by AC Loss (instead of original softmax cross entropy loss), respectively.

| Methods | Normal ACC (%) | Inflammatory ACC (%) | Vascular lesion ACC (%) | Polyp ACC (%) | OA | Cohen's Kappa |
|---|---|---|---|---|---|---|
| DenseNet [4] | 92.69 ± 0.49 | 90.12 ± 0.54 | 93.71 ± 0.52 | 97.59 ± 0.39 | 87.05 ± 0.45 | 82.66 ± 0.60 |
| w/ADB | 93.03 ± 0.40 | 89.94 ± 0.18 | 93.61 ± 0.15 | 97.71 ± 0.27 | 87.14 ± 0.21 | 82.78 ± 0.28 |
| w/AAM | **94.06 ± 0.17** | 91.49 ± 0.81 | 94.47 ± 0.77 | 97.78 ± 0.42 | 88.89 ± 0.52 | 85.13 ± 0.69 |
| w/AC Loss | 93.59 ± 0.30 | 91.20 ± 0.33 | 94.94 ± 0.34 | 97.69 ± 0.46 | 88.70 ± 0.20 | 84.87 ± 0.27 |
| Triple ANet | 94.03 ± 0.09 | **91.73 ± 0.29** | **95.26 ± 0.33** | **97.81 ± 0.20** | **89.41 ± 0.23** | **85.82 ± 0.31** |
| Fan et al. [3] | 85.44 ± 1.43 | 83.09 ± 0.79 | 90.19 ± 0.96 | 95.47 ± 0.89 | 77.10 ± 1.14 | 69.30 ± 1.58 |
| Jia et al. [5] | 86.16 ± 1.07 | 83.37 ± 0.71 | 90.32 ± 0.88 | 95.81 ± 0.59 | 77.83 ± 1.28 | 70.31 ± 1.74 |
| Seguí et al. [7] | 92.11 ± 0.60 | 89.71 ± 0.48 | 94.21 ± 0.57 | 97.31 ± 0.12 | 86.67 ± 0.84 | 82.15 ± 1.12 |
| Yuan et al. [9] | 93.44 ± 0.30 | 90.79 ± 0.26 | 93.91 ± 0.17 | 97.73 ± 0.35 | 87.93 ± 0.07 | 83.84 ± 0.08 |

To individually demonstrate the effectiveness of the proposed ADB, AAM and AC Loss, we conducted several comparison experiments and the results were shown in Table 1 *row* 1–4. In general, it is clear that the proposed ADB, AAM and AC Loss make contribution to the promotion of performance, because involving any of them leads to relatively better performance compared with traditional DenseNet [4]. Especially, AAM and AC Loss show significant improvements. The AAM module was verified to be effective in improving the classification performance, with 1.84%, 2.47% increment in OA and Cohen's Kappa. This increment is due to that AAM captured the long range dependent information and amplified the effects of abnormal regions. We also replaced original softmax cross entropy loss with AC Loss in DenseNet to evaluate the performance of AC Loss, which is denoted as 'w/AC Loss' in Table 1. The great improvement of 1.65%, 2.21% in OA and Cohen's Kappa compared with DenseNet indicates that AC Loss can facilitate the distinction of learned features and strengthen the robustness of Triple ANet.

We further assessed the performance of the our Triple ANet (*row* 5) by comparing it with state-of-the-art methods [3,5,7,9] for WCE image classification. We implemented these methods on our datasets and the comparison results are shown in Table 1 *row* 6–9. The proposed method shows superior performance with an increment of 12.31%, 11.58%, 2.74%, 1.48% in OA, 16.52%, 15.51%, 3.67%, 1.98% in Cohen's Kappa compared with methods [3,5,7,9], respectively. This result validates the proposed Triple ANet possesses superior ability to aggregate abnormal information and extract discriminative features for WCE images.

## 4   Conclusion

Automatic abnormality classification is a challenge task due to the diverse characteristics rendered on WCE images. Our method is fundamentally different from the previous works with traditional convolutional network applications. Instead, we proposed a novel Triple ANet with Adaptive Dense Block (ADB), Abnormal-aware Attention Module (AAM) and Angular Contrastive loss (AC Loss). Our methods can be flexibly transferred to a wide range of medical image classification tasks to extract discriminative features and boost the classification performance.

**Acknowledgments.** This work was supported by Sichuan Provincial Science and Technology Research Grant 2019YJ0632 and TSG 6000690. We gratefully acknowledge the support of NVIDIA Corporation with the donation of the Titan Xp GPU for this research.

# References

1. Deng, J., Guo, J., Xue, N., Zafeiriou, S.: ArcFace: additive angular margin loss for deep face recognition. In: CVPR, pp. 4690–4699 (2019)
2. Dray, X., et al.: Cad-cap: une base de données française à vocation internationale, pour le développement et la validation d'outils de diagnostic assisté par ordinateur en vidéocapsule endoscopique du grêle. Endoscopy **50**(03), 000441 (2018)
3. Fan, S., Xu, L., Fan, Y., Wei, K., Li, L.: Computer-aided detection of small intestinal ulcer and erosion in wireless capsule endoscopy images. Phys. Med. Biol. **63**(16), 165001 (2018)
4. Huang, G., Liu, Z., Van Der Maaten, L., Weinberger, K.Q.: Densely connected convolutional networks. In: CVPR, pp. 4700–4708 (2017)
5. Jia, X., Meng, M.Q.H.: A deep convolutional neural network for bleeding detection in wireless capsule endoscopy images. In: EMBC, pp. 639–642 (2016)
6. Koulaouzidis, A., et al.: Kid project: an internet-based digital video atlas of capsule endoscopy for research purposes. Endosc. Int. Open **5**(06), E477–E483 (2017)
7. Seguí, S., et al.: Generic feature learning for wireless capsule endoscopy analysis. Comput. Biol. Med. **79**, 163–172 (2016)
8. Wang, X., Girshick, R., Gupta, A., He, K.: Non-local neural networks. In: CVPR, pp. 7794–7803 (2018)
9. Yuan, Y., Qin, W., Ibragimov, B., Han, B., Xing, L.: RIIS-DenseNet: rotation-invariant and image similarity constrained densely connected convolutional network for polyp detection. In: Frangi, A.F., Schnabel, J.A., Davatzikos, C., Alberola-López, C., Fichtinger, G. (eds.) MICCAI 2018. LNCS, vol. 11071, pp. 620–628. Springer, Cham (2018). https://doi.org/10.1007/978-3-030-00934-2_69

# Selective Feature Aggregation Network with Area-Boundary Constraints for Polyp Segmentation

Yuqi Fang[1], Cheng Chen[1], Yixuan Yuan[2(✉)], and Kai-yu Tong[1(✉)]

[1] Department of Biomedical Engineering, The Chinese University of Hong Kong, Sha Tin, Hong Kong
kytong@cuhk.edu.hk
[2] Department of Electrical Engineering, City University of Hong Kong, Kowloon Tong, Hong Kong
yxyuan.ee@cityu.edu.hk

**Abstract.** Automatic polyp segmentation is considered indispensable in modern polyp screening systems. It can help the clinicians accurately locate polyp areas for further diagnosis or surgeries. Benefit from the advancement of deep learning techniques, various neural networks are developed for handling the polyp segmentation problem. However, most of these methods neither aggregate multi-scale or multi-receptive-field features nor consider the area-boundary constraints. To address these issues, we propose a novel selective feature aggregation network with the area and boundary constraints. The network contains a shared encoder and two mutually constrained decoders for predicting polyp areas and boundaries, respectively. Feature aggregation is achieved by (1) introducing three up-concatenations between encoder and decoders and (2) embedding Selective Kernel Modules into convolutional layers which can adaptively extract features from different size of kernels. We call these two operations the Selective Feature Aggregation. Furthermore, a new boundary-sensitive loss function is proposed to take into account the dependency between the area and boundary branch, thus two branches can be reciprocally influenced and enable more accurate area predictions. We evaluate our method on the EndoScene dataset and achieve the state-of-the-art results with a Dice of 83.08% and a Accuracy of 96.68%.

## 1 Introduction

Colorectal cancer is the third leading cause of cancer-related deaths. It is estimated that the number of new cases of colorectal cancer in the US will reach 150 thousand in 2019 [1]. Colorectal polyps are believed one of the early symptoms of colorectal cancer. Therefore, regular screening of colorectal polyps is crucial, during which automatic polyp segmentation is considered an indispensable component. It can help clinicians locate the polyp areas for further diagnosis.

In recent years, numerous deep learning based methods are developed for handling polyp segmentation problem [2,3,10,12,13]. The Fully Convolutional

© Springer Nature Switzerland AG 2019
D. Shen et al. (Eds.): MICCAI 2019, LNCS 11764, pp. 302–310, 2019.
https://doi.org/10.1007/978-3-030-32239-7_34

Network (FCN) [5] is a commonly used architecture, which replaces the fully connected layers of traditional Convolutional Neural Networks (CNNs) with convolutional layers, thus preserving the spatial information for segmentation. Brandao et al. [3] adopted the FCN with a pre-trained VGG model to identify and segment polyps from colonoscopy images. Akbari et al. [2] adopted a modified version of FCN, i.e., FCN8s, to further improve the polyp segmentation accuracy. Inspired by FCN, the UNet [10], a more powerful and concise network, is then proposed. It also adopts an encoder-decoder architecture but additionally adds some parallel skip concatenations between the encoder and decoder. Based on UNet, SegNet [12] applied the pooling indices from the encoder to the decoder and UNet++ [13] developed a densely connected encoder-decoder network with deep supervision to further enhance the polyp segmentation performance.

Although these networks achieve high performance, there still exist some defects in their architectures. One problem is that compared with UNet++ [13], the FCN [5], UNet [10], and SegNet [12] do not consider multi-scale features. For instance, skip concatenations in UNet connect encoder layers and decoder layers in a parallel manner, which can only aggregate image features of the same scale. In contrast, UNet++ builds up dense connections for integrating more features at different scales but significantly decrease the training and inference efficiency. Besides, all these networks adopt a fixed size of kernel at each layer. This restricts the network from exploring and leveraging representational features obtained from different receptive fields. As a matter of fact, the fusion of features from different scales and multiple receptive fields can remarkably enlarge the perception dimensions, thus helping the network learn more discriminative representations of the input images. In this work, one of our contributions is to optimize the skip concatenations and enrich the diversity of receptive fields at each layer, namely the selective feature aggregation.

Another problem is that the existing methods neglect the area-boundary constraints, a key factor in improving the segmentation performance. Murugesan et al. [7,8] talked about this issue and proposed to utilize area and boundary information simultaneously in polyp segmentation, but the relationship between the area and boundary is not further explored. Actually, the dependency between areas and boundaries is quite crucial, which is capable of enhancing the area prediction. Specifically, if the predicted area is larger than ground truth, boundary information can constrain the extended areas, while if the predicted area is much smaller than ground truth, boundary information can enlarge the predicted areas. We leverage such relationship to improve the performance of polyp segmentation via a boundary-sensitive loss function in our method.

In this paper, we propose a novel selective feature aggregation network with a boundary-sensitive loss. Three contributions are claimed as follows. (1) We develop a new encoder-decoder network in which multi-scale features of the encoder are selected and concatenated with two decoders, i.e., the area branch and the boundary branch. Moreover, a Selective Kernel Module (SKM) is embedded into convolutional layers to dynamically learn features from different size of kernels, i.e., $3 \times 3$, $5 \times 5$, $7 \times 7$. (2) A boundary-sensitive loss is proposed to leverage the area-boundary constraints, with which the two branches can be mutually improved to produce more accurate predictions. (3) We validate the effectiveness of our method in EndoScene dataset and achieve the state-of-the-art results.

## 2   Method

### 2.1   Network Architecture

In this section, we first present the network architecture, as shown in Fig. 1, then introduce two strategies to select and aggregate the polyp features at different scales or receptive fields. Finally we propose a new boundary-sensitive loss via which the area and boundary branch can be reciprocally affected, thus generating more accurate predictions. Our network is composed of a shared encoder, an area branch, and a boundary branch. Each branch contains four convolutional modules. Each module contains three layers integrated with the SKMs. On top of the area branch, a light-weight UNet is adopted to help detect boundaries of the predicted areas. These boundaries and the contours derived from the boundary branch are used to formalize the boundary-sensitive loss.

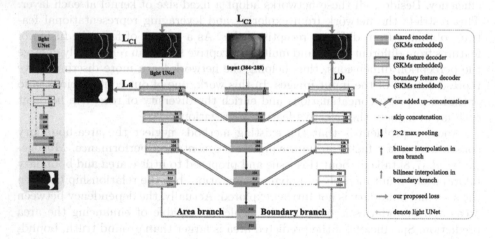

**Fig. 1.** Illustration of the selective feature aggregation network with area-boundary constraints. Numbers in each block represents the number of feature channels. (Color figure online)

### 2.2   Selective Feature Aggregation

**Up-Concatenations.** Inspired by UNet [10] and BESNet [9], we adopt a shared encoder and two decoder branches to assist polyp segmentation, shown in Fig. 1. The shared encoder (middle solid blocks) utilizes five convolutional modules to learn feature representations of the input images. The area branch (left blocks with stripe) is built for area localization while the boundary branch (right hollow blocks) is built for boundary recovery. Different from the architectures in [9, 11, 12], where skip concatenations exist in a parallel manner (black dash lines), three extra up-concatenations are added to both the area and boundary branch (red arrow lines) in our method. In this case, multi-scale feature maps derived from deep layers of the shared encoder are copied to shallow layers of the decoders, which enriches the feature representations and keeps the training and inference process more efficient compared with [13].

**SKM.** Traditionally, most of the convolutional kernels in CNN are with a fixed size, i.e., $3 \times 3$, which cannot simultaneously capture features from other receptive fields. To tackle this problem, we adopt the SKM [4] in our method, which can dynamically aggregate features obtained from different size of kernels. Our work is the first study to embed SKMs into the encoder-decoder networks. As shown in Fig. 2, an input feature map $\mathbf{X} \in \mathbb{R}^{C \times W \times H}$ is first filtered by three respective kernels simultaneously, then followed by a Batch Normalization and a ReLU activation, and outputs three distinct feature maps $X_3$, $X_5$, $X_7$. To regress the weight vectors, we first perform element-wise summation of the three feature maps, $\widetilde{X} = \sum X_k (k \in \{3, 5, 7\})$, then process $\widetilde{X}$ according to the following procedure.

$$f = \mathcal{F}_{fc}\left(\frac{1}{W \times H} \sum_{i=1}^{W} \sum_{j=1}^{H} \widetilde{X}(i,j)\right) \tag{1}$$

$$m_k = e^{W_k f} / \sum e^{W_k f} \quad (k \in \{3, 5, 7\}) \tag{2}$$

where $\mathcal{F}_{fc}$ is a fully connected operation, $f \in \mathbb{R}^C$ denotes the adaptive features, $W_k$ are learnable parameters in $m_k$, and $m_k$ is the weight vector corresponding to $X_k$. With the weight vectors, we are able to adaptively aggregate the feature maps, $\widehat{X} = \sum m_k X_k, k \in \{3, 5, 7\}$.

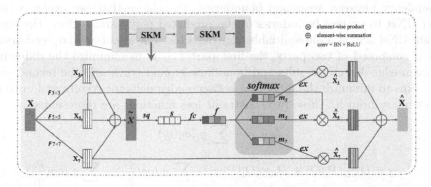

**Fig. 2.** Selective Kernel Module (SKM). sq: squeeze; fc: fully connected; ex: excitation.

## 2.3   Boundary-Sensitive Loss

To make full use of the area-boundary constraints, we propose a joint loss function that can mutually propagate the information between the area branch and boundary branch. As shown in Fig. 1, the loss function is composed of three parts: an area loss $L_a$, a boundary loss $L_b$, and the area-boundary constraint loss, i.e., $L_{C1}$ and $L_{C2}$.

**Area Loss.** $L_a$ consists of a *binary cross-entropy loss* and a *dice loss* [6], which can be represented by the following function.

$$L_a = - \sum_i z_i log(m_i) + (1 - \frac{2 \sum_i m_i z_i + \varepsilon}{\sum_i m_i + \sum_i z_i + \varepsilon}) \tag{3}$$

where $m_i$ indicates the probability of pixel $i$ being categorized into polyp class, $z_i \in \{0, 1\}$ is the corresponding area ground truth label, and $\varepsilon$ is a small positive number used for increasing numerical stabilities. The cross-entropy loss function penalizes pixel classification errors while the dice loss function measures the overlap between the predicted polyp areas and the area ground truth, which can handle the foreground-background imbalance problem.

**Boundary Loss.** $L_b$ measures the difference between outputs of boundary branch and boundary ground truth labels, which can be represented as

$$L_b = - \sum_i y_i log(p_i) \tag{4}$$

where $p_i$ denotes the probability of pixel $i$ being the polyp boundary and $y_i \in \{0, 1\}$ is the corresponding boundary ground truth label.

**Area-Boundary Constraint Loss.** The constraint loss aims to model the dependency between areas and boundaries. To achieve that, we utilize a two-layer UNet to extract boundaries of the predicted polyp areas. Here, the light-weight UNet acts as a differentiable edge detector. The area-boundary constraint loss is composed of two parts, the first part $L_{C1}$ is to minimize the difference between edge detector results and boundary ground truth and the second part $L_{C2}$ aims to minimize the difference between edge detector results and outputs of boundary branch. These two constraint loss functions are represented as

$$L_{C1} = - \sum_i y_i log(q_i) \tag{5}$$

$$L_{C2} = D_{KL}(P\|Q) + D_{KL}(Q\|P) = - \sum_i p_i log(\frac{q_i}{p_i}) - \sum_i q_i log(\frac{p_i}{q_i}) \tag{6}$$

where $q_i$ is the results predicted by the edge detector, i.e., the light-weight UNet, $y_i$ denotes boundary ground truth, and $p_i$ indicates outputs of boundary branch. $D_{KL}$ denotes *Kullback-Leibler divergence* which can measure the distance between two distributions. As a result, minimizing $D_{KL}$ is equivalent to making the final outputs of area and boundary branch closer. Intuitively speaking, $L_{C2}$ tries to make the area and boundary branch internally consistent, thus preventing the two branches deviating from each other too much. Compared with $L_{C1}$ that uses boundary supervision explicitly, $L_{C2}$ can implicitly impose the area-boundary constraints. Due to the consistent training goal of the two branches, the shared encoder can learn more discriminative features and help increase the final segmentation performance. The final loss function is as follows.

$$L_{total} = w_a L_a + w_b L_b + w_{C1} L_{C1} + w_{C2} L_{C2} \tag{7}$$

where $w_a$, $w_b$, and $w_{C1}$ are set to 1, $w_{C2}$ is set to 0.5 by empirical studies.

## 3    Experimental Results

### 3.1    Dataset and Evaluation Metrics

In this work, we adopt the EndoScene dataset [11] which contains 912 images with at least one polyp in each image, acquired from 44 video sequences obtained from 36 subjects. The dataset is divided into a train set, a validation set, and a test set and each sequence is uniquely included in one of the three sets. The area ground truth is provided, while the boundary ground truth is derived by ourselves. The area ground truth is filtered with a 5*5 kernel, where kernel elements are initialized with 0. The element turns to 1 if it overlaps with the area ground truth, otherwise is 0. If kernel elements are not identical, i.e. 0 and 1 exist simultaneously, these elements are regarded as boundary points.

The evaluation metrics we adopt are *Recall, Specificity, Precision, Dice Score, Intersection-over-Union for Polyp* ($IoU_P$), *IoU for Background* ($IoU_B$), *Mean IoU* ($mIoU$), and *Accuracy*. In all experiments, the batch size is set to 4. The initial learning rate is 0.01 and decreases by 10 times after 20 and 100 epochs, respectively. The SGD optimizer is used with a weight decay of 0.0005 and a momentum of 0.9. The models are implemented based on the PyTorch framework and trained on a workstation with Intel Core(TM) i7-9700K@3.60 GHz processors and a NVIDIA GeForce RTX 2080 Ti (11 GB) installed.

### 3.2    Comparative Experiments

The detailed experiment results are presented in Table 1, in which we list the performance of four state-of-the-arts (*row 1–4*) and our proposed method (*row 5*). To further analyze the influence of each component of our method, we conduct several comparative experiments and the results are reported in *row 6–10*. All the results are evaluated on test set, with the checkpoint achieving the highest *Dice Score* on validation set.

As shown in Fig. 3, our method outperforms the four state-of-the-art methods on all the evaluation metrics by a significant increment. Segmentation performance in SegNet [12] and UNet++ [13] is superior to that in FCN8 [3] and

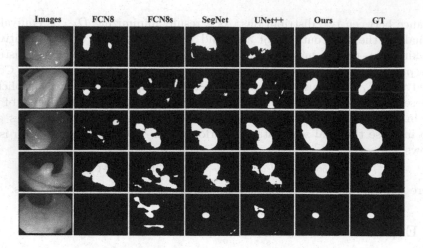

**Fig. 3.** Polyp segmentation results of different methods.

FCN8s [2], which indicates the significance of skip concatenations on accuracy improvement. However, increasing the density of concatenations does not guarantee more improvement on the segmentation performance. We have attempted numerous combinations of concatenations and find that models with complicated concatenations are hard to train and usually cannot give a competitive result. Compared with our up-concatenation model, UNet++ [13] that adopts even more complicated concatenations shows a significant drop in the performance.

Then, we evaluate the performance of the up-concatenations and the SKM components, which are denoted as UNet+Up and UNet+Up+SKM in Table 1. The results show that the UNet with up-concatenations achieves better performance than UNet alone on all the evaluation criteria. This indicates that up-concatenations can effectively transmit multi-scale features from the encoder to the decoder. The SKM component is also verified to be effective in improving the segmentation performance, especially the *Precision* and $IoU_p$ which increase by more than 1.5%. This improvement is achieved by allowing the network to dynamically aggregate features derived from different size of kernels, which is a more appropriate strategy than manually specifying the kernel size.

Further, we evaluate the effectiveness of the boundary-sensitive loss. By comparing the 'UNet+Up+SKM+bd' with 'UNet+Up+SKM' in Table 1, it is apparent that the integration of boundary branch helps improve segmentation accuracy a lot. In particular, the *Recall*, *Precison*, *Dice*, and $IoU_P$ show an increment of more than 1% compared with the model that only contains area branch. This indicates that the boundary information can help improve the representation capability of the shared encoder network via the loss backward propagation mechanism. According to last two rows and *Ours* in Table 1, we can see the area-boundary constraint loss functions also play important roles in improving the segmentation performance. $L_{C1}$ aims to minimize the difference between edge detector results generated by the light-weight UNet and boundary ground truth.

**Table 1.** Comparison with different baselines and other state-of-the-art methods. 'UNet': the typical UNet with area branch; 'Up': up-concatenations; 'SKM': selective kernel module; 'bd': two-branch model with $L_a$ and $L_b$; '$L_{C1}$': the first constraint loss; 'Ours': the two-branch model with total loss, i.e. $L_a$, $L_b$, $L_{C1}$ and $L_{C2}$.

| Methods | $Rec$ | $Spec$ | $Prec$ | $Dice$ | $IoU_P$ | $IoU_B$ | $mIoU$ | $Acc$ |
|---|---|---|---|---|---|---|---|---|
| FCN8 [3] | 53.38 | 98.83 | 78.11 | 55.70 | 45.48 | 93.69 | 69.59 | 93.97 |
| FCN8s [2] | 62.81 | 98.08 | 72.60 | 58.52 | 45.99 | 93.22 | 69.61 | 93.56 |
| SegNet [12] | 81.70 | 99.03 | 85.12 | 79.29 | 70.33 | 95.71 | 83.02 | 95.99 |
| UNet++ [13] | 80.68 | 99.24 | 85.31 | 78.55 | 69.83 | 95.71 | 82.77 | 95.97 |
| *Ours* | **83.84** | 99.43 | 90.19 | **83.08** | **76.23** | **96.44** | **86.33** | **96.68** |
| UNet | 82.29 | 99.08 | 86.13 | 80.45 | 72.10 | 95.84 | 83.97 | 96.12 |
| UNet+Up | 82.53 | 99.18 | 87.13 | 80.85 | 72.74 | 95.88 | 84.31 | 96.16 |
| UNet+Up+SKM | 82.27 | 99.37 | 88.71 | 81.51 | 74.41 | 96.18 | 85.30 | 96.41 |
| UNet+Up+SKM+bd | 83.30 | 99.44 | 90.13 | 82.61 | 75.84 | 96.39 | 86.12 | 96.62 |
| UNet+Up+SKM+bd+$L_{C1}$ | 83.51 | **99.44** | **90.20** | 82.97 | 76.16 | 96.44 | 86.30 | 96.68 |

Since the results of the edge detectors are built upon the area branch, $L_{C1}$ can explicitly backpropagate the boundary supervision information, thus the boundary constraints can be introduced to the area branch. The purpose of $L_{C2}$ is to minimize the difference between edge detector results and outputs of boundary branch. In this way, edge detector results and the outputs of boundary branch can be mutually constrained, thus making area and boundary branch internally consistent. It is worth noting that introduction of either $L_{C1}$ or $L_{C2}$ improves the segmentation accuracy compared with models without any constraint.

## 4  Conclusion

We propose a novel selective feature aggregation network with the area and boundary constraints for polyp segmentation. Up-concatenations and SKMs are used to select multi-scale and multi-receptive-field representations of polyp images. Furthermore, a new loss is proposed to take into account the dependency between the area and boundary branch, thus two branches can be reciprocally influenced and enable more accurate predictions. Experimental results demonstrate that our method shows a superior performance over existing state-of-the-arts and it is capable of enabling more accurate polyp localization. The source code is available at https://github.com/Yuqi-cuhk/Polyp-Seg.

# References

1. American cancer society: Key statistics for colorectal cancer. http://www.cancer. org/cancer/colonandrectumcancer/detailedguide/colorectal-cancer-keystatistics/. Accessed 18 Mar 2019
2. Akbari, M., et al.: Polyp segmentation in colonoscopy images using fully convolutional network. In: 2018 40th Annual International Conference of the IEEE Engineering in Medicine and Biology Society (EMBC), pp. 69–72. IEEE (2018)
3. Brandao, P., et al.: Fully convolutional neural networks for polyp segmentation in colonoscopy. In: Medical Imaging 2017: Computer-Aided Diagnosis, vol. 10134, p. 101340F. International Society for Optics and Photonics (2017)
4. Li, X., et al.: Selective kernel networks. In: Proceedings of the IEEE Conference on Computer Vision and Pattern Recognition, pp. 510–519 (2019)
5. Long, J., Shelhamer, E., Darrell, T.: Fully convolutional networks for semantic segmentation. In: Proceedings of the IEEE Conference on Computer Vision and Pattern Recognition, pp. 3431–3440 (2015)
6. Milletari, F., Navab, N., Ahmadi, S.A.: V-net: Fully convolutional neural networks for volumetric medical image segmentation. In: 2016 Fourth International Conference on 3D Vision (3DV), pp. 565–571. IEEE (2016)
7. Murugesan, B., et al.: Joint shape learning and segmentation for medical images using a minimalistic deep network. arXiv preprint arXiv:1901.08824 (2019)
8. Murugesan, B., et al.: Psi-Net: shape and boundary aware joint multi-task deep network for medical image segmentation. arXiv preprint arXiv:1902.04099 (2019)
9. Oda, H., et al.: BESNet: boundary-enhanced segmentation of cells in histopathological images. In: Frangi, A.F., Schnabel, J.A., Davatzikos, C., Alberola-López, C., Fichtinger, G. (eds.) MICCAI 2018. LNCS, vol. 11071, pp. 228–236. Springer, Cham (2018). https://doi.org/10.1007/978-3-030-00934-2_26
10. Ronneberger, O., Fischer, P., Brox, T.: U-Net: convolutional networks for biomedical image segmentation. In: Navab, N., Hornegger, J., Wells, W.M., Frangi, A.F. (eds.) MICCAI 2015. LNCS, vol. 9351, pp. 234–241. Springer, Cham (2015). https://doi.org/10.1007/978-3-319-24574-4_28
11. Vázquez, et al.: A benchmark for endoluminal scene segmentation of colonoscopy images. J. Healthc. Eng. **2017** (2017)
12. Wickstrøm, K., Kampffmeyer, M., Jenssen, R.: Uncertainty and interpretability in convolutional neural networks for semantic segmentation of colorectal polyps. arXiv preprint arXiv:1807.10584 (2018)
13. Zhou, Z., Rahman Siddiquee, M.M., Tajbakhsh, N., Liang, J.: UNet++: a nested U-Net architecture for medical image segmentation. In: Stoyanov, D., et al. (eds.) DLMIA/ML-CDS -2018. LNCS, vol. 11045, pp. 3–11. Springer, Cham (2018). https://doi.org/10.1007/978-3-030-00889-5_1

# Deep Sequential Mosaicking
# of Fetoscopic Videos

Sophia Bano[1]([✉]), Francisco Vasconcelos[1], Marcel Tella Amo[1], George Dwyer[1],
Caspar Gruijthuijsen[2], Jan Deprest[4], Sebastien Ourselin[3],
Emmanuel Vander Poorten[2], Tom Vercauteren[3], and Danail Stoyanov[1]

[1] Wellcome/EPSRC Centre for Interventional and Surgical Sciences (WEISS)
and Department of Computer Science, University College London, London, UK
sophia.bano@ucl.ac.uk
[2] Department of Mechanical Engineering, KU Leuven University, Leuven, Belgium
[3] School of Biomedical Engineering and Imaging Sciences,
King's College London, London, UK
[4] Department of Development and Regeneration,
University Hospital Leuven, Leuven, Belgium

**Abstract.** Twin-to-twin transfusion syndrome treatment requires fetoscopic laser photocoagulation of placental vascular anastomoses to regulate blood flow to both fetuses. Limited field-of-view (FoV) and low visual
quality during fetoscopy make it challenging to identify all vascular connections. Mosaicking can align multiple overlapping images to generate
an image with increased FoV, however, existing techniques apply poorly
to fetoscopy due to the low visual quality, texture paucity, and hence fail
in longer sequences due to the drift accumulated over time. Deep learning techniques can facilitate in overcoming these challenges. Therefore,
we present a new generalized Deep Sequential Mosaicking (DSM) framework for fetoscopic videos captured from different settings such as simulation, phantom, and real environments. DSM extends an existing deep
image-based homography model to sequential data by proposing controlled data augmentation and outlier rejection methods. Unlike existing
methods, DSM can handle visual variations due to specular highlights
and reflection across adjacent frames, hence reducing the accumulated
drift. We perform experimental validation and comparison using 5 diverse
fetoscopic videos to demonstrate the robustness of our framework.

**Keywords:** Sequential mosaicking · Deep learning · Surgical vision ·
Twin-to-twin transfusion syndrome (TTTS) · Fetoscopy

## 1 Introduction

Twin-to-twin transfusion syndrome (TTTS) can occur during identical twin
pregnancies where abnormal vascular anastomoses in the monochorionic placenta

**Electronic supplementary material** The online version of this chapter (https://
doi.org/10.1007/978-3-030-32239-7_35) contains supplementary material, which is
available to authorized users.

result in uneven blood flow between the fetuses [1]. Fetoscopic laser photocoagulation is the most effective treatment for regulating the blood flow. During treatment, the clinician first visually explores the placenta using fetoscopic video to identify vascular anastomoses, building a mental map and treatment plan. Limited FoV, poor visibility and limited maneuverability of the fetoscope introduce challenges that increase procedural time, can lead to complications and impede verifying completion [14]. Mosaicking can align multiple overlapping images to generate an image with increased FoV. Hence it can provide computer-assisted intervention support to ease the localization of the vascular anastomoses sites.

Mosaicking has recently gained attention to increase the FoV in fetoscopy [3,9–12]. Totz et al. [13] presented a dynamic view expansion and surface reconstruction approach for minimally invasive surgery by analyzing stereo laparoscopy videos. Reeff et al. [10] and Daga et al. [3] utilized a classical image feature-based matching method for creating mosaics from planar placenta images. The relative transformations between pairs of consecutive fetoscopic images are computed and combined in a chain with respect to a reference frame to generate the mosaic. Error in the relative transformations can propagate to introduce large drift in the overall mosaic, where an electromagnetic tracker (EMT) can be integrated within the fetoscope to minimize any drifting errors [11]. However, integrating an EMT sensor with a fetoscope in-vivo is still an open challenge due to limited form-factor of the fetoscope and due to regulation. To this end, an existing registration technique avoided explicit feature correspondence by utilizing pixel-wise alignment of gradient orientations for a single in-vivo fetoscopic video [9]. Fetoscopic videos are captured from monocular cameras and pose challenges for mosaicking due to varying visual quality due to various types of fetoscopes, occlusions, specular highlights, lack of visual texture, poor visibility due to turbid amniotic fluid and non-planar views [6].

Recently, deep image homography estimation methods have been proposed [4,8] that estimate the homography between pairs of image patches extracted from an image. We observe that a full mosaic is generated by computing sequential homographies between adjacent frames, where a fetoscopic video poses challenges such as specular reflections, amniotic fluid particles, and occlusions. This affects the stitching problem, however, such challenges can be tackled when the homography is estimated using multiple pairs of image patches extracted at random from adjacent frames. In this paper, we employ this approach and propose the first generalized Deep Sequential Mosaicking (DSM) framework for creating mosaics with minimum drift from long-range fetoscopic videos captured from various fetoscopes. We adopt the deep image-based homography estimation method [4] to incorporate sequential data by proposing the Controlled Data Augmentation (CDA) and outlier rejection methods. CDA assumes that the transformation between two adjacent frames contains rotation and translation only, and uses a small set of fetoscopic images of varying quality and appearance, for training. To eliminate the error due to varying visual quality and texture paucity between adjacent frames, we propose the outlier rejection method. This increases the robustness by pruning patch-based homography estimates between adjacent

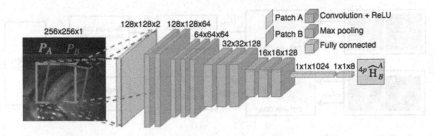

**Fig. 1.** Deep image homography network with controlled data augmentation.

frames. CDA along with the outlier rejection minimize the drift without the use of any external sensors and generate reliable mosaics in this challenging application. Comparison with existing methods and validation on 5 datasets verifies the promising generalization capabilities of our method.

## 2 Homography Estimation with Deep Learning

The Deep Image Homography (DIH) model [4] estimates the relative homography between pairs of image patches extracted from a single image. This model uses the 4-point homography parameterization $^{4p}\mathbf{H}$, instead of the $3 \times 3$ parameterization $\mathbf{H}$, as the rotation and shear components in $\mathbf{H}$ have smaller magnitude compared to the translation, thus have a small effect on the training loss. Let $(u_i, v_i)$ and $(u_i', v_i')$ denote the four corners of image patch $P_A$ and $P_B$. Then the 4-point homography $^{4p}\mathbf{H}$ is given by:

$$^{4p}\mathbf{H} = \begin{bmatrix} \Delta u_1 & \Delta u_2 & \Delta u_3 & \Delta u_4 \\ \Delta v_1 & \Delta v_2 & \Delta v_3 & \Delta v_4 \end{bmatrix}^T, \quad \begin{matrix} \text{where } \Delta u_i = u_i' - u_i, \Delta v_i = v_i' - v_i \\ \text{and } i = 1, 2, 3, 4 \end{matrix} \quad (1)$$

DIH [4] uses a VGG-like architecture, with 8 convolutional and 2 fully connected layers (Fig. 1). The input of the network is $P_A$ and $P_B$, and output is their relative homography. Note that [4] used the MS-COCO dataset for training, where pair of patches were extracted from a single real image, free of artifacts (e.g. specular highlights, amniotic fluid particles) that appear in sequential data.

DIH [4] generated the training data by randomly selecting $P_A$ from a grayscale image and randomly perturbing its corners to obtain $P_B$ and the Ground-Truth (GT). We observe through experimentation that such data augmentation results in scenarios that are challenging for the network to learn, hence results in a large error (Figs. 3(d) and 4). While such errors are acceptable in image-based homography [4], for mosaicking even a small error in pairwise homography accumulates over time resulting in increased drift. Therefore, this data generation approach cannot be used as it is for sequential mosaicking.

## 3 Deep Sequential Mosaicking (DSM)

Mosaic from an image sequence can be generated by finding the pairwise homographies between adjacent frames, followed by computing the relative homo-

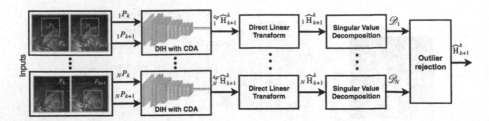

**Fig. 2.** Overview of the proposed Deep Sequential Mosaicking (DSM) method that uses Controlled Data Augmentation (CDA) for training Deep Image Homography (DIH) model and outlier rejection for pruning the homography estimates.

graphies with respect to a reference frame. The GT pairwise homographies are unknown in fetoscopic videos since they are captured from a monocular camera. Therefore, only through visualization, we can observe the error accumulated over time. For minimizing this error, in our proposed DSM, the relative homography is learned between patches that are extracted from a single image following the CDA (Sect. 3.1). Unlike [4], in practice homography is computed between two adjacent frames, having specular highlights and lack of texture, in fetoscopic videos. Therefore, testing by using pairs of patches from two adjacent frames results in varying **H**. To overcome this error, we propose an outlier rejection step (Sect. 3.2) to improve the estimation. During testing (Fig. 2), we compute homographies between pairs of adjacent frames $N$ times by randomly selecting the location of $P_A$. The estimated $^{4p}\mathbf{H}$ is converted to $\mathbf{H}$ by applying Direct Linear Transform (DLT), followed by its decomposition using Singular Value Decomposition (SVD) and outlier rejection for removing inaccurate estimations.

### 3.1  Controlled Data Augmentation (CDA)

Pairwise homography between two consecutive frames $F_k$ and $F_{k+1}$ are related by affine transformations including rotation, translation, scale, and shear. A TTTS procedure is performed at a fixed distance from the placenta, hence the scale remains constant. Fetoscope motion is physically constrained by the incision point (remote center of motion), which makes shear very small in consecutive frames, compared to rotation and translation. Therefore, we neglect the scale and shear components and assume that $F_k$ and $F_{k+1}$ are related by translation and rotation only. This helps to minimize the error in relative homography and consequently reduce the drift in mosaicking. For CDA, given a grayscale image I, an image patch $P_A$ is extracted at a random location with corner points $(u_i, v_i)$, where $i = 1, 2, 3, 4$. Rotation by $\beta$ and translation by $(d_x, d_y)$ is applied:

$$\begin{bmatrix} u_i' \\ v_i' \end{bmatrix} = \begin{bmatrix} cos\beta & sin\beta \\ -sin\beta & cos\beta \end{bmatrix} \begin{bmatrix} u_i \\ v_i \end{bmatrix} + \begin{bmatrix} d_x \\ d_y \end{bmatrix}, \tag{2}$$

to obtain $P_B$, where $\beta$, $d_x$ and $d_y$ are empirically selected. During training, the relative homography is learned between patches that are extracted from a single image following the CDA. Due to lack of texture and poor contrast in fetoscopic videos, homography between two consecutive frames may not be accurate.

## 3.2 Homography Matrix Decomposition and Outlier Rejection

To obtain the most consistent homography matrix, we first decompose the homography matrix by applying SVD [7]:

$$
\begin{bmatrix} \widehat{h}_{11} & \widehat{h}_{12} \\ \widehat{h}_{21} & \widehat{h}_{22} \end{bmatrix} = \begin{bmatrix} cos\widehat{\theta} & sin\widehat{\theta} \\ -sin\widehat{\theta} & cos\widehat{\theta} \end{bmatrix} \begin{bmatrix} \widehat{s}_g & 0 \\ 0 & \widehat{s}_h \end{bmatrix} \begin{bmatrix} cos\widehat{\gamma} & sin\widehat{\gamma} \\ -sin\widehat{\gamma} & cos\widehat{\gamma} \end{bmatrix},
\tag{3}
$$

and $\widehat{t}_x = \widehat{h}_{13}$, $\widehat{t}_y = \widehat{h}_{23}$ are the translation components. By solving Eq. 3, we obtain the decomposed parameters, $\mathscr{D} = \{\widehat{\theta}, \widehat{\gamma}, \widehat{s}_g, \widehat{s}_h\}$ [7]. Next, for $F_k$ and $F_{k+1}$, we compute $_n\widehat{\mathbf{H}}_{k+1}^k$ for $N = 99$ iterations by selecting a new random patch pair $_nP_k$ and $_nP_{k+1}$ at each iteration and obtain $N$ decompose parameters, represented for example as $(\widehat{\theta}_n)_{n=1}^N$. The variations in $(\widehat{s}_{gn})_{n=1}^N$ and $(\widehat{s}_{hn})_{n=1}^N$ are very small due to fixed scale assumption, but are significant in $(\widehat{\theta}_n)_{n=1}^N$ and $(\widehat{\gamma}_n)_{n=1}^N$. Since the first and third matrices in Eq. 3 are orthogonal, $\widehat{\theta}_n = -\widehat{\gamma}_n$, filtering either of the two has the same effect. We apply median filtering, since it is useful for mitigating the effect of the outliers, to $(\widehat{\theta}_n)_{n=1}^N$ to get its argument $i$, giving the most consistent value for $\theta$. This argument is used to obtain $\widehat{\gamma}_i$, $\widehat{s}_{xi}$, $\widehat{s}_{yi}$, $\widehat{t}_{xi}$ and $\widehat{t}_{yi}$, that are then plugged into Eq. 3 to get the consistent $_i\widehat{\mathbf{H}}_{k+1}^k$.

## 4  Experimental Setup and Evaluation Protocol

For experimental analysis, we use 5 fetoscopic videos (Table 1), which include a synthetic video (SYN) - a discontinuous version of this sequence was used in [11], an ex-vivo in water (EX) data reported in [5], a placenta phantom (PHN1), a TTTS phantom[1] in water (PHN2) depicting an in-vivo procedure and an in-vivo TTTS procedure (INVI). Note from Table 1 the variability in visual quality, appearance, resolution, imaging source, camera views and captured motion. These variations pose challenging scenarios for mosaicking methods.

For training, we use 600 frames extracted at random from SYN, PHN1, PHN2, INVI and another ex-vivo still images dataset (not used in testing as it is not a video sequence). EX (Table 1) is not use during training, hence it is an unseen data for testing. We extract square frames, from the circular FoV of fetoscopic videos, to be used as the input to DSM. All images are converted to grayscale and resized to $256 \times 256$ pixels. We use Keras with Tensorflow backend for the implementation and train our network for about 15 h on a Tesla V100 (32 GB) using learning rate of $10^{-4}$ and ADAM optimizer. DIH with CDA is trained for 60,000 epochs with a batch size of 32. In each epoch, pairs of patches are generated by randomly selecting $\beta$ between $(-5, +5)$ *degrees*, and $d_x$ and $d_y$

---

[1] TTTS phantom from Surgical Touch Simulator: https://www.surgicaltouch.com/.

**Table 1.** Main characteristics of the datasets used for the experimental analysis.

| Representative frame | | | | | |
|---|---|---|---|---|---|
| Data type | Synthetic (SYN) | Ex-vivo in water (EX) | Phantom without fetus (PHN1) | TTTS Phantom in water (PHN2) | Invivo TTTS procedure (INVI) |
| Imaging source | - | Stereo | Rigid 30° scope | Rigid scope | Rigid scope |
| No. of frames | 811 | 404 | 681 | 400 | 200 |
| Resolution (pixels) | 385 × 385 | 250 × 250 | 1280 × 960 | 720 × 720 | 470 × 470 |
| Crop resolution (pixels) | 260 × 260 | 250 × 250 | 834 × 834 | 442 × 442 | 312 × 312 |
| Camera view | Planar | Planar | Non-planar | Non-planar heavy occlusions | Non-planar heavy occlusions |
| Motion type | Circular | Spiral | Circular freehand | Exploratory freehand | Exploratory freehand |

between $(-16, 16)$. Same training settings are used for DIH without CDA where each corner point of $P_A$ is perturbed at random between $(-16, 16)$.

We perform comparison of DSM with a feature-based (FEAT) [2] and DIH [4] methods. FEAT extract SURF features from a pair of images and performs an exhaustive search for feature matching to estimate the homography. We report the mean residual error (as detailed in [11]) between the GT and estimated relative homographies for SYN (the only sequence with known GT homographies). For quantitative evaluation, we report the average Root Mean Square Error (RMSE) between pair of image patches with known GT homographies obtained from data augmentation, and average pixel-wise photometric error computed by taking the L1-distance between frame $F_{k+1}$ and reprojected $F_k$ using the estimated homography. We also report qualitative results through visualization.

## 5   Results and Discussion

The visualization and comparison results on one circular loop (360 frames) of the SYN sequence are shown in Fig. 3(a)–(c). Note the small drift in DSM compared to FEAT. Similar behavior is observed from the mean residual error in Fig. 3(d) where the errors are reported for FEAT, DIH and DSM for the complete length of the sequence (811 frames). It can be seen that the error for FEAT starts increasing after approximately 300 frames and the mosaic starts drifting away. DIH error explodes within a few frames due to the random perturbation during training (Sect. 2). On the other hand, the error for DSM is very small and remains bounded. This is further verified from the low RMSE (0.36) and photometric (2.48) errors for DSM (Fig. 4). Comparison of our proposed DSM with FEAT and DIH is presented in Fig. 4. Overall the pairwise homography errors are high for FEAT for all five sequences due to poor visual quality and lack of texture in the fetoscopic videos. The RMSE and photometric errors for DIH are low compared to FEAT but are always higher compared to DSM (e.g. RMSE on EX for DIH (1.64) and DSM (0.38)). In DIH, this error accumulated over time during mosaic generation and resulted in a large drift. For EX, PHN1,

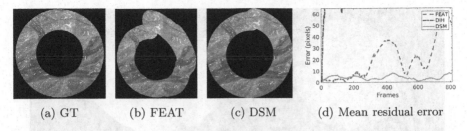

(a) GT          (b) FEAT          (c) DSM          (d) Mean residual error

**Fig. 3.** (a–c) Visualization of mosaics for one circular loop (360 frames) of the SYN sequence. (d) Quantitative comparison of FEAT, DIH and DSM.

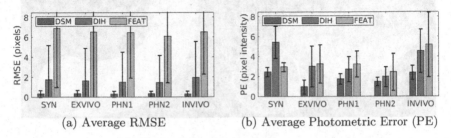

(a) Average RMSE          (b) Average Photometric Error (PE)

**Fig. 4.** Quantitative evaluation and comparison on five diverse fetoscopic videos.

PHN2 and INVI sequences, the average RMSE errors are 0.38, 0.32, 0.35 and 0.34, and photometric errors are 0.98, 1.76, 1.52, 2.42, respectively.

Mosaics generated using the proposed DSM for the EX, PHN1, PHN2 and INVI sequences are shown in Fig. 5. These mosaics are best assessed in the supplemental video that shows the qualitative comparison with respect to FEAT and DIH. DSM created a meaningful mosaic for EX (unseen data) with minimum drift accumulation over time which can be observed from the start and end frames in Fig. 5(a). PHN1 contained non-planar views without occlusions with a freehand circular trajectory. DSM generated reliable mosaics with minimum drift (Fig. 5(b)), however FEAT drifted away due to non-planar views, insufficient feature matches and long-range videos. PHN2 and INVI represent the most challenging scenarios containing highly non-planar views with heavy occlusions, low resolution and texture paucity. We observe from Fig. 5(c) and (d) that although the generated mosaics can serve well for increasing the FoV, yet there is a noticeable drift due to highly challenging conditions. Such errors may be corrected by end-to-end training using the photometric loss [8].

The experimental results show that DSM is capable of handling varying visual quality (varying illumination, specular highlights and low resolution), planar and non-planar views with heavy occlusions. Qualitative evaluation on the unseen EX dataset verified the robustness and generalization capabilities of the proposed DSM. Unlike the existing methods that use external sensors for minimizing the drift [11], DSM relied only on image data and generated meaningful mosaics with minimum drift even for non-planar sequences.

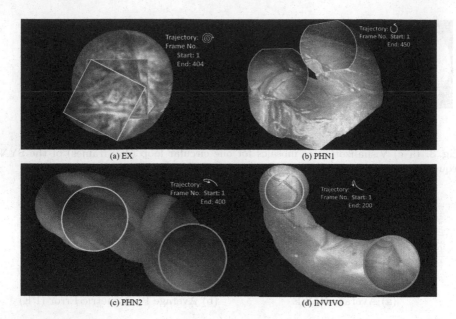

**Fig. 5.** Qualitative results of the proposed DSM on four diverse fetoscopic videos. The motion trajectories, start and end frames are marked for visualization.

## 6    Conclusion

We proposed a deep sequential mosaicking method for fetoscopic videos acquired through various sources which to our knowledge is a first. Our approach used an existing deep image homography network as a backbone for training but performed controlled data augmentation by assuming that there is only a small change in rotation and translation between two consecutive frames. Due to the lack of texture in fetoscopic sequences, varying specular highlights and turbid amniotic fluid, homography estimation varies between consecutive frames when selecting patch location randomly during testing. To overcome this problem, we proposed an outlier rejection step to obtain a reliable prediction in the least squares sense. Experimental evaluation on five diverse fetoscopic sequences showed that, unlike existing methods that drift rapidly in just a few frames, our method produced mosaics with less drift even for long-range sequences.

**Acknowledgments.** This work was supported through an Innovative Engineering for Health award by Wellcome [WT101957]; Engineering and Physical Sciences Research Council (EPSRC) [NS/A000027/1]. It was additionally supported by the Wellcome/EPSRC Centre for Interventional and Surgical Sciences (WEISS) at UCL [203145Z/16/Z] and EPSRC [EP/N027078/1, EP/P012841/1, EP/P027938/1, EP/R004080/1].

# References

1. Baschat, A., et al.: Twin-to-twin transfusion syndrome (TTTS). J. Perinat. Med. **39**(2), 107–112 (2011)
2. Brown, M., Lowe, D.G.: Automatic panoramic image stitching using invariant features. Int. J. Comput. Vis. **74**(1), 59–73 (2007)
3. Daga, P., et al.: Real-time mosaicing of fetoscopic videos using SIFT. In: Medical Imaging: Image-Guided Procedures (2016)
4. DeTone, D., Malisiewicz, T., Rabinovich, A.: Deep image homography estimation. In: RSS Workshop on Limits and Potentials of Deep Learning in Robotics (2016)
5. Dwyer, G., et al.: A continuum robot and control interface for surgical assist in fetoscopic interventions. IEEE Robot. Autom. Lett. **2**(3), 1656–1663 (2017)
6. Gaisser, F., et al.: Stable image registration for in-vivo fetoscopic panorama reconstruction. J. Imaging **4**(1), 24 (2018)
7. Malis, E., Vargas, M.: Deeper understanding of the homography decomposition for vision-based control. Ph.D. thesis, INRIA (2007)
8. Nguyen, T., et al.: Unsupervised deep homography: a fast and robust homography estimation model. IEEE Robot. Autom. Lett. **3**(3), 2346–2353 (2018)
9. Peter, L., et al.: Retrieval and registration of long-range overlapping frames for scalable mosaicking of in vivo fetoscopy. IJCARS **13**(5), 713–720 (2018)
10. Reeff, M., Gerhard, F., Cattin, P., Gábor, S.: Mosaicing of endoscopic placenta images. In: INFORMATIK 2006-Informatik für Menschen, Band 1 (2006)
11. Tella-Amo, M., et al.: Probabilistic visual and electromagnetic data fusion for robust drift-free sequential mosaicking: application to fetoscopy. J. Med. Imaging **5**(2), 021217 (2018)
12. Tella-Amo, M., et al.: Pruning strategies for efficient online globally-consistent mosaicking in fetoscopy. J. Med. Imaging **6**, 035001 (2019)
13. Totz, J., Mountney, P., Stoyanov, D., Yang, G.-Z.: Dense surface reconstruction for enhanced navigation in MIS. In: Fichtinger, G., Martel, A., Peters, T. (eds.) MICCAI 2011. LNCS, vol. 6891, pp. 89–96. Springer, Heidelberg (2011). https://doi.org/10.1007/978-3-642-23623-5_12
14. Vasconcelos, F., et al.: Towards computer-assisted TTTS: laser ablation detection for workflow segmentation from fetoscopic video. IJCARS **13**(10), 1661–1670 (2018)

# Landmark-Guided Deformable Image Registration for Supervised Autonomous Robotic Tumor Resection

Jiawei Ge[1]($\boxtimes$)(iD), Hamed Saeidi[1], Justin D. Opfermann[2], Arjun S. Joshi[3], and Axel Krieger[1]

[1] Department of Mechanical Engineering, University of Maryland,
College Park, MD, USA
jge0@umd.edu
[2] Sheikh Zayed Institute, Children's National Health System, Washington, DC, USA
[3] Division of Otolaryngology - Head and Neck Surgery,
George Washington University, Washington, DC, USA

**Abstract.** Oral squamous cell carcinoma (OSCC) is the most common cancer in the head and neck region, and is associated with high morbidity and mortality rates. Surgical resection is usually the primary treatment strategy for OSCC, and maintaining effective tumor resection margins is paramount to surgical outcomes. In practice, wide tumor excisions impair post-surgical organ function, while narrow resection margins are associated with tumor recurrence. Identification and tracking of these resection margins remain a challenge because they migrate and shrink from pre-operative chemo or radiation therapies, and deform intra-operatively. This paper reports a novel near-infrared (NIR) fluorescent marking and landmark-based deformable image registration (DIR) method to precisely predict deformed margins. The accuracy of DIR predicted resection margins on porcine cadaver tongues is compared with rigid image registration and surgeon's manual prediction. Furthermore, our tracking and registration technique is integrated into a robotic system, and tested using *ex vivo* porcine cadaver tongues to demonstrate the feasibility of supervised autonomous tumor bed resections.

**Keywords:** Medical robotics · Image-guided surgery · Deformable image registration

## 1 Introduction

Oral cavity squamous cell carcinoma (OSCC) and oropharyngeal squamous cell carcinoma (OPSCC) are the two most common cancers in the head and neck region, estimated to account for 420,000 new cases and 228,000 deaths worldwide in 2012 [4]. Surgical resection by electrocauterization is the primary treatment strategy for these cancers, and maintaining tumor-free resection margins is paramount to surgical outcomes. In practice, narrow resection margins are

© Springer Nature Switzerland AG 2019
D. Shen et al. (Eds.): MICCAI 2019, LNCS 11764, pp. 320–328, 2019.
https://doi.org/10.1007/978-3-030-32239-7_36

associated with tumor recurrence while excessive surgical margins will impair post-surgical organ functions.

Today, transoral robotic surgery (TORS) for tumor resection is a prevalent minimal invasive therapy, especially for OPSCC, which is located deeper inside the head and neck than OSCC, and is more difficult to visualize and access [14]. TORS procedures are completed with the aid of robotic assisted surgery (RAS) systems such as the da Vinci Surgical System (Intuitive Surgical, Sunnyvale, California). RAS systems provide surgeons with high dexterity tools, motion scaling, and hand tremor filtering to achieve precise tele-operated tumor resection. Surgeons use visual feedback from endoscopes and remotely control robotic arms with electrosurgical units (ESUs) for OSCC and OPSCC resections. Nevertheless, there are three major limitations when removing oral cancers using TORS. First, surgeons preoperatively mark surgical resection margins with India Ink [11] which are easily obscured by blood and charred tissue intraoperatively. Second, because surgeons mark the tumor margins by mapping preoperative computed tomography (CT) or magnetic resonance (MR) images onto visual cues which migrate and shrink from preoperative chemo or radiation therapies, the intraoperative margins do not precisely reflect the original tumor beds. Third, for robotic assisted but still manually operated surgeries, tissue motion and complex tumor shapes require prolonged and concentrated cutting following the inked tumor margins, thus placing burdens on surgeons and leading to inconsistent resection margins.

In this paper, we address these issues by performing supervised autonomous tumor resection with our smart tissue autonomous robot (STAR) system, guided by long-lasting NIR fluorescent markers. As our first contribution, we report a novel near-infrared fluorescent marking and landmark-based deformable image registration (DIR) method to precisely predict deformed tumor beds. In our previous work, we developed a NIR marker with features of (i) strong tissue penetration of the NIR light, (ii) high signal to noise ratio, (iii) durability and (iv) bio-compatibility [3,6]. The NIR markers can be tracked intraoperatively regardless of blood and charred tissue interference. They have been used to guide robot moving along simple convex polygonal paths as vertices but not for complex and irregular trajectories [9]. In this paper, we dispense the markers on irregular-shaped tumor bed contours, imitate tumor shrinkage and deformation caused by preoperative and intraoperative therapies, and demonstrate submillimeter accuracy at predicting deformed tumor beds using the landmark-based DIR technique based on elastic body spline (EBS). Moreover, the DIR accuracy is also compared with the results from rigid image registration and experienced surgeon's manual prediction. Our second contribution is integrating the proposed marking and registration technique into the robotic system, and performing supervised autonomous tumor resection following registered tumor bed contours using the experimental setup shown in Fig. 1a. The porcine cadaver tongues are cut by an electrocautery tool and the robot cutting accuracy is evaluated.

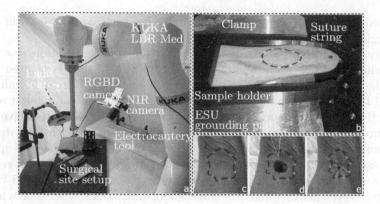

**Fig. 1.** Pictures of (a) robotic testbed, (b) surgical site setup, (c) pseudotumor contours and placed markers on samples, (d) imitated tumor shrinkage by cutting a hole, and (e) applied purse-string suture.

## 2    Methods

### 2.1    Testbed

Figure 1a demonstrates our robotic system, which is comprised of four components, (i) a 7-DOF robotic manipulator (KUKA LBR Med, KUKA, Augsburg, Germany), (ii) a monopolar electrocautery tool (DRE ASG-300 ESU, DRE Veterinary, Louisville, KY) as well its grounding pad, (iii) a dual camera system, (iv) and the control system. More specifically, the dual camera system is comprised of a low-cost off-the-shelf RGBD camera (Intel Corp., Santa Clara, California), a NIR camera (Basler Inc., Exton, PA) and a 760 nm high power light-emitting diode (North Coast Technical Inc., Chesterland, OH). The NIR light source excites the fluorescence of the NIR markers and the NIR camera detects 2D marker positions, while the RGBD camera captures the 3D tongue surface information.

As for our test sample setup shown in Fig. 1b, a clamp, a holder, a surgical suture, and a linear motion stage (Thorlabs Inc., Newton, NJ) are used to imitate human tongue OSCC resection surgeries.

### 2.2    Landmark-Based Tumor Bed Registration

In order to realize a precise tumor bed resection via the supervised autonomous robotic system, we need to accurately track and predict tumor bed locations during the surgery based on the pre-chemotherapy diagnosis. The intraoperative tumor beds tracking method developed in this paper relies on two main components, (i) a bio-compatible and durable tissue marking method to use as descriptive landmarks for tumor beds, and (ii) a soft tissue deformation tracking algorithm that allows reconstructing tumor bed regions via the descriptive landmarks during the surgery. Firstly, the tumor bed contours were drawn on

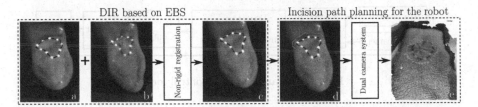

**Fig. 2.** NIR images of (a) cadaver porcine tongue with drawn pseudotumor contours and NIR markers, (b) elongated tongue with a imitated shrunk tumor, (c) estimated tumor bed after landmark based registration, and (d) 2D incision path with 5 mm offset generated from segmented pseudotumor contours; and (e) point cloud image of overlayed 3D path for robotic incision.

every sample tissue using black ink. Then, for the first component, we mixed FDA-approved NIR fluorophore Indocyanine Green (ICG), cyanoacrylate (Permabond) and acetone to get liquid marker solution, and then dispensed a few drops of it with syringes evenly separated on drawn contours. When the solution drops contacted tissue, they quickly hardened into flat disks, maintained their positions, and the NIR signals were captured by the NIR camera as shown in Fig. 2a [6]. Before the DIR, we imitated tumor shrinkage by cutting a hole on each sample tissue, and closing it with the purse-string suture (PSS) technique. Additionally, the intraoperative tumor deformation was imitated by pulling the tongue tip with a stay suture, similarly as during real surgery. Figure 1b, c, d, and e show the applied deformations to the tongues to mimic tumor shrinkage after chemotherapy and surgical setup.

For the registration, we selected a DIR algorithm based on EBS to predict deformed contours owing to its good performance for a limited number of landmarks. Because the NIR markers have a certain size, only a limited number of them can be placed to trace tumor beds. EBS achieved similar registration accuracy with fewer landmarks compared to thin plate spline (TPS) [2]. The EBS is based on a mechanical model of an elastic body, which is the Navier equilibrium partial differential equations. This physics-based model depicts the tissue displacement fields subjected to applied loads. Unlike TPS, the point forces are converted to smooth global force fields to avoid singularities. Based on every pair of landmark positions before and after tissue deformation, there's one displacement solution for all the points in the image before deformation. The final displacement fields can be yielded by a linear combination of them. In addition, we created a simple GUI allowing the operator to manually pair the landmarks. This algorithm was integrated into Insight Segmentation and Registration Toolkit (ITK) to track tumor bed contours, while the Poisson's ratio was preset to be 0. An example of implementing this EBS algorithm with our NIR marking technique to track tumor bed contours solely based on detected NIR markers' center positions, is shown in Fig. 2.

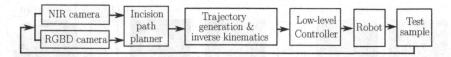

**Fig. 3.** The autonomous control loop.

## 2.3 Autonomous Control System

Figure 3 shows the block diagram of the autonomous controller used for the robotic tests in this paper. In the first place, we performed a standard hand-eye calibration using a checkerboard for both cameras and robot in order to acquire their relative positions. And the real-time video frames from the RGBD and NIR cameras were collected and processed to detect the NIR makers on the target tissue and also find the 3D coordinates of the desired incision path. The path planning algorithm developed in this paper utilized landmark-based DIR based on EBS, detailed earlier in Sect. 2.2, and calculated a warped sample image (Fig. 2c). Then, the path planner detected disconnected black tumor bed contour segments, and connected the closest two points between adjacent segments with straight lines to recover the full tumor bed contours. Finally, the path planner added a 5 mm offset to the full contours as the minimal margin needed to adequately resect diseased tissue (Fig. 2d) [10], downsampled them to forty 2D points, and projected the corresponding 3D path on the point cloud model of the tissue surface (Fig. 2e). The path projection method relies on the real-time ray tracing of the waypoints of the planned path via the dual camera system as detailed in [3]. The resulting 3D reference waypoints are converted to the joint-space trajectories via Kinematics and Dynamics Library (KDL) of Open Robot Control Systems (OROCOS) [12]. A low-level closed-loop robot controller implemented via IIWA stack [7] ensures that the robot follows the desired joint-space trajectories and hence the 3D incision path on the tissue.

## 3 Experiments and Results

### 3.1 Accuracy Evaluation and Comparison of the Deformable Image Registration

**Tasks and Evaluation.** In the first experiment, we aimed to (i) determine the ideal number of NIR markers needed for DIR registration, and (ii) compare the prediction accuracy of DIR with rigid image registration and experienced surgeon's prediction.

The contour of one of three tumor beds was drawn on the center of a clamped cadaver porcine tongue ($N = 6$) using black ink and UV visible ink (MaleDen Inc.) for image registrations and manual predictions, respectively. The contour shapes were modeled from case reports of OSCC [1,5,13], while the contour diameter was the average size of T2-stage OSCC. Ten markers were then evenly

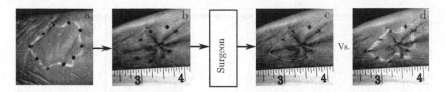

**Fig. 4.** Steps of surgeon's tumor bed predictions: (a) Original tongue sample with tumor bed marked by UV marker and India Ink landmarks, (b) deformed sample with UV light off, (c) surgeon's drawn tumor bed prediction, and d) ground truth of deformed tumor bed contour.

placed on each contour. This maximum number of markers per contour were determined experimentally avoiding mutual interference between NIR markers on tongues.

To simulate intraoperative tissue deformation caused by surgical staging, the base of each tongue was clamped and the tip of the tongue pulled to 120% of the original length (Fig. 1b). Preoperative tissue deformation induced by chemo and radiotherapy was simulated by removing 30% of the tumor bed tissue, and closing the resulting defect using the PSS technique (Fig. 1c, d, and e). Before and after tongue pulling and combined pulling and shrinking, the centroid of each marker was detected from a NIR image and used as a landmark for DIR and rigid image registration. The ground truth was found by black color segmentation on each tongue sample before and after each deformation, and using Matlab to segment the tumor bed contour. The prediction error for each sample (N = 3 to 10 markers) was calculated by finding the average minimum distance between either DIR or rigid registration and the ground truth. The error was calculated for each point on the ground truth (GT) contour by finding the closest point on the registration (Reg) contour (i.e. measured as $\min_j \|\mathbf{GT}_i - \mathbf{Reg}_j\|_2$ for point $i$ on the ground truth contour).

To calculate the human prediction error, ten India Ink markers were evenly placed on the same tumor bed contours used prior (N = 6). UV visible marking was used to draw the contours for ground truth measurement. Before and after images of the tissue deformations were provided to an experienced otolaryngologist, who was blinded to the UV contours post-deformation. The expert surgeon was then instructed to draw their predicted tumor bed contour in the post deformation image using Fig. 4b. A UV light was used to illuminate the tissue sample revealing the ground truth tumor bed. The ground truth contour was segmented using Matlab as before, and the human prediction error was calculated by finding the average minimum distance between the surgeon's prediction and the ground truth.

**Results.** Figure 5 presents tumor contour registration and prediction errors. For tissue pulling tests, it was observed that both DIR and rigid image registration predict millimeter accuracy contours (Fig. 5a). However, when tumor shrinkage

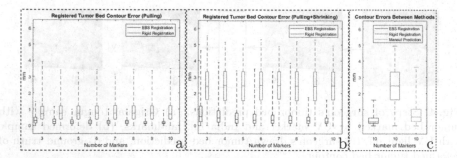

**Fig. 5.** Tumor contour registration and prediction errors: Box plots of registration errors for (a) pulling test, (b) combined pulling and shrinking, and (c) comparison of DIR, rigid registration, and surgeon's prediction using 10 markers.

Result 1: 4.28±0.69 mm    Result 2: 4.84±1.09 mm    Result 3: 4.65±0.94 mm

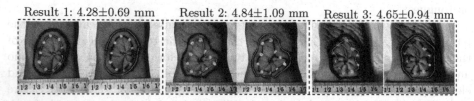

**Fig. 6.** Robotic resection results. Drawn tumor contours and performed cuts were highlighted in green in the left and right images for three samples, respectively. (Color figure online)

was induced as well, DIR performed better than rigid registration (Fig. 5b). We noted that registration errors for our DIR technique decreased as markers were added to tumor bed contours. This decrease was noticed up to N = 10 markers, which we defined as the optimal number of markers needed for accurate DIR registration. When using ten markers to identify tumor bed contours, contour errors were calculated as 0.36 ± 0.30 mm, 2.45 ± 1.09 mm, 0.75 ± 0.64 mm for DIR, rigid registration, and surgeon's prediction, respectively (Fig. 5c).

### 3.2    Supervised Autonomous Tumor Resection

**Surgical Tasks and Evaluation.** OSCC tumor bed contours based on Sect. 3.1 were drawn on porcine cadaver tongues (N = 3) and marked with ten evenly spaced NIR markers. The shrinking & pulling combined tissue deformation was applied to the samples. Using a GUI, an operator took NIR pictures of porcine tongues before and after the deformation, and manually selected the NIR markers. Then the registered tumor bed contours, offset margins, 2D and 3D incision waypoints were generated automatically as illustrated in Sect. 2.3 and Fig. 2. The 3D incision waypoints were passed to the robot controller, and the electrocautery tool tip followed the paths to cut tongues. Finally, using the same Matlab contour comparison codes, the actual incision paths were compared with drawn tumor contours on tongues as the ground truth, and the expected difference should be our predefined offset, which was 5 mm.

**Results.** The resulting electrosurgical contour was manually segmented and compared to the marked tumor contour drawn as ground truth (Fig. 6). The average minimum distance between the cut edge and tumor contour, computed in Matlab, was measured to be $4.28 \pm 0.69$ mm, $4.84 \pm 1.09$ mm, and $4.65 \pm 0.94$ mm for the first, second, and third OSCC geometries, respectively.

## 4   Discussion and Conclusions

In this work, we proposed a near-infrared fluorescent marking and landmark-based DIR method to predict OSCC contours in submillimeter accuracy. It was a considerable achievement of our registration method to outperform an experienced otolaryngologist by 0.39 mm on average. Comparing the maximum error from surgeon predictions of 3.63 mm to our DIR predictions of 1.59 mm further underscored the improvement (Fig. 5c). Moreover, we also successfully performed supervised autonomous pseudotumor resections following resection paths generated by the proposed method. In the current work, we only implemented 2D DIR, but the proposed method can be extended to 3D DIR for more accurate results in the future. Furthermore, we are currently developing a 3D laparoscopic camera system [8], which will enable us to translate our current work towards clinical usage with oral space limitations.

**Acknowledgments.** This work is supported by the National Institutes of Health under award numbers 1R01EB020610 and R21EB024707. The content is solely the responsibility of the authors and does not necessarily represent the official views of the National Institutes of Health.

## References

1. Credé, A., Locher, M., Bredell, M.: Tongue cancer in young patients: case report of a 26-year-old patient. Head Neck Oncol. **4**, 20 (2012)
2. Davis, M.H., Khotanzad, A., Flamig, D.P., Harms, S.E.: A physics-based coordinate transformation for 3-D image matching. IEEE Trans. Med. Imaging **16**(3), 317–328 (1997)
3. Decker, R.S., Shademan, A., Opfermann, J.D., Leonard, S., Kim, P.C., Krieger, A.: Biocompatible near-infrared three-dimensional tracking system. IEEE Trans. Bio-Med. Eng. **64**(3), 549–556 (2017)
4. Ferlay, J., et al.: Cancer incidence and mortality worldwide: sources, methods and major patterns in GLOBOCAN 2012. Int. J. Cancer **136**(5), E359–E386 (2015)
5. Ferreira, J.C.B., Oton-Leite, A.F., Guidi, R., Mendonça, E.F.: Granular cell tumor mimicking a squamous cell carcinoma of the tongue: a case report. BMC Res. Notes **10**, 14 (2017)
6. Ge, J., Opfermann, J.D., Saeidi, H., Krieger, A., Joshi, A.S.: A novel biocompatible marker for image guided transoral robotic surgery. In: 2019 American Head and Neck Society (AHNS) Annual Meeting, Austin, Texas, May 2019

7. Hennersperger, C., et al.: Towards MRI-based autonomous robotic US acquisitions: a first feasibility study. IEEE Trans. Med. Imaging **36**(2), 538–548 (2017)
8. Le, H.N.D., et al.: Demonstration of a laparoscopic structured-illumination three-dimensional imaging system for guiding reconstructive bowel anastomosis. J. Biomed. Opt. **23**(5), 056009 (2018)
9. Leonard, S., Wu, K.L., Kim, Y., Krieger, A., Kim, P.C.: Smart tissue anastomosis robot (STAR): a vision-guided robotics system for laparoscopic suturing. IEEE Trans. Biomed. Eng. **61**(4), 1305–1317 (2014)
10. Nahhas, A.F., Scarbrough, C.A., Trotter, S.: A review of the global guidelines on surgical margins for nonmelanoma skin cancers. J. Clin. Aesthetic Dermatol. **10**(4), 37–46 (2017)
11. Sarode, S.C., Sarode, G.S., Patil, S., Mahajan, P., Anand, R., Patil, A.: Comparative Study of Acrylic Color and India Ink for their use as a surgical margin inks in oral squamous cell carcinoma. World J. Dent. **6**, 26–30 (2015)
12. Smits, R.: KDL: Kinematics and Dynamics Library. http://www.orocos.org/kdl
13. Stanko, P., et al.: Squamous cell carcinoma and piercing of the tongue - a case report. J. Cranio-Maxillofac. Surg. **40**(4), 329–331 (2012)
14. Weinstein, G.S., et al.: Transoral robotic surgery: a multicenter study to assess feasibility, safety, and surgical margins. Laryngoscope **122**(8), 1701–1707 (2012)

# Multi-view Learning with Feature Level Fusion for Cervical Dysplasia Diagnosis

Tingting Chen[1,2], Xinjun Ma[1,2], Xuechen Liu[1,2], Wenzhe Wang[1,2],
Ruiwei Feng[1,2], Jintai Chen[1,2], Chunnv Yuan[5], Weiguo Lu[4], Danny Z. Chen[3],
and Jian Wu[1,2(✉)]

[1] College of Computer Science and Technology, Zhejiang University,
Hangzhou 310027, China
wujian2000@zju.edu.cn
[2] Real Doctor AI Research Centre, Zhejiang University, Hangzhou, China
[3] Department of Computer Science and Engineering, University of Notre Dame,
Notre Dame, IN 46556, USA
[4] Department of Gynecologic Oncology, Women's Hospital, School of Medicine,
Zhejiang University, Hangzhou, China
[5] Women's Reproductive Health Laboratory of Zhejiang Province, Women's
Hospital, School of Medicine, Zhejiang University, Hangzhou, China

**Abstract.** In this paper, we propose a novel multi-view deep learning approach for cervical dysplasia diagnosis (CDD), using multi-views of image data (acetic images and iodine images) from colposcopy. In general, a major challenge to analyzing multi-view medical image data is how to effectively exploit meaningful correlations among such views. We develop a new *feature level fusion* (FLF) method, which captures comprehensive correlations between the acetic and iodine image views and sufficiently utilizes information from these two views. Our FLF method is based on attention mechanisms and allows one view to assist another view or allows both views to assist mutually to better facilitate feature learning. Specifically, we explore deep networks for two kinds of FLF methods, *uni-directional fusion* (UFNet) and *bi-directional fusion* (BFNet). Experimental results show that our methods are effective for characterizing features of cervical lesions and outperform known methods for CDD.

## 1 Introduction

Cervical cancer is the second most common type of cancer in the female reproductive system [7], devastating lives and seriously affecting the life quality of patients. Screening can help prevent cervical cancer by detecting Squamous

---

T. Chen, X. Ma and X. Liu—Equal contribution.

---

**Electronic supplementary material** The online version of this chapter (https://doi.org/10.1007/978-3-030-32239-7_37) contains supplementary material, which is available to authorized users.

© Springer Nature Switzerland AG 2019
D. Shen et al. (Eds.): MICCAI 2019, LNCS 11764, pp. 329–338, 2019.
https://doi.org/10.1007/978-3-030-32239-7_37

Intraepithelial Lesions (SIL)[1], which have two groups: the Low-grade SIL (LSIL) and High-grade SIL (HSIL) [3]. In clinical practice, an important goal of screening is to differentiate HSIL from Normal/LSIL for early detection of cervical cancer, since the majority (60%) of LSIL will regress back to normal spontaneously while lesions in HSIL require treatment [8].

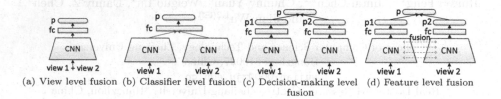

(a) View level fusion  (b) Classifier level fusion  (c) Decision-making level fusion  (d) Feature level fusion

**Fig. 1.** Four types of multi-view fusion methods (p = predicted values).

Colposcopy, a commonly-used cervical cancer screening method, takes multiple pictures of the cervix after applying 5% acetic acid and Lugol iodine solution to the cervix epithelium [4]. Acetic images[2] capture the response to the acetic acid (aceto-whitening), and iodine images show the degree of Lugol non-staining [4]. Considering each type of images as one view of data, we propose a multi-view learning framework to model the problem of cervical dysplasia diagnosis.

Previous cervical dysplasia analysis methods often extracted hand-crafted features from acetic images and utilized Support Vector Machine (SVM) [12], Adaboost [11], or Random Forest [12] to classify Normal/LSIL and HSIL. The work in [8,10] combined acetic images with some clinical test results (e.g., HPV and Pap tests)[3], and used SVM [10] or K-Nearest Neighbor [8] to compute the decision score for each modality separately. Then, they integrated the decision scores of all modalities to form the final decision. Xu *et al.* [13] proposed a deep learning network to model non-linear relations between acetic images and some clinical test results (also called non-image data in this paper). Note that these cervical dysplasia analysis methods used only one image view (i.e., acetic images), which may be insufficient to characterize cervical lesions. In practice, clinicians often analyze acetic images and iodine images together to identify potential lesions for more accurate diagnosis [5]. This is because both acetic and iodine images often contain highly relevant information. For example, aceto-whitening regions in acetic images can be treated as a complementary support of Lugol non-staining regions in iodine images (and vice versa). To better capture lesion features and conform with real diagnostic practice, we design our multi-view learning framework to explore the fusion of acetic and iodine images.

---

[1] SIL is a precancerous lesion and abnormal growth of squamous cells on cervix surface.

[2] Also called Cervigrams if the screening method used is digital cervicography. Colposcopy and cervicography both apply 5% acetic acid to the cervix epithelium.

[3] HPV tests examine whether the cervix is infected by Human Papilloma Virus; Pap tests check whether cervical cells have abnormal changes related to HPV infection. No matter HPV or Pap test result is abnormal or not, colposcopy will be performed.

However, fusing different views of image data to recognize and analyze lesions is a big challenge in medical image analysis. A simple solution is to fuse multi-view features at the view level [1] (Fig. 1(a)). It concatenates (in channel dimension) multiple image views into a 3D tensor, and puts the tensor to a Convolution Neural Network (CNN) to learn multimodal features. Since view level fusion (VLF) learns all features in a single network and does not include other branches, it has a relatively small computational cost for model training. But VLF sometimes suffers unstable performance and decreased robustness if any image view is damaged or lesions are not well presented [1]. Some other multi-view learning methods, such as classifier level fusion (CLF) (Fig. 1(b)) and decision-making level fusion (DMLF) (Fig. 1(c)), can reduce the limitations of VLF and are widely used in many multimodal scenarios [8,10,13–15]. Rather than learning all the features together, these methods first extract view-specific features, and then fuse features of each view in the classifier level [13–15] or the final decision-making layers [8,10]. Compared to VLF, they can learn at least one set of useful features if one or more views are informative [1]. But, since they extract features of each modality separately (with no interaction between one another), it may already incur loss of some useful information among the multiple views, which can be a big drawback of such methods.

To address the drawbacks of the known image fusion methods and better capture cervical lesions, we propose a new approach, called *feature level fusion* (FLF), that fuses features of two views during the feature extraction process (Fig. 1(d)). The main contributions of our work are summarized as follows: (1) introducing a new multi-view (acetic view and iodine view) learning framework for cervical dysplasia diagnosis; (2) proposing a feature level fusion method using features of different Conv layers via attention mechanisms; (3) visualizing and verifying the effectiveness of two FLF methods: uni-directional fusion and bi-directional fusion; (4) achieving diagnosis for cervical dysplasia with 80.74% accuracy and 83.17% sensitivity on a large dataset (and 83.51% accuracy and 85.10% sensitivity if including clinical test data), outperforming known methods using any single source of information alone and known multi-view frameworks.

## 2    Proposed Method

Our FLF approach is designed based on attention mechanisms, and we explore two kinds of FLF methods: uni-directional fusion and bi-directional fusion. Our uni-directional FLF method allows the acetic view to assist the iodine view (or vice versa), and our bi-directional method allows both views to assist mutually, to better characterize cervical lesions. In the subsections below, we elaborate the networks with uni-directional fusion (denoted by UFNet) and bi-directional fusion (denoted by BFNet), respectively.

### 2.1    Uni-Directional Fusion Network

Figure 2 shows the overall architecture of UFNet. It takes a pair of acetic and iodine ROI image regions (we use Faster R-CNN [6] to detect one cervix region of interest (ROI) in each colposcopic image) as input, and outputs the predicted classes from two pathways. The construction of UFNet consists of bottom-up pathways, assistant modules, and residual fusion, which are described below.

**Bottom-Up Pathways.** There are two bottom-up pathways corresponding to the two image views we have: the acetic view and iodine view. We call the pathway that provides complementary information (or attention) as *auxiliary pathway* and the other as *primary pathway*. To maintain consistency of the network structure, we use two identical backbones, ResNet-50 [2], for the two pathways. ResNet-50 consists of five groups of convolutional layers, e.g., Conv1, Conv2, Conv3, Conv4, and Conv5. We choose only the output feature maps of the last layer of each group to participate in the fusion. This choice is mainly for efficiency and practicality considerations. In Fig. 2, the four square blocks of each bottom-up pathway correspond to Conv2, Conv3, Conv4, and Conv5 in ResNet-50, and these square blocks are drawn as getting smaller along the pathway to indicate that they produce semantically stronger features. We denote the feature activation output of each group's last layer as $\{C_2, C_3, C_4, C_5\}$. For the auxiliary pathway, we use its feature maps $\{C_2^a, C_3^a, C_4^a, C_5^a\}$ to generate attention features for the primary pathway and merge with the corresponding feature maps $\{C_2^p, C_3^p, C_4^p, C_5^p\}$ of the primary pathway. We do not use Conv1 to join the fusion due to its too shallow and modality-specific features.

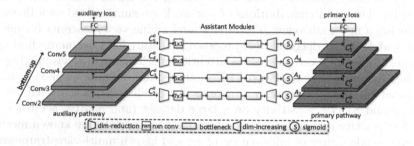

**Fig. 2.** The overall architecture of UFNet (FC denotes fully connected layer).

**Assistant Modules.** The middle part of Fig. 2 shows the structures of the assistant modules, which have different detailed designs for different Conv groups (since the semantics of the feature maps in these Conv groups are from low to high levels). For a set of $\{C_2^a, C_3^a, C_4^a, C_5^a\}$, they first undergo a $1 \times 1$ convolutional layer to reduce the channel dimension (i.e., $N$ to $d$), so as to reduce the number of parameters and model complexity. $N$ is the number of the original channels, and we set $d = 256$. Then, as features in lower layers of the auxiliary pathway are shallow and have less semantics, we apply larger kernel convolution and more bottleneck blocks [2] to them to obtain larger receptive fields (cover more contextual information) and better facilitate the feature learning ability of the primary pathway. These operations allow the auxiliary pathway to provide more global information for the primary pathway. For features in deeper layers, since they already have strong semantics and the receptive fields are large, we use smaller kernel convolution and less bottleneck blocks on them. Specifically, a convolutional kernel size (CKS) of $7 \times 7$ with 4 bottleneck blocks, a CKS of $5 \times 5$ with 3 bottleneck blocks, a CKS of $3 \times 3$ with 2 bottleneck blocks, and a CKS of $1 \times 1$ with 1 bottleneck block are applied to these $C_i^a$'s, respectively. Finally, a sigmoid layer normalizes the output range to $[0, 1]$ after increasing the channel dimension to the original size (i.e., $d$ to $N$). We denote the outputs of the assistant modules from different Conv groups as $\{A_2, A_3, A_4, A_5\}$, each having the same shape as the feature map output (i.e., $\{C_2^p, C_3^p, C_4^p, C_5^p\}$) of corresponding Conv group of the primary pathway.

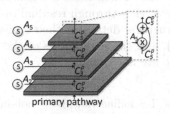

**Fig. 3.** Residual fusion (also see Fig. 2).

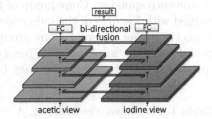

**Fig. 4.** Network structure of BFN.

**Residual Fusion.** To maintain the activation of deep layers [9], we merge the outputs of the assistant modules with the feature maps from the primary pathway via multiplication and addition (see Fig. 3), which can be described as:

$$C_i^{p'} = (1 + A_i) \times C_i^p \tag{1}$$

where $A_i$ is the feature weights (ranging in $[0, 1]$) obtained from the $i$-th Conv group's assistant module, $i \in \{2, 3, 4, 5\}$, and $C_i^p$ is the feature map output of the $i$-th Conv group of the primary pathway. Then, the fused features $C_i^{p'}$ are fed to the next layer.

**Loss Function.** We express the loss function of UFNet as:

$$L = (1 - \lambda)L_a + \lambda L_p \tag{2}$$

where $L_a$ and $L_p$ are the Cross-Entropy (CE) losses for the auxiliary pathway and primary pathway, respectively, and $\lambda$ is a hyper-parameter that controls the relative importance of $L_a$ and $L_p$. We set $\lambda = 0.75$, since $L_p$ is the main optimization metric in UFNet and $L_a$ is an auxiliary loss for optimizing the auxiliary pathway to provide more informative features to the primary pathway and better assist the primary pathway.

## 2.2   Bi-directional Fusion Network

Bi-directional fusion uses two directions of fusion and employs information from both the acetic view and iodine view, which means that the acetic view and iodine view are both auxiliary view and primary view. A sketch of the structure of our bi-directional fusion network (BFNet) is shown in Fig. 4.

**Assistant Modules.** Bi-directional fusion has two assistant modules for each Conv group of the two bottom-up pathways. Specifically, for the feature output of a Conv group, there is one assistant module using features of the acetic view to generate attention features for the corresponding Conv group of the iodine view. Simultaneously, there is another structurally identical but directionally opposite assistant module using features of the iodine view to generate attention features for the corresponding Conv group of the acetic view. Then, these attentions are merged with features of the iodine view and acetic view through residual fusion, respectively. For different Conv groups, the structural details of their assistant modules are the same as in UFNet (see Fig. 2), and the parameters of the two opposite assistant modules for each Conv group are not shared.

**Table 1.** Performance comparison. A = acetic view, I = iodine view, NI = non-image data and #Para = number of parameters. Arrows give the directions of fusion.

| Methods | Accuracy (%) | Sensitivity (%) | Specificity (%) | AUC (%) | #Para (M) |
|---|---|---|---|---|---|
| A-only | $77.91 \pm 0.92$ | $76.25 \pm 4.38$ | $79.66 \pm 2.84$ | $85.50 \pm 0.78$ | 23.512 |
| I-only | $76.48 \pm 0.70$ | $78.38 \pm 6.36$ | $74.47 \pm 5.27$ | $83.75 \pm 0.58$ | 23.512 |
| **UFNet(I→A)** | $79.58 \pm 0.75$ | $78.11 \pm 6.16$ | $\mathbf{81.13 \pm 0.50}$ | $86.21 \pm 0.50$ | 55.213 |
| **UFNet(A→I)** | $78.18 \pm 0.89$ | $80.44 \pm 1.18$ | $75.81 \pm 2.68$ | $85.94 \pm 0.40$ | 55.213 |
| **BFNet(A⇌I)** | $\mathbf{80.74 \pm 0.51}$ | $\mathbf{83.17 \pm 0.84}$ | $78.19 \pm 1.77$ | $87.60 \pm 0.29$ | 63.410 |
| VLF [1] (Fig. 1(a)) | $75.62 \pm 0.65$ | $74.58 \pm 1.37$ | $76.72 \pm 1.55$ | $83.57 \pm 0.16$ | 73.860 |
| CLF [1] (Fig. 1(b)) | $78.22 \pm 1.34$ | $81.37 \pm 3.86$ | $74.89 \pm 1.84$ | $85.22 \pm 1.74$ | 114.145 |
| DMLF [1] (Fig. 1(c)) | $79.04 \pm 0.45$ | $82.17 \pm 3.24$ | $75.73 \pm 2.60$ | $\mathbf{88.11 \pm 0.85}$ | 147.720 |
| Xu et al. (A+NI) [13] | $81.32 \pm 0.49$ | $83.30 \pm 1.93$ | $79.24 \pm 3.05$ | $89.27 \pm 0.40$ | 25.749 |
| **BFNet(A⇌I)+NI** | $\mathbf{83.51 \pm 0.83}$ | $\mathbf{85.10 \pm 2.85}$ | $\mathbf{81.84 \pm 4.16}$ | $\mathbf{90.72 \pm 0.56}$ | 67.884 |

**Loss Function.** In BFNet, the final decision is obtained by averaging the outputs from both the two pathways, rather than mainly depending on the result of the primary pathway as in UFNet. We consider the two pathways as of equal importance. Thus, the loss function of BFNet is the same as that of UFNet, except that the hyper-parameter $\lambda$ for BFNet is set to 0.5.

## 3   Experiments

**Dataset.** We evaluate the performance of our approach on a cervical dataset, provided by a local hospital, which contains one acetic image, one iodine image and other clinical test data (e.g., Pap and HPV tests) for each patient during each visit. The annotation is based on pathology interpretations on each biopsy taken during a visit, which is a commonly used gold standard to define the ground truth diagnosis. In total, our visit-level dataset has 1503 positives (HSIL) and 1426 negatives (Normal: 939, LSIL: 487).

**Evaluation Metrics.** For all our experiments, we conduct 5-fold cross-validation and report the average results and standard deviation, and evaluate the classification performance in terms of accuracy, sensitivity, specificity and area under the receiver operator characteristic curve (AUC).

**Implementation.** All the models are trained using SGD with a momentum = 0.9 and a gradually decreasing learning rate starting at 0.001. For data augmentation, we apply random rotations, followed by restrained random crops. With random brightness and mirror used, the images are scaled to size $512 \times 512$. Particularly, the random state is set as the same, which ensures that the augmented data of the two image views are kept synchronous during training.

**Evaluation and Results.** Table 1 shows the performance of the single-view methods (1st block), our multi-view fusion methods (2nd block), known multi-view methods (3rd block), and the previous CDD methods (4th block). For fair comparison, all the methods are based on the backbone of ResNet-50 [2]. All the known methods we compare with are implemented based on the original papers.

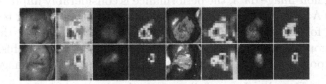

**Fig. 5.** Visualization results of BFNet(A⇌I). From left to right: acetic images, acetic features, masked acetic images, assisted acetic features, iodine images, iodine features, masked iodine images, and assisted iodine features.

As shown in the first two blocks of Table 1, the methods using multiple views are generally superior to the methods using only one single view. For example, compared to the "A-only", our method with the iodine view as auxiliary view (UFNet(I→A)) achieves improvements of 1.67%, 1.86%, 1.47%, and 0.71% in accuracy, sensitivity, specificity, and AUC, respectively. The performance of UFNet(A→I) with the acetic view as auxiliary view is also better than the one using the iodine view alone. This confirms the effectiveness of fusing multiple image views. With competitive results achieved by UFNets, bi-directional fusion (BFNet(A⇌I)) further improves performance by 1.16% and 2.56% in accuracy, 5.06% and 2.73% in sensitivity, and 1.39% and 1.66% in AUC, respectively. It shows that, by adding another direction of fusion, BFNet can take advantage of more information from multiple views and better exploit the complex correlations between these views. We also observe that the acetic view has a better specificity and the iodine view has a better sensitivity. These two views can well assist each other to produce better results.

We use BFNet when comparing with known multi-view methods (3rd block). One can see that BFNet outperforms all the three methods (VLF, CLF, and DMLF) and exceeds the best result (DMLF) by a margin of 1.7%, 1%, and 2.46% in accuracy, sensitivity, and specificity, respectively. However, DMLF yielded a slightly better AUC score than BFNet, with an improvement of 0.51%. We also give the number of parameters of all the methods in the paper. Comparing with the known multi-view methods, our proposed assistant modules for uni-directional and bi-directional methods do not introduce too many parameters (8.819M and 16.386M), and the UFNet and BFNet have less parameters.

Furthermore, the studies in [8,10,13] showed that other clinical test results (e.g., HPV and Pap) are helpful for CDD. Similar to [13], we also combine our BFNet with some clinical test results to better learn cervical lesion features and conform with actual clinical practice. When including clinical test results, our "BFNet(A$\rightleftharpoons$I)+NI" model improves the accuracy by 2.77%, sensitivity by 1.93%, specificity by 3.65%, and AUC by 3.12% over BFNet(A$\rightleftharpoons$I). It is also better than the method in [13] (4th block), which fuses features of acetic images and non-image data. Note that we did not find any known deep learning models that use multiple views of acetic-iodine images and clinical test results as in our "BFNet(A$\rightleftharpoons$I)+NI" model for comparison. Our results in Table 1 show that, compared with a single image view, our methods are all helpful for CDD. Further, when adding non-image data, the performance is considerably improved (by both our "BFNet(A$\rightleftharpoons$I)+NI" and [13]). This shows that other clinical tests are also quite useful for CDD. Since the work in [13] already explored the fusion of images and non-image data and our focus is on multi-view image fusion, we will not discuss too much about the fusion of image views and non-image view.

**Visualization Results.** In our fusion methods, the acetic and iodine views can assist one another to help the multi-view feature learning. To examine the effect of our fusion methods, we visualize the feature maps (following the method in [16]) of the Conv5 group in BFNet. As shown in Fig. 5, we choose two paired acetic and iodine images, and visualize their feature maps with the weighted summation activation magnitude. It is observed that, compared with the original acetic and iodine feature maps, the assisted feature maps can repress noise or other suspicious but non-lesion regions, and focus more attention on the regions that both views show high activation. We give visualization results of all the Conv groups (Conv2–Conv5) of UFNet and BFNet in *Supplementary Material.*

## 4    Conclusions

In this paper, we proposed a novel multi-view deep learning framework for the task of CDD. By introducing new FLF methods, our model well explores inherent correlations between two different image views (acetic and iodine images). Further, by developing new uni-directional fusion and bi-directional fusion methods, the multi-view feature learning process is directly facilitated. Experiments on colposcopic image data validated the effectiveness of our new methods. In the future, we will seek to improve and generalize our methods to more complex situations such as with three or even more views or multiple views providing very different information (not as closely related as acetic and iodine images).

**Acknowledgment.** The research of D.Z. Chen was supported in part by NSF Grant CCF-1617735. The research of the Real Doctor AI Research Centre was partially supported by the Subject of the Major Commissioned Project "Research on China's Image in the Big Data" of Zhejiang Province's Social Science Planning Advantage Discipline "Evaluation and Research on the Present Situation of China's Image" No. 16YSXK01ZD-2YBMinistry of Education of China under grant No. 2017PT18, the Zhejiang University Education Foundation under grants No. K18-511120-004, No. K17-511120-017, and No. K17-518051-021, the Major Scientific Project of Zhejiang Lab under grant No. 2018DG0ZX01, the National Natural Science Foundation of China under grant No. 61672453, and the Key Laboratory of Medical Neurobiology of Zhejiang Province.

# References

1. Guo, Z., Li, X., Huang, H., et al.: Medical image segmentation based on multi-modal convolutional neural network: Study on image fusion schemes. In: ISBI, pp. 903–907 (2018)
2. He, K., Zhang, X., Ren, S., et al.: Deep residual learning for image recognition. In: CVPR, pp. 770–778 (2015)
3. Jusman, Y., Ng, S.C., Abu Osman, N.A.: Intelligent screening systems for cervical cancer. Sci. World J. **2014**(2), Article ID 810368 (2014)
4. Khan, M.J., Werner, C.L., Darragh, T.M., et al.: ASCCP colposcopy standards: role of colposcopy, benefits, potential harms, and terminology for colposcopic practice. J. Lower Genital Tract Dis. **21**(4), 223 (2017)
5. Longatto-Filho, A., Naud, P., Derchain, S.F., et al.: Performance characteristics of Pap test, VIA, VILI, HR-HPV testing, cervicography, and colposcopy in diagnosis of significant cervical pathology. Virchows Arch. **460**(6), 577–585 (2012)
6. Ren, S., He, K., Girshick, R., Jian, S.: Faster R-CNN: towards real-time object detection with region proposal networks. In: NIPS, pp. 91–99 (2015)
7. Siegel, R.L., Miller, K.D., Jemal, A.: Cancer statistics, 2017. CA Cancer J. Clin. **67**(1), 7–30 (2017)
8. Song, D., Kim, E., Huang, X., et al.: Multimodal entity coreference for cervical dysplasia diagnosis. IEEE TMI **34**(1), 229–245 (2015)
9. Wang, F., Jiang, M., Qian, C., et al.: Residual attention network for image classification. In: CVPR, pp. 6450–6458 (2017)
10. Xu, T., Huang, X., Kim, E., et al.: Multi-test cervical cancer diagnosis with missing data estimation. In: Medical Imaging: CAD, vol. 9414, p. 94140X (2015)
11. Xu, T., Kim, E., Huang, X.: Adjustable AdaBoost classifier and pyramid features for image-based cervical cancer diagnosis. In: ISBI, pp. 281–285 (2015)
12. Xu, T., et al.: A new image data set and benchmark for cervical dysplasia classification evaluation. In: Zhou, L., Wang, L., Wang, Q., Shi, Y. (eds.) MLMI 2015. LNCS, vol. 9352, pp. 26–35. Springer, Cham (2015). https://doi.org/10.1007/978-3-319-24888-2_4

13. Xu, T., Zhang, H., Huang, X., Zhang, S., Metaxas, D.N.: Multimodal deep learning for cervical dysplasia diagnosis. In: Ourselin, S., Joskowicz, L., Sabuncu, M.R., Unal, G., Wells, W. (eds.) MICCAI 2016. LNCS, vol. 9901, pp. 115–123. Springer, Cham (2016). https://doi.org/10.1007/978-3-319-46723-8_14

14. Yang, X., et al.: Joint detection and diagnosis of prostate cancer in multi-parametric MRI based on multimodal convolutional neural networks. In: Descoteaux, M., Maier-Hein, L., Franz, A., Jannin, P., Collins, D.L., Duchesne, S. (eds.) MICCAI 2017. LNCS, vol. 10435, pp. 426–434. Springer, Cham (2017). https://doi.org/10.1007/978-3-319-66179-7_49

15. Yoo, Y., et al.: Hierarchical multimodal fusion of deep-learned lesion and tissue integrity features in brain MRIs for distinguishing neuromyelitis optica from multiple sclerosis. In: Descoteaux, M., Maier-Hein, L., Franz, A., Jannin, P., Collins, D.L., Duchesne, S. (eds.) MICCAI 2017. LNCS, vol. 10435, pp. 480–488. Springer, Cham (2017). https://doi.org/10.1007/978-3-319-66179-7_55

16. Zhou, B., Khosla, A., Lapedriza, A., et al.: Learning deep features for discriminative localization. In: CVPR, pp. 2921–2929 (2016)

# Real-Time Surface Deformation Recovery from Stereo Videos

Haoyin Zhou and Jayender Jagadeesan[✉]

Surgical Planning Laboratory, Brigham and Women's Hospital,
Harvard Medical School, Boston, MA 02115, USA
jayender@bwh.harvard.edu

**Abstract.** Tissue deformation during the surgery may significantly decrease the accuracy of surgical navigation systems. In this paper, we propose an approach to estimate the deformation of tissue surface from stereo videos in real-time, which is capable of handling occlusion, smooth surface and fast deformation. We first use a stereo matching method to extract depth information from stereo video frames and generate the tissue template, and then estimate the deformation of the obtained template by minimizing ICP, ORB feature matching and as-rigid-as-possible (ARAP) costs. The main novelties are twofold: (1) Due to non-rigid deformation, feature matching outliers are difficult to be removed by traditional RANSAC methods; therefore we propose a novel 1-point RANSAC and reweighting method to preselect matching inliers, which handles smooth surfaces and fast deformations. (2) We propose a novel ARAP cost function based on dense connections between the control points to achieve better smoothing performance with limited number of iterations. Algorithms are designed and implemented for GPU parallel computing. Experiments on *ex-* and *in vivo* data showed that this approach works at an update rate of 15 Hz with an accuracy of less than 2.5 mm on a NVIDIA Titan X GPU.

**Keywords:** Tissue deformation recovery · Feature matching outliers · GPU parallel computation

## 1 Background

Tissue visualization during surgery is typically limited to the anatomical surface exposed to the surgeon through an optical imaging modality, such as laparoscope, endoscope or microscope. To identify the critical structures lying below the tissue surface, surgical navigation systems need to register the intraoperative data to preoperative MR/CT imaging before surgical resection. However, during surgery, tissue deformation caused by heartbeat, respiration and instruments interaction may make the initial registration results less accurate. The ability to compensate for tissue deformation is essential for improving the accuracy of surgical navigation. In this paper, we propose an approach to recover the deformation of tissue surface from stereo optical videos in real-time.

© Springer Nature Switzerland AG 2019
D. Shen et al. (Eds.): MICCAI 2019, LNCS 11764, pp. 339–347, 2019.
https://doi.org/10.1007/978-3-030-32239-7_38

In recent years, several groups have investigated methods to recover tissue deformation from optical videos, and most methods are based on the minimization of non-rigid matching and smoothing costs [1]. For example, Collins et al. proposed a monocular vision-based method that first generated the tissue template and then estimated the template deformation by matching the texture and boundaries with a non-rigid iterative closet points (ICP) method [2]. In this method, the non-rigid ICP-based boundary matching algorithm significantly improves the accuracy. However, during surgery, only a small area of the target tissue may be exposed and the boundaries are often invisible, which makes it difficult to match the template. Object deformation recovery in the computer vision field is also a suitable approach to recover tissue deformation. For example, Zollhfer et al. proposed to generate the template from an RGB-D camera and then track the deformation by minimizing non-rigid ICP, color and smoothing costs [3]. Newcombe et al. have developed a novel deformation recovery method that does not require the initial template and uses sparse control points to represent the deformation [4]. Guo et al. used forward and backward $L_0$ regularization to refine the deformation recovery results [5]. To date, most deformation recovery methods [6,7] are based on the non-rigid ICP alignment to obtain matching information between the template and the current input, such as monocular/stereo videos or 3D point clouds from RGB-D sensors. However, non-rigid ICP suffers from a drawback that it cannot track fast tissue deformation and camera motion, and obtain accurate alignment in the tangential directions on smooth tissue surfaces. During surgery, the endo/laparoscope may move fast or even temporally out of the patient for cleaning, which makes non-rigid ICP difficult to track the tissue. In addition, smoke and blood during the surgery may cause significant occlusion and interfere with the tracking process. Hence, the ability to match the template and the input video when non-rigid deformation exists is essential for intraoperative use of deformation recovery methods.

A natural idea to obtain additional information is to match the feature points between the template and the input video. Among many types of feature descriptors, ORB [8] has been widely used in real-time applications due to its efficiency. To handle feature matching outliers, RANSAC-based methods have proven effective in rigid scenarios but are difficult to handle non-rigid deformation [9]. Another common method to address outliers is to apply robust kernels to the cost function, which cannot handle fast motion. In this paper, we propose a novel method that combines 1-point-RANSAC and reweighting methods to handle matching outliers in non-rigid scenarios. In addition, we propose a novel as-rigid-as-possible (ARAP) [10] method based on dense connections to achieve better smoothing performance with limited number of iterations.

## 2   Method

As shown in Fig. 1, we proposed a GPU-based stereo matching method, which includes several efficient post-processing steps to extract 3D information from stereo videos in real-time. Readers may refer to Ref. [11] for more details on this stereo matching method.

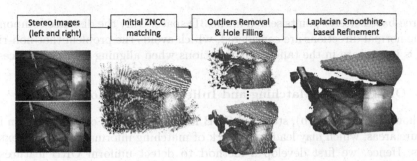

**Fig. 1.** The process of our stereo matching method with a pair of stereo microscopy images captured during neurosurgery.

In our system, the initial template of the tissue surface is generated by the stereo matching method, then we track the deformation of the template by representing the non-rigid deformation with sparse control points on the template, and estimating the parameters of the control points to make the deformed template match the output of the GPU-based stereo matching method. The algorithms are parallelized and run on the GPU. Similar to DynamicFusion [4], we employ dual-quaternion to represent deformation and each control point $i$ is assigned a dual-quaternion $W_i^t$ to represent its warp function at time $t$, and the template points are deformed according to the interpolation of neighboring control points. Then, the deformation recovery problem is to estimate $W_i^t$, $i = 1, \ldots, N$, and we use the Levenberg-Marquardt algorithm to minimize the following cost function

$$f_{\text{Total}}(W_i^t) = f_{\text{ICP}} + w_{\text{ORB}} f_{\text{ORB}} + w_{\text{ARAP}} f_{\text{ARAP}}, \tag{1}$$

where $f_{\text{ICP}}$ and $f_{\text{ORB}}$ are based on non-rigid ICP and ORB matches between the template and the current stereo matching results respectively. The as-rigid-as-possible (ARAP) cost $f_{\text{ARAP}}$ smoothes the estimated warp functions $W_i^t$, which is especially important for the estimation of occluded areas. $w_{\text{ORB}}$ and $w_{\text{ARAP}}$ are user defined weights. In our experiments, we use $w_{\text{ORB}} = 10.0$ and $w_{\text{ARAP}}$ is dynamically adjusted due to the varying number of valid points in $f_{\text{ICP}}$ and ORB matching inliers in $f_{\text{ORB}}$. We sum up the related weights of ICP and ORB terms for each $W_i^t$, and scale up or down $w_{\text{ARAP}}$ accordingly.

A GPU-based parallel Levenberg-Marquardt (LM) algorithm was developed to minimize the cost (1). We update each $W_i^t$ independently in the LM iterations. For the computation of the Jacobian matrix $\mathbf{J}$ related to each $W_i^t$, multiple parallel GPU threads are launched to compute rows of $\mathbf{J}$, then we perform Cholesky decomposition to update $W_i^t$, $i = 1, \ldots, N$.

The non-rigid ICP term $f_{\text{ICP}}$ is determined by the distances between the deformed template and the stereo matching results. The Tukey's penalty function is employed to handle outliers. We have developed a rasterization process that re-projects the template points to the imaging plane to build correspondences between template points and the stereo matching results, which is parallelized to each template point and runs on the GPU. This rasterization step is faster than kd-tree-based closest points search in the 3D space. Only the distance component in the normal directions are considered, which avoids the problem that non-rigid ICP is inaccurate in the tangential directions when aligning smooth surfaces.

## 2.1    ORB Feature Matching and Inliers Pre-selection

As shown in Fig. 2(a)–(b), standard ORB feature detection concentrates on rich texture areas, which may lead to the lack of matching information at low texture areas. Hence, we first develop a method to detect uniform ORB features to improve the accuracy of deformation recovery, which uses GPU to detect FAST corners and suppresses those if a neighboring pixel has larger corner response in parallel. Then, the ORB features of the initial template are matched to the live video frames. Two corresponding 3D point clouds are obtained, which may include incorrect matches.

Since at least three matches are needed to determine the rigid relative pose between two 3D point clouds, traditional RANSAC methods only work when the three matches are all inliers and have similar deformation [9]. Another common method to handle outliers is to apply robust kernels to the cost function, which is effective but cannot handle fast camera motion or tissue deformation. Under a reasonable assumption that local deformations at small areas of the tissue surface are approximate to rigid transforms, we propose a novel 1-point-RANSAC and reweighting method to pre-select potential matching inliers following the idea of Ref. [12], as shown in Fig. 2(c). Denoting the two sets of corresponding 3D ORB features as $o_k^1$ and $o_k^2$, $k = 1, \ldots, N$, a random match $k_0$ is selected as the reference, and rectify the coordinates with respect to $k_0$ by

$$\mathbf{S}_{k0}^l = \left[ o_1^l - o_{k0}^l, \cdots, o_N^l - o_{k0}^l \right]_{3 \times N}, l = 1, 2. \tag{2}$$

For a reference $k_0$, we denote the local rigid transform as $o_{k0}^2 = \mathbf{R}o_{k0}^1 + \mathbf{T}$, where $\mathbf{R} \in SO(3)$ is the rotation matrix and $\mathbf{T}$ is the translation vector. Rigid transform for a neighboring match inlier $k$ should satisfy

$$\mathbf{S}_{k0}^2(k) \approx \mathbf{R}\mathbf{S}_{k0}^1(k), \tag{3}$$

where $\mathbf{S}_{k0}(k)$ is the $k$th column of $\mathbf{S}_{k0}$, and $\mathbf{R}$ can be obtained from matches that satisfy (3). We propose a reweighting method to eliminate the impacts of other matches, that is

$$d_k = \left\| \mathbf{S}_{k0}^2(k) - \mathbf{R}\mathbf{S}_{k0}^1(k) \right\|, w_k = \min \left( H/d_k, 1 \right), \tag{4}$$

where $d_k$ is the distance related to the $k$th match. $w_k$ is the weight of the $k$th ORB match and if the $k$th match is either an outlier, or an inlier that does not satisfy (3), $w_k$ is small. $H$ is a predefined threshold. With a selected reference $k_0$, we alternatively update $\mathbf{R}$ from weighted $\mathbf{S}_{k0}^1$ and $\mathbf{S}_{k0}^2$, and update $w_k$ according to (4). In experiments we perform 10 iterations with each $k_0$. A small sum of $w_k$ suggests that few matches satisfy (3) and $k_0$ may be an outlier, and we omit the

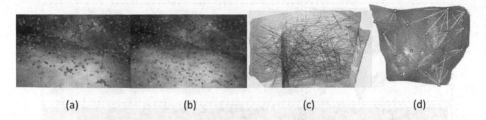

(a)          (b)          (c)          (d)

**Fig. 2.** (a)–(b) ORB feature detection results on laparoscopy images captured during a lung surgery using (a) OpenCV (b) Our method. (c) Matching inliers pre-selection results with a deforming phantom. The blue lines are selected inliers and black lines are identified as outliers. (d) Dense connections between control points with a silicon heart phantom. (Color figure online)

results with reference $k_0$. In our experiments, we randomly select 30 different matches as the reference $k_0$.

We first apply this 1-point-RANSAC + reweighting method to assign weights to ORB matches, the results of which will be used in the subsequent LM algorithm to minimize term $f_{ORB}$ in (1). It should be clarified that we are not implying that this 1-point-RANSAC + reweighting method is able to find all inliers. To take into account all inliers, in the LM algorithm we assign the pre-selected matches the same weight as $w_k$, and assign other ORB matches weight according to $w_k = -1/(5H)d_k + 1$, $w_k \in [0, 1]$.

## 2.2 As-Rigid-As-Possible Smoothing

Traditional ARAP methods are based on sparse connections, such as triangular meshes. This type of connection is too sparse to propagate the smoothing impact fast enough, and in practice we found that it cannot perform well with the limited number of iterations in the LM algorithm. Hence, we propose to use dense connections as shown in Fig. 2(d). The weights of connections in traditional ARAP methods are sensitive and need to be specifically designed based on the angles of the triangular mesh [10], hence the ARAP cost function has to be redesigned to handle the dense connections as follows:

$$f_{ARAP} = \sum_{i1,i2} w_{i1,i2} \left( f_{length,i1i2} + w_{angle} f_{angle,i1i2} + w_{rotation} f_{rotation,i1i2} \right) \quad (5)$$

where $i_1$ and $i_2$ are two control points. $w_{i1,i2}$ is the weight of connection between $i_1$ and $i_2$, and a smaller distance between points $i_1$ and $i_2$ at time 0 suggests larger $w_{i1,i2}$. We use $w_{angle} = 20.0$ and $w_{rotation} = 100.0$.

For control points $i_1$ and $i_2$,

$$f_{length,i1i2} = \left( \|p_{i2}^t - p_{i1}^t\| - \|p_{i2}^0 - p_{i1}^0\| \right)^2$$
$$f_{angle,i1i2} = acos(W_{i1}^t(p_{i2}^0) - p_{i1}^t, p_{i2}^t - p_{i1}^t) \quad (6)$$
$$f_{rotation,i1i2} = \|W_{i1}^t(1,2,3,4) - W_{i2}^t(1,2,3,4)\|^2$$

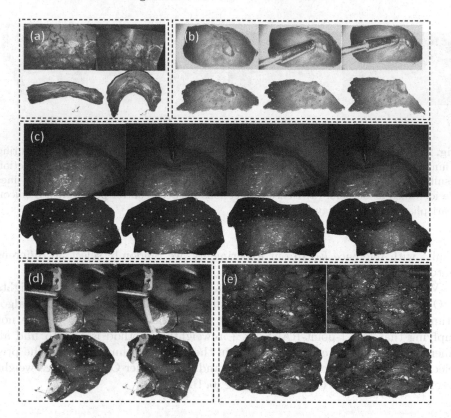

**Fig. 3.** Qualitative experiments. First row: input video frames. Second row: the deformed template and the control points (green dots). (a) Phantom. (b) *Ex vivo* porcine liver. (c) Hamlyn *in vivo* data with deformation caused by instrument interaction (d) Hamlyn *in vivo* data with respiration and heartbeat. (e) *In vivo* kidney data with deformation caused by respiration. (Color figure online)

where $p_i^t$ is the coordinate of point $i$ at time $t$. $f_{angle,i1i2}$ equals to the angle between the normalized vectors $W_{i1}^t(p_{i2}^0) - p_{i1}^t$ and $p_{i2}^t - p_{i1}^t$, where $W_{i1}^t(p_{i2}^0)$ suggest to apply $W_{i1}^t$ to $p_{i2}^0$. $f_{rotation,i1i2}$ is introduced because $W_i^t$ has 6-DoFs, which is determined by the differences between the first four components of dual-quaternion $W_{i1}^t$ and $W_{i2}^t$.

## 3   Experiments

Algorithms were implemented with CUDA C++ running on a desktop with Intel Xeon 3.0 GHz CPU and NVIDIA Titan X GPU. We first conducted qualitative experiments on *ex*- and *in vivo* data. As shown in Fig. 3(a), we deformed a smooth phantom with lung surface texture and captured $960 \times 540$ stereo videos with a KARL STORZ stereo laparoscope. We removed intermediate video frames between the two frames in Fig. 3(a) to simulate fast deformation, and our method

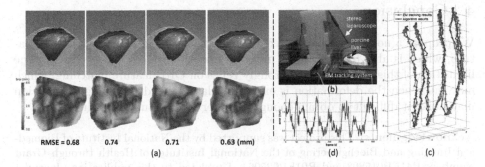

**Fig. 4.** Quantitative experiments. (a) Hamlyn heart Phantom data. First row: colored models are the deformed templates, white points are the ground truth. Second row: distance maps. Average runtime: stereo matching 3.8 ms, ORB feature detection and matching 10.6 ms, inliers pre-selection 4.1 ms, LM 14.2 ms. (b)–(d) Experiment with the EM tracking system. (b) Hardware. (c) 3D trajectories. (d) Errors. Average runtime: stereo matching 17.6 ms, ORB feature detection and matching 11.6 ms, inliers pre-selection 3.1 ms, LM 30.7 ms. (Color figure online)

is capable of tracking the large deformation. The second experiment was conducted with *ex vivo* porcine liver as shown in Fig. 3(b). The deformation was caused by instrument interaction, and our method is able to handle instrument occlusion. For the *in vivo* experiments shown in Fig. 3(c)–(e), we used both the Hamlyn data [13] and our data, in which the videos have camera motion and tissue deformation. We generated the tissue template before instrument interaction and then track the deformation of the template. The algorithm detected key inlier ORB features on the reconstructed surface and tracked these template features robustly in spite of respiratory and pulsatile motions, and instrument occlusions. These results highlight the robustness of tracking in spite of physiological motions and varying illumination.

We conducted two quantitative experiments. The first experiment was conducted on Hamlyn data as shown in Fig. 4(a). The Hamlyn data consists of stereo video images of a silicon phantom simulating heartbeat motion and corresponding ground truth was obtained using CT scan. The template was generated from the first video frame. Results show an RMSE of less than 1 mm and the average runtime of 32.7 ms per frame. In the second experiment, we used the EM tracking system (medSAFE Ascension Technologies Inc.) as the ground truth, as shown in Fig. 4(b)–(d). The porcine liver was placed in an abdominal phantom (The Chamberlain Group) and a medSAFE EM sensor was attached to the liver surface. We deformed the liver manually and recorded the EM sensor measurements and compared it with that of the our method. Deformation estimation results on 420 video frames (Fig. 4(c)–(d)) show a mean error of 1.06 mm and standard deviation of 0.56 mm. As shown in Fig. 4(c), the maximum distance between the trajectory points is 15.7 mm. The average runtime was 63.0 ms per frame.

# 4 Conclusion

We propose a novel deformation recovery method that integrates the ORB feature, which is able to handle fast motion, smooth surfaces and occlusion. The limitation of this work is that it strongly relies on ORB feature matching, which may fail when the deformation is extremely large and different light reflection may make it difficult to obtain enough number of ORB matching inliers.

**Acknowledgments.** This project was supported by the National Institute of Biomedical Imaging and Bioengineering of the National Institutes of Health through Grant Numbers P41EB015898 and R01EB025964. Unrelated to this publication, Jayender Jagadeesan owns equity in Navigation Sciences, Inc. He is a co-inventor of a navigation device to assist surgeons in tumor excision that is licensed to Navigation Sciences. Dr. Jagadeesans interests were reviewed and are managed by BWH and Partners Health-Care in accordance with their conflict of interest policies.

# References

1. Schoob, A., Kundrat, D., Kahrs, L.A., Ortmaier, T.: Stereo vision-based tracking of soft tissue motion with application to online ablation control in laser microsurgery. Med. Image Anal. **40**, 80–95 (2017)
2. Collins, T., Bartoli, A., Bourdel, N., Canis, M.: Robust, real-time, dense and deformable 3D organ tracking in laparoscopic videos. In: Ourselin, S., Joskowicz, L., Sabuncu, M.R., Unal, G., Wells, W. (eds.) MICCAI 2016. LNCS, vol. 9900, pp. 404–412. Springer, Cham (2016). https://doi.org/10.1007/978-3-319-46720-7_47
3. Zollhfer, M., Matthias, N., Shahram, I., et al.: Real-time non-rigid reconstruction using an RGB-D camera. ACM Trans. Graph. **33**(4), 156 (2014)
4. Newcombe, R.A., Fox, D., Seitz, S.M.: DynamicFusion: reconstruction and tracking of non-rigid scenes in real-time. In: CVPR, pp. 343–352 (2015)
5. Guo, K., Xu, F., Wang, Y., Liu, Y., Dai, Q.: Robust non-rigid motion tracking and surface reconstruction using L0 regularization. In: ICCV, pp. 3083–3091 (2015)
6. Modrzejewski, R., Collins, T., Bartoli, A., Hostettler, A., Marescaux, J.: Soft-body registration of pre-operative 3D models to intra-operative RGBD partial body scans. In: Frangi, A.F., Schnabel, J.A., Davatzikos, C., Alberola-López, C., Fichtinger, G. (eds.) MICCAI 2018. LNCS, vol. 11073, pp. 39–46. Springer, Cham (2018). https://doi.org/10.1007/978-3-030-00937-3_5
7. Petit, A., Lippiello, V., Siciliano, B.: Real-time tracking of 3D elastic objects with an RGB-D sensor. In: IROS (2015)
8. Rublee, E., Rabaud, V., Konolige, K., Bradski, G.: ORB: an efficient alternative to SIFT or SURF, pp. 2564–2571 (2011)
9. Tran, Q.-H., Chin, T.-J., Carneiro, G., Brown, M.S., Suter, D.: In defence of RANSAC for outlier rejection in deformable registration. In: Fitzgibbon, A., Lazebnik, S., Perona, P., Sato, Y., Schmid, C. (eds.) ECCV 2012. LNCS, vol. 7575, pp. 274–287. Springer, Heidelberg (2012). https://doi.org/10.1007/978-3-642-33765-9_20
10. Sorkine, O., Alexa, M.: As-rigid-as-possible surface modeling. In: Symposium on Geometry Processing, vol. 4, pp. 109–116 (2007)

11. Zhou, H., Jagadeesan, J.: Real-time dense reconstruction of tissue surface from stereo optical video. IEEE Trans. Med. Imaging (2019, early access)
12. Zhou, H., Zhang, T., Jayender, J.: Re-weighting and 1-Point RANSAC-Base PnP solution to handle outliers. IEEE TPAMI (2018, early access)
13. Mountney, P., Stoyanov, D., Yang, G.Z.: Three-dimensional tissue deformation recovery and tracking. IEEE Signal Process. Mag. **27**(4), 14–24 (2010)

# Microscopy

# Rectified Cross-Entropy and Upper Transition Loss for Weakly Supervised Whole Slide Image Classifier

Hanbo Chen[1(✉)], Xiao Han[1], Xinjuan Fan[2], Xiaoying Lou[2],
Hailing Liu[2], Junzhou Huang[1], and Jianhua Yao[1]

[1] Tencent AI Lab, Shenzhen, China
hanbochen@tencent.com
[2] Sixth Affiliated Hospital of Sun Yat-sen University, Guangzhou, China

**Abstract.** Convolutional neural network (CNN) has achieved promising results in classifying histopathology images so far. However, most clinical data only has label information for the whole tissue slide and annotating every region of different tissue type is prohibitively expensive. Hence, computer aided diagnosis of whole slide images (WSIs) is challenging due to: (1) a WSI contains tissues with different types but it is classified by the most malignant tissue; (2) the gigapixel size of WSIs makes loading the whole image and end-to-end CNN training computationally infeasible. Previous works tended to classify WSI patch-wisely using the whole slide label and overlooked one useful information: it is an error to classify a patch as higher-grade classes. To address this, we propose a rectified cross-entropy loss as a combination of soft pooling and hard pooling of discriminative patches. We also introduce an upper transition loss to restrain errors. Our experimental results on colon polyp WSIs showed that, the two new losses can effectively guide the CNN optimization. With only WSI class information available for training, the patch-wise classification results on the testing set largely agree with human experts' domain knowledge.

**Keywords:** Whole slide histopathology image · Weakly supervised classifier · Rectified cross-entropy · Upper transition loss

## 1 Introduction

Histopathology image analysis plays a critical role in the cancer diagnosis [1]. The emerging whole slide scan technique is now changing pathologists' workflow with the assistance of computer-aided diagnosis (CAD) system [2]. The growing amount of digital histopathology images also brings opportunity of training machine learning algorithms for automatic cancer classification and segmentation [3].

As the state-of-art image classifier of today, convolutional neural network (CNN) has achieved remarkable performance in many medical image analysis tasks and has been widely applied in CAD systems [4]. However, in our view, there are two challenges limiting the direct use of CNN in training classifiers for whole slide tissue images (WSIs). First, although a WSI contains tissues of various degrees of abnormality, clinical reports usually only focus on the most severe type of abnormality tissue

© Springer Nature Switzerland AG 2019
D. Shen et al. (Eds.): MICCAI 2019, LNCS 11764, pp. 351–359, 2019.
https://doi.org/10.1007/978-3-030-32239-7_39

observed. In extreme cases, it is possible that only less than 1% cells on a WSI are cancerous while the rest are normal. Second, the gigapixel size of WSIs makes loading the whole image and end-to-end training computationally infeasible.

One solution is to manually annotate the regions of interest (ROIs) of different tissue types and acquire training samples in those ROIs. However, it requires comprehensive domain knowledge and is labor-intensive, which makes it hard to scale up the scope of the study. Another critical problem is that since different types of cells could be mixed, it is not an intuitive task to draw a clear boundary to delineate them.

Another way is to first sample patches on WSIs, and then train machine learning algorithms to automatically identify the discriminative regions associated with each class. For instance, Hou et al. [5] proposed to assign the label of an WSI to all the patches extracted from it and train a CNN to classify patches. In the training loop of CNN, all patches are initially taken as training samples and then the patches with lower classification probability are iteratively eliminated from the training set. In [6], the authors extended this approach by first clustering patches by its appearance and then cluster-wisely excluding the patches that are less discriminative for the classification task. Those approaches are simple and effective to learn patch-wise features of WSI classification. However, they all used hard sampling method, which makes a binary decision when selecting training samples. In practice, the samples on the boundary between classes could have a prediction probability around 50%. These samples play a critical role in delineating the class boundary. Simply excluding them from training samples may affect training performance.

In addition, we notice an overlooked information that could help improve the WSI classification – the label of WSIs are defined in a hierarchical way. In clinical data, the label of a WSI is usually assigned by the most severe phenotype that can be observed. For instance, a WSI of colon histopathology tissue will be classified as adenocarcinoma when related cancerous cells are observed and other less important findings such as adenoma may not be reported. We think the hierarchical relation between WSI classes could potentially improves the performance of WSI classifiers.

Given those observations, in this paper, we propose two new losses for weakly supervised training of WSI classifier. (1) We introduce rectified cross-entropy loss to create a soft-weighted zone for samples close to the decision boundary. (2) We design an upper transition loss to penalize the classifier when a training sample is classified as a higher tier phenotype than it should be. Our experimental result showed that, with the new losses, CNN could be more effectively trained to classify the patches by using WSI label only and could be a potential tool to unveil properties in large WSIs.

## 2   Methods

Our proposed method is outlined in Fig. 1. The training objective is to correctly classify WSI foreground patches with only WSI-level label information. Formally, each WSI is taken as a bag $X_i$ and the foreground patches extracted from it are taken as instances: $X_i = \{x_{i,1}, x_{i,2}, \ldots, x_{i,N_i}\}$. In training data, only the class of WSI is known: $\langle X_i, Y_i \rangle$, and two assumptions stand: (1) it is not necessary for all $x_{ij} \ni X_i$ to be classified as $Y_i$, but at least a certain $\rho$ percent of $X_i$ should be classified as $Y_i$: $\sum_{x_{i,j} \ni X_i} P(Y_i|x_{i,j})/N_i > \rho$. (2) The classes are hierarchical ordered such that the patches should not be classified into higher-level class than it actually belongs to, i.e., $P(y, x_{i,j}) = 0$ when $Y_i < y$. Classifying low-level class patch into high-level class is called upper transition and is taken as an error. To meet the first assumption, we design rectified cross-entropy loss $L_{RCE}$. For the second assumption, upper transition loss $L_{UT}$ is introduced to regulate the training. The objective function of optimization is then summarized below:

$$(\theta) = \text{argmin}_\theta L_{RCE} + \lambda L_{UT} \tag{1}$$

where $\theta$ is classifier parameters and $\lambda$ is the trade-off value. In the following sections, we will introduce in detail: (Sect. 2.1) the data preprocessing pipeline, (Sect. 2.2) rectified cross-entropy loss $L_{RCE}$, and (Sect. 2.3) upper transition loss $L_{UT}$.

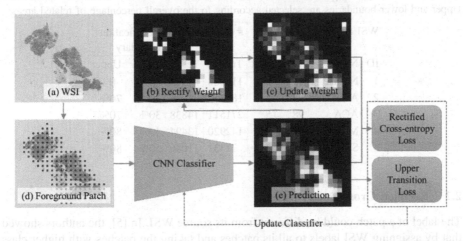

**Fig. 1.** Illustration of our proposed method. WSI foreground patches are classified by CNN separately. The classification result is then used to update sample weight to compute rectified cross-entropy loss. The upper transition loss prevents classifier from errors. (Color figure online)

## 2.1 Experimental Data

400 WSIs of H&E stained colon polyp histopathology sections are collected for this study. 5 types of colon polyps are considered: (1) normal (including hyperplastic polyp), (2) adenoma, (3) adenocarcinoma (ACA), (4) mucinous adenocarcinoma (MACA), and (5) signet ring cell carcinoma (SRCCA). The classes are ordered in the way that the class of a WSI sets an upper bound for its patch labels. For instance, for a WSI classified as adenoma, part of the tissue could be normal while no cancerous cell should be observed on this slide and thus the patches extracted from it can only be classified as either (1) normal or (2) adenoma.

WSIs are acquired by Hamamatsu NanoZoomer 2.0-RS scanner in 40 × magnification scale (229 nm/pixel). 24 WSIs are randomly selected as testing data. Since global appearance of tissue is important for diagnosis, pathologist usually prefer 10 × magnification to balance global and local view. Thus to increase receptive field and computational efficiency, our analysis is conducted in 10 × magnification scale after downsampling. Before analysis, foreground patches are extracted by a heuristic method. Since in H&E stain, foreground tissue is usually in purple, red, or blue color while background is usually white (empty) or dark gray (shadow), we simply take the colorful pixels as foreground pixels. In practice, when the difference between the maximum and the minimum RGB values is larger than 24: $\max(r, g, b) - \min(r, g, b) > 24$, we take the pixel as foreground. A sliding window of size 512 and stride 256 screens the WSI and when the percentage of foreground pixels is larger than 1/64, the patch is kept as a foreground patch. The number of WSIs and patches are summarized in Table 1.

**Table 1.** Summary of experimental data and the rectification boundary selection for each class. Upper and lower boundaries are selected according to the overall percentage of related areas.

| WSI class | | # of WSIs | | # of patches | | Rectification boundary | |
|---|---|---|---|---|---|---|---|
| ID | Name | Train | Test | Train | Test | Lower | Upper |
| 1 | Normal | 95 | 5 | 116208 | 4495 | 0% | 0% |
| 2 | Adenoma | 95 | 5 | 180112 | 7719 | 30% | 70% |
| 3 | ACA | 98 | 5 | 271511 | 14838 | 30% | 70% |
| 4 | MACA | 57 | 5 | 142920 | 13494 | 40% | 80% |
| 5 | SRCCA | 28 | 4 | 71331 | 11086 | 50% | 80% |

## 2.2 Rectified Cross-Entropy Loss

The label of a patch could be different from its source WSI. In [5], the authors showed that by assigning WSI labels to all its patches and taking the patches with higher class probability as training set, CNN prediction is close to interobserver agreement between pathologists. However, with only hard pooling, this approach is less efficient in dealing with samples close to the decision boundary. We improve this method by combining hard pooling with soft pooling. In practice, we rank the patches from a WSI $X_i$ in ascending order by their discriminative score $s_{i,j}$. The patches are then split into three groups based on their rank $r_{i,j}$: (1) muted, (2) soft pool, (3) hard pool (Fig. 2). A rectified weight $w_{i,j}$ is assigned according to their group to scale cross-entropy loss:

$$L_{RCE} = - \sum_{x_{i,j} \in X_i} w_{i,j} \log(P(Y_i | x_{i,j}, \theta)) \tag{2}$$

$$w_{i,j} = \begin{cases} 0 & r_{i,j} < \beta_l \\ (r_{i,j} - \beta_l)/(\beta_u - \beta_l) & \beta_l \le r_{i,j} < \beta_u \\ 1 & \beta_u \le r_{i,j} \end{cases} \tag{3}$$

where $\beta_l$ and $\beta_u$ are lower and upper boundary respectively. The upper boundary is the minimum percent of possible abnormal tissues among all tissues and the lower boundary is the average percent of abnormal tissues. Notably, the discriminative score $s_{i,j}$ is initially set to 1 and then iteratively updated during training by the classifier:

$$s_{i,j,t+1} = (1 - \mu)s_{i,j,t} + \mu P(Y_i | x_{i,j}, \theta_t) \tag{4}$$

where $t$ is the training epoch number, and $\mu \in [0, 1]$ is the decay parameter. As will be discussed later, since we also need to compute $L_{UT}$ for the patches even if it is not discriminative for the class it is assigned to, the patches with $w_{i,j} = 0$ will not be excluded in our training process.

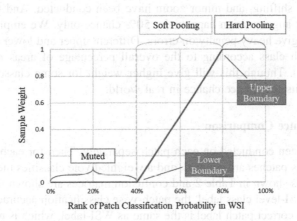

**Fig. 2.** Illustration of rectified sample weight.

## 2.3 Upper Transition Loss

Given the observation that a patch shouldn't be assigned a class label that is of higher-grade than its WSI class, heavy penalty should be given when a patch is falsely classified as higher-level classes. $L_{UT}$ is designed to enforce such penalty. To simplify the training process, $L_{UT}$ is designed in the similar form of cross-entropy:

$$L_{UT} = - \sum_{x_{i,j} \in X_i} \sum_{y_k > Y_i} \log(1 - P(y_k | x_{i,j}, \theta)) \tag{5}$$

where $y_k$ is the class that is higher than $Y_i$. $L_{UT}$ can also be viewed as the loss of multi-instance classification task. Here, $1 - P(y_k | x_{i,j}, \theta)$ is the predicted probability that the instance $x_{i,j}$ must not belongs to class $y_k$.

# 3  Results

## 3.1  Implementation

Our proposed method is implemented with TensorFlow (https://www.tensorflow.org/) and Python. To evaluate the performance, two well-established CNN architectures, Resnet50 [7] and Densenet169 [8] have been tested. We also tried to train classifier without $L_{UT}$ and compared the result. Adam optimizer with 0.0001 initial learning rate is used to update the CNN parameters. To balance the number of training samples between classes, samples are randomly picked from each class in turn such that the same number of samples of each class are fed to the training process. To avoid overfitting, random online augmentation including image flip, hue shifting, brightness scaling, channel shifting, and minor zoom have been conducted. And to stabilize the training process, augmentation happens by 50% chance only. We empirically set $\lambda$ in Eq. (1) to 10 to give heavy penalty on errors. Different upper and lower boundaries are selected for each class according to the overall percentage of areas related to WSI classes (Table 1). Though this will give higher weight for some classes, the value is consistent with its occurrence chance in real world.

## 3.2  Performance Comparison

Prediction has been conducted on each patch separately. Then for each WSI, the predicted class of its patches are counted, and a weighted vote classifies the WSI. A summary of results is shown in Table 2 and confusion matrices are shown in Fig. 3. Since we only have WSI-level class label, the patch-wise classification accuracy is computed by assuming the correct patch label is the same as WSI-label, which is not precise. For more accurate analysis, we also analyze the reliable part of the data. Specifically, we computed upper transition rate – the percentage of patches wrongly classified as higher-level classes, and normal recall – the percent of normal patches correctly classified. Because the number of patches in testing set is significantly different between classes, for fair comparison, different weights are assigned to patches from different classes such that the sum of weighted samples is the same among classes.

**Table 2.** Summary of the performance of different methods

| Method | Patch-wise analysis | | | WSI-wise analysis | |
|---|---|---|---|---|---|
| | Accuracy | Transition rate | Normal recall | 5-class accuracy | 3-class accuracy |
| Resnet50 | 55.5% | 15.90% | 35.82% | 56% | 76% |
| Densenet169 | 62.23% | 14.96% | 72.41% | 80% | 96% |
| Resnet50+$L_{RCE}$ | 58.54% | 21.03% | 34.62% | 52% | 72% |
| Densenet169+$L_{RCE}$ | 63.48% | 13.24% | 71.64% | 76% | 96% |
| Resnet50+$L_{RCE}$+$L_{UT}$ | 57.66% | 6.42% | 81.74% | 72% | 100% |
| Densenet169+$L_{RCE}$+$L_{UT}$ | 60.94% | 8.13% | 81.27% | 76% | 100% |

Reduced transition rate and increased normal recall suggesting that $L_{UT}$ is effective in preventing error. Though the patch-wise accuracy decreased, visual inspection further suggested that the classification result is closer to human knowledge by using $L_{UT}$. As highlighted by red arrows in Fig. 4(a–c), a large area of adenoma has been wrongly classified as ACA when $L_{UT}$ is absent. Though the sample's WSI label is ACA, the classifier trained with $L_{UT}$ is more accurate. Another example of adenoma WSI is shown in Fig. 4(d–f). The normal tissues have been mistakenly classified as adenoma, ACA, and even SRCCA without $L_{UT}$ regulating the training.

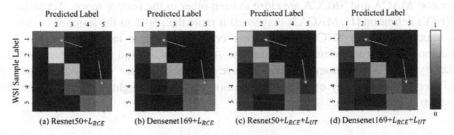

**Fig. 3.** Confusion matrix of test patch prediction by different classifiers. Each row counts the WSI label of patches and each column counts their predicted labels. Green arrows highlighted the major occurrence of transition error (normal VS. adenoma, MACA VS. SRCCA). For visualization purpose, the matrices are normalized such that each row sum up to 1. Color bar shows on the right. (Color figure online)

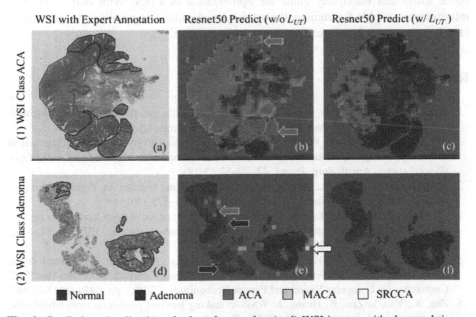

**Fig. 4.** Prediction visualization of selected examples. (a, d) WSI images with abnormal tissues outlined by expert. (b, c, e, f) Class probability color-coded prediction results overlaid on top of WSI images. Color-codes are in the bottom. (Color figure online)

By inspecting the confusion matrix of different classifiers (Fig. 3), it is intriguing that the chance of classifying a patch as the class adjacent to its WSI class is relatively high. This is in consensus with the progressive relationships between classes. For instance, it has been shown that most adenomas develop together with hyperplastic polyp [9] and carcinoma sometimes arises from adenoma [10]. Notably, the major transition error occurs either (1) between normal class and adenoma, or (2) between MACA and SRCCA (green arrows in Fig. 3). The first type of error is because most of the hyperplastic polyps in our normal samples are relatively small and thus the variation of normal tissues is not sufficient and biased. As for the second type of error, it is because MACA and SRCCA are close to each other in the feature space. According to WHO's definition [1], MACA is diagnosed if more than 50% of the lesion is composed of mucin while for SRCCA, signet-ring cells could occur in the mucin pools of mucinous adenocarcinoma. If we combine ACA, MACA, and SRCCA together and classify them as carcinoma (3-class accuracy in Table 2), our proposed method can achieve 100% accuracy on WSI classification task by a weighted voting on the histogram of patch labels.

## 4  Discussion and Conclusion

In this work, we proposed two new losses: rectified cross-entropy loss and upper transition loss for weakly supervised training of CNN for patch-wise WSI classification. Our experimental results on colon polyp WSIs showed that, the two newly proposed losses can effectively guide the optimization of CNN. With only WSI class information available for training, the patch-wise classification results on the testing set largely agrees with human experts' domain knowledge.

## References

1. Hamilton, S.R., Aaltonen, L.A.: Pathology and Genetics of Tumours of the Digestive System. International Agency for Research on Cancer Press, Lyon (2000)
2. Mukhopadhyay, S., et al.: Whole slide imaging versus microscopy for primary diagnosis in surgical pathology: a multicenter blinded randomized noninferiority study of 1992 cases (Pivotal study). Am. J. Surg. Pathol. **42**, 39–52 (2018)
3. Madabhushi, A., Lee, G.: Image analysis and machine learning in digital pathology: challenges and opportunities. Med. Image Anal. **33**, 170–175 (2016)
4. Greenspan, H., van Ginneken, B., Summers, R.M.: Guest editorial deep learning in medical imaging: overview and future promise of an exciting new technique. IEEE Trans. Med. Imaging **35**, 1153–1159 (2016)
5. Hou, L., Samaras, D., Kurc, T.M., Gao, Y., Davis, J.E., Saltz, J.H.: Patch-based convolutional neural network for whole slide tissue image classification. In: The IEEE Conference on Computer Vision and Pattern Recognition (CVPR), pp. 2424–2433 (2016)
6. Zhu, X., Yao, J., Zhu, F., Huang, J.: WSISA: making survival prediction from whole slide histopathological images. In: The IEEE Conference on Computer Vision and Pattern Recognition (CVPR), pp. 7234–7242 (2017)

7. He, K., Zhang, X., Ren, S., Sun, J.: Deep residual learning for image recognition. In: The IEEE Conference on Computer Vision and Pattern Recognition (CVPR), pp. 770–778 (2016)
8. Huang, G., Liu, Z., Weinberger, K.Q., van der Maaten, L.: Densely connected convolutional networks. In: The IEEE Conference on Computer Vision and Pattern Recognition (CVPR), pp. 4700–4708 (2017)
9. Ferrandez, A., Samowitz, W., DiSario, J.A., Burt, R.W.: Phenotypic characteristics and risk of cancer development in hyperplastic polyposis: case series and literature review. Am. J. Gastroenterol. **99**, 2012–2018 (2004)
10. Jass, J.R.: Do all colorectal carcinomas arise in preexisting adenomas? World J. Surg. **13**, 45–51 (1989)

# From Whole Slide Imaging to Microscopy: Deep Microscopy Adaptation Network for Histopathology Cancer Image Classification

Yifan Zhang[1,2], Hanbo Chen[2], Ying Wei[2], Peilin Zhao[2], Jiezhang Cao[1],
Xinjuan Fan[3], Xiaoying Lou[3], Hailing Liu[3], Jinlong Hou[2], Xiao Han[2],
Jianhua Yao[2], Qingyao Wu[1(✉)], Mingkui Tan[1(✉)], and Junzhou Huang[2(✉)]

[1] South China University of Technology, Guangzhou, China
{qyw,mingkuitan}@scut.edu.cn
[2] Tencent AI Lab, Shenzhen, China
jzhuang@uta.edu
[3] Sixth Affiliated Hospital of Sun Yat-sen University, Guangzhou, China

**Abstract.** Deep learning (DL) has achieved remarkable performance on digital pathology image classification with whole slide images (WSIs). Unfortunately, high acquisition costs of WSIs hinder the applications in practical scenarios, and most pathologists still use microscopy images (MSIs) in their workflows. However, it is especially challenging to train DL models on MSIs, given limited image qualities and high annotation costs. Alternatively, directly applying a WSI-trained DL model on MSIs usually performs poorly due to huge gaps between WSIs and MSIs. To address these issues, we propose to exploit deep unsupervised domain adaptation to adapt DL models trained on the labeled WSI domain to the unlabeled MSI domain. Specifically, we propose a novel Deep Microscopy Adaptation Network (DMAN). By reducing domain discrepancies via adversarial learning and entropy minimization, and alleviating class imbalance with sample reweighting, DMAN can classify MSIs effectively even without MSI annotations. Extensive experiments on colon cancer diagnosis demonstrate the effectiveness of DMAN and its potential in customizing models for each pathologist's microscope.

**Keywords:** Histopathology image classification · Unsupervised domain adaptation · Deep learning · Microscopy image · While slide image

## 1 Introduction

Histopathology image is a gold standard for clinical diagnosis of cancer [1,2]. By examining processed tissue slides, pathologists are able to identify abnormal

---

Y. Zhang, H. Chen and Y. Wei are co-first authors.

© Springer Nature Switzerland AG 2019
D. Shen et al. (Eds.): MICCAI 2019, LNCS 11764, pp. 360–368, 2019.
https://doi.org/10.1007/978-3-030-32239-7_40

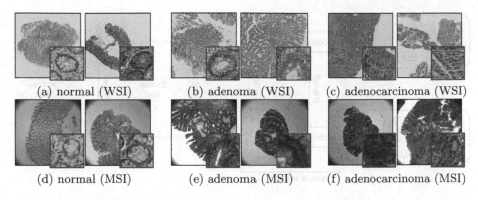

(a) normal (WSI)          (b) adenoma (WSI)          (c) adenocarcinoma (WSI)

(d) normal (MSI)          (e) adenoma (MSI)          (f) adenocarcinoma (MSI)

**Fig. 1.** Examples of the inter-domain discrepancy between WSIs (a–c) and MSIs (d–f), and the intra-domain discrepancy in each category. Bottom right of each subfigure shows the zoomed view.

tissues, pinpoint cancer types, and differentiate cancer stages at the cell level. Notably, this task is highly labor intensive and requires extensive expertise. Hence, computer-aided diagnosis (CAD) has been in great demand [3–5].

Despite success of deep learning (DL) [6–8] in medical image analysis, it hinges on massive annotated images for training [2]. Thanks to digital slide scan devices and hence a growing number of labeled whole slide images (WSIs), remarkable performance has been achieved on digital pathology image classification (DPIC) tasks, such as colon cancer diagnosis [9] and survival analysis [10].

However, due to high acquisition costs of WSIs, pathologists still largely rely on microscopes in their workflows. This brings the need for CAD systems for microscopy images (MSIs), where MSIs captured by digital cameras are fed into computers as a stream for analysis. Unfortunately, it is even more challenging to train DL models on MSIs due to: (1) variances of microscope devices in, *e.g.,* light sources, scope shades and view fields; (2) varied preferences of pathologists, *e.g.,* some pathologists prefer darker light; (3) wild imaging environments with white noises, motion blurs and losses of focus. To combat these challenges, one attractive option is to customize models for each pathologist with a small number of MSIs gathered on his or her own device. However, annotation costs for such customized MSIs are inevitably expensive. To this end, we are motivated to leverage labeled data in the WSI domain to improve the performance in the unlabeled MSI domain. This problem, known as deep unsupervised domain adaptation (DUDA) [11–13], remains largely unexplored for MSIs [1].

DUDA from WSIs to MSIs poses three challenges. As shown in Fig. 1, the first challenge is the inter-domain discrepancy, mainly derived from different imaging devices and techniques [1]. In this regard, directly applying a WSI-trained model to MSIs tends to perform poorly and be impractical. The second challenge lies in the intra-domain discrepancy, which originates from inconsistent data preparations, such as tissue collections, sectioning and staining [14]. Such inconsistency would result in intra-class inhomogeneity and raise the difficulty

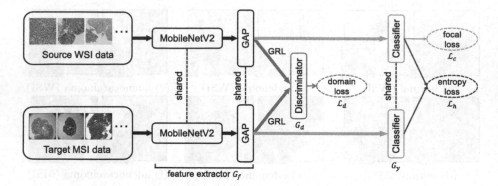

**Fig. 2.** The scheme of Deep Microscopy Adaptation Network, where GAP means Global Average Pooling [6] and GRL denotes Gradient Reverse Layer [11]. Considering the practical requirement of low computational cost and high inference speed, we implement MobileNetV2 [6], a highly efficient deep convolutional network, to extract features and predict classes.

of DPIC [15]. Lastly, class imbalance makes it particularly difficult to classify minor but important categories [2], *e.g.*, the adenocarcinoma in Fig. 1. However, most DUDA methods for general images [11–13] and for WSIs [14,16,17] neglect the intra-domain discrepancy and class imbalance, hence performing poorly in this task.

To solve these challenges, we propose a novel Deep Microscopy Adaptation Network (DMAN) algorithm. Specifically, we minimize both domain discrepancies via adversarial learning and entropy minimization, while alleviating class imbalance with sample reweighting. In this way, DMAN is able to learn domain-invariant and discriminative features which contribute to DPIC of MSIs with only labeled WSIs. Notably, this approach eliminates the need for annotating MSIs and helps to customize models for each pathologist's microscope, thus showing great potential for real-world applications.

## 2   Method

### 2.1   Problem Definition

This paper studies deep unsupervised domain adaptation (DUDA) from WSIs to MSIs. In this case, WSIs are well-labeled as the source domain, while the target domain (*i.e.*, MSIs) is fully unlabeled. Formally, we formulate source data as $\mathcal{D}_s = \{\mathbf{x}_i^s, y_i^s\}_{i=1}^{n_s}$, where $\mathbf{x}_i^s$ denotes the $i$-th WSI with $y_i^s$ as its label, and $n_s$ is the total number of WSIs. Meanwhile, target data is denoted as $\mathcal{D}_t = \{\mathbf{x}_j^t\}_{j=1}^{n_t}$, where $\mathbf{x}_j^t$ is the $j$-th MSI and $n_t$ is the number of unlabeled MSIs. Both domains have the same label space with $C$ classes. The goal of this paper is to learn a deep neural network, $G_y(G_f(\mathbf{x})) \to y$, which learns domain-invariant features $G_f(\mathbf{x})$ for both domains, so that the classifier $G_y(\cdot)$ trained with labeled WSIs can also apply to unlabeled MSIs. To this end, we propose a novel Deep Microscopy Adaptation Network (DMAN).

## 2.2 Deep Microscopy Adaptation Network

As shown in Fig. 2, DMAN consists of three key components: a deep convolutional network $G_f$ for feature representation, a classifier $G_y$ for prediction, and a domain discriminator $G_d$ to discriminate features of WSIs from those of MSIs.

To overcome the three challenges described in Sect. 1, i.e., inter-domain discrepancy, intra-domain discrepancy, and class imbalance for classification, we train DMAN with the following three strategies, respectively. First, we adopt domain adversarial learning [13] to enforce $G_f$ to learn domain-invariant features, so that the inter-domain discrepancy is minimized. On one hand, a domain discriminator $G_d$ is trained by minimizing a domain classification loss $\mathcal{L}_d$ to adequately distinguish feature representations between WSIs and MSIs; on the other hand, the feature extractor $G_f$ is trained to confuse the discriminator by maximizing $\mathcal{L}_d$. Following [11,14], we implement the adversarial optimization with a gradient reversal layer (GRL) which reverses the gradient $\nabla\mathcal{L}_d$ when backpropagating $\nabla\mathcal{L}_d$ to $G_f$. Second, to alleviate the intra-domain discrepancy and encourage intra-class homogeneity, we train the base network $(G_f, G_y)$ by minimizing the prediction entropy $\mathcal{L}_h$. Third, we also exploit a class classification loss $\mathcal{L}_c$, namely focal loss, to train the imbalance-aware and discriminative base network $(G_f, G_y)$. We summarize the overall optimization procedure as follows:

$$(\hat{\theta}_f, \hat{\theta}_y) = \underset{\theta_f, \theta_y}{\text{argmin}}\ \underbrace{-\alpha\mathcal{L}_d}_{\text{domain loss}}\ +\ \underbrace{\beta\mathcal{L}_h}_{\text{entropy loss}}\ +\ \underbrace{\mu\mathcal{L}_c}_{\text{focal loss}}\ ,$$

$$(\hat{\theta}_d) = \underset{\theta_d}{\text{argmin}}\ \underbrace{\alpha\mathcal{L}_d}_{\text{domain loss}}\ , \tag{1}$$

where $\theta_f$, $\theta_y$ and $\theta_d$ indicate parameters of $G_f$, $G_y$ and $G_d$, respectively. Moreover, $\alpha$, $\beta$ and $\mu$ are trade-off parameters. Note that the whole training process can be implemented with standard backpropagation in an end-to-end manner.

We next detail domain classification loss $\mathcal{L}_d$ in Sect. 2.3, entropy loss $\mathcal{L}_h$ in Sect. 2.4 and class classification loss $\mathcal{L}_c$ in Sect. 2.5.

## 2.3 Adversarial Learning for Inter-domain Adaptation

Diverse imaging devices and techniques intrinsically result in huge domain discrepancies between WSIs and MSIs. To resolve the discrepancies, as we mentioned above, we resort to domain adversarial learning. Specifically, as shown in Eq. (1), the key is to train the domain discriminator $G_d$ and the feature extractor $G_f$ via a minimax optimization problem regarding the domain loss. To this end, most existing methods [11,13] adopt the generative adversarial loss [7] as the domain classification loss $\mathcal{L}_d$:

$$-\frac{1}{n_t}\sum_{\mathbf{x}_j^t \in \mathcal{D}_t} \log\left(G_d(G_f(\mathbf{x}_j^t))\right) - \frac{1}{n_s}\sum_{\mathbf{x}_i^s \in \mathcal{D}_s} \log\left(1 - G_d(G_f(\mathbf{x}_i^s))\right), \tag{2}$$

where the domain label of the source domain is 0, and that of the target domain is 1. Such a loss with sigmoid cross-entropy only evaluates domain classification correctness but fails to measure the domain distance [18]. As a result, maximizing this loss may not guarantee an effective $G_f$ capable of learning highly domain-invariant features. Instead, inspired by LSGAN [18], we propose to use the least square loss for inter-domain adaptation:

$$\mathcal{L}_d = \frac{1}{n_t} \sum_{\mathbf{x}_j^t \in \mathcal{D}_t} \left(G_d(G_f(\mathbf{x}_j^t))-1\right)^2 + \frac{1}{n_s} \sum_{\mathbf{x}_i^s \in \mathcal{D}_s} \left(G_d(G_f(\mathbf{x}_i^s))\right)^2. \tag{3}$$

This loss, directly matching a domain label with the prediction without sigmoid, preserves domain distance. In this sense, it not only improves domain confusion but also stabilizes training, thus boosting performance of DUDA.

## 2.4   Entropy Minimization for Intra-class Homogeneity

Color, scale, resolution and intensity variations are common in WSIs and MSIs. These variations intrinsically lead to intra-class inhomogeneity in DPIC [14], and thus degrade performance of existing deep algorithms [2]. To solve this issue, we propose to impose the following entropy loss:

$$\mathcal{L}_h = -\frac{1}{n_t + n_s} \sum_{\mathbf{x}_i \in \mathcal{D}_s, \mathcal{D}_t} \sum_{k=1}^{C} G_y^k(G_f(\mathbf{x}_i)) \log \left(G_y^k(G_f(\mathbf{x}_i))\right), \tag{4}$$

where $C$ denotes the class number and $G_y^k(G_f(\cdot))$ indicates the predicted probability of class $k$. Note that, the conditional entropy is a measure of class overlaps, so minimizing entropy encourages small overlaps among classes but high compactness within a class [19], and thus alleviate intra-class inhomogeneity.

## 2.5   Focal Loss for Class-Imbalance Classification

We next detail class classification loss $\mathcal{L}_c$ based on only labeled WSIs $(\mathbf{x}_i^s, y_i^s)$. Most existing DL models for medical image classification adopt cross-entropy:

$$-\frac{1}{n_s} \sum_{(\mathbf{x}_i^s, y_i^s) \in \mathcal{D}_s} \sum_{k=1}^{C} y_{i,k}^s \log \left(G_y^k(G_f(\mathbf{x}_i^s))\right), \tag{5}$$

where $y_{i,k}^s$ means the label of the $i$-th source sample regarding class $k$. Although cross-entropy performs well in many class-balanced classification tasks, it ignores the class-imbalance issue, which is quite common in DPIC [1]. One possible solution to this issue is cost-sensitive learning, which assigns uneven misclassification costs for different classes. One critical problem here is how to define costs for multiple classes, since the ground-truth distribution of classes is unknown and complicated in real-world DPIC tasks.

Our solution is motivated by an observation that class imbalance intrinsically makes classification of minority classes more difficult. As a result, the predicted probabilities of minority classes would be lower than those of majority classes [8]. Hence, if we assign higher costs for the predictions with low probabilities but assign low costs for those with high probabilities, we can redress the imbalance better. Inspired by this observation, we propose to use the focal loss [8] as follows:

$$\mathcal{L}_c = -\frac{1}{n_s} \sum_{(\mathbf{x}_i^s, y_i^s) \in \mathcal{D}_s} \sum_{k=1}^{C} y_{i,k}^s (1 - G_y^k(G_f(\mathbf{x}_i^s)))^\gamma \log\left(G_y^k(G_f(\mathbf{x}_i^s))\right), \quad (6)$$

where $\gamma$ is a hyperparameter to determine the degree to which classification focuses on minority classes. To avoid excessive cost mitigation on majority classes, a balanced value of $\gamma$ is expected. By minimizing this loss, DMAN focuses more on minority classes and thus deals with class imbalance better.

## 3    Experimental Results

We evaluate our method on the following settings.

**Dataset:** 303 H&E stained histopathology slides, diagnosed as 3 types of colon polyps (normal, adenoma, and adenocarcinoma), are provided by the Sixth Affiliated Hospital of Sun Yat-sen University. WSI of each slide is acquired in 40× magnification scale (229 nm/pixel) by the Hamamatsu NanoZoomer 2.0-RS scanner. ROIs corresponding to the 3 types are then annotated by experts on WSI scans with our in-house tool. MSIs of 30 slides are acquired with microscope in 10× magnification scale (FOV: 2.73 × 2.73 mm$^2$, matrix size: 2048 × 2048). Specifically, we focus on 10× magnification scale, since it is the preferred scale for pathologist's diagnosis. For consistency, WSIs are down-sampled to the same resolution as MSIs. Then, a sliding window crops MSIs and annotated WSI regions into patches of size 512. The label of each patch is defined by the annotation in its center. WSI and MSI patches acquired from 15 slides are taken as the testing set, and the rest serves as the training set. Data statistics are shown in Table 1.

**Table 1.** Statistics of dataset

| Domain | Training set | | | | Test set | | | |
|---|---|---|---|---|---|---|---|---|
| | normal | adenoma | adenocarcinoma | Total | normal | adenoma | adenocarcinoma | Total |
| WSI | 36,047 | 3,627 | 3,080 | 42,754 | 1,944 | 201 | 223 | 2,368 |
| MSI | 2,696 | 1,042 | 1,084 | 4,822 | 1,110 | 487 | 713 | 2,310 |

**Baselines:** We first compare DMAN with two baselines directly trained on WSIs, including **Source-only-C** (with cross-entropy loss) and **Source-only** (with focal loss). We also evaluate two other baselines that harness the collective power of WSIs and annotated MSIs, including **Fine-tuning** (finetuning the model on WSIs with 500 labeled MSIs), and **Mix** (training with a mixture of WSIs and 500 labeled MSIs). We also compare DMAN with several state-of-the-art DUDA methods, including **DDC** [12], **DANN** [11], and **ADDA** [13]. For fair comparison, all methods employ the same network structure to DMAN but with different losses and optimization rules. For completeness, we also evaluate two variants of DMAN, *i.e.*, **DMAN-F** (using focal loss as the domain loss) and **DMAN-H** (without the entropy loss).

**Implementation Details and Metrics:** We implement DMAN with Tensorflow. The discriminator consists of three fully connected layers with 1024, 1024 and 1 hidden units, respectively. We use Adam optimizer with the batch size 16 and fixed learning rate $10^{-5}$ on a single GPU. Moreover, we set $\mu = 1$, $\gamma = 2$, $\alpha = 0.1$ and $\beta = 0.1$. Ablation studies are not included due to space limit. We use Accuracy, mean Precision, mean Recall and F1-measure as the **metrics**.

### 3.1 Evaluation on Digital Pathology Image Classification

From the results in Table 2, we are able to draw several conclusions. **First,** we observe apparent discrepancies between WSIs and MSIs, evidenced by the performance gap between testing Source-only on WSIs and on MSIs. Moreover, the superiority of Source-only over Source-only-C on MSIs confirms the effectiveness of the focal loss in alleviating class imbalance. **Second,** fine-tuning with limited labeled MSIs improves slightly over Source-only due to over-fitting. Although Mix performs better than Fine-tuning, it also suffers from over-fitting and performs unsatisfactorily. **Third,** all DUDA methods outperform Source-only. Notably, DMAN and DANN (without labeled MSIs) even outperform Mix (with labeled MSIs). These observations demonstrate positive contributions of DUDA to DPIC tasks. **Lastly,** DMAN-based methods outperform all other baselines. This validates not only the superiority of our method but also its potential for customizing to each pathologist's microscope. Moreover, the improvement of DMAN over DMAN-F and DMAN-H validates the necessity of least square domain loss and entropy loss.

### 3.2 Visualization of Feature Representations

We visualize t-SNE embeddings of learned features after the GAP layer. Take the adenoma class as an example. Figure 3(a) displays the domain discrepancy between WSIs and MSIs. Figure 3(b–c) show that DDC and DANN fail to reduce the inter-domain discrepancy and suffer from intra-class inhomogeneity. Figure 3(d) displays that DMAN can well resolve both inter-domain and intra-domain discrepancies.

**Table 2.** Comparisons on DPIC in terms of four metrics (%), where Labeled Set and Test Set indicate the labeled set for training and evaluation, respectively.

| Methods | Labeled set | Test set | Accuracy | Precision | Recall | F1-measure |
|---|---|---|---|---|---|---|
| Source-only | WSI | WSI | 93.67 | 83.77 | 93.03 | 87.16 |
| Source-only-C | WSI | MSI | 82.21 | 87.78 | 76.15 | 78.55 |
| Source-only | WSI | MSI | 83.72 | 88.48 | 78.59 | 81.10 |
| Fine-tuning | Both | MSI | 85.02 | 83.47 | 85.40 | 84.15 |
| Mix | Both | MSI | 87.53 | 86.68 | 87.16 | 86.91 |
| DDC | WSI | MSI | 87.14 | 85.96 | 88.60 | 86.96 |
| ADDA | WSI | MSI | 85.11 | 86.55 | 83.51 | 84.72 |
| DANN | WSI | MSI | 88.01 | 88.60 | 87.17 | 87.82 |
| DMAN-F | WSI | MSI | 88.57 | 89.27 | 87.83 | 88.50 |
| DMAN-H | WSI | MSI | 89.09 | 90.17 | 88.21 | 89.10 |
| DMAN | WSI | MSI | **90.48** | **90.67** | **90.35** | **90.50** |

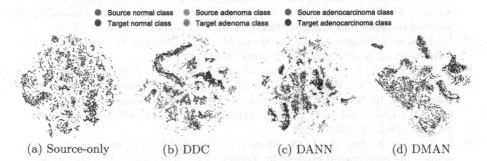

● Source normal class   ● Source adenoma class   ● Source adenocarcinoma class
● Target normal class   ● Target adenoma class   ● Target adenocarcinoma class

(a) Source-only        (b) DDC        (c) DANN        (d) DMAN

**Fig. 3.** t-SNE plots in terms of classes and domains, where clusters of the adenoma are circled. The closer samples across domains with the same class are, the more effective domain adaptation is.

## 4   Conclusion

We have proposed the novel DMAN[1] for adapting WSI-trained networks to predict MSIs. In detail, we propose to reduce inter-domain discrepancy with adversarial learning and diminish intra-domain discrepancy using entropy minimization. Moreover, we exploit the focal loss to effectively alleviate the class-imbalance issue. In this way, DMAN conduct DPIC of MSIs effectively based on only labeled WSIs. Promising experiments demonstrate the effectiveness of DMAN and its potential in customizing models to each pathologist's microscope.

---

[1] This work was partially supported by National Natural Science Foundation of China (NSFC) (61876208, 61502177 and 61602185), Guangdong Provincial Scientific and Technological Fund (2017B090901008, 2017A010101011, 2017B090910005, 2018B010107001), Pearl River S&T Nova Program of Guangzhou 201806010081, CCF-Tencent Open Research Fund RAGR20170105, Program for Guangdong Introducing Innovative and Entrepreneurial Teams 2017ZT07X183.

# References

1. Xing, F., Xie, Y., Su, H., Liu, F., Yang, L.: Deep learning in microscopy image analysis: a survey. TNNLS **29**, 1–19 (2018)
2. Litjens, G., Kooi, T., Bejnordi, B.E., Setio, A., Ciompi, F., Snchez, C.I.: A survey on deep learning in medical image analysis. Med. Image Anal. **42**, 60–88 (2017)
3. Becker, C., et al.: Domain adaptation for microscopy imaging. TMI **34**, 1125–1139 (2015)
4. Bermúdez-Chacón, R., Becker, C., Salzmann, M., Fua, P.: Scalable unsupervised domain adaptation for electron microscopy. In: Ourselin, S., Joskowicz, L., Sabuncu, M.R., Unal, G., Wells, W. (eds.) MICCAI 2016. LNCS, vol. 9901, pp. 326–334. Springer, Cham (2016). https://doi.org/10.1007/978-3-319-46723-8_38
5. Heimann, T., Mountney, P., John, M., Ionasec, R.: Learning without labeling: domain adaptation for ultrasound transducer localization. In: Mori, K., Sakuma, I., Sato, Y., Barillot, C., Navab, N. (eds.) MICCAI 2013. LNCS, vol. 8151, pp. 49–56. Springer, Heidelberg (2013). https://doi.org/10.1007/978-3-642-40760-4_7
6. Sandler, M., Howard, A., Zhu, M., Zhmoginov, A., Chen, L.C.: MobileNetV2: inverted residuals and linear bottlenecks. In: CVPR, pp. 4510–4520 (2018)
7. Goodfellow, I., Pouget-Abadie, J., Mirza, M., Xu, B., Bengio, Y.: Generative adversarial nets. In: NeurIPS, pp. 2672–2680 (2014)
8. Lin, T.Y., et al.: Focal loss for dense object detection. In: ICCV (2017)
9. Armin, M.A., et al.: Visibility map: a new method in evaluation quality of optical colonoscopy. In: Navab, N., Hornegger, J., Wells, W.M., Frangi, A.F. (eds.) MICCAI 2015. LNCS, vol. 9349, pp. 396–404. Springer, Cham (2015). https://doi.org/10.1007/978-3-319-24553-9_49
10. Li, R., Yao, J., Zhu, X., Li, Y., Huang, J.: Graph CNN for survival analysis on whole slide pathological images. In: Frangi, A.F., Schnabel, J.A., Davatzikos, C., Alberola-López, C., Fichtinger, G. (eds.) MICCAI 2018. LNCS, vol. 11071, pp. 174–182. Springer, Cham (2018). https://doi.org/10.1007/978-3-030-00934-2_20
11. Ganin, Y., Lempitsky, V.: Unsupervised domain adaptation by backpropagation. In: ICML, pp. 1180–1189 (2015)
12. Tzeng, E., Hoffman, J., Zhang, N., Saenko, K., Darrell, T.: Deep domain confusion: maximizing for domain invariance. arXiv:1412.3474 (2014)
13. Tzeng, E., et al.: Adversarial discriminative domain adaptation. In: CVPR (2017)
14. Lafarge, M.W., Pluim, J.P.W., Eppenhof, K.A.J., Moeskops, P., Veta, M.: Domain-adversarial neural networks to address the appearance variability of histopathology images. In: Cardoso, M.J., et al. (eds.) DLMIA/ML-CDS 2017. LNCS, vol. 10553, pp. 83–91. Springer, Cham (2017). https://doi.org/10.1007/978-3-319-67558-9_10
15. Mangin, J.F.: Entropy minimization for automatic correction of intensity nonuniformity. In: Workshop on MMBIA (2000)
16. Wollmann, T., Eijkman, C.S., Rohr, K.: Adversarial domain adaptation to improve automatic breast cancer grading in lymph nodes. In: ISBI, pp. 582–585 (2018)
17. Ren, J., Hacihaliloglu, I., Singer, E.A., Foran, D.J., Qi, X.: Adversarial domain adaptation for classification of prostate histopathology whole-slide images. In: Frangi, A.F., Schnabel, J.A., Davatzikos, C., Alberola-López, C., Fichtinger, G. (eds.) MICCAI 2018. LNCS, vol. 11071, pp. 201–209. Springer, Cham (2018). https://doi.org/10.1007/978-3-030-00934-2_23
18. Mao, X., et al.: Least squares generative adversarial networks. In: ICCV (2017)
19. Grandvalet, Y., Bengio, Y.: Semi-supervised learning by entropy minimization. In: NeurIPS (2005)

# Multi-scale Cell Instance Segmentation with Keypoint Graph Based Bounding Boxes

Jingru Yi[1][(✉)], Pengxiang Wu[1], Qiaoying Huang[1], Hui Qu[1], Bo Liu[2],
Daniel J. Hoeppner[3], and Dimitris N. Metaxas[1]

[1] Department of Computer Science, Rutgers University, Piscataway, NJ 08854, USA
{jy486,pw241,qh55,hq43,dnm}@cs.rutgers.edu
[2] JD Digits, Mountain View, CA 94043, USA
[3] Lieber Institute for Brain Development, Baltimore, MD 21205, USA

**Abstract.** Most existing methods handle cell instance segmentation problems directly without relying on additional detection boxes. These methods generally fails to separate touching cells due to the lack of global understanding of the objects. In contrast, box-based instance segmentation solves this problem by combining object detection with segmentation. However, existing methods typically utilize anchor box-based detectors, which would lead to inferior instance segmentation performance due to the class imbalance issue. In this paper, we propose a new box-based cell instance segmentation method. In particular, we first detect the five pre-defined points of a cell via keypoints detection. Then we group these points according to a keypoint graph and subsequently extract the bounding box for each cell. Finally, cell segmentation is performed on feature maps within the bounding boxes. We validate our method on two cell datasets with distinct object shapes, and empirically demonstrate the superiority of our method compared to other instance segmentation techniques. Code is available at: https://github.com/yijingru/KG_Instance_Segmentation.

**Keywords:** Instance segmentation · Detection · Cell segmentation

## 1 Introduction

Instance segmentation plays an important role in biomedical tasks such as cell migration study [9] and cell nuclei detection [11]. This problem requires not only classifying the objects, but also separating them from the neighboring instances. The main challenges in cell instance segmentation involve low contrast of cell boundaries, background impurities, cell adhesion and cell clustering.

To handle cell instance segmentation, one representative class of methods focus on segmenting the cell instances directly without the aid of bounding boxes. These box-free methods generally fail to separate the touching cells due

© Springer Nature Switzerland AG 2019
D. Shen et al. (Eds.): MICCAI 2019, LNCS 11764, pp. 369–377, 2019.
https://doi.org/10.1007/978-3-030-32239-7_41

to the lack of global understanding of the objects. For example, DCAN [1] proposes to extract cell instances by overlapping their contours onto the semantic segmentation results. While being efficient, DCAN tends to produce over-segmentation due to the fuzzy contours between the touching cells. STARDIST [11] suggests using convex polygons to separate cells, but with an assumption that the cell shape should be convex. CosineEmbedding [9] proposes to retrieve the cell instance by clustering the pixel embeddings. However, it tends to incur large number of false positives due to the separate clustering results for each individual cell.

To overcome the weakness of box-free instance segmentation, recent studies have sought to incorporate object detection into segmentation. These box-based methods first localize the cells via bounding boxes, and then perform individual cell segmentation on the regions defined by the bounding boxes. One major advantage of such methods is that they are able to distinguish cells based on their global object features instead of the local pixel-level information (e.g., boundary). As a result, box-based instance segmentation is more powerful in separating touching cells compared to the box-free strategies.

For box-based methods, a good object detector plays a critical role in the instance segmentation performance. However, previous methods (e.g., FCIS [6] and Mask R-CNN [3]) generally adopt anchor box-based detectors, which suffer from a severe imbalance between the number of positive and negative anchor boxes [5]. Recently, keypoints-based detectors are developed to solve the aforementioned problem. As one representative example, CornerNet [5] proposes to detect the top-left and bottom-right points of an object for the generation of bounding box proposals, and achieves better accuracy than the anchor box-based detectors. However, such design also makes CornerNet prone to losing box proposals due to the missing detection of any corner points.

In this paper, we propose a new box-based cell instance segmentation method. In particular, we detect the top-left, top-right, bottom-left, bottom-right, and the center points of a cell rectangle using keypoints detection. Our motivation is that a bounding box can be represented by any three points or any pair of diagonal points among the five points. In this way, we effectively increase the probability of retrieving bounding boxes even when some keypoints are undetected. To generate bounding boxes, we group these points for each cell instance according to a keypoint graph. To further improve the detection accuracy, we use multi-scale feature maps to detect cells of different sizes. Cell segmentation is subsequently performed on feature maps cropped by the bounding box. We evaluate our method on two different cell datasets, and demonstrate its superiority in the instance segmentation of cells with different shapes.

## 2   Method

The overview of our box-based instance segmentation framework is shown in Fig. 1. We use a ResNet-50 Conv1-4 [4] as the backbone network. The framework comprises two branches: keypoints detection branch (Fig. 1a) and individual cell segmentation branch (Fig. 1b). We illustrate the flowchart of generating cell bounding boxes in Fig. 1c.

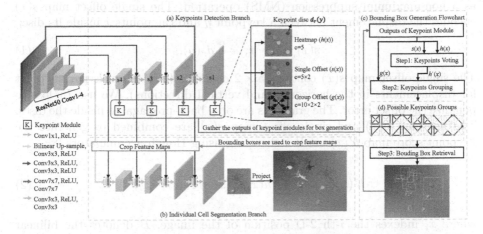

**Fig. 1.** Multi-scale cell instance segmentation framework. We use a ResNet-50 Conv1-4 [4] as the backbone network. The framework contains two branches: (a) keypoints detection branch and (b) individual cell segmentation branch. The keypoint module outputs the heatmap $h(x)$, single offset map $s(x)$, and group offset map $g(x)$ that will be used for bounding box generation. $x$ represents a 2-D position in the map, $y$ is a 2-D position of the keypoint, $c$ indicates the channel of the map and $s$ denotes the scales. The red, blue, pink, green, yellow circles on these maps indicate the top-left, top-right, bottom-left, bottom-right and center points, respectively. (c) shows the bounding box generation flowchart, where $h'(x)$ is the keypoint score map. (d) illustrates the possible keypoints groups that are used for box retrieval. (Color figure online)

## 2.1 Bounding Box Generation

To obtain the bounding boxes of cells, we propose to detect the top-left, top-right, bottom-left, bottom-right, and the center points of a cell rectangle using keypoints detection. The keypoints detection branch is shown in Fig. 1a, which outputs the heatmap $h(x)$, the single offset map $s(x)$ and the group offset map $g(x)$ at each scale $s_i, i = 1, 2, 3, 4$, for keypoints voting and grouping. $x$ represents a 2-D position (horizontal and vertical coordinates) in the image maps. Bounding boxes are then extracted according to the flowchart of Fig. 1c.

*Step1: Keypoints voting.* The keypoints voting takes two maps as input: the heatmap $h(x)$ and the single offset map $s(x)$. Heatmap is commonly applied in human pose estimation [7,8] to predict the possibility of keypoints locations, which is a binary classification problem. To create the heatmap, we place a disc $d_r(y) = \{x : ||x-y|| \leq r\}$ around each keypoint $y$ (see Fig. 1a), where $y$ denotes a 2-D position of a keypoint, and $r = 5$ is the radius of the disc. The heatmap $h(x)$ contains 5 channels (one channel per keypoint), where $h(x) = 1$ for $x \in d_r(y)$, otherwise $h(x) = 0$. We use binary cross entropy loss to optimize the parameters. After obtaining the heatmap of the keypoints, we use a single offset map $s(x)$ [8] to extract the local maxima for each heatmap disc on $h(x)$. This can be viewed as a non-maximum suppression (NMS) operation. The single offset map $s(x)$ encodes the displacement between a keypoint $y$ and the points $x$ inside its disc:

$$s(x) = y - x, \ x \in d_r(y). \tag{1}$$

The single offset map $s(x)$ contains $5 \times 2$ channels (two channels per keypoint for displacements in the horizontal and vertical directions). We use $L_1$ loss to penalize the offset error. The gradients are only back-propagated inside the discs. The heatmap $h(x)$ and single offset map $s(x)$ are combined to generate the keypoint score map $h'(x)$ via Hough voting using Hough accumulators [8]:

$$h'(x) = \frac{1}{\pi r^2} \sum_{i=1}^{N} h(x_i) B(x_i + s(x_i) - x), \tag{2}$$

where $x_i$ indexes the $i$-th 2-D position of the image, $B$ denotes the bilinear interpolation kernel.

*Step2: Keypoints grouping.* The local maxima in the keypoint score map $h'(x)$ represent the candidate positions of the keypoints. We apply a maximum filter to $h'(x)$ and extract the keypoint locations via a peak threshold (0.004). After obtaining the keypoints, our next step is to group the keypoints for each cell instance. We propose a keypoint graph to group the keypoints, where the five types of keypoints are the vertices of the keypoint graph. We use a group offset to connect each pair of keypoints bi-directionally. In particular, for a pair of keypoints $(k, l)$ of a particular cell instance, the group offset from the $k$-th keypoint to the $l$-th keypoint is given by

$$g_{k,l}(x) = (y_l - x), x \in d_r(y_k). \tag{3}$$

The group offset map $g(x)$ has $10 \times 2 \times 2$ channels (two channels per pair of keypoints for displacements in the horizontal and vertical directions). The same to single offset map, we compute the $L_1$ loss to optimize the parameters and only back-propagate the loss at locations inside the keypoint discs. To group the keypoints, we first put all the detected keypoints into a queue and sort them according to their scores on $h'(x)$. Then we pop the keypoint out of the queue in a descending order iteratively, and greedily connect the $(k, l)$ pair of keypoints using $g(x)$. At each iteration, we reject a repetitive detection by checking if the positions of two keypoints are within a disc.

*Step3: Bounding box retrieval.* After aggregating the keypoint groups at scales $s_1, s_2, s_3, s_4$, our next step is to generate the bounding box for each cell instance. Figure 1d shows the possible keypoint groups that can be transformed to a full box. It can be seen that any three points or any pair of diagonal points in the keypoint graph can retrieve a box, which decreases the possibility of losing box proposals due to undetected points. We avoid detecting the same object multiple times by applying NMS.

## 2.2   Cell Segmentation

After obtaining the bounding boxes for all cell instances in the input images, we perform the individual cell segmentation for each cell instance. Motivated by U-net [10], we combine the feature maps from the shallow layers with the feature maps from the deep layers to take advantage of both high-level semantics and low-level image details. Specifically, we crop the multi-scale feature maps from the backbone network (see Fig. 1b) and then perform a bottom-up segmentation for the cropped cell patches. Note that we intentionally employ an individual cell segmentation branch (Fig. 1b) for cell segmentation instead of directly reusing the feature map at $s_1$ (Fig. 1a). Our motivation is to use the branch to guide the model to eliminate the interference from neighboring cells and learn an objectness concept especially for cells with irregular shapes (see Fig. 3).

## 3   Experiments

*Datasets.* We evaluate our method on a neural cell dataset with irregular shapes and sizes and another cell nuclei dataset with regular shapes. The neural cell dataset contains 644 images that are sampled from a collection of time-lapse microscopic videos of rat CNS stem cells. The image size is 640 × 512. We randomly select 386 image for training, 129 for validation and 129 for testing. For the cell nuclei dataset, we use the public training data of 2018 Data Science Bowl. This dataset is acquired under a variety of conditions and varies in the image size, cell type, magnification and imaging modality. From the total of 670 images, we randomly select 402 images for training, 134 images for validation and 134 images for testing. The input images are resized to 512 × 512 in our experiments.

*Implementation Details.* We use the ground-truth bounding boxes to train the segmentation branch of Fig. 1b. In testing, we perform the individual segmentation with the bounding boxes generated from keypoints detection. The training images are augmented using random expanding, cropping, flipping, contrast distortion and brightness distortion. We train the network for 100 epochs and stop when the validation loss does not decrease significantly. The weights of the backbone network are pre-trained from ImageNet. Other weights of the network are initialized from a standard Gaussian distribution. The model is implemented with PyTorch on NVIDIA K80 GPUs.

*Evaluation Metrics.* We use the average precision (AP) at box-level IOU (intersection over union) [2] at threshold of 0.5 and 0.7 to evaluate the detection performances. We use the AP at mask-level IOU [3,6] at threshold of 0.5 and 0.7 to evaluate the instance segmentation performances. We also report the mean mask-level IOU [12] between the predicted segmentation masks and the ground truth masks at threshold of 0.5 and 0.7.

**Table 1.** Cell instance segmentation evaluation results. Seg $s_1$ means directly performing individual cell segmentation from feature map $s_1$. Seg branch refers to the individual cell segmentation branch in Fig. 1b.

| Model | Neural cell | | | | DSB2018 | | | |
|---|---|---|---|---|---|---|---|---|
| | AP@0.5 | AP@0.7 | IOU@0.5 | IOU@0.7 | AP@0.5 | AP@0.7 | IOU@0.5 | IOU@0.7 |
| DCAN [1] | 45.03 | 10.76 | 64.49 | 75.91 | 51.88 | 23.45 | 74.08 | 82.56 |
| CosineEmbedding [9] | 25.93 | 9.09 | 62.22 | 75.07 | 17.87 | 3.41 | 64.14 | 76.84 |
| Mask R-CNN [3] | 66.02 | 32.10 | 72.10 | 79.30 | 69.88 | 54.69 | 80.57 | 84.83 |
| Ours (seg $s_1$) | 78.49 | 50.97 | 75.51 | **80.42** | 71.38 | 59.38 | 83.10 | 86.10 |
| Ours (seg branch) | **88.03** | **63.08** | **77.04** | 79.94 | **71.58** | **59.81** | **83.29** | **86.22** |

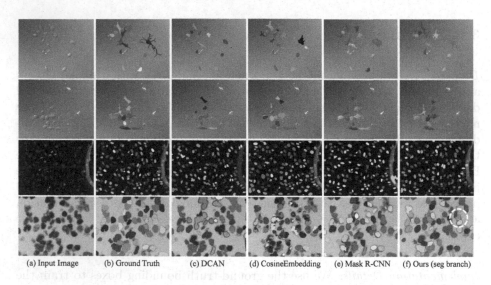

(a) Input Image    (b) Ground Truth    (c) DCAN    (d) CosineEmbedding    (e) Mask R-CNN    (f) Ours (seg branch)

**Fig. 2.** Qualitative cell instance segmentation results on neural cells (top two rows) and cell nuclei (bottom two rows). We compare our instance segmentation method with DCAN [1], CosineEmbedding [9] and Mask R-CNN [3]. The white dotted circle shows an example where our method separates the touching cells.

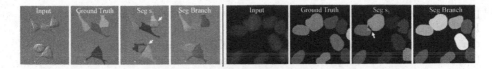

**Fig. 3.** Comparison between individual cell segmentation from feature map $s_1$ (seg $s_1$) and from individual cell segmentation branch (seg branch). The left four columns are neural cells. The right four columns are cell nuclei. The yellow arrows point to the over-segmentations of method seg $s_1$. (Color figure online)

**Table 2.** Detection evaluation results. Single-scale dec means the keypoints detection at $s_1$ (see Fig. 1), while multi-scale dec means the detection at $s_1, s_2, s_3, s_4$

| Model | Neural cell | | DSB2018 | |
|---|---|---|---|---|
| | AP@0.5 | AP@0.7 | AP@0.5 | AP@0.7 |
| DCAN [1] | 13.85 | 9.09 | 52.86 | 31.02 |
| CosineEmbedding [9] | 27.45 | 10.99 | 11.93 | 1.30 |
| Mask R-CNN [3] | 64.65 | 17.76 | 69.93 | 45.25 |
| CornerNet [5] | 60.42 | 39.75 | 47.99 | 38.35 |
| Ours (single-scale dec) | 60.97 | 46.69 | **80.39** | **69.11** |
| Ours (multi-scale dec) | **79.30** | **55.18** | 80.14 | 67.60 |

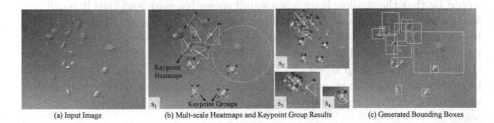

(a) Input Image    (b) Mult-scale Heatmaps and Keypoint Group Results    (c) Generated Bounding Boxes

**Fig. 4.** Visualization of heatmap predictions and keypoint groups overlaid on the input images. We show the heatmaps at four scales $s_i, i = 1, 2, 3, 4$. The circles illustrate an example that a large cell is unrecognized at scale $s_1$ but is captured at scale $s_4$.

## 4   Results and Discussion

We compare our instance segmentation method with DCAN [1], CosineEmbedding [9] and Mask R-CNN [3]. The quantitative and qualitative results are reported in Table 1 and Fig. 2. As can be seen from Fig. 2, DCAN tends to remove the details along with the cell boundaries for neural cells. For nuclei dataset, it is unable to differentiate the touching cells due to the unclear cell boundaries. CosineEmbedding [9] clusters the pixel embeddings to segment the cell instances. However, the clustering usually generates multiple separate clusters for the same cell instance. Therefore, it suffers from huge false positives and achieves inferior performance in detection, especially for crowded nuclei dataset (Table 2). Mask R-CNN [3] is superior in cell detection, but it cannot predict the long and slender structures of the cells because of its ROI align mechanism. Compared to these methods, our keypoints detection-based cell instance segmentation performs well in both capturing the long and slender cell structures and separating the touching cells. Moreover, from the last two rows of Table 1 and from Fig. 3 we can observe that the individual cell segmentation branch (Fig. 1b) performs better than segmentation based solely on feature map $s_1$ (Fig. 1a), especially for neural cells. The reason would be that the model lacks an object concept for cells when segmenting them only using feature map $s_1$. As a result, it is difficult for the model to filter out the interference of neighboring cells (see Fig. 3). In contrast, the individual cell segmentation branch is able to provide guidance for the network to eliminate the unrelated cell parts for each cell ROI patch.

We also report the cell detection comparison results in Table 2 to analyze the detection ability of our keypoint graph-based detection. We add the comparison between our method and the keypoint-based detector CornerNet [5] in Table 2. It can be seen that our keypoint graph-based detector achieves better accuracy in capturing the bounding boxes of the cells, compared to the other methods. Besides, the multi-scale detection performs better than single-scale detection for neural cell dataset. To illustrate the reason, we visualize the heatmap predictions and the keypoint groups in Fig. 4. As can be seen, the model can hardly detect the keypoints of cells with large sizes on the shallow layers. One possible reason would be that the shallow layer has a small receptive field, and thus it is difficult for the model to recognize a large object on the shallow layers. This defect also brings difficulty in predicting the correct displacement between two keypoints pairs for large cells, due to the loss of objectness concept. Compared to the shallow layers, the deep layers are able to detect the large cells because of their large receptive fields, as shown in Fig. 4. For cell nuclei, we do not observe obvious superiority for multi-scale cell detections since the sizes of nuclei are at a similar scale.

## 5   Conclusion

In this paper, we propose a new instance segmentation method that combines the keypoint-based detector with the individual cell segmentation. In particular, we propose a novel keypoint-based detector that is more effective in generating bounding box proposals. The experimental results demonstrate the advantages of our method in segmenting the cell instances with both regular and irregular shapes, compared to the other instance segmentation methods.

## References

1. Chen, H., Qi, X., Yu, L., Heng, P.A.: DCAN: deep contour-aware networks for accurate gland segmentation. In: CVPR, pp. 2487–2496 (2016)

2. Everingham, M., Van Gool, L., Williams, C.K., Winn, J., Zisserman, A.: The PASCAL visual object classes (VOC) challenge. IJCV **88**(2), 303–338 (2010)
3. He, K., Gkioxari, G., Dollár, P., Girshick, R.: Mask R-CNN. In: ICCV, pp. 2961–2969 (2017)
4. He, K., Zhang, X., Ren, S., Sun, J.: Deep residual learning for image recognition. In: CVPR, pp. 770–778 (2016)
5. Law, H., Deng, J.: CornerNet: detecting objects as paired keypoints. In: Ferrari, V., Hebert, M., Sminchisescu, C., Weiss, Y. (eds.) Computer Vision – ECCV 2018. LNCS, vol. 11218, pp. 765–781. Springer, Cham (2018). https://doi.org/10.1007/978-3-030-01264-9_45
6. Li, Y., Qi, H., Dai, J., Ji, X., Wei, Y.: Fully convolutional instance-aware semantic segmentation. In: CVPR, pp. 2359–2367 (2017)
7. Newell, A., Yang, K., Deng, J.: Stacked hourglass networks for human pose estimation. In: Leibe, B., Matas, J., Sebe, N., Welling, M. (eds.) ECCV 2016. LNCS, vol. 9912, pp. 483–499. Springer, Cham (2016). https://doi.org/10.1007/978-3-319-46484-8_29
8. Papandreou, G., Zhu, T., Chen, L.-C., Gidaris, S., Tompson, J., Murphy, K.: PersonLab: person pose estimation and instance segmentation with a bottom-up, part-based, geometric embedding model. In: Ferrari, V., Hebert, M., Sminchisescu, C., Weiss, Y. (eds.) Computer Vision – ECCV 2018. LNCS, vol. 11218, pp. 282–299. Springer, Cham (2018). https://doi.org/10.1007/978-3-030-01264-9_17
9. Payer, C., Štern, D., Neff, T., Bischof, H., Urschler, M.: Instance segmentation and tracking with cosine embeddings and recurrent hourglass networks. In: Frangi, A.F., Schnabel, J.A., Davatzikos, C., Alberola-López, C., Fichtinger, G. (eds.) MICCAI 2018. LNCS, vol. 11071, pp. 3–11. Springer, Cham (2018). https://doi.org/10.1007/978-3-030-00934-2_1
10. Ronneberger, O., Fischer, P., Brox, T.: U-Net: convolutional networks for biomedical image segmentation. In: Navab, N., Hornegger, J., Wells, W.M., Frangi, A.F. (eds.) MICCAI 2015. LNCS, vol. 9351, pp. 234–241. Springer, Cham (2015). https://doi.org/10.1007/978-3-319-24574-4_28
11. Schmidt, U., Weigert, M., Broaddus, C., Myers, G.: Cell detection with star-convex polygons. In: Frangi, A.F., Schnabel, J.A., Davatzikos, C., Alberola-López, C., Fichtinger, G. (eds.) MICCAI 2018. LNCS, vol. 11071, pp. 265–273. Springer, Cham (2018). https://doi.org/10.1007/978-3-030-00934-2_30
12. Yi, J., Wu, P., Jiang, M., Huang, Q., Hoeppner, D.J., Metaxas, D.N.: Attentive neural cell instance segmentation. Med. Image Anal. **55**, 228–240 (2019)

# Improving Nuclei/Gland Instance Segmentation in Histopathology Images by Full Resolution Neural Network and Spatial Constrained Loss

Hui Qu[1]([✉]), Zhennan Yan[2], Gregory M. Riedlinger[3], Subhajyoti De[3], and Dimitris N. Metaxas[1]

[1] Department of Computer Science, Rutgers University, Piscataway, USA
hui.qu@cs.rutgers.edu
[2] SenseTime Research, Shanghai, China
[3] Rutgers Cancer Institute of New Jersey, New Brunswick, USA

**Abstract.** Image segmentation plays an important role in pathology image analysis as the accurate separation of nuclei or glands is crucial for cancer diagnosis and other clinical analyses. The networks and cross entropy loss in current deep learning-based segmentation methods originate from image classification tasks and have drawbacks for segmentation. In this paper, we propose a full resolution convolutional neural network (FullNet) that maintains full resolution feature maps to improve the localization accuracy. We also propose a variance constrained cross entropy (varCE) loss that encourages the network to learn the spatial relationship between pixels in the same instance. Experiments on a nuclei segmentation dataset and the 2015 MICCAI Gland Segmentation Challenge dataset show that the proposed FullNet with the varCE loss achieves state-of-the-art performance. The code is publicly available (https://github.com/huiqu18/FullNet-varCE).

**Keywords:** Nuclei segmentation · Gland segmentation · Deep learning

## 1 Introduction

Histopathology image analysis is often one of the first steps in diagnosis, stratification, and clinical management of diseases such as cancer. The size, shape, and some other morphological appearances of image structures like nuclei and glands are highly related to the presence and severity of diseases [3]. Trained pathologists typically examine such images manually, which is laborious and subjective. Therefore, computational methods [3,5,13,21] have been developed for the quantitative and objective analyses of histopathology images. Image segmentation, which extracts the cells, nuclei, or glands from the histopathology images, goes before all analyses, and thus is a key step in the whole pipeline.

D. Shen et al. (Eds.): MICCAI 2019, LNCS 11764, pp. 378–386, 2019.
https://doi.org/10.1007/978-3-030-32239-7_42

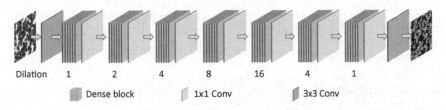

Dilation    1        2        4        8        16        4        1

Dense block          1x1 Conv              3x3 Conv

**Fig. 1.** Network structure of the FullNet. Dense blocks are utilized to reduce the number of feature maps. Each dense block has different dilation factor (the digit under each block) to ensure the receptive field is large enough for recognition.

Current state-of-the-art nuclei/gland segmentation methods [1,2,9,10,15,16, 18] adopt fully convolutional network (FCN) [7] and its variants, which extract features using an encoder and recover high resolution prediction from low resolution feature maps. They have achieved good segmentation performance compared to traditional methods. The encoder part of FCNs is inspired by structures originally designed for image classification. The pooling operation can greatly increase the receptive field to distill more-abstract features. However, such downsampling may reduce the localization accuracy of boundaries in segmentation tasks. Another issue in these methods is the cross entropy loss used for training. The loss only cares about if the classification of individual pixel is correct or not, and pays no attention to the spatial relationship between pixels. Although the deep neural networks can learn some high-level features like object's prior from ground-truth labels, the segmentation results are still not satisfactory when the objects have various colors, textures and shapes, especially in medical images.

To solve these issues, in this paper we propose a full resolution neural network (FullNet) to improve the localization accuracy and a variance constrained cross entropy (varCE) loss to enhance the learning of pixels' spatial relationship. The FullNet consists of densely connected layers [4] and doesn't contain any pooling or up-sampling layers. All feature maps and output have the same full resolution as the input image, thus keeping the information (e.g., edges) as much as possible to improve segmentation performance. For each convolution layer, dilated convolution [19] is utilized to increase the receptive field, similar to the effect of pooling operations in classification networks. The varCE loss combines the regular cross entropy term with a variance term. The cross entropy term performs classification for each pixel. The variance term aims to reduce the variance of pixels' probabilities within each instance. It works as a spatial constraint on pixels belonging to the same instance, and helps the network to better understand the shapes of objects. The combination of FullNet and varCE loss is able to achieve state-of-the-art performance on nuclei segmentation and gland segmentation.

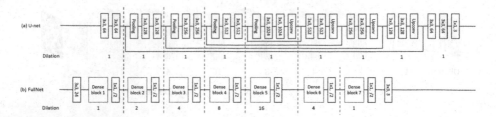

**Fig. 2.** Dilation factors in (a) U-net and (b) FullNet. Each red dash line represents a change of dilation factor in FullNet or a down-sampling of feature maps in U-net. (Color figure online)

## 2    Methods

### 2.1    FullNet Structure

The structure of our FullNet is shown in Fig. 1. It consists of a $3 \times 3$ convolutional layer, seven blocks of densely connected layers with different dilation factors, a $1 \times 1$ convolutional layer after each block, and a final $3 \times 3$ convolutional layer.

There are no pooling layers in the network, thus the feature maps retain the same resolution as the input to avoid the loss of details by pooling. The potential memory problem caused by the large number and size of feature maps is solved by the dense block structure. As in [4], each layer in a dense block takes all preceding feature maps as input, and outputs a fixed number of feature maps. This can enhance the feature reuse and strengthen feature propagation, thus achieving good performance with fewer feature maps. Different from the original dense blocks, we adopt *Conv-LeakyReLU-BN* instead of *BN-ReLU-Conv* structure for each dense layer. Putting BN after convolution in a dense layer can significantly reduce the memory requirements of intermediate feature maps, because for each dense layer the number of input feature maps is often much larger than that of outputs. LeakyReLU is preferred due to its benefit of solving "dying ReLU" problem [8]. The $1 \times 1$ convolution layer right after each dense block can further compress the number of features by half.

In order to ensure the large receptive field for recognition, we employ dilated convolution [19] in dense blocks, and decide the dilation factors by taking the U-net [11] as reference. In the U-net, each pooling layer reduces the size of feature maps by half, which doubles the effective receptive field since the filter size keeps the same. In the FullNet, to compensate for the shrinkage of receptive field after removing pooling layers, we use ordinary convolution in the first block and double the dilation factor for each subsequent block until block 5. In other words, the dilation factors are $\mathbf{d} = (1, 2, 4, 8, 16)$ for the first five blocks of FullNet, shown in Fig. 2. The last two blocks with dilation 4 and 1 are added to ameliorate the gridding artifacts caused by large dilation factors, as mentioned in [20]. The hybrid dilation factor strategy [14] is also adopted within each block to reduce the artifacts further.

The network outputs three-class probability maps: inside object areas, edges and background areas. The predicted edges are beneficial to separate the crowded and touching nuclei/glands.

## 2.2 Variance Constrained Cross Entropy Loss

In segmentation tasks, cross entropy loss is most widely used to classify each pixel into the correct class. The cross entropy loss for $M$ classes is defined as

$$\mathcal{L}_{CE}(y,t,w) = -\frac{1}{N} \sum_{i=1}^{N} \sum_{m=1}^{M} w_i t_i^{(m)} \log y_i^{(m)} \tag{1}$$

where $N$ is the number of all pixels, $y_i^{(m)}$ is the probability of pixel $i$ belonging to class $m$, $t_i^{(m)} \in \{0,1\}$ is the corresponding groundtruth label of class $m$, $w_i$ is the optional weight for pixel $i$.

The cross entropy loss doesn't consider the spatial relationship between pixels. When an object in the image has non-uniform color or texture, the network often fails to segment the whole object using cross entropy loss. To address the problem, we add a variance term to the cross entropy loss:

$$\mathcal{L}_{var}(y,t) = \frac{1}{C} \sum_{c=1}^{C} \frac{1}{|S_c|} \sum_{i=1}^{|S_c|} (\mu_c - \hat{y}_i)^2 \tag{2}$$

where $C$ is the number of instances, $S_c$ is the set of pixels that belong to instance $c$, $|S_c|$ is the number of pixels in set $S_c$, $\hat{y}_i$ is the probability of the correct class for pixel $i$, and $\mu_c$ is the mean value of pixels' probabilities $\hat{y}_i$ in set $S_c$: $\mu_c = \frac{1}{|S_c|} \sum_{i=1}^{|S_c|} \hat{y}_i$. Note that the variance is computed within each instance, thus placing a local constraint for pixels belonging to the same instance. Ideally, if the variance is zero for a certain instance, pixels in the range of this instance have the same probabilities $\hat{y}_i$, resulting in consistent predictions for those pixels.

The final variance constrained cross entropy (varCE) loss can be written as

$$\mathcal{L}_{varCE} = \mathcal{L}_{CE} + \alpha \mathcal{L}_{var} \tag{3}$$

where $\alpha$ is a parameter that adjusts the weight of the variance term. In the varCE loss, the variance term pulls the pixels in each instance towards the same class and meanwhile the cross entropy term drives these pixels to the correct class. As a result, the segmentation performance will be enhanced.

## 2.3 Post-processing

With the trained model, we get a three-class segmentation map for a test image. The map corresponding to inside object areas is selected as the initial segmentation map. Morphological operations including connected component labeling, small areas removal and dilation with a disk filter are performed to obtain the

**Table 1.** Nuclei segmentation results on Multi-Organ dataset using different methods.

| Method | Same organ test set | | | | Different organ test set | | | |
|---|---|---|---|---|---|---|---|---|
| | F1 | Dice | H | AJI | F1 | Dice | H | AJI |
| CNN3 [6] | 0.8222 | 0.7301 | 7.39 | 0.5154 | 0.8327 | 0.8051 | **8.03** | 0.4989 |
| U-net [11] | 0.8510 | 0.7962 | 6.89 | 0.5815 | 0.8401 | 0.7732 | 10.57 | 0.5481 |
| FCN-pooling | 0.8521 | 0.7278 | 8.42 | 0.5038 | 0.8245 | 0.7178 | 11.24 | 0.4778 |
| FullNet | 0.8519 | 0.7914 | 6.92 | 0.5862 | 0.8637 | 0.7983 | 8.15 | 0.5995 |
| FullNet & varCE | **0.8552** | **0.8007** | **6.54** | **0.5946** | **0.8639** | **0.8054** | 8.16 | **0.6164** |

**Table 2.** Gland segmentation results on GlaS dataset using different methods. Rank of each entry is listed for clear comparison.

| Method | testA | | | | | | testB | | | | | | Rank sum |
|---|---|---|---|---|---|---|---|---|---|---|---|---|---|
| | F1 | Rank | $Dice_{obj}$ | Rank | $H_{obj}$ | Rank | F1 | Rank | $Dice_{obj}$ | Rank | $H_{obj}$ | Rank | |
| CUMedVision [1] | 0.912 | 6 | 0.897 | 7 | 45.42 | 6 | 0.716 | 9 | 0.781 | 9 | 160.35 | 9 | 46 |
| Xu et al. (a) [15] | 0.858 | 9 | 0.888 | 8 | 54.20 | 8 | 0.771 | 8 | 0.815 | 7 | 129.93 | 8 | 48 |
| Xu et al. (b) [16] | 0.893 | 7 | 0.908 | 4 | 44.13 | 4 | 0.843 | 6 | 0.833 | 6 | 116.82 | 6 | 33 |
| Yan et al. [17] | **0.924** | 1 | 0.902 | 6 | 49.88 | 7 | 0.844 | 4 | 0.840 | 4 | 106.08 | 5 | 27 |
| MILD-Net [2] | 0.914 | 4 | 0.913 | 2 | 41.54 | 3 | 0.844 | 4 | 0.836 | 5 | 105.89 | 4 | 22 |
| Yang et al. [18] | 0.921 | 3 | 0.904 | 5 | 44.74 | 5 | **0.855** | 1 | **0.858** | 1 | 96.98 | 2 | 17 |
| FCN-pooling | 0.869 | 8 | 0.844 | 9 | 71.78 | 9 | 0.825 | 7 | 0.810 | 8 | 124.94 | 7 | 48 |
| FullNet | 0.914 | 4 | 0.909 | 3 | 40.38 | 2 | **0.855** | 1 | 0.853 | 3 | 99.46 | 3 | 16 |
| FullNet & varCE | **0.924** | 1 | **0.914** | 1 | **37.28** | 1 | 0.853 | 3 | 0.856 | 2 | **88.75** | 1 | **9** |

final segmentation results. Because the predicted edges are often thicker than true edges, which help to separate touching objects, the initial prediction of the inside is not the exact mask of objects. In order to include the periphery areas, the dilation operation is necessary.

## 3 Experiments

We evaluate the proposed method on two benchmark datasets for nuclei segmentation and gland segmentation, and compare it with state-of-the-art approaches.

### 3.1 Datasets and Evaluation Metrics

**Datasets.** The Multi-Organ nuclei segmentation dataset [6] consists of 30 H&E stained histopathology image of size $1000 \times 1000$. They are taken from multiple hospitals and include a diversity of nuclear appearances from seven organs. Images in the train and same organ test sets are from four organs while those in the different organ test set are from the other three organs. The MICCAI 2015 gland segmentation challenge dataset (GlaS) [12] consists of 165 images that come from 16 H&E stained histological sections of colorectal adenocarcinoma.

They are separated into train, testA and testB parts, containing 80, 65 and 20 images, respectively. Train and testA parts have both benign and malignant cases, while testB set is mostly malignant cases.

**Evaluation Metrics.** For nuclei segmentation, we use the same metrics in [6]: F1-score, average Dice coefficient, average Hausdorff distance, and the Aggregated Jaccard Index (AJI) proposed in that paper. For gland segmentation, three official provided metrics in the MICCAI 2015 Challenge are used: F1-score, object-level Dice coefficient and object-level Hausdorff distance.

## 3.2 Implementation Details

In consideration of the memory usage and the model effectiveness, we set the number of dense layers in each block as 6 and the number of output feature maps for each layer as 24. During training, we randomly crop images of $208 \times 208$ pixels with the batch size of 8 as input. It requires two 12 GB GPUs for training with the above configuration. The FullNet is trained using Adam optimizer. The weight for variance term in the loss function is set to $\alpha = 1$ for both datasets. The learning rate and training epoch are 0.001 and 300 for nuclei segmentation, and 0.0005 and 1000 for gland segmentation. Since both datasets are not large enough, we perform data augmentations like random scale, flip, rotation, affine and elastic transformation. Test time augmentations are utilized for more accurate predictions.

## 3.3 Results and Comparison

The quantitative results are presented in Tables 1 and 2. Typical qualitative results are shown in Fig. 3. The FCN-pooling is the same structure as FullNet except that there are pooling layers (2x) after the first four dense blocks and up-sampling layers (4x) before the last two blocks, and no dilated convolution. It is used to illustrate the effect of full resolution feature maps in the FullNet.

For nuclei segmentation, we compare the FullNet with two methods on the Multi-Organ dataset. One is the patch-based CNN3 method [6], which uses a small patch to predict the central pixel's class and utilizes region growing as post-processing to refine the segmentation results. The other one is the U-net, the reference structure of our FullNet. From the results in Table 1, it is obvious that FullNet outperforms CNN3 on both test sets. Compared to U-net, the plain FullNet achieves equal performance on the same organ test set, but have better generalization performance on the different organ test set. With the varCE loss, the segmentation accuracies are improved for nearly all metrics.

For gland segmentation, we compare our method with state-of-the-arts [1, 2, 15–18]. In the results of Table 2, the proposed FullNet with varCE loss obtains the best performance on four columns, while has very similar performance on the other two. The improvement on the Hausdorff distance is especially large, revealing the good localization performance of our method. The rank sum of

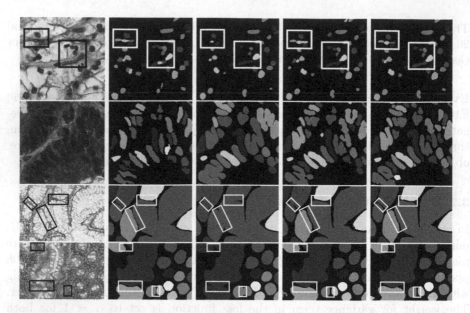

**Fig. 3.** Typical results of nuclei segmentation (top two rows) and gland segmentation (bottom two rows). For each row, from left to right are original image, ground-truth instance label, segmentation results of FCN-pooling, FullNet without varCE and FullNet with varCE loss, respectively. Distinct colors in the images indicate different instances. Rectangles are drawn for clear comparison.

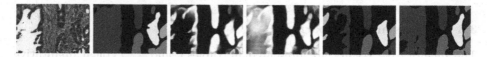

**Fig. 4.** The effect of the varCE loss. From left to right: image, ground-truth label, probability maps without and with varCE loss, segmentation results without and with varCE loss.

all evaluation metrics illustrates that our approach achieves the best overall performance.

***The Effect of Full Resolution Feature Maps.*** For both tasks, the FullNet has much better performance than FCN-pooling, because FCN-pooling cannot produce accurate shapes and edges while the full resolution maps in FullNet are able to, as shown in Fig. 3. The accurate localization of edges is beneficial for separating touching nuclei and glands.

***The Effect of varCE Loss.*** Both quantitative and qualitative results have proven that the variance term in the loss function can enhance the segmentation performance. We take an example in Fig. 4 to illustrate why it works. The gland in the left part of the image is hard for the network to recognize due to its large lumen and incomplete contour. Without the variance term, the pixels in the lumen part have pretty low probabilities, thus are classified as background pixels. With the variance term, it correlates the pixels belonging to the lumen part to pixels of the boundary part by minimizing the variance of probabilities inside the gland. As a result, the pixels' probabilities in the lumen part increase and most pixels of the gland are classified correctly.

### 3.4 Inference Time

It takes 0.268 s for a forward pass of our proposed FullNet on images of size $500 \times 500$ on an NVIDIA TITAN X GPU. For comparison, the time of the FCN-pooling and U-net is 0.085 s and 0.061 s, respectively. The measurements were averaged over 100 individual forward passes.

## 4 Conclusion and Future Work

We propose a full resolution convolutional network (FullNet) and a variance constrained cross entropy (varCE) loss for nuclei and gland segmentation in histopathology images. The FullNet removes all pooling layers in the fully convolutional network and takes advantages of densely connected layers and dilated convolutions to resolve memory and small receptive field problems. The varCE loss places a spatial constraint on pixels that assists the network to learn the shape of objects. The proposed framework achieves state-of-the-art segmentation results of both nuclei and glands in H&E stained histopathology images. In future work, we consider to explore the performance of deeper FullNets, and the possibility of reducing the computational cost while retaining the performance.

## References

1. Chen, H., Qi, X., Yu, L., Heng, P.A.: DCAN: deep contour-aware networks for accurate gland segmentation. In: Proceedings of CVPR, pp. 2487–2496 (2016)
2. Graham, S., et al.: MILD-Net: minimal information loss dilated network for gland instance segmentation in colon histology images. Med. Image Anal. **52**, 199–211 (2019)
3. Gurcan, M.N., Boucheron, L., Can, A., Madabhushi, A., Rajpoot, N., Yener, B.: Histopathological image analysis: a review. IEEE Rev. Biomed. Eng. **2**, 147 (2009)
4. Huang, G., Liu, Z., Van Der Maaten, L., Weinberger, K.Q.: Densely connected convolutional networks. In: Proceedings of CVPR, vol. 1, p. 3 (2017)
5. Janowczyk, A., Madabhushi, A.: Deep learning for digital pathology image analysis: a comprehensive tutorial with selected use cases. J. Pathol. Inform. **7**, 29 (2016)
6. Kumar, N., Verma, R., Sharma, S., Bhargava, S., Vahadane, A., Sethi, A.: A dataset and a technique for generalized nuclear segmentation for computational pathology. IEEE Trans. Med. Imaging **36**(7), 1550–1560 (2017)
7. Long, J., Shelhamer, E., Darrell, T.: Fully convolutional networks for semantic segmentation. In: Proceedings of CVPR, pp. 3431–3440 (2015)
8. Maas, A.L., Hannun, A.Y., Ng, A.Y.: Rectifier nonlinearities improve neural network acoustic models. In: Proceedings of the ICML, vol. 30, p. 3 (2013)

9. Qu, H., et al.: Joint segmentation and fine-grained classification of nuclei in histopathology images. In: ISBI 2019, pp. 900–904. IEEE (2019)
10. Qu, H., et al.: Weakly supervised deep nuclei segmentation using points annotation in histopathology images. In: MIDL 2019, pp. 390–400 (2019)
11. Ronneberger, O., Fischer, P., Brox, T.: U-Net: convolutional networks for biomedical image segmentation. In: Navab, N., Hornegger, J., Wells, W.M., Frangi, A.F. (eds.) MICCAI 2015. LNCS, vol. 9351, pp. 234–241. Springer, Cham (2015). https://doi.org/10.1007/978-3-319-24574-4_28
12. Sirinukunwattana, K., et al.: Gland segmentation in colon histology images: the glas challenge contest. Med. Image Anal. **35**, 489–502 (2017)
13. Su, H., Xing, F., Kong, X., Xie, Y., Zhang, S., Yang, L.: Robust cell detection and segmentation in histopathological images using sparse reconstruction and stacked denoising autoencoders. In: Navab, N., Hornegger, J., Wells, W.M., Frangi, A.F. (eds.) MICCAI 2015. LNCS, vol. 9351, pp. 383–390. Springer, Cham (2015). https://doi.org/10.1007/978-3-319-24574-4_46
14. Wang, P., et al.: Understanding convolution for semantic segmentation. In: 2018 IEEE Winter Conference on Applications of Computer Vision (WACV), pp. 1451–1460. IEEE (2018)
15. Xu, Y., Li, Y., Liu, M., Wang, Y., Lai, M., Chang, E.I.-C.: Gland instance segmentation by deep multichannel side supervision. In: Ourselin, S., Joskowicz, L., Sabuncu, M.R., Unal, G., Wells, W. (eds.) MICCAI 2016. LNCS, vol. 9901, pp. 496–504. Springer, Cham (2016). https://doi.org/10.1007/978-3-319-46723-8_57
16. Xu, Y., et al.: Gland instance segmentation using deep multichannel neural networks. IEEE Trans. Biomed. Eng. **64**(12), 2901–2912 (2017)
17. Yan, Z., Yang, X., Cheng, K.-T.T.: A deep model with shape-preserving loss for gland instance segmentation. In: Frangi, A.F., Schnabel, J.A., Davatzikos, C., Alberola-López, C., Fichtinger, G. (eds.) MICCAI 2018. LNCS, vol. 11071, pp. 138–146. Springer, Cham (2018). https://doi.org/10.1007/978-3-030-00934-2_16
18. Yang, L., Zhang, Y., Chen, J., Zhang, S., Chen, D.Z.: Suggestive annotation: a deep active learning framework for biomedical image segmentation. In: Descoteaux, M., Maier-Hein, L., Franz, A., Jannin, P., Collins, D.L., Duchesne, S. (eds.) MICCAI 2017. LNCS, vol. 10435, pp. 399–407. Springer, Cham (2017). https://doi.org/10.1007/978-3-319-66179-7_46
19. Yu, F., Koltun, V.: Multi-scale context aggregation by dilated convolutions. In: ICLR 2016 (2016)
20. Yu, F., Koltun, V., Funkhouser, T.A.: Dilated residual networks. In: Proceedings of CVPR, vol. 2, p. 3 (2017)
21. Zhang, X., Xing, F., Su, H., Yang, L., Zhang, S.: High-throughput histopathological image analysis via robust cell segmentation and hashing. Med. Image Anal. **26**(1), 306–315 (2015)

# Synthetic Augmentation and Feature-Based Filtering for Improved Cervical Histopathology Image Classification

Yuan Xue[1], Qianying Zhou[1], Jiarong Ye[2], L. Rodney Long[3], Sameer Antani[3], Carl Cornwell[3], Zhiyun Xue[3], and Xiaolei Huang[1](✉)

[1] College of Information Sciences and Technology, Pennsylvania State University, University Park, PA, USA
suh972@psu.edu
[2] Department of Statistics, Pennsylvania State University, University Park, PA, USA
[3] National Library of Medicine, National Institutes of Health, Bethesda, MD, USA

**Abstract.** Cervical intraepithelial neoplasia (CIN) grade of histopathology images is a crucial indicator in cervical biopsy results. Accurate CIN grading of epithelium regions helps pathologists with precancerous lesion diagnosis and treatment planning. Although an automated CIN grading system has been desired, supervised training of such a system would require a large amount of expert annotations, which are expensive and time-consuming to collect. In this paper, we investigate the CIN grade classification problem on segmented epithelium patches. We propose to use conditional Generative Adversarial Networks (cGANs) to expand the limited training dataset, by synthesizing realistic cervical histopathology images. While the synthetic images are visually appealing, they are not guaranteed to contain meaningful features for data augmentation. To tackle this issue, we propose a synthetic-image filtering mechanism based on the divergence in feature space between generated images and class centroids in order to control the feature quality of selected synthetic images for data augmentation. Our models are evaluated on a cervical histopathology image dataset with limited number of patch-level CIN grade annotations. Extensive experimental results show a significant improvement of classification accuracy from 66.3% to 71.7% using the same ResNet18 baseline classifier after leveraging our cGAN generated images with feature based filtering, which demonstrates the effectiveness of our models.

## 1 Introduction

Cervical cancer is the fourth-most frequently diagnosed cancer among women all over the world [1]. The diagnosis of cervical cancer and its precancerous stages can be accomplished through assessment of histopathology slides of cervical tissue by pathologists. An important outcome of the assessment is the

© Springer Nature Switzerland AG 2019
D. Shen et al. (Eds.): MICCAI 2019, LNCS 11764, pp. 387–396, 2019.
https://doi.org/10.1007/978-3-030-32239-7_43

cervical intraepithelial neoplasia (CIN) grade, an important indicator for abnormality assessment identified by the abnormal growth of cells on the surface of the cervix. CIN grade can be divided into CIN1, CIN2, and CIN3 with increased severity from mild to severe. Thus, accurate assessment of CIN grade is crucial for diagnosis and treatment planning of cervical cancer.

Considering the shortage of pathologists, an automatic cervical histopathology image classification system has great potential in under developed regions for its low cost and accessibility. Moreover, such a system can help pathologists with diagnosis and potentially mitigate the inter- and intra- pathologist variation. Existing literature [2,6] have studied various supervised learning methods for nuclei-based cervical cancer classification. Chankong et al. [2] proposed automatic cervical cancer cell segmentation and classification using fuzzy C-means (FCM) clustering and various types of classifiers. Guo et al. [6] designed handcrafted nuclei-based features for fusion-based classification on digitized epithelium histopathology slides with linear discriminant analysis (LDA) and support vector machines (SVM) classifier. While accomplishments have been achieved with fully-supervised learning methods, they require large amounts of expert annotations of cervical whole slide images. Since the annotation process can be tedious and time-consuming, it often results in limited number of labeled data available for supervised learning models.

Recently, several works have leveraged unsupervised learning methods, more specifically, Generative Adversarial Networks (GANs) [4] in medical image analysis to mitigate the small dataset sizes and limited annotations [3,10,14]. Frid-Adar et al. [3] investigated conditional GANs (cGANs) [11] to generate synthetic CT images and improved the performance of CNN in liver lesion classification, by adding generated images into the training data as data augmentation. Similarly, Madani et al. [10] found GAN based data augmentation achieved higher accuracy than traditional augmentation in Chest X-ray classification. Ren et al. [14] explored a method to classify the prostate histopathology images by domain adaptation so that knowledge learned in the source domain can be transferred to the target dataset without annotation. Although the GANs in previous applications can generate visually appealing synthetic images, the feature quality of generated images varies among examples and not all of them are guaranteed to contain meaningful features to improve the model performance in the original task.

In this paper, we study the 4-class (normal, CIN 1–3) cervical histopathology image classification problem based on a ResNet18 [7] baseline classifier. We run and evaluate our models on a heterogeneous epithelium image dataset with limited number of patch-level annotations. Images in the dataset have various color, shapes and texture which makes the classification very challenging. While the capability of the baseline model is limited by the number of training data, we propose a cGAN based image synthesis model to generate high-fidelity synthetic epithelium histopathology patches to expand the training data. To improve the diversity of synthetic images, we incorporate the minibatch discrimination [15] to reduce the closeness between examples inside a minibatch. Moreover, unlike previous works which directly added the generated data into the training set, we apply a feature based filtering mechanism to further improve the feature quality of the synthetic images added. We first pre-train a feature extractor using baseline ResNet18 model and calculate feature centroids for each class as the average feature of all training images. The generated images are then filtered based on the distance to the corresponding centroid in the feature space. Experimental results show that our proposed cGAN model along with the feature based filtering significantly outperform the baseline ResNet18 model and the traditional augmentation methods.

## 2   Methodology

An overall illustration of our proposed data augmentation pipeline can be found in Fig. 1. In traditional fully-supervised training, the model is trained on training images and the inference is done by feeding the test data to the trained model. In previous GAN-based augmentation works [3,10], a GAN model is first trained to generate some synthetic images based on the training data, then the generated images are added to the original training data as a data augmentation strategy. However, since the discriminator in GAN only outputs a high level judgement (0 or 1) of the fidelity of generated images, such pipeline cannot guarantee that the generated data have similar features to the real images which contribute to the classification task. To tackle this issue, we propose a feature based filtering mechanism to further improve the feature quality and fidelity of the synthetic images. We first introduce the cGAN model used in our framework.

### 2.1   Theoretical Preliminaries

The conventional cGANs [11] have an objective function defined as:

$$\min_{\theta_G} \max_{\theta_D} \mathcal{L}_{\text{cGAN}} = \mathbb{E}_{x \sim p_{\text{data}}}[\log D(x \mid c)] + \mathbb{E}_{z \sim \mathcal{N}}[\log(1 - D(G(z \mid c)))]. \quad (1)$$

In the objective function above, $\theta_G$ and $\theta_D$ represent the parameters for the generator $G$ and discriminator $D$ in cGAN, respectively. $x$ represents the real data from an unknown distribution $p_{\text{data}}$ and $c$ is the conditional label (e.g., CIN grades). $z$ is a random vector for the generator $G$, drawn from a normal distribution $\mathcal{N}(0, 1)$. $G$ is trained to fool the discriminator with synthetic data by minimizing the objective. Meanwhile, $D$ that takes both $z$ and $c$ as input is trained to maximize the objective, aiming to distinguish real data and synthetic images generated by $G$.

During the experiments, we observe that the intra-class diversity of the generated images greatly affects the data augmentation performance. Consider a mode-collapse GAN model which only generates very limited number of modes, all generated images will look similar. In such case, no matter how many examples are added to the training data, only few of them contribute to the data augmentation. To this end, we incorporate the minibatch discrimination module [15] into our discriminator to reduce the homogeneity between generated

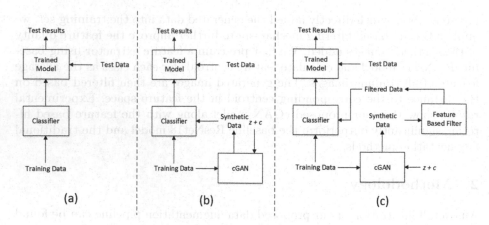

**Fig. 1.** Illustration and comparison between different training processes. (a) Traditional training pipeline; (b) Conditional GAN augmented training pipeline; (c) Our proposed cGAN augmentation with feature based filtering. The input to the cGAN are noise vector $z$ and label condition vector $c$.

examples inside a minibatch. Let $f(x_i) \in R^A$ denote a feature vector for input $x_i$ from an intermediate layer in the discriminator, where $A =$ out channels $\times$ weight $\times$ height. We multiply $f(x_i)$ by a transformation matrix $T \in R^{A \times B \times C}$ to compute a matrix $M_i \in R^{B \times C}$, where $B$ represents the number of output features of the minibatch discriminator, and $C$ refers to the number of kernel dimension which is set to 3 by default in our experiments. The similarity of the image $x_i$ with the rest of images $x_j$ in the same batch is computed as

$$o(x_i)_b = \sum_{j=1}^{n} \exp(-||M_{i,b} - M_{j,b}||_{L_1}), \tag{2}$$

and $o(x_i) = [o(x_i)_1, o(x_i)_2, \ldots, o(x_i)_B] \in R^B$. Then the similarity $o(x_i)$ is concatenated with $f(x_i)$ and fed into the next layer of the discriminator. Minibatch discrimination penalizes the generator if mode is collapsing and encourages the model to generate diverse images. With minibatch discrimination, our cGAN models can generate more diverse images which can be effectively added to the training data for augmentation.

We then introduce the feature based filtering method after generating synthetic images from our trained cGAN model. One of the advantages of GANs is that the input is drawn from a distribution and one can generate an infinite number of images with a trained GAN. Thus, any filtering methods will not affect the number of images available to be added to the training data. We first pre-train a feature extractor using the baseline classifier on the original training set to extract visual features of the input images. The features consist of activations produced by different layers in the feature extractor. The feature distance between image $x$ and centroid $c$ is then defined as

$$D_f(x,c) = \sum_l \frac{1}{H_l W_l} ||\hat{\phi}_l(x) - \hat{\phi}_l(c)||_2^2, \tag{3}$$

where $\hat{\phi}_l$ is the unit-normalized activation in the channel dimension $A_l$ of the $l$th layer of a feature extraction network with shape $H_l \times W_l$. This $\ell_2$ distance between unit-normalized activation can be regarded as a cosine distance in the feature space.

The centroid $c$ is calculated as the average feature of all training images in the same class. For class $i$, its centroid $c_i$ is represented by

$$c_i = [\frac{1}{N_i} \sum_{j=1}^{N_i} \phi_1(x_j), \frac{1}{N_i} \sum_{j=1}^{N_i} \phi_2(x_j), \ldots, \frac{1}{N_i} \sum_{j=1}^{N_i} \phi_L(x_j)], \tag{4}$$

where $N_i$ denotes the number of training samples in $i$th class and $x_j$ is the $j$th training sample. Similar to Eq. 3, $\phi_l$ is the activation extracted from the $l$th layer of the feature extraction network. $L$ is the total number of layers utilized in the feature based filtering.

## 2.2   Implementation Details

Our GAN model is built upon the DCGAN [13] and WGAN-GP [5] with several alterations. The conditional generator consists of 8 convolutional blocks, where the first block consists of two separate transpose convolutional blocks for conditional labels $c$ and random vector $z$. After the first block, the activations of $c$ and $z$ are concatenated along the channel dimension and fed into the next layer of the generator. Different from DCGAN which uses transpose convolution for upsampling, our convolutional block consists of a bilinear upsampling with factor 2 except for the first shared block which has factor $2 \times 1$, a $3 \times 3$ convolution with stride 1, a batch normalization layer and a ReLU activation. The final block is a $7 \times 7$ convolution followed by a tanh activation.

The conditional discriminator consists of 7 convolutional blocks, where the first block includes two separate convolutional blocks for conditional labels $c$ and random vector $z$ with no batch normalization as in DCGAN. The activations of $c$ and $z$ are concatenated and fed into the rest of convolutional blocks. Each of the rest of the convolutional blocks contains a $4 \times 4$ convolutional layer, a batch normalization layer and a LeakyRelu activation. Each convolution has stride 2 except for the 6th and 7th block which has stride $2 \times 1$ and 1, respectively. Activations of the last convolutional block are then fed into the minibatch discrimination layer as described in Eq. 2. After the minibatch discrimination, a fully connected layer outputs the final logits of discriminator.

Our cGAN model is trained with WGAN-GP loss with batchsize 100, fixed learning rate $2e-4$ and 700 training epochs. The baseline classifier is the widely used ResNet18 [7] which has shown promising performance in various vision tasks. All classification models are trained using the same baseline classification model with batchsize 64 by Adam optimizer [8] with weight decay $2e-5$ and the

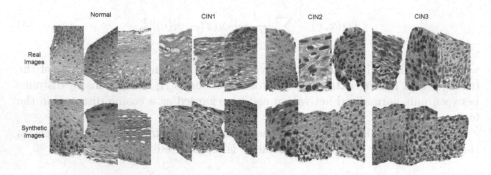

**Fig. 2.** Examples of real and synthetic images for all CIN grades.

cross-entropy loss. The initial learning rate of all classification models is $1e-3$ and is reduced by factor 0.2 when the validation accuracy has stopped being improved for 5 epochs.

## 3   Experiments

The experimental dataset is a cervical histopathology image dataset collected from a collaborating health sciences center. It contains multiple data sources, all of which are annotated by the same pathologist. The data processing follows [6] by dividing an annotated image into patches according to the medial axis of the epithelium tissue in that image. We first divide the medial axis into several straight segments, and crop the patches with each containing one straight segment. The cropped patches are then rotated such that all their medial axes align horizontally after rotation. The cropped patches are resized to a unified size of $256 \times 128$. In total, there are $1,112$ normal, 181 CIN1, 463 CIN2, 454 CIN3 patches. Examples of the images can be found in the first row of Fig. 2. All evaluations are done based on the patch-level ground truth annotations. We randomly split the dataset, by patients, into training, validation, and test sets, with ratio 7:1:2 and keep the ratio of image classes almost the same among different sets. All evaluations and comparisons reported in this section are done on the test set.

We report quantitative evaluation scores between all baseline models and our models including the accuracy, area under the ROC curve (AUC), sensitivity and specificity to provide a comprehensive comparison. All models are run for 5 rounds with random initialization for fair comparison. The mean and standard deviation results of 5 runs are illustrated in Table 1. We use the same baseline classifier with same hyperparameters setting in all experiments to ensure differences only come from the augmentation mechanisms.

We first conduct experiments with the baseline ResNet18 [7] classifier trained on the original training data and the data with traditional data augmentation. The traditional data augmentation used in our experiments includes random horizontal and vertical flipping, random adjustment of brightness, contrast and

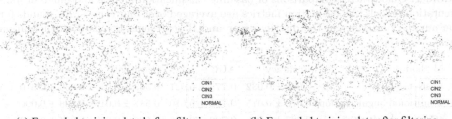

(a) Expanded training data before filtering    (b) Expanded training data after filtering

**Fig. 3.** t-SNE visualization of extracted image features of expanded training data. The ratio of synthetic images to the original training images is set to 2 for both before and after filtering ($R = 2$).

saturation to serve as a color based augmentation. From the first two rows of Table 1, one can see that there are no obvious improvements from leveraging traditional data augmentation, which further indicates that traditional augmentation methods do not perform well on such classification problem. Since we cannot ensure the feature quality of the traditional augmentation, we only train all our GAN models using the original training data.

Examples of the synthetic images generated by our cGAN models compared to the real images in the training set are shown in Fig. 2. As one can observe from Fig. 2, our generated images are realistic and keep important features such as color, shape and location of nuclei, and texture information so that the generated images can be used to extend the original training set.

While the synthetic images are visually appealing, high realism is not equivalent to meaningful features for improving classification results. We further explore the distribution of generated images in the feature space in Fig. 3 to ensure they are separable. We use the t-SNE [9] dimension reduction algorithm which can convert the embedding of high-dimensional data into a two-dimensional space for better visualization. After training a baseline ResNet18 classifier with the original training data, we use the pre-trained ResNet18 model as the feature extractor to extract features from the last convolutional layer in the ResNet18 model. We use the same feature extractor for both the expanded training data without and with feature based filtering in Fig. 3(a) and (b), respectively. Although overall there are overlapping between classes in the feature space which indicates the difficulty of such classification problem, the new training data with feature based filtering clearly have more distinguishable features than the ones without the feature filtering, which supports our claim and is in accord with the improvements in classification performance.

In all GAN-based augmentation models, the generated synthetic images are added into the original training set in equal proportion and we use ratio $R$ to represent the number of synthetic images to the number of real images. We keep the same proportion between classes as in the original set to make sure synthetic images generated from minority classes are meaningful for augmentation. We

**Table 1.** Quantitative comparisons of baseline classification models and different augmentation models. All evaluation metrics are averaged over four classes. AC stands for the auxiliary classifier in the discriminator and R represents the data augmentation ratio.

| Method | Accuracy | AUC | Sensitivity | Specificity |
|---|---|---|---|---|
| ResNet18 [7] | $0.663 \pm 0.032$ | $0.775 \pm 0.021$ | $0.553 \pm 0.019$ | $0.866 \pm 0.010$ |
| Traditional augmentation | $0.670 \pm 0.015$ | $0.780 \pm 0.010$ | $0.587 \pm 0.016$ | $0.868 \pm 0.006$ |
| cGAN + AC R = 0.5 | $0.687 \pm 0.009$ | $0.792 \pm 0.006$ | $0.596 \pm 0.009$ | $0.874 \pm 0.003$ |
| cGAN + AC R = 2 | $0.660 \pm 0.020$ | $0.773 \pm 0.014$ | $0.551 \pm 0.032$ | $0.862 \pm 0.011$ |
| Ours w/o filtering R = 0.5 | $0.695 \pm 0.009$ | $0.796 \pm 0.006$ | $0.559 \pm 0.032$ | $0.874 \pm 0.006$ |
| Ours w/o filtering R = 2 | $0.705 \pm 0.010$ | $0.804 \pm 0.007$ | $0.555 \pm 0.019$ | $0.872 \pm 0.005$ |
| Ours w/ filtering R = 0.5 | $0.716 \pm 0.009$ | $0.810 \pm 0.005$ | $\mathbf{0.611 \pm 0.012}$ | $\mathbf{0.886 \pm 0.006}$ |
| Ours w/ filtering R = 2 | $\mathbf{0.717 \pm 0.008}$ | $\mathbf{0.811 \pm 0.006}$ | $0.608 \pm 0.009$ | $0.882 \pm 0.003$ |

start with a cGAN model with an auxiliary classifier (AC) [12] which is similar to [3]. The auxiliary classifier is added to the last layer of the discriminator network to output the class labels for both real and synthetic images. While cGAN with AC works fine when the ratio is 0.5, the same model with ratio being 2 significantly degrades the classification performance, resulting in even worse scores than the baseline model with no augmentation. One possible reason is that the auxiliary classifier is trained on both real and synthetic images (mainly trained on synthetic images when $R > 1$), the features learned in the training process may not represent the original real data very well. Rather, if a feature extractor is trained only on the real data, the learned features could be more meaningful to the original data.

Following this idea, we provide an ablation study of our cGAN models with and without the feature filtering. For feature based filtering, we first generate 5,000 images for each class, then the images with lowest distance to the corresponding centroids will be kept. Retained quantity is calculated based on the ratio $R$. As shown in Table 1, our no filtering cGAN model with different ratios all show improvements in classification performance. Meanwhile, the feature filtering brings obvious benefits to all evaluation metrics, and our full models with different number of synthetic images added to the training data achieved best performance in all metrics. More importantly, the quality levels of generated images from our full models are very stable. Classification performances are similar among different ratios and during different runs, with consistently high mean and low std, which demonstrates that the feature qualities of generated images after filtering are superior to images generated by other models or without filtering.

## 4   Conclusions

In this paper, we investigate a novel GAN based augmentation pipeline for cervical histopathology image classification problem. We mainly focus on one of the major limitations of using GAN for augmentation: one cannot measure and control the quality of the synthetic images. While traditional GANs try to improve the fidelity of synthetic images, an augmentation system should try to generate images which have better feature quality rather than visual realism. By introducing a feature based filtering mechanism, our model boosts the performance of baseline classifier significantly on a challenging cervical histopathology dataset. As an attempt to make better use of GAN based augmentation models in medical imaging, our proposed pipeline has great potentials in other medical imaging applications where the number of labeled data is limited.

**Acknowledgements.** This research was supported in part by the Intramural Research Program of the National Institutes of Health (NIH), National Library of Medicine (NLM), and Lister Hill National Center for Biomedical Communications (LHNCBC), under Contract # HHSN276201800170P. We gratefully acknowledge the invaluable medical assistance from Dr. Rosemary Zuna, M.D., of the University of Oklahoma Health Sciences Center, and the work of Dr. Joe Stanley of Missouri University of Science and Technology which made the data collection possible.

# References

1. Bray, F., Ferlay, J., Soerjomataram, I., Siegel, R.L., Torre, L.A.D.L., Jemal, A.: Global cancer statistics 2018: GLOBOCAN estimates of incidence and mortality worldwide for 36 cancers in 185 countries. CA: A Cancer J. Clin. **68**(6), 394–424 (2018)
2. Chankong, T., Theera-Umpon, N., Auephanwiriyakul, S.: Automatic cervical cell segmentation and classification in PAP smears. Comput. Methods Programs Biomed. **113**(2), 539–556 (2014)
3. Frid-Adar, M., Diamant, I., Klang, E., Amitai, M., Goldberger, J., Greenspan, H.: GAN-based synthetic medical image augmentation for increased cnn performance in liver lesion classification. Neurocomputing **321**, 321–331 (2018)
4. Goodfellow, I., et al.: Generative adversarial nets. In: NeurIPS, pp. 2672–2680 (2014)
5. Gulrajani, I., Ahmed, F., Arjovsky, M., Dumoulin, V., Courville, A.C.: Improved training of wasserstein GANs. In: NeurIPS, pp. 5767–5777 (2017)
6. Guo, P., et al.: Nuclei-based features for uterine cervical cancer histology image analysis with fusion-based classification. IEEE J. Biomed. Health Inform. **20**(6), 1595–1607 (2016)
7. He, K., Zhang, X., Ren, S., Sun, J.: Deep residual learning for image recognition. In: CVPR, pp. 770–778 (2016)
8. Kingma, D.P., Ba, J.: Adam: a method for stochastic optimization. arXiv preprint arXiv:1412.6980 (2014)
9. van der Maaten, L., Hinton, G.: Visualizing data using t-SNE. J. Mach. Learn. Res. **9**(Nov), 2579–2605 (2008)
10. Madani, A., Moradi, M., Karargyris, A., Syeda-Mahmood, T.: Chest x-ray generation and data augmentation for cardiovascular abnormality classification. In: Medical Imaging 2018: Image Processing, vol. 10574, p. 105741M. International Society for Optics and Photonics (2018)
11. Mirza, M., Osindero, S.: Conditional generative adversarial nets. arXiv preprint arXiv:1411.1784 (2014)

12. Odena, A., Olah, C., Shlens, J.: Conditional image synthesis with auxiliary classifier GANs. In: ICML, pp. 2642–2651 (2017)
13. Radford, A., Metz, L., Chintala, S.: Unsupervised representation learning with deep convolutional generative adversarial networks. arXiv preprint arXiv:1511.06434 (2015)
14. Ren, J., Hacihaliloglu, I., Singer, E.A., Foran, D.J., Qi, X.: Adversarial domain adaptation for classification of prostate histopathology whole-slide images. In: Frangi, A.F., Schnabel, J.A., Davatzikos, C., Alberola-López, C., Fichtinger, G. (eds.) MICCAI 2018. LNCS, vol. 11071, pp. 201–209. Springer, Cham (2018). https://doi.org/10.1007/978-3-030-00934-2_23
15. Salimans, T., Goodfellow, I., Zaremba, W., Cheung, V., Radford, A., Chen, X.: Improved techniques for training GANs. In: NeurIPS, pp. 2234–2242 (2016)

# Cell Tracking with Deep Learning for Cell Detection and Motion Estimation in Low-Frame-Rate

Junya Hayashida[✉] and Ryoma Bise

Kyushu University, Fukuoka, Japan
junya.hayashida@human.ait.kyushu-u.ac.jp

**Abstract.** Cell behavior analysis in high-throughput biological experiments is important for research and discovery in biology and medicine. To perform the high-throughput experiments, it requires to capture images in low frame rate in order to record images on multi-points. In such a low frame rate image sequence, movements of cells between successive frames are often larger than distances to nearby cells, and thus current methods based on proximity do not work properly. In this study, we propose a cell tracking method that enables to track cells in low frame rate by simultaneously estimating all of the cell motions in successive frames. In the experiments under dense conditions in low frame rate, our method outperformed the other methods.

**Keywords:** Cell tracking · Microscopy image analysis

## 1 Introduction

Cell behavior analysis is important in biology and medicine. To analyze the quantitative cell behavior metrics, hundreds of cells are tracked in populations. However, it is time-consuming and tedious to track a large number of cells manually. Automatic cell tracking is required for this reason.

High-throughput biological experiments require multi-point scanning to monitor the entire cell population in a wide view with monitoring a high magnification on individual cell's details. To obtain high-resolution images on multi-points, we have to capture the time-lapse images with low frame rate. In such a low frame rate image sequence, movements of cells between successive frames are often larger than distances to nearby cells. This makes it almost impossible to associate cells between frames based on proximity.

On the other hand, a human can predict the individual cell positions and motions from the positional relationship of nearby cells empirically. It indicates

**Electronic supplementary material** The online version of this chapter (https://doi.org/10.1007/978-3-030-32239-7_44) contains supplementary material, which is available to authorized users.

that the motion *i.e.*, the association of cells between successive frames can be estimated by a data-driven approach.

In this paper, we propose a cell tracking method that can directly predict cell motion (association) called Cell Motion Field (CMF) by data-driven using deep learning. This enables cell tracking at low frame rates. In addition, it may terminate tracking cells in the middle of the entire trajectory when false negatives occur for several frames. To address this problem, our method first generates small trajectories (tracklets) and then associates the tracklets using CMF that can estimate the cell motion between the frames the miss-detection occurrence, where CMFs are trained for motion estimation in several interval frames. We evaluated the effectiveness of the proposed method with several current tracking methods using data-sets that cells are cultured in dense conditions. In this comparison, our method achieved the best performance.

## 2   Related Work

Many cell tracking methods have been proposed. Recently, current methods take a detection-and-association approach that first detect cells in each frame, and then associates detected cells between successive frames [1,8]. To detect cell regions at each frame, many cell detection/segmentation methods have been proposed, such as Graph-cut [1], deep learning [10]. To associate cells, optimization for associating cells between successive frames is solved by linear programming [8]. Graph-based optimization methods have been proposed that represent an entire image sequence as a graph, where a cell is a node and an association hypothesis is an edge, and then the method solves the global solutions [3,11]. However, these methods use the proximity of the cell positions as the association scores, and thus these methods do not work at low frame rate when cells move largely.

Recently, data-driven approaches for estimating cell motion or optical flow using deep neural networks have been proposed. He *et al.* [7] estimate the label of motion, such that the direction of cell motion, enlargement and reduction of cell shape. However, it does not work the case when many cells appear in dense since this method was developed to track a single object. Several CNN-based methods for estimating optical flow have been proposed such as FlowNet [6]. However, it remains as challenges how to prepare the ground-truth of the flow in cell images, and even though it can be estimated, it is not obvious how to use the flow for tracking multiple cells in dense condition. Unlike these existing methods, we propose a method to simultaneously estimate multiple cell motions in an image by end-to-end learning and use it for tracking.

## 3   Cell Tracking with Cell Motion Estimation

Figure 1 shows the overview of the proposed method. The method first estimates cell positions and the Cell Motion Field (CMF) that represents the motion of

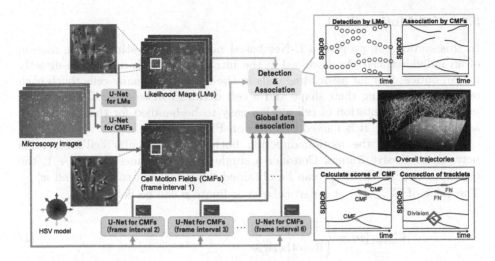

**Fig. 1.** Overview of proposed method.

cells between successive frames. Next, short trajectories (tracklets) are generated by associating the detected cells between successive frames using CMF as association scores. In general, a tracklet terminates when a false negative of cell detection occurs, where the false negatives may continue several frames. Then, to obtain the final cell trajectories with the lineage information, global data association associates the tracklets using CMF that can estimate the cell motion between the several frames the miss-detection occurs, where CMFs were trained for motion estimation in several interval frames.

### 3.1 Cell Position Estimation by Regression

The proposed method first estimates cell positions by U-Net [10] that has been widely used for segmentation tasks. In general, a segmentation task requires pixel-level annotation as training data that segments a boundary of each cell. To reduce the annotation costs, instead, we use cell centroid positions as training data. Since the human annotation is not strict and has gaps from the true position, we design the cell position estimation problem as a regression problem that estimates likelihood map, where an annotated cell position becomes a peak and the value gradually decreases with a Gaussian distribution (Fig. 1). To train the position estimation U-Net from the input of the original image, we use the mean of squared error (MSE) between the original image and the estimated likelihood map. This trains the U-Net as a regressor. In the test, the trained U-Net estimates the likelihood map and then the peaks on the map are detected as cell centroid positions. The estimated cell positions are used for the next processes.

## 3.2   Cell Motion Field

In this section, we propose a U-Net based network that estimates the motion of an individual cell. As discussed in the introduction, it is difficult to directly use an optical flow for associating cells in the cases when many cells touch each other with changing their shape and a cell divides to two cells. Therefore, we propose a representation of cell motion easy to be handled for the association, as shown in Fig. 1. It is named Cell Motion Field (CMF).

CMF encodes the motion direction between a particular cell's centroids between successive frames. Consider a single cell $i$ in frames $t$ and $t + 1$, the corresponding CMF $\mathbf{C}^i_{t,t+1}$ can be obtained using cell centroids $\boldsymbol{x}^i_t$, and $\boldsymbol{x}^i_{t+1}$. The value of $\mathbf{C}^i_{t,t+1}(\boldsymbol{p})$ at a particular coordinate $\boldsymbol{p}$ can be defined as:

$$\mathbf{C}^i_{t,t+1}(\boldsymbol{p}) = \begin{cases} \boldsymbol{v} & \text{if } \boldsymbol{p} \in \boldsymbol{L} \\ \boldsymbol{0} & \text{otherwise,} \end{cases} \tag{1}$$

$$L = \{\forall \boldsymbol{p} \text{ s.t. } 0 \le \boldsymbol{v} \cdot (\boldsymbol{p} - \boldsymbol{x}^i_t) \le ||\boldsymbol{x}^i_{t+1} - \boldsymbol{x}^i_t||_2,$$
$$|\boldsymbol{v}_\perp \cdot (\boldsymbol{p} - \boldsymbol{x}^i_t)| \le \sigma_c\}, \tag{2}$$

where $\boldsymbol{v} = (\boldsymbol{x}^i_{t+1} - \boldsymbol{x}^i_t)/||\boldsymbol{x}^i_{t+1} - \boldsymbol{x}^i_t||_2$ is the unit vector in the direction of the motion flow between the cell's centroids between $t$ and $t + 1$ and $\boldsymbol{v}_\perp$ is a unit vector perpendicular to $\boldsymbol{v}$. The CMF is an image that has two channels, where a channel indicates the motion of x and y coordinates, respectively. Here, $\boldsymbol{L}$ indicates the rectangle region whose endpoints are the centroids $\boldsymbol{x}^i_t, \boldsymbol{x}^i_{t+1}$, the length is $||\boldsymbol{x}^i_{t+1} - \boldsymbol{x}^i_t||_2$, and the wide is the $2\sigma_c$, where $\sigma_c$ is a hyperparameter that is set as the half of the mean of cell radius. When the cell $i$ divided to two cells $j$ and $k$, we generate the two motion flows ($\boldsymbol{x}^i_t$ to $\boldsymbol{x}^j_{t+1}$) and ($\boldsymbol{x}^i_t$ to $\boldsymbol{x}^k_{t+1}$) with similar manner to the single cell migration. The CMF $\mathbf{C}_{t,t+1}$ that aggregates all the individual CMFs is defined as:

$$\mathbf{C}_{t,t+1}(\boldsymbol{p}) = \frac{\sum_i \mathbf{C}^i_{t,t+1}(\boldsymbol{p})}{||\sum_i \mathbf{C}^i_{t,t+1}(\boldsymbol{p})||_2}. \tag{3}$$

One of the advantages of this representation is that it only requires the cell centroid positions of two successive frames that are the same with the training data for detection.

Given such ground-truth of CMF, a U-Net is trained using the loss function that is the mean squared error between the training data and the estimated data. In the test data, the trained U-Net can produce all of the cell motion flow in the input image as CMF.

## 3.3   Tracklet Generation by Joint Solving Detection and Association

In this step, the proposed method generates short trajectories (tracklets) using the cell position likelihood map and CMF. Since the tracking process usually heavily depends on the detection results, i.e., detection errors directly propagate to the tracking step, to avoid such error propagation, cell detection and association simultaneously determined frame-by-frame using binary programming, similar to [2].

First, cell position candidates are obtained by thresholding for the cell position likelihood map with multiple thresholds since the center of a cell has high values and then the value gradually decreases as far from the center. If two cells touch with blurry boundaries, the candidates include the three candidate regions; two cell regions and a region contain these two cells.

Next, a set of all association hypotheses between the cell region candidates and tracking results at the previous frame is listed up. Then the corresponding scores are calculated using the cell position likelihood map and CMF for each hypothesis. Let the coordinates of the centroid of the $i$-th detected region at frame $t-1$ be $p_{t-1}^i$, that of the $j$-th detected region at frame $t$ be $p_t^j$, the maximum likelihood value of the $j$-th region be $l_t^j$, and CMF between frames $t-1$ and $t$ be $C_{t-1,t}$, the score $\rho_{t-1,t}^{i,j}$ is defined as:

$$\rho_{t-1,t}^{i,j} = l_t^j D_{t-1,t}^{i,j} I_{t-1,t}^{i,j} \tag{4}$$

$$D_{t-1,t}^{i,j} = \exp\left(-\frac{\|p_t^j - p_{t-1}^i\|_2^2}{\lambda}\right) \tag{5}$$

$$I_{t-1,t}^{i,j} = \int_0^1 C_{t-1,t}(r(u)) \cdot \frac{(p_t^j - p_{t-1}^i)}{\|p_t^j - p_{t-1}^i\|_2} du \tag{6}$$

$$r(u) = (1-u)p_{t-1}^i + up_t^j \tag{7}$$

where $r(u)$ interpolates the position of the two centroids $p_{t-1}^i$ and $p_t^j$. $l_t^i$ indicates the likelihood that the detected candidates is a true cell, $D_{t-1,t}^{i,j}$ indicates the proximity of two positions between the $i$-th cell at $t-1$ and the $j$-th candidate at $t$, $I_{t-1,t}^{i,j}$ is the linear integral over the corresponding CMF, along the line segment connecting the centroid of the cell at $t$ and that of the candidate at $t+1$, where $D_{t-1,t}^{i,j} I_{t-1,t}^{i,j}$ indicates the likelihood of the association.

The optimization for selecting the optimal set of association hypotheses can be solved by binary programming that has constraints to avoid conflict association. The optimization is formulized as:

$$y^* = \arg\max_{y} \rho^T y \tag{8}$$

$$\text{subject to } A^T y \leq 1, \ y \in \{0,1\},$$

where vector $\rho$ stores the score of every possible hypothesis and matrix $A$ stores the constraints to avoid conflict hypotheses, where $A$ is defined with the similar manner to [2]. $y$ is a $H \times 1$ binary vector where $H$ is the number of hypotheses. $y_k = 1$ means the $k$-th hypothesis is selected in the optimal solution. If the hypothesis ($p_t^i$ moves to $p_{t+1}^j$) is selected in the optimal solution, the $j$-th candidate $p_{t+1}^j$ is selected as a cell region and also associated to $p_t^i$. This frame-by-frame association is iteratively done for all the frames. If a false negative detection occurs at $t+1$ near the cell $x_t^i$, the tracklet is terminated.

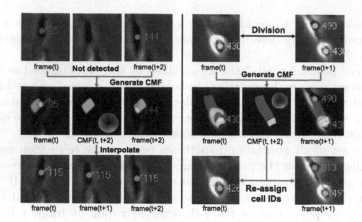

**Fig. 2.** Examples of CMFs used for global association. Left: example when a miss-detection occurs at $t + 1$. Right: example when a cell divided two cells.

### 3.4 Global Association Using CMF

Given the set of tracklet, we associate tracklets to obtain the final tracking results with cell division information by global data association. In this process, we also use CMF for computing the score of the association hypothesis between tracklets. False negatives may occur during several frames between two split tracklets. To estimate the motion flow between the interval of several frames, we train the multiple CMF estimation U-Net for the different intervals in advance as shown in Fig. 1. In addition, when a cell divides to two cells, the CMF estimation U-Net can simultaneously estimate the two flows to the daughter cells. Similar to [3], tracklet association hypotheses are listed up. To compute the scores of the hypotheses, CMF is also used. If the frame interval between two tracklets is $a$, the CMF estimation network for $a$ frame intervals is selected and the method computes the hypothesis score using the estimated CMF, where the score is $I_{t-1,t}^{i,j}$ (Eq. 6). Then, the optimal hypothesis set is optimized by binary programming that maximizes the sum of scores. Using the optimal association, the method re-assigns the cell ID, interpolates coordinates between tracklets, and identifies the parent-daughter relationships when a cell division occurs to obtain the final cell trajectories.

## 4   Experiments

In the experiments, we evaluated the effectiveness of the proposed method compared with several methods in challenging open data-sets [9], where mouse myoblast cells (C2C12) were cultured under 4 different media conditions; (1) control (no growth factor), (2) fibroblast growth factor 2 (FGF2), (3) bone morphogenetic protein 2 (BMP2), and (4) FGF2 + BMP2. Each dataset includes 4 or 5 image sequences (total is 18), where the cells were captured by phase contrast

**Table 1.** Performance of compared methods.

| Metric | Data | *Bensh* [1] | *Chalfoun* [5] | *Bise* [3] | *Ours w/o CMF* | Proposed |
|---|---|---|---|---|---|---|
| Association accuracy | 1 | 0.556 | 0.748 | 0.841 | 0.865 | **0.883** |
| | 2 | 0.458 | 0.639 | 0.727 | 0.866 | **0.894** |
| | 3 | 0.746 | 0.724 | 0.915 | 0.963 | **0.971** |
| | 4 | 0.602 | 0.785 | 0.820 | 0.934 | **0.951** |
| | Average | 0.584 | 0.720 | 0.816 | 0.909 | **0.927** |
| Target effectiveness | 1 | 0.448 | 0.564 | 0.809 | 0.729 | **0.832** |
| | 2 | 0.395 | 0.450 | 0.642 | 0.712 | **0.813** |
| | 3 | 0.589 | 0.460 | 0.834 | 0.914 | **0.958** |
| | 4 | 0.453 | 0.588 | 0.722 | 0.796 | **0.895** |
| | Average | 0.466 | 0.512 | 0.736 | 0.787 | **0.875** |

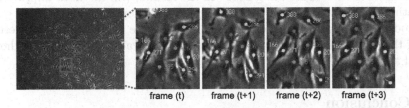

frame (t)        frame (t+1)        frame (t+2)        frame (t+3)

**Fig. 3.** Examples of tracking results by our method under culture condition 3 (BMP2).

microscopy at every 5 min over 780 frames with the resolution of $1040 \times 1392$. Since our target is to track cells in low frame rate, the frame rate of the dataset was reduced to one-fifth of the original (*i.e.*, the interval is 25 min). 3 fully annotated sequences (the total is 980 frames) were used for training the detection and CMF estimation networks, and 15 sequences were used for test data, where 10% of the initial number of cells are randomly selected in the initial frame and their progeny cells are manually tracked. The appearance of C2C12 changes drastically under the different conditions [8] due to the characteristic of differentiation, such as bone muscles and myotubes. It is a challenging task to track cells under such various conditions (Fig. 3).

The left images of Fig. 2 show the examples of CMFs in the case, where a miss detection occurs at frame $t + 1$ and the tracklet of ID85 was terminated at $t$ and a new tracklet of ID144 starts to track the same cell. Since the interval between tracklets is 2 ($t$ to $t+2$), the CMF estimation U-Net for the intervals of 2 frames was performed to estimate the CMF. This successfully estimated the cell motion and the tracklets were connected with the linear interpolation with the re-assigned ID. The right images show examples in the case, where a cell divided into two cells. In this case, the CMF estimation U-Net also succeeded to estimate both cell motions of these two daughter cells, and the cell division information was registered.

To demonstrate the efficacy of our method quantitatively, we compared our method with three methods; Bensch [1], Chalfoun [5] and Bise [3]. In addition, to demonstrate the effectiveness of CMF, the proposed method without CMF was also evaluated. To evaluate the performance, we used two quantitative metrics; association accuracy and target effectiveness [4]. Association accuracy indicates the number of true associations divided by the total number of associations. The target effectiveness is computed as the number of the assigned track observations over the total number of frames of the target, where each target (human annotated) is assigned to a track (computer-generated) that contains the most observations from that ground-truth.

Table 1 shows the tracking performances in the comparison. Our methods achieved the best performance under all culture conditions. One of the reasons that our methods outperformed the other methods is that our cell detection and global association approach improved the performance much. To demonstrate the effectiveness of the proposed CMF, we also evaluated the improvement of the proposed method without using CMF. In the results, Our methods improved the targeting effectiveness over 9% on average. In addition, the performance of our method using a low frame rate was better than those of the compared methods using the original frame rate. It demonstrated the practicality of our method in a real application.[1]

## 5    Conclusion

In this paper, we proposed a cell tracking method that can directly predict cell motion (association) using deep learning. This enables cell tracking in low frame rates. We evaluated the effectiveness of the proposed method with several current tracking methods using data-sets that cells are cultured in dense conditions. These experiments demonstrated the effectiveness of the proposed method to track cells that are densely located and often touch each other in a low frame rate, where our method outperforms the other methods.

**Acknowledgement.** This work was supported by JSPS KAKENHI Grant Number 18H04738 and 18H05104.

## References

1. Bensch, R., Ronneberger, O.: Cell segmentation and tracking in phase contrast images using graph cut with asymmetric boundary costs. In: ISBI, pp. 1220–1223 (2015)
2. Bise, R., Maeda, Y., Kim, M., Kino-oka, M.: Cell tracking under high confluency conditions by candidate cell region detection-based-association approach. In: Biomedical Engineering (2013)
3. Bise, R., Yin, Z., Kanade, T.: Reliable cell tracking by global data association. In: ISBI, pp. 1004–1010 (2011)
4. Blackman, S.S.: Multiple-target tracking with radar applications (1986)

---

[1] The supplementary video is on http://human.ait.kyushu-u.ac.jp/~bise/researches-bise-CIA-en.html.

5. Chalfoun, J., Majurski, M., Dima, A., et al.: Lineage mapper: a versatile cell and particle tracker. Sci. Rep. **6**(1), 36984 (2016)
6. Dosovitskiy, A., Fischer, P., et al.: FlowNet: learning optical flow with convolutional networks. In: ICCV (2015)
7. He, T., Mao, H., Guo, J., Yi, Z.: Cell tracking using deep neural networks with multi-task learning. Image Vis. Comput. **60**, 142–153 (2017). Regularization Techniques for High-Dimensional Data Analysis
8. Kanade, T., Yin, Z., Bise, R., et al.: Cell image analysis: algorithms, system and applications. In: WACV, pp. 374–381 (2011)
9. Ker, D., Eom, S., Sanami, S., et al.: Phase contrast time-lapse microscopy datasets with automated and manual cell tracking annotations. Sci. Data **5**, 180237 (2018)
10. Ronneberger, O., Fischer, P., Brox, T.: U-Net: convolutional networks for biomedical image segmentation. In: Navab, N., Hornegger, J., Wells, W.M., Frangi, A.F. (eds.) MICCAI 2015. LNCS, vol. 9351, pp. 234–241. Springer, Cham (2015). https://doi.org/10.1007/978-3-319-24574-4_28
11. Schiegg, M., Hanslovsky, P., Kausler, B.X., et al.: Conservation tracking. In: ICCV, pp. 2928–2935 (2013)

# Accelerated ML-Assisted Tumor Detection in High-Resolution Histopathology Images

Nikolas Ioannou[1]([✉]), Milos Stanisavljevic[1], Andreea Anghel[1],
Nikolaos Papandreou[1], Sonali Andani[1], Jan Hendrik Rüschoff[2], Peter Wild[3],
Maria Gabrani[1], and Haralampos Pozidis[1]

[1] IBM Research – Zurich, Rüschlikon, Switzerland
{nio,ysm,aan,npo,son,mga,hap}@zurich.ibm.com
[2] Institute of Pathology and Molecular Pathology, University Hospital Zurich,
Zurich, Switzerland
[3] Dr. Senckenberg Institute of Pathology, University Hospital Frankfurt,
Frankfurt, Germany

**Abstract.** Color normalization is one of the main tasks in the processing pipeline of computer-aided diagnosis (CAD) systems in histopathology. This task reduces the color and intensity variations that are typically present in stained whole-slide images (WSI) due to, e.g., non-standardization of staining protocols. Moreover, it increases the accuracy of machine learning (ML) based CAD systems. Given the vast amount of gigapixel-sized WSI data, and the need to reduce the time-to-insight, there is an increasing demand for efficient ML systems. In this work, we present a high-performance pipeline that enables big data analytics for WSIs in histopathology. As an exemplary ML inference pipeline, we employ a convolutional neural network (CNN), used to detect prostate cancer in WSIs, with stain normalization preprocessing. We introduce a set of optimizations across the whole pipeline: (i) we parallelize and optimize the stain normalization process, (ii) we introduce a multi-threaded I/O framework optimized for fast non-volatile memory (NVM) storage, and (iii) we integrate the stain normalization optimizations and the enhanced I/O framework in the ML pipeline to minimize the data transfer overheads and the overall prediction time. Our combined optimizations accelerate the end-to-end ML pipeline by 7.2× and 21.2×, on average, for low and high resolution levels of WSIs, respectively. Significantly, it allows for a seamless integration of the ML-assisted diagnosis with state-of-the-art whole slide scanners, by reducing the prediction time for high-resolution histopathology images from ∼30 min to under 80 s.

## 1 Introduction

Histopathology image analysis based on machine learning (ML) has become a valuable tool in computational pathology for assisting the work of pathologists towards efficient decision support [13,15]. With the advent of whole slide

© Springer Nature Switzerland AG 2019
D. Shen et al. (Eds.): MICCAI 2019, LNCS 11764, pp. 406–414, 2019.
https://doi.org/10.1007/978-3-030-32239-7_45

imaging technology and the advances in deep learning, there has been research, recently, towards building efficient architectures that achieve high accuracy in many applications related to medical image analysis [9]. At the same time, given the large size and computational requirements of high-resolution whole-slide images (WSIs), there is a stringent need to build high-performance pipelines that enable large-scale and high-resolution medical image processing. In particular, when considering the ML inference task, the end-to-end pipeline should deliver high-accuracy results with minimum latency; otherwise the computing system for diagnosis support may become a bottleneck instead of a valuable asset.

The multi-resolution format of WSIs, along with the typical preprocessing specific to hematoxylin and eosin (H&E) stained WSIs, make the computational requirements of ML-based histopathology image analysis challenging. Due to the giga-pixel size of high-resolution WSIs, the preprocessing stages of an end-to-end ML pipeline may become a significant burden during inference, and thus adversely affect the time-to-insight. A popular WSI preprocessing method used in histopathological diagnosis is stain normalization (SN). This preprocessing step reduces the color variations present in WSIs due to differences in the exposure time of the tissue glass slide before scanning, staining and storage procedures, H&E concentration, type of scanners etc. Such variations can decrease the performance of ML-based systems for image analysis.

In this paper, we present a high-performance pipeline for SN preprocessing that enables big data analytics for WSIs in histopathology. The proposed pipeline uses a state-of-the-art unsupervised method based on stain-vector estimation [11]. Furthermore, the standard image loading/storing library (libtiff) used in conventional tools (OpenSlide [1]), has significant performance overheads for high-resolution images. Therefore, we also introduce a novel I/O backend to the libtiff library, that is optimized for fast non-volatile memory (NVM) storage. Our framework enables efficient image I/O and delivers significantly higher performance on fast NVM storage compared to the default library. On top of this enhanced I/O backend, we present a multi-threaded image loading/storing architecture that further accelerates the WSI ingestion process. Last, we integrate the fast SN pipeline and the optimized I/O system in a complete ML inference pipeline to minimize the overheads of data transfer across stages and the overall prediction time. As an exemplary ML pipeline for computational pathology, we employ a Tensorflow-based convolutional neural network (CNN) with stain normalization preprocessing for prostate cancer detection in WSIs. Compared to the state-of-the-art ML pipeline, our optimizations reduce the inference time by more than 7×, on average, for low-resolution and by more than 21× for high-resolution WSIs. To put this into perspective, it brings down the prediction time from 27.2 min to 77 s for high-resolution WSIs, drastically reducing the time-to-insight for pathologists. This improved end-to-end ML inference time allows for a seamless integration of the ML diagnosis pipeline with state-of-the-art whole slide scanners (60 s scan time [2]).

## 2    Background

***Histopathology WSI Preprocessing: Stain Normalization.*** In this work we focus on a well-known normalization algorithm [11] which is based on the principle that the color of each pixel (RGB channels) is a linear combination of the two stain vectors – hematoxylin and eosin (H&E). The algorithm estimates the stain vectors of the image by using a singular-value decomposition-based method (SVD) on the non-background pixels. Stain normalization has been shown to be critical for ML-based image analysis pipelines. Ciompi et al. [3] demonstrate that the accuracy of an ML system can be improved by 20% when using stain-normalized input.

One of the main challenges of the normalization method under study [11] is its scalability to large-scale WSIs, e.g. 40X resolution. Typical implementations of this method are not system-aware: the multi-core processors and memory of the running system are not efficiently used to allow fast loading and processing of WSIs. Moreover, the loading of a WSI relies on external libraries for reading and writing Tagged Image File Format files (libtiff/OpenSlide). These libraries are not optimized for modern parallel architectures, thus they can significantly slow down the WSI processing run-time.

***ML Pipelines for Histopathology WSIs.*** Zerhouni et al. [16] propose an ML architecture for mitosis detection in breast histopathology WSIs. The approach uses stain normalized patches of the image in 40X resolution to train a Wide Residual Network. Cireşan et al. [4] propose an ML-based pipeline also for mitosis detection in breast histopathology images. The study uses H&E-stained WSIs split into patches that feed the training engine of an 11-layer CNN model. Be it nuclei detection and classification or segmentation medical tasks, many of their corresponding ML approaches have a common basic architecture: (1) split the input WSI into patches, (2) preprocess (e.g., staining normalization) each patch and store on disk, (3) load the normalized patches and train an ML model, and (4) run prediction using the trained model. ML inference pipelines working on WSIs often operate on large datasets of hundreds of images. With high-resolution WSIs, this may translate to a tera-byte scale volume of data (e.g., 100 images in 40X resolution results in 2 TB of uncompressed data), which requires an optimized and scalable ML architecture. The training and inference engines are typically accelerated by using GPU technologies. WSI preprocessing (stain normalization) however also needs to be scalable and fast enough to handle large WSIs. Moreover, every part of the ML system that involves image loading/storing should be highly-optimized to remove any I/O bottlenecks.

## 3    Optimized ML Pipeline Architecture

Figure 1 depicts the overall system architecture for an end-to-end inference pipeline. It starts by loading the WSI, then performs the stain normalization ($A$ to $C$), writes out the normalized image, which is in turn picked up by the inference engine, where patch extraction and inference evaluation are performed.

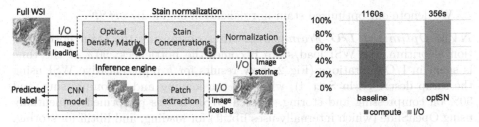

**Fig. 1.** System architecture overview.

**Fig. 2.** Breakdown of stain normalization time.

***Stain Normalization.*** As a reference baseline implementation of the stain normalization algorithm (Macenko et al. [11]) we use a publicly available MATLAB code [14]. The processing blocks $A$, $B$, and $C$ in Fig. 1 correspond to optical density matrix (ODM [12]) calculation, computation of stain concentrations and their robust maximums, and pixels normalization with transformation back to RGB space, respectively. Even when ported to C++, the reference code suffers from high memory consumption and long processing times for 40X WSIs. We denote this C++ reference implementation by *baseline*. To enable and speed-up the processing of such WSIs we perform the following optimizations:

(a) After image loading only RGB pixel values are stored in memory. Since staining normalization typically operate in optical density (OD) space, conversion is performed on non-background pixels only, on-the-fly, in the processing blocks $A$, $B$ and $C$. A look-up table method is used for the conversion from RGB to OD space instead of the log function in order to speed-up computation.

(b) In blocks $A$ and $B$, which are benchmarked as the most time-consuming steps, we use partial sorting that runs 2–3x faster compared to full sorting.

(c) For the exponential function in the processing block $C$, we use the fast exponentiation library [5] since it performs 5–10x faster compared to the corresponding function in the standard C library.

(d) Since the processing blocks $A$, $B$, and $C$ perform many independent operations on individual pixels, their execution is parallelized across all available CPU threads using the OpenMP library.

(e) Given that the processing blocks $A$ and $B$ are the most time-consuming due to the difficulty of parallelizing the sorting operation, we perform another optimization that is using a Monte Carlo sampling technique [6]. In this method, a sample of non-background pixels is randomly chosen from the set of all non-background pixels in order to estimate the required robust extremes [11].

We denote our optimized stain normalization engine by *optSN*.

***NVM-Optimized I/O Framework.*** After optimizing the stain normalization algorithm, the WSI load/store becomes the bottleneck: 90% of the time is spent in I/O operations (Fig. 2 show results for a representative WSI using the setup described in Sect. 4), with 40% on loading and decompressing, and 50% on compressing and storing. Typical WSIs I/O is performed sequentially using OpenSlide (which internally uses libtiff) for loading, and libtiff for storing. This approach does not efficiently utilize the multi-core architectures of modern CPUs, nor the inherent parallelism of high-performance NVM storage devices. This is due to the following performance limitations of the libtiff I/O backend: (i) it uses non-thread safe I/O system calls (`read`, `write`), (ii) it is not scalable with respect to decompressing (compressing) an image for reading (writing) as it keeps internal non thread-safe state, and (iii) it uses buffered I/O that uses the OS page cache, which leads to uncontrolled memory consumption as well as it has limited scalability when concurrently accessing the page cache from multiple cores [17].

To accelerate the medical image ingestion process, we need to load and store WSIs in parallel. To this end, we introduce a new I/O backend to the libtiff library optimized for modern NVM devices and multi-core CPUs that (i) is thread-safe and scalable allowing for a large I/O parallelism, and (ii) accesses the storage directly (`O_DIRECT`), bypassing the page cache. We achieve this by extending the C++ I/O API of libtiff (`tiffio.hxx`) to provide a new interface that utilizes a fast NVM-optimized key-value store [8] – a persistent data store that uses a hash-table index plus log-structured data allocation [7].

Furthermore, we build an efficient multi-threaded I/O framework around the extended libtiff that provides C++/Python APIs for WSI loading and storing. Multi-threaded loading is enabled by using one TIFF file handle per thread (`TIFFOpen`); each thread independently loads and de-compresses a separate part of the image. To enable multi-threaded image storing, we disable image compression, and use the optimized I/O backend which allows for parallel writes. This new I/O framework delivers higher performance on multi-core systems and fast NVM storage compared to the default I/O backend and is used in both the stain normalization and the inference engine pipeline stages. Note that the parallel image compression and de-compression optimizations are applicable to any multi-core system, irrespective of the underlying storage hardware.

Ultimately, our I/O framework supports images of most common scanner formats: Aperio, Philips, Ventana, and Hamamatsu. These formats are typically single-file pyramidal TIFF or BigTIFF-like formats with proprietary metadata.

***ML Inference Pipeline.*** To predict on an unseen WSI, we run inference using a trained model of a VGG-inspired [10] architecture as shown in Fig. 3. The model input consists of WSI patches loaded in a user-defined image resolution. The model output is the predicted label for the specific task. For this study, we train two models for tumor detection, one for patches of size $512 \times 512$ pixels extracted from 10X resolution (model A) and one for patches of size $2048 \times 2048$ pixels extracted from 40X resolution (model B). For inference on 10X patches, we first load 10X image from an WSI. To avoid running inference on background patches, we perform binary thresholding to obtain the mask of the tissue region. The thresholding can be time-consuming in 10X, thus we perform it at 2.5X. From the tissue region of the 10X image, we extract non-overlapping patches of size 512 × 512 and perform prediction for each patch using model A. The 40X inference pipeline is similar to that of the 10X case, except for (1) the patch size which is 2048 × 2048, and (2) the prediction is performed using model B.

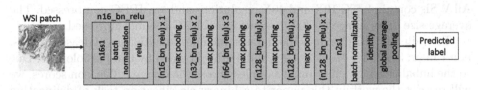

**Fig. 3.** CNN architecture overview. A convolution layer with 16 3 × 3 filters, and a stride of 1 × 1 is denoted by n16s1. The same, followed by a batch normalization layer (yellow) and a RELU non-linearity (green) is denoted by n16_bn_relu. The learning rate used for training is 0.001, the optimizer SGD with momentum 0.9 and the batch size 16. (Color figure online)

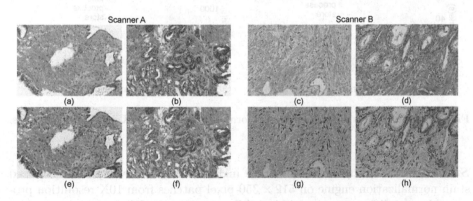

**Fig. 4.** Original patches (a)–(d) and their normalized versions (e)–(h) after applying our optimized stain normalization algorithm *optSN* described in Sect. 3.

**Putting it All Together.** The *baseline* ML pipeline (Fig. 1) comprises of stain normalization using a C++ implementation of the publicly available MATLAB code [14], OpenSlide C/libtiff library for loading/storing respectively, and an inference engine using the VGG-inspired CNN and the OpenSlide Python library for loading. We modify this baseline to (i) incorporate the parallelized and high-performance stain normalization (*optSN*) and (ii) utilize the NVM-optimized I/O framework across the pipeline stages: loading WSIs for normalization, writing out normalized images, and feeding them to the inference engine (*optIO*).

## 4  Evaluation

**Setup.** For the evaluation we use a server with two 10-core Intel® Xeon® E5-2630v4 CPUs, 125 GiB RAM, running a 4.4 Linux kernel (Ubuntu 16.04). The machine has 10 Intel® Flash NVMe Solid State Drives (SSD, P3600 400 GB 2.5in PCIe), and an NVIDIA® GTX 1080 GPU with 8 GiB of GDDR5 memory.

We use 20 H&E-stained needle-based biopsy WSIs of prostate cancer tissue. These images were digitized using a Ventana scanner and are in BigTIFF format. All WSIs contain 2.5X, 10X and 40X resolutions and are JPEG compressed. The average size of an image at 40X resolution is 21.7 GiBs uncompressed.

To train our ML pipeline, the dataset includes annotations (Gleason scores: non-tumor, $3 + 3$, $3 + 4$, $4 + 3$, $4 + 4$ and $4 + 5$) provided by two pathologists. Due to the imbalanced distribution of samples across the different Gleason scores, we will restrict the work in this paper to a binary classification task of delineating tumor and non-tumor regions. All regions with a Gleason score higher than or equal to $3 + 3$ will be considered as tumor and the remaining as non-tumor.

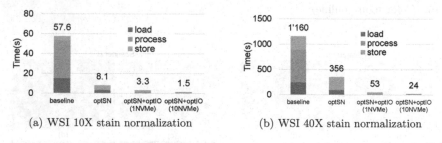

(a) WSI 10X stain normalization        (b) WSI 40X stain normalization

**Fig. 5.** Baseline SN vs. optimized SN: performance results for 10X and 40X resolutions.

**Stain Normalization.** We illustrate in Fig. 4 the effectiveness of optimized stain normalization engine on $512 \times 350$-pixel patches from 10X resolution produced by two different scanners (A and B, respectively). While the input images (top row) show significant color variation, the normalized ones show more uniform color contrast as a result of the normalization process.

Next, we focus on the performance of the stain normalization preprocessing step. Images are first loaded and decompressed using libtiff. Stain normalization is then performed on the in-memory uncompressed image, and, finally, the normalized image is written out (compressed or uncompressed). Figure 5 depicts the average results over all 20 images at two resolutions: 10X (Fig. 5a) and 40X (Fig. 5b). The results compare the *baseline* sequential stain normalization implementation that uses OpenSlide vs. our optimizations: (i) the high-performance stain normalization (*optSN*) and (ii) optimized I/O framework (*optSN+optIO*) on two different storage devices (1 and 10 NVMe SSDs). Our optimized SN provides a speedup of 7.1× and 3.2× (for 10X and 40X resolution, respectively) over

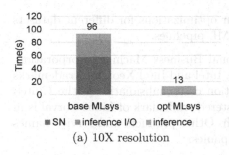 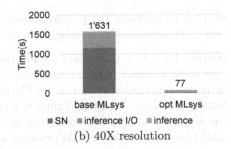

(a) 10X resolution                    (b) 40X resolution

**Fig. 6.** End-to-end inference pipeline performance on 10X and 40X WSIs, with time broken down into preprocessing, loading for inference, and inference execution.

the baseline. The optimized I/O backend provides an additional 2.4× speedup (6.7× for 40X); faster storage devices (10 instead of 1 NVMe SSD) result in additional 2.2× improvement, bringing the total speedup over the baseline to 39× and 49.3×, for 10X and 40X resolution, respectively. Note that without the improved I/O backend, it does not make a notable difference whether we use fast or slow storage devices: loading (storing) the WSIs is CPU-bound when performed sequentially and when decompression (compression) is used.

*End-to-End ML Inference Pipeline Performance.* The next results are obtained using the end-to-end inference pipeline presented in Sect. 3, including the stain normalization engine. We compare the baseline ML system vs. our optimized ML system that combines preprocessing and inference acceleration. The average results across the 20 WSIs are depicted in Fig. 6, for 10X and 40X. Our combined optimizations in preprocessing and image I/O improve the end-to-end inference latency of a WSI by 7.2× and 21.2×, for 10X and 40X, respectively. This is due to a dramatic reduction in the stain normalization time, but also by reducing the time taken to load the preprocessed images for inference. The run-time of inference model loading and patch extraction is independent of the image size, and thus takes a larger percentage of time on 10X than on 40X (33% vs. 6%); this explains the relatively lower speedup for 10X resolution compared to 40X. Across the whole WSI dataset the total prediction time is reduced, on average, from 96 s to 13 s for 10X, and from 27.2 min to 77s for 40X.

## 5  Conclusion

We presented an efficient ML pipeline for computational pathology, incorporating a parallel and highly-efficient stain normalization engine and a multithreaded NVM-optimized I/O framework. Our optimized pipeline holds great promise to improve the performance of ML pipelines designed for tumor detection. Indeed we showed that for a given medical task and ML pipeline, our optimizations can dramatically reduce the time needed for an ML-assisted tumor detection. For the particular biopsy dataset, the per-image run-time of the end-to-end ML inference pipeline is reduced from 30 min to under 80 s. As future work we plan to evaluate the performance of our optimizations for different datasets and to investigate the scalability to other ML pipelines.

**Notes:** IBM is a trademark of International Business Machines Corporation, registered in many jurisdictions worldwide. Intel and Intel Xeon are trademarks or registered trademarks of Intel Corporation or its subsidiaries in the United States and other countries. Linux is a registered trademark of Linus Torvalds in the United States, other countries, or both. Other products and service names might be trademarks of IBM or other companies.

# References

1. OpenSlide is a C library that provides a simple interface to read whole-slide images. https://openslide.org/
2. Ultra Fast Scanner (Digital pathology slide scanner). www.usa.philips.com/healthcare
3. Ciompi, F., et al.: The importance of stain normalization in colorectal tissue classification with convolutional networks. In: ISBI (2017)
4. Cireşan, D.C., Giusti, A., Gambardella, L.M., Schmidhuber, J.: Mitosis detection in breast cancer histology images with deep neural networks. In: Mori, K., Sakuma, I., Sato, Y., Barillot, C., Navab, N. (eds.) MICCAI 2013. LNCS, vol. 8150, pp. 411–418. Springer, Heidelberg (2013). https://doi.org/10.1007/978-3-642-40763-5_51
5. Fast approximate function of exponential function exp and log. https://github.com/herumi/fmath
6. Harrison, R.L.: Introduction to Monte Carlo simulation. In: American Institute of Physics Conference Series (2010)
7. Ioannou, N., et al.: Elevating commodity storage with the SALSA host translation layer. In: IEEE MASCOTS (2018)
8. Kourtis, K., et al.: Reaping the performance of fast NVM storage with uDepot. In: FAST (2019)
9. Litjens, G., et al.: A survey on deep learning in medical image analysis. Med. Image Anal. **42**, 60–88 (2017)
10. Liu, S., Deng, W.: Very deep convolutional neural network based image classification using small training sample size. In: ACPR (2015)
11. Macenko, M., et al.: A method for normalizing histology slides for quantitative analysis. In: ISBI (2009)
12. Ruifrok, A.C., Johnston, D.A.: Quantification of histochemical staining by color deconvolution. Anal. Quant. Cytol. Histol. **23**(4), 291–299 (2001)
13. Veta, M., et al.: Breast cancer histopathology image analysis: a review. IEEE Trans. Biomed. Eng. **61**(5), 1400–1411 (2014)
14. Staining unmixing and normalization. https://github.com/mitkovetta/staining-normalization
15. Wernick, M.N., et al.: Machine learning in medical imaging. IEEE Sig. Process. Mag. **27**(4), 25–38 (2010)
16. Zerhouni, E., et al.: Wide residual networks for mitosis detection. In: ISBI (2017)
17. Zheng, D., et al.: A parallel page cache: IOPS and caching for multicore systems. In: HotStorage (2012)

# Pre-operative Overall Survival Time Prediction for Glioblastoma Patients Using Deep Learning on Both Imaging Phenotype and Genotype

Zhenyu Tang[1,2], Yuyun Xu[3], Zhicheng Jiao[2], Junfeng Lu[4], Lei Jin[4], Abudumijiti Aibaidula[4], Jinsong Wu[4], Qian Wang[5], Han Zhang[2(✉)], and Dinggang Shen[2(✉)]

[1] Beijing Advanced Innovation Center for Big Data and Brain Computing, Beihang University, Beijing, China
[2] Department of Radiology and BRIC, University of North Carolina at Chapel Hill, Chapel Hill, NC, USA
{hanzhang, dgshen}@med.unc.edu
[3] Hangzhou Medical College, Hangzhou, Zhejiang, China
[4] Neurosurgery Department of Huashan Hospital, Shanghai, China
[5] The Medical Image Computing Lab, Shanghai Jiao Tong University, Shanghai, China

**Abstract.** Glioblastoma (GBM) is the most common and deadly malignant brain tumor with short yet varied overall survival (OS) time. Per request of personalized treatment, accurate pre-operative prognosis for GBM patients is highly desired. Currently, many machine learning-based studies have been conducted to predict OS time based on pre-operative multimodal MR images of brain tumor patients. However, tumor genotype, such as MGMT and IDH, which has been proven to have strong relationship with OS, is completely not considered in pre-operative prognosis as the genotype information is unavailable until craniotomy. In this paper, we propose a new deep learning based method for OS time prediction. It can derive genotype related features from pre-operative multimodal MR images of brain tumor patients to guide OS time prediction. Particularly, we propose a multi-task convolutional neural network (CNN) to accomplish tumor genotype and OS time prediction tasks. As the network can benefit from learning genotype related features toward genotype prediction, we verify upon a dataset of 120 GBM patients and conclude that the multi-task learning can effectively improve the accuracy of predicting OS time in personalized prognosis.

**Keywords:** Overall survival time prediction · Glioblastoma · Genetic information

## 1 Introduction

Glioblastoma (GBM) is the most common grade IV malignant brain tumor. It accounts for about 30% of all primary brain tumors [1], with about 12,760 cases of GBM confirmed in the USA in 2018 [2], and 13,000 patients die each year [4]. GBM is the

© Springer Nature Switzerland AG 2019
D. Shen et al. (Eds.): MICCAI 2019, LNCS 11764, pp. 415–422, 2019.
https://doi.org/10.1007/978-3-030-32239-7_46

most deadly malignant tumors with a median survival time of merely 18–24 months [3]. Traditional treatment of GBM is surgical resection followed by radiation therapy and/or chemotherapy [5]. However, the inherent heterogeneity of GBM often causes varying prognosis, resulting in large variability of overall survival (OS) time across individuals [6]. Therefore, accurate individual pre-operative prognosis for GBM patients is highly desired for personalized treatment and precision medicine.

Recently, many deep learning (DL) based methods for pre-operative prognosis of brain tumor patients have been proposed [7, 8]. Most of them adopt the convolutional neural network (CNN) to predict OS time from pre-operative multimodal MR brain images. However, the tumor genotype (i.e., genomic biomarkers), which has been proven to be strongly related to the patient OS time, is often not considered in these studies. For example, the O-6-methylguanine-DNA methyltransferase (MGMT) promoter methylation (met) was found to be a positive factor of good prognosis of GBM patients [9], and Long-term OS time was reported to be related to the mutation (mut) of the isocitrate dehydrogenase 1/2 (IDH) [10]. Besides MGMT and IDH, which have been already recognized, other genomic biomarkers, such as the chromosomes 1p/19q and the telomerase reverse transcriptase (TERT), were also found to be related to OS time [11, 12]. The main reason of no tumor genotype considered in current pre-operative image based prognosis studies is straightforward – the tumor genotype information is unavailable until craniotomy (open-skull operation) is conducted.

In order to use the strong relationship between tumor genotype and patient prognosis for learning prognosis-related features effectively, in this paper, we propose a new DL based pre-operative OS time prediction method for GBM. The input of our method is still the pre-operative multi-modal MR brain images of GBM patients. However, in addition to outputting OS prediction, our method is unique to simultaneously derive tumor genotype in order to learn more effective prognosis-related features for better OS prediction. The joint predictions of tumor genotype and OS time are achieved by a multi-task CNN in particular. Experimental results with a single-center GBM bio-bank dataset show that our method outperforms both the state-of-the-art DL based and radiomics based pre-operative OS time prediction methods.

## 2    Method

We attain joint predictions of four tumor genotype (i.e., targeting the genomic biomarkers of MGMT, IDH, 1p/19q and TERT) and OS time through an integrated multi-task CNN. The features are jointly learned for accurate predictions of both the tumor genotype and OS time. Particularly, each tumor genotype prediction task is designed to predict a corresponding genomic biomarker based on the input pre-operative multi-modal MR brain images. For each genomic biomarker, there are two possible types: MGMT is either methylation (met) or unmethylation (unmet), IDH is either mutation (mut) or wild type (wt), 1p/19q is either co-deletion (cd) or wild type (wt), and TERT is either mutation (mut) or wild type (wt). The tumor genotype related features that are learned from pre-operative images are then used in the OS time prediction task, leading to much improved OS time prediction accuracy.

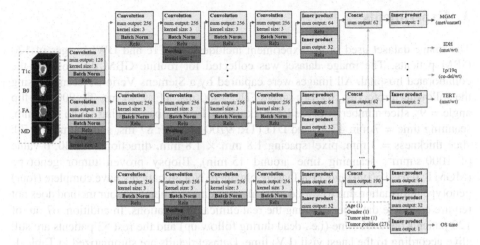

**Fig. 1.** The structure of the multi-task CNN. There are five tasks in the network: four tasks for tumor genotype prediction (only two of them are drawn in the figure) and one task for the pre-operative OS time prediction. The tumor genotype related features learned from tumor genotype prediction tasks are fed to the FC layer of the OS time prediction task.

The structure of our network is shown in Fig. 1. The network input is a 3D multi-modal MR image patch containing a complete tumor (i.e., pre-operation). The currently used MR modalities are T1 contrast enhanced (T1c) image, and three diffusion weighted imaging (DWI) derived MR modalities (i.e., B0, FA and MD, representing different aspects of intra-tumor contents). Creating 3D multimodal MR image patches for training and testing will be presented in the experiment. In the network, after the first two common convolutional blocks, the network is split into five branches, each of which corresponds to a tumor genotype or the OS time prediction task. In the multi-task CNN, the tumor genotype related features learned from the four tumor genotype prediction tasks are fed to the fully connected (FC) layer of the OS time prediction task. Moreover, some essential clinical features, including patient age, gender, tumor size and position, are fed to the FC layer of each task. It is worth noting that the feature of tumor position is encoded by 27 binary digits (i.e., 0 or 1 at each digit). Specifically, we divide each brain into $3 \times 3 \times 3$ non-overlap blocks. If the tumor extends to a certain block, then the corresponding digit for this block is 1, and otherwise 0.

In the training phase, labels of tumor genotype and patient OS time (in days) are known for each input 3D multimodal MR image patch. Based on the labels, the softmax loss is applied to each tumor genotype prediction task (binary prediction), while the loss function of the OS time prediction task is the Euclidean loss with respect to the clinical follow-ups (regression). It is worth noting that, in the testing phase, no tumor genotype information is needed, as our network can derive tumor genotype related features from the input images directly. In this way, we can apply our method to real scenario, as tumor genotype information is unavailable before surgery.

## 3   Experiments

The image dataset used in the experiment includes MR T1c and DWI images of 120 GBM patients. The image dataset was collected for routine GBM diagnosis in the collaborated hospital. All images were captured by a Siemens Verio 3T scanner using the following protocols: 3D T1c image (TR: 1900 ms, TE: 2.93 ms, TI: 900 ms, flip angle = 9°, slice number = 176, slice thickness = 1 mm, pixel spacing 1 mm × 1 mm, scanning time = 7 min 47 s), and DTI (TR: 9700 ms, TE: 87 ms, slice number = 70, slice thickness = 3 mm, pixel spacing 1.8 mm × 1.8 mm, direction = 20/30, b-value of 1000 s/mm$^2$, scanning time around 15 min). Biopsy proven tumor genotype (MGMT, IDH, 1p/19q, and TERT) were obtained. Not all patients have complete (four) genotype information due to varied clinical requirement. Therefore, our method does not require complete data, better fitting the real clinical applications. In addition, 67 out of 120 patients have OS time (i.e., dead during follow up) and the rest 53 patients are still alive according to the latest visit (LV) time. Dataset details are summarized in Table 1.

**Table 1.** Image dataset of 120 GBM patients.

| Age (years) | Gender | OS (days) | LV (days) |
|---|---|---|---|
| 51.6 ± 14.6 | 42 (F)/78 (M) | 439.0 ± 221.5 | 627.4 ± 327.1 |
| | | 67 patients | 53 patients |
| MGMT | IDH | 1p/19q | TERT |
| 63 (unmet) | 86 (wt) | 50 (wt) | 50 (wt) |
| 42 (met) | 7 (mut) | 9 (cd) | 56 (mut) |
| 15 (unknown) | 27 (unknown) | 61 (unknown) | 14 (unknown) |

As aforementioned, four image modalities (T1c, B0, FA and MD) are currently used in our study. Considering that most of the DWI-derived metrics need to be calculated in the DWI native space, in current study, images of different modalities are aligned to the corresponding B0 image (in DWI native space) using a rigid transformation. Moreover, the brain tumor mask including tumor entity and edema for each patient is manually labeled based on T1c and B0 by a senior neuro-radiologist. Examples of the four image modalities and the brain tumor mask of a GBM patient are shown in Fig. 2.

T1c          B0          FA          MD          Mask

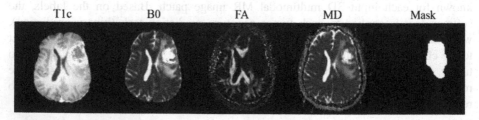

**Fig. 2.** Examples of the four modalities (T1c, B0, FA and MD) and the corresponding brain tumor mask of a GBM patient.

The training and testing data of our network are 3D multimodal MR image patches containing a complete tumor cropped from the image data of GBM patients. Since we have tumor mask images for all patients, the center of each tumor and the bounding box can be calculated. By analyzing the tumor bounding boxes of all patients, the size of the 3D image patch is set to $64 \times 64 \times 32$ voxels, which is large enough to contain complete brain tumor of each patient. Each 3D multimodal MR image patch is centered at the tumor center. For the training data, the corresponding genotype label for MGMT, IDH, 1p/19q or TERT is set to 0 (unmet or wt), 1 (met, mut or co-deletion) and $-1$ (unknown), respectively. The OS label is the patient OS time in days, or $-1$ for patients who are alive at the latest LV. To augment the training data, we rotate tumors in axial direction around the tumor center in the range of $0°-360°$ (step size of $10°$) to get corresponding 3D multimodal MR image patches and mirror patches. Moreover, to solve the imbalanced data of IDH (86 wt to 7 mut) and 1p/19q (50 wt to 9 cd), rotation step size of $2°$ is used for IDH of mut and 1p/19q of cd. In this way, 12,672 3D multimodal MR image patches are available. It is worth noting that, some image patches have incomplete labels (i.e., unknown genotype or no OS time). In this case, no back propagation is proceeded in the corresponding multi-task CNN branches during the training.

We perform 10-fold cross validation to evaluate our method. In each time, 3D multimodal MR image patches with corresponding labels of 108 patients are used for training (90 patients) and validation (18 patients). The original 3D multimodal MR image patches (with no augmentation) of the remained 12 patients are used as the testing data. In addition, five mono-task CNNs, each of which handles one of the tumor genotype and OS time prediction tasks, are evaluated for comparison. The topologies of these five mono-task CNNs are the same as the branch in our multi-task CNN (see Fig. 3).

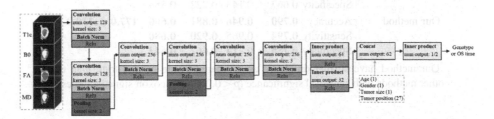

**Fig. 3.** Mono-task CNN for tumor genotype and OS time prediction.

Besides deep learning based methods, radiomics (RD) with random forest (RF) based method is also compared here (denoted as RD-RF). Particularly, radiologic features of input images are first extracted using Pyradiomics [13] and then refined by feature selection with $\ell_1$ regularization [14]. Finally, the selected features are fed to RF for classification (tumor genotype prediction) and regression (OS time prediction), respectively. In our experiment, five RD-RFs, each of which contains 100 decision trees in RF, are trained to predict four tumor genotype and the OS time. The same 10-fold cross validation is adopted for fair comparison. The training data here are the 3D multimodal MR image patches used in mono-task CNN and our method. As RF requests complete data, we exclude patients who have missing labels of tumor genotype or OS time. In this way, image data of 105 patients are available for MGMT, 93 for IDH, 59 for 1p/19q, 106 for TERT and 67 for OS time, respectively. For each modality in the 3D multimodal MR image patch, 93 radiologic features of first-order statistics, gray-level co-occurrence matrix, gray-level size zone matrix, and gray-level run length matrix are calculated. Furthermore, 16 shape features derived from the corresponding 3D mask image and 4 clinical features (age, gender, tumor size and location) are also adopted. As a summary, each training data contains 392 features (i.e., 93 × 4 + 16 + 4). Finally, after feature selection, 47 features are preserved for MGMT, 1p/19q, and TERT, 59 features for IDH, and 62 features for OS time prediction.

The evaluation results are summarized in Table 2. The OS time of 67 patients with known OS time are predicted by different methods and compared in accordance to the root mean squared error (RMSE). The predicted tumor genotype results of 120 patients using each method under comparison are evaluated by Accuracy, Sensitivity and Specificity. We use Wilcoxon signed rank test [15] over the OS time predicted by all methods under comparison. Our method is better than the mono-task CNN ($p = 0.003$) and the RD-RF ($p = 0.034$).

**Table 2.** Evaluation results of mono-task CNN, RD-RF and our method.

|  |  | MGMT | IDH | 1p/19q | TERT | OS (RMSE) |
|---|---|---|---|---|---|---|
| Mono-task CNN | Accuracy | 0.724 | 0.925 | 0.814 | 0.632 | 261.0 ± 175.0 |
|  | Sensitivity | 0.730 | 0.965 | 0.880 | 0.640 |  |
|  | Specificity | 0.714 | 0.429 | 0.444 | 0.625 |  |
| RD-RF | Accuracy | 0.676 | 0.925 | 0.763 | 0.575 | 225.0 ± 136.0 |
|  | Sensitivity | 0.683 | **0.988** | 0.860 | 0.560 |  |
|  | Specificity | 0.667 | 0.143 | 0.222 | 0.589 |  |
| Our method | Accuracy | **0.790** | **0.946** | **0.881** | **0.660** | **177.0 ± 130.0**[*] |
|  | Sensitivity | **0.794** | 0.965 | **0.920** | **0.680** |  |
|  | Specificity | **0.786** | **0.714** | **0.667** | **0.643** |  |

[*]Our method have smaller difference as compared to the ground truth than the other methods with statistical significance ($p < 0.05$ of Wilcoxon signed rank test).

Figure 4 illustrates the predicted OS times of 67 patients with known OS time using each method. The predicted result from our method is more compact in distribution and better fits the diagonal line than the other methods. In addition, we also predict the OS time for the other 53 patients with LV time (still alive). The numbers of "successful" predictions (i.e., the number of LV-only patients with predicted OS time longer than their LV time) are larger using our method than using other methods. Specifically, based on our method, 32 out of 53 patients have longer predicted OS time than their LV time, while such numbers based on mono-task CNN and RD-RF are reduced to 18 and 20, respectively.

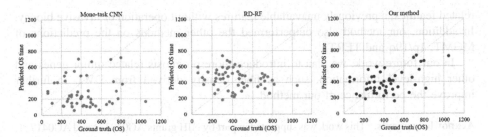

**Fig. 4.** Predicted OS time of 67 patients who have ground truth OS time (already dead) using mono-task CNN (left), RD-RF (middle) and our method (right).

The survival curves (Kaplan-Meier plot) [16] of all the 120 patients are calculated and shown in Fig. 5. Compared to the RMSE that requires all patients to have determined OS time, survival curves can be drawn using all patients with or without known OS time. Therefore, it serves a good evaluation. The survival curves calculated based on the predicted results using mono-task CNN (Fig. 5 left), RD-RF (Fig. 5 middle) and our method (Fig. 5 right) are compared with the ground truth (the red curves), respectively. The predicted survival curve of our method is much closer to the ground truth than the other two methods. Particularly, the corresponding $p$ values from the Log-rank (Mantel-Cox) test [17] are 0.0425 (mono-task CNN), 0.1925 (RD-RF) and 0.5152 (our method). These $p$ values can partly indicate that both the predicted survival curve based on our method is less different from (or more similar with) the ground truth compared to the other two methods.

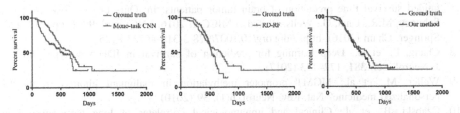

**Fig. 5.** Survival curves of 120 patients. The survival curves of mono-task CNN, RD-RF and our method are marked in blue (left), green (middle) and purple (right), respectively. Each of them is compared with the ground truth marked in red. (Color figure online)

## 4 Conclusions

We proposed a new multi-task convolutional neural network (CNN) based pre-operative overall survival (OS) time prediction method, which predicts tumor genotype as separate tasks to guide feature learning for OS time prediction. Within this framework, both imaging phenotype and genotype information could be jointly learned for more accurate OS time prediction for GBM patients. Our method outperformed both the conventional mono-task CNN based method and the state-of-the-art, radiomics based random forest method. This is mainly because of the usage of tumor genotype related features, a previously unavailable features without operation or invasive biopsy. In addition, our method also outperformed the other methods on the predictions of MGMT, 1p/19q and TERT.

In our future work, we plan to introduce more prognosis related tumor genes and other high-level information, such as fiber density derived from DWI, to further improve the performance of our method.

**Acknowledgements.** This work was supported in part by NIH grants AG049371 and AG041721.

# References

1. Anil, R., Colen, R.R.: Imaging genomics in glioblastoma multiforme: a predictive tool for patients prognosis, survival, and outcome. Magn. Reson. Imaging Clin. **24**(4), 731–740 (2016)
2. Ostrom, Q.T., et al.: CBTRUS statistical report: primary brain and other central nervous system tumors diagnosed in the United States in 2010–2014. Neuro-Oncol. **19**(suppl_5), v1–v88 (2017)
3. Chow, D., et al.: Imaging genetic heterogeneity in glioblastoma and other glial tumors: review of current methods and future directions. Am. J. Roentgenol. **210**(1), 30–38 (2018)
4. International RadioSurgery Association (2018). http://www.irsa.org/glioblastoma.html
5. Lefranc, F., et al.: Present and potential future issues in glioblastoma treatment. Expert Rev. Anticancer Ther. **6**(5), 719–732 (2006)
6. Sottoriva, A., et al.: Intratumor heterogeneity in human glioblastoma reflects cancer evolutionary dynamics. Proc. Natl. Acad. Sci. **110**(10), 4009–4014 (2013)
7. Nie, D., Zhang, H., Adeli, E., Liu, L., Shen, D.: 3D deep learning for multi-modal imaging-guided survival time prediction of brain tumor patients. In: Ourselin, S., Joskowicz, L., Sabuncu, M.R., Unal, G., Wells, W. (eds.) MICCAI 2016. LNCS, vol. 9901, pp. 212–220. Springer, Cham (2016). https://doi.org/10.1007/978-3-319-46723-8_25
8. Chang, P., et al.: Deep learning for prediction of survival in IDH wild-type gliomas. J. Neurol. Sci. **381**, 172–173 (2017)
9. Weller, M., et al.: MGMT promoter methylation in malignant gliomas: ready for personalized medicine? Nat. Rev. Neurol. **6**(1), 39 (2010)
10. Czapski, B., et al.: Clinical and immunological correlates of long term survival in glioblastoma. Contemp. Oncol. **22**(1A), 81 (2018)
11. Hill, C., Hunter, S.B., Brat, D.J.: Genetic markers in glioblastoma: prognostic significance and future therapeutic implications. Adv. Anat. Pathol. **10**(4), 212–217 (2003)
12. Lee, Y., et al.: The frequency and prognostic effect of TERT promoter mutation in diffuse gliomas. Acta Neuropathol. Commun. **5**(1), 62 (2017)
13. van Griethuysen, J.J., et al.: Computational radiomics system to decode the radiographic phenotype. Cancer Res. **77**(21), e104–e107 (2017)
14. Liu, J., Chen, J., Ye, J.: Large-scale sparse logistic regression. In: Proceedings of the 15th ACM SIGKDD International Conference on Knowledge Discovery and Data Mining. ACM (2009)
15. Woolson, R.: Wilcoxon signed-rank test. Wiley Encyclopedia of Clinical Trials, pp. 1–3 (2007)
16. Kaplan, E.L., Meier, P.: Nonparametric estimation from incomplete observations. J. Am. Stat. Assoc. **53**(282), 457–481 (1958)
17. Mantel, N.: Evaluation of survival data and two new rank order statistics arising in its consideration. Cancer Chemother. Rep. **50**, 163–170 (1966)

# Pathology-Aware Deep Network Visualization and Its Application in Glaucoma Image Synthesis

Xiaofei Wang[1]📧, Mai Xu[1,2(✉)]📧, Liu Li[1]📧, Zulin Wang[1], and Zhenyu Guan[1]

[1] School of Electronic and Information Engineering, Beihang University,
Beijing, China
MaiXu@buaa.edu.cn

[2] Hangzhou Innovation Institute, Beihang University, Beijing, China

**Abstract.** The past few years have witnessed the great success of applying deep neural networks (DNNs) in computer-aided diagnosis. However, little attention has been paid to provide pathological evidence in the existing DNNs for medical diagnosis. In fact, feature visualization in DNNs is able to help understanding how the computer make decisions, and thus it shows promise on finding pathological evidence from computer-aided diagnosis. In this paper, we propose a novel pathology-aware visualization approach for DNN-based glaucoma classification, which is used to locate the pathological evidence from fundus images for glaucoma. Besides, we apply the visualization framework to the glaucoma images synthesis task, through which specific pathological areas of synthesized images can be enhanced. Finally, experimental results show that the visualization heat maps can pinpoint different glaucoma pathologies with high accuracy, and that the generated glaucoma images are more pathophysiologically clear in rim loss (RL) and retinal neural fiber layer damage (RNFLD), which is verified by the ophthalmologist.

**Keywords:** Deep neural networks · Visualization · Glaucoma ·
Image synthesis

## 1 Introduction

The recent success of deep neural networks (DNNs) has benefitted medical diagnosis [1], especially for automatically detecting glaucoma in fundus images [2]. In addition to improving the classification accuracy, visualizing the DNNs have also attracted a lot of attention. In automatic medical diagnosis, it is critical to explain the behavior of a machine learning model and to make medical experts know the machine diagnosis. An effective visualization method should be able to point out all possible reasons for making decisions in DNNs, since many diseases have more than one typical pathologies, e.g., rim loss (RL) and retinal neural fiber layer damage (RNFLD) for glaucoma. However, in glaucoma image classification, there are only binary labels (positive or negative) annotated by

© Springer Nature Switzerland AG 2019
D. Shen et al. (Eds.): MICCAI 2019, LNCS 11764, pp. 423–431, 2019.
https://doi.org/10.1007/978-3-030-32239-7_47

medical experts, which limits the existing visualization methods to pinpoint different pathological evidence hidden behind DNNs. To address such a problem, we propose a novel pathology-aware visualization method for glaucoma classification network. Firstly, feature maps of the classification network are selected by their activation values, through which the features with tiny activation values are screened out to reduce the noise effects in the visualization result. Secondly, the features are further screened and divided into two groups by their centroid-centric moment of inertia (CMI) values, consistent with the property of RL and RNFLD in glaucoma fundus images. Finally, the selected features are combined in a gradient-based weight to generate the final visualization heat map. Experimental results show that our pathology-aware visualization method can pinpoint both the RL and RNFLD area in glaucoma fundus images with high accuracy.

In addition, we further use feature visualization to glaucoma image synthesis, such that pathological area can be easily distinguished. Specifically, we propose combining the traditional generative adversarial network (GAN) and our pathology-aware visualization, called pathology-based GAN (Patho-GAN). The key idea of Patho-GAN is to enforce the synthesized images of GAN to have the similar visualization results to the reference image. After training the Patho-GAN, one can obtain the synthesized glaucoma images with pathophysiologically clearer RL and RNFLD, which are verified by the ophthalmologist.

The main contributions of this paper are: (1) we propose a novel pathology-aware visualization method to find different pathological evidence (RL and RNFLD) for glaucoma classification network; (2) we propose Patho-GAN to apply the feature visualization to the glaucoma image synthesis task, thus enhancing RL and RNFLD of the synthesized glaucoma images.

## 2    Literature Review

**Visualization Methods:** Recently, many visualization methods have been proposed to explain the reasoning behind the DNNs' decisions [3–7]. Specifically, in natural image domain, [3] proposed the occlusion experiment (Occ), in which they obtain a region-relevance heat map by occluding different portions of the input image and monitoring the output of the classifier. Zhou et al. [5] focused on the last convolutional layer and proposed Class Activation Map (CAM) method to combine the feature maps and generate the visualization heat map, while [4] aimed to find the evidence in the input space and proposed the guided backpropagation (GBP) method. Meanwhile, in medical domain, some specially designed visualization methods have also been proposed to better adapt the medical image properties. For instance, [7] modified the Occ by occluding the known pathologies of Alzheimer disease, while [6] focused on the intermediary feature maps and visualized the evidence for skin lesions. Nevertheless, the existing visualization methods are not able to pinpoint different kinds of decision evidence of DNNs with only simply annotated labels (positive or negative). To address such a problem, we propose a pathology-aware visualization method to find and visualize different pathological evidence for glaucoma classification network.

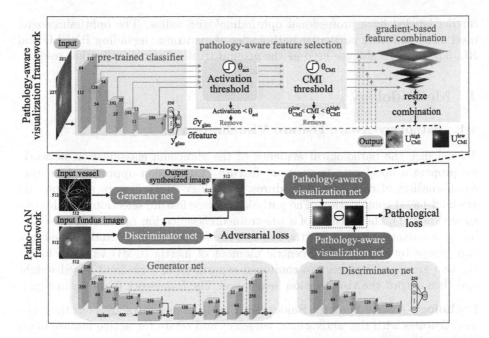

**Fig. 1.** Framework of pathology-aware visualization (top row) and Patho-GAN (bottom row).

**Applications of Feature Visualization:** Due to the good performance in finding pathological evidence of DNNs, feature visualization has recently been applied to many tasks, such as weakly supervised image classification [8], disease lesion localization [9], image registration [10] and segmentation [11]. However, different from the existing applications, we apply feature visualization to the medical image synthesis task, particularly for glaucoma in this paper, such that the pathological area can be further enhanced for the synthesized images.

## 3 Preliminaries

**Database:** The fundus images used to train the DNNs in this paper were obtained from the Large-scale Attention based Glaucoma (LAG) database [12]. The LAG database contains 5,824 fundus images with 2,392 positive and 3,432 negative glaucoma samples, which are randomly divided into training (4,792 images), validation (200 images) and test (832 images) sets. In a preprocessing step, the images are downscaled to a resolution of $280 \times 280$ pixels, and the RGB values are normalized between 0 and 1. We augment the training set by taking random crops of $227 \times 227$ pixels, and further augment each crop by rotating (angle sampled uniformly between 0 and $2\pi$).

**Ground Truth for Visualization:** To evaluate the visualization results, 350 positive glaucoma images were randomly selected from the LAG test set and further labeled by a professional ophthalmologist online. The ophthalmologist used boxes to locate particular pathologies of glaucoma, including RNFLD and RL. The label results are used as the ground truth of our visualization results.

# 4 Methodology

## 4.1 Pathology-Aware Feature Visualization

To visualize the pathological evidence of the glaucoma classification network, we propose a novel pathology-aware feature visualization approach. Our approach consists of two main procedures: pathology-aware feature selection and gradient-based combination. The pathology-aware feature selection includes two subprocess: (1) The features of a pre-trained classification network are selected by their activation values; (2) the features are further screened and divided into two groups by their centroid-centric moment of inertia (CMI) values. Finally, the two groups of features are combined separately in a gradient-based weight and then output the visualization heat maps. The framework is shown in Fig. 1.

**Pathology-Aware Feature Selection:** Firstly, in order to screen out the "useless" features with tiny activations, we select and retain the active feature maps $\mathbf{A}^{k,l} \in \mathbb{R}^{M^l \times N^l}$ (the $k$-th feature in the $l$-th layer, with height $M^l$ and width $N^l$) in set $\mathbf{U}^l_{\text{act}}$:

$$\mathbf{U}^l_{\text{act}} = \{\mathbf{A}^{k,l} \mid \|\mathbf{A}^{k,l}\|_1 > \theta_{\text{act}} \cdot \max_n \|\mathbf{F}^{n,l}\|_1\}, \tag{1}$$

where $\mathbf{F}^{n,l}$ denotes the $n$-th feature in layer $l$ and $\theta_{\text{act}}$ is a threshold of the activation value. Secondly, the features are further selected according to their CMI value, which measures the geometric distortion and brightness distortion of feature maps. Given a feature map $\mathbf{A}^{k,l}$, the CMI value is defined as $J_{k,l}$:

$$J_{k,l} = \sum_{i=1}^{M^l} \sum_{j=1}^{N^l} [(i - i_c^{k,l})^2 + (j - j_c^{k,l})^2] \mathbf{A}_{i,j}^{k,l}, \tag{2}$$

where $(i_c^{k,l}, j_c^{k,l})$ is the centroid coordinate of $\mathbf{A}^{k,l}$. Based on the CMI value, the features are divided into two sets: $\mathbf{U}^{\text{high}}_{\text{CMI}}$ and $\mathbf{U}^{\text{low}}_{\text{CMI}}$, in which the CMI values of the features are higher than $\theta^{\text{high}}_{\text{CMI}}$ and lower than $\theta^{\text{low}}_{\text{CMI}} (< \theta^{\text{high}}_{\text{CMI}})$ respectively.

**Gradient-Based Feature Combination:** After feature selection, we first compute the gradient of the score for positive glaucoma, $y^{\text{glau}}$ (before the softmax), with respect to the selected feature maps $\mathbf{A}^{k,l}$, i.e., $\frac{\partial y^{\text{glau}}}{\partial \mathbf{A}^{k,l}}$. Then, these gradients flowing back are global-average-pooled (GAP) to obtain the feature importance weight $w^{k,l}$:

$$w^{k,l} = \frac{1}{N^l \times M^l} \sum_{i=1}^{M^l} \sum_{j=1}^{N^l} \frac{\partial y^{\text{glau}}}{\partial \mathbf{A}_{ij}^{k,l}}. \tag{3}$$

Weight $w^{k,l}$ captures the "importance" of the map of the $k$-th feature in the $l$-th layer for positive glaucoma. Finally, we perform a gradient-weighted combination of forward activation maps to obtain the visualization map $\mathbf{V}$ for an input glaucoma image $\mathbf{I}$:

$$\mathbf{V}(\mathbf{I}) = \sum_{\mathbf{A}^{k,l} \in \mathbf{U}} w^{k,l} \mathbf{A}^{k,l}, \tag{4}$$

where $\mathbf{U}$ is the feature set $\mathbf{U}_{\text{CMI}}^{\text{high}}$ or $\mathbf{U}_{\text{CMI}}^{\text{low}}$.

## 4.2 Visualization-Based Fundus Image Synthesis

In this section, we design the Patho-GAN to synthesize glaucoma fundus images enhanced in RNFL and RL. The Patho-GAN is achieved by combining a basic GAN and our visualization system. The framework of Patho-GAN is shown in Fig. 1. The overall structure of Patho-GAN consists of three subnets: generator net, discriminator net and pathology-aware visualization net. Given the vessel segmentation image (generated by the method proposed in [13]) and a noise code as input, the generator tries to synthesize images, while the discriminator net tries to tell apart the synthesized images from the real ones. The visualization net enforces the synthesized image to have the similar visualization results to the reference image.

**Generator Net:** We use the U-Net [14] structure for the generator network. Taking a segmentation image $\mathbf{Y} \in \{0,1\}^{W \times H}$ with a noise code $\mathbf{z} \in \mathbb{R}^Z$ as input, the network outputs a synthesized glaucoma fundus image $\mathbf{X}_{\text{syn}} \in \mathbb{R}^{W \times H \times 3}$, where 3 means the three channels of RGB. Mathematically, the image synthesis process can be expressed as $G_\theta(\mathbf{X}_{\text{syn}}) : (\mathbf{Y}, \mathbf{z}) \mapsto \mathbf{X}_{\text{syn}}$, where $\theta$ is the learnable parameters.

**Discriminator Net:** We can also define a discriminant function $D_\gamma : (\mathbf{X}_{\text{real}}) \mapsto p \in [0,1]$. When input with a real image $\mathbf{X}_{\text{real}}$, $p$ should tend to 1; when input with a synthesized image $\mathbf{X}_{\text{syn}}$, $p$ need to tend to 0. We follow the GAN's strategy and solve the following optimization problem that characterizes the interplay between $G$ and $D$:

$$\max_\theta \min_\gamma L(G_\theta, D_\gamma) = \mathbb{E}\left[ L_{\text{adv}}(\theta, \gamma) + \lambda L_{\text{patho}}(\theta) \right]. \tag{5}$$

In the above equation, $L_{\text{adv}} = \log D_\gamma(\mathbf{X}_{\text{real}}) + \log(1 - D_\gamma(G_\theta(\mathbf{Y}, \mathbf{z})))$ is the adversarial loss and $L_{\text{patho}}$ is the pathological loss, with $\lambda > 0$ being a trade-off constant.

**Pathology-Aware Visualization Net:** To enhance the synthesized glaucoma images in specific pathological area, we enforce the synthesized image to have the similar visualization heat map to the reference input image. In this way, the Patho-GAN can generate glaucoma fundus images with clearer pathologies (e.g., RL and RNFL). The $L_{\text{patho}}$ is defined as:

$$L_{\text{patho}} = \|\mathbf{V}(\mathbf{X}_{\text{real}}) - \mathbf{V}(\mathbf{X}_{\text{syn}})\|_1. \tag{6}$$

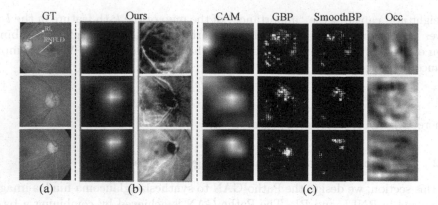

**Fig. 2.** (a) The ground truth of RNFL and RL. (b) The visualization results of our visualization method. The left column shows visualization results of features in $\mathbf{U}_{\mathrm{CMI}}^{\mathrm{high}}$ and the right one shows results of $\mathbf{U}_{\mathrm{CMI}}^{\mathrm{low}}$. (c) The visualization results of other methods.

## 5   Experiments and Results

### 5.1   Setting

In our experiments, the classification network is trained on the training set of LAG database for 500 epochs, with mini-batches of size 8 and the learning rate of 0.001 with Adam optimizer [15]. We have evaluated the performance of the network on the test set of LAG. Our network achieves a classification accuracy of 0.89 and AUC of 0.84. Note that the main scope of this paper is about the visualization method, not optimizing the DNN. In visualization, the selection thresholds $\theta_{\mathrm{act}}$, $\theta_{\mathrm{CMI}}^{\mathrm{low}}$ and $\theta_{\mathrm{CMI}}^{\mathrm{high}}$ are set to 0.1, 0.1 and 0.9 respectively.

In training the Patho-GAN, The input images are upscaled from 500 to 512 (pixels), with values scaled to the range of $[0, 1]$. The batch size is set to 1, and random rotation is performed on the input. The training is done using the SGD optimizer and the learning rate is set to 0.0002. We update the generator twice and then update discriminator once. During training, the noise code is sampled element-wise from zero-mean Gaussian with standard deviation of 0.01 and the trade-off constant $\lambda$ is set to 1000. The training finishes after 240,000 mini-batches, and the inference speed of Patho-GAN is 13 ms per image on a computer with a GPU of Nvidia GeForce GTX 1080.

### 5.2   Pathology-Aware Visualization Results

In our experiment, we compare the visualization performance between our method and 4 other commonly used methods: CAM [5], GBP [4], SmoothBP [16] and Occ [3]. The visualization results are shown in Fig. 2. As can be seen, our pathology-aware visualization performs better in locating both the RL and RNFLD areas. Besides, CAM creates the heat maps similar to ours but more dispersedly. Occ produces the heat maps highlighting large areas but without any clear emphasis. Although GBP and SmoothBP can show part of the RL and RNFLD, there exists strong noise that makes the pathological regions not be highlighted.

**Table 1.** RL and RNFLD localization accuracy (mean ± std %) for our and 4 other methods on the LAG test set.

| Accuracy | Ours | CAM | GBP | SmoothBP | Occlusion |
|---|---|---|---|---|---|
| RL | **31.8 ± 0.3** | 21.3 ± 0.2 | 11.2 ± 0.4 | 13.3 ± 0.8 | 4.2 ± 0.2 |
| RNFLD | **41.2 ± 0.5** | 3.8 ± 0.1 | 7.6 ± 0.8 | 6.3 ± 0.7 | 23.6 ± 0.3 |

Moreover, to quantitatively evaluate the visualization methods, we calculate the average pathology localization accuracy of these methods. The localization accuracy of a heat map is defined as $\text{Acc} = \frac{\sum_{(i,j) \in \text{GT}} I_{i,j}}{\sum_{(i,j)} I_{i,j}}$, where $I_{i,j}$ indicates the value of pixel $(i, j)$ at the heat map. The localization results are shown in Table 1. Compared to other methods, our pathology-aware visualization reaches a much higher accuracy in both RL and RNFLD localization. Thus, we can conclude that our pathology-aware visualization method can pinpoint different pathological evidence for the glaucoma classification network.

### 5.3 Synthesized Glaucoma Images of Patho-GAN

After training the Patho-GAN with the pathological constrain from the feature set $\mathbf{U}_{\text{CMI}}^{\text{high}}$ and $\mathbf{U}_{\text{CMI}}^{\text{low}}$, we obtain the synthesized glaucoma fundus images enhanced in RL and RNFLD areas. The training results are shown in Fig. 3. As can be seen in Fig. 3(a), the synthesized images with enhancement in RL can highlight the turning point of blood vessels from the optic cup to the optic disc, and thus the rim is more clear. In Fig. 3(b), the synthesized images with enhancement in RNFLD show a clearly shading boundary than the baseline, making the RNFLD more evident.

To further verify our method, we conducted an evaluation experiment with the assistance of a professional ophthalmologist. In the experiment, the ophthalmologist was asked to evaluate the randomly shuffled fundus images synthesized by our Patho-GAN and the baseline. For each image, he rated two scores (ranged 1–5, higher indicates better): (1) clarity of RL, and (2) clarity of RNFLD. Finally, we collected valid scores on 240 synthesized images and calculated the average scores in RL and RNFLD. In RL, Patho-GAN scores **4.19** while the baseline score is 3.90; in RNFLD, Patho-GAN scores **3.14**, while the baseline obtain the score of 2.05. The $p$ value of T-test is $3.30 \times 10^{-3}$ and $6.90 \times 10^{-7}$ for RL and RNFLD clarity, respectively, i.e., our mean score is higher than the baseline. Thus, we can conclude that the Patho-GAN can synthesize glaucoma images with pathophysiologically clearer RL and RNFLD.

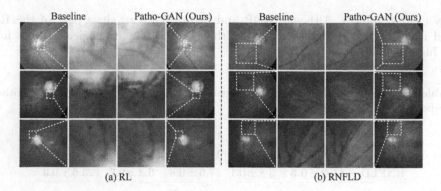

**Fig. 3.** Details comparison between Patho-GAN and the baseline method (without pathological constrain) in RL (a) and RNFLD (b).

## 6  Summary

In this paper, we have proposed a novel pathology-aware visualization method that pinpoints different pathological evidence for glaucoma classification network, by pre-selecting the feature maps and combining them in a gradient-based weight. Visualization results showed that our method can well locate the RL and RNFLD in the glaucoma fundus images with high accuracy. Moreover, we proposed the Patho-GAN, which applied our visualization method to the glaucoma image synthesis task. The experimental results showed that our Patho-GAN can synthesize glaucoma images with pathophysiologically clearer RL and RNFLD.

**Acknowledgments.** This work was supported by the NSFC projects 61876013, 61922009, 61573037, and by BMSTC under Grant Z181100001918035.

## References

1. Esteva, A., et al.: Dermatologist-level classification of skin cancer with deep neural networks. Nature **542**(7639), 115 (2017)
2. Chen, X., Xu, Y., Wong, D.W.K., Wong, T.Y., Liu, J.: Glaucoma detection based on deep convolutional neural network. In: EMBC 2015, pp. 715–718. IEEE (2015)
3. Zeiler, M.D., Fergus, R.: Visualizing and understanding convolutional networks. In: Fleet, D., Pajdla, T., Schiele, B., Tuytelaars, T. (eds.) ECCV 2014. LNCS, vol. 8689, pp. 818–833. Springer, Cham (2014). https://doi.org/10.1007/978-3-319-10590-1_53
4. Springenberg, J.T., Dosovitskiy, A., Brox, T., Riedmiller, M.: Striving for simplicity: the all convolutional net. arXiv preprint arXiv:1412.6806 (2014)
5. Zhou, B., Khosla, A., Lapedriza, A., Oliva, A., Torralba, A.: Learning deep features for discriminative localization. In: CVPR 2016, pp. 2921–2929 (2016)
6. Van Molle, P., De Strooper, M., Verbelen, T., Vankeirsbilck, B., Simoens, P., Dhoedt, B.: Visualizing convolutional neural networks to improve decision support for skin lesion classification. In: Stoyanov, D., et al. (eds.) MLCN/DLF/IMIMIC

-2018. LNCS, vol. 11038, pp. 115–123. Springer, Cham (2018). https://doi.org/10.1007/978-3-030-02628-8_13

7. Rieke, J., Eitel, F., Weygandt, M., Haynes, J.-D., Ritter, K.: Visualizing convolutional networks for MRI-based diagnosis of alzheimer's disease. In: Stoyanov, D., et al. (eds.) MLCN/DLF/IMIMIC -2018. LNCS, vol. 11038, pp. 24–31. Springer, Cham (2018). https://doi.org/10.1007/978-3-030-02628-8_3

8. Wang, X., et al.: Weakly supervised learning for whole slide lung cancer image classification. In: MIDL (2018)

9. Gondal, W.M., Köhler, J.M., Grzeszick, R., Fink, G.A., Hirsch, M.: Weakly-supervised localization of diabetic retinopathy lesions in retinal fundus images. In: ICIP, pp. 2069–2073. IEEE (2017)

10. Hu, Y., et al.: Label-driven weakly-supervised learning for multimodal deformarle image registration. In: ISBI (2018)

11. Kervadec, H., Dolz, J., Tang, M., Granger, E., Boykov, Y., Ayed, I.B.: Constrained-cnn losses for weakly supervised segmentation. MIA **54**, 88–99 (2019)

12. Li, L., Xu, M., Wang, X., Jiang, L., Liu, H.: Attention based glaucoma detection: a large-scale database with a CNN model. arXiv preprint arXiv:1903.10831 (2019)

13. Xiancheng, W., et al.: Retina blood vessel segmentation using a U-net based convolutional neural network. In: ICDS 2018, Beijing, China, 8–9 June 2018 (2018)

14. Ronneberger, O., Fischer, P., Brox, T.: U-Net: convolutional networks for biomedical image segmentation. In: Navab, N., Hornegger, J., Wells, W.M., Frangi, A.F. (eds.) MICCAI 2015. LNCS, vol. 9351, pp. 234–241. Springer, Cham (2015). https://doi.org/10.1007/978-3-319-24574-4_28

15. Kingma, D.P., Ba, J.: Adam: a method for stochastic optimization. arXiv preprint arXiv:1412.6980 (2014)

16. Smilkov, D., Thorat, N., Kim, B., Viégas, F., Wattenberg, M.: SmoothGrad: removing noise by adding noise. arXiv preprint arXiv:1706.03825 (2017)

# CORAL8: Concurrent Object Regression for Area Localization in Medical Image Panels

Sam Maksoud[✉], Arnold Wiliem, Kun Zhao, Teng Zhang, Lin Wu, and Brian Lovell

School of Information Technology and Electrical Engineering,
The University of Queensland, Brisbane, QLD, Australia
s.maksoud@uqconnect.edu.au

**Abstract.** This work tackles the problem of generating a medical report for multi-image panels. We apply our solution to the Renal Direct Immunofluorescence (RDIF) assay which requires a pathologist to generate a report based on observations across eight different whole slide images (WSI) in concert with existing clinical features. To this end, we propose a novel attention-based multi-modal generative recurrent neural network (RNN) architecture capable of dynamically sampling image data concurrently across the RDIF panel. The proposed methodology incorporates text from the clinical notes of the requesting physician to regulate the output of the network to align with the overall clinical context. In addition, we found the importance of regularizing attention weights for the word generation processes. This is because the system can ignore the attention mechanism by assigning equal weights for all members. Thus, we propose two regularizations to encourage efficient use of the attention mechanism. Experiments on our novel collection of RDIF WSIs provided by Sullivan Nicolaides Pathology demonstrate that our framework offers significant improvements over existing methods.

## 1 Introduction

Automatic image captioning [17] is an important topic in the medical research area as it frees pathologists from manual medical image interpretation and reduces the cost significantly [5]. Typically this involves conditioning a recurrent neural network (RNN) on image features encoded by a convolutional neural network (CNN). This method has shown great promise in non-specific image captioning tasks but has not generalized well to the complex domain of medical images [18,19].

**Electronic supplementary material** The online version of this chapter (https://doi.org/10.1007/978-3-030-32239-7_48) contains supplementary material, which is available to authorized users.

A common solution is to employ a pathologist to annotate training data [19]. However, even with access to annotated image features and medical reports, the overall clinical context is still important in medical image interpretation. This is because certain pathologies may be morphologically indistinguishable. One such case is the differential diagnoses of immunotactoid glomerulonephritis and diabetic nephropathy. In the Renal Direct Immunofluorescence (RDIF) assay, both conditions can present with linear accentuation of the glomerualar basement membrane for IgG; the significance of this pattern cannot be determined without clinical confirmation/exclusion of diabetes mellitus [1]. For this reason, image captioning models conditioned solely on image data may not be the ideal solution for tasks in the medical domain.

The second major challenge of image captioning tasks in the medical domain is correlating information from multiple images. For example, a pathologist must interpret a set of 8 different renal biopsy sections of the same patient to report the RDIF assay. Several methods have been proposed to enable captioning of multiple images by assuming images in the set exhibit temporal dependence [3] or contain multiple views/instances of the same object [18]. These assumptions are unsuitable for the multi-object temporally independent RDIF set. We refer to this as the ordered set to sequence problem: it must be an ordered set to preserve the identity of the antibody in the RDIF panel.

To address the problems outlined above, we describe a novel framework to overcome the clinical context bias and generate a RDIF medical report. The contributions of this paper are listed as follows:

1. To our knowledge, we are the first work to solve the ordered set to sequence problem by proposing a novel attention based architecture which provides concurrent access to all images at each step and models the clinical notes as priors to regulate clinical contexts.
2. We also introduce two novel regulators, Salient Alpha (SAL) and Time Distributed Variance (TDVAR), to discourage uniform attention weights.
3. Finally, we will release a novel RDIF dataset with quantitative baseline results provided using metrics from BLEU [13], ROUGE [11] and METEOR [10].

## 2   Renal Direct Immunoflourescence Dataset

The novel RDIF dataset used in this paper was assembled from routine clinical samples in collaboration with Sullivan Nicolaides Pathology; a subsidiary of Sonic Healthcare Limited. To prepare the RDIF slides, eight separate sections of renal biopsy tissue are treated with fluorescein isothiocyanate (FITC) conjugated antibodies to one of either IgG, IgA, IgM, Kappa, Lambda, C1q, C3 or Fibrinogen antibodies. The dataset comprises of 144 patient samples split into 99 training, 15 validation and 30 test sets. Each sample contains the eight WSI's, the clinical notes of the requesting physician, and the medical report. This dataset can be accessed at https://github.com/cradleai/rdif.

## 3   Proposed Method - CORAL8

### 3.1   Architecture

As illustrated in Fig. 1, the main aim of CORAL8 is to generate a medical report, $\mathcal{R}$ from an ordered set of images $\mathcal{I}$ and clinical notes $\mathcal{Q}$. To this end, we train a sentence generator $\phi_s$ which receives a report context vector and local image features vector as input and generates sequence of words. There are several desirable properties that we enforce in the sentence generator:

1. It must generate coherent sentences;
2. The generated sentences must be in concert with the clinical contexts described in the clinical notes;
3. The attention mechanism must produce diverse representations of local image features for the report generation. The mechanism must also ensure that local features from each image in the set are equally represented in the generative sequence.

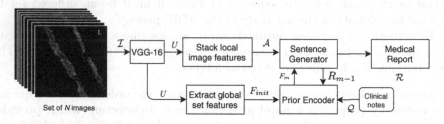

**Fig. 1.** This image illustrates the framework of the proposed CORAL8 architecture.

To generate coherent sentences, we train a neural network called the prior encoder $\phi_p$ which extracts context features $F_m$; where $m$ is the index of the sentence. The context features are a joint representation of; (1) previous sentence features; and (2) previous context features. To encourage agreement between the generated report and the clinical context, we feed the prior encoder with; (1) clinical notes features and (2) global image set features. This can be interpreted as forming a general impression of the image features with respect to the clinical context. The context features will then be fed into the sentence generator. Finally, to ensure that the model attends to each image in the set, we use a regulated attention mechanism to generate a dynamic local image features conditioning vector $L_t$ used to generate the next word in the sentence. We describe these components in detail below.

**Image Encoder** encodes an ordered set of images $\mathcal{I} = \{I_1, .., I_N\}$ into the set of local image features $\mathcal{A}$ and the global image features $F_{init}$. More specifically, we first extract the $14 \times 14 \times 512$ features $U$ from the 4th max-pool layer of the pre-trained VGG-16 network [16]. Then the extracted features $U$

are concatenated and flattened to compute the local image representations, $\mathcal{A} = \{A_1, \ldots, A_a\}, A_i \in \mathbb{R}^{N \times d}$ where $a = 196$ and $d = 512$ are the dimensions of the flattened image and feature channels respectively. Meanwhile, in order to produce a global representation for $\mathcal{I}$, we apply an FC layer to $U$ to extract $F_{init}$ with 1x$H$ fixed dimensions. Then, $\mathcal{A}$ and $F_{init}$ are fed into the following attention and context encoder networks.

**Prior Encoder** extracts the context vector $F_m$ to represent features from the clinical notes and previously generated sentence $R_{m-1}$. More specifically, for each sentence we first use a word embedding to produce fixed vector representations $\mathcal{S} = \{s_1, \ldots, s_C\}, s_t \in \mathbb{R}^{V \times E}$ and $\mathcal{Q} = \{q_1, \ldots, q_C\}, q_i \in \mathbb{R}^{V \times E}$ for the set of words in the previous sentence and clinical notes respectively; where, $V$ is the size of the vocabulary, $C$ is the number of words in each sentence, $E = 512$ is the word embedding space and $q_i$ and $s_t$ are both 1-of-$V$ encoded words. $R_{m-1}$ is then fed into a bidirectional LSTM [4] and followed by an FC layer to encode a fixed 1x$H$ representation $J_m$. We then concatenate $J_m$ and $F_{m-1}$ and apply an FC layer to encode $F_m$ with 1x$H$ fixed dimensions. At $m = 0$, the output of the image encoder $F_{init}$ and the embed clinical notes $\mathcal{Q}$ are used in place of $F_{m-1}$ and $R_{m-1}$ respectively.

**Sentence Generator** is an RNN that generates a sentence $\hat{R}_m$ word by word conditioned on the outputs of image encoder $\mathcal{A}$ and prior encoder $F_m$. After a sentence is generated, the prior encoder receives it as input to generate $F_{m+1}$ which is then fed back to the sentence generator to generate the next sentence: this is repeated until the entire medical report is generated. More specifically, the attention network first computes a probability distribution over $\mathcal{A}$ using the deterministic soft attention methods described in [17] to compute $\kappa_{ti}$. $\kappa_{ti}$ is then used to compute the weighted inter-image features vector $\mathcal{Z}_t = \phi(\{A_i\}, \{\kappa_i\}) = \sum_i^a \kappa_i A_i$. The network then computes a second probability distribution $\alpha_{ti}$ in the same way over $\mathcal{Z}_t = \{z_1, \ldots, z_N\}, z_i \in \mathbb{R}^d$. The second soft attention weighted inter-image feature vector $L_t = \phi(\alpha(\{z_i\}, \{\alpha_i\})) = \sum_i^N \alpha_i z_i$ serves as the 1x$d$ local features conditioning vector used to generate $s_{t+1}$. $L_t$ and $h_t$ are then passed through to a visual sentinel. The visual sentinel multiplies $L_t$ and $F_m$ by gating scalars $\beta_L$ and $\beta_F$. Both gating scalars; are computed as follows

$$\beta_x = Sigmoid(w_x h_t + b_x) \tag{1}$$

where $w_x$ and $b_x$ are hyper-parameters to be learned by the network. This allows the network to judge the importance of $L_t$ and $F_m$ features when generating $s_{t+1}$. $\beta_L L_t$, $\beta_F F_m$ and $s_t$ are concatenated and fed into a LSTM. A deep multilayer perceptron output layer (MLP) [14] then computes $\mathcal{X}_{prob} = \{p_i, \ldots, p_V\}$; the probability distribution over the vocabulary of V words using the 1x$H$ hidden state $h_t$ output of the LSTM. Specifically, MLP takes $s_t$, $L_t$, $h_t$ and $F_m$ as input and computes the probability distribution for $s_t$ as:

$$p(S_t | S_{t-1}, L_t, F_m) = \tanh(W_v(S_{t-1} + W_h h_t + W_L L_t + W_F F_m)) \tag{2}$$

Where $W_v \in \mathbb{R}^{V \times E}$, $W_h \in \mathbb{R}^{H \times E}$, $W_L \in \mathbb{R}^{E \times d}$, $W_f \in \mathbb{R}^{E \times H}$ are all parametrized by the neural network. We then apply an *argmax* function to

$\mathcal{X}_{prob}$ to generate the next word in the sentence. This process is repeated for all words in the sentence.

## 3.2 Attention Regularization

When weights of the attention mechanism are not regularized, there is a possibility that the network will assign each data point equal attention weights. In this scenario, the attention mechanism does not offer any advantage over average pooling of image features. To this end, we apply a set of regularizations on the attention weights to enforce selectivity and attend only to image features that contribute to the model's predictions at a given time step.

**Xu's et al.** We first apply the regularization proposed by Xu et al. [17] to ensure that all the attention weights sum to one for both the temporal direction and spatial direction of the alpha attention matrix. More specifically, Xu et al. encourage a doubly stochastic property on the attention matrix which contains attention weights for visual features localisation at each time step. The loss function for Xu et al. is defined as:

$$C_{xu} = \sum_{i}^{N} (1 - \sum_{t}^{C} \alpha_{ti})^2 \tag{3}$$

**Salient Alpha (SAL).** The aim for SAL regularization is to increase the distance between the maximum weight and the average weight to force the network to be highly selective when attending to image regions. We define SAL as follows.

$$C_{SAL} = \frac{1}{C} \sum_{t=0}^{C} \left( \frac{max_i(\alpha_{ti}) - mean_i(\alpha_{ti})}{mean_i(\alpha_{ti})} \right) \tag{4}$$

Where $max_i$ is the maximum value and $mean_i$ is the mean along the column axis.

**Time Distributed Variance (TDVAR).** The TDVAR aims to increase the variance of the attention weights. This will enforce the network to assign different attention weights for each generated word and enforces high variability in the attended features when generating the text sequence. We define TDVAR as follows:

$$C_{TD} = \frac{1}{N} \sum_{i=0}^{N} \left( \frac{std_t(\alpha_{ti})}{mean_t(\alpha_{ti})} \right) \tag{5}$$

Where $std_t$ is the standard deviation and $mean_t$ is the mean along the row axis of $\alpha_{ti}$. We then combine these three regularization terms to produce $C_{alpha}$ as follows:

$$C_{alpha} = \lambda_1 C_{xu} + \frac{\lambda_2}{max(\delta, C_{SAL})} + \frac{\lambda_3}{max(\delta, C_{TD})} \tag{6}$$

where $\lambda_1$, $\lambda_2$ and $\lambda_3$ are hyperparameters to scale the representation of each term. $\delta$ is used to avoid zero division and exploding gradients in the initial training steps.

### 3.3    Training Protocol

We use random initialisation for neural network weights and zero initialisation for biases. The embedding matrix $\mathbb{R}^{V \times E}$ is randomly initialised with values between $-1$ and $+1$. During training, the input to the network is $\mathcal{D}_t = \{\mathcal{I}, \mathcal{R}, \mathcal{Q}\}_i^{D_t} = 0$. The cost function used to train the network is as follows;

$$\textbf{Cost} = -\log(P(\mathcal{R}|\mathcal{I} \cap \mathcal{Q})) + C_{alpha} \tag{7}$$

We update the gradients of the network using truncated backpropagation through time (TBTT) with $\tau = 2\,m$ [12] and ADAM optimisation [8] *i.e.* The error is computed over the generated sentence, and the prior encoded previous sentence of lengths $m$. We implement the norm clipping strategy of [15] to stabilize the network and prevent exploding gradients. During inference, the inputs to the network are $\mathcal{D}_{in} = \{\mathcal{I}, \mathcal{Q}\}_{i=0}^{D_{in}}$. **NEWLINE** tokens serve as the initial word inputs to the sentence generator; which generates the sentence word by word. Sentences are then generated one by one until the entire medical report sequence is complete.

## 4    Experiments and Results

**Table 1.** This table provides the quantitative evaluations metrics for the machine generated texts.

| Architecture | BLEU-1 | BLEU-2 | BLEU-3 | BLEU-4 | ROUGE | METEOR |
|---|---|---|---|---|---|---|
| CORAL8 | **0.49** | **0.35** | **0.28** | **0.23** | **0.39** | **0.31** |
| Recurrent attention [18] | 0.36 | 0.26 | 0.21 | 0.17 | 0.30 | 0.29 |
| Xu *et al.* [17] | 0.44 | 0.30 | 0.23 | 0.19 | 0.35 | 0.30 |
| VANNILA | 0.31 | 0.19 | 0.12 | 0.07 | 0.30 | 0.29 |
| CORAL8 w/o clinical notes | 0.44 | 0.29 | 0.22 | 0.17 | 0.34 | 0.29 |
| CORAL8 w/o TDVAR | 0.42 | 0.22 | 0.17 | 0.17 | 0.37 | 0.26 |
| CORAL8 w/o Xu's regularization | 0.42 | 0.30 | 0.23 | 0.19 | 0.36 | 0.29 |
| CORAL8 w/o SAL | 0.41 | 0.29 | 0.22 | 0.18 | 0.36 | 0.29 |
| CORAL8 w/o attention regularization | 0.44 | 0.31 | 0.25 | 0.20 | 0.37 | 0.28 |

We prepare the dataset by resizing all images to $224 \times 224 \times 3$ pixels in order to make use of a VGG-16 network pre-trained on ImageNet [2]. All words from the medical reports and clinical notes are tokenized and we replace any word that occurs less than two times in the dataset with a special **UNK** token. This creates the vocabulary of 596 words. **NEWLINE** and **EOS** tokens are added to every sentence to indicate the start and end of the sentence respectively. Each sentence is padded to a fixed length of 40 word with **NULL** tokens. Finally, each medical report is padded to a fixed length of seven sentences.

We trained our model for 30 epochs using a learning rate of 0.001, $\lambda_1 = 1$, $\lambda_2 = 0.5$, $\lambda_3 = 0.5$ and $\delta = 0.001$. Then, the performance was evaluated using BLEU [13], ROUGE [11], and METEOR [10]. We use an implementation of [18] to serve as the baseline for our experiment; we refer to this method as **Recurrent Attention**. As the authors of [18] did not publish the source code for their model, we include validation experiments for our implementation in the supplementary materials. The alpha regularization method proposed in [17] applied to our CORAL8 model is also compared as a baseline. We conduct ablation studies to evaluate the contributions of each proposed component to the overall performance of our model. To determine the significance of clinical note features, we train a model that omits the initial prior encoder step and uses $F_{init}$ to represent the context vector for the first sentence i.e. $F_0 = F_{init}$. Examples of generated reports with and without clinical notes can be found in Table 2. To asses the effects of each alpha regularization term; we train a model that omits it from the cost function. Visualizations of the effects these omissions have on the attention mechanism are provided in the supplementary materials. We also include a vanilla implementation where the sentence generator consists of LSTM conditioned only on $S_t$ and $F_{init}$. The quantitative results for all models are provided in Table 1.

**Table 2.** This table contains examples of machine generated reports. Due to space constraints, we only include the final sentence of the report as it contains the overall impressions. Unabridged examples are included in the supplementary materials. Key words are highlighted in bold.

|  | Example 1 | Example 2 | Example 3 |
|---|---|---|---|
| Clinical notes | Renal biopsy. For IF and histology. Creatinine 250. Proteinuria, haematuria, **suspected IgA nephropathy** | histopathology, IF. Renal failure. Urine protein -/blood positive. **ANCA positive. ?ANCA vasculitis.** ? Crescentic necrotising GN | Renal Bx. Diabetic. **Hypertensive.** eGFR 23. Proteinuria |
| Ground truth | iga UNK oxford classification s1 t2 UNK and UNK are UNK due to UNK tissue UNK | pauci immune anca related focal segmental necrotising glomerulonephritis | arterionephrosclerosis with UNK UNK interstitial fibrosis and hypertensive vascular disease glomerulomegaly consistent with grade 1 diabetic glomerulopathy widespread low grade tubular epithelial injury with some atn |
| CORAL8 with clinical notes | iga nephropathy oxford classification m0 t0 | focal segmental necrotising and crescentic pauci immune glomeruli nephritis | acute on chronic thrombotic microangiopathy tma UNK a history of UNK hypertension |
| CORAL8 without clinical notes | fsgs | there is equivocal reactivity for igg igm c3 and c1q of the glomeruli with a similar intensity | there is no |

# 5    Discussion and Future Direction

Table 1 shows that removing any component of the proposed model decreases performance across all quantitative metrics. This suggests that SAL, TDVAR and clinical notes all contribute to the final model performance. It is important to note that these metrics only measure the alignment of machine generated and ground truth texts, they do not provide sufficient means to validate the utility of these models in a clinical setting. However, as this is a pilot study in the application of deep learning for automatic reporting of the RDIF assay, these metrics are useful in establishing a quantitative baseline for measuring the relative performance in terms of generating narrative texts.

Insights into how clinical data improves accuracy can be inferred from Table 2. The first example refers to a case of IgA nephropathy; oxford classification S1 T1. S1 indicates that some glomeruli are segmentally sclerosed; this is a feature of IgA nephropathy and focal segmental glomerular sclerosis (FSGS). The model without clinical notes concluded the image was FSGS, but the presence of *suspected IgA nephropathy* in the clinical notes resulted in the proposed model predicting IgA nephropathy. In the second example, the proposed model accurately predicts pauci immune glomeruli nephritis. This condition is often referred to as Anti-neutrophil cytoplasmic antibody (ANCA) associated vasculitis, due to its strong association with ANCA antibodies [6]. The presence of *ANCA positive ?ANCA vasculitis* in the clinical notes suggests that the proposed model is capturing the associations between the clinical context and the pathologist impressions of the RDIF assay. Example 3 illustrates an incorrect impression generated by the CORAL8 model. Despite being incorrect, the example demonstrates how conditions with similar clinical features are modelled by the network. The underlying pathophysiology for arterionephrosclerosis and the predicted condition (thrombotic microangiopathy) can be due to the observed hypertension [7,9]. This indicates that clinical notes may help stratify candidate medical conditions into groups with shared clinical features.

These results indicate that, although the proposed model architecture is foremost in a relative sense, generating narrative style medical reports continues to be a challenging obstacle to overcome. By releasing the dataset to the community, we hope to encourage further research into developing models to generate narrative medical reports for these multi-image medical panels. We advocate the inclusion of the additional clinical data in such models in order to accommodate the ethos of stratified medicine in the modern clinical landscape. When we achieve non-relative proficiency in generating narrative medical texts, in future works we will explore additional quantitative methods of validating the clinical utility of the machine generated reports for this task.

**Acknowledgements.** This research was funded by the Australian Government through the Australian Research Council and Sullivan Nicolaides Pathology under Linkage Project LP160101797.

# References

1. Alsaad, K., Herzenberg, A.: Distinguishing diabetic nephropathy from other causes of glomerulosclerosis: an update. J. Clin. Pathol. **60**(1), 18–26 (2007). https://doi. org/10.1136/jcp.2005.035592
2. Deng, J., Dong, W., Socher, R., Li, L.J., Li, K., Fei-Fei, L.: ImageNet: a large-scale hierarchical image database. In: CVPR, pp. 248–255. IEEE (2009). https://doi. org/10.1109/cvprw.2009.5206848
3. Donahue, J., et al.: Long-term recurrent convolutional networks for visual recognition and description. In: CVPR, pp. 2625–2634 (2015). https://doi.org/10.1109/ cvpr.2015.7298878
4. Graves, A., Schmidhuber, J.: Framewise phoneme classification with bidirectional lstm and other neural network architectures. Neural Netw. **18**(5–6), 602–610 (2005). https://doi.org/10.1016/j.neunet.2005.06.042
5. Ho, J., et al.: Can digital pathology result in cost savings? A financial projection for digital pathology implementation at a large integrated health care organization. J. Pathol. Inform. **5**(1), 33 (2014). https://doi.org/10.4103/2153-3539.139714
6. Kallenberg, C.G., Heeringa, P., Stegeman, C.A.: Mechanisms of disease: pathogenesis and treatment of ANCA-associated vasculitides. Nat. Rev. Rheumatol. **2**(12), 661 (2006). https://doi.org/10.1038/ncprheum0355
7. Khanal, N., Dahal, S., Upadhyay, S., Bhatt, V.R., Bierman, P.J.: Differentiating malignant hypertension-induced thrombotic microangiopathy from thrombotic thrombocytopenic purpura. Ther. Adv. Hematol. **6**(3), 97–102 (2015). https://doi. org/10.1177/2040620715571076
8. Kingma, D.P., Ba, J.: Adam: a method for stochastic optimization. arXiv preprint arXiv:1412.6980 (2014)
9. Kopp, J.B.: Rethinking hypertensive kidney disease. Curr. Opin. Nephrol. Hypertens. **22**(3), 266–272 (2013). https://doi.org/10.1097/mnh.0b013e3283600f8c
10. Lavie, A., Agarwal, A.: Meteor. In: StatMT. Association for Computational Linguistics (2007). https://doi.org/10.3115/1626355.1626389
11. Lin, C.Y.: ROUGE: a package for automatic evaluation of summaries. In: Text Summarization Branches Out (2004)
12. Mikolov, T., Karafiát, M., Burget, L., Černockỳ, J., Khudanpur, S.: Recurrent neural network based language model. In: Eleventh Annual Conference of the International Speech Communication Association (2010)
13. Papineni, K., Roukos, S., Ward, T., Zhu, W.J.: BLEU. In: ACL. Association for Computational Linguistics (2001). https://doi.org/10.3115/1073083.1073135
14. Pascanu, R., Gulcehre, C., Cho, K., Bengio, Y.: How to construct deep recurrent neural networks. arXiv preprint arXiv:1312.6026 (2013)
15. Pascanu, R., Mikolov, T., Bengio, Y.: On the difficulty of training recurrent neural networks. In: ICML, pp. 1310–1318 (2013)
16. Simonyan, K., Zisserman, A.: Very deep convolutional networks for large-scale image recognition. arXiv preprint arXiv:1409.1556 (2014)
17. Xu, K., et al.: Show, attend and tell: neural image caption generation with visual attention. In: ICML, pp. 2048–2057 (2015)

18. Xue, Y., et al.: Multimodal recurrent model with attention for automated radiology report generation. In: Frangi, A.F., Schnabel, J.A., Davatzikos, C., Alberola-López, C., Fichtinger, G. (eds.) MICCAI 2018. LNCS, vol. 11070, pp. 457–466. Springer, Cham (2018). https://doi.org/10.1007/978-3-030-00928-1_52
19. Zhang, Z., Xie, Y., Xing, F., McGough, M., Yang, L.: MDNet: a semantically and visually interpretable medical image diagnosis network. In: CVPR, pp. 6428–6436 (2017). https://doi.org/10.1109/cvpr.2017.378

# ET-Net: A Generic Edge-aTtention Guidance Network for Medical Image Segmentation

Zhijie Zhang[1], Huazhu Fu[2(✉)], Hang Dai[2], Jianbing Shen[2], Yanwei Pang[1], and Ling Shao[2]

[1] School of Electrical and Information Engineering, Tianjin University, Tianjin, China
[2] Inception Institute of Artificial Intelligence, Abu Dhabi, UAE
huazhu.fu@inceptioniai.org

**Abstract.** Segmentation is a fundamental task in medical image analysis. However, most existing methods focus on primary region extraction and ignore edge information, which is useful for obtaining accurate segmentation. In this paper, we propose a generic medical segmentation method, called Edge-aTtention guidance Network (ET-Net), which embeds edge-attention representations to guide the segmentation network. Specifically, an edge guidance module is utilized to learn the edge-attention representations in the early encoding layers, which are then transferred to the multi-scale decoding layers, fused using a weighted aggregation module. The experimental results on four segmentation tasks (*i.e.*, optic disc/cup and vessel segmentation in retinal images, and lung segmentation in chest X-Ray and CT images) demonstrate that preserving edge-attention representations contributes to the final segmentation accuracy, and our proposed method outperforms current state-of-the-art segmentation methods. The source code of our method is available at https://github.com/ZzzJzzZ/ETNet.

## 1 Introduction

Medical image segmentation is an important procedure in medical image analysis. The shapes, size measurements and total areas of segmentation outcomes can provide significant insight into early manifestations of life-threatening diseases. As a result, designing an efficient general segmentation model deserves further attention. Existing medical image segmentation methods can mainly be divided into two categories: edge detection and object segmentation. The edge detection methods first identify object boundaries utilizing local gradient representations, and then separate the closed loop regions as the objects. These methods, which aim to obtain highly localized image information, can achieve high accuracy in boundary segmentation, and are adequate for simple structures. For example, the level-set technique is employed to minimize an objective function for estimating tumor segmentation based on shape priors [16]. The

D. Shen et al. (Eds.): MICCAI 2019, LNCS 11764, pp. 442–450, 2019.
https://doi.org/10.1007/978-3-030-32239-7_49

template matching method is proposed to obtain optic disc boundary approximations with the Circular Hough Transform in retinal images [1]. Other edge detection methods are employed to extract blood vessels in retinal images [6,11]. However, these edge detection methods depend on local edge representations and lack object-level information, which leads to trivial segmentation regions and discontinuous boundaries. By contrast, object segmentation methods [7,18] utilize global appearance models of foregrounds and backgrounds to identify the target regions, which preserves the homogeneity and semantic characteristics of objects, and reduces the uncertainties in detecting the boundary positions. A common way of doing this is to classify each pixel/patch in an image as foreground or background. For example, a superpixel classification method was proposed to segment the optic disc and cup regions for glaucoma screening [4]. However, without utilizing edge information, several object segmentation methods need to refine the initial coarse segmentation results using additional post-processing technologies (e.g., Conditional Random Field and shape fitting), which is time-consuming and less related to previous segmentation representations.

Recently, the success of U-Net has significantly promoted widespread applications of segmentation on medical images, such as cell detection from 2D image [12], vessel segmentation from retinal images [6] and lung region extraction from chest X-Ray and CT images [10]. However, there are still several limitations when applying Deep Convolutional Neural Networks (DCNNs) based on a U-Net structure. In medical image segmentation, different targets sometimes have similar appearances, making it difficult to segment them using a U-Net based DCNN. Besides, inconspicuous objects are sometimes over-shadowed by irrelevant salient objects, which can confuse the DCNNs, since it cannot extract discriminative context features, leading to false predictions. In addition, target shapes and scale variations are difficult for DCNNs to predict. Although U-Net proposes to aggregate high-level and low-level features to address this problem, it only slightly alleviates it, since it aggregates features of different scale without considering their different contributes. Herein, we propose a novel method to extract discriminative context features and selectively aggregate multi-scale information for efficient medical image segmentation.

In this paper, we integrate both edge detection and object segmentation in one deep learning network. To do so, we propose a novel general medical segmentation method, called Edge-aTtention guidance Network (ET-Net), which embeds edge-attention representations to guide the process of segmentation. In our ET-Net, an edge guidance module (EGM) is provided to learn the edge-attention representations and preserve the local edge characteristics in the early encoding layers, while a weighted aggregation module (WAM) is designed to aggregate the multi-scale side-outputs from the decoding layers and transfer the edge-attention representations to high-level layers to improve the final results. We evaluate the proposed method on four segmentation tasks, including optic disc/cup segmentation and vessel detection in retinal images, and lung segmentation in Chest X-Ray and CT images. Results demonstrate that the proposed ET-Net outperforms the state-of-the-art methods in all tasks.

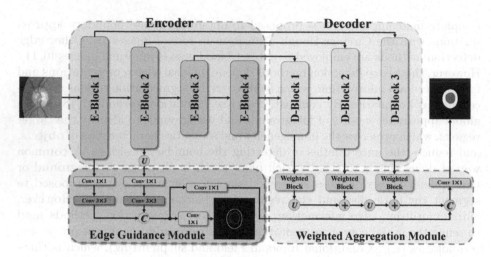

**Fig. 1.** Illustration of our ET-Net architecture, which includes the main encoder-decoder network with an edge guidance module and weighted aggregation module. 'Conv' denotes the convolutional layer, while 'U', 'C', and '+' denote the upsampling, concatenation, and addition layers, respectively.

## 2    Method

Figure 1 illustrates the architecture of our ET-Net, which is primarily based on an encoder-decoder network, with the EGM and WAM modules appended on the end. The ResNet-50 [8] is utilized as the encoder network, which comprises of four Encoding-Blocks (E-Blocks), one for each different feature map resolution. For each E-Block, the inputs first go through a feature extraction stream, which consists of a stack of $1 \times 1 - 3 \times 3 - 1 \times 1$ convolutional layers, and are then summed with the shortcut of inputs to generate the final outputs. With this residual connection, the model can generate class-specific high-level features. The decoder path is formed from three cascaded Decoding-Blocks (D-Blocks), which are used to maintain the characteristics of the high-level features from the E-Blocks and enhance their representation ability. As shown in Fig. 2(a), the D-Block first adopts a depth-wise convolution to enhance the representation of the fused low-level and high-level features. Then, a $1 \times 1$ convolution is used to unify the number of channels.

### 2.1    Edge Guidance Module

As stated in Sect. 1, edge information provides useful fine-grained constraints to guide feature extraction during segmentation. However, only low-level features preserve sufficient edge information. As such, we only apply the EGM at the top of early layers, *i.e.*, E-Block 1 and 2, of the decoding path, as shown in Fig. 1. The EGM has two main fashions: (1) it provides an edge-attention representation to

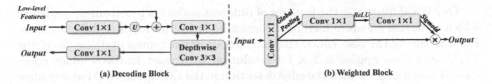

**Fig. 2.** Illustration of the E-Block and Weighted Block. 'U', '+' and '×' denote upsampling, addition, and multiplication layers, respectively.

guide the process of segmentation in the decoding path; (2) it supervises the early convolutional layers using the edge detection loss.

In our EGM, the outputs of E-Block 2 are upsampled to the same resolution as the outputs of E-Block 1, and then fed into the $1 \times 1 - 3 \times 3$ convolutional layers and concatenated together. After that, the concatenated features go through one of two branches: a $1 \times 1$ convolutional layer to act as the edge guidance features in the decoding path, or another $1 \times 1$ convolutional layer to predict the edge detection results for early supervision. The Lovász-Softmax loss [2] is used in our EGM, since it performs better than cross entropy loss for class imbalanced problems. It can be formulated as:

$$\mathcal{L} = \frac{1}{C} \sum_{c \in C} \overline{\Delta_{J_c}}(m(c)), \quad \text{and} \quad m_i(c) = \begin{cases} 1 - p_i(c) & \text{if } c = y_i(c), \\ p_i(c) & \text{otherwise,} \end{cases} \quad (1)$$

where $C$ denotes the class number, and $y_i(c) \in \{-1, 1\}$ and $p_i(c) \in [0, 1]$ are the ground truth label and predicted probability of pixel $i$ for class $c$, respectively. $\overline{\Delta_{J_c}}$ is the Lovász extension of the Jaccard index [2]. With the edge supervision, the transmitted edge features are better able to guide the extraction of discriminative features in high-level layers.

## 2.2 Weighted Aggregation Module

In order to adapt to the shape and size variations of objects, existing methods tend to sum up multi-scale outputs along the channel dimension for final predictions (*e.g.*, [5,19]). However, not all features in high-level layers are activated and benefit the recovery of objects. Aiming to address this, we develop the WAM to emphasize the valuable features, and aggregate multi-scale information and edge-attention representations to improve the segmentation performance. As shown in Fig. 1, outputs of each D-Block are fed into the Weighted Blocks to highlight the valuable information. The structure of a Weighted Block is shown in Fig. 2(b). In this block, global average pooling is first employed to aggregate the global context information of inputs, and then two $1 \times 1$ convolutional layers with different non-linearity activation functions, *i.e.*, ReLU and Sigmoid, are applied to estimate the layer relevance and generate the weights along the channel dimension. After that, the generated weights are multiplied with the outputs to yield more representative features.

Our WAM integrates the features of different scales via a bottom-up pathway, which generates a feature hierarchy consisting of feature maps of different sizes. Finally, the WAM also concatenates edge-attention representations from the EGM, and then applies a $1 \times 1$ convolution to extract features under edge-guided conditions. As with the edge detection in the EGM, our WAM also utilizes the Lovász-Softmax loss as the segmentation loss function. Thus, the total loss function of our ET-Net is defined as: $\mathcal{L}_{total} = \alpha \cdot \mathcal{L}_{seg} + (1 - \alpha) \cdot \mathcal{L}_{edge}$, where $\mathcal{L}_{edge}$ and $\mathcal{L}_{seg}$ denote the losses for edge detection in EGM and segmentation in WAM, respectively. In our experiments, weight $\alpha$ is empirically set to 0.3.

### 2.3   Implementation Details

For data augmentation, we apply a *random mirror*, *random scale*, which ranges from 0.5 to 2, and *random rotation* between $-10$ and $10°$, for all datasets. *random color jitters* with a probability of 0.5 are also applied to the data. All input images are randomly cropped to $512 \times 512$.

The initial weights of the encoder network come from ResNet-50 [8] pre-trained on ImageNet, and the parameters of the other layers are randomly initialized. A dilation strategy is used in E-Block 4, with an output stride of $1/16$. During training, we set the *batch_size* to 16 with synchronized batch normalization, and adopt 'poly' learning rate scheduling $lr = base\_lr \times (1 - \frac{iters}{total\_iters})^{power}$, in which the power is set to 0.9 and *base_lr* is 0.005. The *total_iters* is calculated by the *num_images* $\times$ *epochs*/*batch_size*, where *epochs* is set to 300 for all datasets. Our deep models are optimized using the Adam optimizer with a momentum of 0.9 and a weight decay of 0.0005. The whole ET-Net framework is implemented using PyTorch. Training (300 epochs) requires approximately 2.5 h on one NVIDIA Titan Xp GPU. During testing, the segmentation results, including edge detection and object segmentation, are produced within 0.015 s. per image.

## 3   Experiments

We evaluate our approach on three major types of medical images: retinal images, X-Ray and CT images. For convenience comparison, we select the evaluation metrics that are highly related to generic segmentation.

**Optic Disc and Cup Segmentation in Retinal Images:** We evaluate our method on optic disc and cup segmentation in retinal images, which is a common task in glaucoma detection. Two public datasets are used in this experiment: the REFUGE[1] dataset, which consists of 400 training images and 400 validation images; the Drishti-GS [14] dataset, which contains 50 training images and 51 validation images. Considering the negative influence of non-target areas in fundus images, we first localize the disc centers following the existing automatic

---

[1] https://refuge.grand-challenge.org/.

**Table 1.** Optic disc/cup segmentation results on retinal fundus images.

| Method | REFUGE | | | Drishti-GS | | |
|---|---|---|---|---|---|---|
| | $Dice_{OC}$ (%) | $Dice_{OD}$ (%) | mIoU (%) | $Dice_{OC}$ (%) | $Dice_{OD}$ (%) | mIoU (%) |
| FCN [13] | 84.67 | 92.56 | 82.47 | 87.95 | 95.69 | 83.92 |
| U-Net [12] | 85.44 | 93.08 | 83.12 | 88.06 | 96.43 | 84.87 |
| M-Net [5] | 86.48 | 93.59 | 84.02 | 88.60 | 96.58 | 85.88 |
| Multi-task [3] | 86.74 | 94.01 | 84.36 | 88.96 | 96.55 | 85.94 |
| $p$OSAL [17] | 87.50 | 94.60 | - | 90.10 | 97.40 | - |
| Our ET-Net | **89.12** | **95.29** | **86.70** | **93.14** | **97.52** | **87.92** |

**Table 2.** Segmentation results on retinal fundus, X-Ray and CT images.

| Method | DRIVE | | MC | | LUNA | |
|---|---|---|---|---|---|---|
| | Acc. (%) | mIoU (%) | Acc. (%) | mIoU (%) | Acc. (%) | mIoU (%) |
| FCN [13] | 94.13 | 74.55 | 97.35 | 90.53 | 96.18 | 93.82 |
| U-Net [12] | 94.45 | 75.46 | 97.82 | 91.64 | 96.63 | 94.79 |
| M-Net [5] | 94.58 | 75.81 | 97.96 | 91.95 | 97.27 | 94.92 |
| Multi-task [3] | 94.97 | 76.21 | 98.13 | 92.24 | 97.82 | 94.96 |
| Our ET-Net | **95.60** | **77.44** | **98.65** | **94.20** | **98.68** | **96.23** |

disc detection method [5], and then transmit the localized images into our network. The proposed approach is compared with the classic segmentation methods (*i.e.*, FCN [13] U-Net [12], M-Net [5], and Multi-task [3] (it predicts edge and object predictions on the same features.), and the state-of-the-art segmentation method $p$OSAL [17], which achieved first place for the optic disc and cup segmentation tasks in the REFUGE challenge. The dice coefficients of optic disc ($Dice_{OD}$) and cup ($Dice_{OD}$), as well as mean intersection-over-union (mIoU), are employed as evaluation metrics. As shown in Table 1, our ET-Net achieves the best performance on both the REFUGE and Drishti-GS datasets. Our model achieves particularly impressive results for optic cup segmentation, which is an especially difficult task, achieving 2% improvement of $Dice_{OC}$ over the next best method.

**Vessel Segmentation in Retinal Images:** We evaluate our method on vessel segmentation in retinal images. DRIVE [15], which contains 20 images for training and 20 for testing, is adopted in our experiments. The statistics in Table 2 show that our proposed method achieves the best performance, with 77.44% mIoU and 95.60% accuracy, when compared with classical methods (*i.e.*, U-Net [12], M-Net [5], FCN [13] and Multi-task [3]).

**Lung Segmentation in X-Ray Images:** We conduct lung segmentation experiments on Chest X-Rays, which is an important component for computer-aided diagnosis of lung health. We use the Montgomery County (MC) [9] dataset, which contains 80 training images and 58 testing images. We compare our ET-Net with FCN [13], U-Net [12], M-Net [5] and Multi-task [3], in terms of mIoU and accuracy (Acc.) scores. Table 2 shows the results, where our method achieves the state-of-the-art performance, with an Acc. of 98.65% and mIoU of 94.20%.

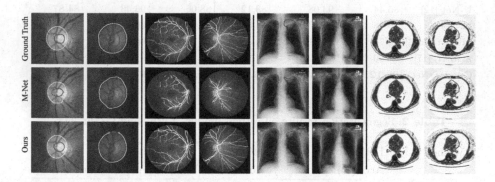

**Fig. 3.** Visualization of segmentation results. From left to right: optic disc/cup, and vessel segmentation in retinal fundus images, lung segmentation in Chest X-Ray and CT images.

**Table 3.** Ablation study of optic disc/cup segmentation on the Drishti-GS *test* set

| Method | $Dice_{OC}$ (%) | $Dice_{OD}$ (%) | mIoU (%) |
|---|---|---|---|
| Base network | 90.11 | 95.77 | 84.41 |
| Base network + EGM | 91.24 | 97.17 | 86.49 |
| Base network + WAM | 91.49 | 97.07 | 86.62 |
| Base network + EGM + WAM | **93.14** | **97.52** | **87.92** |

**Lung Segmentation in CT Images:** We evaluate our method on lung segmentation from CT images, which is fundamental for further lung nodule disease diagnosis. The Lung Nodule Analysis (LUNA) competition dataset[2] is employed, which is divided into 214 images for training and 53 images for testing. As with the lung segmentation from Chest X-Ray images, we compare our method with FCN [13], U-Net [12], M-Net [5], and Multi-task [3], in terms of mIoU and Acc. scores. The randomly cropped images are fed into the proposed network. As shown in Table 2, our ET-Net outperforms previous state-of-the-art methods, obtaining an Acc. of 98.68% and mIoU of 96.23%.

In addition to quantitative results, we provide qualitative segmentation results, shown in Fig. 3. As can be seen, our results are close to the ground truth. When compared with the predictions of other methods, it is clear that our results are better, especially, in the edge regions.

---

[2] https://www.kaggle.com/kmader/finding-lungs-in-ct-data/data.

## 3.1 Ablation Study

To evaluate the contributions of each component of the proposed method, we conduct experiments with different settings on the Drishti-GS dataset. As shown in Table 3, we choose the encoder-decoder network shown in Fig. 1 as the base network, which achieves 90.11%, 95.77% and 84.41% in terms of $Dice_{OC}$, $Dice_{OD}$ and mIoU, respectively. When we append the proposed EGM, it yields results of 91.24%/97.17%/86.49% ($Dice_{OC}$/$Dice_{OD}$/mIoU). This dramatically outperforms the base network, with only a small addition to the computational cost, proving that edge information is of vital importance for segmentation. To study the effect of the WAM, we append the WAM to the base network, without concatenating the edge features to base network. With the same training settings, this approach achieves performances of 91.49%/97.07%/86.62%, compared to the base network. The obvious performance gains for all three metrics illustrate the efficiency of the proposed the WAM. Finally, our whole ET-Net, with both EGM and WAM, obtains the best performance on the Drishti-GS *test* set.

## 4 Conclusion

In this paper, we propose a novel Edge-aTtention Guidance network (ET-Net) for general medical image segmentation. By assuming that edge detection and region segmentation are mutually beneficial, we have proposed the Edge Guidance Module to detect object edges and generate edge-attention representations that contain sufficient edge information. Moreover, a Weighted Aggregation Module has been employed to highlight the valuable features of high-level layers, which are combined with the edge representations, to guide the final segmentation. Experiments on various medical imaging tasks have demonstrated the superiority of our proposed ET-Net compared to other state-of-the-art methods. In future work, we will extend our approach to 3D segmentation on CT and MRI volumes.

## References

1. Aquino, A., Gegundez-Arias, M.E., Marin, D.: Detecting the optic disc boundary in digital fundus images using morphological, edge detection, and feature extraction techniques. IEEE TMI **29**(11), 1860–1869 (2010)
2. Berman, M., Rannen Triki, A., Blaschko, M.B.: The Lovász-Softmax loss: a tractable surrogate for the optimization of the intersection-over-union measure in neural networks. In: CVPR (2018)
3. Chen, H., Qi, X., et al.: DCAN: deep contour-aware networks for accurate gland segmentation. In: CVPR (2016)
4. Cheng, J., Liu, J., et al.: Superpixel classification based optic disc and optic cup segmentation for glaucoma screening. IEEE TMI **32**(6), 1019–1032 (2013)
5. Fu, H., Cheng, J., et al.: Joint optic disc and cup segmentation based on multi-label deep network and polar transformation. IEEE TMI **37**(7), 1597–1605 (2018)

6. Fu, H., Xu, Y., Lin, S., Kee Wong, D.W., Liu, J.: DeepVessel: retinal vessel segmentation via deep learning and conditional random field. In: Ourselin, S., Joskowicz, L., Sabuncu, M.R., Unal, G., Wells, W. (eds.) MICCAI 2016. LNCS, vol. 9901, pp. 132–139. Springer, Cham (2016). https://doi.org/10.1007/978-3-319-46723-8_16

7. Gu, Z., et al.: CE-Net: context encoder network for 2D medical image segmentation. IEEE TMI (2019, in press). https://doi.org/10.1109/TMI.2019.2903562

8. He, K., Zhang, X., et al.: Deep residual learning for image recognition. In: CVPR (2016)

9. Jaeger, S., Candemir, S., et al.: Two public chest X-ray datasets for computer-aided screening of pulmonary diseases. QIMS 4(6), 475–477 (2014)

10. Mansoor, A., Bagci, U., et al.: Segmentation and image analysis of abnormal lungs at CT: current approaches, challenges, and future trends. Radiographics 35(4), 1056–1076 (2015)

11. Moccia, S., Momi, E.D., et al.: Blood vessel segmentation algorithms - review of methods, datasets and evaluation metrics. CMPB 158, 71–91 (2018)

12. Ronneberger, O., Fischer, P., Brox, T.: U-Net: convolutional networks for biomedical image segmentation. In: Navab, N., Hornegger, J., Wells, W.M., Frangi, A.F. (eds.) MICCAI 2015. LNCS, vol. 9351, pp. 234–241. Springer, Cham (2015). https://doi.org/10.1007/978-3-319-24574-4_28

13. Shelhamer, E., Long, J., Darrell, T.: Fully convolutional networks for semantic segmentation. TPAMI 39(4), 640–651 (2017)

14. Sivaswamy, J., Krishnadas, S.R., et al.: Drishti-GS: retinal image dataset for optic nerve head (ONH) segmentation. In: IEEE ISBI (2014)

15. Staal, J., Abràmoff, M.D., et al.: Ridge-based vessel segmentation in color images of the retina. IEEE TMI 23(4), 501–509 (2004)

16. Tsai, A., Yezzi, A., et al.: A shape-based approach to the segmentation of medical imagery using level sets. IEEE TMI 22(2), 137–154 (2003)

17. Wang, S., Yu, L., et al.: Patch-based output space adversarial learning for joint optic disc and cup segmentation. IEEE TMI (2019, in press). https://doi.org/10.1109/TMI.2019.2899910

18. Wang, W., Lai, Q., et al.: Salient object detection in the deep learning era: an in-depth survey. arXiv:1904.09146 (2019)

19. Wang, W., Shen, J., Ling, H.: A deep network solution for attention and aesthetics aware photo cropping. IEEE PAMI 41(7), 1531–1544 (2019)

# Instance Segmentation of Biomedical Images with an Object-Aware Embedding Learned with Local Constraints

Long Chen, Martin Strauch, and Dorit Merhof[✉]

Institute of Imaging & Computer Vision, RWTH Aachen University,
Aachen, Germany
{long.chen,martin.strauch,dorit.merhof}@lfb.rwth-aachen.de
https://www.lfb.rwth-aachen.de/

**Abstract.** Automatic instance segmentation is a problem that occurs in many biomedical applications. State-of-the-art approaches either perform semantic segmentation or refine object bounding boxes obtained from detection methods. Both suffer from crowded objects to varying degrees, merging adjacent objects or suppressing a valid object. In this work, we assign an embedding vector to each pixel through a deep neural network. The network is trained to output embedding vectors of similar directions for pixels from the same object, while adjacent objects are orthogonal in the embedding space, which effectively avoids the fusion of objects in a crowd. Our method yields state-of-the-art results even with a light-weighted backbone network on a cell segmentation (BBBC006 + DSB2018) and a leaf segmentation data set (CVPPP2017). The code and model weights are public available (https://github.com/looooongChen/instance_segmentation_with_pixel_embeddings/).

**Keywords:** Instance segmentation · CNN · Object embedding

## 1 Introduction

Many biomedical applications, such as phenotyping [1] and tracking [2], rely on instance segmentation, which aims not only to group pixels in semantic categories but also to segment individuals from the same category. This task is challenging because objects of the same class can get crowded together without obvious boundary clues.

A prevalent class of approaches used for biomedical images is based on semantic segmentation, obtaining instances through per-pixel classification [3, 4]. Although this approach generates good object coverage, crowded objects are often mistakenly regarded as one connected region. DCAN [4] predicts the object

This work was supported by the Deutsche Forschungsgemeinschaft (Research Training Group 2416 MultiSenses-MultiScales).

contour explicitly to separate touching glands. However, segmentation by contours is very unreliable in many cases, since a few misclassified pixels can break a continuous boundary.

Another major class of approaches, such as Mask-RCNN [7], refine the bounding boxes obtained from object detection methods [5,6]. Object detection methods rely on non-maximum suppression (NMS) to remove duplicate predictions resulting from exhaustive search. This becomes problematic when bounding boxes of two objects overlap with a large ratio: one valid object will be suppressed. A finer shape representation star-convex polygons is used by [8] with the intention of reducing false suppression. However, it is only suitable for roundish objects [8,9].

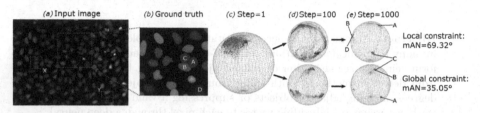

**Fig. 1.** *(a)* In images of repeated patterns, different pixels, such as X and Y, can have similar content in their receptive fields. *(c)–(e)* demonstrate the convergence of the embedding loss on image (a) in a 3 dimensional space (background ignored). In *(e)*, both local and global constraints form 3 clusters which are orthogonal to each other. While adjacencies A, B and C are well separated under local constraints, B and C belong to the same cluster under global constraints. The better discriminative property of local constraints is also reflected by the mean angle of neighbors ($mAN$). In addition, distant objects, such as B and D, occupying the same space is a desired property.

In this work, we propose to get instances by grouping pixels based on an object-aware embedding. A deep neural network is trained to assign each pixel an embedding vector. Pixels of the same object will have similar directions in the embedding space, while spatially close objects are orthogonal to each other. Since our method performs pixel-level grouping, it is not affected by different object shape and it does not suffer from the false suppression problem. On the other hand, it avoids the fusion of adjacent objects like the semantic segmentation based methods.

Some recent research [10,12,13] proposes the use of embedding vectors to distinguish individual objects in the driving scene and natural images. These approaches force each object to occupy a different part of the embedding space. The global constraint is actually not necessary, and could even be detrimental, for biomedical images that often contain repeated local patterns. For example, content in the receptive fields of pixel X and Y (Fig. 1(a)) are very similar, both with one object above and one below. The network has no clear clue to assign X and Y different embeddings. Forcing them to be different is likely to hinder training. Furthermore, the global constraint is inefficient in terms of embedding space utilization. There is no risk of distant objects being merged, thus they could share the same embedding space, such as B and D in Fig. 1.

The main contributions of our work are as follows: (1) we propose to train the embedding mapping only constraining adjacent objects to be different, (2) a novel loss of a good geometrical explanation (adjacent instances live in orthogonal space), (3) a multi-task network head for embedding training and obtaining segmentations from embeddings, which can be applied to any backbone networks.

Our method is compared with several strong competing approaches. It yields comparable or better results on two data sets: a combined fluorescence microscopy data set of BBBC06[1] and the part of DSB2018[2] used by [8] and the CVPPP2017[3] leaf segmentation data set.

## 2   Method

Our approach has has two output branches taking the same feature map as input: the embedding branch and the distance regression branch (Fig. 2). Both consist of two convolutional layers. The last layer of the embedding branch uses linear activation and each filter outputs one dimension of the embedding vector.

The distance regression branch has a single layer output with relu activation. We regress the distance from an object pixel to the closest boundary pixel (normalized within each object). The distance map is used to help obtain segmentations from the embedding map, details are depicted in Sect. 2.2.

The background is treated as a standalone object that is adjacent to all other objects. For distance regression, background pixels are set to zero. It is worth mentioning that the distance map alone provides enough cue to separate objects. But we argue that it is not optimal to obtain accurate segmentations since both object and background pixels are of small values around the boundaries, which is ambiguous and sensitive to small perturbations. In this work, the distance regression plays the role of roughly locating the objects.

### 2.1   Loss Function

The training loss consists of two parts: $L_{reg}$ and $L_{emb}$, which supervise the learning of the distance regression branch and the embedding branch separately. We use $\lambda_1 = 5$ to give more emphasis on the embedding training.

$$L = L_{reg} + \lambda_1 L_{emb}$$

We minimize the mean squared error for the distance regression, with each pixel weighted to balance the foreground and background frequency.

---

[1]   https://data.broadinstitute.org/bbbc/BBBC006/.
[2]   https://www.kaggle.com/c/data-science-bowl-2018.
[3]   https://www.plant-phenotyping.org/CVPPP2017-challenge.

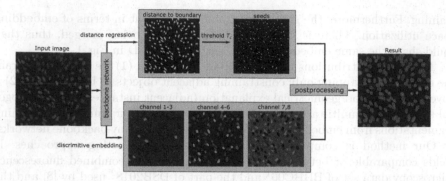

**Fig. 2.** Our framework consists of two branches: the distance regression branch predicts the normalized distance from a pixel to the closest boundary, the embedding branch is responsible for mapping the feature map to the embedding space. The distance map and embedding map are combined to get segmentations (Sect. 2.2). We demonstrate the embedding as RGB images for every 3 channels. (Color figure online)

Intuitively, embeddings of the same object should end up at similar positions in the embedding space, while different objects should be discriminable. So naturally, the embedding loss is formulated as the sum of two terms: the consistency term $L_{con}$ and the discriminative term $L_{dis}$.

To give a specific formula, we have to determine how "similarity" is measured. While euclidean distance is used by many works [10,11], we construct the loss with cosine distance, which decouples from the output range of different networks: $D(e_i, e_j) = 1 - \frac{e_i^T e_j}{\|e_i\|_2 \|e_j\|_2}$, where $e_i, e_j \in \mathbb{R}^D$ are embeddings of pixel $i$ and $j$. The outcome of cosine distance ranges from 0 meaning exactly the same direction, to 2 meaning the opposite, with 1 indicating orthogonality.

Instead of pushing each object pair as far as possible [10,11,13] in the embedding space (global constraint), we only push adjacent objects into each other's orthogonal space (local constraint). As shown in Fig. 1, far away objects can occupy the same position in the embedding space, which uses the space more effectively. In the embedding map in Fig. 2, only a few colors appears repeatedly, still ensuring that adjacent objects have different colors.

Let's say that there are K objects within an image with $(M_1, M_2, \ldots, M_K)$ pixels respectively. The loss can be written as follows:

$$L_{center} = \frac{1}{\sum_{k=1}^{K} M_k} \sum_{k=1}^{K} \sum_{p=1}^{M_k} w_p (d_p - \widehat{d}_p)^2$$

$$L_{emb} = L_{con} + L_{dis}$$

$$= \frac{1}{\sum_{k=1}^{K} M_k} \sum_{k=1}^{K} \sum_{p=1}^{M_k} w_p D(e_p, u_k) + \frac{1}{K} \sum_{k=1}^{K} \frac{1}{|N_d(k)|} \sum_{n \in N_d(k)} |1 - D(u_k, u_n)|,$$

where $d_p$ and $\widehat{d}_p$ are the regression output and ground truth of pixel p, $e_p$ is the embedding of pixel $p$, $u_k$ is the mean embedding (normalized) of object $k$, $w_p$ is the factor for balancing the foreground and background frequency. $N_d(k)$ indicates the neighbors of object $k$. An object is considered as a neighbor if its shortest distance to object k is less than $d$.

## 2.2 Postprocessing

Since objects form clusters in the embedding space, a clustering method that does not require to specify the number of clusters (e.g. mean shift [14]) can be employed to obtain segmentations from the embedding. However, due to the time complexity of mean shift, even processing medium-size images takes tens of seconds. Since our embedding space has a good geometric explanation, we propose a simple but effective way to obtain segmentations:

1. Threshold the distance map to get the central region of an object. We use $T_c = 0.7$ in our experiment.
2. Compute the mean embedding $u_k$ of each seed region.
3. Iteratively perform morphological dilation with a $3 \times 3$ kernel. Frontier pixels $e_i$ are included into the object, if it is not assigned to other objects and $D(e_i, u_k)$ is smaller than $T_e = 0.3$.
4. Stop when no new pixels are included.

Threshold $T_e$ is determined based on the fact that a pixel embedding should be closer to the ground truth object than any others in terms of angle. Thus, we set the midpoint 45° as the boundary, $T_e = 1 - cos(45°) \approx 0.3$.

# 3   Results

## 3.1   Data Sets and Evaluation Metrics

In order to compare different methods, we chose two data sets that reflect typical phenomena in biomedical images:

**BBBC006 + PartDSB2018:** We combined the fluorescence microscopy images of cells used by [8] (part of DSB2018[3]) and BBBC0006[2]. BBBC006 is a larger data set containing more densely distributed cells. We removed a small number of images without objects or with obvious labeling mistakes. The data were randomly split into 1003 training images and 230 test images. The evaluation metric was the *average precision* (AP) over a range of *IoU* (intersection over union) thresholds from 0.5 to 0.95 (see footnote 2).

**CVPPP2017:** Compared to the roundish cells, the leaves in CVPPP2017 have more complex shapes and exhibit more overlap or contact. We randomly sampled 648 images for training and 162 images for testing. The results were evaluated in terms of symmetric best dice (SBD), foreground-background dice (FBD), difference in count (DiC) and absolute DiC [1].

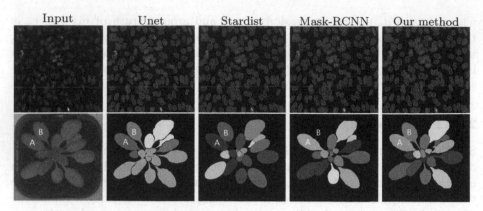

**Fig. 3.** Qualitative results of the cell segmentation and leaf segmentation for four approaches. In the first row, correct matches ($IoU = 0.6$) are highlighted in blue, while false positives are marked in red. The second row shows the leaf segmentation results with color-coded instances. (Color figure online)

## 3.2   Competing Methods

**Unet:** We employed the widely used Unet [3] to perform 3-label segmentation (object, contour, background). Since many objects are in contact, we introduced a 2-pixel boundary to separate them.

**Mask-RCNN:** Mask-RCNN [7] localizes objects by proposal classification and non-max suppression (NMS). Afterwards, segmentation is performed on each object bounding box. We generated 1000 proposals with anchor scales (8, 16, 32, 64, 128) for the cell data set and 50 proposals with scales (16, 32, 64, 128, 256) for the leaf data set. The NMS threshold was set to 0.9 for both data sets.

**Stardist:** Star-convex polygons are used by [8] as a finer shape representation. Without an explicit segmentation step, the final segmentation is obtained by combining distances from center to boundary in 32 radial directions. The final step of Stardist consists of NMS to suppress overlapping polygons.

For comparability, all methods except Mask-RCNN used a simplified U-net [8] (3 pooling and 3 upsampling) as the backbone network and trained from scratch. Mask-RCNN (ResNet-101 [15] backbone) was fine-tuned on the basis of a model pretrained with the MS COCO data set[4].

## 3.3   Results and Discussion

Th Unet had the lowest mean $AP$ in Table 1. The $AP$ value decreased rapidly with increasing $IoU$ because of the false fusion of adjacent cells. Both Stardist and Mask-RCNN can handle most adjacent objects, but when a few cells form a tight roundish cluster, both methods are likely to fail. Mask-RCNN yielded the

---

[4] http://cocodataset.org/#home.

**Table 1.** Average precision $(AP)$ for different $IoU$ thresholds on the cell data set. Different $d$ for defining neighbors (Sect. 2.1) are tested (-d10, -d30 and -d100). To highlight the effect of local constraint, a 4-dimensional embedding is trained additionally.

| $IoU$ | 0.5 | 0.55 | 0.6 | 0.65 | 0.7 | 0.75 | 0.8 | 0.85 | 0.9 | Mean $AP$ |
|---|---|---|---|---|---|---|---|---|---|---|
| Unet9 | .8302 | .8152 | .7994 | .7816 | .7609 | .7206 | .6216 | .4478 | .2332 | .6678 |
| Stardist | .8178 | .8015 | .7880 | .7733 | .7552 | .7304 | .6910 | .6225 | .4749 | .7172 |
| Mask-RCNN | .8820 | .8636 | .8492 | .8354 | **.8231** | **.8030** | **.7728** | **.7095** | .5483 | **.7874** |
| ours-d10-dim16 | **.9108** | **.8858** | **.8611** | **.8428** | .7936 | .7518 | .7031 | .6466 | **.5528** | .7720 |
| ours-d30-dim16 | .9039 | .8727 | .8480 | .8169 | .7776 | .7305 | .6805 | .6272 | .5311 | .7543 |
| ours-d100-dim16 | .9007 | .8765 | .8507 | .8212 | .7812 | .7354 | .6842 | .6256 | .5190 | .7549 |
| ours-d10-dim4 | .9040 | .8786 | .8533 | .8130 | .7723 | .7203 | .6778 | .6254 | .5386 | .7537 |
| ours-d30-dim4 | .8925 | .8637 | .8339 | .8003 | .7525 | .7043 | .6624 | .6047 | .4878 | .7335 |
| ours-d100-dim4 | .6289 | .6090 | .5871 | .5567 | .5166 | .4828 | .4494 | .4082 | .3181 | .5063 |

best score in the high $IoU$ range, which is the benefit of an explicit segmentation step: masks are better aligned with the object boundary. Qualitative results in Fig. 3 show that our method is better at distinguishing objects that are in contact. This is also reflected by the highest $AP$ of our method for $IoU < 0.7$.

The leaf segmentation results better reflect the characteristics of each approach. As shown in Fig. 3, the Unet outlines the leaves accurately, but merges several instances into one (green and yellow). All other approaches proved to be object-aware. However, Mask-RCNN missed leaf B, because the bounding box of B is almost identical to that of A. Stardist avoids such false suppression by using a better shape representation, which comes at the expense of losing finer structures, such as the petioles. This is easy to understand, since Stardist obtains a mask by fitting a polygon based on discrete radial directions. In contrast, our method does not only avoids misses, but also produces a good contour.

**Local vs. Global Constraint:** To demonstrate the effect of local constraint, we tested the method with different $d$: larger $d$ treats more objects as neighbors (large enough $d$ is equivalent to the global constraint). The best result is always achieved at $d = 10$, which only takes objects in contact or almost in contact as neighbors. In the case of dimension 4, the performance drop on the cell data set is especially significant at $d = 100$ due to the inefficient use of embedding space. The same drop happens at $d = 30$ on the leaf segmentation data set.

**Incomplete Object Mask:** Inconsistent embeddings within an object (Fig. 4) sometimes occurs near the boundary, leading to incomplete segmentations. This is why our method performs not as good as Mask-RCNN in high $IoU$ range. The reason of the inconsistence deserves further study.

**Table 2.** Evaluation results on CVPPP2017 data set. See Table 2 caption for method name abbreviations.

| Metric | $SBD$ | $FBD$ | $DiC$ | $|DiC|$ |
|---|---|---|---|---|
| Unet9 | 0.5456 | 0.9045 | −3.9259 | 5.0370 |
| Stardist | 0.8019 | 0.9327 | 1.9506 | 2.6543 |
| Mask-RCNN | 0.7972 | 0.9060 | −0.1543 | 1.080 |
| ours-dist10-dim16 | **0.8307** | **0.9417** | −0.1790 | **0.7346** |
| ours-dist30-dim16 | 0.8159 | 0.9303 | −0.2160 | 0.7593 |
| ours-dist100-dim16 | 0.8101 | 0.9312 | −0.2593 | 0.9259 |
| ours-d10-dim4 | 0.8005 | 0.9377 | −0.6605 | 1.0185 |
| ours-d30-dim4 | 0.7163 | 0.3338 | −0.6358 | 0.9444 |
| ours-d100-dim4 | 0.7095 | 0.3495 | −0.5432 | 1.0741 |

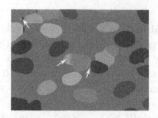

**Fig. 4.** Embeddings within the same object are not completely consistent (white arrows) in some cases. (Color figure online)

## 4    Conclusion and Outlook

Our proposed approach can not only outline objects accurately, but also is free from false object suppression and object fusion. The local constraint (orthogonality of neighboring objects) makes full use of the embedding space and gives a good geometric interpretation. Our method is especially attractive for images containing a large number of objects that are repeated and in contact and yields state-of-the-art results even with a light-weighted backbone network.

Since our approach generates embeddings that live in orthogonal spaces, if this space can be aligned with the standard space by rotating, segmentations can directly obtained from embeddings. An alternative approach to bypass postprocessing would be to add sparsity constraints on the embedding vector during training. We will test the feasibility of these two methods in the future.

## References

1. Scharr, H., et al.: Leaf segmentation in plant phenotyping: a collation study. Mach. Vis. Appl. **27**(4), 585–606 (2016)
2. Ulman, V., et al.: An objective comparison of cell-tracking algorithms. Nat. Methods **14**, 1141–1152 (2017)
3. Ronneberger, O., Fischer, P., Brox, T.: U-Net: convolutional networks for biomedical image segmentation. In: Navab, N., Hornegger, J., Wells, W.M., Frangi, A.F. (eds.) MICCAI 2015. LNCS, vol. 9351, pp. 234–241. Springer, Cham (2015). https://doi.org/10.1007/978-3-319-24574-4_28
4. Chen, H., Qi, X., Yu L., Dou, Q., Qin, J., Heng, P.A.: DCAN: deep contour-aware networks for accurate gland segmentation. In: 2016 CVPR, pp. 2487–2496 (2016)
5. Ren, S., He, K, Girshick, R., Sun, J,: Faster R-CNN: towards real-time object detection with region proposal networks. In: 28th NIPS, pp. 91–99 (2015)
6. Liu, W., et al.: SSD: single shot multibox detector. In: Leibe, B., Matas, J., Sebe, N., Welling, M. (eds.) ECCV 2016. LNCS, vol. 9905, pp. 21–37. Springer, Cham (2016). https://doi.org/10.1007/978-3-319-46448-0_2
7. He, K., Gkioxari, G., Dollár, P., Girshick, R.: Mask R-CNN. In: 2017 ICCV, pp. 2980-2988 (2017)

8. Schmidt, U., Weigert, M., Broaddus, C., Myers, G.: Cell detection with star-convex polygons. In: Frangi, A.F., Schnabel, J.A., Davatzikos, C., Alberola-López, C., Fichtinger, G. (eds.) MICCAI 2018. LNCS, vol. 11071, pp. 265–273. Springer, Cham (2018). https://doi.org/10.1007/978-3-030-00934-2_30

9. Jetley, S., Sapienza, M., Golodetz, S., Torr, P.H.: Straight to shapes: real-time detection of encoded shapes. In: 2017 CVPR, pp. 4207–4216 (2017)

10. De Brabandere, B., Neven, D., Van Gool, L.: Semantic instance segmentation with a discriminative loss function. CoRR (2017)

11. Fathi, A., et al.: Semantic instance segmentation via deep metric learning. CoRR (2017)

12. De Brabandere, B., Neven, D., Van Gool, L.: Semantic instance segmentation for autonomous driving. In: 2017 CVPR Workshop, pp. 478–480 (2017)

13. Kong, S., Fowlkes, C.C.: Recurrent pixel embedding for instance grouping. In: CVPR, pp. 9018–9028 (2018)

14. Comaniciu, D., Meer, P.: Mean shift: a robust approach toward feature space analysis. IEEE Trans. Pattern Anal. Mach. Intell. **24**(5), 603–619 (2002)

15. He, K., Zhang, X., Ren, S., Sun, J.: Deep residual learning for image recognition. In: 2016 CVPR, pp. 770–778 (2016)

# Diverse Multiple Prediction on Neuron Image Reconstruction

Ze Ye[1]($\boxtimes$), Cong Chen[2], Changhe Yuan[2], and Chao Chen[1]

[1] Stony Brook University, Stony Brook, NY 11794, USA
{ze.ye,chao.chen.1}@stonybrook.edu
[2] The City University of New York, New York, NY, USA
{cong.chen,changhe.yuan}@qc.cuny.edu

**Abstract.** Neuron reconstruction from anisotropic 3D Electron Microscopy (EM) images is a challenging problem. One often considers an input image as a stack of 2D image slices, and consider both intra and inter slice segments information. In this paper, we present a new segmentation algorithm which builds a unified energy function and jointly optimize the per-slice segmentation and the inter-slice consistency. To find an optimal solution from the huge solution space, we propose a novel diverse multiple prediction method which also encourages diversity in partial solutions. We demonstrate the strength of our method in several public datasets.

## 1  Introduction

Thanks to recent technology breakthrough, the new serial-section Electron Microscope is able to collect high resolution neuron images from insects or animals' nerve tissue. Such *neuron images* contain detailed geometric information of the densely packed neuronal structures, e.g., dendrites and axons. Reconstructing these 3D neuronal structures helps neuroscientists characterizing different types of neurons and analyzing how they collaborate to achieve different functionalities.

A majority of publicly available neuron images are *anisotropic*, i.e., having fine resolution in two spatial dimensions, but a coarse resolution in the third dimension, e.g., $4 \times 4 \times 50\,\text{nm}^3$ [1] or $3 \times 3 \times 30\,\text{nm}^3$ resolution [2]. An automatic reconstruction algorithm often considers such an anisotropic image as a stack of high-resolution 2D slices, and takes a two-stage approach. First, it partitions, or say segments, each 2D slice into regions corresponding to different neuronal structures. Second, regions of consecutive slices are linked to each other based on their geometric consistency to form 3D structures. See Fig. 1 for an illustration.

To segment each 2D slice into neuronal regions, one needs to identify the boundaries of the neurons, i.e., membranes. Different classifiers, such as random forests or Convolutional Neural Networks (CNNs), have been trained to classify each pixel as either belonging to the membranes or not [4,5,11]. While for 3D linking, one predicts the links between regions of consecutive slices based on

© Springer Nature Switzerland AG 2019
D. Shen et al. (Eds.): MICCAI 2019, LNCS 11764, pp. 460–468, 2019.
https://doi.org/10.1007/978-3-030-32239-7_51

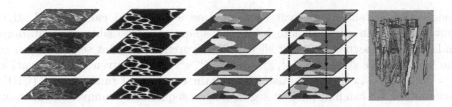

**Fig. 1.** From left to right, raw images, likelihood map, segmentation of each slices, linked segmented images, reconstructed neurons.

their geometric information. Various methods have been proposed to solve this 3D linking problem effectively [8, 9, 13].

A common issue of these existing approaches is the loose coupling of the two stages. Algorithms for the first stage only use the limited 2D observations, and thus fail to fully leverage the 3D information. In this paper, we propose a new method to jointly segment all 2D slices while considering their geometric consistency. We formulate the problem as a simple chain graphical model problem with huge state-space, i.e., all possible segmentations for each slice. To solve the problem, we progressively find segmentation candidates of each slice conditioned on those of previous slices.

At each slice, we maintain top $B$ candidate segmentations to increase the chance of finding a better solution. The huge state-space makes it challenging to find high quality solution even with top $B$ solutions per slice. We propose a novel *diverse multiple prediction* method to explore the top $B$ *diverse* solutions as candidates. Underlying the algorithm is another graphical model so that the prediction of top $B$ diverse solutions is tractable.

Instead of complicated geometric constraints [8, 9, 13], we use a computation friendly surrogate scoring function, namely, the Rand Index (RI), to model the geometric consistency between segmentations of consecutive slices. The RI effectively penalizes topological changes such as merge/split, while being robust to shifting. Thanks to the decomposability of RI, we turn each prediction step, i.e., finding the top $B$ diverse segmentations of each slice, into another Markov random field problem and thus can solve it efficiently.

In summary, our contribution is twofold.

- Propose a simple chain graphical model for the reconstruction problem. The unified principled framework is easier to tune and to generalize.
- Propose a *diverse multiple prediction* algorithm to solve the inference problem. It efficiently searches the solution space and finds a high-quality solution.

Experiments on several public datasets prove the advantage of our method. Further ablation studies show the benefits of different technical contributions.

## 2 Method

We create a unified chain graphical model to take both 2D slice information and 3D geometric consistency into consideration. Given an anisotropic neuron image with $M$ slices, we treat each slice as a node and each pair of adjacent slices as an edge. Denote by $S$ the space of all possible segmentations and $s^j \in S$ a segmentation of slice $j$. We search for a joint segmentation of the whole image stack $\mathbf{s} = (s^1, s^2, \cdots, s^{M-1}, s^M) \in S^M$ given the observation $\mathbf{x} = (x^1, x^2, \cdots, x^{M-1}, x^M)$. Using the chain conditional random field (CRF) formulation, we can find the best segmentation sequence by computing the maximum a posteriori (MAP):

$$\mathrm{argmax}_{\mathbf{s} \in S^M} P(\mathbf{s}|\mathbf{x}) = \mathrm{argmin}_{\mathbf{s} \in S^M} \exp(-E(\mathbf{s}; \mathbf{x}))/Z(x), \qquad (2.1)$$

$$E(\mathbf{s}; \mathbf{x}) = \sum_{j=1}^{M} E_j(s^j; x^j) + \sum_{j=1}^{M-1} E_{j,j+1}(s^j, s^{j+1}), \qquad (2.2)$$

where $Z(\mathbf{x}) = \sum_{\mathbf{s} \in S^M} \exp(-E(\mathbf{s}; \mathbf{x}))$ is the partition function. The energy $E(\mathbf{s}; \mathbf{x})$ is a sum of unary and binary energy terms: $E_j(s^j; x^j)$ measures how likely slice $j$ has segmentation $s^j$ given $x^j$. $E_{j,j+1}(s^j, s^{j+1})$ measures the geometric similarity between segmentations of slices $j$ and $j+1$. Note that there is no observation term in binary term since the geometric similarity is independent to observation $\mathbf{x}$. For convenience, we drop the observation term $\mathbf{x}$ or $x^j$ when referring to energy term $E_j(s^j; x^j)$ for the rest of the paper.

**Energy Terms.** We adapt the tree-structured CRF [12] to express the unary term in Eq. (2.2): $E_j(s^j) = E_j(y^j) = \sum_{(u,v) \in \mathcal{E}} \theta_{u,v}(y_u^j, y_v^j) + \sum_{u \in \mathcal{V}} \theta_u(y_u^j)$. Here $\mathcal{V}$ and $\mathcal{E}$ are the node set and edge set of a *hierarchical merging tree*, i.e., a tree constructed by running a watershed region merging algorithm over the likelihood map trained on CNNs [5]. Nodes of the tree correspond to regions in the image. Edges decide how different regions are merged into larger ones during the watershed merging process. We use $\theta$ to express the energy term of each node $u$ or edge$(u, v)$ while the value of $y$ indicates whether the corresponding node is a correct segment. See Fig. 2 for an illustration. Note each tree-structured CRF is constructed based on a given likelihood of slice $j$, while the parameters in the model is trained over all training slices. The tree-structured CRF provides an energy for each segmentation $s^j$ and is treated as the unary energy term of our overall chain CRF (Eq. (2.2)).

We use RI to represent binary term: $E_{j,j+1}(s^j, s^{j+1}) = -\eta RI(s^j, s^{j+1})$. The RI can explicitly enforce geometric consistency between two consecutive segmentations and it can be calculated very efficiently. Here the $\eta$ is the weight of the binary term (inter-slice weight) that indicates how strong the model seeks to enforce inter-slice geometry similarity.

**Inference.** Equation (2.1) has a huge solution space, $S^M$; it is exponential to the number of slices, $M$, and the space of segmentations $S$ is exponential to the size of each slice. Finding the global optimal solution from such huge solution space is infeasible. Instead, we propose an efficient prediction algorithm to find a high quality solution. We first propose to use a multiple prediction method to solve the problem (Sect. 2.1). However, during the multiple prediction, only a limited number of partial solutions are maintained. To further improve the quality of these partial solutions, and thus the final prediction, we propose a

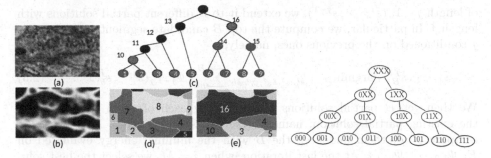

**Fig. 2.** (a) Raw image patch. (b) Membrane probability map. (c) Merging tree which black nodes are undersegment and blue nodes are oversegment. (d) Nine segments corresponded to leaf nodes. (e) Final segmentation. (Color figure online)

**Fig. 3.** A search tree for a 3-node chain graph, with each node having two possible values (0 and 1). An example beam search with $B = 2$ is highlighted with red. (Color figure online)

novel *diverse multiple prediction* method (Sect. 2.2). In each prediction step, the diverse multiple prediction finds the top solutions that are not only high in scores, but also *diverse*.

## 2.1   Prediction Algorithms

We iteratively determine the values $s^1, s^2, \cdots, s^M$. At each step, we find preferred $s^j$ given solutions of previous nodes $s^1, \cdots, s^{j-1}$. To introduce our final algorithm in the next section, we first propose a few baseline multiple prediction methods.

Rewrite Eq. (2.2) as $E(\mathbf{s}) = E_1(s^1) + \sum_{j=2}^{M} \Psi_{j-1,j}(s^{j-1}, s^j; x^j)$, where $\Psi_{j-1,j}(s^{j-1}, s^j; x^j) = E_{j-1,j}(s^{j-1}, s^j) + E_j(s^j; x^j)$. To compute the optimal segmentation $\widehat{\mathbf{s}} = (\widehat{s}^1, \cdots, \widehat{s}^M)$, a straightforward algorithm, called the *greedy search (GRE)*, starts by finding the $s^1$ optimizing $E_1$, i.e., $\widehat{s}^1 = \operatorname{argmin}_{s^1} E_1(s^1; x^1)$. Next, it iteratively finds the optimal $s^j$ conditioned on $\widehat{s}^{j-1}$ that has already been determined, i.e., $\widehat{s}^j = \operatorname{argmin}_{s^j} \Psi_{j-1,j}(\widehat{s}^{j-1}, s^j; x^j)$. Figure 3 shows a *search tree* in which each internal *search node* corresponds to a partial solution and each leaf search node corresponds to a complete solution. The greedy algorithm finds a leaf search node using a greedy method: starts from the root. At each internal search node, it finds the best child and continues, until a leaf is reached.

**Multiple Prediction.** The idea of multiple prediction is to keep track of $B > 1$ many top partial solutions until the last level. Note this is the same as the well-known beam search method. We start by finding the top $B$ solutions of $E_1(s^1; x^1)$. At the $j$-th iteration, using partial solutions from the $(j-1)$-th iteration, we find the top $B$ partial solutions with length $j$. For each partial solution of length $j - 1$, $(\widehat{s}^1, \cdots, \widehat{s}^{j-1})$, we extend it to $B$ different partial solutions with length $j$. In particular, we compute the top $B$ candidate segmentations for slice $j$ conditioned on the previous ones, namely,

$$\widehat{s}_1^j, \cdots, \widehat{s}_B^j = \text{argmin}_{s_1^j, \cdots, s_B^j : s_b^j \neq s_{b'}^j, \forall b \neq b'} \sum_{b=1}^{B} \Psi_{j-1,j}(\widehat{s}^{j-1}, s_b^j; x^j). \qquad (2.3)$$

We then get $B$ partial solutions by appending each of them to the end of the existing partial solution, namely, $\{(\widehat{s}^1, \cdots, \widehat{s}^{j-1}, \widehat{s}_b^j) \mid b = 1, \cdots, B\}$. We compare all of them and keep the $B$ with the minimal energy evaluated on $E_1, \Psi_{1,2}, \cdots, \Psi_{j-1,j}$. At the last iteration, when $j = M$, we select the best solution. Figure 3 illustrates the beam search with $B = 2$ on the search tree.

## 2.2   Diverse Multiple Prediction

Although efficient, aforementioned prediction algorithms are not necessarily optimal. As we could only keep $B$ partial solutions at each step, the multiple prediction algorithm may end up with a suboptimal solution. To address this issue, we propose to enforce that the partial solutions are not only low in energy, but also high in *diversity*. By enforcing diversity, the partial solutions have a better chance to include a high-quality one.

We propose a new method: *diverse multiple prediction*. At each iteration, instead of the top $B$ solution, we compute the top $B$ solution that are sufficiently diverse. We adapt the *m-diverse best* formulation by Batra *et al.* [3]. First, we find the best solution, then the second best which is at least $\delta$ away from the best. The $b$-th solution is the best with at least $\delta$ dissimilarity from the previously $b - 1$ chosen solutions. Using the Hamming distance measure between two segmentations $\text{dist}(\cdot, \cdot)$, the $b$-th solution is:

$$\widehat{s}_b^j = \text{argmin}_{s^j \in S} \text{cost}(s^j) \qquad \text{s.t.} \quad \text{dist}(s^j, \widehat{s}_{b'}^j) \geq \delta, \forall b' \in \{1, \cdots, b-1\} \quad (2.4)$$

Here the cost function $\text{cost}(s^j)$ is $E_1(s^1)$ when $j = 1$ and $\Psi_{j-1,j}(\widehat{s}^{j-1}, s^j)$ otherwise. The problem can be reduced into a sequence of $B$ many MAP inference tasks [3]. A hyperparameter $\lambda$ tunes the weights of diversity.

It is essential that the cost function can be written as a tractable graphical model, so that its MAP inference can be computed efficiently. Using Rand Index as binary term, we can rewrite the cost function $\Psi_{j-1,j}$ as a tree-structured graphical model energy. Therefore, the m-diverse-best solutions can be solved efficiently. For convenience, we denote by the top $B$ diverse solution as $\text{mdiv}(E_1; x^j)$ or $\text{mdiv}(\Psi_{j-1,j}; x^j, \widehat{s}^{j-1})$ depending on the relevant energy term. The pseudocode of our diverse multiple prediction algorithm is given in Algorithm 1.

## 3   Experiments

In this section, we validate our proposed method using public datasets. We also use ablation study to closely inspect the behavior of our prediction method.

---

**Algorithm 1.** Diverse Multiple Prediction

---

**Require:** Input image $\mathbf{x}$
**Ensure:** Segmentation $\mathbf{s}$
1: $(\widehat{s}_1^1, \cdots, \widehat{s}_B^1) \leftarrow \text{mdiv}(E_1; x^j)$        ▷ The top $B$ diverse solutions for slice # 1.
2: $S \leftarrow \{(\widehat{s}_1^1), \cdots, (\widehat{s}_B^1)\}$        ▷ The top $B$ partial solutions with length 1.
3: **for** $j = 2$ **to** $M$ **do**
4:      $S' \leftarrow \emptyset$
5:      **for** $(\widehat{s}^1, \cdots, \widehat{s}^{j-1}) \in S$ **do**
6:          $(\widehat{s}_1^j, \cdots, \widehat{s}_B^j) \leftarrow \text{mdiv}(\Psi_{j-1,j}; x^j, \widehat{s}^{j-1})$     ▷ For each length $j-1$ partial solution in $S$, compute the top $B$ diverse solution conditioned on $\widehat{s}^{j-1}$ and $x^j$.
7:          **for** $b = 1$ **to** $B$ **do**
8:             $S' \leftarrow S' \cup \{(\widehat{s}^1, \cdots, \widehat{s}^{j-1}, \widehat{s}_b^j)\}$ ▷ Add $B$ length $j$ partial solutions into $S'$.
9:          **end for**
10:      **end for**
11:      Resize $S'$. Only keep top $B$ partial solutions in $S'$ with the minimal partial energy $E_1(\widehat{s}^1; x^1) + \sum_{j'=2}^{j} \Psi(\widehat{s}^{j'-1}, \widehat{s}^{j'}; x^{j'})$.
12:      $S \leftarrow S'$
13: **end for**
14: **return** The solution $\widehat{\mathbf{s}} \in S$ with the minimal energy $E(\mathbf{s}; \mathbf{x})$.

---

**Datasets.** We use two public datasets: the Drosophila first instar larva ventral nerve cord (VNC) [1] and mouse cortex (MOU) [2]. Both datasets were used as public challenges. So their test sets do not have ground truth annotation. We use their training sets for evaluation. VNC contains 30 consecutive slices for training, each of size $512 \times 512$. The resolution is $4 \times 4 \times 50 \, \text{nm}^3$. We use a three-fold cross validation and report the mean performance over the validation sets. Due to the nature of the problem, the validation set needs to be consecutive slices rather than random slices. For fold 1, we use slices 1–10 for validation and 11–30 for training. Similarly, for folds 2 and 3, we use 11–20 and 21–30 to validate, respectively. MOU has 100 consecutive training slices, each with size $1024 \times 1024$ (resolution $3 \times 3 \times 30 \, \text{nm}^3$). We use a three-fold cross validation and report the mean performance, using slices 1–33, 34–66, and 67–100 as validation sets, respectively.

**Table 1.** ARE of all methods on the two datasets.

|         | DMP        | MP     | GRE    | CRF    | LIU    |
|---------|------------|--------|--------|--------|--------|
| VNC     | **0.0172** | 0.0191 | 0.0197 | 0.0235 | 0.0244 |
| MOU     | **0.0271** | 0.0275 | 0.0279 | 0.037  | 0.0375 |
| MOU-3D  | **0.0863** | 0.0894 | 0.090  | 0.1147 | 0.1151 |

**Baselines.** We compare our method, diverse multiple prediction (DMP), with two state-of-the-arts. LIU [10] prunes the hierarchical merging tree in a greedy manner. CRF [12] constructs and trains tree-structured CRF on hierarchical merging trees, but ignores inter-slice geometric constraints. We also compare with two baselines that have been introduced in this paper: greedy search (GRE) and multiple prediction (MP). Note we focus on the segmentation task, so we do not compare with various methods on computing better boundary likelihood maps [4–7]. Instead, we assume a same boundary likelihood map for all methods. We use the boundary likelihood map from [4] for VNC, and the one from [5] for MOU. The hyperparameters of all methods are fine-tuned to ensure fairness.

For our own method, we choose the inter-slice weight $\eta = 600$ and set the upper bound of solution candidate $B = 6$. For diverse multiple prediction method, we set the diversity weight $\lambda = 0.1$.

**Experiment Setting.** All compared methods output joint segmentations of all slices. We directly evaluate the performance by comparing the 2D segmentation with ground truth annotation over all slices and aggregate. The goal is to show that using inter-slice geometric consistency and advanced search strategy, we can improve the per-slice segmentation quality. We report the results on both VNC and MOU. Furthermore, since the segmentations can be linked together to reconstruct the 3D neurons (Fig. 1), we may evaluate all the methods by applying a common 3D linking tool [9] and compare the 3D reconstruction results. We report the results only on MOU (called MOU-3D), as such 3D reconstruction ground truth annotation is not available for VNC.

We measure the performance using the standard Adaptive Rand Error (ARE) score, which ranges between 0 and 1 (the smaller the better). [1] The results of all methods over VNC, MOU, and MOU 3D linking are reported in Table 1. A qualitative example is also shown in Fig. 4. Highlighted areas are where the difference occurs. We observe that MP improves upon GRE, while DMP achieves even better results.

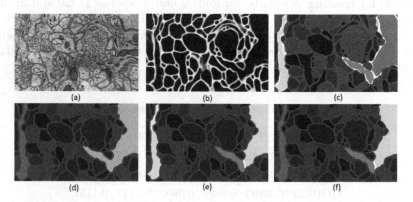

**Fig. 4.** (a) Raw image. (b) Membrane probability map. (c) Ground truth. (d) GRE. (e) MP. (f) DMP.

---

[1] ARE is closely related to Rand index but is the corrected-for-chance version, and thus is not decomposable like RI.

**Ablation Study.** To further investigate the behavior of our method, we carry out the ablation study on three hyperparameters: number of partial solutions to memorize $B$, inter-slice energy weight $\eta$, and diversity weight $\lambda$ on VNC dataset [1]. Figure 5(a) shows the ARE scores of three proposed methods with regard to the $B$ values. Note that all three methods are equivalent when $B = 1$. DMP converges to the best score even with a small $B$. MP needs a larger $B = 6$.

The second parameter we study is the inter-slice weight $\eta$. Figure 5(b) shows those three ARE scores with $\eta$ ranged from 0 to 1200. Note that all three methods are equivalent to CRF when $\eta = 0$ since inter-slice consistency is no longer in effect and three methods eventually generate local best solution in each slice.

The last parameter is $\lambda$ which measures the diversity in our diverse multiple prediction method. Figure 5(c) shows the performance of our method (DMP) with regard to $\lambda$.

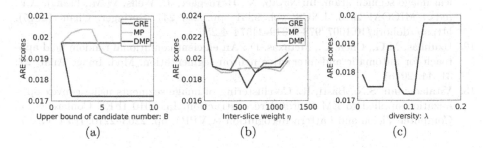

**Fig. 5.** Ablation study on three parameters: $B$, $\eta$ and $\lambda$.

**Acknowledgements.** This work was partially supported by NSF IIS-1855759, CCF-1855760 and IIS-1829560.

# References

1. Arganda-Carreras, I., Seung, H., Cardona, A., Schindelin, J.: Segmentation of neuronal structures in EM stacks challenge–ISBI 2012 (2012)
2. Arganda-Carreras, I., Seung, H., Vishwanathan, A., Berger, D.: 3D segmentation of neurites in EM images challenge-ISBI 2013 (2013)
3. Batra, D., Yadollahpour, P., Guzman-Rivera, A., Shakhnarovich, G.: Diverse M-best solutions in Markov random fields. In: Fitzgibbon, A., Lazebnik, S., Perona, P., Sato, Y., Schmid, C. (eds.) ECCV 2012. LNCS, vol. 7576, pp. 1–16. Springer, Heidelberg (2012). https://doi.org/10.1007/978-3-642-33715-4_1
4. Ciresan, D., Giusti, A., Gambardella, L.M., Schmidhuber, J.: Deep neural networks segment neuronal membranes in electron microscopy images. In: Advances in Neural Information Processing Systems, pp. 2843–2851 (2012)
5. Fakhry, A., Peng, H., Ji, S.: Deep models for brain em image segmentation: novel insights and improved performance. Bioinformatics **32**(15), 2352–2358 (2016)
6. Fakhry, A., Zeng, T., Ji, S.: Residual deconvolutional networks for brain electron microscopy image segmentation. IEEE Trans. Med. Imaging **36**(2), 447–456 (2017)

7. Funke, J., et al.: Large scale image segmentation with structured loss based deep learning for connectome reconstruction. IEEE Trans. Pattern Anal. Mach. Intell. **41**, 1669–1680 (2018)
8. Kaynig, V., Fuchs, T.J., Buhmann, J.M.: Geometrical consistent 3D tracing of neuronal processes in ssTEM data. In: Jiang, T., Navab, N., Pluim, J.P.W., Viergever, M.A. (eds.) MICCAI 2010. LNCS, vol. 6362, pp. 209–216. Springer, Heidelberg (2010). https://doi.org/10.1007/978-3-642-15745-5_26
9. Liu, T., Jones, C., Seyedhosseini, M., Tasdizen, T.: A modular hierarchical approach to 3D electron microscopy image segmentation. J. Neurosci. Methods **226**, 88–102 (2014)
10. Liu, T., Seyedhosseini, M., Ellisman, M., Tasdizen, T.: Watershed merge forest classification for electron microscopy image stack segmentation. In: Proceedings/IEEE International Conference on Computer Vision. IEEE International Conference on Computer Vision, vol. 2013, p. 4069. NIH Public Access (2013)
11. Ronneberger, O., Fischer, P., Brox, T.: U-Net: convolutional networks for biomedical image segmentation. In: Navab, N., Hornegger, J., Wells, W.M., Frangi, A.F. (eds.) MICCAI 2015. LNCS, vol. 9351, pp. 234–241. Springer, Cham (2015). https://doi.org/10.1007/978-3-319-24574-4_28
12. Uzunbas, M.G., Chen, C., Metaxas, D.: An efficient conditional random field approach for automatic and interactive neuron segmentation. Med. Image Anal. **27**, 31–44 (2016)
13. Vitaladevuni, S.N., Basri, R.: Co-clustering of image segments using convex optimization applied to EM neuronal reconstruction. In: 2010 IEEE Conference on Computer Vision and Pattern Recognition (CVPR), pp. 2203–2210. IEEE (2010)

# Deep Segmentation-Emendation Model for Gland Instance Segmentation

Yutong Xie[1], Hao Lu[2], Jianpeng Zhang[1], Chunhua Shen[2], and Yong Xia[1,3(✉)]

[1] National Engineering Laboratory for Integrated Aero-Space-Ground-Ocean
Big Data Application Technology, School of Computer Science and Engineering,
Northwestern Polytechnical University, Xi'an 710072, China
yxia@nwpu.edu.cn
[2] School of Computer Science, University of Adelaide,
Adelaide, SA 5005, Australia
[3] Research & Development Institute of Northwestern Polytechnical University
in Shenzhen, Shenzhen 518057, China

**Abstract.** Accurate and automated gland instance segmentation on histology microscopy images can assist pathologists to diagnose the malignancy degree of colorectal adenocarcinoma. To address this problem, many deep convolutional neural network (DCNN) based methods have been proposed, most of which aim to generate better segmentation by improving the model structure and loss function. Few of them, however, focus on further emendating the inferred predictions, thus missing a chance to refine the obtained segmentation results. In this paper, we propose the deep segmentation-emendation (DSE) model for gland instance segmentation. This model consists of a segmentation network (Seg-Net) and an emendation network (Eme-Net). The Seg-Net is dedicated to generating segmentation results, and the Eme-Net learns to predict the inconsistency between the ground truth and the segmentation results generated by Seg-Net. The predictions made by Eme-Net can in turn be used to refine the segmentation result. We evaluated our DSE model against five recent deep learning models on the 2015 MICCAI Gland Segmentation challenge (GlaS) dataset and against two deep learning models on the colorectal adenocarcinoma (CRAG) dataset. Our results indicate that using Eme-Net results in significant improvement in segmentation accuracy, and the proposed DSE model is able to substantially outperform all the rest models in gland instance segmentation on both datasets.

## 1 Introduction

Colorectal adenocarcinoma is one of the most common cancers in the world [1]. Accurate segmentation of the gland instances on histology images is an effective means to assess the gland morphology, which is essential for pathologists to determine the malignancy degree of colorectal adenocarcinoma [2,3]. Manual annotation of gland instances, however, requires a high degree of concentration and

© Springer Nature Switzerland AG 2019
D. Shen et al. (Eds.): MICCAI 2019, LNCS 11764, pp. 469–477, 2019.
https://doi.org/10.1007/978-3-030-32239-7_52

expertise and is time-consuming due to the myriad size of histology images [4]. Therefore, automated gland instance segmentation is of crucial importance in clinical practice to improve the efficiency as well as objectivity and to reduce the workload of pathologists. The automation of this task is challenging since (1) the heterogeneous glandular morphology between benign and malignant makes it difficult to delineate the glands from the background, and (2) the tiny gaps between adjacent glands render more difficulties in separating each gland from others. Two examples that illustrate both issues are displayed in Fig. 1.

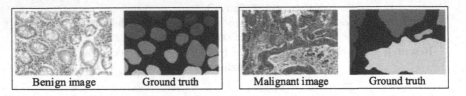

**Fig. 1.** Two examples of gland instance segmentation in benign and malignant cases. Individual glands are denoted by different colors. (Color figure online)

Recently, deep convolutional neural networks (DCNNs) have achieved remarkable success in image segmentation [2,4–7], which inspires many researchers to apply DCNNs to gland instance segmentation. Chen *et al.* [5] proposed a multi-task deep neural network that employs multi-level contextual features to separate the glands from the background and also explores the contour information to delineate individual glands. Grahama *et al.* [2] presented a minimal information loss dilated network to retain maximum information during feature extraction, aiming to improve the segmentation of individual glands. Xu *et al.* [6] developed a deep multi-channel network that uses three channels to learn gland regions, contours, and location cues, respectively, to segment the glands and separate individual ones. Yan *et al.* [4] proposed a shape-preserving loss to learn gland segmentation and contour detection simultaneously. These methods aim to generate better predictions through improving the segmentation model, such as designing advanced network architectures, defining novel losses, and supplementing additional contour detection modules. Different from these attempts, we focus on refining the inferred segmentation results (i.e. emendating the under-segmentation or over-segmentation regions), which is beneficial to further improve the segmentation of gland instances.

In this paper, we propose a deep segmentation-emendation (DSE) model for the gland instance segmentation on histology images. This model is composed of two networks: a segmentation network (Seg-Net) and an emendation network (Eme-Net). The Seg-Net predicts the segmentation mask (MaskSeg) of an input image, and the Eme-Net learns an emendation mask (MaskEme) that represents the inconsistency between the predicted MaskSeg and the corresponding ground truth. In the inference stage, each test image is fed to both trained Seg-Net and Eme-Net, and the predicted MaskEme is used to emendate the predicted

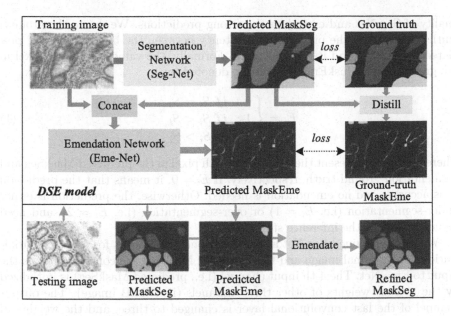

**Fig. 2.** The technical pipeline of our proposed DSE model.

MaskSeg for an improved segmentation performance. We evaluated the proposed DSE model against several existing approaches on two benchmark datasets.

The contributions of this work include: (1) supplemented the Seg-Net with the Eme-Net, which is able to predict the over- and under-segmentation resulted from the Seg-Net; (2) employed such predictions to emendate the segmentation results produced by the Seg-Net; and (3) reported the state-of-the-art gland instance segmentation performance on two benchmark datasets.

## 2   Method

The pipeline of our DSE model consists of offline training of both Seg-Net and Eme-Net and online inference, in which the predicted MaskEme is employed to emendate the MaskSeg predicted by Seg-Net for refinement (see Fig. 2).

**Segmentation Network:** We employ the advanced semantic segmentation network Deeplabv3+ [8] pre-trained on MS-COCO [9] and PASCAL VOC 2012 datasets [10], as the backbone of Seg-Net. To adapt Deeplabv3+ to our segmentation task, we remove its last convolutional layer, and then add a new convolutional layer with two output channels and a softmax layer for prediction. The weights attached to new layers are randomly initialized. We optimize the Seg-Net by minimizing the cross-entropy loss.

**Emendation Network:** To further improve the quality of the inferred MaskSeg, we design the Eme-Net that learns a MaskEme to estimate the segmentation quality of Seg-Net and emendate the wrong predictions. We define the ground-truth MaskEme as the pixel-wise consistency between the binary MaskSeg predicted by Seg-Net and its ground truth. Formally, the value of the $i$-th pixel in the ground-truth MaskEme, $\hat{E}_i$, can be denoted by:

$$\hat{E}_i = \begin{cases} 0 & if \ S_i = \hat{S}_i \\ 1 & if \ S_i < \hat{S}_i \\ 2 & if \ S_i > \hat{S}_i \end{cases} \tag{1}$$

where $S_i$ and $\hat{S}_i$ represent the value of the $i$-th pixel in the predicted MaskSeg and segmentation ground truth, respectively. If $\hat{E}_i = 0$, it means that the prediction $S_i$ is accurate and no emendation is needed. Otherwise, the prediction is either under-segmentation (i.e. $\hat{E}_i = 1$) or over-segmentation (i.e. $\hat{E}_i = 2$), and need be emendated in the inference stage.

We use the trained Seg-Net as the backbone of Eme-Net for a better initialization. The original image and the predicted MaskSeg are concatenated as the input to Eme-Net. The 4-th input channel (i.e., predicted MaskSeg) is initialized by the average weights of other three channels (i.e., RGB image). The output channel of the last convolutional layer is changed to three, and the weights of the modified convolutional layer are randomly initialized.

Different from training Seg-Net, training Eme-Net suffers from extremely severe class-imbalance, since the number of pixels with a value of 1 or 2 accounts for only about 1% of the pixels with a value of 0 in each ground-truth MaskEme. To address this issue, we jointly optimize the weighted multi-class Dice loss and the cross-entropy (ce) loss during the process of training Eme-Net. The combined loss can be expressed as:

$$\mathcal{L} = \mathcal{L}_{Dice} + \mathcal{L}_{ce} = \frac{1}{C} \sum_{c=1}^{C} \omega_c \left[ 1 - \frac{2 \sum_{i=1}^{V} \hat{E}_i^c E_i^c}{\sum_{i=1}^{V} (\hat{E}_i^c + E_i^c) + \varepsilon} \right] - \frac{1}{V} \sum_{v=1}^{V} \sum_{c=1}^{C} \omega_c \hat{E}_i^c log E_i^c \tag{2}$$

where $C$ is the number of categories, $V$ denotes the number of pixels, $E_i^c$ indicates the prediction of $i$-th pixel belonging to the class $c$, $\hat{E}_i^c$ represents the target value of $i$-th pixel in the MaskEme, $\varepsilon$ is a smoothing factor, and $\omega_c$ is the weight of the class $c$. The weight $\omega_c$ can be formulated as $\omega_c = log \frac{V}{V^c}$, where $V^c$ denotes the number of pixels belonging to the class $c$.

**Inference Process:** The predicted MaskEme can be used to emendate the wrong predictions (i.e. the over- and under-segmentation regions) inferred by the Seg-Net in inference stage for refinement. The value of $i$-th pixel for the refined MaskSeg $S_i'$ can be formulated as:

$$S_i' = \begin{cases} S_i & if \ E_i = 0 \\ 1 & if \ E_i = 1 \\ 0 & if \ E_i = 2 \end{cases} \tag{3}$$

where $S_i$ and $E_i$ represent the value of $i$-th pixel of the predicted MaskSeg and MaskEme, respectively. If $E_i = 1$, we emendate the prediction $S_i$ as the gland class $\{1\}$. If $E_i = 2$, we emendate the prediction $S_i$ as the background class $\{0\}$.

## 3   Datasets

We evaluated the proposed DSE model on two benchmark datasets: the 2015 MICCAI Gland Segmentation (GlaS) Challenge dataset [11] and the colorectal adenocarcinoma gland (CRAG) dataset [2,12]. The GlaS dataset contains 85 training and 80 test images (60 in Part A and 20 in Part B). The image size ranges from $567 \times 430$ to $775 \times 522$. The CRAG dataset has 173 training and 40 test images, mostly having a size of $1512 \times 1516$. All training images in both datasets are equipped with the ground-truth masks for instance segmentation, which were manually annotated by pathologists.

## 4   Experiments and Results

**Implementation Details:** During training, we randomly cropped patches from each training image as the input of both Seg-Net and Eme-Net to not only reserve as much information as possible but also weigh the balance of segmentation performance and computational cost. The patch size was set to $416 \times 416$ on the GlaS dataset and $512 \times 512$ on the CRAG dataset. To alleviate the overfitting of deep neural networks, we employed the online data argumentation techniques, including random rotation, shear, shift, zoom of width and height, whitening, horizontal and vertical flips, and color normalization, to enlarge the training set. We optimized both networks using the standard SGD with a batch size of 4, an initial learning rate of 0.001, and the maximum epoch of 1000, and also set 20% of the training set aside to monitor the performance of both networks. In the inference stage, we extracted patches of the same size from each test image with a stride of 256 pixels. The final segmentation of a whole image is generated by recomposing and averaging the predictions of those patches.

**Evaluation Metrics:** We evaluated the segmentation results using three metrics provided by the GlaS Challenge[1], including (1) accuracy of the detection of individual glands (Object F1 Score), (2) volume-based accuracy of the segmentation of individual glands (Object Dice), and (3) shape similarity between the segmentation result and its ground truth (Object Hausdorff Distance). For the overall results, each method will be assigned three ranking numbers based on the three metrics. The sum of these numbers will be used for the final ranking.

**Results on the GlaS Challenge Dataset:** We compared the proposed DSE model against the minimal information loss dilated network (MILD-Net) [2], the deep network with shape-preserving loss (SPL-Net) [4], the deep multi-channel network (DMCN) [6], the deep contour-aware network (DCAN) [5], and the

---

[1] https://warwick.ac.uk/fac/sci/dcs/research/tia/glascontest/.

**Table 1.** Comparison with five methods on the GlaS Challenge dataset. S and R denote score and rank, respectively

| Methods | Object F1 | | | | Object Dice | | | | Object Hausdorff | | | | Rank sum |
|---|---|---|---|---|---|---|---|---|---|---|---|---|---|
| | Part A | | Part B | | Part A | | Part B | | Part A | | Part B | | |
| | S | R | S | R | S | R | S | R | S | R | S | R | |
| DSE model (Ours) | 0.926 | 1 | 0.862 | 1 | 0.927 | 1 | 0.871 | 1 | 31.209 | 1 | 80.509 | 1 | 6 |
| MILD-Net [2] | 0.914 | 3 | 0.844 | 2 | 0.913 | 2 | 0.836 | 3 | 41.540 | 2 | 105.890 | 2 | 14 |
| SPL-Net [4] | 0.924 | 2 | 0.844 | 2 | 0.902 | 4 | 0.840 | 2 | 49.881 | 5 | 106.075 | 3 | 18 |
| DMCN [6] | 0.893 | 5 | 0.843 | 4 | 0.908 | 3 | 0.833 | 4 | 44.129 | 3 | 116.821 | 4 | 23 |
| DCAN [5] | 0.912 | 4 | 0.716 | 5 | 0.897 | 5 | 0.781 | 6 | 45.418 | 4 | 160.347 | 6 | 30 |
| MPCNN [11] | 0.891 | 6 | 0.703 | 6 | 0.882 | 6 | 0.786 | 5 | 57.413 | 6 | 145.575 | 5 | 34 |

**Table 2.** Comparison with two methods on the CRAG dataset.

| Methods | Object F1 | | Object Dice | | Object Hausdorff | | Rank sum |
|---|---|---|---|---|---|---|---|
| | S | R | S | R | S | R | |
| DSE model (Ours) | 0.835 | 1 | 0.889 | 1 | 120.127 | 1 | 3 |
| MILD-Net [2] | 0.825 | 2 | 0.875 | 2 | 160.140 | 2 | 6 |
| DCAN [5] | 0.736 | 3 | 0.794 | 3 | 218.76 | 3 | 9 |

**Table 3.** Performance of the Seg-Net and our DSE model on two datasets.

| Datasets | Method | Object F1 | Object Dice | Object Hausdorff |
|---|---|---|---|---|
| GlaS Part A | Seg-Net | 0.888 | 0.908 | 41.009 |
| | DSE model | 0.926 | 0.927 | 31.209 |
| GlaS Part B | Seg-Net | 0.827 | 0.855 | 89.090 |
| | DSE model | 0.862 | 0.871 | 80.509 |
| CRAG | Seg-Net | 0.774 | 0.850 | 155.430 |
| | DSE model | 0.835 | 0.889 | 120.127 |

multi-path convolutional neural network (MPCNN) [11] on the GlaS dataset. The obtained average performance of these models was listed in Table 1. It shows that our DSE model achieves the highest accuracy in terms of all performance metrics on both parts of testing data. Specifically, our model improves the Object F1 by 0.2%, Object Dice by 1.4%, and Object Hausdorff Distance by 10.331 over the second best performance on the Part A of testing data. The results on the Part B are generally lower than that on Part A, since Part B contains a majority of malignant images with more complex morphology that increases the difficulty of gland instance segmentation. Nevertheless, our model exhibits an even more obvious performance improvement on the Part B (i.e. 1.8% in Object F1, 3.1% in Object Dice, and 25.381 in Object Hausdorff Distance) than on Part A. It evidences that our model can improve the accuracy of gland instance segmentation and shape detection on both easy and difficult cases.

**Results on the CRAG Dataset:** We also evaluated the proposed DSE model against MILD-Net [2] and DCAN [5] methods on the CRAG dataset. The obtained average performance in Table 2 reveals that our DSE model consistently surpasses other two methods by large margins over all metrics, which is in line with the conclusion we drew on the GlaS dataset. The superior performance on both datasets also suggests that our model is robust to handle different datasets.

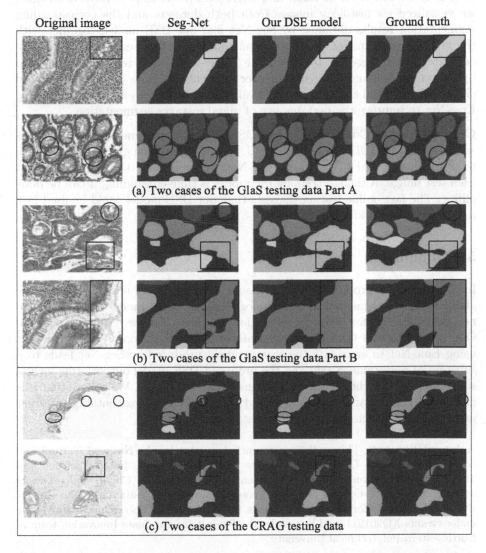

Original image    Seg-Net    Our DSE model    Ground truth

(a) Two cases of the GlaS testing data Part A

(b) Two cases of the GlaS testing data Part B

(c) Two cases of the CRAG testing data

**Fig. 3.** Visualization of gland segmentation results of six cases selected from the GlaS and CRAG datasets. Multiple gland instances are highlighted by different colors. (Color figure online)

**Ablation Study:** The major uniqueness of our DSE model is to use the newly designed Eme-Net to emendate the wrong predictions made by Seg-Net. To validate the performance improvement resulted from Eme-Net, we compared our model to Seg-Net, which does not use Eme-Net for emendation, on both GlaS and CRAG datasets. The average performance of both models was shown in Table 3. It reveals that using Eme-Net to emendate the segmentation results produced by Seg-Net improves substantially the Object Dice by 1.9%, 1.6%, and 3.9% on the Part A of GlaS, Part B of GlaS, and CRAG datasets, respectively. Meanwhile, we visualized six histology images from both datasets and the corresponding segmentation results obtained by Seg-Net and our DSE model, together with the ground truth, in Fig. 3. It shows that our model can segment glands more accurately than Seg-Net, by filling the under-segmented regions (highlighted by red rectangles) and removing the over-segmented regions (highlighted by red circles). Both visual and quantitative evaluation proves the effectiveness of using Eme-Net to improve the performance of gland instance segmentation.

**Computational Complexity:** The DSE model was trained using the Keras software on a NVIDIA Tesla P100 GPU. In our experiments, it took about 12 h to train Seg-Net and 24 h to train Eme-Net, and cost only 0.5 to 2 s to segment each test image. Although training the model is time-consuming, it can be done offline. The fast online testing suggests that our DSE model could be used in a routine clinical workflow.

## 5    Conclusion

In this paper, we proposed the DSE model, a segment-and-refine paradigm, for gland instance segmentation on histology images. This model consists of two networks: Seg-Net for image segmentation and Eme-Net for result emendation. Our results on the GlaS Challenge dataset and CRAG dataset suggest that using Eme-Net to emendate the segmentation produced by Seg-Net leads to a substantial performance gain and the proposed DSE model outperforms several state-of-the-art methods by large margins on both datasets. We believe that this method is general and can be extended to the instance segmentation of other medical images, such as nuclear segmentation.

**Acknowledgment.** This work was supported in part by the National Natural Science Foundation of China under Grants 61771397, in part by the Science and Technology Innovation Committee of Shenzhen Municipality, China, under Grants JCYJ20180306171334997, in part by Synergy Innovation Foundation of the University and Enterprise for Graduate Students in Northwestern Polytechnical University under Grants XQ201911, and in part by the Project for Graduate Innovation team of Northwestern Polytechnical University.

# References

1. Fleming, M., Ravula, S., Tatishchev, S.F., Wang, H.L.: Colorectal carcinoma: pathologic aspects. J. Gastrointest. Oncol. **3**(3), 153 (2012)
2. Graham, S., et al.: MILD-Net: minimal information loss dilated network for gland instance segmentation in colon histology images. Med. Image Anal. **52**, 199–211 (2019)
3. Washington, M.K., et al.: Protocol for the examination of specimens from patients with primary carcinoma of the colon and rectum. Archiv. Pathol. Lab. Med. **133**(10), 1539–1551 (2009)
4. Yan, Z., Yang, X., Cheng, K.-T.T.: A deep model with shape-preserving loss for gland instance segmentation. In: Frangi, A.F., Schnabel, J.A., Davatzikos, C., Alberola-López, C., Fichtinger, G. (eds.) MICCAI 2018. LNCS, vol. 11071, pp. 138–146. Springer, Cham (2018). https://doi.org/10.1007/978-3-030-00934-2_16
5. Chen, H., Qi, X., Yu, L., Heng, P.A.: DCAN: deep contour-aware networks for accurate gland segmentation. In: CVPR, pp. 2487–2496 (2016)
6. Xu, Y., et al.: Gland instance segmentation using deep multichannel neural networks. IEEE Trans. Biomed. Eng. **64**(12), 2901–2912 (2017)
7. Chen, Z., Zhang, J., Tao, D.: Progressive lidar adaptation for road detection. IEEE/CAA J. Automatica Sinica **6**(3), 693–702 (2019)
8. Chen, L.C., Zhu, Y., Papandreou, G., Schroff, F., Adam, H.: Encoder-decoder with atrous separable convolution for semantic image segmentation. In: ECCV (2018)
9. Lin, T.Y., et al.: Microsoft COCO: common objects in context. In: Fleet, D., Pajdla, T., Schiele, B., Tuytelaars, T. (eds.) ECCV 2014. LNCS, vol. 8693, pp. 740–755. Springer, Cham (2014). https://doi.org/10.1007/978-3-319-10602-1_48
10. Everingham, M., Van Gool, L., Williams, C.K., Winn, J., Zisserman, A.: The pascal visual object classes (VOC) challenge. Int. J. Comput. Vis. **88**(2), 303–338 (2010)
11. Sirinukunwattana, K., et al.: Gland segmentation in colon histology images: the glas challenge contest. Med. Image Anal. **35**, 489–502 (2017)
12. Awan, R., et al.: Glandular morphometrics for objective grading of colorectal adenocarcinoma histology images. Sci. Rep. **7**(1), 16852 (2017)

# Fast and Accurate Electron Microscopy Image Registration with 3D Convolution

Shenglong Zhou, Zhiwei Xiong$^{(\boxtimes)}$, Chang Chen, Xuejin Chen, Dong Liu,
Yueyi Zhang, Zheng-Jun Zha, and Feng Wu

University of Science and Technology of China, Hefei, China
zwxiong@ustc.edu.cn

**Abstract.** We propose an unsupervised deep learning method for serial electron microscopy (EM) image registration with fast speed and high accuracy. Current registration methods are time consuming in practice due to the iterative optimization procedure. We model the registration process as a parametric function in the form of convolutional neural networks, and optimize its parameters based on features extracted from training serial EM images in a training set. Given a new series of EM images, the deformation field of each serial image can be rapidly generated through the learned function. Specifically, we adopt a spatial transformer layer to reconstruct features in the subject image from the reference ones while constraining smoothness on the deformation field. Moreover, for the first time, we introduce the 3D convolution layer to learn the relationship between several adjacent images, which effectively reduces error accumulation in serial EM image registration. Experiments on two popular EM datasets, Cremi and FIB25, demonstrate our method can operate in an unprecedented speed while providing competitive registration accuracy compared with state-of-the-art methods, including learning-based ones.

**Keywords:** Unsupervised learning · Serial-section EM · Image registration · 3D convolution

## 1 Introduction

Electron microscopy (EM) at nanometer resolution plays an important role in biomedical science, which is usually adopted to resolve tiny structures for various analysis purposes, e.g., neuron reconstruction [5,8]. Typically, a standard pipeline to obtain large-scale EM data is embedding specimen into a block of solid medium, cutting it into a series of sections, and then staining and imaging sections individually. Serial section scanning avoids the penetration problem during staining and imaging, but introduces non-linear deformation between adjacent sections at the same time, such as tissue shrinkage, compression, or expansion. To reconstruct the 3D volume, serial EM images need to be aligned, but artifacts caused by deformation could affect the subsequent analysis seriously if not properly handled. Therefore, serial EM image registration is necessary to alleviate

© Springer Nature Switzerland AG 2019
D. Shen et al. (Eds.): MICCAI 2019, LNCS 11764, pp. 478–486, 2019.
https://doi.org/10.1007/978-3-030-32239-7_53

the deformation artifacts and reproduce the 3D volume as close as possible to the original specimen.

Although there has been tremendous advancement in medical image registration [2] as well as optical flow estimation [4], serial EM image registration still remains challenging. Different from videos and common medical images such as 3D MRI data, EM data has not only complicated tissue deformation but also obvious drifting for long image series. Moreover, each image in a serial has individual content, especially due to the fact that the axis resolution is usually much lower than the lateral resolution during imaging. Therefore, simply warping one image to another by aggressively maximizing pixel-wise correlation, as performed in common registration methods, would restrict each image to be exactly identical and thus degrade the fidelity of registration.

Traditional EM registration methods intend to address the challenging deformation using elaborate regularization. Arganda-Carreras et al. [1] added a consistency term on the basis of a standard registration method to generate the elastic deformation field suitable for each image pair. However, this method does not consider more adjacent sections so it is sensitive to error accumulation. Saalfeld et al. [9] applied a global elastic constraint with more adjacent sections to reconstruct the continuous 3D volume, avoiding error accumulation to a large extent. However, it is time consuming for large-scale data due to its high complexity of optimization. Moreover, these two methods need complicated parameter tuning which is undesirable in practical applications. Recently, learning-based methods appeared to handle EM registration. Yoo et al. [11] proposed a combination of a spatial transformer network [7] and an autoencoder [6] that generated a deformation field for entire image registration. Instead of using previous constraint terms, this method involved a feature-based image similarity measure and used the back-propagation algorithm to finetune the deformation field automatically. The latter operation reduces the burden of parameter tuning. Nevertheless, this learning-based method is still slow due to its iterative optimization for each independent image pair. For example, it would take 26 h to align a 3D volume sized $520 \times 520 \times 520$. This speed is unacceptable if we want to deal with even larger scale EM data.

In this paper, we propose an unsupervised deep learning method for serial EM image registration, which models the registration process as a parametric function based on feature-level similarity. Rather than imposing a computational intensive optimization as in previous methods, we learn a global optimization function during the training phase instead. Then EM registration can be achieved rapidly through inference of the learned function when unseen serial EM images are given during the testing phase. This registration function is realized using convolutional neural networks (CNNs), which takes serial EM images as input and outputs a deformation field between them. Meanwhile, we use a pre-trained autoencoder to extract high-level features from each image as the similarity measure, which gets rid of pixel-wise correlation and ensures the independence of image content. More importantly, to alleviate the error accumulation problem, we introduce the 3D convolution for the first time to learn the relationship

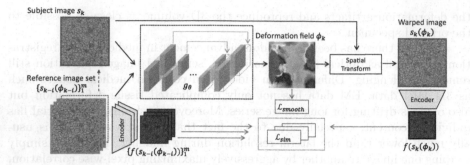

**Fig. 1.** Framework of our method. We learn parameters for the function $g_\theta$ composed of a 3D CNN that registers the subject image $s_k$ to a reference image set $\{s_{k-i}(\phi_{k-i})\}_1^m$. During training, we warp $s_k$ with $\phi_k$ using a spatial transformer layer. The loss function compares $s_k(\phi_k)$ and $\{s_{k-i}(\phi_{k-i})\}_1^m$ based on high-level features $f$ from a pre-trained autoencoder which shares weight for each image and enforces smoothness of $\phi_k$.

between several adjacent images, making use of richer global information when generating the deformation field. Evaluated on two popular EM datasets, our method significantly improves the registration speed while providing competitive accuracy compared with existing methods, which greatly facilitates the 3D volumetric reconstruction of EM images as well as subsequent analysis.

## 2  Method

A deformation field is usually required in the image registration task to warp a subject image to its reference image(s). Let $S = \{s_1, s_2, ..., s_k, ..., s_N\}$ denote a serial EM image set, where $s_1$ denotes the starting image. The goal of registration is to generate a deformation field set $\Phi = \{\phi_2, ..., \phi_k, ..., \phi_N\}$, which can warp $S$ to the registered image set $S(\phi(p)) = \{s_1, s_2(\phi_2(p)), ..., s_k(\phi_k(p)), ..., s_N(\phi_N(p))\}$, where $\phi(p)$ represents the location after registration for each pixel $p$ in an image and $s_k(\phi_k(p))$ ($s_k(\phi_k)$ for short) represents the registered $s_k$.

A straightforward method to obtain $\Phi$ is to decompose this group registration problem into a sequential one, i.e., obtaining $\phi_k$ in order from front to back using paired images. However, in this case, only a single registered image $s_{k-1}(\phi_{k-1})$ is adopted as the reference when performing registration on the subject image $s_k$, which may easily result in the accumulation of error. To address this issue, we take $m$ previously registered images $\{s_{k-i}(\phi_{k-i}(p)) \mid i = 1, ....., m\}$ ($\{s_{k-i}(\phi_{k-i})\}_1^m$ for short) into consideration to compose a reference image set when performing registration on $s_k$. We demonstrate in experiments that this operation can effectively alleviate the error accumulation.

We model a function $\phi_k = g_\theta(\{s_{k-i}(\phi_{k-i})\}_1^m, s_k)$ using a 3D CNN, where $\phi_k$ denotes the deformation field of the subject image $s_k$ and $\theta$ denotes the learnable

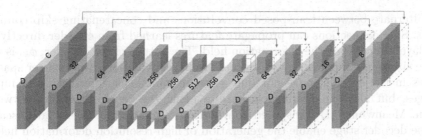

**Fig. 2.** The detailed architecture of our 3D CNN. $D$ denotes the depth dimension, $C$ denotes the channel dimension of feature maps. The spatial dimensions are reduced in half after each convolution. Dotted cubes denote concatenating skip connections.

parameter set of $g$. The framework of our method is shown in Fig. 1. The network takes $m$ serial images $\{s_{k-i}(\phi_{k-i})\}_1^m$ and $s_k$ as input, and generates $\phi_k$ based on a set of parameters $\theta$ in the form of 3D convolution kernels. Then we warp $s_k$ to $s_k(\phi_k)$ using a spatial transformer layer. Considering the independence of the EM image content, we extract features $f$ from input images using a pre-trained autoencoder, to evaluate the similarity between $f(s_k(\phi_k))$ and $\{f(s_{k-i}(\phi_{k-i}))\}_1^m$ and update $\theta$. Relying on an external training dataset, we adopt the Adam solver to find the optimal parameter set $\hat{\theta}$ by minimizing a loss function $\mathcal{L}$ as follows

$$\hat{\theta} = \arg\min_{\theta} \mathcal{L}(\{f(s_{k-i}(\phi_{k-i}))\}_1^m, f(s_k), g_\theta) \tag{1}$$

Given an unseen serial EM images $S$ during test time, the deformation field set $\Phi$ can be rapidly generated through the inference of $g$ in order. In essence, we replace the computational intensive optimization with a CNN to generate a deformation field in one pass, without parameter tuning during test time, which accelerates the registration speed significantly. Note that the training dataset need not to be registered in advance so the proposed method is unsupervised in essence. In conjunction with the newly introduced 3D convolution, our method gives high registration accuracy at the same time.

**3D CNN Architecture.** The implementation of $g$ is based on a hierarchical U-net structure, consisting of an encoder and a decoder with skip connections. Figure 2 depicts the detailed architecture of this network. First, we feed $\{s_{k-i}(\phi_{k-i})\}_1^m$ and $s_k$ as the input of the network. Then, we apply 3D convolutions followed by Leaky ReLU activations in both the encoder and decoder stages, with shrinking kernel size $(Depth \times Height \times Width)$ of $3 \times 7 \times 7$, $3 \times 5 \times 5$, and $3 \times 3 \times 3$ in the encoder stage and the inverse in the decoder stage.

In the encoder, we use strided convolutions to reduce the spatial dimensions, while retaining the depth dimension with padding. The receptive field of the last layer in the encoder should be no smaller than the maximal displacement occuring in serial images, and thus convolutions are applied over $(1/64)^2$ the size of the input for the last layer based on our empirical observation. In the decoder, we alternate between transposed convolutions and concatenating skip connections. Skip connections can propagate features learned from encoder directly to the layers generating the deformation field. The output of the decoder, $\phi_k$, is the same size as the input image $s_k$. Successive 3D convolutions over coarser spatial scales in the encoder stage not only capture multi-scale information of input images, but also exploit the relationship along the depth dimension between them. Meanwhile, 3D transposed convolutions operating on finer spatial scales in the decoder stage enable the generation of high-resolution deformation fields.

**Spatial Transformation Layer.** To minimize the dissimilarity between the warped image and the reference images, we conduct a differentiable transformation operation inspired by spatial transformer networks [7] to compute $s_k(\phi_k)$. For each pixel $p$, we first compute a subpixel location $\phi_k(p)$ in $s_k$. Then, we linearly interpolate the values at four neighboring pixels. Benefiting from its differentiable characteristic, we can backpropagate similarity errors using standard gradient-based methods during optimization.

**Feature Extractor.** To ensure the independence of image content as much as possible, we evaluate the similarity based on image features $f$ extracted from an autoencoder. The autoencoder consists of an encoder comprised of seven 2D convolutional layers with $3 \times 3$ kernel followed by ReLU activations and a decoder which is symmetrical to the encoder. Input of the autoencoder is any 2D image $s_k$ and output is the corresponding reconstructed image $\hat{s}_k$. By minimizing the $\ell_2$ distance between $s_k$ and $\hat{s}_k$, the encoder can generate representative high-level features $f(s_k)$ of image $s_k$, which is $(1/16)^2$ of the input size.

**Loss Function.** We formulate a differentiable loss function $\mathcal{L}$ in Eq. (1), consisting of two components: $\mathcal{L}_{sim}$ that penalizes the dissimilarity between image features, and $\mathcal{L}_{smooth}$ that penalizes local variations in $\phi_k$. We set $\mathcal{L}_{sim}$ to the weighted sum of $\ell_2$ distances between the warped subject image feature $f(s_k(\phi_k))$ and every reference image feature $f(s_{k-i}(\phi_{k-i}))$ as

$$\mathcal{L}_{sim}(\{f(s_{k-i}(\phi_{k-i}))\}_1^m, f(s_k(\phi_k))) = \sum_{i=1}^{m} w_i \, \|f(s_k(\phi_k)) - f(s_{k-i}(\phi_{k-i}))\|_2^2 \quad (2)$$

where $w_i$ is the weight that is inversely proportional to the distance between the subject image and the reference image in the series. Solely minimizing $\mathcal{L}_{sim}$ may generate a discontinuous $\phi_k$, so we promote the smoothness of $\phi_k$ by imposing a regularizer on its spatial gradients as

$$\mathcal{L}_{smooth}(\phi_k) = \|\nabla \phi_k(p)\|_2^2 \quad (3)$$

The complete loss is therefore

$$\mathcal{L} = \mathcal{L}_{sim}(\{f(s_{k-i}(\phi_{k-i}))\}_1^m, f(s_k(\phi_k))) + \lambda \mathcal{L}_{smooth}(\phi_k) \quad (4)$$

where $\lambda$ is a regularization parameter.

# 3   Experiments and Results

In this section, we compare our method with several state-of-the-art EM registration algorithms, i.e., elastic [9] (also known as TrakEM2 [3]) and bUnwarpJ [1] which are representative and widely-adopted traditional methods, and ssEMnet [11] which belongs to the emerging deep learning category. Two popular serial EM datasets, Cremi[1] and FIB25 [10], are used for evaluation.

The training images are from the FAFB dataset [12], the first whole brain EM dataset of drosophila. We select 200 serial EM images at a $3072 \times 3072$ resolution without precise registration as the training data. Due to the GPU storage limit, we set the input size of our network as $1024 \times 1024$, and apply random crop on the training images before feeding them into network. The GPU used in experiments is an NVIDIA V100, and we also use an E5-2667 Intel Xeon CPU for testing the speed of different methods where GPU is not applicable. We set $m = 1$, $\lambda = 2.0$ in our 2D model, and $m = 3$, $\lambda = 3.0$ in our 3D model.

**Evaluation on Cremi Paired Images.** The Cremi dataset is cut out from FAFB, which is a well-known benchmark in the MICCAI 2017 Challenge on Circuit Reconstruction from EM Images. Part of this dataset has been registered manually with neuron segmentation labels. To be roughly consistent with the settings of the ssEMnet, we use a registered volume ($1180 \times 1180 \times 32$) of this dataset as ground-truth to quantitatively evaluate the registration performance based on the neuron labels. We apply random deformation on each ground-truth image and its label using a thin plate spline defined by random vectors on random positions, where the random vectors are sampled from a normal distribution with zero mean and the random positions are uniformly distributed over the image grid. The same random operations are applied on the training data.

To verify the effectiveness of the proposed method, we first investigate image pair registration in serial EM images. Specifically, an image pair is composed of one ground-truth image and one randomly deformed image adjacent to it. In this setting, error accumulation would not happen, and 3D convolution will be simplified to 2D convolution. We perform four registration methods, bUnwarpJ, elastic, ssEMnet-2D and our 2D model. To measure the registration accuracy, we select the 50 largest neurons and calculate the average Dice Similarity Coefficient (DSC). Also, we calculate the total running time of 31 image pairs. As can be seen from Table 1, while our method gives the highest accuracy, it performs more than 5 times faster than bUnwarpJ, more than 10 times faster than elastic, and more than 1300 times faster than ssEMnet.

**Evaluation on Cremi Serial Images.** We have verified the effectiveness of our simplified 2D model, but generating the deformation field in order from front to back based on each image pair will introduce error accumulation in practice. We now investigate our 3D model which involves more serial images during

---

[1] https://cremi.org/.

**Table 1.** Quantitative results and running time on the Cremi test set.

|        | Methods          | DSC (%)         | CPU time (s)      | GPU time (s)       |
|--------|------------------|-----------------|-------------------|--------------------|
| Paired | bUnwarpJ [1]     | 88.1 ± 2.9      | 376.0 ± 132.1     | –                  |
|        | elastic [9]      | 87.5 ± 3.9      | 946.0 ± 96.6      | –                  |
|        | ssEMnet-2D [11]  | 90.2 ± 3.1      | –                 | 2579.1 ± 1492.6    |
|        | ours(2D)         | **91.1 ± 2.3**  | **87.7 ± 0.7**    | **1.9 ± 0.1**      |
| Serial | bUnwarpJ [1]     | 65.9 ± 10.4     | 422               | –                  |
|        | elastic [9]      | 78.3 ± 6.6      | 1439              | –                  |
|        | ssEMnet-3D [11]  | **80.0 ± 2.8**  | –                 | 5699.5 ± 3356.1    |
|        | ours-2D          | 78.6 ± 3.0      | **130.2 ± 1.0**   | **2.5 ± 0.7**      |
|        | ours-3D          | 80.0 ± 3.0      | 457.4 ± 10.6      | 7.9 ± 0.4          |

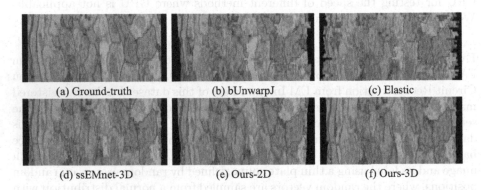

(a) Ground-truth    (b) bUnwarpJ    (c) Elastic

(d) ssEMnet-3D    (e) Ours-2D    (f) Ours-3D

**Fig. 3.** Vertical view of the registered results on the Cremi test set. Red contours mark the edges of neurons in ground-truth. Each neuron is assigned a unique color. (Color figure online)

registration, to verify that the 3D convolution can effectively reduce the error accumulation. Using the same Cremi test set, we perform five methods, including bUnwarpJ, elastic, ssEMnet-3D which also uses several adjacent images, our 2D model and our 3D model. Table 1 provides the DSC results and the running time of 32 serial images. It can be seen that our 3D model gives competitive registration accuracy to ssEMnet but performs at a speed more than 700 times faster. Compared with traditional methods including our 2D model, our 3D model gives notably higher accuracy while still maintaining high efficiency.

Figure 3 shows the vertical cross section of each result. From the visual results, bUnwarpJ shows an obvious drifting and elastic cannot register the vertical membrane well. At the same time, our 2D model shows some drifting of the leftmost neuron compared with our 3D model, which is comparable to ssEMnet. Based on the numerical and visualization results, our 3D model does alleviate the error accumulation and achieves a competitive registration performance.

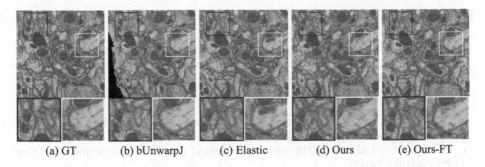

(a) GT          (b) bUnwarpJ          (c) Elastic          (d) Ours          (e) Ours-FT

**Fig. 4.** Vertical view of the registered results of the FIB25 test set. The execution time: (b) 1.6 h, (c) 3.3 h, and (d, e) 75 s.

**Evaluation on FIB25 Serial Images.** To further evaluate the generalizability of our method as well as its robustness for long serial image registration, we apply the 3D model trained on the FAFB dataset on a sub-volume ($520 \times 520 \times 520$) from the registered FIB25 dataset. Different from Cremi, FIB25 is the isotropic data from the brain of drosophila. Again we randomly deform the registered serial images to generate the test data. We perform three methods (bUnwarpJ, elastic, and our 3D model) on the FIB25 test data. Meanwhile, to explore the potential of our method on FIB25, we select another sub-volume ($1280 \times 1280 \times 100$) from FIB25 and finetune our 3D model pre-trained on FAFB. Figure 4 shows the vertical cross section of the registration results. The overall quality of the direct generalization of our method is comparable to elastic and better than bUnwarpJ, while our finetuned model further improves the registration accuracy, as indicted by less artifacts compared with the ground-truth image and more continuous structures. Compared with the representative elastic algorithm, our method reduces the execution time from 3.3 h to 75 s.

## 4 Conclusions

In this paper, we presented an unsupervised deep learning method for serial EM image registration with fast speed and high accuracy. A global registration function composed of 3D CNNs is learned during the training phase, which can be inferenced rapidly to generate the deformation field of serial EM images during the testing phase. Experimental results validate the unprecedented speed and competitive performance of our method compared with state-of-the-arts.

**Acknowledgment.** We acknowledge funding from Natural Science Foundation of China under Grant 91732304, Anhui Provincial Natural Science Foundation No.1908085QF256, and the Fundamental Research Funds for the Central Universities under Grant WK2380000002.

# References

1. Arganda-Carreras, I., Sorzano, C.O.S., Marabini, R., Carazo, J.M., Ortiz-de-Solorzano, C., Kybic, J.: Consistent and elastic registration of histological sections using vector-spline regularization. In: Beichel, R.R., Sonka, M. (eds.) CVAMIA 2006. LNCS, vol. 4241, pp. 85–95. Springer, Heidelberg (2006). https://doi.org/10.1007/11889762_8
2. Balakrishnan, G., et al.: An unsupervised learning model for deformable medical image registration. In: CVPR (2018)
3. Cardona, A., et al.: TrakEM2 software for neural circuit reconstruction. PloS One 7(6), e38011 (2012)
4. Dosovitskiy, A., et al.: FlowNet: learning optical flow with convolutional networks. In: ICCV (2015)
5. Funke, J., et al.: Large scale image segmentation with structured loss based deep learning for connectome reconstruction. IEEE Trans. Pattern Anal. Mach. Intell. 41, 1669–1680 (2018)
6. Hinton, G.E., et al.: Reducing the dimensionality of data with neural networks. Science 313(5786), 504–507 (2006)
7. Jaderberg, M., et al.: Spatial transformer networks. In: NIPS (2015)
8. Januszewski, M., et al.: High-precision automated reconstruction of neurons with flood-filling networks. Nat. Methods 15(8), 605 (2018)
9. Saalfeld, S., et al.: Elastic volume reconstruction from series of ultra-thin microscopy sections. Nat. Methods 9(7), 717 (2012)
10. Takemura, S.Y., et al.: Synaptic circuits and their variations within different columns in the visual system of drosophila. Proc. Natl. Acad. Sci. 112(44), 13711–13716 (2015)
11. Yoo, I., Hildebrand, D.G.C., Tobin, W.F., Lee, W.-C.A., Jeong, W.-K.: ssEMnet: serial-section electron microscopy image registration using a spatial transformer network with learned features. In: Cardoso, M., et al. (eds.) DLMIA/ML-CDS - 2017. LNCS, vol. 10553, pp. 249–257. Springer, Cham (2017). https://doi.org/10.1007/978-3-319-67558-9_29
12. Zheng, Z., et al.: A complete electron microscopy volume of the brain of adult drosophila melanogaster. Cell 174(3), 730–743 (2018)

# PlacentaNet: Automatic Morphological Characterization of Placenta Photos with Deep Learning

Yukun Chen[1]([⊠]), Chenyan Wu[1], Zhuomin Zhang[1], Jeffery A. Goldstein[2], Alison D. Gernand[1], and James Z. Wang[1]

[1] The Pennsylvania State University, University Park, PA, USA
yzc147@psu.edu
[2] Northwestern Memorial Hospital, Chicago, IL, USA

**Abstract.** Analysis of the placenta is extremely useful for evaluating health risks of the mother and baby after delivery. In this paper, we tackle the problem of automatic morphological characterization of placentas, including the tasks of placenta image segmentation, umbilical cord insertion point localization, and maternal/fetal side classification. We curated an existing dataset consisting of around 1,000 placenta images taken at Northwestern Memorial Hospital, together with their pixel-level segmentation map. We propose a novel pipeline, PlacentaNet, which consists of three encoder-decoder convolutional neural networks with a shared encoder, to address these morphological characterization tasks by employing a transfer learning training strategy. We evaluated its effectiveness using the curated dataset as well as the pathology reports in the medical record. The system produced accurate morphological characterization, which enabled subsequent feature analysis of placentas. In particular, we show promising results for detection of retained placenta (*i.e.*, incomplete placenta) and umbilical cord insertion type categorization, both of which may possess clinical impact.

**Keywords:** Placenta · Convolutional neural network · Segmentation · Transfer learning

This work was supported primarily by the Bill & Melinda Gates Foundation. The computation was support by the NVIDIA Corporation's GPU Grant Program. Discussions with William Tony Parks have been helpful. Celeste Beck, Dolzodmaa Davaasuren, and Leigh A. Taylor assisted in dataset curation.
A. D. Gernand and J. Z. Wang have equal contributions.

**Electronic supplementary material** The online version of this chapter (https://doi.org/10.1007/978-3-030-32239-7_54) contains supplementary material, which is available to authorized users.

D. Shen et al. (Eds.): MICCAI 2019, LNCS 11764, pp. 487–495, 2019.
https://doi.org/10.1007/978-3-030-32239-7_54

# 1   Introduction

The placenta is a window into the events of a pregnancy and the health of the mother and baby [12]. Yet, a very small percentage of placentas around the world are ever examined by a pathologist. Even in developed countries like the U.S., placentas are examined and characterized by a pathologist only when it is considered necessary and resources are available. Full pathological examination is expensive and time consuming. In placenta examination, pathologists complete a report that contains various measurements (*e.g.*, the weight, the disc diameter) and diagnoses (*e.g.*, completeness or retained placenta, cord insertion type, shape category). These measurements and placental diagnoses are extremely useful for the short- and long-term clinical care of the mother and baby.

Automated placenta analysis based on photographic imaging can potentially allow more placentas to be examined, reduce the number of normal placentas sent for full pathological examination, and provide more accurate and timely morphological and pathological measurements or analyses. Typical photographs of the placentas capture the umbilical cord inserting into the fetal side of the disc, as well as the maternal side appearance. Two example images of placentas can be found later in Fig. 1(a). This paper focuses on a fully automated system for morphological characterization of placentas. Such systems will be the cornerstone for automated pathological analyses because segmentation of disc and cord, location of cord insertion point, and determination of fetal/maternal side are important first steps before further analyses can be done.

**Related Work.** Existing placenta imaging research can be roughly categorized into two types: those using microscopic images of slices of the placentas [6,15] and those using the macroscopic images of the placentas taken by cameras [17] or by MRI [1]. A comprehensive overview of both microscopic and macroscopic placenta pathology can be found in a book by Benirschke *et al.* [3]. To our knowledge, there has not been an automated approach to analyze placenta photographs. We believe such an approach has the potential to be adopted widely because it requires no specialized hardware beyond an ordinary camera or a camera phone.

In this paper, we propose a transfer learning (TL) approach to tackle the associated tasks of morphological characterization rather than employing one independent model for each task. TL promises performance gain and robustness enhancement through representation sharing for closely related tasks [10]. Specifically, we transfer the learned representation of the encoder from the segmentation task to the other two tasks, *i.e.* disc side classification and insertion point localization. Our network architecture design takes inspiration from the recent deep learning advances on classification [4], image segmentation [7,13], and key-point localization [9]. In particular, the design of our segmentation module follows the practice of concatenating feature maps in encoder with feature maps in decoder, such as performed in the U-Net [13]; and the design of our insertion point module follows the practice of regressing a Gaussian heat map, rather than using the coordinate values, as the ground truth, which has been shown to be successful in human key-point/joint localization tasks [3,9,11,16]. Tompson *et al.* first showed the importance of intermediate supervision to improving localization accuracy [9]. We take their idea in our design by considering two heat map predictions in the final loss—one from the final feature layer and one from the intermediate feature layer.

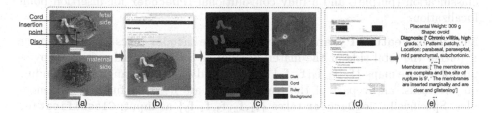

**Fig. 1.** Data curation process. (a–c): collecting pixel-level segmentation map for cord, disc, and ruler, insertion point location, and classification of whether an image captures fetal or maternal side placenta through our web-based labeling tool. (d–e): extracting diagnoses and measurements from unidentified pathological report in PDF format.

## 2  The Dataset

We obtained a dataset consisting of 1,003 placenta images, of which 430 are fetal-side images and 573 are maternal-side images[1], from Northwestern Memorial Hospital, a large urban academic medical center. We also have the complete pathology report for each placenta, written in natural language by the pathologist who originally examined the placenta. Pathology classification is standardized and pathologist are perinatal experts. Figure 1 shows our data curation process. We developed a web-based tool (Fig. 1(b)) to collect (i) the pixel-wise segmentation maps, (ii) the side-type label as fetal side or maternal side, and (iii) the cord insertion point (only for fetal side, visualized as a Gaussian heat map centered at the marked coordinate in (Fig. 1(c))) so that multiple trained labelers can annotate this dataset concurrently. We also extract diagnoses from the pathology reports.

We divide the dataset into training and testing sets with the ratio of 0.8:0.2. Because the insertion point can only be observed from the fetal side, we only use the 430 fetal-side images for insertion point prediction, with the same training-testing ratio as aforementioned.

---

[1] The numbers of fetal-side and maternal-side images are uneven because some of the collected images did not meet our image quality standard (*e.g.* disc occluded by irrelevant object such as scissors) and we had to discard them from the dataset. We plan to release our dataset in the future after substantial expansion.

## 3   The Method

The proposed PlacentaNet model, as illustrated in Fig. 2, consists of an Encoder for feature pyramid extraction (blue), which is shared among all tasks, a fully convolutional SegDecoder for placenta image segmentation on both fetal- and maternal-side images (red), a Classification Subnet for fetal/maternal-side classification (purple), and a fully convolutional IPDecoder for insertion point localization.

**Encoder as Feature Pyramid Extractor.** The Encoder takes a placenta image $x$ (either the fetal side or the maternal side) as the input and outputs a pyramid of feature maps $\{f_1, f_2, f_3, f_4, f_5\}$ (represented as blue rectangles). Depending on the tasks, all or part of the feature maps are used by further task modules. Specifically, SegDecoder takes $\{f_1, f_2, f_3, f_4, f_5\}$ as input; Classification Subnet takes $\{f_5\}$ as input; and IPDecoder takes $\{f_3, f_4, f_5\}$ as input. The Conv-1 and Conv-2 blocks both consist of a Conv-BatchNorm-Relu layer. The difference, however, is that the Conv layer in Conv-1 block has stride 1, while the Conv layer in Conv-2 block has stride 2. The Res conv blocks are residual blocks with two convolutional layers with stride 2 and 1, respectively, and the same kernel size $3 \times 3$, each of which spatially downsamples the input feature maps to half of its size and doubles the number of feature channels. The residual structure has been shown especially helpful for training deep architectures by He *et al.* [4].

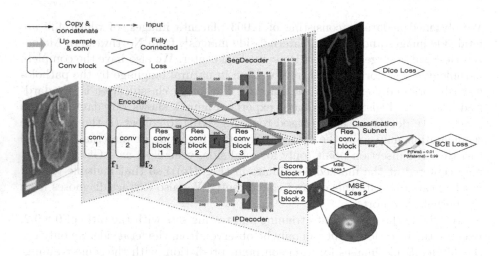

**Fig. 2.** The architecture of PlacentaNet: a multi-task convolutional neural network for placenta image segmentation, cord insertion point localization, and placenta disc side classification. "Up sample & Conv" is implemented by a transposed convolution layer. "Res conv blocks" are residual blocks with two convolutional layers with stride 2 and 1, respectively, and the same kernel size $3 \times 3$. "Score blocks" are convolutional layers with kernel size $1 \times 1$ and the number of output channel 1. The soft-max layers are omitted. We use dice loss, BCE loss and MSE loss for the segmentation, classification, and insertion point localization, respectively. (Color figure online)

**SegDecoder for Segmentation.** Our `SegDecoder` module consists of four expanding fully convolutional blocks, each of which takes the concatenation of a copy of the corresponding feature map $\mathbf{f}_i, i \in \{1, 2, 3, 4\}$, and transposes a convoluted (up-scaling factor 2) output feature map of the last layer. Finally, we apply soft-max to predict the probability of pixel $(i, j)$ being of class $k$, denoted as $\mathbf{p}(i, j, k)$. To overcome the problem of highly imbalanced number of pixels for different categories, we use dice loss [8] instead of the common cross entropy loss. Since we have four classes rather than two classes in [8], we adjust the dice loss to suit the 4-class scenario:

$$L^{\mathrm{seg}} = 1 - \frac{\sum_{i,j} \sum_{k=0}^{3} \mathbf{p}(i, j, k) \cdot \mathbf{g}(i, j, k)}{\sum_{i,j} \sum_{k=0}^{3} (\mathbf{p}(i, j, k) + \mathbf{g}(i, j, k))}, \tag{1}$$

where $i, j$ run over the row and column indexes of an image, respectively; $\mathbf{p}(i, j, k)$ and $\mathbf{g}(i, j, k)$ denote the predicted probability of the pixel at location $(i, j)$ and the 0/1 ground truth of that pixel belonging to class $k$, respectively.

**Classification Subnet for Fetal/Maternal Side Classification.** Because the fetal/maternal side can be inferred from the "disc" region of a placenta alone, we crop the full placenta image $\mathbf{x}$ by a rectangle including the region of disc and resize the cropped image to $512 \times 512$ pixels as the input to the `Encoder`, which we denote as $\mathbf{x}_c$. The cropping is based on the ground truth segmentation map during training and on the predicted segmentation map at inference. Our `Classification Subnet` consists of a Res conv block, two fully connected layers, and a soft-max layer. At the end, a binary cross entropy (BCE) loss is applied to supervise the network.

**IPDecoder for Insertion Point Localization.** Because the insertion point is always located within or adjacent to the "disc" region, we use cropped disc region image $\mathbf{x}_c$, by the same way as we perform cropping in `Classification Subnet`, as the input to the `Encoder`. Our `IPDecoder` is also fully convolutional and consists of two expanding fully convolutional blocks, the structure of which are the same as in the first two convolutional blocks in `SegDecoder`. The similarity of `IPDecoder`'s structure with `SegDecoder`'s helps us to ensure that the shared encoder representation could also be readily utilized here. Inspired by the success of intermediate supervision [9], we predict the insertion point localization heat map after each expanding convolutional block by a convolutional layer with kernel size $1 \times 1$ (denoted as "Score block" in Fig. 2) and use the MSE loss to measure the prediction error:

$$L_k^{\mathrm{ip}} = \sum_{i,j} ||\mathbf{h}(i, j) - \hat{\mathbf{h}}(i, j)||^2, \quad k \in \{1, 2\}, \tag{2}$$

where $\mathbf{h}(i, j)$ and $\hat{\mathbf{h}}(i, j)$ are the ground truth (Gaussian) heat map and the predicted heat map, respectively. And the final loss for insertion point is $L^{\mathrm{ip}} = L_1^{\mathrm{ip}} + L_2^{\mathrm{ip}}$. During inference, the predicted insertion point location is determined by $(i, j) = \arg\max_{i,j} \hat{\mathbf{h}}(i, j)$.

**Training and Testing.** We use mini-batched stochastic gradient descent (SGD) with learning rate 0.1, momentum 0.9, and weight decay 0.0005 for all training. We use a batch size of 2 for all segmentation training and a batch size of 10 for all insertion point localization and fetal/maternal side classification training. The procedures of training are as follows. We first train the `SegDecoder` + `Encoder` from scratch with parameters initialized to zero. Next, we fix the learned weights for the `Encoder` and train `Classification Subnet` and `IPDecoder` subsequently (in other words, the `Encoder` only acts as a fixed feature pyramid extractor at this stage). The rationale for making such choices is that the training for segmentation task consumes all images we have gathered and makes use of pixel-wise dense supervision, which is much less likely to lead to an overfitting problem. In contrast, the training of `Classification Subnet` takes binary value as ground truth for each image and the training of `IPDecoder` only uses around half of the whole dataset (only fetal-side images). To alleviate the lack of labels and to make the model more robust, we use common augmentation techniques including random rotation ($\pm 30°$), and horizontal and vertical flipping for all training images.

**Implementation.** We implemented the proposed pipeline in PyTorch and ran experiments on an NVIDIA TITAN Xp GPU. For segmentation training, all images are first resized to $768 \times 1024$, which is of the same aspect ratio as the original placenta images. For insertion point localization and fetal/maternal side classification training, we resize all cropped "disc" region images to $512 \times 512$, which is natural because the cropped "disc" regions often have a bounding box close to a square.

## 4   Experiments and Evaluation

**Segmentation.** We compared our approach with two fully convolutional encoder-decoder architectures, the U-Net [13] and the SegNet [2]. The results are shown in Fig. 3(a–d). We report the segmentation performance using standard segmentation metrics pixel accuracy, mean accuracy, and mean IoU. In Fig. 3 (b, c, and d), we compare pixel-wise prediction confusion matrices of our approach, U-Net, and Segnet, respectively, which reflects more detail about segmentation performance for different categories. We also show a few segmentation examples in Fig. 3(e) for qualitative comparison. Our approach yields the best segmentation results, especially for differentiating the cord and the ruler classes.

**Fetal/Maternal Side Classification.** We achieve an overall fetal/maternal side classification accuracy of 97.51% on our test set. Without the shared encoder representation, we can only achieve 95.52% by training `Encoder` + `Classification Subnet` from scratch. We also compare their confusion matrices in Fig. 1 in the supplementary material.

**Insertion Point Localization.** We use Percentage of Correct Keypoints (PCK) as the evaluation metric. PCK measures the percentage of the predictions falling

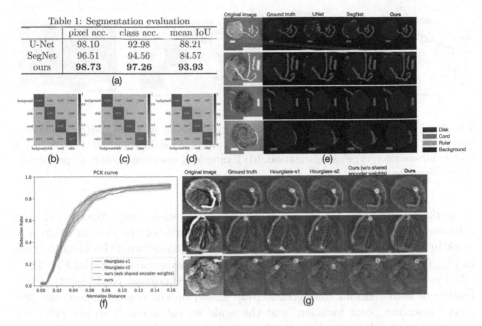

Table 1: Segmentation evaluation

|        | pixel acc. | class acc. | mean IoU |
|--------|------------|------------|----------|
| U-Net  | 98.10      | 92.98      | 88.21    |
| SegNet | 96.51      | 94.56      | 84.57    |
| ours   | **98.73**  | **97.26**  | **93.93**|

(a)

(b)    (c)    (d)    (e)

(f)    (g)

**Fig. 3.** Evaluation results. (a) Segmentation evaluation accuracy. (b–d) Confusion matrices of our approach, U-Net, and SegNet, respectively. (e) Example segmentation results. We show both fetal-side results (top two rows) and maternal-side results (bottom two rows). (f) Quantitative evaluation of insertion point localization with PCK curves. (g) Examples of insertion point heat map prediction. (Color figure online)

within a circle of certain radius centered at the ground truth location. We compare our approach (both with and without shared encoder weights) to the Hourglass model (with number of stacks 1 and 2), which shows competitive results in human keypoint localization [9]. Figure 3(f) shows the PCK curves, with the $x$-axis being the radius normalized by the diameter of the placenta. Each curve in Fig. 3(f) is the average of the results for five models trained with different seeds, and the light-colored band around each curve (viewable when the figure is enlarged) shows the standard deviation of the results. Our approach with shared Encoder consistently gives the best results, especially when the normalized distance is from 0.2 to 0.6. We show a few qualitative examples of the insertion point heat maps predicted by each model, along with the ground truth (Fig. 3(g)).

**Placenta Feature Analysis.** The predictions of PlacentaNet enable us to conduct automatic placenta feature analysis by subsequent models/procedures.
*(1) Detection of retained placenta.* Retained placenta is a cause of postpartum hemorrhage and, if prolonged, it can serve as a nidus for infection [14]. Pathologists judge if there could be retained placenta by carefully inspecting the maternal surface of a placenta's disc. We identified 119 out of 573 maternal side placenta images in our dataset with possible "retained placenta" based on the pathology reports and we asked a perinatal pathologist (coauthor) to annotate where the possible missing parts are for each of them. We trained two neural

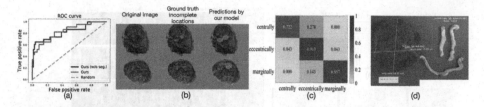

**Fig. 4.** (a) ROC curve for retained placenta classification. AUC for red(blue) curve is 0.836(0.827). (b) Example of retained placenta problem localization. (c) The confusion matrix for insertion type categorization. (d) Example of insertion point type prediction. (Color figure online)

networks for this task, for classification and localization, respectively, and both achieved promising results. We show the ROC curve of the classification network in Fig. 4(a) and example localization results along with the ground truth in Fig. 4(b). (More localization results are in supplementary material Fig. 3).

*(2) Umbilical cord insertion type categorization.* Abnormal cord insertion is a feature of fetal vascular malperfusion [5]. Based on the segmentation, the predicted insertion point location, and the scale we extracted from the ruler, we can measure the distance from the insertion point to the nearest margin of the disc, and the lengths of the long and short axes of the disc (all in centimeters). Further, we classify the cord insertion type into "centrally", "eccentrically", and "marginally", based on the ratio between *the distance from the insertion point to its closest disc margin* and *the average between the lengths of the long and short axes.* We achieve an overall 88% test accuracy. We show the classification confusion matrix in Fig. 4(c). One qualitative example of our prediction is shown in Fig. 4(d). Detailed procedures and more qualitative examples of measurement and classification are in supplementary material Figs. 1 and 2.

## 5    Conclusions and Future Work

We proposed a novel, compact multi-head encoder-decoder CNN to jointly solve placenta morphological characterization tasks. We showed that our approach can achieve better performance than competitive baselines for each task. We showed that the representation learned from segmentation task could benefit insertion point localization and fetal/maternal side classification task. In the future, it would be interesting to explore if these tasks could mutually benefit each other. The use of this method in automated prediction of pathological indicators is the next direction we will pursue.

## References

1. Alansary, A., et al.: Fast fully automatic segmentation of the human placenta from motion corrupted MRI. In: Ourselin, S., Joskowicz, L., Sabuncu, M.R., Unal, G., Wells, W. (eds.) MICCAI 2016. LNCS, vol. 9901, pp. 589–597. Springer, Cham (2016). https://doi.org/10.1007/978-3-319-46723-8_68

2. Badrinarayanan, V., et al.: SegNet: a deep convolutional encoder-decoder architecture for image segmentation. IEEE T-PAMI **39**(12), 2481–2495 (2017)
3. Benirschke, K., Burton, G.J., Baergen, R.N.: Pathology of the Human Placenta, 6th edn. Springer, Heidelberg (2012). https://doi.org/10.1007/978-3-642-23941-0
4. He, K., et al.: Deep residual learning for image recognition. In: The IEEE CVPR, pp. 770–778 (2016)
5. Khong, T.Y., et al.: Sampling and definitions of placental lesions: Amsterdam placental workshop group consensus statement. Archiv. Pathol. Lab. Med. **140**(7), 698–713 (2016)
6. Kidron, D., et al.: Automated image analysis of placental villi and syncytial knots in histological sections. Placenta **53**, 113–118 (2017)
7. Long, J., et al.: Fully convolutional networks for semantic segmentation. In: The IEEE CVPR, pp. 3431–3440 (2015)
8. Milletari, F., et al.: V-Net: fully convolutional neural networks for volumetric medical image segmentation. In: International Conference on 3D Vision (3DV), pp. 565–571. IEEE (2016)
9. Newell, A., Yang, K., Deng, J.: Stacked hourglass networks for human pose estimation. In: Leibe, B., Matas, J., Sebe, N., Welling, M. (eds.) ECCV 2016. LNCS, vol. 9912, pp. 483–499. Springer, Cham (2016). https://doi.org/10.1007/978-3-319-46484-8_29
10. Pan, J., et al.: A survey on transfer learning. IEEE TKDE **22**(10), 1345–1359 (2009)
11. Payer, C., et al.: Integrating spatial configuration into heatmap regression based cnns for landmark localization. Med. Image Anal. **54**, 207–219 (2019)
12. Roberts, D.J., et al.: Placental pathology, a survival guide. Archiv. Pathol. Lab. Med. **132**(4), 641–651 (2008)
13. Ronneberger, O., Fischer, P., Brox, T.: U-Net: convolutional networks for biomedical image segmentation. In: Navab, N., Hornegger, J., Wells, W.M., Frangi, A.F. (eds.) MICCAI 2015. LNCS, vol. 9351, pp. 234–241. Springer, Cham (2015). https://doi.org/10.1007/978-3-319-24574-4_28
14. Silver, R.: Abnormal placentation: placenta previa, vasa previa, and placenta accreta. Obstet. Gynecol. **126**(3), 654–668 (2015)
15. Thomas, K.A., Sottile, M.J., Salafia, C.M.: Unsupervised segmentation for inflammation detection in histopathology images. In: Elmoataz, A., Lezoray, O., Nouboud, F., Mammass, D., Meunier, J. (eds.) ICISP 2010. LNCS, vol. 6134, pp. 541–549. Springer, Heidelberg (2010). https://doi.org/10.1007/978-3-642-13681-8_63
16. Tompson, J., et al.: Joint training of a convolutional network and a graphical model for human pose estimation. In: NIPS, pp. 1799–1807 (2014)
17. Yampolsky, M., et al.: Centrality of the umbilical cord insertion in a human placenta influences the placental efficiency. Placenta **30**(12), 1058–1064 (2009)

# Deep Multi-instance Learning for Survival Prediction from Whole Slide Images

Jiawen Yao, Xinliang Zhu, and Junzhou Huang[✉]

Department of Computer Science and Engineering,
The University of Texas at Arlington, Arlington, TX 76019, USA
jzhuang@uta.edu

**Abstract.** Recent image-based survival models rely on discriminative patch labeling, which are both time consuming and infeasible to extend to large scale cancer datasets. Different from the existing works on learning using key patches or clusters from WSIs, we take advantages of a deep multiple instance learning to encode all possible patterns from WSIs and consider the joint effects from different patterns for clinical outcomes prediction. We evaluate our model in its ability to predict patients' survival risks across the Lung and Brain tumors from two large whole slide pathological images datasets. The proposed framework can improve the prediction performances compared with existing state-of-the-arts survival analysis approaches. Results also demonstrate the effectiveness of the proposed method as a recommender system to provide personalized recommendations based on an individual's calculated risk.

## 1 Introduction

Recent technological innovations are enabling scientists to capture big whole slide pathological images (WSIs) at increasing speed and resolution for diagnosis. The high resolution of image data greatly benefits survival analysis with more precise information. However, it also brings critical computational bottlenecks from the unprecedented scale and complexity of these data. Instead of handling original WSIs, classical image-based survival methods adopted several discriminative patches from manually annotated Region Of Interests (ROIs) and then extracted hand-crafted features for predictions [12,13,16–18]. However, these approaches have very high risks to ignore survival-discriminative patterns if only select several tiles from very heterogeneous whole pathological image slides.

To address this issue and fully exploit whole slide pathological images, several WSI-based survival models are proposed [5,10,20]. Zhu et al. [20] proposed a patch-based two-stage framework to predict patients' survival outcomes. Patches are first sampled from the WSIs and clustered to different clusters according to their visual appearances (phenotypes). During training, the first stage selects key phenotypes based on patch-wise survival prediction results from DeepConvSurv

This work was partially supported by US National Science Foundation IIS-1718853 and the NSF CAREER grant IIS-1553687.

models [19]. The second stage aggregates the selected phenotypes to perform patient-level prediction. Although this framework has practical merits to consider important patch clusters, it treats each cluster within a patient as independent of each other and doesn't consider the joint effects from different clusters could contribute to clinical outcomes. Figure 1 shows two whole slide images from lung cancer patients. Patches framed in red represent tumor regions and those in blue show low-grade tumor or non-tumor regions. Patient B has much worse clinical outcome than patient A and one distinct pattern in patient A is that the biopsy sample has more non-tumor tissue regions. This observation reminds us that the joint effects of phenotypes could be used to better predict patients' survival status.

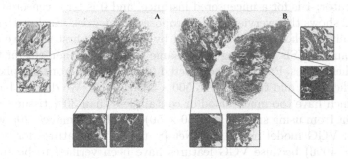

**Fig. 1.** Gigapixel Whole Slide Histopathological Images of two lung cancer patients (best viewed in color).

In this paper, we view the problem of survival prediction as a form of the multi-instance learning. The primary motivation of using multi-instance learning (MIL) is because of its ability to learn discriminative patterns based on a training set of bags, where each bag contains multiple feature vectors known as discriminative instances. This enables us to identify patients' survival outcomes without any instance-level (patch-level) labels. Different from recent survival models that treated and trained patch clusters independently, our model relaxes this strong assumption by combining local and global representation, and thus can efficiently exploit all possible patterns from WSIs. Extensive experimental results verify the effectiveness of the proposed framework on two serious cancer diseases—our method can efficiently exploit and utilize all discriminative patterns in whole slide pathological images to perform accurate patients' survival predictions.

## 2   Methodology

Given a set of $N$ patients, $\{x_i\}, i = 1 \ldots N$, each patient has the label $(t_i, \delta_i)$ indicating the survival status. The observation time $t_i$ is either a survival time $(O_i)$ or a censored time $(C_i)$ for each data instance. If and only if $t_i = \min(O_i, C_i)$

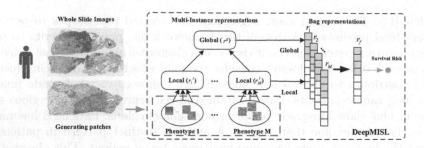

**Fig. 2.** An overview of the proposed model.

can be observed during the study, the dataset is said to be right-censored [7]. $\delta_i$ is the indicator: 1 is for a uncensored instance, and 0 is for a censored instance.

Figure 2 shows the overview of the proposed framework. Each patient $x_i$ may contain multiple whole slides. Motivated by [20], at the first step, we extracted patches from all WSIs belonging to the same patient and then cluster them into different phenotypes. Patches are extracted from 5X (2 microns per pixel) objective magnifications and then fixed to $500 \times 500 \times 3$ size. We discard background patches which have too much blood or contain less than 30% tissue sections.

Different from using smaller size ($50 \times 50$) thumbnail images [20], we use the pre-trained VGG model from ImageNet [8] to extract features for each image patch ($d = 4096$) because VGG features have been verified to be suitable for stratification of complex tissue patterns [1]. Then we adopt K-means to cluster patches based on their VGG features. By clustering different patches from all patients into several distinguished phenotype groups, we will have different phenotype groups with various prediction powers on patients' survival. The proposed method takes phenotypes as multiple inputs and considers their connections for predicting survival status. The output of the network is the risk function to indicate the survival risk of this patient.

**Local Representations via MI-FCN.** After clustering, one patient $x$ is denoted by different phenotype groups as $[(1 \times m_1 \times d), (1 \times m_2 \times d), ..., (1 \times m_M \times d)]$ and $M$ is the number of phenotypes, $m_i$ means the number of patches in $i$-th phenotype. For each phenotype, the input is a set of $m_i$ patches, can be organized as $1 \times m_i \times d$ ($d$ is the feature dimension or channel). Then we used the Multi-Instance Fully Convolutional Networks (MI-FCN) [14] to learn local representation. The reason to use the fully convolutional networks (FCN) without including any fully connected layers is that FCN is more flexible and can handle any spatial resolution, which is needed for the considered problem since the number of patches in each phenotype varies. Figure 3 shows the basic architecture of MI-FCN. The network consists of two layer-pairs of $1 \times 1$ conv layer and ReLU layer. The global max-pooling layer will be added at the end. For $j$-th phenotype, the local representation is denoted as $\mathbf{r_j}^l$. The combination of multiple layers of fully convolutional layers and non-linear activation functions has proven to be a powerful non-linear feature mapping in Multi-Instance problem [14].

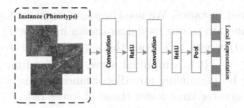

**Fig. 3.** The network architecture in each phenotype.

**Bag Representations.** Local representations from different phenotypes are then concatenated to construct patient-level global representation $\mathbf{r}^g$. Such global information encodes representations across all phenotypes. $\mathbf{r}^g$ captures the information across all the phenotypes within the bag. Then we concatenate the global feature $\mathbf{r}_g$ with the corresponding local representation $\mathbf{r}^l$ to form the combined representation $\mathbf{r}$. If we take $j$-th phenotype as the example, then the combined representation is denoted as $\mathbf{r}_j = \mathbf{r}_j^l \oplus \mathbf{r}^g$ where $\oplus$ is the concatenation operator. Each of combined representations $\mathbf{r}_1, \ldots, \mathbf{r}_M$ will go through a fully connected layer and then will be aggregated together to form the final bag representation $\mathbf{r}_f$. Different from the classification task whose positive labels rely on independent positive instances, patient's survival status is observed and judged by the joint effects of phenotypes. Intuitively, the global feature encodes holistic information of the patient and disambiguating polysemy encoded in local representation from phenotype. Since the instances actually correspond to the phenotypes from WSIs, the bag representation is capable of capturing the complex relationship between phenotypes and thus form global representations for the survival prediction at patient level. Table 1 shows the architecture of the proposed network.

**Table 1.** The architecture of the proposed network

| Layer | Input | Output size |
|---|---|---|
| MI-FCN $i$ | $1 \times m_j \times d$ | $256\ (r_j^l)$ |
| Concatenation | $r_j^l$ | $256 * M\ (r^g)$ |
| Concate. $j$ | $r^g \oplus r_j^l$ | $256 \times (1 + M)\ (r_j)$ |
| Fully-Connect $j$ | $r_j$ | $1\ (r_j)$ |
| Concate. | $r_{conca}$ | $M\ (r_f)$ |
| Fully-Connect | $r_f$ | $1$ (risk) |

**Loss Function.** The network aggregates those features from each phenotype by fully connected network to make a final survival prediction. For $i$-th patient sample passing through the proposed model, the output of this patient's survival score is denoted as $\mathbf{o}_i$. Assume the label of the $i$-th patient as $(t_i, \delta_i)$ where $t_i$ is the observed time, $\delta_i$ is the indicator, 1 is for a uncensored instance (death), and 0 is for a censored instance. We use the same negative log partial likelihood in [20] as the loss function in our model as shown in below $L(\mathbf{o}_i) = \sum_i \delta_i(-\mathbf{o}_i + \log \sum_{j:t_j >= t_i} \exp(\mathbf{o}_j))$ where $j$ is from the set whose survival time is equal or larger than $t_i$ ($t_j \geq t_i$). In a simplified view, the loss function contributes to overall concordance by penalizing any discordance in any values of higher risk patients if they are greater than lower those of lower risk.

## 3    Experiments

**Dataset Description and Baselines.** We focus on the lung and brain cancer in our study and used two cancer survival datasets with high resolution whole slide pathological images. To evaluate models, 2/3 patients were randomly selected as training set and the rest 1/3 patients were used as testing set. We split parts of training data as validation set (20%) in our setting to perform early stop training. **Lung Cancer**: Lung Adenocarcinoma (ADC) is one major subtype lung cancer (30%). The dataset used is the National Lung Screening Trial (NLST)[1]. In this dataset, we have 153 patients with 241 WSIs. The number of sampling patches is 33,046. **GBM**: Glioblastoma multiforme (GBM) is the most common malignant brain tumor. We collected 156 patients with 285 WSIs from The Cancer Genome Atlas (TCGA) cohort[2]. The number of patches from GBM is 53,662.

Following the recent framework [18], we extracted dense image patches from ROIs and calculated hand-crafted features using CellProfiler [2] which serves as a state-of-the-art medical image feature extracting and quantitative analysis tool. These types of image features include cell shape, size, texture of the cells and nuclei, as well as the distribution of pixel intensity in the cells and nuclei. Then average calculation is performed patient-wise to get patient-level features from patch-level features. The comparison method includes the most popular regularized Cox proportional hazards models: (LASSO-Cox) [11] and elastic-net penalized Cox (EN-Cox) [15], Parametric censored regression models with Weibull, Logistic distribution [4], Random Survival Forest (RSF) [3], Multi-Task Learning model for Survival Analysis (MTLSA) [6] and one WSI-based survival model WSISA [20].

**Implementation Details.** For training, we use stochastic gradient descent with momentum 0.9 and weight decay $5 \times 10^{-4}$ with a mini-batch size of 32. The learning rate is set to $10^{-4}$ at first and then decreased to $10^{-5}$ after 20 epochs. The training monitors the loss on validation dataset and it will early stop if the loss increases too much. Experiments were conducted on a single NVIDIA GeForce GTX 1080 GPU with 8 GB memory.

**Results and Discussions.** We report the C-index value as our main evaluation metric. C-index serves as a standard evaluation metric in survival analysis [9]. It shows the prediction power of the proposed method compared with different survival models. The value of C-index ranges from 0 to 1. The larger the value is,

---

[1] https://biometry.nci.nih.gov/cdas/nlst/.

[2] https://tcga-data.nci.nih.gov/docs/publications/tcga/.

the better the model predicts. We tested a few possible numbers of phenotypes, such as $\{1, 3, 5, 7\}$ on TCGA-GBM dataset. The corresponding C-Index values are $0.503, 0.611, 0.657$ and $0.576$. Note that when the number of phenotypes is 1, all patches in the bag will be organized together and no clustering is used. That means the model without using phenotypes is unable to achieve good results. The reason is patches in one bag actually are very heterogeneous. It is difficult to learn survival-related representations from unorganized patches. This validates the effectiveness of the consideration of phenotypes in our model. Results suggest the number of 5 achieves slightly better predictions. Thus, we decide to choose to cluster 5 phenotypes in our model.

Table 2 shows the C-index values from various survival regression methods on two datasets. One can see that the proposed method achieves the highest C-index values which presents the best prediction performance among all methods. From the table, ROI based models (methods before WSISA) perform not well due to two reasons: (1) the limitation of local information provided by the patches extracted from the ROI; (2) the non-effective way to represent the heterogeneity of tumor using hand-crafted features. Instead of using a small set of patches and human-designed features, the proposed method can effectively learn complex deep bag representation from phenotypes to predict patient survival outcomes.

**Table 2.** Performance comparison of the proposed methods and other existing related methods using C-index values on two datasets. The larger C-index value is better.

| Model | Lung-ADC | GBM |
|---|---|---|
| LASSO-Cox [11] | 0.552 | 0.496 |
| EN-Cox [15] | 0.547 | 0.501 |
| RSF [3] | 0.486 | 0.539 |
| Weibull [4] | 0.531 | 0.521 |
| Logistic [4] | 0.542 | 0.539 |
| MTLSA [6] | 0.549 | 0.577 |
| WSISA [20] | 0.612 | 0.585 |
| **Proposed** | **0.678** | **0.657** |

From the table, WSISA shows the good representative ability of features for survival prediction. However, WSISA needs a separate stage to train several DeepConvSurv models independently and will discard some phenotypes in the final stage, the performance actually depends on how well to select important clusters. Instead of selecting phenotypes, our proposed method incorporates phenotypes not into separate learning paradigm which is more favorable to solving survival problem. Because all phenotypes have various power to provide information for survival analysis and it is useful to consider all connections among them instead of separately treating one as independent of each other.

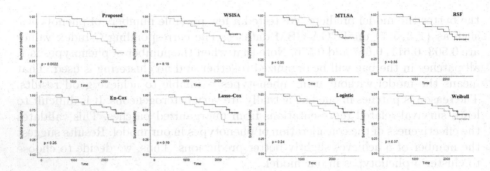

**Fig. 4.** Kaplan-Meier survival curves of different models for NLST dataset. High risk (great than median) groups are plotted as green lines, and low risk (less than or equal to median) groups are plotted as red lines. The x axis shows the time in days and y axis presents the probability of overall survival. Log rank $p$ value is shown on each figure. "+" means the censored patient. (Color figure online)

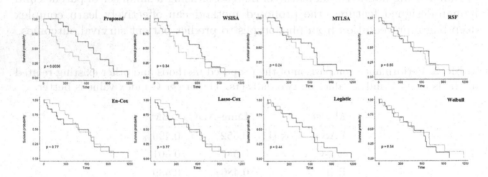

**Fig. 5.** Kaplan-Meier survival curves of different models for GBM dataset.

Given the trained survival models, we can use the estimated testing risk scores to classify patients into low or high-risk group for personalized treatments. Two groups are classified by the median of predicted risk score. Patients with longer survival time should be classified into low risk group and vice versa. We evaluate if those models can correctly classify patients into two groups. We plot Kaplan-Meier survival curves in Fig. 4 on NLST-LungADC data set and Fig. 5 on TCGA-GBM data set. The log rank test is conducted to test the difference of two curves and can evaluate how well the model classify testing patients into low and high risk groups. It is shown that the proposed method can achieve the most significant log rank test outcome while some of others do not reach statistical significances. Kaplan-Meier curves suggest that the proposed comprehensive prediction model can offer better personalized risk scores which can accurately group individuals into two groups. The proposed model has a significant impact on population survival times. It can be used as a recommendation system for offering personalized treatments by determining the relationship between a patient's whole slide pathological images and his or her risk of an event (death).

## 4   Conclusion

We proposed a deep multi-instance model to directly learn survival patterns from gigapixel images without annotations which make it more easily applicable in large scale cancer dataset. Compared to existing image-based survival models, the developed framework can handle various numbers and sizes whole slide images among different patients. It can learn holistic information of the patient using bag representations and achieve much better performance compared to state-of-the-art methods. Future research will focus on how clustering can be integrated into the framework as phenotype clusters are fixed in the current model during training.

**Acknowledgments.** The authors would like to thank the National Cancer Institute for access to NCI's data collected by the National Lung Screening Trial. The statements contained herein are solely of the authors and do not represent or imply concurrence or endorsement by NCI.

## References

1. Bychkov, D., et al.: Deep learning based tissue analysis predicts outcome in colorectal cancer. Sci. Rep. **8**(1), 3395 (2018)
2. Carpenter, A.E., et al.: CellProfiler: image analysis software for identifying and quantifying cell phenotypes. Genome Biol. **7**(10), R100 (2006)
3. Ishwaran, H., Gerds, T.A., Kogalur, U.B., Moore, R.D., Gange, S.J., Lau, B.M.: Random survival forests for competing risks. Biostatistics **15**(4), 757–773 (2014)
4. Lee, E.T., Wang, J.: Statistical Methods for Survival Data Analysis, vol. 476. Wiley, Hoboken (2003)
5. Li, R., Yao, J., Zhu, X., Li, Y., Huang, J.: Graph CNN for survival analysis on whole slide pathological images. In: Frangi, A.F., Schnabel, J.A., Davatzikos, C., Alberola-López, C., Fichtinger, G. (eds.) MICCAI 2018. LNCS, vol. 11071, pp. 174–182. Springer, Cham (2018). https://doi.org/10.1007/978-3-030-00934-2_20
6. Li, Y., Wang, J., Ye, J., Reddy, C.K.: A multi-task learning formulation for survival analysis. In: Proceedings of the 22nd ACM SIGKDD International Conference on Knowledge Discovery and Data Mining, KDD 2016 (2016)
7. Reddy, C.K., Li, Y.: A review of clinical prediction models. In: Healthcare Data Analytics, pp. 343–378. Chapman and Hall/CRC (2015)
8. Simonyan, K., Zisserman, A.: Very deep convolutional networks for large-scale image recognition. arXiv preprint arXiv:1409.1556 (2014)
9. Steck, H., Krishnapuram, B., Dehing-Oberije, C., Lambin, P., Raykar, V.C.: On ranking in survival analysis: bounds on the concordance index. In: Advances in Neural Information Processing Systems, pp. 1209–1216 (2008)
10. Tang, B., Li, A., Li, B., Wang, M.: CapSurv: capsule network for survival analysis with whole slide pathological images. IEEE Access **7**, 26022–26030 (2019)

11. Tibshirani, R., et al.: The lasso method for variable selection in the cox model. Stat. Med. **16**(4), 385–395 (1997)
12. Wang, H., Xing, F., Su, H., Stromberg, A., Yang, L.: Novel image markers for non-small cell lung cancer classification and survival prediction. BMC Bioinform. **15**(1), 310 (2014). http://www.biomedcentral.com/1471-2105/15/310
13. Wang, S., Yao, J., Xu, Z., Huang, J.: Subtype cell detection with an accelerated deep convolution neural network. In: Ourselin, S., Joskowicz, L., Sabuncu, M.R., Unal, G., Wells, W. (eds.) MICCAI 2016. LNCS, vol. 9901, pp. 640–648. Springer, Cham (2016). https://doi.org/10.1007/978-3-319-46723-8_74
14. Yang, H., Zhou, J.T., Cai, J., Ong, Y.S.: MIML-FCN+: multi-instance multi-label learning via fully convolutional networks with privileged information. In: CVPR, pp. 1577–1585 (2017)
15. Yang, Y., Zou, H.: A cocktail algorithm for solving the elastic net penalized cox's regression in high dimensions. Stat. Interface **6**(2), 167–173 (2012)
16. Yao, J., Wang, S., Zhu, X., Huang, J.: Imaging biomarker discovery for lung cancer survival prediction. In: Ourselin, S., Joskowicz, L., Sabuncu, M.R., Unal, G., Wells, W. (eds.) MICCAI 2016. LNCS, vol. 9901, pp. 649–657. Springer, Cham (2016). https://doi.org/10.1007/978-3-319-46723-8_75
17. Yao, J., Zhu, X., Zhu, F., Huang, J.: Deep correlational learning for survival prediction from multi-modality data. In: Descoteaux, M., Maier-Hein, L., Franz, A., Jannin, P., Collins, D.L., Duchesne, S. (eds.) MICCAI 2017. LNCS, vol. 10434, pp. 406–414. Springer, Cham (2017). https://doi.org/10.1007/978-3-319-66185-8_46
18. Yu, K.H., et al.: Predicting non-small cell lung cancer prognosis by fully automated microscopic pathology image features. Nat. Commun. **7**, 12474 (2016)
19. Zhu, X., Yao, J., Huang, J.: Deep convolutional neural network for survival analysis with pathological images. In: 2016 IEEE International Conference on Bioinformatics and Biomedicine (BIBM), pp. 544–547. IEEE (2016)
20. Zhu, X., Yao, J., Zhu, F., Huang, J.: WSISA: making survival prediction from whole slide histopathological images. In: CVPR, pp. 7234–7242 (2017)

# High-Resolution Diabetic Retinopathy Image Synthesis Manipulated by Grading and Lesions

Yi Zhou[✉], Xiaodong He, Shanshan Cui, Fan Zhu, Li Liu, and Ling Shao

Inception Institute of Artificial Intelligence, Abu Dhabi, UAE
yi.zhou@inceptioniai.org

**Abstract.** Diabetic retinopathy (DR) is a complication of diabetes that severely affects eyes, and can be graded into five levels according to international protocol. However, optimizing a grading model with strong generalization ability requires large balanced training data, which is difficult to collect in general but particularly for the high severity levels. Typical data augmentation methods, including flip and rotation cannot generate data with high diversity. In this paper, we propose a diabetic retinopathy generative adversarial network (DR-GAN) to synthesize high-resolution fundus images, which can be manipulated with arbitrary grading and lesion information. Thus, large-scale generated data can be used for more meaningful augmentation to train a DR grading model. The proposed retina generator is conditioned on vessel and lesion masks, and adaptive grading vectors sampled from the latent grading space, which can be adopted to control the synthesized grading severity. Moreover, multiscale discriminators are designed to operate from large to small receptive fields, and joint adversarial losses are adopted to optimize the whole network in an end-to-end manner. With extensive experiments evaluated on the EyePACS dataset connected to Kaggle, we validate the effectiveness of our method, which can both synthesize highly realistic (1280 × 1280) controllable fundus images and contribute to the DR grading task.

## 1 Introduction

Diabetic retinopathy (DR) is a common disease that causes vision damage among people with diabetes. Ophthalmologists usually identify DR severity based on the type and number of related lesions. According to the international protocol [4], the DR severity can be graded into five levels: normal, mild, moderate, severe non-proliferative diabetic retinopathy (NPDR) and PDR. [8,14,16] proposed state-of-the-art deep models to implement DR grading, which obtained significant improvement over conventional methods. Training an effective deep CNN model usually requires a large amount of diverse and balanced data. However, the distribution of DR data over different grades is extremely imbalanced

**Electronic supplementary material** The online version of this chapter (https://doi.org/10.1007/978-3-030-32239-7_56) contains supplementary material, which is available to authorized users.

since the abnormal fundus images only take up a small portion. For example, in EyePACS [1], which is the largest public DR dataset, cases with DR level 3 and 4 only account for 2.35% and 2.16% of images, respectively, while the normal images of level 0 account for 73.67%. Adopting such imbalanced data for training will make a model less sensitive to the samples with higher DR severity levels and lead to overfitting. Although common data augmentation methods such as flip, random crop and rotation, can mitigate the problem, the less diversity of samples still limits a model's performance. Thus, we propose a generative model to synthesize more miscellaneous DR images with different grading levels.

Generative Adversarial Network (GAN) [3], which consists of a generative model $G$ and a discriminative model $D$ competing against each other in a min-max game, have led to great progress in synthesizing photo-realistic images. It has also been explored for synthesizing retinal fundus images. Costa *et al.* [2] and Zhao *et al.* [15] adopted U-Net architectures to transfer vessel segmentation masks to fundus images using a vanilla GAN architecture. However, the generated samples have block defects and do not have controllable grading information. Recently, Niu *et al.* [9] attempted to generate fundus images given the pathological descriptors and vessel segmentation masks. The position and quantity of lesions can be adjusted. However, the synthesized images still needs to be evaluated by ophthalmologists to determine whether or not they are gradable for benefiting grading model. In this work, our generative model can be manipulated with arbitrary grading and lesion information during synthesis; thus, the generated samples can be directly exploited to help train the DR grading model and improve the grading accuracy.

Specifically, our proposed model consists of a high-resolution retina image generator conditioned on vessel and lesion masks, multi-scale discriminators with multi-task learning losses, and an adaptive grading manipulation module to control the severity level of the synthesized DR images. The **main contributions** of our method are highlighted as follows: **1.** A conditional high-resolution image generator is proposed to synthesize retina images with controllable lesion and grading information. In addition to the normal encoder-decoder design, a fine-grained generative design aims to progressively synthesize better and more realistic local details. Moreover, multi-scale discriminators are optimized by the adversarial loss, feature matching loss and grading loss simultaneously. **2.** Adopting real DR images with available grading annotations, we learn different latent grading spaces for randomly sampling adaptive grading vectors. These vectors can be regarded as grading embeddings that help manipulate multi-scale synthesis blocks for more effective generation.

## 2   Proposed Methods

### 2.1   High-Resolution DR Image Generation

To generate high-resolution images [13], we design a two-stage encoder-decoder model that synthesizes $1280 \times 1280$ images. As illustrated in Fig. 1, the building blocks of the retina generator (shown in blue and denoted as $G_m$) aim to

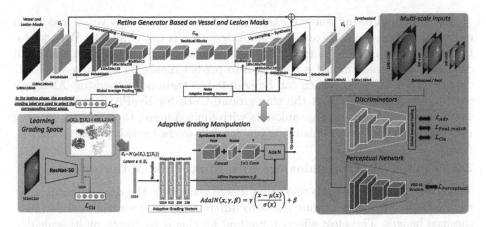

**Fig. 1.** Overview of DR-GAN. A retina generator employs a two-stage encoder-decoder architecture to generate fundus images, which is conditioned on the inputs of vessel and lesion masks. The optimization of the generator is based on an adversarial learning framework with a proposed multi-scale discriminator, which combines multi-task losses for training. Moreover, to better manipulate the grading information of the synthesized image, we propose to learn adaptive grading vectors and embed them into image synthesis blocks to control the appearance of generated lesions. We also found the adaptive grading manipulation can increase the diversity of the synthesized data due to the effective random sampling from the pre-learned latent grading spaces. (Color figure online)

generate images of resolution of $640 \times 640$. Then, the blocks in color of yellow, denoted as $G_l$, can further synthesize better and more realistic local details to increase the resolution to $1280 \times 1280$. **(1)** $G_m$ consists of three parts: encoding blocks, residual blocks and synthesis blocks. The encoding blocks employ a fully-convolutional module with four $Conv$ layers. The kernel size is set to 7 for the first $Conv$ and 3 for the others. We configure a $Conv$ operation with stride 2 rather than using pooling, for downsampling. The padding type is set as the same and a ReLU activation and batch normalization are adopted after each layer. The residual blocks component increases the depth of the network and is proposed to learn better transformation functions and representations through a deeper perceptron. Finally, the synthesis blocks part embedded with an adaptive grading manipulation operation also form a significant component of our model, which is explained in Sect. 2.3. **(2)** $G_l$ has a much simpler design, only including two $Conv$ layers and two corresponding transposed $Conv$ layers. The input for the first transposed $Conv$ layer is the element-wise sum of the feature maps of the last $Conv$ layer of $G_l$ and the feature maps of the last transposed $Conv$ layer of $G_m$. Such a design helps the $G_l$ directly inherit the learned global features from the $G_m$ and further progressively synthesize the local details based on the mask inputs, with a larger resolution. Please note that the $G_m$ is first pre-trained and then the $G_l$ is added for fine-tuning.

The proposed retina generator is conditioned on the input of vessel and lesion masks, since large-scale pixel-level annotated data is not available. We adopt a U-Net architecture [11] to train the segmentation models based on the small dataset. The trained model is then used to predict masks on the large-scale DR dataset (EyePACS [1]), which can be adopted to train our generator. Although the predicted masks are not the true ground-truth for EyePACS data, because they can be produced in large amounts with limited noise, they are nevertheless valuable for training and enhancing our model's overall synthesis performance.

## 2.2 Multi-scale Discriminators with Multi-task Optimization

To better optimize the high-resolution image generator, the discriminator must have receptive fields of various scales to differentiate between the real and synthesized images. The most effective method for this is to design multi-scale discriminators with the identical network structures. In this work, we adopt the original image of size $1280 \times 1280$, as well two downsampled versions of sizes $640 \times 640$ and $320 \times 320$. The three scales of images are passed through three different discriminators $D_n, n \in \{1, 2, 3\}$. The discriminator applied to the smallest scale image provides the largest receptive field to focus on holistic fundus image structure and big lesion patterns. In contrast, the one applied to the largest scale image provides the smallest receptive field to generate more local details and, particularly, small lesion regions. Global average pooling is configured at the end for fitting different scales.

In this work, a multi-task loss is carefully designed to train the generator and discriminator within an adversarial learning architecture. In addition to the normal adversarial loss $\mathcal{L}_{Adv}$ which maximizes the output of the discriminator for generated data, a feature matching loss $\mathcal{L}_{Feat\_match}$ is also adopted to optimize the generator to match the statistics of features in the intermediate layers of the discriminator. Moreover, we also incorporate an auxiliary classification loss $\mathcal{L}_{Cls}$ (adopting focal loss $\mathcal{L}_{focal}$ [7] due to the imbalanced data distribution) to enable the discriminator to learn discriminative representations for DR grading on both the synthesized and real data. For the largest scale input, $\mathcal{L}_{Perceptual}$ is also adopted to equip the model with an additional perceptual network $F$ based on the VGG-19 backbone, which enables more efficient training.

We integrate the input vessel and lesion masks for the generator $G$, which combines $G_m$ and $G_l$, into one conditional map, denoted as $\mathbf{c}$. The corresponding real fundus image and grading label are indicated as $\mathbf{x}$ and $\mathbf{y}$, respectively. The overall training loss is defined in the following equation:

$$\min_G \left( \left( \sum_{n=1,2,3} \max_{D_n} \mathcal{L}_{Adv}(\mathbf{c}, \mathbf{x}) \right) + \lambda_1 \sum_{n=1,2,3} \mathcal{L}_{Feat\_match}(\mathbf{c}, \mathbf{x}) \right) \tag{1}$$

$$+ \lambda_2 \min_{G,F} \mathcal{L}_{Perceptual}(\mathbf{c}, \mathbf{x}) + \lambda_3 \sum_{n=1,2,3} \min_{D_n} \mathcal{L}_{Cls}(\mathbf{c}, \mathbf{x}, \mathbf{y})$$

$$= \min_G \left( \left( \sum_{n=1,2,3} \max_{D_n} (\mathbb{E}[\log D_n(\mathbf{c}, \mathbf{x})] + \mathbb{E}[\log(1 - D_n(\mathbf{c}, G(\mathbf{c})))] \right. \right.$$

$$+ \lambda_1 \sum_{n=1,2,3} (\mathbb{E}[||D_n^p(\mathbf{c}, \mathbf{x}) - D_n^p(\mathbf{c}, G(\mathbf{c}))||_1])) + \lambda_2 \min_{G,F} \mathbb{E}[||F^q(\mathbf{x}) - F^q(G(\mathbf{c}))||_1]$$

$$+ \lambda_3 \sum_{n=1,2,3} \min_{D_n}(\mathcal{L}_{focal}(D_n(\mathbf{x}), \mathbf{y}) + \mathcal{L}_{focal}(D_n(G(\mathbf{c})), \mathbf{y})),$$

where $p$ and $q$ denote the $p^{th}$ and $q^{th}$ intermediate layer in $D_n$ and $F$, respectively. During implementation, we compute all the layers for the feature matching and perceptual loss. $\lambda_1$, $\lambda_2$ and $\lambda_3$ controls the weights of different losses and are set as 10, 10 and 1 for the best result. Finally, a channel-wise concatenation of the conditional maps and the real/synthesized images is conducted on the input of the discriminator.

## 2.3   Adaptive Grading Manipulation

Our ultimate aim is to generate fundus images with controllable DR severity levels, which can be used to augment images and improve the performance of the DR grading model. In this paper, we propose to learn adaptive grading vectors for manipulation in the synthesis blocks. The overall idea is illustrated in the bottom part of Fig. 1. The adaptive grading vectors are learned and sampled from the latent grading spaces. We first employ ResNet-50 to train a DR grading model based on the fundus images, to extract discriminative features. Based on the feature visualization, we can clearly obtain five clusters, each representing one of the five DR grading levels. $X_i, i \in [0, 1, 2, 3, 4]$ defines the five feature sets, where $X = f_{ResNet-50}(\mathbf{x})$. For each set of a particular grading level, we compute the mean $\mu(X_i)$ and variance $\Sigma(X_i)$ to model the corresponding normal distribution space. Once the five latent grading distributions are learned, we randomly sample latent vectors $\mathbf{z} \in \mathcal{Z}_i$, where $\mathcal{Z}_i$ is subject to $\mathcal{N}(\mu(X_i), \Sigma(X_i))$. During the training phase, based on the grading ground-truth of an input pair of mask and real image, a latent vector $\mathbf{z}$ is sampled from the corresponding space. Inspired by [6], a four-layer non-linear mapping network is first devised to encode $\mathbf{z}$ via affine transformations, which can benefit the generator manipulated by grading. We take the latent grading vectors as inputs for the synthesis blocks. In each synthesis block, the feature maps $Feat$ are first concatenated with a random noise whose number of channels is quarter that of $Feat$. Then, a $1 \times 1$ $Conv$ is applied to fuse the features. Adaptive instance normalization (AdaIN) [5] embeds the grading vectors, as shown in Fig. 1. A fused feature $x$ is normalized individually. $\gamma$ and $\beta$ are the scale and bias vectors learned from the adaptive grading vectors. In each synthesis block with different channel-wise dimension of feature maps, the corresponding grading vector is split into the $\gamma$ and $\beta$.

**Testing Phase.** Based on the input vessel and lesion masks from the testing phase, we need to select which grading distribution to sample the latent vector from for grading manipulation. To address this problem, an additional convolution and global average pooling are inserted after the last encoding block to further train the grading function. During testing, the predicted grading label is used for the selection. Moreover, once the whole model is trained, we can automatically imitate multiple lesion masks for one vessel mask to synthesize various fundus images with controllable grading labels.

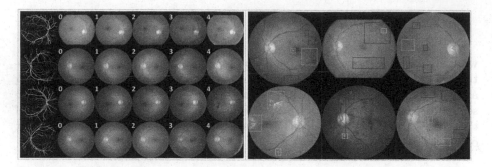

**Fig. 2.** Examples of synthesized images (**1280** × **1280**, best viewed zoomed in). Left: for a given an input vessel, the corresponding DR images with five different grading levels are generated. Right: the detailed synthesized lesion patterns are demonstrated. The red, yellow, green and blue bounding-boxes indicate the hemorrhages, hard exudates, soft exudates and microaneurysms, respectively. (Color figure online)

## 3   Experimental Evaluation

### 3.1   Evaluation of Image Synthesis

**Datasets.** To train the whole DR-GAN model, large-scale data with pixel-wise annotated vessels and lesion masks are required. However, the **EyePACS** [1] only contains grading labels. Thus, we adopt the small-scale DRIVE [12] and IDRID [10] datasets, which include pixel-level annotations to train the vessel and lesion segmentation models, respectively, and then perform inference on EyePACS to obtain masks that can be coarsely used as the weak ground-truths for training the DR-GAN.

Before evaluating the quantitative improvement of the DR grading performance by data augmentation with synthesized data, we first qualitatively demonstrate the generated image fidelity and evaluate the controllability under different grading and lesion conditions. In this work, we mainly adopt the training samples from the EyePACS, as well as the extracted vessel and lesion masks, to train the model. Once this is done, for each vessel mask, we can arbitrarily control the quantity and position of the lesion spots within the corresponding masks to synthesize images with different degrees of DR. Specifically, by manipulating the lesion masks, the corresponding grading labels can be coarsely predicted. Thus, we synthesize 10,000 images for each grading level to augment the data. The left part of Fig. 2 provides the examples of various vessel structures and their corresponding synthesized images exhibiting different degrees of DR. We find that the fidelity of generated images and the manipulation performance by lesion and grading are highly promising. For example, only microaneurysms will appear in the grade 0 and 1 in most of the cases. Hard exudates will be increasingly more with the more severe DR level. Hemorrhages and soft exudates will mainly appear in the 3 and 4. The right of Fig. 2 shows more detailed examples of synthesized lesion appearances, such as microaneurysms, hemorrhages, soft and hard exudates. More examples can be found in the supplementary document.

To conduct a quantitative evaluation of image synthesis, we deploy the Freshet Inception Distance (FID) to evaluate the quality. In FID, we use the Inception network to extract features from an intermediate layer. Then we model the data distribution for these features using a multivariate Gaussian distribution with mean $\mu$ and covariance $\Sigma$. The results are reported in the supplementary file.

## 3.2 Data Augmentation by Synthesis for DR Grading

Our biggest concern is to evaluate whether or not the synthesized data can mitigate the unbalanced data distribution over different grading levels and be beneficial for training the grading models. We train the baselines for the grading model, which adopt three different classic backbones (VGG-16, ResNet-50 and Inception-v3), with and without using the synthesized data for augmentation. Some state-of-the-art approaches are also re-implemented and compared.

**Table 1.** Evaluation of augmentation by synthesized data.

| Settings | Tr-Real Te-Fake | | Tr-Real Te-Real | | Tr-Real & Fake Te-Real | |
|---|---|---|---|---|---|---|
| Backbones | Acc. | Kappa | Acc. | Kappa | Acc. | Kappa |
| VGG-16 | 87.52 | 86.14 | 84.92 | 82.13 | 86.15 | 84.45 |
| ResNet-50 | 89.16 | 87.93 | 86.24 | 83.82 | 87.84 | 85.76 |
| Inception-v3 | 88.23 | 87.09 | 85.80 | 83.44 | 87.41 | 85.23 |
| Zoom-in [14] | 89.54 | 88.23 | 86.51 | 85.19 | 88.23 | 86.45 |
| AFN [8] | 90.20 | 88.96 | 87.64 | 85.78 | 88.97 | 86.92 |

**Table 2.** Evaluation of the effectiveness of each designed module.

| Settings | Tr-Real Te-Fake | | Tr-Real & Fake Te-Real | |
|---|---|---|---|---|
| Baselines-Res50 | Acc. | Kappa | Acc. | Kappa |
| ResNet-50 | 89.16 | 87.93 | 87.84 | 85.76 |
| w/o Lesion Masks | 76.27 | 72.31 | 84.16 | 80.55 |
| w/o AGM | 86.35 | 84.28 | 86.45 | 84.09 |
| w/o $\mathcal{L}_{Perceptual}$ | 87.24 | 86.42 | 86.97 | 84.78 |
| w/o $\mathcal{L}_{Cls}$ in D | 87.45 | 86.03 | 86.73 | 83.92 |

We configure two experimental settings. For the first setting, we train the grading models only using the real samples from the EyePACS training set and test on the synthesized data. For the second one, we combine the training set of EyePACS and the synthesized data for training, and evaluate on the testing set of EyePACS. As illustrated in the Table 1, both the classification accuracy and the quadratic weighted kappa metric [1] are adopted for evaluation. First, the model trained on the real data with grading ground-truths, achieves a highly promising grading performance on the synthesized data. The best classification accuracy 90.20% and the kappa value 88.96% are obtained by the AFN [8] model. Under the second setting, where real test images from EyePACS are supplemented with synthesized data during training, results show that consistent improvement is achieved across all five approaches. The accuracy increases on average by 1.50% and the kappa is increased by 1.69%. We believe that once we obtain more training data with more accurate lesion masks, the proposed DR-GAN will be further enhanced and contribute to the grading performance more significantly.

## 3.3   Ablation Studies

To separately evaluate the effectiveness of manipulation using lesion and grading information, as well as the contribution of the multi-loss training, we conducted four ablation studies based on the baseline ResNet-50. **Without (w/o) Lesion Masks:** We first study the effect of removing the input lesion masks and only use the grading manipulation module by arbitrarily selecting the latent grading space. **w/o adaptive grading manipulation (AGM):** Similarly, we investigate the effectiveness of the AGM module by detaching it while keeping the input lesion masks. **w/o** $\mathcal{L}_{Perceptual}$ and **w/o** $\mathcal{L}_{Cls}$ are also explored for their respective contributions to the overall loss functions. Table 2 compares the grading performance of each baseline. We find that dropping the input of the lesion masks significantly affects the grading performance due to the poor quality of synthesized lesion patterns. Thus, augmentation by the generated data cannot contribute to the grading model. Besides, compared to the model without AGM, this design can increase the grading result by a margin of 1.67% in terms of kappa. The AGM can improve the fidelity and diversity of the synthesized lesion appearances within the corresponding grading levels. Moreover, dropping either the $\mathcal{L}_{Perceptual}$ or $\mathcal{L}_{Cls}$ in the multi-loss training will both reduce the performance. Specifically, for the discriminator without the embedded $\mathcal{L}_{Cls}$, the grading accuracy decreases by 1.11%, while the kappa value decreases by 1.84%.

## 4   Conclusion

In this paper, we proposed an effective high-resolution DR image generation model that is conditioned on the grading and lesion information. The synthesized data can be used for data augmentation, particularly for those abnormal images with severe DR levels, to improve the performance of grading models. Moreover, the synthesized data can be also used for training junior ophthalmologists. In the future work, more real annotated pixel-level lesion masks will be added for training DR-GAN better.

## References

1. Kaggle diabetic retinopathy detection competition. https://www.kaggle.com/c/diabetic-retinopathy-detection
2. Costa, P., et al.: Towards adversarial retinal image synthesis. arXiv preprint arXiv:1701.08974 (2017)
3. Goodfellow, I., et al.: Generative adversarial nets. In: NIPS, pp. 2672–2680 (2014)
4. Gulshan, V., et al.: Development and validation of a deep learning algorithm for detection of diabetic retinopathy in retinal fundus photographs. JAMA **316**(22), 2402–2410 (2016)
5. Huang, X., Belongie, S.: Arbitrary style transfer in real-time with adaptive instance normalization. In: IEEE ICCV, pp. 1501–1510 (2017)
6. Karras, T., Laine, S., Aila, T.: A style-based generator architecture for generative adversarial networks. arXiv preprint arXiv:1812.04948 (2018)

7. Lin, T.Y., Goyal, P., Girshick, R., He, K., Dollár, P.: Focal loss for dense object detection. In: IEEE ICCV, pp. 2980–2988 (2017)
8. Lin, Z., et al.: A framework for identifying diabetic retinopathy based on anti-noise detection and attention-based fusion. In: Frangi, A.F., Schnabel, J.A., Davatzikos, C., Alberola-López, C., Fichtinger, G. (eds.) MICCAI 2018. LNCS, vol. 11071, pp. 74–82. Springer, Cham (2018). https://doi.org/10.1007/978-3-030-00934-2_9
9. Niu, Y., et al.: Pathological evidence exploration in deep retinal image diagnosis. arXiv preprint arXiv:1812.02640 (2018)
10. Porwal, P., et al.: Indian diabetic retinopathy image dataset (IDRID): a database for diabetic retinopathy screening research. Data 3(3), 25 (2018)
11. Ronneberger, O., Fischer, P., Brox, T.: U-Net: convolutional networks for biomedical image segmentation. In: Navab, N., Hornegger, J., Wells, W.M., Frangi, A.F. (eds.) MICCAI 2015. LNCS, vol. 9351, pp. 234–241. Springer, Cham (2015). https://doi.org/10.1007/978-3-319-24574-4_28
12. Staal, J., Abràmoff, M.D., Niemeijer, M., Viergever, M.A., Van Ginneken, B.: Ridge-based vessel segmentation in color images of the retina. IEEE Transactions on Medical Imaging 23(4), 501–509 (2004)
13. Wang, T.C., Liu, M.Y., Zhu, J.Y., Tao, A., Kautz, J., Catanzaro, B.: High-resolution image synthesis and semantic manipulation with conditional GANs. In: IEEE CVPR, pp. 8798–8807 (2018)
14. Wang, Z., Yin, Y., Shi, J., Fang, W., Li, H., Wang, X.: Zoom-in-Net: deep mining lesions for diabetic retinopathy detection. In: Descoteaux, M., Maier-Hein, L., Franz, A., Jannin, P., Collins, D.L., Duchesne, S. (eds.) MICCAI 2017. LNCS, vol. 10435, pp. 267–275. Springer, Cham (2017). https://doi.org/10.1007/978-3-319-66179-7_31
15. Zhao, H., Li, H., Maurer-Stroh, S., Cheng, L.: Synthesizing retinal and neuronal images with generative adversarial nets. Med. Image Anal. 49, 14–26 (2018)
16. Zhou, Y., et al.: Collaborative learning of semi-supervised segmentation and classification for medical images. In: IEEE CVPR (2019)

# Deep Instance-Level Hard Negative Mining Model for Histopathology Images

Meng Li, Lin Wu[✉], Arnold Wiliem, Kun Zhao, Teng Zhang, and Brian Lovell

School of ITEE, The University of Queensland, Brisbane, QLD 4072, Australia
{meng.li,lin.wu,k.zhao1,patrick.zhang}@uq.edu.au,
arnold.wiliem@ieee.org, lovell@itee.uq.edu.au

**Abstract.** Histopathology image analysis can be considered as a Multiple instance learning (MIL) problem, where the whole slide histopathology image (WSI) is regarded as a bag of instances (*i.e.*, patches) and the task is to predict a single class label to the WSI. However, in many real-life applications such as computational pathology, discovering the key instances that trigger the bag label is of great interest because it provides reasons for the decision made by the system. In this paper, we propose a deep convolutional neural network (CNN) model that addresses the primary task of a bag classification on a histopathology image and also learns to identify the response of each instance to provide interpretable results to the final prediction. We incorporate the attention mechanism into the proposed model to operate the transformation of instances and learn attention weights to allow us to find key patches. To perform a balanced training, we introduce adaptive weighing in each training bag to explicitly adjust the weight distribution in order to concentrate more on the contribution of hard samples. Based on the learned attention weights, we further develop a solution to boost the classification performance by generating the bags with hard negative instances. We conduct extensive experiments on colon and breast cancer histopathology data and show that our framework achieves state-of-the-art performance.

## 1 Introduction

Deep learning has become increasingly popular in the medical imaging area. However, due to high computational cost, working on whole slide histopathology images (WSIs) with gigapixel resolution is challenging. As a consequence, some approaches attempt to divide WSIs into small patches [5], and predict the final diagnosis of a WSI without providing the pixel-level annotations. To alleviate the annotation efforts, multiple instance learning (MIL) is introduced and explored for weakly annotated WSIs [21], where a WSI is considered as a bag, and the patches of that WSI are regarded as instances. Hence, the problem is cast as dealing with a bag of instances for which a single class label is assigned to

**Electronic supplementary material** The online version of this chapter (https://doi.org/10.1007/978-3-030-32239-7_57) contains supplementary material, which is available to authorized users.

© Springer Nature Switzerland AG 2019
D. Shen et al. (Eds.): MICCAI 2019, LNCS 11764, pp. 514–522, 2019.
https://doi.org/10.1007/978-3-030-32239-7_57

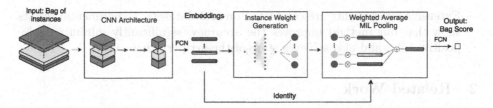

**Fig. 1.** The architecture of the end-to-end deep CNN model with adaptive attention mechanism. The input is the bag of instances (patches of each WSI), which are fed into a CNN model to produce the latent representation of each instance. Then the embeddings of instances go through a fully connected network with the attention weights generated. The learned weights are multiplied with the embeddings of instances in element-wise to be classified by the classifier.

the WSI. However, providing insights into the contribution of each instance to the bag label is crucial to medical diagnosis. Furthermore, if the features of the negative instances are not well learned, the model will be prone to predict a bag with many negative instances to be a positive bag because of the bias issue [4]. In Liu et al.'s work [11], the concept of key instances is discussed, which indicates that in the MIL task, discovering the key instances that trigger the bag label is critical. Thus, one reason for a model to make a wrong prediction about a negative bag is that some challenging instances mislead the model. This will affect decision making of a medical diagnosis model, as a single challenging instance in a WSI may lead to a wrong diagnosis result. The challenging instances herein are referred to as **hard negative patches (instances)** which are incorrectly classified as positive by the prediction model. The other prominent challenge in training a deep model for WSIs is the training imbalance, which means the model tends to become biased towards learning from limited negative patches together with many positive patches.

To address these challenges, we propose an approach that generates the hard negative instances in histopathology images based on instance-level adaptive weighting. Specifically, we incorporate the attention mechanism into the training model, which is computed with adaptive weight loss to explicitly assign larger weights to hard negative instances. The selected instances are used to constitute hard training bags through a bag generation algorithm to further improve the training accuracy. The overview of our framework is shown in Fig. 1. The major contributions of this paper are summarised below.

- We propose a MIL model that incorporates adaptive attention mechanism into an end-to-end deep CNN to detect key instances for histopathology image analysis.
- We present a strategy that is able to address the training imbalance issue through adaptive weighting distribution on negative samples.
- We develop a bag generation algorithm based on the selected hard negative instances and compose the hard bags for the improved classification training.

– Extensive experiments are conducted on real datasets. Experimental results show that our method improves the accuracy, significantly minimizes false positive rate, and also achieves state-of-the-art performance.

## 2   Related Work

**MIL on Histopathology Images.** Different MIL approaches were proposed to work on medical images [2,5,7,10]. A two-stage Expectation Maximization based algorithm combined with a deep convolutional neural network (CNN) works well to classify instances on multiple medical datasets [5]. In Kandemir et al.'s work [7], a Gaussian process with relational learning is introduced to exploit the similarity between instances of Barrett's cancer dataset. To relate the instances and the bags, different permutation-invariant pooling approaches with CNN have been proposed. One solution is noisy-and pooling function with CNN, which has achieved promising results on medical images [10]. Couture et al. [2] adopt an instance-based approach and aggregate the predictions of patches by using a quantile function on breast cancer. In this paper, our work aims to augment the CNN training with attention mechanism to attentively select hard samples, which achieves state-of-the-art performance on colon cancer and breast cancer dataset [7,16].

**Instance-Level Weights.** The attention mechanism has become well known in deep learning, especially for natural language processing tasks and image representation learning [8,9,22–24]. For MIL problems, attention is represented by the weights of each instance in a bag, a higher weight means more attention. The method to obtain instance weights was first proposed in Pappas and Popescu-Beliss's work [13], where the weights of instances were trained in a linear regression model. They improved the previous method by using a single layer neural network [14]. A more recent solution was introduced, where the weights were learned by a two-layer neural network [6]. However, these works did not further analyze the generated attention weights. In this work, we propose a method that exploits the relation among the weights and reuses them to improve the model performance.

**Hard Negative Mining.** The main idea of hard negative mining is to repeatedly bootstrap negative examples by selecting false positives which the detector incorrectly classifies [3]. Hard negative mining is originally used in object detection tasks, where the datasets usually involve overwhelming easy examples [15]. Recently, this simple but effective technique is commonly used in the medical domain. Difficult negative regions are extracted from the training set to boost model performance on lymph nodes [19] and breast cancer WSIs [1]. Whilst these works make advances in this domain, to our knowledge, there is no work which addresses hard negative mining for MIL tasks. In this paper, we propose an approach which is able to detect hard negative instances by utilizing the attention weight given for each instance in a bag. Based on this, we propose several hard negative bag generation algorithms. As shown in the experiment, our proposed approach achieves significant improvement in comparison with the baselines.

## 3  Our Method

Given a histology image (bag) $\mathbf{X_i}$ with its label $C \in \{0,1\}$, and its instances $X_{ij} \in \mathbf{X_i}$, $j = 1, 2, ..., N_i$, our goal is to identify a set of hard negative instances from negative bags $\mathbf{X_i}$ with $C_i = 0$. We define $\hat{\mathbf{X}}_i = \{\mathbf{h_1}, \mathbf{h_2}, ..., \mathbf{h_M}\}$ as the set of hard negative instances identified from the negative bags. We generate hard negative bags from $\hat{\mathbf{X}}_i$ and use these bags in the training step to improve accuracy. To this end, we develop an instance-level, attention-based CNN model which determines the instance weights by inspecting their corresponding response to contribute the final prediction outcome. The attention selection of key instances allows us to detect the hard negative instances leading to false positives. Then, we propose a bag generation algorithm which produces new bags with selected hard negative patches for retraining.

**Instance-Level Adaptive Weighing Attention.** We implement a neural network $f_\phi(\cdot)$ to transform the $j$-th instance in the $i$-th bag into a low-dimensional embedding $g_{ij} = f_\phi(X_{ij})$, where $g_{ij} \in \mathbb{R}^M$. To get the bag representation which is permutation-invariant, a max or a mean aggregation is usually used in the MIL problem [10]. However, neither of them can be trained to get the instance weights which are needed in our case. As a result, a weighted average aggregation method is used. Given the embedding-based instances $G_i = \{g_{i1}, g_{i2}, ..., g_{iN_i}\}$, the weighted average is shown as follows:

$$z_i = \sum_{j=1}^{N_i} w_{ij} g_{ij}, \quad w_{ij} = \frac{\exp(\mathbf{v}_i^\top \frac{U_i g_{ij}^\top}{1+|U_i g_{ij}^\top|})}{\sum_{j=1}^{N_i} \exp(\mathbf{v}_i^\top \frac{U_i g_{ij}^\top}{1+|U_i g_{ij}^\top|})} \tag{1}$$

In (1), $\mathbf{v}_i \in \mathbb{R}^{L \times 1}$ and $\mathbf{U}_i \in \mathbb{R}^{L \times M}$ are the attention network weight parameters. A softsign activation function is implemented to ensure proper gradient flow. We normalize the weights $w_{ij}$ through a softmax function so that all the weights sum to 1. However, the weights defined in (1) are not constrained and could make all the instances receive uniformly distributed weights, which would make it difficult to identify hard negative instances. To this end, we introduce an adaptive weighting method to explicitly enlarge the weights difference between the positive and negative instances:

$$z_i = \sum_{j=1}^{N_i - N_{in}} w_{ij} g_{ij} + \lambda \sum_{j=1}^{N_{in}} w_{ij} g_{ij}, \tag{2}$$

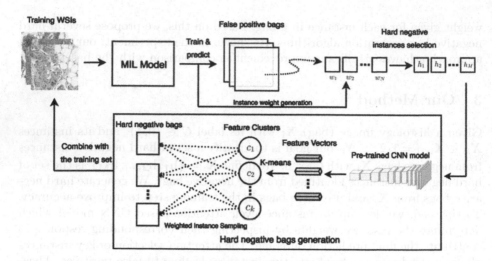

**Fig. 2.** The proposed novel hard negative mining process. The training images are first fed into the deep MIL model with balanced training to select instances to constitute the false positive bags. We learn attention weights for instances, which can be used to select the hard instances that fool the model to make the wrong prediction. Next, the hard negative instances are grouped to form the new hard negative bags by a bag generation algorithm. The patches firstly go through a pre-trained CNN model without the last layer to produce the feature vectors. A K-means clustering is then used to group features into clusters from which hard negative bags are produced by randomly sampling instances across feature clusters dynamically. Finally, the training is augmented with hard negative bags for improved accuracy.

where $N_{in} = |\{X_{ij}|j \in pseudo\ negative\ instances\}|$ is the number of pseudo negative instances. In each iteration, the instances are treated as pseudo negative by thresholding on the average weights in each cycle. The balancing hyper-parameter $\lambda$ is empirically set to 2 in our paper. We note that when $\lambda$ is set $> 1$, the weights of the pseudo negative instances will be reduced. This will increase the differences between the positive instance and the negative instances. After obtaining the weighted embeddings, we use a CNN layer for classification. In the end, the weights of instances are learned so that we can make use of them to mine the hard negative instances.

**Hard Negative Instance Mining.** After the training process finishes, we obtain the false positive bags $\{B_1, B_2, ..., B_N\}$, where each bag $B_l$ has the corresponding weights of instances as $\{w_{l1}, w_{l2}, ..., w_{lN_l}\}$, via selecting the hard negative instances through attention weights:

$$H_l = \{w_{li} \mid w_{li} \geq \sigma_l + \overline{w_l}\} \tag{3}$$

where $\sigma_l$ is the standard deviation and $\overline{w_l}$ is the mean of the weights in the $l$-th bag. We group all hard negative instances from all false positive bags together and obtain the bag $\hat{X}_i = \{\mathbf{h_1}, \mathbf{h_2}, ..., \mathbf{h_M}\}$.

**Hard Negative Bag Generation.** In this stage, new hard negative bags are generated for re-training the network to further improve the bag prediction accuracy. As histology images contain a variety of patterns in negative regions [20], we propose to select diverse patches into each negative bag such that the deep model will learn features comprehensively. The overview of the bag generation process is shown in Fig. 2. The hard negative instances first go through a pre-trained CNN model to convert to feature vectors. The features are then clustered by the K-means algorithm into $c$ feature groups $C_1, C_2, ..., C_c$, which contain $N_1, N_2, ..., N_c$ items. To conform to the training set bag size, we empirically generate the $i$-th new bag $B_i$ which has a Gaussian random size with $\sigma$ and $\mu$, where $\sigma$ is the standard deviation and $\mu$ is the mean of all training bag sizes. We limit the size from $Z_{min}$ to $Z_{max}$ where $Z_{min}$ and $Z_{max}$ are the minimum and maximum bag size respectively of the training set. We follow a weighted sampling strategy that randomly selects instances from each cluster and puts in $B_i$. The possibility to designate a cluster to sample instance is denoted as $P_j = \frac{N_j}{\sum_{j=1}^{c} N_j}$.

## 4    Experiments

**Datasets.** We conduct experiments on two public datasets: Colon Cancer dataset [16] and UCSB dataset [7]. Colon Cancer dataset involves 100 Hematoxylin and Eosin stained (H&E) images from 9 patients at $0.55\mu$m/pixel resolution. The histology images include multiple tissue appearance that belongs to both normal and malignant regions, and can be either used for detection or classification. In total, 22,444 nuclei are annotated in four classes, $i.e.$ epithelial, inflammatory, fibroblast, and miscellaneous. A histology image is positive if it consists of at least one epithelial nucleus. We divide each image into 27 × 27 patches. The UCSB dataset contains 58 H&E stained image excerpts (26 malignant, 32 benign) from breast cancer patients. The histology image size is 896 × 768 and we divide each image into 32 × 32 patches. To reduce the noisy patches, each image is converted from the RGB color space to the HSV space, and an Otsu algorithm is used to select the optimal threshold values in each channel to filter the patches [12]. The patches are randomly flipped and rotated for augmentation. Finally, the color normalization (histogram equalization) is performed on each patch.

**Implementation Details.** We adopt a deep CNN architecture [16] and a MIL pooling layer [6] to extract features and a fully connected layer to make the classification. More detailed treatment for the architecture can be found in the supplementary material. We follow the work [6], and train the network using an Adam optimizer with $\beta_1 = 0.9$ and $\beta_2 = 0.999$. A cross-entropy loss function is used for regression. For the Colon Cancer/UCSB dataset, we set the learning rate

**Table 1.** Evaluation of different methods for colon cancer data. The average of five experiments with its corresponding standard error is reported. SB: single bag hard negative mining, MB: multiple bags with random sampling, FMB: multiple bags with features clustering sampling, AUC: area under the curve, FPR: false positive rate.

| Method | Accuracy | Precision | Recall | F-score | AUC | FPR |
|---|---|---|---|---|---|---|
| MIL model [6] | $0.904 \pm 0.011$ | $0.953 \pm 0.014$ | $0.855 \pm 0.017$ | $0.901 \pm 0.011$ | $0.968 \pm 0.009$ | NA |
| Our model | $0.906 \pm 0.007$ | $0.912 \pm 0.010$ | $0.916 \pm 0.012$ | $0.905 \pm 0.008$ | $0.952 \pm 0.012$ | $0.104 \pm 0.012$ |
| Our model+SB | $0.922 \pm 0.004$ | $0.937 \pm 0.011$ | $0.920 \pm 0.014$ | $0.920 \pm 0.005$ | $0.979 \pm 0.004$ | $0.084 \pm 0.012$ |
| Our model+MB | $0.942 \pm 0.005$ | $0.963 \pm 0.010$ | $\mathbf{0.928 \pm 0.017}$ | $0.939 \pm 0.006$ | $0.982 \pm 0.009$ | $0.052 \pm 0.010$ |
| Our model+FMB | $\mathbf{0.948 \pm 0.004}$ | $\mathbf{0.980 \pm 0.003}$ | $\mathbf{0.920 \pm 0.006}$ | $\mathbf{0.945 \pm 0.004}$ | $\mathbf{0.983 \pm 0.004}$ | $\mathbf{0.036 \pm 0.007}$ |

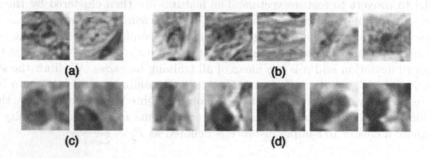

**Fig. 3.** Positive and hard negative examples: (a) Colon data: instances that include malignant regions. (b) Colon data: detected hard negative instances that mislead the model to predict a normal bag into a malignant result. (c) UCSB data: instances that include malignant regions. (d) UCSB data: detected hard negative instances that mislead the model to predict a normal bag into a malignant result.

$= 5 \times 10^{-5}/5 \times 10^{-6}$ and weight decay $= 5 \times 10^{-4}/1 \times 10^{-4}$. Each experiment runs for $120/300$ epochs, and the epoch with the lowest loss is chosen for evaluation. We evaluate our method using 10-fold/4-fold cross-validation and five repetitions for each experiment. To ensure fair comparison, we test on the same set of bags in each fold for the methods.

**Results and Discussion.** Tables 1 and 2 show the results of our method against different baselines on two datasets. We compare different hard negative mining strategies, *i.e.*, the single hard negative bag generation (SB), the randomly generated multiple bags (MB), and the features clustering bags (FMB). Among these methods, the proposed FMB solution has an overall better result than the others and sets the new state-of-the-art result for colon cancer dataset. For the UCSB dataset, We achieve the same area under the curve (AUC) result as the state-of-the-art method in Song et al.'s work [17]. Figure 3 demonstrates the detected hard negative instances by our solution. It is noticeable that compared to the baseline method, the false positive rate (FPR) is significantly decreased, and the recall is increased by including hard negative mining, which is particularly essential in histopathology image diagnosis because both false positive and

**Table 2.** Evaluation of different methods for the UCSB dataset. The average of five experiments with its corresponding standard error is reported. SB: single bag hard negative mining, MB: multiple bags with random sampling, FMB: multiple bags with features clustering sampling, AUC: area under the curve, FPR: false positive rate.

| Method | Accuracy | Precision | Recall | F-score | AUC | FPR |
|---|---|---|---|---|---|---|
| MIL model [6] | $0.755 \pm 0.016$ | $0.728 \pm 0.016$ | $0.731 \pm 0.042$ | $0.725 \pm 0.023$ | $0.799 \pm 0.020$ | NA |
| SDR+SVM [17] | **0.983** | NA | NA | NA | **0.999** | NA |
| Our model | $0.821 \pm 0.006$ | $0.870 \pm 0.032$ | $0.800 \pm 0.038$ | $0.806 \pm 0.011$ | $0.942 \pm 0.008$ | $0.220 \pm 0.058$ |
| Our model+SB | $0.893 \pm 0.001$ | $0.920 \pm 0.012$ | $0.886 \pm 0.024$ | $0.887 \pm 0.015$ | $0.949 \pm 0.006$ | $0.140 \pm 0.019$ |
| Our model+MB | $0.936 \pm 0.004$ | $0.936 \pm 0.011$ | $0.943 \pm 0.014$ | $0.935 \pm 0.005$ | $0.967 \pm 0.004$ | $0.100 \pm 0.016$ |
| Our model+FMB | $\mathbf{0.975 \pm 0.008}$ | $\mathbf{0.975 \pm 0.012}$ | $\mathbf{0.979 \pm 0.009}$ | $\mathbf{0.975 \pm 0.007}$ | $\mathbf{0.999 \pm 0.001}$ | $\mathbf{0.040 \pm 0.019}$ |

false negative could result in severe consequences for patients. It is also critical that the AUC is increased, as this indicates that the generated hard negative bags do not cause class imbalance issues.

## 5  Conclusions

In this paper, we introduce an effective approach to MIL tasks on histopathology data that incorporates the attention mechanism with adaptive weighing into the deep CNNs for balanced training. To further improve the training accuracy, we develop a novel hard negative mining strategy by generating the bags with hard negative instances. Experimental results demonstrate that our approach makes a decent improvement from the baseline method and achieves state-of-the-art performance. In future work, we plan to evaluate our model on the larger WSIs. Moreover, we intend to generalize our model to the multi-class task not limited in the binary classification.

**Acknowledgement.** This research was funded by the Australian Government through the Australian Research Council and Sullivan Nicolaides Pathology under Linkage Project LP160101797.

## References

1. Bejnordi, B.E., et al.: Deep learning-based assessment of tumor-associated stroma for diagnosing breast cancer in histopathology images. In: ISBI (2017)
2. Couture, H.D., Marron, J.S., Perou, C.M., Troester, M.A., Niethammer, M.: Multiple instance learning for heterogeneous images: training a CNN for histopathology. In: Frangi, A.F., Schnabel, J.A., Davatzikos, C., Alberola-López, C., Fichtinger, G. (eds.) MICCAI 2018. LNCS, vol. 11071, pp. 254–262. Springer, Cham (2018). https://doi.org/10.1007/978-3-030-00934-2_29
3. Dalal, N., Triggs, B.: Histograms of oriented gradients for human detection. In: CVPR (2005)
4. Han, Y., et al.: Avoiding false positive in multi-instance learning. In: NIPS (2010)
5. Hou, L., et al.: Patch-based convolutional neural network for whole slide tissue image classification. In: CVPR (2016)

6. Ilse, M., Tomczak, J., Welling, M.: Attention-based deep multiple instance learning. In: ICML (2018)
7. Kandemir, M., Zhang, C., Hamprecht, F.A.: Empowering multiple instance histopathology cancer diagnosis by cell graphs. In: Golland, P., Hata, N., Barillot, C., Hornegger, J., Howe, R. (eds.) MICCAI 2014. LNCS, vol. 8674, pp. 228–235. Springer, Cham (2014). https://doi.org/10.1007/978-3-319-10470-6_29
8. Wu, L., Wang, Y., Gao, J., Li, X.: Where-and-when to look: deep Siamese attention networks for video-based person re-identification. IEEE Trans. Multimed. (2019)
9. Lin, W., Wang, Y., Li, X., Gao, J.: Deep attention-based spatially recursive networks for fine-grained visual recognition. IEEE Trans. Cybern. **49**(5), 1791–1802 (2019)
10. Kraus, O.Z., Ba, J.L., Frey, B.J.: Classifying and segmenting microscopy images with deep multiple instance learning. In: Bioinformatics (2016)
11. Liu, G., Wu, J., Zhou, Z.-H.: Key instance detection in multi-instance learning. In: ACML (2012)
12. Otsu, N.: A threshold selection method from gray-level histograms. In: SMCS (1979)
13. Pappas, N., Popescu-Belis, A.: Explaining the stars: weighted multiple-instance learning for aspect-based sentiment analysis. In: EMNLP (2014)
14. Pappas, N., Popescu-Belis, A.: Explicit document modeling through weighted multiple-instance learning. In: JAIR (2017)
15. Shrivastava, A., Gupta, A., Girshick, R.: Training region-based object detectors with online hard example mining. In: CVPR (2016)
16. Sirinukunwattana, K., et al.: Locality sensitive deep learning for detection and classification of nuclei in routine colon cancer histology images. In: T-MI (2016)
17. Song, Y., Li, Q., Huang, H., Feng, D., Chen, M., Cai, W.: Low dimensional representation of fisher vectors for microscopy image classification. In: T-MI (2017)
18. Sun, M., Han, T.X., Liu, M.C., Khodayari-Rostamabad, A.: Multiple instance learning convolutional neural networks for object recognition. In: ICPR (2016)
19. Wang, D., et al.: Deep learning for identifying metastatic breast cancer. arXiv preprint arXiv:1606.05718 (2016)
20. Xu, Y., et al.: Multiple clustered instance learning for histopathology cancer image classification, segmentation and clustering. In: CVPR, June 2012
21. Xu, Y., et al.: Deep learning of feature representation with multiple instance learning for medical image analysis. In: ICASSP (2014)
22. Wu, L., Wang, Y., Gao, J., Li, X.: Deep adaptive feature embedding with local sample distributions for person re-identification. Pattern Recogn. **73**, 275–288 (2018)
23. Lin, W., Wang, Y., Li, X., Gao, J.: Deep attention-based spatially recursive networks for fine-grained visual recognition. IEEE Trans. Cybern. **49**(5), 1791–1802 (2019)
24. Wu, L., Wang, Y., Shao, L.: Cycle-consistent deep generative hashing for cross-modal retrieval. IEEE Trans. Image Process. (2019)

# Synthetic Patches, Real Images: Screening for Centrosome Aberrations in EM Images of Human Cancer Cells

Artem Lukoyanov[1,2], Isabella Haberbosch[1,3], Constantin Pape[1], Alwin Krämer[3], Yannick Schwab[1], and Anna Kreshuk[1(✉)]

[1] European Molecular Biology Laboratory (EMBL), Heidelberg, Germany
anna.kreshuk@embl.de
[2] Smart Engines, Moscow, Russia
[3] Clinical Cooperation Unit Molecular Hematology/Oncology,
German Cancer Research Center (DKFZ), Heidelberg, Germany

**Abstract.** Recent advances in high-throughput electron microscopy imaging enable detailed study of centrosome aberrations in cancer cells. While the image acquisition in such pipelines is automated, manual detection of centrioles is still necessary to select cells for re-imaging at higher magnification. In this contribution we propose an algorithm which performs this step automatically and with high accuracy. From the image labels produced by human experts and a 3D model of a centriole we construct an additional training set with patch-level labels. A two-level DenseNet is trained on the hybrid training data with synthetic patches and real images, achieving much better results on real patient data than training only at the image-level. The code can be found at https://github.com/kreshuklab/centriole_detection.

**Keywords:** Synthetic images · Electron microscopy · Screening

## 1 Introduction

Centrosomes consist of a pair of centrioles embedded in pericentriolar material and act as the major microtubule organizing centers of eukaryotic cells. They are pivotal for several fundamental cellular processes, including formation of bipolar mitotic spindles, a process essential for accurate chromosome segregation. Centrosome aberrations are a hallmark of cancer and have been described in virtually all malignancies examined. Surprisingly, with very few exceptions, no electron microscopy (EM) data on aberrant centrosomes in primary tumor tissues are available. As a consequence, next to nothing is known with regard to ultrastructure, biogenesis and functional consequences of specific types of centrosome aberrations. The main roadblock of such studies has long been on the image acquisition side, since high-throughput EM imaging is technically very difficult to orchestrate. The situation has recently been alleviated by the introduction of software tools for targeted electron microscopy [11], which allow for

© Springer Nature Switzerland AG 2019
D. Shen et al. (Eds.): MICCAI 2019, LNCS 11764, pp. 523–531, 2019.
https://doi.org/10.1007/978-3-030-32239-7_58

automated imaging of a large number (1000–2000) of cells on thin resin sections. These cells then need to be screened for centrosome/centriole abnormalities. The screening - a time consuming, tedious task with a hit rate of 2 to 5% - is currently performed manually. This contribution proposes an algorithm for automatic centriole detection and thus closes the last methodological gap on the way to fully automated screening for centrosome aberrations within a cancer cell population.

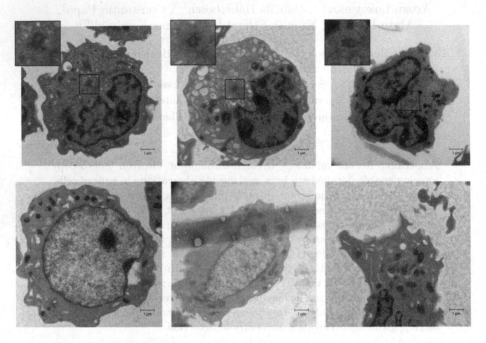

**Fig. 1.** Examples of positive (top) and negative (bottom) images from the screening. The centrioles of the positive images are shown in more detail in the top left corners.

During screening, experts mark which images contain a centriole to trigger reimaging at higher magnification or with TEM tomography for detailed study of the ultrastructure. The task we intend to solve is thus one of image classification, as no labels are placed on the centrioles themselves and their location in the positive images is not known. Figure 1 shows several example images from the screening, illustrating the challenges of the classification task. Centrioles are fairly small and, to an untrained eye, look very similar to other ultrastructure elements. Besides, since cell sectioning is done without seeing the centrioles, they can be positioned at any orientation to the cutting plane. Consequently, their appearance - roughly cylindrical in 3D - can range from a circle to two parallel lines (Fig. 1, top row). Finally, the screening images are not artifact-free (Fig. 1, bottom center) and can differ significantly in their intensity distribution (Fig. 1, bottom left and right).

The task of automated centriole detection has, to the best of our knowledge, not been addressed before in EM images. The state-of-the-art algorithms for detection of other objects in EM images rely on dense object-level labels [1,5,14] as input for training a convolutional neural network (CNN). We intend to use a CNN as well, but we are limited to much weaker image-level labels. Numerous image classification CNNs developed for natural image processing could provide a good fit, but did not work in practice. Their lack of performance can perhaps be explained by the relatively very small size of the object in question. Specialized algorithms for the detection of small objects have been proposed in the remote sensing domain [10,15], but they again rely on object-level labels.

Besides direct image classification, the screening problem can also be addressed in the framework of multiple instance learning [8]. This approach is often used in computer-aided diagnostics, with image patches serving as instances and complete images as bags. The main drawback for our application is the intentional removal of spatial context between the patches.

Artificial image generation is a popular means to augment insufficient training data, used both in medical [9] and natural image domains [13]. For object detection in particular, several suggestions have been made on how an object can be consistently pasted into an empty background scene [2,3]. Inspired by this work, we propose to limit the synthesis to image patches and create synthetic groundtruth by pasting slices of a 3D centriole model into patches of a few negatively labeled training images. The combined hybrid groundtruth of synthetic patches and real images is used to train a special two-level neural network. The training begins from the first patch-level sub-network. After this network is trained (on synthetic patches), we freeze its weights and attach the image-level sub-network to be trained on real images.

The hybrid groundtruth of synthetic patches and real images has several advantages over existing approaches: (i) we avoid the difficult task of generating whole cell images with correct placement of all the organelles; (ii) we can train a powerful network on the patch level and capture all the fine ultrastructure in the patch necessary to recognize centrioles from other similar objects; (iii) we can preserve spatial context between the patches for the image-level prediction.

Our complete model and training procedure are described in detail in the next section. In Sect. 3, we apply the network to real patient data and show that it achieves sufficiently high accuracy for fully automated screening. Finally, in Sect. 4 we discuss other possible applications of our hybrid training setup.

## 2  Methods

### 2.1  Generation of Synthetic Patches

We start from a simplified 3D model of a centriole which at this resolution can be described as two orthogonal hollow cylinders roughly 250 nm in diameter and 500 nm in length. Transmission Electron Microscopy works by detecting electrons which pass through a sample - in this case, a 200 nm section of a cell. To simulate this process, we perform three random rotations of the model around three axes, pick a random length value and take a 10-pixel slice out of the model at this position. The slice is then summed into a 2D image along the depth axis and Gaussian blur is applied. Our 3D model and sample images are shown in Fig. 2.

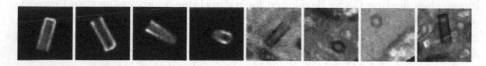

**Fig. 2.** Left: artificially generated slices of the cylinder model of a centriole. Right: model slices painted into background cell patches.

The generated model slices need to be combined with realistic cell background patches. Instead of generating them ad-hoc, we select patches from the negative training samples since those were labeled not to contain a centriole. The screening images contain multiple cells and the negative label of the whole image only refers to the central one. We select the central cell by a combination of smoothing, binarization, morphological erosion, connected components filtering and dilation. Since large intensity shifts are present between the screening images, we choose an adaptive binarization threshold of $0.9 \times \mathbb{E}(I)$, where $\mathbb{E}(I)$ stands for average intensity of the image.

Once the cell image without centrioles is selected, we proceed to choose a patch inside the cell. We prefer relatively empty patches without other organelles in the middle, as we do not want to paste the centriole on top of a different object. We generate a set of $60 \times 60$ boxes covering the cell and randomly select from the patches of this set, weighing the probability for the patch to be selected by the standard deviation of the intensity inside it: $P_{selected} = 1/(N_{patches} * \sigma^4)$.

The final step consists of painting the model slice into the background patch. Since image formation in TEM depends on the scattering of electrons while they pass through the specimen, we propose to subtract the model slice image from the background patch. Additionally, the generated patch needs to remain within the real image intensity range. Let $I_{bg}$ be the background image patch, $S$ the model slice, $Q_5$ the 5% quantile. We combine the background and the model slice into the final image $I$ by the following formula:

$$I = \max(Q_5(I_{bg}),\ I_{bg} - \alpha * \sigma * S * \epsilon)$$

Here, $\alpha$ is a scaling factor, $\sigma$ the standard deviation of the background patch and $\epsilon$ a random number between 0.9 and 1.1. A few examples of generated patches are shown in Fig. 2.

## 2.2   Neural Network and Hybrid Training

We use the synthetic patches described above to train a convolutional neural network for patch classification. Once the training on synthetic patches is finished, we incorporate the trained network into a bigger one which is then trained on real images with image-level labels.

On the patch level, we use a DenseNet [6] with a growth rate of 32, three dense blocks with depths 6, 12 and 32, three fully connected layers with 1280, 80 and 16 input channels.

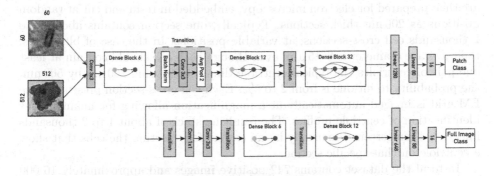

**Fig. 3.** The architecture of the proposed two-level network. The full network is based on DenseNet-B, i.e. a DenseNet with a bottleneck $1 \times 1$ convolution layer. Activation layers are omitted for clarity. Code will be made publicly available.

The network architecture is illustrated in Fig. 3. We construct the image-level network by extending the patch-level one. In more detail, we keep the first three dense blocks, remove the fully connected layers, add two more convolutional layers and two more dense blocks of depth 6 and 12, and finally add three fully connected layers with 648, 80 and 16 channels. The weights of the first three dense blocks are frozen at the values that were obtained during patch-level training. The new layers of the network are trained on real images for the task of image classification. After the training converges, we un-freeze the weights of the first three blocks and continue the training end-to-end until convergence.

Our motivation for the 3-step training procedure is as follows: the goal of the first training step is to tune the low-level filters in the first blocks to the problem of centriole detection. The second step learns to combine the patch-level filter responses with the global image context. Finally, the third step trains the complete network end-to-end and learns to recognize centrioles in real images and classify them even better.

Besides the hybrid patch/image model above, we investigate two simpler alternatives. Both start from the patch-level network trained on synthetic data. We apply the network to the whole image in a sliding window manner with a stride of 10 pixels. For each pixel we obtain a score for the probability of the patch centered at this pixel to contain a centriole. In the first approach we then threshold the probabilities and assign the image a positive label if at least one area of the image remains above the threshold (there is at least one strong centriole detection). The second approach uses the probability map as input to another neural network. Note that unlike the hybrid network neither of these methods allow for retraining the patch-level neural network.

# 3    Experiments

## 3.1    Dataset Description

For imaging in TEM, patient cells are collected, fixed and pelleted. The pellets are then prepared for electron microscopy, embedded in resin and cut at random positions as 200 nm thick sections. Typically, one section contains about 1 to 2 thousands cell cross-sections, at variable positions. In the case of blast cells, their average diameter is 8–15 μm; even though each cell should contain at least one pair of centrioles the typical centriole dimensions being 200 nm by 500 nm, the probability to hit one is from 2 to 5%. Each cell cross-section present on the EM grid is imaged automatically at a magnification allowing for unambiguous identification of centriole profiles. The resulting stack of about 1 to 2 thousands images is then screened manually by an expert for selecting the cells that show a centriole on that specific section.

In total the dataset contains 742 positive images and approximately 16 000 negative images, from 6 to 147 positive images for each of 14 patients. For each patient, we randomly sample the negative images to obtain a balanced training and test set. The performance of the screening algorithms is measured as accuracy of image label assignment.

## 3.2    State-of-the-art Image Classification Models

First we apply the standard image classification networks, namely VGG [12], ResNet [4], DenseNet and DenseNet with additional skip connections between dense blocks. The best result on a balanced test set was at 58% accuracy. All models overfit very quickly even when regularization is used. Augmenting the dataset with synthetic images generated by the same procedure as we use for patches did not improve the performance.

The next experiment was based on multiple instance learning, where we implemented the attention-based model of [7]. Since at most one centriole is visible, the positive bags only had a single positive instance and the network never achieved accuracy above 54%.

## 3.3    Hybrid Training

The patch-level network operated on 60 × 60 patches. In total, approximately 20 000 (18 000 for train and 2000 for test) patches were generated for its training in each experiment. The network achieved the accuracy of 98.7% on synthetic patches. A few examples of its predictions on real images are shown in Fig. 4. The fourth image is correctly predicted as negative and the rest as positive. However, spurious predictions as shown in the second image are often present at objects similar to centrioles, and also inside the nucleus which resembles the empty background we used in the positive samples.

We compare several approaches to aggregating patch-level information for image-level prediction. In the first one, the patch level predictions are thresholded at 50% and the whole image is assigned to positive class if at least one

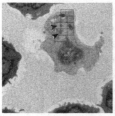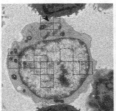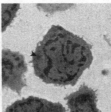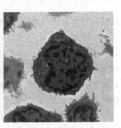

**Fig. 4.** Real images with patch network predictions (red boxes) and real centrioles positions (blue arrowheads). The first 3 images contain centrioles which are detected correctly. In the 2nd image false positive detections are present along with the correct centriole patch. The 4th image does not contain a centriole and is correctly predicted as negative. (Color figure online)

patch is positive. In the second, we train a DenseNet on the predictions of the patch network. For the proposed hybrid training, we evaluate a 2-step and a 3-step training procedure. In the 2-step training the weights of the first three dense blocks remain frozen after the training of the patch-level sub-network. We perform 4-fold cross validation on the patient level, using 75% of the images from 9 patients for training and the other for validation. Five unseen patients are used for testing. The results on different folds are very consistent. As the final experiment, we unfreeze the weights of the first three dense blocks for the network trained on one of the folds and continue training end-to-end until convergence. The results of our experiments are summarized in Table 1.

The hyperparameters were set as follows: Adam optimizer with $betas = (0.9, 0.999)$, $eps = 10^{-8}$, $learning\ rate = 10^{-3}$ and scheduler which reduces learning rate by 5% each 10 epochs if the validation does not improve. We perform the standard data augmentation: random flips, random translation at 10%, random re-scale at 10%, random rotation around arbitrary axes.

**Table 1.** Accuracy of the algorithms on a balanced test set from unseen patients

| Threshold patch predictions | Train from patch predictions | Hybrid network 2-step training | Hybrid network 3-step training |
|---|---|---|---|
| 68 | 64 | 80.36 ± 1.18 | 87.23 |

## 4   Discussion and Future Work

We have proposed an algorithm for automated centriole screening in EM images which can be trained, by using a 3D model of a centriole to generate synthetic patches, purely from image-level manual labels. On a test dataset of real patient data the algorithm demonstrates high accuracy and stability across folds in cross-validation. High-throughput screening is fairly tolerant to detection errors: as long as a sufficient number of centrioles are detected to draw statistical conclusions, a small number of false positives or false negatives are considered a reasonable price to pay for reduction in manual labor. The accuracy achieved by our algorithm was judged to be sufficient for fully automated screening.

The main drawback of our approach comes from its main strength - it relies on the 3D model of a centriole to train the patch-level classifier. We show in Table 1 that the image-level classifier can learn to correct patch-level errors. Still, centrosome aberrations which lead to a significant change in centriole appearance will likely be confusing for the algorithm. These, however, would be challenging for a human expert as well.

Outside the original application of screening for centriole presence, the hybrid training approach would apply equally well to other organelles of uniform shape, such as various coated vesicles. At even higher resolution it can be extended to large single molecules, while at much lower resolution in the natural image domain it can be applied to problems of defect detection and quality control.

# References

1. Beier, T., et al.: Multicut brings automated neurite segmentation closer to human performance. Nat. Methods **14**(2), 101 (2017)
2. Dwibedi, D., Misra, I., Hebert, M.: Cut, paste and learn: surprisingly easy synthesis for instance detection. In: ICCV 2017, pp. 1301–1310. IEEE (2017)
3. Gupta, A., Vedaldi, A., Zisserman, A.: Synthetic data for text localisation in natural images. In: CVPR 2016, pp. 2315–2324. IEEE (2016)
4. He, K., Zhang, X., Ren, S., Sun, J.: Deep residual learning for image recognition. In: CVPR 2016, pp. 770–778 (2016)
5. Heinrich, L., Funke, J., Pape, C., Nunez-Iglesias, J., Saalfeld, S.: Synaptic cleft segmentation in non-isotropic volume electron microscopy of the complete *Drosophila* brain. In: Frangi, A.F., Schnabel, J.A., Davatzikos, C., Alberola-López, C., Fichtinger, G. (eds.) MICCAI 2018. LNCS, vol. 11071, pp. 317–325. Springer, Cham (2018). https://doi.org/10.1007/978-3-030-00934-2_36
6. Huang, G., Liu, Z., van der Maaten, L., Weinberger, K.Q.: Densely connected convolutional networks. In: CVPR 2017, pp. 2261–2269 (2017)
7. Ilse, M., Tomczak, J.M., Welling, M.: Attention-based deep multiple instance learning. In: ICML 2018 (2018)
8. Kandemir, M., Hamprecht, F.A.: Computer-aided diagnosis from weak supervision: a benchmarking study. Comput. Med. Imaging Graph. **42**, 44–50 (2015)
9. Mahmood, F., Chen, R., Durr, N.J.: Unsupervised reverse domain adaptation for synthetic medical images via adversarial training. IEEE Trans. Med. Imaging **37**(12), 2572–2581 (2018)
10. Pang, J., Li, C., Shi, J., Xu, Z., Feng, H.: R2-CNN: fast tiny object detection in large-scale remote sensing images. IEEE Trans. Geosci. Remote Sens. 1–13 (2019)
11. Schorb, M., Haberbosch, I., Hagen, W., Schwab, Y., Mastronarde, D.: Software tools for automated transmission electron microscopy. bioRxiv, p. 389502, August 2018. https://doi.org/10.1101/389502

12. Simonyan, K., Zisserman, A.: Very deep convolutional networks for large-scale image recognition. In: ICLR (2015)
13. Tremblay, J., et al.: Training deep networks with synthetic data: bridging the reality gap by domain randomization. In: CVPR 2018 (2018)
14. Xiao, C., et al.: Automatic mitochondria segmentation for EM data using a 3D supervised convolutional network. Frontiers Neuroanat. **12**, 92 (2018)
15. Yang, X., Sun, H., Fu, K., Yang, J., Sun, X., et al.: Automatic ship detection of remote sensing images from google earth in complex scenes based on multi-scale rotation dense feature pyramid networks. Remote Sens. **10**(1), 132 (2018)

# Patch Transformer for Multi-tagging Whole Slide Histopathology Images

Weijian Li[1(✉)], Viet-Duy Nguyen[1], Haofu Liao[1], Matt Wilder[2], Ke Cheng[2], and Jiebo Luo[1]

[1] Department of Computer Science, University of Rochester, Rochester, USA
{wli69,hliao6,jluo}@cs.rochester.edu, vnguy14@u.rochester.edu
[2] HistoWiz Inc., 760 Parkside Avenue, Brooklyn, NY 11226, USA
ke@histowiz.com

**Abstract.** Automated whole slide image (WSI) tagging has become a growing demand due to the increasing volume and diversity of WSIs collected nowadays in histopathology. Various methods have been studied to classify WSIs with single tags but none of them focuses on labeling WSIs with multiple tags. To this end, we propose a novel end-to-end trainable deep neural network named *Patch Transformer* which can effectively predict multiple slide-level tags from WSI patches based on both the correlations and the uniqueness between the tags. Specifically, the proposed method learns patch characteristics considering (1) patch-wise relations through a patch transformation module and (2) tag-wise uniqueness for each tagging task through a multi-tag attention module. Extensive experiments on a large and diverse dataset consisting of 4,920 WSIs prove the effectiveness of the proposed model.

## 1 Introduction

Whole slide images (WSIs) contain rich information about the morphological and functional characteristics of biological systems, which facilitate clinical diagnosis and research [12]. To better represent image contents, pathologists frequently examine and correct the attribute tags that are inconsistent or missing for the collected WSIs. However, this tag assignment process is time-consuming and can be biased by subjective judgments, making it essential to automatically and accurately assign tags to these digital histopathology images.

To achieve this goal, several patch-based methods have been proposed for automated WSI tagging. For example, previous work [1,14] proposes to use convolutional neural networks (CNNs) to classify and retrieve WSIs with patch-level information. Hou et al. [5] also introduce several patch-based deep models but to address a slide-level WSI classification task with a novel two-steps learning schema. A more recent work by Mercan et al. [9] investigate a multi-instance based model on a multiple label classification task. Their model extracts hand-crafted features from prelocated Regions of Interest (ROIs) and learns slide-level labels with weakly supervised learning. The results of these studies indicate a

© Springer Nature Switzerland AG 2019
D. Shen et al. (Eds.): MICCAI 2019, LNCS 11764, pp. 532–540, 2019.
https://doi.org/10.1007/978-3-030-32239-7_59

great benefit of integrating detailed patch contents for slide-level decision making. However, their integration approaches are preliminary and constrained.

A better way to integrate patch-level information and to automatically locate ROIs is to leverage an attention mechanism that considers the importance of each patch. Ilse et al. [6] propose an attention mechanism under a multi-instance learning to highlight the patch instances that contribute the most to slide-level colon cancer classification. Li et al. [8] propose a graph convolutional network (GCN) based method to learn attention weights for each patch. However, their method requires a large number of patch nodes and detailed graph structure knowledge to construct a complete graph representation for effective GCN training. Therefore, a method that can adaptively learn slide-level representations with limited prior knowledge is needed.

One of the options is to adopt the "Scaled Dot-Product Attention" (SDPA), which is a self-attention mechanism introduced in the Transformer model [11] for Neural Machine Translation. It constructs rich instance-level representations considering the pairwise relationships of all given instances without higher-level structural knowledge. However, SDPA may not be the best choice considering different instance contexts between words and WSI patches. The differences in tasks themselves should also lead to different attention designs. Therefore, it is necessary to investigate and construct an appropriate attention mechanism to extract informative patch features for WSI tagging.

In summary, our contributions are as follows: (1) A novel patch based deep model *Patch Transformer* is designed for multi-tagging whole slide images. To the best of our knowledge, *this is the first multi-tagging approach for WSIs*. The proposed model is trained end-to-end under a multi-task learning scheme where each task is a multi-class classification problem. (2) A *Patch Transformation Module* extracts patch characteristics considering global context with limited prior structural knowledge through a multi-head attention mechanism. (3) A *Multi-Tag Attention Module* constructs tag-specific representations by aggregating weighted patch features. (4) Extensive experiments on a large and diverse dataset containing 4,920 WSIs demonstrate the improved performance of the proposed model compared to the state-of-the-art methods.

## 2    Methods

Given a WSI dataset $I = \{I_1, ..., I_n\}$ where each $I_n$ is a whole slide image, we have bags of patches $B = \{B_1, ..., B_n\}$ where each $B_n$ is a bag of $M$ sampled patches from the non-background regions of $I_n$. We have $K$ sets of tags $C_k$ each has multiple classes. For the whole slide images $I$, their corresponding $k$th tags can be represented as $L_k = \{L_{k1}, ..., L_{kn}\}$, where $L_{kn} \in C_k$. Our goal is to correctly assign all $K$ tags for each image.

**Patch Transformation Module.** Inspired by the Transformer model [11], we introduce a patch transformation module to effectively learn patch characteristics by considering global patch contexts. As depicted in Fig. 1, the proposed

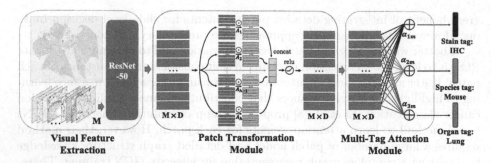

**Fig. 1.** Overview of the proposed Patch Transformer. The proposed model mainly consists of three parts: (1) *Visual Feature Extraction:* capturing the visual feature of each patch from the original WSI; (2) *Patch Transformation Module:* producing the characteristic enhanced patch representations by an attention aggregation mechanism; (3) *Multi-Tag Attention Module:* constructing tag-related global slide representations for final prediction leveraging the extracted patch features following the same attention format as (2).

module takes as inputs from the latent visual embeddings extracted by a ResNet-50 [4] network. It then maps each patch feature into different attention domains through multi-head attentions. The final feature outputs are the aggregation of the obtained representations. Concretely, for the visual embedding $V \in \mathbb{R}^{M \times D}$, the output of the module can be represented by

$$V' = \sigma(V + W^T[\mathbf{f}_1, ..., \mathbf{f}_h]), V' \in \mathbb{R}^{M \times D}, W \in \mathbb{R}^{(h \times D) \times D} \tag{1}$$

where $h$ represents the $h$th head in the module, $\sigma(\cdot)$ is the ReLU non-linear activation function and $D$ is the feature dimension. Each $\mathbf{f}_h$ is a feature extracted by an attention unit which we will detail later. Different from the original task [11], here different patches share the same attribute tags. Selecting the most informative patches that contribute the most to the slide level prediction becomes the main challenge. To address this issue, we formulate the multi-head computation as an attention aggregation process to obtain characteristic-enhanced feature representations for informative patch selection. The original "Scaled Dot-Product Attention" [11] is not appropriate due to its designed patch-wise feature mix and fusion property which would diminish unique characteristics. Instead, for the extracted patch feature matrix $V$, we perform element-wise multiplication between $V$ and multi-head patch attention matrices, i.e., $\mathbf{f}_h = V \odot A_h$, $V, A_h \in \mathbb{R}^{M \times D}$. The attention matrix $A_h$ can be written as $A_h = [\mathbf{a}_h, \mathbf{a}_h, ..., \mathbf{a}_h]$, where each column $\mathbf{a}_h \in \mathbb{R}^{M \times 1}$ is a duplicate of the attention vector for the patch features. Each weight in $\mathbf{a}_h$ is calculated by

$$a_{hm} = \text{Softmax}(W_h^T \tanh(U_h^T v_m)), W_h \in \mathbb{R}^{D' \times 1}, U_h \in \mathbb{R}^{D \times D'}, v_n \in \mathbb{R}^{D \times 1} \tag{2}$$

where $D'$ represent the transformed feature dimension. We adopt a similar attention mechanism to the one proposed in [6] for effective patch selection. But we

**Table 1.** Tag distribution of the dataset.

| Stain | H&E | IHC | Special | | | | | |
|---|---|---|---|---|---|---|---|---|
| Count | 2803 | 1672 | 445 | | | | | |
| Species | Human | Monkey | Mouse | Pig | Rat | Zebrafish | | |
| Count | 816 | 29 | 3435 | 33 | 439 | 168 | | |
| Organ | Bone | Brain | Breast | Cecum | Colon | Heart | Skin | Skin Dorsal |
| Count | 89 | 238 | 264 | 119 | 338 | 160 | 752 | 67 |
| Organ | Intestine | Kidney | Liver | Lung | Pancreas | Prostate | Spleen | Skin Ventral |
| Count | 186 | 335 | 901 | 644 | 347 | 202 | 204 | 74 |

do not follow the conventional attention mechanisms by reducing the feature matrix to a unified vector. Instead, we add a residual connection from the input to the output and directly aggregate it with each patch's weighted representations (Eq. 1). In this way, we explicitly expose each patch feature's distinct characteristics while at the same time preserving its original feature representation. The final output is obtained by applying the ReLU non-linear activation function.

**Multi-tag Attention Module.** Our goal is to extract the most informative slide-level features for tag classifications. Based on our observation, there exists correlations among different tags, e.g. most Zebrafish slides are H&E stained, which makes multi-task learning an appropriate approach. Meanwhile, different tags focus not only on common regions but also on tag-specific regions which results in different potential ROIs. To learn each tag's ROI adaptively and to form tag-related slide level representations, we propose a multi-tag attention module. The proposed module adopts the same attention mechanism as used in the previously introduced patch transformation module except that the output is obtained by aggregating weighted patch features. This consistent design helps our model leverage the previously learned patch characteristics to assign tag-related weights. Formally, the tag-specific representations can be represented by $t_k = \sum_{m=1}^{M} \alpha_{km} \times v'_m$ where $k$ represents the $k$th tag. $v'_n \in \mathbb{R}^{D' \times 1}$ is a patch feature in $V'$, $\alpha_{kn} \in \mathbb{R}^{1 \times 1}$ is a tag-related weight scalar and is computed following the same format in Eq. (2). The prediction probability for each tag of each WSI is computed by

$$\hat{l}_k = \text{Softmax}(W_k^T t_k), W_k \in \mathbb{R}^{D' \times D_k}, t_k \in \mathbb{R}^{D' \times 1} \tag{3}$$

where $D_k$ equals to the number of classes in $C_k$. The model is end-to-end trained with a combination of multi-class cross entropy losses (CE) for each tag weighted by $\lambda_k$

$$\mathcal{L} = \sum_{k=1}^{K} \lambda_k \mathcal{L}_k = \sum_{k=1}^{K} \lambda_k \frac{1}{N} \sum_{n=1}^{N} \text{CE}(l_{kn}, \hat{l}_{kn}) \tag{4}$$

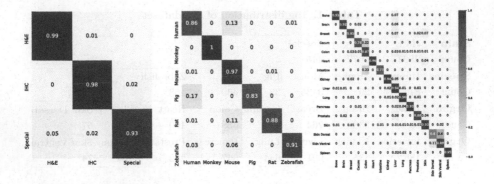

**Fig. 2.** Normalized confusion matrices of the proposed PT-3head-MTA model for Stain tag, Species tag and Organ tag.

## 3   Experiments and Results

**Dataset and Settings.** The dataset used in this study contains 4,920 WSIs provided by a histopathology service company. On average, the size of each image file is 1.17GB. The dataset contains three slide level tags, namely: *Stain*, *Species*, and *Organ*. In total, there are 3 stain tags, 6 species tags and 16 organ tags. Stain tag indicates the type of dye used in the histopathology staining process. Species tag indicates the type of species that the slide comes from. Organ tag indicates the organ type the slide contains. All other information is not included in the experiment except the three attribute tags mentioned above. Detailed tag distribution can be found in Table 1.

We first randomly split our dataset into training and testing sets with an 8:2 ratio. Then 10% of the training data are randomly picked and are kept as the validation set for model and parameter tuning. For each whole slide image, we use 40x resolution and apply the widely adopted Otsu [10] method on the grayscale image to remove background regions. During training, $M = 32$ non-overlapping image patches of size $512 \times 512$ from the non-background regions are randomly extracted. Due to the class imbalance problem and the variety of the samples, we conduct rich data augmentation operations including random cropping, left-right/bottom-up flipping, and rotating. The final patch inputs are of size $224 \times 224$. The 2048 dimensional outputs of `conv5_3` of the `ResNet_50` [4] are used as the latent visual embeddings. `ResNet_50` is pretrained on ImageNet [3] and finetuned during the training process. The model is implemented based on Tensorflow and is trained with the Adam optimizer with $lr = 0.0001$, $\beta_1 = 0.9$, $\beta_2 = 0.999$. $\lambda_1 = \lambda_2 = \lambda_3 = 1$.

**Comparison Methods.** We compare our model with the state-of-the-art methods in: (1) whole slide image classification tasks; (2) multiple-instance learning tasks. Patch based methods [5] follow a two-step learning process. They use the patch-level predictions for the final slide-level prediction. For GCN [7], we con-

**Table 2.** Quantitative results. PT: the proposed Patch Transformation module; MTA: the proposed Multi-Tag Attention module; SDPA: replacing our attention mechanism with the "Scaled Dot-Product Attention" introduced in [11].

| Model | Macro F1 | | | | Micro F1 | | | |
|---|---|---|---|---|---|---|---|---|
| | Stain | Species | Organ | Avg. | Stain | Species | Organ | Avg. |
| Patchbased-LR [5] | 0.937 | 0.477 | 0.378 | 0.597 | 0.972 | 0.857 | 0.556 | 0.795 |
| Patchbased-SVM [5] | 0.951 | 0.754 | 0.371 | 0.692 | 0.975 | **0.951** | 0.531 | 0.819 |
| GCN [7] | 0.961 | 0.832 | 0.822 | 0.872 | 0.981 | 0.921 | 0.881 | 0.927 |
| DeepMIL [13] | 0.962 | 0.863 | 0.850 | 0.892 | 0.981 | 0.932 | 0.904 | 0.939 |
| TwoBranches [2] | **0.976** | 0.845 | 0.866 | 0.895 | **0.988** | 0.932 | 0.908 | 0.942 |
| MTA | 0.961 | 0.836 | 0.824 | 0.873 | 0.981 | 0.932 | 0.879 | 0.931 |
| PT-1head | 0.957 | 0.848 | 0.850 | 0.885 | 0.981 | 0.933 | 0.904 | 0.939 |
| PT-1head-MTA | 0.962 | 0.846 | 0.872 | 0.893 | 0.982 | 0.933 | 0.908 | 0.941 |
| PT-3head (SDPA)-MTA | 0.951 | 0.830 | 0.866 | 0.882 | 0.975 | 0.916 | 0.901 | 0.930 |
| PT-3head-MTA | 0.962 | **0.889** | **0.879** | **0.910** | 0.982 | 0.939 | **0.912** | **0.944** |

sider WSI as a graph where each patch is a node. Graph edges are defined based on patch-to-patch spatial distance. Maxpooling is adopted as instance aggregation method. For DeepMIL [13], we adopt the structure that only contains visual features. To examine the effect of patch-level labels, we adopt the Two-Branches [2] model where the additional branch targets patch-level predictions. Each patch has the same labels as the original WSI. The total loss is a combination of patch-level and slide-level cross-entropy losses. We adopt the publicly available implementation of GCN [7][1] and reimplement the other baseline models.

For fair comparison, we keep all patch extraction and prepossessing steps the same. All models adopt the same pretrained ResNet-50 structure as feature extractor. If the original model aims at single tag classification, we append additional tag classification heads to obtain a model with the same structure as used in our model. To further investigate the effect of the two proposed modules, we conduct several ablation studies.

**Quantitative Results.** Our quantitative evaluation results can be found in Table 2. Considering the class imbalance distribution of our dataset, we adopt both Macro F1 and Micro F1 scores as our evaluation metrics. For Macro F1 score, the final result is calculated by the class average values of Precision and Recall. Thus, Macro F1 score indicates an unweighted average result over all classes. It shows how our model performs in each class under the tags. For Micro F1 score, the final result is calculated based on overall predictions without considering the class categories. It shows how our model performs over the entire dataset. The confusion matrices of our best model PT-3head-MTA for the three

---

[1] https://github.com/tkipf/gcn.

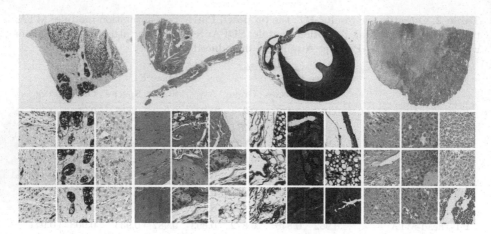

**Fig. 3.** Multi-Tag Attention Module's attention result visualization. Each WSI has three columns. Each of the three columns belongs to one of the three tags: *Stain*, *Species*, and *Organ* from left to right. Patches in the columns are sorted by attention weights in the corresponding tag from the top to the bottom. The ground truth tags for the four WSIs are respectively: (IHC, Human, Liver), (H&E, Mouse, Bone), (Special Stain, Rat, Kidney), (H&E, Mouse, Liver). (Color figure online)

tags are also computed and can be found in Fig. 2. In general, our model accurately assigns the three tags to the WSIs to prove its effectiveness.

As is shown in Table 2, our model outperforms most previous methods for all three tagging tasks on both Macro F1 and Micro F1 metrics. The proposed full model under a three-heads setting leads to the best overall average performance. Comparing to the two-step based models [5], the other models have relatively better and more stable performance across three tasks which indicates the benefit of learning the patch features jointly. GCN [7] and PT-3head (SDPA)-MTA [11] achieve higher scores than patch-based methods but lower scores than TwoBranches and our proposed models. We consider the reason is the degradation of patch characteristics by the weighted combination of the other patches. This can be seen more clearly by comparing PT-3head (SDPA)-MTA with PT-3head-MTA where the proposed attention module is replaced in PT-3head (SDPA)-MTA with the "Scaled Dot-Product Attention". The Two-Branches [2] model adopts both slide level and patch level classification losses and thus uses extra knowledge. This extra knowledge helps their model achieve the best F1 scores for stain tagging because of the similar color patterns shared by different patches. On the other hand, due to the large variance in patch textures, this strategy inhibits the performances of species and organ tagging which are more sensitive to the variations of image textures. By examining the ablations of our models, we find that combining the MTA and PT modules gives better performance than MTA or PT alone, indicating a mutual promotional effect of the two proposed modules. Furthermore, increasing the attention heads also brings additional benefit for extracting patch characteristics which results in higher F1 scores.

**Qualitative Results.** To visually validate the effect of multi-tag attention module, we collect and examine the attention weights as well as their corresponding patch images. Here we show four groups of examples in Fig. 3. As depicted, each attention head focuses on different patch patterns. For instance, the attention head that aims at tagging stain labels has higher interest on patches with simpler textures but larger tissue areas. These patches mainly contain apparent color patterns such as the blue dots for IHC, red and pink regions for H&E. While for the species and organ attention heads, patches with relatively complex structures and textures are assigned higher attention weights as they provide more contextual information for tagging species and organ labels.

## 4  Conclusions and Future Work

We present a novel framework to assign multiple attribute tags for the whole slide histopathology images. Two modules are introduced, namely a patch transformation module which adopts a multi-head attention mechanism to extract and integrate patch level characteristics, and a multi-tag attention module which adaptively weights and aggregates patch features into a global slide representation for slide-level predictions targeting different tags. The proposed framework is validated on a 4,920 WSI dataset with overall improved performance over the state-of-the-art methods. More importantly, the insights on the tagging decisions can be gained effectively by visualizing the patches with the highest attention weights. Future work includes adopting extra information, e.g., multi-resolutions into the framework and developing multi-resolution fusion mechanisms to improve species and organ tag learning. Furthermore, the learned slide-level features can be explored for WSI retrieval tasks.

**Acknowledgement.** This work is supported in part by NSF through award IIS-1722847, NIH through the Morris K. Udall Center of Excellence in Parkinson's Disease Research, and our corporate sponsor HistoWiz.

## References

1. Babaie, M., et al.: Classification and retrieval of digital pathology scans: a new dataset. In: CVPR-Workshops, pp. 8–16 (2017)
2. Das, K., Conjeti, S., Roy, A.G., Chatterjee, J., Sheet, D.: Multiple instance learning of deep convolutional neural networks for breast histopathology whole slide classification. In: ISBI, pp. 578–581. IEEE (2018)
3. Deng, J., Dong, W., Socher, R., Li, L.J., Li, K., Fei-Fei, L.: ImageNet: a large-scale hierarchical image database. In: CVPR, pp. 248–255. IEEE (2009)
4. He, K., Zhang, X., Ren, S., Sun, J.: Deep residual learning for image recognition. In: CVPR, pp. 770–778 (2016)

5. Hou, L., Samaras, D., Kurc, T.M., Gao, Y., Davis, J.E., Saltz, J.H.: Patch-based convolutional neural network for whole slide tissue image classification. In: CVPR, pp. 2424–2433 (2016)
6. Ilse, M., Tomczak, J., Welling, M.: Attention-based deep multiple instance learning. In: ICML, pp. 2132–2141 (2018)
7. Kipf, T.N., Welling, M.: Semi-supervised classification with graph convolutional networks. arXiv preprint arXiv:1609.02907 (2016)
8. Li, R., Yao, J., Zhu, X., Li, Y., Huang, J.: Graph CNN for survival analysis on whole slide pathological images. In: Frangi, A.F., Schnabel, J.A., Davatzikos, C., Alberola-López, C., Fichtinger, G. (eds.) MICCAI 2018. LNCS, vol. 11071, pp. 174–182. Springer, Cham (2018). https://doi.org/10.1007/978-3-030-00934-2_20
9. Mercan, C., Aksoy, S., Mercan, E., Shapiro, L.G., Weaver, D.L., Elmore, J.G.: Multi-instance multi-label learning for multi-class classification of whole slide breast histopathology images. TMI 37(1), 316–325 (2018)
10. Otsu, N.: A threshold selection method from gray-level histograms. IEEE Trans. Syst. Man Cybern. 9(1), 62–66 (1979)
11. Vaswani, A., et al.: Attention is all you need. In: NeurIPS, pp. 5998–6008 (2017)
12. Wang, F., Oh, T., Vergara-Niedermayr, C., Kurc, T., Saltz, J.: Managing and querying whole slide images. In: Proceedings of SPIE-the International Society for Optical Engineering, vol. 8319. NIH Public Access (2012)
13. Wu, J., Yu, Y., Huang, C., Yu, K.: Deep multiple instance learning for image classification and auto-annotation. In: CVPR, pp. 3460–3469 (2015)
14. Zeng, T., Ji, S.: Deep convolutional neural networks for multi-instance multi-task learning. In: ICDM, pp. 579–588. IEEE (2015)

# Pancreatic Cancer Detection in Whole Slide Images Using Noisy Label Annotations

Han Le[1]([✉]), Dimitris Samaras[1], Tahsin Kurc[2], Rajarsi Gupta[2,3],
Kenneth Shroyer[3], and Joel Saltz[2]

[1] Department of Computer Science,
Stony Brook University, Stony Brook, NY, USA
hdle@cs.stonybrook.edu
[2] Department of Biomedical Informatics,
Stony Brook Medicine, Stony Brook, NY, USA
[3] Department of Pathology,
Stony Brook University Hospital, Stony Brook, NY, USA

**Abstract.** We propose an approach to accurately predict regions of pancreatic cancer in whole-slide images (WSIs) by leveraging a relatively large, but noisy, dataset. We employ a noisy label classification (NLC) method (called the *NLC model*) that utilizes a small set of clean training samples and assigns the appropriate weights to training samples to deal with sample noise. The weights are assigned online so that the network loss approximates the loss for the clean samples. This method results in a 9.7% performance improvement over the baseline non-NLC method (the *Baseline-Noisy model*). We use both methods in an ensemble setup to generate labels for a large training dataset to train a classifier. This classifier outperforms a classifier trained with manually annotated data by 2.94%–3.74% in terms of AUC for testing patches in WSIs.

**Keywords:** Pancreas · Pancreatic cancer · Whole slide image

## 1 Introduction

We target the problem of automatically detecting regions of pancreatic cancer in WSIs. Segmentation of cancer regions is a fundamental operation in digital pathology image analysis [7,9]. Pancreatic cancer segmentation is particularly important since it can be utilized to characterize immune responses that have been shown to affect survival outcomes and treatment response in pancreatic cancer patients [3]. A challenge to using deep learning in this task is the difficulty of generating detailed and large training datasets. In pancreatic cancer, malignant cells are typically arranged in irregularly shaped and poorly formed glands that infiltrate surrounding tissues. There is a wide spectrum of heterogeneity in the appearance of tumor cells, combined with the fact that a majority

© Springer Nature Switzerland AG 2019
D. Shen et al. (Eds.): MICCAI 2019, LNCS 11764, pp. 541–549, 2019.
https://doi.org/10.1007/978-3-030-32239-7_60

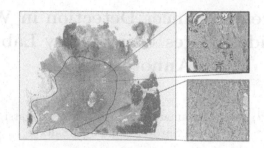

**Fig. 1.** A WSI with human annotation. The red box indicates a true positive patch; the blue box indicates a false positive patch extracted from the tumor annotated regions. (Please zoom in on a digital device). (Color figure online)

of the cancer region is comprised of non-cancer stromal and immune cells [5]. This morphologic complexity significantly limits highly detailed and fine-grained annotations because the annotation process is too laborious and time consuming.

*In order to address this challenge, we propose an approach that formulates the cancer region detection problem as a noisy label classification problem.* Annotated cancer regions are considered noisy due to the lack of specific delineation and labeling of the cancer and non-cancer components within the cancer region. Our approach uses a small amount of high-quality ground truth data (*clean data*), a larger volume of *noisy data*, and an ensemble of deep learning models to generate a large training dataset for a deep learning classifier.

Studies [1] have shown that the performance of a deep learning network can be adversely affected when it is trained with a noisy dataset. Numerous methods have been proposed to cope with noisy label classification for natural images [6,10–12,14]. Ren et al. [11] propose a technique to assign weights to training samples by using an additional clean validation set. Their intuition is to apply smaller weights to noisy samples and increase the weights of clean training samples to improve the gradient update. There is relatively limited work on the development and application of noisy label classification methods in medical imaging data [2,4,13]. Dgani et al. [4] model label noise as a part of the deep learning network to recover true labels of noisy samples for the task of classifying breast micro-calcifications in multi-view mammograms.

We make the following contributions: **(1)** Our approach is the first method for detection of pancreatic cancer regions in WSIs by using a large, but noisy, training dataset combined with the noisy label classification (NLC) technique of Ren et al. [11]; **(2)** We propose a pipeline to generate a large training dataset from moderately-sized and noisy annotated data; **(3)** Using this pipeline, we have generated a training dataset of 353,000 patches from 190 WSIs in The Cancer Genome Atlas (TCGA) repository. Our experiments show that a classifier trained with this larger noisy dataset outperforms a classifier trained with fewer clean ground truth data only. Our approach provides a viable mechanism for generating a large training dataset from moderately-sized and noisy annotated

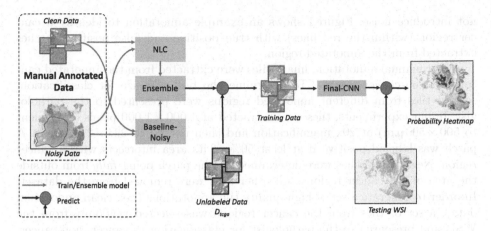

**Fig. 2.** Proposed training data generation pipeline. The NLC and the Baseline-Noisy models are trained with limited manually annotated data. The Ensemble model generates labels for patches extracted from 190 TCGA WSIs, $D_{tcga}$.

data. The training dataset and our prediction results on 190 TCGA WSIs are publicly available for use in other imaging studies[1].

## 2    Noisy Label Classification Approach

We propose a patch-based classification model to detect and classify cancer and non-cancer regions. This method partitions a WSI into tiles (or patches) of $P \times P$ pixels and predicts a class label for each tile. The classification model is trained with a set of tiles from cancer and non-cancer regions. In this section, we describe the process of generating a set of training tiles from a relatively small amount of high-quality annotated data (*clean data*) and a larger set of weakly annotated data (*noisy data*). The overall framework is illustrated in Fig. 2.

### 2.1    Tumor Region Annotation and Tile Extraction

Cancer and non-cancer regions in WSIs are manually segmented by pathologists. Pathologists are normally asked to carefully draw accurate contours around all of the cancer and non-cancer regions after histologic examination at intermediate and high-magnification. As a result, they often have to spend hours to generate high-quality and error-free ground-truth training datasets. In this work, the pathologist was asked to mark the boundaries of the cancer region in each WSI at low- to intermediate-magnification. This reduced manual annotation time but introduced noise because non-cancer components within the cancer regions could not be delineated at low-magnification. Note that the regions that lie outside of the annotated cancer regions were guaranteed to be non-cancer regions and did

---

[1] https://github.com/SBU-BMI/quip_paad_cancer_detection.

not introduce noise. Figure 1 shows an example annotation to identify a cancer region (within the red lines) with true positive and false positive patches extracted from the annotated region.

After manual annotation, image tiles were extracted from the annotated cancer and non-cancer regions. To determine the best tile size for classification, several tiles from different annotated regions were presented to the pathologist. In our experiments, tiles were extracted at $1,000 \times 1,000$ pixels (equivalent to $500 \times 500 \mu m$) at 20x magnification and then resized to $224 \times 224$ pixels. A patch was labeled positive if at least 50% of its area intersects with a cancer region. Negative patches were determined by the patch being *fully* from outside the area of the cancer regions. All other tiles were removed from the dataset. In order to generate a set of high-quality tile annotations (i.e., clean annotation data), a set of tiles from the cancer regions was selected randomly from the WSIs and presented to the pathologist for classification as cancer, non-cancer, or undecided. If the pathologist could not classify a tile, the tile was labeled as *undecided* and removed from the clean annotation dataset.

## 2.2   NLC Model: Noisy Label Classification Model

The manual annotation process ensures that tiles outside of cancer regions are true negative samples (non-cancer tiles). Tiles extracted from cancer regions are labeled positive, but this set contains both true and false positive samples (noisy training samples, i.e., non-cancer tiles that represent immune and stromal cells within the cancer region). To address this issue, we have adapted the noisy label classification method proposed by Ren et al. [11] with a modification on how to construct the subset of clean samples. Instead of selecting random clean samples from all regions in the WSIs, we choose samples in cancer regions only. In our experiments, we generated 100 clean samples per class via this strategy.

Let $(x, y)$ be a (tile, label) tuple, and let $D_n$ and $D_c$ be the set of noisy and clean samples, respectively. The network parameters, $\theta$, can be computed by minimizing the training loss over the training data: $\min_\theta \sum_{d_i \in D_n} w_i \mathcal{L}_i(d_i, \theta)$, where $w_i$ is the importance weight of sample $x_i$ and $\mathcal{L}_i$ is the loss function associated with $x_i$. The weights $\{w_i\}_{i=1}^N$ are treated as hyperparameters. They are computed by minimizing the loss over the clean dataset: $\min_{w \geq 0} \sum_{d_i \in D_c} \mathcal{L}_i(d_i, \theta^*(w))$. For computational efficiency, the update of the weights is computed in an online manner for each batch of training samples.

## 2.3   Ensemble Model of NLC and Baseline-Noisy Models

The Baseline-Noisy model is the same CNN architecture used for the NLC model, but it is trained with the noisy and clean samples without NLC. In our experiments (see Sect. 3.2), we observed that the NLC model is better than the Baseline-Noisy model at classifying patches in cancer regions, whereas the Baseline-Noisy model is better at classifying patches in non-cancer regions. To utilize the strengths of both models, an Ensemble Model computes the final prediction for a tile by averaging the prediction probabilities from the NLC and

**Table 1.** Dataset statistics. $D_n$ and $D_c$ were used in training the NLC and the Baseline-Noisy models. The Unlabeled Data, $D_{tcga}$, was used to generate the training set for the Final-CNN model. $T_{seer}$, $T_{seer2}$, and $T_{tcga}$ are test sets.

| Purpose | ID | #WSIs | #Positive | #Negative | #Total |
|---------|-----|-------|-----------|-----------|--------|
| Noisy training | $D_n$ | 50 | 21,805 | 47,640 | 69,445 |
| Clean set | $D_c$ | 14 | 100 | 100 | 200 |
| Unlabeled Data | $D_{tcga}$ | 190 | - | - | 353,000 |
| Testing | $T_{seer}$ | 14 | 1,700 | 1,700 | 3,400 |
| Testing | $T_{seer2}$ | 14 | 850 | 2,550 | 3,400 |
| Testing | $T_{tcga}$ | 190 | 1,051 | 2,003 | 3,054 |

Baseline-Noisy models. We used the Ensemble model to generate labels for a large training dataset for the Final-CNN model in Fig. 2.

# 3   Experimental Evaluation

## 3.1   Experimental Setup

**Datasets.** We used high-resolution WSIs of pancreatic adenocarcinoma (PAAD) scanned at 40x magnification (approximately 0.25 microns per pixel) from SEER[2] (64 WSIs) and TCGA[3] (190 diagnostic WSIs). A pathologist manually annotated cancer and non-cancer regions in 50 WSIs that were randomly selected from the SEER dataset to generate the *noisy* annotation data. This process yielded a total of 69,445 tiles; 21,805 positive/cancer tiles and 47,640 negative/non-cancer tiles. We generated a manually annotated *clean* dataset of 100 positive and 100 negative tiles from the remaining 14 SEER images. The noisy and clean data comprised the "Manually Annotated Dataset" in Fig. 2. This dataset is used to train the NLC and the Baseline-Noisy models. We randomly extracted 353,000 tiles from 190 TCGA WSIs. This dataset, $D_{tcga}$, was used as part of the training dataset for the Final-CNN in Fig. 2.

We created three test datasets: $T_{seer}$, $T_{seer2}$, and $T_{tcga}$. $T_{seer}$ consists of 1700 positive tiles and 1700 negative tiles from 14 SEER WSIs. We initially extracted a total of 3,960 patches from cancer regions in these images for pathologist review and classification as positive or negative. The pathologist labeled 1,829 patches (46.2%) as positive, 1,833 patches (46.3%) as negative, and 298 patches (7.5%) as undecided. From the clean samples (1,829 positive and 1,833 negative patches), we randomly selected 3,400 patches to create $T_{seer}$ and 200 patches for $D_c$. The second set, $T_{seer2}$, contains a subset of 850 negative and 850 positive samples from $T_{seer}$, and 1,700 negative samples randomly extracted in the non-tumor regions from 14 SEER WSIs. The third test dataset, $T_{tcga}$, is made up of 3,054

---

[2] https://seer.cancer.gov/.
[3] https://portal.gdc.cancer.gov/.

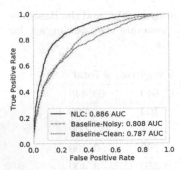
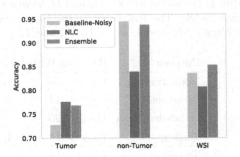

**Fig. 3.** Area Under the Curve (AUC) of the NLC, the Baseline-Noisy, and the Baseline-Clean evaluated on $T_{seer}$.

**Fig. 4.** Accuracy of the proposed models in tumor and non-tumor regions, and in WSIs as evaluated on $T_{seer2}$.

patches from 190 TCGA WSIs. Table 1 shows the number of patches extracted for the training and test datasets.

**Baseline-Clean: Baseline Model on Clean Data.** To evaluate the contribution of the clean dataset to the performance of the network, we trained the Baseline-Clean model by using the clean set only. The model is optimized by minimizing the following training loss: $\min_\theta \sum_{d_i \in D_c} \mathcal{L}_i(d_i, \theta)$.

**Implementation.** We used the Preact-Resnet-34 architecture [8] for all of the models: NLC, Baseline-Noisy, Baseline-Clean and the Final-CNN model. Preact-Resnet is a common CNN that is used in many medical imaging applications. We trained the NLC, Baseline-Noisy, and Baseline-Clean models with the same training process starting with an initial learning rate of 0.001, a momentum of 0.9 and a weight decay of 0.0001. The learning rate was decreased by a factor of 10 at the $100^{th}$ and $125^{th}$ epochs. The network weights of the models were initialized randomly and the models were trained until convergence (which took 150 epochs). We used the cross entropy loss function to compute the loss for each training sample: $\mathcal{L}_i = -y_i log(\hat{y}_i) - (1 - y_i)log(1 - \hat{y}_i)$, where $y_i = 1$ if the sample is positive and $y_i = 0$ otherwise. $\hat{y}_i$ is the prediction score of the network after the sigmoid function is applied.

We trained the two Final-CNN classification models with $D_{tgca}$: one model with labels generated by the Baseline-Noisy model and the other with labels by the Ensemble model. We used the same training procedure as for the Baseline-Noisy model apart from starting with a learning rate of 0.01. We decreased the learning rate by 10 at the $10^{th}$ epoch. We initialized the CNNs with the weights of the Baseline-Noisy model and trained for 15 epochs.

## 3.2  Results

We used the area under the ROC (Receiver Operating Characteristic) curve, or simply AUC, as our performance metric. Figure 3 shows the AUC values of

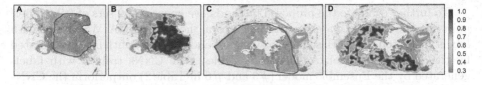

**Fig. 5.** Prediction probability maps with example WSIs generated using the Final-CNN model trained with $D_{tcga}$ with labels generated by the Ensemble model. Images A, C show the ground truth cancer regions (red lines) segmented by pathologists. Images B, D display the probability maps as heatmaps on two unseen testing SEER WSIs. (Color figure online)

the NLC, Baseline-Noisy, and Baseline-Clean models tested against $T_{seer}$. The Baseline-Clean model shows the worst performance with an AUC of 0.787. We attribute this to the fact that it was trained with a small training dataset. The NLC model outperforms the Baseline-Noisy model by 9.7% in the tumor regions, where the performance improvement is due to the use of the NLC method.

The experiments show that the NLC model generally performs well in tumor regions, whereas the Baseline-Noisy model performs better than the NLC model in non-tumor regions. We believe that this is because of the training process. The NLC model is regularized by clean data (however limited) that guides the network to better distinguish between positive and negative samples in tumor regions. In contrast, there is no clear guidance from tumor regions for the Baseline-Noisy model during training. The performance suffered in tumor regions because negative and positive patches inside a tumor region are not explicitly distinguished from one another. Because the number of negative samples is larger than the number of positive samples, the Baseline-Noisy model likely learned to better detect negative samples in non-tumor regions. This observation led to the implementation of the Ensemble as shown in Fig. 2. Figure 4 shows the performance of the NLC, Baseline-Noisy, and Ensemble models with test patches in tumor regions, test patches in non-tumor regions, and all of the test patches in the test dataset $T_{seer2}$.

**Table 2.** AUC values of CNNs trained with SEER data with human annotation (#1 and #4), and with $D_{tcga}$ with labels generated by the Baseline-Noisy model (#2 and #5), or by the Ensemble model (#3 and #6). Models are evaluated on 2 test sets: $T_{tcga}$ (#1 – #3) and $T_{seer2}$ (#4 – #6).

| # | Trainset | Label source | Testset | AUC |
|---|----------|--------------|---------|-----|
| 1 | $D_n \cup D_c$ | Human | $T_{tcga}$ | 0.829 |
| 2 | $D_{tcga}$ | Baseline-Noisy | $T_{tcga}$ | 0.832 |
| 3 | $D_{tcga}$ | Ensemble | $T_{tcga}$ | **0.860** |
| 4 | $D_n \cup D_c$ | Human | $T_{seer2}$ | 0.917 |
| 5 | $D_{tcga}$ | Baseline-Noisy | $T_{seer2}$ | 0.928 |
| 6 | $D_{tcga}$ | Ensemble | $T_{seer2}$ | **0.944** |

To further evaluate the proposed methods, we generated 2 sets of (tile, label) pairs for the 353,000 patches extracted from the 190 TCGA WSIs: one with labels generated by the Baseline-Noisy model and the other with labels generated by the Ensemble model. As shown in Table 2, the CNNs trained with labels generated by the Ensemble model (#3 and #6 in Table 2) outperform the CNNs trained with manually generated labels (#1 and #4) by 3.74% on $T_{tcga}$ and by 2.94% on $T_{seer2}$ testset in terms of AUC. They also slightly outperform the CNNs trained with labels generated by the Baseline-Noisy model. Figure 5 shows probability heatmaps of two SEER WSIs classified by the Final-CNN model trained with $D_{tcga}$ and patch labels generated by the Ensemble model.

## 4   Conclusions

Generating large training sets for pancreatic cancer region detection is very challenging due to the complexity and heterogeneity of tumor regions. Our approach involves collecting a relatively small set of clean data in cancer regions and applying a technique for assigning weights to training samples. Our results show that this approach can generate large training sets from noisy datasets. Given the high cost of generating ground truth data, we believe that methods which work with weakly-labeled, noisy data will be crucial to the broader adoption of deep learning in digital pathology. We plan to investigate additional sampling and noise reduction techniques to improve the quality of weakly-labeled training datasets and cancer region detection accuracy.

**Acknowledgement.** This work was supported in part by 1U24CA180924-01A1, 3U24CA215109-02, and 1UG3CA225021-01 from the NCI, R01LM011119-01 and R01LM009239 from the NLM. This work leveraged resources from XSEDE, which is supported by NSF ACI-1548562 grant, including the Bridges system (NSF ACI-1445606) at the Pittsburgh Supercomputing Center. We thank Vu Nguyen for meaningful discussions.

## References

1. Arpit, D., et al.: A closer look at memorization in deep networks. In: Proceedings of the 34th International Conference on Machine Learning-Volume 70, pp. 233–242. JMLR.org (2017)
2. Azizi, S., et al.: Learning from noisy label statistics: detecting high grade prostate cancer in ultrasound guided biopsy. In: Frangi, A.F., Schnabel, J.A., Davatzikos, C., Alberola-López, C., Fichtinger, G. (eds.) MICCAI 2018. LNCS, vol. 11073, pp. 21–29. Springer, Cham (2018). https://doi.org/10.1007/978-3-030-00937-3_3
3. Balachandran, V.P., et al.: Identification of unique neoantigen qualities in long-term survivors of pancreatic cancer. Nature **551**(7681), 512 (2017)
4. Dgani, Y., Greenspan, H., Goldberger, J.: Training a neural network based on unreliable human annotation of medical images. In: 2018 IEEE 15th International Symposium on Biomedical Imaging (ISBI 2018), pp. 39–42. IEEE (2018)
5. Feig, C., Gopinathan, A., Neesse, A., Chan, D.S., Cook, N., Tuveson, D.A.: The pancreas cancer microenvironment. Clin. Cancer Res. **18**, 4266–4276 (2012)

6. Ghosh, A., Kumar, H., Sastry, P.: Robust loss functions under label noise for deep neural networks. In: Thirty-First AAAI Conference on Artificial Intelligence (2017)
7. Golatkar, A., Anand, D., Sethi, A.: Classification of breast cancer histology using deep learning. In: Campilho, A., Karray, F., ter Haar Romeny, B. (eds.) ICIAR 2018. LNCS, vol. 10882, pp. 837–844. Springer, Cham (2018). https://doi.org/10.1007/978-3-319-93000-8_95
8. He, K., Zhang, X., Ren, S., Sun, J.: Identity Mappings in Deep Residual Networks. In: Leibe, B., Matas, J., Sebe, N., Welling, M. (eds.) ECCV 2016. LNCS, vol. 9908, pp. 630–645. Springer, Cham (2016). https://doi.org/10.1007/978-3-319-46493-0_38
9. Kong, B., Sun, S., Wang, X., Song, Q., Zhang, S.: Invasive cancer detection utilizing compressed convolutional neural network and transfer learning. In: Frangi, A.F., Schnabel, J.A., Davatzikos, C., Alberola-López, C., Fichtinger, G. (eds.) MICCAI 2018. LNCS, vol. 11071, pp. 156–164. Springer, Cham (2018). https://doi.org/10.1007/978-3-030-00934-2_18
10. Patrini, G., Rozza, A., Krishna Menon, A., Nock, R., Qu, L.: Making deep neural networks robust to label noise: a loss correction approach. In: Proceedings of the IEEE Conference on Computer Vision and Pattern Recognition, pp. 1944–1952 (2017)
11. Ren, M., Zeng, W., Yang, B., Urtasun, R.: Learning to reweight examples for robust deep learning. In: Proceedings of the 35th International Conference on Machine Learning (2018)
12. Tanaka, D., Ikami, D., Yamasaki, T., Aizawa, K.: Joint optimization framework for learning with noisy labels. In: Proceedings of the IEEE Conference on Computer Vision and Pattern Recognition, pp. 5552–5560 (2018)
13. Xue, C., Dou, Q., Shi, X., Chen, H., Heng, P.A.: Robust learning at noisy labeled medical images: applied to skin lesion classification. In: IEEE International Symposium on Biomedical Imaging (2019)
14. Zhang, Z., Sabuncu, M.: Generalized cross entropy loss for training deep neural networks with noisy labels. In: Advances in Neural Information Processing Systems, pp. 8778–8788 (2018)

# Encoding Histopathological WSIs Using GNN for Scalable Diagnostically Relevant Regions Retrieval

Yushan Zheng[1,2]($\boxtimes$), Bonan Jiang[3], Jun Shi[4], Haopeng Zhang[1,2], and Fengying Xie[1,2]

[1] Beijing Advanced Innovation Center for Biomedical Engineering, Beihang University, Beijing 100191, China
yszheng@buaa.edu.cn
[2] Image Processing Center, SA, Beihang University, Beijing 100191, China
[3] Beijing-Doblin International College,
Beijing University of Technology, Beijing 100124, China
[4] School of Software, Hefei University of Technology, Hefei 230601, China

**Abstract.** The research on content-based histopathological image retrieval (CBHIR) has become popular in recent years. CBHIR systems provide auxiliary diagnosis information for pathologists by searching for and returning regions that are contently similar to the region of interest (ROI) from a pre-established database. To retrieve diagnostically relevant regions from a database that consists of histopathological whole slide images (WSIs) for query ROIs is challenging and yet significant for clinical applications. In this paper, we propose a novel CBHIR framework for regions retrieval from WSI-database based on hierarchical graph neural networks (GNNs). Compared to the present CBHIR framework, the structural information of WSI is preserved by the proposed model, which makes the retrieval framework more sensitive to regions that are similar in tissue distribution. Moreover, benefited from the hierarchical GNN structures, the proposed framework is scalable for both the size and shape variation of ROIs. It allows the pathologist defining the query region using free curves. Thirdly, the retrieval is achieved by binary codes and hashing methods, which makes it very efficient and thereby adequate for practical large-scale WSI-database. The proposed method is validated on a lung cancer dataset and compared to the state-of-the-art methods. The proposed method achieved precisions above 82.4% in the irregular region retrieval task, which are superior to the state-of-the-art methods. The average time of retrieval is 0.514 ms.

**Keywords:** Digital pathology · Histopathological image analysis · GNN · CBIR · ACDC-LungHP

**Electronic supplementary material** The online version of this chapter (https://doi.org/10.1007/978-3-030-32239-7_61) contains supplementary material, which is available to authorized users.

# 1    Introduction

With the development of whole slide imaging techniques for digital pathology, the computer aided cancer diagnosis methods based on histopathlogical image analysis (HIA) have been widely studied. Content-based histopathological image retrieval (CBHIR) is an emerging approach in this domain [1]. CBHIR searches a pre-established WSI database for the regions the pathologist concerned and provides contently similar regions to the pathologists for reference. Compared to the typical HIA methods based on image segmentation and classification [2], CBHIR methods can provide more valuable information including the diagnostically similar regions, the meta-information, and the diagnosis reports of experts stored along with the cases in the digital pathology system.

The present studies for CBHIR are generally on databases consist of image blocks or patches in a fixed size. However, the practical histopathological databases generally consist of digital whole slide images and the query regions created by the pathologists are in different sizes and shapes. It is challenging to efficiently retrieve regions from large-scale database containing WSIs in very high pixel-resolutions and accurately return the similar cases the pathologists needed. To meet the efficiency requirement for large-scale histopathological database retrieval, the binary encoding and hashing techniques have been successfully introduced to accelerate the process of retrieval [1,3]. To index WSIs for region-level retrieval, the WSIs are commonly divided into small patches following the sliding window paradigm. However, the diagnosis of cancer with tissue sections not only depends on the local nuclei features but also the contextual information from a broad region surrounding the nuclei. Several retrieval strategies have been developed to improve the scalability of the retrieval framework to size variation of query regions [4–6]. These methods mainly applied feature vector quantification approach, e.g. pooling operations, to embed the features of local patches, which is a convenient to generate uniform representation for irregular tissue regions. However, the adjacent relationship of different type of biopsy objects are lost during the feature quantification, for which the structure similarity between tumor regions are difficult to recognize in the procedure of retrieval.

In this paper, we propose a novel framework for histopathological image retrieval from large-scale WSI-database based on graph neural network (GNN) [8] and hashing method. The proposed framework for CBHIR is illustrated in Fig. 1. The WSIs are first divided into patches and converted into image features using a pre-trained convolutional neural networks (CNN). Then, graphs of tissue are established based on spatial relationships and feature distances of patches. Finally, the tissue-graphs are fed into the designed GNN-Hash model to obtain the indexes for retrieval. The retrieval strategy proposed in this paper is scalable for both the size and shape of query ROIs, which makes the proposed method more applicable than the present methods.

The novelty and contribution of this paper to the problem is two-fold. To our knowledge, we are the first to introduce GNN for histopathological image retrieval. Besides the local features of tissue regions, the distribution of tissue

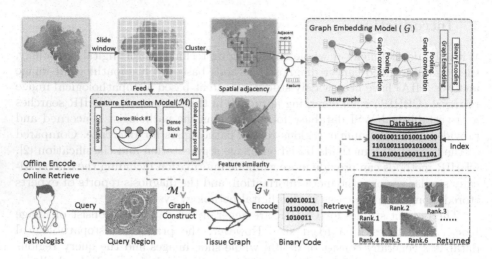

**Fig. 1.** The proposed CBHIR framework. In the offline stage, tissue graphs are first constructed based on the spatial adjacency and feature similarity of patches. Then, the graphs are embedded into binary codes and stored to the retrieval database. When retrieving, the region the pathologist queries are converted into a binary code and then the diagnostically relevant regions are retrieved and returned to pathologists.

is considered and preserved in the process of WSI encoding. The accuracy and scalability of the CBHIR framework has been improved. Secondly, we combined the GNN structure with binary encoding and designed a GNN-Hash model. The GNN-Hash model is trained end-to-end from graphs with variable number of nodes to the binary-like codes, which makes the retrieval framework both structural-preserving and time-saving. It determines that the proposed method is applicable for practical large-scale WSI database.

The remainder of this paper is organized as follows. Section 2 introduces the methodology of the proposed method. The experiment is presented in Sect. 3. Section 4 summarizes the contributions.

## 2    Methods

Motivated by the development of graph information analysis (e.g. protein structure recognition and social network analysis), we propose to establish graph structures to depict the adjacent relationship of local regions in WSIs. The details of the proposed methods are introduced in this section.

### 2.1    Tissue Graph Construction

A graph $G$ can be represented as $(\mathbf{A}, \mathbf{X})$. $\mathbf{A} \in \mathbb{R}^{n \times n}$ is an adjacent matrix that defines the connectivity of the $n$ nodes in $G$, where $a_{ij} = 1, a_{ij} \in \mathbf{A}$ represents

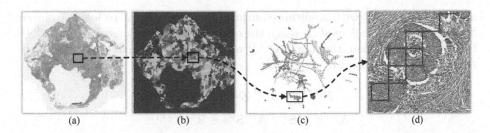

(a)　　　　　　　(b)　　　　　　　(c)　　　　　　　(d)

**Fig. 2.** The flowchart of tissue graphs, where (a) is a digital WSI, (b) illustrates the sub-regions, (c) shows the graphs established on sub-regions, and (d) jointly presents a graph and its corresponding regions where the nodes are drawn on the centroids of patches.

the $i$-th and the $j$-th node in the graph are connected, and $a_{ij} = 0$, otherwise. $\mathbf{X} \in \mathbb{R}^{n \times d}$ denotes the node feature matrix assuming each node is represented as a $d$-dimensional column vector. In this paper, the sub-regions in the WSI are described by graphs. The flowchart to construct graphs for a WSI is presented in Fig. 2. First, the WSI is divided into non-overlapping patches using a sliding window. Then, the patches are fed into a pre-trained convolutional neural network (CNN) to extract patch features $\mathbf{X}$. Considering that the tumor regions in a WSI varies in shape and size, we propose mosaicking the adjacent patches into irregular sub-regions. Specifically, the agglomerative hierarchical clustering algorithm [7] is employed to merge the patches based on the similarities between patch features. To ensure the sub-regions are spatially connected, only the 4-connected patches are allowed to be mosaicked. After the clustering, a set of graphs $\{G_i\}$ can be established (Fig. 2(c)). The set $\{G_i\}$ can cover the entire content of the WSI and thereby can be used to index the WSI for retrieval.

## 2.2 GNN-Hash for Graph Encoding

To establish the retrieval indexes, the graphs are needed to be encoded into vectors in equal dimensions. It is challenging to simultaneously embed the node attributes and edge information into an uniform representation. Graph neural network (GNN) [8] is an emerging techniques for graph information embedding, which has been proven effective in histopathological image analysis [9]. Generally, GNNs can be represented following message-passing architecture $\mathbf{H}^{(k)} = M(\mathbf{A}, \mathbf{H}^{(k-1)} : \theta^{(k)})$, where $H^{(k)} \in \mathbb{R}^{n \times d}$ denotes the embeddings on the $k$-th step of passing, $M$ is the message propagation function [10–12] that depends on the adjacent matrix $\mathbf{A}$, the output of the previous step $\mathbf{H}^{(k-1)}$, and the set of trainable parameters $\theta^{(k)}$. $\mathbf{H}^{(0)}$ is the original attributes of the nodes, i.e., the CNN features of patches $\mathbf{X}$ in our method. For simplicity, a GNN module with multiple steps of embeddings can be represented as $\mathbf{Z} = GNN(\mathbf{A}, \mathbf{X})$. Multiple GNNs can be stacked to learn deep representations of graphs. Recently, Ying et al. [13] proposed a differentiable graph pooling module (DiffPool), which enables the hierarchical GNNs to be trained in end-to-end fashion. Specifically, an additional GNN with a softmax output layer is designed to learn a matrix $\mathbf{S} \in \mathbb{R}^{n_l \times n_{l+1}}$, which is used to assign the output representations of the $l$-th GNN to $n_{l+1}$ clusters. Then, the input $\mathbf{X}^{(l+1)}$ and the adjacent matrix $\mathbf{A}^{(l+1)}$ for the next GNN are obtained by equations:

$$\mathbf{X}^{(l+1)} = \mathbf{S}^{(l)\mathrm{T}}\mathbf{Z}^{(l)} \in \mathbb{R}^{n_{l+1} \times n_l}$$
$$\mathbf{A}^{(l+1)} = \mathbf{S}^{(l)\mathrm{T}}\mathbf{A}^{(l)}\mathbf{S}^{(l)} \in \mathbb{R}^{n_{l+1} \times n_{l+1}}$$

In our method, the network is used to learn representations that are effective for data retrieval. To ensure the framework is applicable to practical large-scale pathological database, we modified the output of the hierarchical GNNs to generate a GNN-Hash structure. Specifically, a binary encoding layer is defined based on the last graph embeddings $\mathbf{Z}^{(L)} \in \mathbb{R}^{N \times d}$: $\mathbf{Y} = \tanh(\mathbf{Z}^{(L)}\mathbf{W} + \mathbf{b})$, where $\mathbf{W}$ and $\mathbf{b}$ are the weights and bias for a linear projection. $\mathbf{Y} \in (-1, 1)^{N \times d_h}$ is the network outputs that can be simply converted into binary codes by equation $\mathbf{B} = sign(\mathbf{Y}) \in \{-1, 1\}^{N \times d_h}$, where $N$ is the number of graphs and $d_h$ is the dimension of binary codes. The loss function for training the GNN-Hash is defined as

$$J = \frac{1}{N}\|\frac{1}{d_h}\mathbf{Y}^{\mathrm{T}}\mathbf{Y} - \mathbf{C}\|_F^2 + \lambda\|\mathbf{W}^{\mathrm{T}}\mathbf{W} - \mathbf{I}\|_F^2$$

where $\mathbf{C} \in \{-1, 1\}^{N \times N}$ is the pair-wise label matrix in which $c_{ij} = 1$ represents the $i$-th and $j$-th tissue graphs are relevant and $c_{ij} = -1$ otherwise, and $\lambda$ is a weight coefficient. Finally, the proposed GNN-Hash structure is trained end-to-end from the input graph $G$ with CNN-features to the output $\mathbf{Y}$.

### 2.3    Retrieval Using Binary Codes

For each WSI in the retrieval database, a set of binary codes ($\mathbf{B}$) that represent the graphs in the WSI can be obtained using the trained model. When retrieving, the region the pathologist queries is divided into patches and converted into binary code using the same model. Then, the similarities between the query code and those in the database are measure using Hamming distance. After ranking the similarities, the top-ranked regions are retrieved and finally returned to the pathologist.

## 3    Experiments

### 3.1    Experimental Setting

The experiments were conducted on the ACDC-LungHP dataset[1] [14], which contains 150 WSIs within lung cancer regions annotated by pathologists. In the evaluation, 30 WSIs were randomly selected as the testing dataset and the

---

[1] The dataset is accessible at https://acdc-lunghp.grand-challenge.org/. Since the annotations of testing part of the data set are not yet published, only the 150 training WSIs of the data were used in this paper.

**Table 1.** Comparison of retrieval performance with the state-of-the-art methods.

| Methods | P@50 | P@200 | MAP@50 | MAP@200 | Complexity | Time |
|---|---|---|---|---|---|---|
| Shi et al. [3] | 0.726* | 0.723* | 0.747* | 0.733* | $\mathcal{O}(n)$ | 180 ms |
| Zheng et al. [16] | 0.759 | 0.745 | 0.781 | 0.761 | $\mathcal{O}(m \log n)$ | 86.1 ms |
| Ma et al. [4] | 0.735 | 0.726 | 0.756 | 0.736 | $\mathcal{O}(n)$ | 0.507 ms |
| Jimenez et al. [6] | 0.750 | 0.745 | 0.770 | 0.753 | $\mathcal{O}(mn)$ | 4.97 s |
| GNN-LR** | 0.797 | 0.794 | 0.812 | 0.802 | $\mathcal{O}(n)$ | 1.20 ms |
| GNN-Hash | **0.826** | **0.824** | **0.838** | **0.833** | $\mathcal{O}(n)$ | 0.514 ms |

*This is result for fixed-size-patch ($224 \times 224$ pixels) retrieval task. Because there are 489,330 patches in the retrieval database, the average running time of this method is much longer than other methods with $\mathcal{O}(n)$ complexity.
**This is the retrieval result based on the last representation (LR) of the designed hierarchical GNNs structure but trained using the classification loss proposed in [13].

remainders were used to train the retrieval models and establish the retrieval database. To evaluate the scalability to size and shape variations of query ROIs, the WSIs were divided into irregular sub-regions under 40× lenses using the clustering approach introduced in Sect. 2.1. Consequently, 2894 query regions are generated and 16261 regions are created to establish the retrieval database. The number of patches in each region ranges from 1 to 136 with a median number of 37.

The DenseNet-121 structure [15] pre-trained for classification task within the training WSIs was used as the feature extractor of patches. Two GNN modules within three embedding steps and two DiffPool modules were stacked to generate the GNN-Hash structure. The dimension of node embeddings was tuned from 60 to 120 with a step of 20 on the training set and determined as 100. The bit number of the output binary code was set $d_h = 32$. The proposed method was implemented in python with pytorch. All the experiments were conducted on a computer with an Intel Core i7-7700k CPU of 4.2 GHz and a GPU of Nvidia GTX 1080Ti.

## 3.2  Results and Discussion

The proposed method is compared with 4 state-of-the-art-methods [3,4,6,16] proposed for histological image retrieval. For fair comparison, the backbones of the compared methods are the same DenseNet-121 structure used in our model. In the evaluation, the graphs that contain more than 10% cancerous pixels referring to the pathologists' annotation are defined as *cancerous graph*, and the remainders are defined as *non-cancerous graph*. The retrieval precision (P@R) and the mean average precision (MAP@R) of the top $R$ returned graphs are used as the evaluation metrics. The experimental results are summarized in Table 1.

Overall, the proposed method achieved the best retrieval performance. The query regions and the database regions in [3] are limited to square patches in a

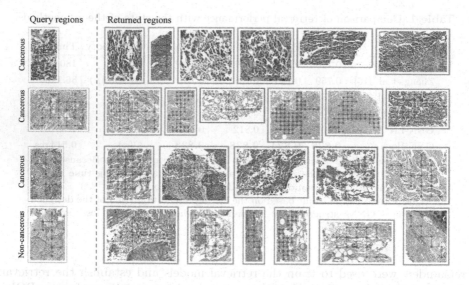

**Fig. 3.** Visualization of the retrieval performance of the proposed method, where the first column provides 4 query regions, the top-returned regions are ranked on the right, the relevant return regions (has the same label with the query region) are framed in green and the irrelevant regions are in red. The locations of the graph are meanwhile displayed. A high-quality copy of this picture is submitted as supplemental material.

fixed size. Hence, we regarded the patches in graphs as the retrieval instances and reported the patch-level retrieval performance for this method. Besides, the other methods are scalable to the size variation of query regions. Ma et al. [4] proposed quantifying the patch features in a region using max-pooling operation and calculating the similarities between regions based on the pooled representations. The percentage of patches of different tissue types is ignored by the pooling operation, which has reduced the retrieval accuracy. Zheng et al. [16] and Jimenez et al. [6] proposed measuring the similarity of two regions by an ensemble of feature distances of all the patch pairs across the two regions. The local similarities between the regions are considered in the two methods, which has improved the MAP@200 to 0.761 and 0.753, respectively. The main drawback of the two methods is that the adjacent relationship of tissue objects cannot be effectively described, which has severely affected the performance of retrieval. In contrast, the proposed method constructed graphs within tissue regions. The information of tissue allocation has been sufficiently described and well preserved via the hierarchical embeddings of the proposed GNN-Hash model. It contributes to a significant improvement of MAP@200 from 0.761 to 0.833, compared to that obtained by Zheng et al. [16]. The retrieval results obtained by the proposed framework are visualized in Fig. 3. It presents that the proposed model can adapt to the variation of size and shape of query regions and the diagnostically relevant regions to the query regions are successfully retrieved.

The efficiency is also important for CBHIR system. The computational complexity (by $\mathcal{O}$ notation) relevant to the pixel size of query region $m$ and the scale of the database $n$ for the compared methods are given in Table 1. Correspondingly, the average time consumption for retrieval are also compared (the feature extraction time is not involved). In our method, the computation for retrieval is irrelevant to the size of query region after the encoding and thereby the complexity is $\mathcal{O}(n)$. Moreover, benefiting from the binary encoding, the similarity measurement is time-saving than those (e.g. GNN-LR) based on float-type high-dimensional features. When the order of magnitudes of WSI in database increases and the content in the database is abundant, a hashing table will be pre-established. Then, the retrieval can be easily achieved by a table-lookup operation, for which the complexity of retrieval can be further reduced to $\mathcal{O}(1)$.

## 4   Conclusion

In this paper, we proposed a novel histopathological image retrieval framework for large-scale database consisting of WSIs. The instances in the database are defined based on graphs and are converted into binary codes by the designed GNN-Hash model. The experimental results have demonstrated that the proposed model achieves the state-of-the-art retrieval performance and is scalable to size and shape variations of query regions and can effectively retrieve relevant regions that contain similar content and structure of tissue. It allows pathologists to create query regions by free-curves on the digital pathology platform. Benefiting from hashing structure, the retrieval process is completed based on hamming distance, which is very time-saving. Overall, the proposed method is effective, efficient and practical for large-scale WSI database retrieval.

**Acknowledgment.** This work was supported by the National Natural Science Foundation of China (No. 61771031, 61371134, 61471016, and 61501009), China Postdoctoral Science Foundation (No. 2019M650446) and Motic-BUAA Image Technology Research Center.

## References

1. Li, Z., Zhang, X., Müller, H., et al.: Large-scale retrieval for medical image analytics: a comprehensive review. Med. Image Anal. **43**, 66–84 (2018)
2. Bejnordi, B.E., Veta, M., Van Diest, P.J., et al.: Diagnostic assessment of deep learning algorithms for detection of lymph node metastases in women with breast cancer. JAMA **318**(22), 2199–2210 (2017)
3. Shi, X., Sapkota, M., Xing, F., et al.: Pairwise based deep ranking hashing for histopathology image classification and retrieval. Pattern Recogn. **81**, 14–22 (2018)
4. Ma, Y., Jiang, Z., Zhang, H., et al.: Generating region proposals for histopathological whole slide image retrieval. Comput. Methods Programs Biomed. **159**, 1–10 (2018)
5. Zheng, Y., Jiang, Z., Zhang, H., et al.: Histopathological whole slide image analysis using context-based CBIR. IEEE Trans. Med. Imaging **37**(7), 1641–1652 (2018)

6. Jimenez-del-Toro, O., Otálora, S., Atzori, M., Müller, H.: Deep multimodal case-based retrieval for large histopathology datasets. In: Wu, G., Munsell, B., Zhan, Y., Bai, W., Sanroma, G., Coupé, P. (eds.) Patch-MI 2017. LNCS, vol. 10530, pp. 149–157. Springer, Cham (2017). https://doi.org/10.1007/978-3-319-67434-6_17
7. Day, W.H.E., Edelsbrunner, H.: Efficient algorithms for agglomerative hierarchical clustering methods. J. Classif. 1(1), 7–24 (1984)
8. Wu, Z., Pan, S., Chen, F., et al.: A comprehensive survey on graph neural networks. arXiv:1901.00596 (2019)
9. Li, R., Yao, J., Zhu, X., Li, Y., Huang, J.: Graph CNN for survival analysis on whole slide pathological images. In: Frangi, A.F., Schnabel, J.A., Davatzikos, C., Alberola-López, C., Fichtinger, G. (eds.) MICCAI 2018. LNCS, vol. 11071, pp. 174–182. Springer, Cham (2018). https://doi.org/10.1007/978-3-030-00934-2_20
10. Gilmer, J., Schoenholz, S.S., Riley, P.F., et al.: Neural message passing for quantum chemistry. In: Proceedings of the 34th International Conference on Machine Learning (ICML), pp. 1263–1272 (2017)
11. Hamilton, W., Ying, Z., Leskovec, J.: Inductive representation learning on large graphs. In: Proceedings of Advances in Neural Information Processing Systems (NeurIPS), pp. 1024–1034 (2017)
12. Kipf, T.N., Welling, M.: Semi-supervised classification with graph convolutional networks. In: Proceedings of International Conference on Learning Representations (ICLR) (2017)
13. Ying, Z., You, J., Morris, C., et al.: Hierarchical graph representation learning with differentiable pooling. In: Proceedings of Advances in Neural Information Processing Systems (NeurIPS), pp. 4805–4815 (2018)
14. Li, Z., Hu, Z., et al.: Computer-aided diagnosis of lung carcinoma using deep learning - a pilot study. arXiv:1803.05471v1 (2018)
15. Huang, G., Liu, Z., Van Der Maaten, L., et al.: Densely connected convolutional networks. In: Proceedings of the IEEE Conference on Computer Vision and Pattern Recognition (CVPR), pp. 4700–4708 (2017)
16. Zheng, Y., Jiang, Z., Zhang, H., et al.: Size-scalable content-based histopathological image retrieval from database that consists of WSIs. IEEE J. Biomed. Health Inf. 22(4), 1278–1287 (2018)

# Local and Global Consistency Regularized Mean Teacher for Semi-supervised Nuclei Classification

Hai Su[1], Xiaoshuang Shi[1], Jinzheng Cai[1], and Lin Yang[1,2]([✉])

[1] Department of Biomedical Engineering,
University of Florida, Gainesville, FL 32611, USA
{hsu224,xsshi2015,jimmycai}@ufl.edu
[2] Department of Electrical and Computer Engineering,
University of Florida, Gainesville, FL 32611, USA
lin.yang@bme.ufl.edu

**Abstract.** Nucleus classification is a fundamental task in pathology diagnosis for cancers, *e.g.*, Ki-67 index estimation. Supervised deep learning methods have achieved promising classification accuracy. However, the success of these methods heavily relies on massive manually annotated data. Manual annotation for nucleus classification are usually time consuming and laborious. In this paper, we propose a novel semi-supervised deep learning method that can learn from small portion of labeled data and large-scale unlabeled data for nucleus classification. Our method is inspired by the recent state-of-the-art self-ensembling (SE) methods. These methods learn from unlabeled data by enforcing consistency of predictions under different perturbations while ignoring local and global consistency hidden in data structure. In our work, a label propagation (LP) step is integrated into the SE method, and a graph is constructed using the LP predictions that encode the local and global data structure. Finally, a Siamese loss is used to learn the local and global consistency from the graph. Our implementation is based on the state-of-the-art SE method *Mean Teacher*. Extensive experiments on two nucleus datasets demonstrate that our method outperforms the state-of-the-art SE methods, and achieves $F_1$ scores close to the supervised methods using only 5%–25% labeled data.

**Keywords:** Nucleus classification · Semi-supervised learning · Deep learning

## 1 Introduction

Nucleus type information is essential in many pathology diagnoses [4,9]. In many settings, the presence and portion of certain types of nucleus are used to assess the proliferation rate, subtypes or grade of the diseases [4,13]. Traditionally, nucleus classification is treated as a supervised classification problem [3,4,9]

© Springer Nature Switzerland AG 2019
D. Shen et al. (Eds.): MICCAI 2019, LNCS 11764, pp. 559–567, 2019.
https://doi.org/10.1007/978-3-030-32239-7_62

and deep neural networks have achieved rather satisfactory performance. However, the superiority of supervised deep learning usually heavily relies on the availability of massive manually annotated data. As well known that large- scale annotation for medical data is expensive and time consuming, *e.g.*, diagnostic pathology images, while large-scale unlabeled data are relatively easy to obtain. To alleviate the high demand for manual annotation, semi-supervised deep learning (SSDL) has been developed to learn from a small portion of labeled data and large-scale unlabeled data. Recently, self-ensembling (SE) based semi-supervised learning has attracted broad attention [7,8,11]. The intuition of SE method is to enforce a prediction consistency for each training sample under different perturbations. Such consistency is not dependent on label information, and is able to extract extra semantic information from the unlabeled data. One of the successful SE method is called *temporal ensembling* (TE) [5]. In TE, for each unlabeled sample, an exponential moving average (EMA) of the prediction within multiple previous training epochs is computed as the proxy target. A mean square error (MSE) between the predictions and the proxy targets is used as the consistency loss. The proxy targets are the ensembled predictions of those from many previous epochs, thus serve as stronger proxy labels that provide extra semantic information in addition to the labeled data. However, TE requires to maintain a matrix of size $N \times C$, where $N$ denotes the number of training samples, including labeled and unlabeled data, and $C$ is the number of classes. This requirement makes TE model heavy when learning on large datasets. To alleviate this problem, *Mean Teacher* (MT) [10] utilizes two models (student and teacher models). Instead of maintaining the EMA of the proxy labels, MT method maintains a teacher model as the EMA of the student model. In each minibatch evaluation, the output of the teacher model is used as the proxy target. Since such proxy target is generated by the EMA model aggregated from many student models, it provides better proxy targets.

One aspect ignored by the aforementioned SE methods is the intrinsic structure of data. That is the local and global consistency widely existing in many datasets [2,12]. Local consistency refers to that samples from the same class are likely to lie in the same vicinity in the feature space. Global consistency means that samples from the same global structure are likely to share the same label. To enforce the local and global consistency, in this paper, we propose a novel loss function that is computed over a graph constructed via label propagation (LP) [14]. Specifically, we utilize the LP algorithm to iteratively propagate the label information from the labeled samples to the unlabeled ones based on the local structure until a global stable state is reached, then construct a graph based on the LP predicted labels. Next, Siamese loss is employed to pull the data from same class closer and push those from different classes further away. Therefore, the two consistencies are enforced. Experiments on two nucleus classification datasets illustrate the superior performance of the proposed method over the recent state-of-the-art SE methods.

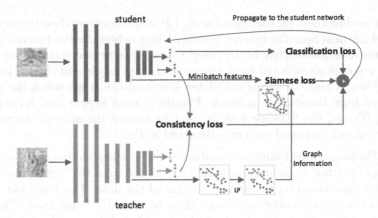

**Fig. 1.** Each minibatch consists of both labeled and unlabeled samples. The LP predicted labels and the ground truth labels are used to construct a graph capturing the local and global structure of the data. A Siamese loss is computed based on the graph. The student network is updated by a hybrid loss consisting of classification loss, consistency loss and the Siamese loss.

## 2 Mean Teacher with Label Propagation

### 2.1 Preliminaries

Since our method is based on mean teacher (MT) [10], we first briefly introduce mean teacher in this subsection. Let $\mathcal{X}_l = \{x_1, x_2, \cdots, x_n\} \subset \mathbb{R}^m$ denote the labeled data and $\mathcal{X}_u = \{x_{n+1}, x_{n+2}, \cdots, x_N\} \subset \mathbb{R}^m$ denote the unlabeled data. The system consists of two networks, *i.e.*, the student network and the teacher network. The parameters of the teacher network is the EMA of the student network computed by: $\theta'_\tau = \alpha\theta'_{\tau-1} + (1-\alpha)\theta_\tau$, where $\alpha$ denotes the EMA coefficient, and $\theta$ and $\theta'$ represent the parameters of the student model and the teacher model, respectively. $\tau$ represents the global training iteration. The student network is updated by the following loss:

$$Loss_{mt} = \frac{1}{n}\sum_i^n (-y_i \log f_\theta(x_i)) + w(\tau)\lambda_{EMA}\mathbb{E}_{x,\eta,\eta'}[\|f_{\theta'}(x_j, \eta') - f_\theta(x_j, \eta)\|],$$

$$(1)$$

where $\lambda_{EMA}$ is the coefficient controlling the strength of consistency between predictions of the same sample under different perturbations represented by $\eta$ and $\eta'$. $w(\tau)$ is a ramp function of the global iterations $\tau$. The first term is the cross-entropy loss for the labeled data and the second term enforces the consistency between the predictions of the student network $f_\theta(x, \eta)$ and the teacher network $f_{\theta'}(x, \eta')$. The consistency term is computed on all the data.

### 2.2 Local and Global Consistency Regularized Mean Teacher

As mentioned before, the MT method ignores the connection between the samples thus fails to extract more semantic information from the unlabeled data. In the proposed method, for each minibatch, LP is first conducted on the intermediate level features from the teacher network. This is because the teacher network is an ensemble model that is supposed to generate better feature embedding. Then a graph is constructed using the ground truth labels and the LP predicted labels. Next, a Siamese loss is calculated based on the graph using the features generated from the student network. Finally, a novel hybrid loss, including the loss Eq. (1) and the Siamese loss, is used to update the student network. An overview of our proposed system is depicted in Fig. 1.

**Label Propagation:** Label propagation [14] is a transductive semi-supervised learning algorithm. It propagates label information from the labeled data to the unlabeled data based on the affinity matrix of the data. The basic idea is that the data close to each other are more likely to share the same label. Therefore, the LP procedure computes the label of an unlabeled data as the weighted sum of the labels of its neighbors. Through an iterative procedure, the label can be propagated from the labeled data to their neighbors, and the neighbors of neighbors. Finally, the unlabeled data are assigned labels that respect the global structure of the data. The LP algorithm is proven to converge. More details of the proof can be found in [14].

**Graph Based Clustering Loss:** With the LP predicted labels for the unlabeled data, the pairwise connection information between the data points are known. With this information a graph can be built by:

$$A_{ij} = \begin{cases} 1, & \text{if } y_i = y_j, \\ 0, & \text{otherwise,} \end{cases} \tag{2}$$

where $y_i$ denotes the LP predicted labels for unlabeled data ($j \le n < i \le N$) and the ground truth labels for the labeled data ($i, j \le n$). To enforce the local and global consistencies, we propose to use the contrastive Siamese loss [1] to pull the samples within the same class closer and push those from different classes further away:

$$L_s = \begin{cases} \|z_i - z_j\|^2, & \text{if } A_{ij} = 1, \\ \max(0, m - \|z_i - z_j\|^2), & \text{if } A_{ij} = 0, \end{cases} \tag{3}$$

where $z_i$ represents the feature vector from the intermediate layers of the student network and $m$ is a hyperparameter. The final proposed loss function is:

$$L_{total} = Loss_{mt} + w(\tau)(\lambda_{g1} \sum_{x_i, x_j \in \mathcal{X}_l} L_{s1} + \lambda_{g2} \sum_{x_i \in \mathcal{X}_l, x_j \in \mathcal{X}_u} L_{s2}), \tag{4}$$

where $\lambda_{g1}$ denotes the weight of the Siamese loss computed on the labeled samples, and $\lambda_{g2}$ represents the weight of the Siamese loss computed on both unlabeled and labeled data. Since the LP does not change the labels of the labeled samples, the Siamese loss $L_{s1}$ ensures that there is always some correct information for learning. Note that we do not compute Siamese loss between the unlabeled samples. This is because the LP-predicted labels are very noisy. Including them in the loss could harm the training.

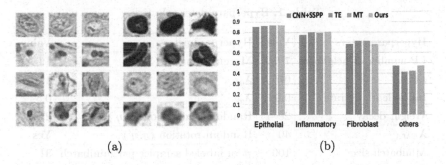

(a)                                    (b)

**Fig. 2.** (a) Some sample nuclei from the two datasets. (b) The $F_1$ scores of each class in the MoNuseg data obtained using 25% training data.

## 3   Experiments

To evaluate our method, we conduct experiments on two datasets, including the MoNuseg dataset [9] and our own Ki-67 nucleus dataset. In the MoNuseg dataset, there are four types of nucleus, (*i.e.*, Epithelial, Inflammatory, Fibroblast, Miscellaneous). In the Ki-67 dataset, there are also four types of nucleus, including immunopositive (non-)tumor nucleus and immunonegative (non-)tumor nucleus. The MoNuseg dataset contains 22462 nuclei and the Ki-67 dataset contains 17516 nuclei. For both datasets, 80% nuclei images are used for training, 20% of the training data is used for validation, and the rest are used for testing. A few samples of each type of nucleus are shown in Fig. 2(a).

We compare our method against two state-of-the-art SSDL methods, *i.e.*, TE [5] and MT [10], and a baseline fully supervised training method using the labeled data only. For each comparison, we train the different methods using only $x\%$ ($x = \{5, 10, 25, 50\}$ for the MoNuseg dataset, and $x = \{1, 5, 10\}$ for the Ki-67 dataset) of the training data as labeled data and the rest as unlabeled data. In fully supervised setting, the same network is trained using the labeled data only. Additionally, since the MoNuseg dataset is a publicly available dataset, we also show two results reported in [9], *i.e.*, CNN-SSPP and CNN-NEP. These two methods are fully supervised methods. In all the comparisons, weighted average $F_1$ score is used as evaluation metric. For the semi-supervised settings, and we report the average $F_1$ scores and their standard deviations of 5 runs on the testing data. In each of the 5 runs, a different set of labeled data are randomly selected.

### 3.1   Implementation Details

**Network Architecture.** In this paper, we adopt a network similar to the one used in [10]. The difference is the kernel size of the last two convolutional layers are set to 3. The input noise layer, ZCA layer, mean-only batch normalization are omitted. The advantage of our choice is that every component in our network can be implemented using standard Pytorch functions and scikit-learn package.

**Table 1.** Hyperparameter selection.

| Hyperparameters | Value | Hyperparameters | Value |
|---|---|---|---|
| LP number of neighbors | 7–10 | Margin $m$ in Eq. (3) | 1.0 |
| LP $\alpha$ | 0.7 | $\lambda_{g1}$ | 1.0 |
| Initial learning rate | 0.001 | $\lambda_{g2}$ | 0.5 |
| Weight decay | $2e$-4 | Random translation $(\eta, \eta')$ | 2 |
| $\lambda_{EMA}$ | 40 | Random rotation $(\eta, \eta')$ | Yes |
| Minibatch size | 100 | # of labeled samples per minibatch | 31 |
| LP iteration $k$ | 30 | # of classes $C$ | 4 |

The features used in label propagation and Siamese loss are extracted from the intermediate layer (Fig. 1). Such design is chosen empirically. LP is conducted for each minibatch to build a connection graph. The Siamese loss based on the graph is computed in two terms Eq. (4). Specifically, the summation on $L_{s1}$ is computed on 30 labeled data, and the summation on $L_{s2}$ is from this 30 labeled data and 30 randomly selected unlabeled data. The coefficients for these two terms are shown in Table 1. The time complexity of LP is $k\mathcal{O}(CN^2)$, where $k$ denotes the number of iterations, and $C$ denotes the number of classes, and $N$ denotes the minibatch size. With such overhead, our model can still be trained within 6 h on a GTX 1080 Ti GPU.

**Hyperparameter Selection.** Mostly we follow the parameter settings used in MT method [10]. The learning rate and the ramp function $w(\tau)$ are ramped up and down during the 150000 global steps. Specifically, they are ramped up in the first 40000 global steps, then kept constant for the following 85000 global steps, and finally decreased to 0 in the last 25000 global steps. We use $w(\tau) = e^{-5(1-\tau/150000)^2}$ as the ramp-up function and $w(\tau) = e^{-12.5(\tau/150000)^2}$ as the ramp-down function. The other parameter setting in our method are shown in Table 1.

## 3.2    Results and Analysis

Tables 2 and 3 illustrate that our method outperforms the state of the arts, especially when using less labeled data. For the MoNuseg dataset (Table 2), our method achieves around 2% higher $F_1$ scores compared to MT and TE methods when using 5% and 10% of the training data. Along with the increase of labeled data used, the performance of all the semi-supervised methods converges. In comparison with the baseline fully supervised method using labeled data only, our performance is higher by large margin. In contrast to the results reported in [9], our method outperforms CNN-SSPP using only 5% labeled data and achieves the performance close to CNN-NEP using only 25% labeled data. It is worth note that our method and CNN-SSPP take the nucleus patch as the sole

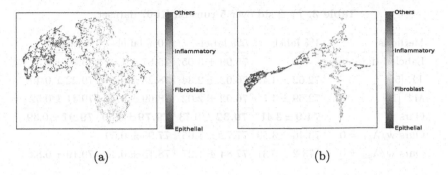

(a)                                                    (b)

**Fig. 3.** Embeddings of the MoNuseg testing data projected to 2D space using UMAP [6]. (a) The feature embedding obtained by MT. (b) The embedding obtained by our method.

input while CNN-NEP takes into account the contextual information around the nucleus. This means CNN-NEP is actually using more labeled data. Moreover, the contextual information around the nucleus may not be a general approach for all nucleus classification problems. CNN-SSPP and CNN-NEP are both fully supervised methods. They are listed in the column 50% labels in Table 2, because they are based on two-fold cross validation [9]. Since the MoNuseg dataset is an imbalanced dataset, we show a comparison of the $F_1$ scores for each class in Fig. 2(b). Finally, to demonstrate the effect of the graph based clustering loss, we show the feature embedding of the MoNuseg testing data in Fig. 3.

For the Ki-67 dataset, we observed similar behavior. Our method outperforms the MT, TE and fully supervised method. Ablation studies are designed to show the effect of our proposed graph based clustering loss. Since the graph based clustering loss consists of two parts: (i) $L_{s1}$ computed on the labeled data only; and (ii) $L_{s2}$ computed between the unlabeled data and the labeled data. We train our model with one of the two losses removed and show the performance in Table 3. It can be seen that the performance drops if either one of them is removed. This shows the advantage of learning from a graph constructed on both labeled and unlabeled data.

**Table 2.** $F_1 \pm$ std over 5 runs on MoNuseg dataset [9].

| Supervised methods | 5% labels | 10% labels | 25% labels | 50% labels | All labels |
|---|---|---|---|---|---|
| Labeled data only | $63.21 \pm 1.92$ | $64.97 \pm 1.72$ | $73.04 \pm 0.54$ | $74.5 \pm 0.72$ | $78.15 \pm 0.25$ |
| CNN-SSPP [9] | - | - | - | 74.8 | - |
| CNN-NEP [9] | - | - | - | 78.4 | - |
| Semi-supervised | 5% labels | 10% labels | 25% labels | 50% labels | All labels |
| TE [5] | $73.2 \pm 0.51$ | $74.01 \pm 0.85$ | $76.46 \pm 0.24$ | $76.48 \pm 0.21$ | $76.57 \pm 0.26$ |
| MT [10] | $73.07 \pm 0.56$ | $74.35 \pm 0.54$ | $76.42 \pm 0.56$ | $76.59 \pm 0.33$ | $78.1 \pm 0.29$ |
| Ours | $\mathbf{75.02 \pm 0.55}$ | $\mathbf{75.79 \pm 0.23}$ | $\mathbf{76.72 \pm 0.17}$ | $\mathbf{76.89 \pm 0.25}$ | $\mathbf{78.3 \pm 0.23}$ |

**Table 3.** $F_1 \pm$ std over 5 runs on Ki-67 dataset.

| Methods | 1% labels | 5% labels | 10% labels | All labels |
|---|---|---|---|---|
| Labeled data only | - | $75.99 \pm 3.05$ | $75.87 \pm 1.02$ | $79.06 \pm 0.37$ |
| TE [5] | $72.62 \pm 4.47$ | $76.02 \pm 2.34$ | $78.25 \pm 0.48$ | $79.22 \pm 0.49$ |
| MT [10] | $72.69 \pm 4.7$ | $76.92 \pm 2.02$ | $78.69 \pm 0.47$ | $79.41 \pm 0.52$ |
| Ours | $\mathbf{74.9 \pm 3.41}$ | $\mathbf{79.32 \pm 0.73}$ | $\mathbf{79.79 \pm 0.59}$ | $\mathbf{79.91 \pm 0.39}$ |
| Ours w/$\lambda_{g1} = 0$ | $73.46 \pm 3.59$ | $77.72 \pm 1.65$ | $77.95 \pm 0.59$ | - |
| Ours w/$\lambda_{g2} = 0$ | $73.2 \pm 3.31$ | $77.84 \pm 1.27$ | $78.15 \pm 0.46$ | $79.19 \pm 0.83$ |

## 4   Conclusion

In this paper, we presented a novel semi-supervised deep learning method for nucleus classification. The proposed method is a type of self-ensembling based deep learning methods with additional regularization from the local and global consistency criteria. The consistencies enable the framework to learn a better distance metric such that the resultant model outperforms the state-of-the-art self-ensembling methods on two nucleus classification datasets. The proposed approach is general for image classification, thus can be easily adapted for many other image classification tasks.

## References

1. Bromley, J., Guyon, I., LeCun, Y., Säckinger, E., Shah, R.: Signature verification using a "Siamese" time delay neural network. In: Advances in Neural Information Processing Systems (NIPS), pp. 737–744 (1994)
2. Chapelle, O., Weston, J., Schölkopf, B.: Cluster kernels for semi-supervised learning. In: Advances in Neural Information Processing Systems (NIPS), pp. 601–608 (2003)
3. Chen, H., Dou, Q., Wang, X., Qin, J., Heng, P.A., et al.: Mitosis detection in breast cancer histology images via deep cascaded networks. In: AAAI, pp. 1160–1166 (2016)
4. Cireşan, D.C., Giusti, A., Gambardella, L.M., Schmidhuber, J.: Mitosis detection in breast cancer histology images with deep neural networks. In: Mori, K., Sakuma, I., Sato, Y., Barillot, C., Navab, N. (eds.) MICCAI 2013. LNCS, vol. 8150, pp. 411–418. Springer, Heidelberg (2013). https://doi.org/10.1007/978-3-642-40763-5_51
5. Laine, S., Aila, T.: Temporal ensembling for semi-supervised learning. arXiv preprint arXiv:1610.02242 (2016)
6. McInnes, L., Healy, J.: UMAP: uniform manifold approximation and projection for dimension reduction. arXiv preprint arXiv:1802.03426 (2018)
7. Miyato, T., Maeda, S.I., Ishii, S., Koyama, M.: Virtual adversarial training: a regularization method for supervised and semi-supervised learning. IEEE Trans. Pattern Anal. Mach. Intell. (TPAMI) (2018)

8. Rasmus, A., Berglund, M., Honkala, M., Valpola, H., Raiko, T.: Semi-supervised learning with ladder networks. In: Advances in Neural Information Processing Systems (NIPS), pp. 3546–3554 (2015)
9. Sirinukunwattana, K., Raza, S.E.A., Tsang, Y.W., Snead, D.R., Cree, I.A., Rajpoot, N.M.: Locality sensitive deep learning for detection and classification of nuclei in routine colon cancer histology images. IEEE Trans. Med. Imaging (TMI) 35(5), 1196–1206 (2016)
10. Tarvainen, A., Valpola, H.: Mean teachers are better role models: weight-averaged consistency targets improve semi-supervised deep learning results. In: Advances in Neural Information Processing Systems (NIPS), pp. 1195–1204 (2017)
11. Valpola, H.: From neural PCA to deep unsupervised learning. In: Advances in Independent Component Analysis and Learning Machines, pp. 143–171. Elsevier (2015)
12. Weston, J., Ratle, F., Mobahi, H., Collobert, R.: Deep learning via semi-supervised embedding. In: Montavon, G., Orr, G.B., Müller, K.-R. (eds.) Neural Networks: Tricks of the Trade. LNCS, vol. 7700, pp. 639–655. Springer, Heidelberg (2012). https://doi.org/10.1007/978-3-642-35289-8_34
13. Xing, F., Su, H., Neltner, J., Yang, L.: Automatic Ki-67 counting using robust cell detection and online dictionary learning. IEEE Trans. Biomed. Eng. (TBME) 61(3), 859–870 (2014)
14. Zhou, D., Bousquet, O., Lal, T.N., Weston, J., Schölkopf, B.: Learning with local and global consistency. In: Advances in Neural Information Processing Systems (NIPS), pp. 321–328 (2004)

# Perceptual Embedding Consistency for Seamless Reconstruction of Tilewise Style Transfer

Amal Lahiani[1,2]([⊠]), Nassir Navab[2], Shadi Albarqouni[2], and Eldad Klaiman[1]

[1] Pathology and Tissue Analytics, Pharma Research and Early Development,
Roche Innovation Center Munich, Penzberg, Germany
amal.lahiani@roche.com
[2] Computer Aided Medical Procedures,
Technische Universität München, Munich, Germany

**Abstract.** Style transfer is a field with growing interest and use cases in deep learning. Recent work has shown Generative Adversarial Networks (GANs) can be used to create realistic images of virtually stained slide images in digital pathology with clinically validated interpretability. Digital pathology images are typically of extremely high resolution, making tilewise analysis necessary for deep learning applications. It has been shown that image generators with instance normalization can cause a tiling artifact when a large image is reconstructed from the tilewise analysis. We introduce a novel perceptual embedding consistency loss significantly reducing the tiling artifact created in the reconstructed whole slide image (WSI). We validate our results by comparing virtually stained slide images with consecutive real stained tissue slide images. We also demonstrate that our model is more robust to contrast, color and brightness perturbations by running comparative sensitivity analysis tests.

**Keywords:** Style transfer · Generative Adversarial Networks · Embedding consistency · Whole slide images · Digital pathology

## 1 Introduction

In the field of pathology tissue staining is used to examine biological structures in tissue. Tissue staining is a complex, expensive and time consuming process. Additionally, tissue samples are scarce and expensive. As a result, different state of the art style transfer based methods have been applied in order to synthesize virtually stained images from other modalities. Style transfer is a field with

---

S. Albarqouni and E. Klaiman—Shared senior authorship.

**Electronic supplementary material** The online version of this chapter (https://doi.org/10.1007/978-3-030-32239-7_63) contains supplementary material, which is available to authorized users.

growing interest and use cases in deep learning allowing to render an image in a new style while preserving its original semantic content. One of the main challenges of style transfer applications is the necessity to distinguish between style features (e.g. color) and content features (e.g. semantic structures) [5]. Recent deep learning based style transfer works have shown that using perceptual losses instead of or along with pixel level losses can help the network learn relevant high level style and content features and thus generate high quality stylized images [7,13]. Deep learning based style transfer has been used to generate augmented faces [3], virtual artwork with specific artist styles [18] and recently also virtually stained histopathological whole slide images (WSIs) [4,8].

Some groups used approximative and empirical methods in order to virtually generate H&E images from fluorescence images [6,9,16]. In the field of deep learning, generative Adversarial Networks (GANs) have been used in [1,2,11,12] in order to predict brightfield images from autofluorescence of unstained tissue, H&E from unstained lung hyperspectral tissue image, immunofluorescence from H&E and H&E stained whole slide images from non-stained prostate biopsies respectively. In [4] and [10], a neural network has been used in order to predict fluorescent labels from transmitted light images. The training of these supervised methods is based on spatially registered image pairs of the input and output modalities. As generating paired slide images with different stainings is a complex task involving the use of consecutive tissue sections or a stain-wash-stain technique, unsupervised deep learning methods have been used in virtual staining [8] and stain normalization applications [15]. In [8], CycleGAN [18] has been used in order to virtually generate duplex Immunohistochemistry (IHC) stained images from real stained images.

Another important challenge in digital pathology computer aided applications is the size of high resolution WSIs. For this reason, tile based analysis is usually used in order to deal with memory limitations. Inference of trained generators on WSIs in a tilewise manner when instance normalization modules are used has been shown to present tiling artifacts in the reconstructed WSI [8]. While instance normalization has been proven to be crucial in style transfer applications GAN training [17], it makes a pixel in the output image depend not only on the network and the receptive field area but also on the statistics of the entire input image. This results in applying different functions to adjacent pixels belonging to different adjacent tiles. Using large overlap for the tiles during inference can mitigate this problem [8] but still presents some residual tiling and is very costly.

In order to make virtual staining of WSIs more efficient and robust for real world use cases, we aim to better address this instance normalization induced tiling artifact in a way that does not require superfluous processing. We introduce a novel and new perceptual embedding loss function into the CycleGAN network architecture during training aimed at regularizing the effect of input image contrast, color and brightness perturbations in the generator latent space. We apply our proposed method to train a network to generate a virtual brightfield IHC fibroblast activation protein (FAP) - cytokeratin (CK) duplex tissue

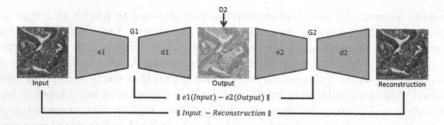

**Fig. 1.** Proposed model. G, D, e and d denote generator, discriminator, encoder and decoder respectively. The objective function includes three loss types: adversarial loss, cycle consistency loss and color invariant embedding consistency loss.

staining images from stained H&E tissue images. We validate our results by comparing the virtually generated images to their corresponding real consecutive stained slides. We also perform a comparative sensitivity analysis to validate our hypothesis that the introduced perceptual embedding loss helps train a generator network that is more contrast, brightness and color perturbation robust.

## 2    Proposed Approach

We propose a novel approach to generate seamless high quality virtual staining WSIs and specifically address the image reconstruction tiling artifact by introducing a perceptual embedding consistency loss to the CycleGAN network during training. CycleGAN model is built under the assumption that translating one image from domain X to Y then back from Y to X should result in the original input image. It consists of two mapping generators and two discriminators aiming at distinguishing between the real and generated images. The addition of the perceptual embedding loss allows to minimize the difference between the latent features in the two generators of the CycleGAN (Fig. 1). We use L2-norm to calculate the distance between the latent features in the generators bottlenecks and add this loss multiplied by a weight to the total loss of the network architecture alongside the reconstruction and adversarial losses.

The combination of these different losses helps the network learn meaningful feature-level representations in an unsupervised fashion in order to capture the semantics and styles of input and output histology staining domains, thus allowing us to learn a meaningful mapping between both domains and to obtain a more homogeneous contrast in virtual WSIs after tilewise inference. We hypothesize that forcing bottleneck features in both generators to be similar forces color and contrast invariance. Color and contrast invariant features that could successfully enable generation of virtual histopathological staining while maintaining the capability to cycle back to the original image could consist of condensed anatomical information, e.g. cell shapes, nuclear density, tissue textures, etc. Under this assumption, adjacent pixels belonging to different tiles would be more homogeneously mapped to the output space.

The objective function for our network includes three loss types. In addition to the adversarial loss and the cycle consistency loss described in [18] we add a perceptual embedding consistency loss (Eq. 1) between the two generator embeddings. This perceptual loss forces the generators in the network to learn a semantic content and contrast free features in the latent space, allowing a homogenization of the output contrast when the new style is added to the semantic features in the decoder block. We introduce the embedding consistency loss as:

$$L_{embd}(G_1, G_2) = \mathbb{E}_{X \sim \mathbb{P}_X}[\|e_1(x) - e_2(G_1(x))\|_2] + \mathbb{E}_{Y \sim \mathbb{P}_Y}[\|e_2(y) - e_1(G_2(y))\|_2], \tag{1}$$

where $X$ and $Y$ correspond to the two domains. $G_1$ and $G_2$ correspond to the generators of the model, $e_1$ and $e_2$ correspond to the encoders of the first and second generator respectively and $\|.\|_2$ is the $L2$ distance. The combined objective function is then:

$$L = L_{GAN}(G_1, D_2, X, Y) + L_{GAN}(G_2, D_1, Y, X) + \omega_{cyc}L_{cyc} + \omega_{embd}L_{embd}, \tag{2}$$

where $D_1$ and $D_2$ correspond to both discriminators, $L_{GAN}(G_1, D_2, X, Y)$ and $L_{GAN}(G_2, D_1, Y, X)$ to the adversarial losses of both mappings and $L_{cyc}$ to the cycle consistency loss. $\omega_{cyc}$ and $\omega_{embd}$ correspond to the weights of the cycle and embedding consistency losses respectively.

## 3    Experiments and Results

We use the described approach to train a network to virtually stain biopsy tissue WSIs with a duplex FAP-CK IHC stain from H&E stained slide images. CK is a marker for tumor cells and (FAP) is expressed by cancer-associated fibroblasts in the stroma of solid tumor. H&E is widely used for cancer diagnosis and tissue assessment, so our application could leverage existing H&E images to generate new and otherwise unattainable information about these biopsies.

### 3.1    Dataset

Our dataset consists of a selected set of WSIs from surgical specimen of Colorectal Carcinoma metastases in liver tissue from our internal pathology image database. The dataset includes 25 tissue blocks from different patients, each with 2 consecutive slides stained with H&E and FAP-CK respectively. We divide the total of the 50 WSIs into training and testing sets with 10 WSIs and 40 WSIs respectively. Our training set consists of 5 H&E stained WSIs and 5 FAP-CK stained WSIs from 5 patients tissue blocks. Due to memory limitations, all high resolution training images were split into $512 \times 512$ tiles with 128 overlap at 10x magnification factor. After tiling, our training dataset contains 7592 H&E $512 \times 512$ RGB tiles and 7550 FAP-CK $512 \times 512$ RGB tiles. We validate our method on a dedicated test dataset consisting of 20 paired WSIs from consecutive tissue sections of the same tissue blocks stained with H&E and FAP-CK. The testing images are taken from different patients than those of the training set.

## 3.2  Implementation Details

We trained the proposed model and a baseline CycleGAN model [8] for 20 epochs with ResNet-6 generator architectures and $70 \times 70$ PatchGANs discriminators. Hyperparameters are chosen similarly to [18] and we fix the embedding weight $\omega_{embd}$ to be equal to the cycle consistency loss weight $\omega_{cyc}$ ($\omega_{embd} = \omega_{cyc} = 10$). The training was distributed on 8 v100 GPUs using the Pytorch distributed computing library and the stochastic synchronous ADAM algorithm. We train the model on the Roche Pharma High Performance Computing (HPC) Cluster in Penzberg. The training lasted 9 h.

## 3.3  Evaluation Metric

We evaluate and compare our method to the CycleGAN architecture described in [8] by measuring the complex wavelet structural similarity index CWSSIM [14] between the virtually generated FAP-CK images and their corresponding consecutive real stained FAP-CK images. In order to use the CWSSIM as an evaluation metric, we registered the consecutive slide images using a geometric point set matching method.

CWSSIM is an extension of the structural similarity index (SSIM) to the complex wavelet domain. The CWSSIM index is a number bounded between 0 and 1 where 0 means highly dissimilar images and 1 means perfect matching. The choice of the CWSSIM as a measure to assess the performance is based on the fact that this metric, unlike other metrics, is robust to small translations and rotations. Actually, as explained in [14], small image distortions result in consistent phase changes in the local wavelet coefficients which does not affect the structural content of the image. Since our validation paired real/virtual data are not obtained from the same section but from consecutive sections of the same tissue block, even after careful registration of the paired images, mismatched areas in the tissue could still exist in some regions of the images. This fact made the use of other intensity and geometric based indices not necessarily very well correlated to the visual similarity between the images.

## 3.4  Ablation Test and Comparison

In order to visualize the effect of our proposed perceptual embedding consistency loss, we conduct an ablation study where we train the same model using the same generators and discriminators architectures, the same hyperparameters and the same number of epochs with and without the perceptual embedding consistency loss. We notice that both models learn a reasonable mapping between domains

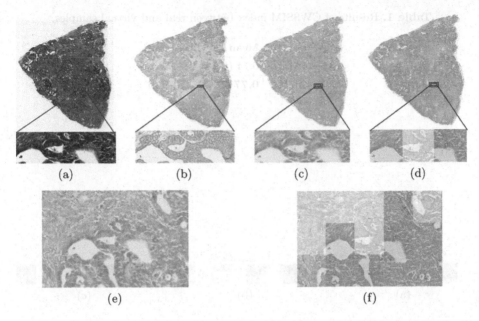

(a)          (b)          (c)          (d)

(e)                              (f)

**Fig. 2.** (a), (b), (c) and (d) correspond to an input H&E image from the testing set, the corresponding consecutive registered real stained FAP-CK, the virtual FAP-CK image obtained with our model and the virtual FAP-CK image obtained with the baseline CycleGAN. (e) and (f) correspond to zooms of the blue boxes in (c) and (d) respectively. We can clearly see the effect of the embedding consistency loss in homogenising the contrast of the reconstructed WSI. (Color figure online)

in the field of view level and the semantic content of the images is generally preserved. However, when we consider the reconstructed WSIs, we notice that our approach yields a significantly more continuous image with substantially less tiling artifacts than the baseline method (Fig. 2). An additional example of virtual FAP-CK WSIs from the testing set obtained after tilewise inference and image reconstruction with the baseline method and our approach is presented in the supplementary material.

Virtual and consecutive real images are first registered and tiled to 1024 × 1024 fields of views. The 20 testing blocks yielded 1236 virtual tiles and their corresponding 1236 real tiles. Then we compute the similarity index between the real and virtual tiles for the models trained with and without the embedding consistency loss. The results are summarized in Table 1. The median CWSSIM for all patients is equal to 0.79 and 0.74 with our approach and CycleGAN respectively, reflecting 6.75% of relative improvement. Additionally, we measure the CWSSIM per patient and we observe higher average CWSSIM for 85% of the patients (see supplementary material for the box plot representation of the CWSSIM index per patient).

**Table 1.** Results of CWSSIM index between real and virtual samples.

| Method | Mean (median) ± Std |
|---|---|
| CycleGAN [8] | 0.74 (0.74) ± 0.153 |
| Ours | **0.77 (0.79) ± 0.146** |

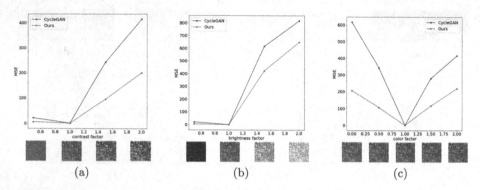

(a)              (b)              (c)

**Fig. 3.** Average MSE between the embeddings of the original and perturbed tiles for the 100 selected tiles. (a), (b) and (c) correspond to contrast, brightness and color perturbations respectively. The blue and red curves correspond to the results obtained for CycleGAN and our approach respectively. (Color figure online)

## 3.5 Sensitivity Analysis

In order to verify our assumptions about the effect of the perceptual embedding consistency loss on learning semantic content and a more color, contrast and brightness invariant embedding, we perform a comparative sensitivity analysis. The analysis includes insertion of color, brightness and color perturbations into the generator input and comparison of the effect of that perturbation on the generator embeddings between our approach and plain CycleGAN.

For this, we randomly select a subset of 100 (512 × 512) tiles from the testing dataset. We perform an inference with the model's generator on each tile followed by inference of the same generator on different perturbed versions of the tile. Then we calculate the Mean Square Error (MSE) between the embeddings of the original tiles and embeddings of each of the corresponding perturbed versions of the tiles. Figure 3 shows the average MSE values of the 100 selected tiles obtained from contrast, brightness and color perturbations of the generator input. We report on the results obtained with our approach compared with the baseline CycleGAN. All graphs clearly show that our approach results in smaller MSE values in the latent space for the different perturbations. This shows that the perceptual embedding loss drives the network to learn image embeddings that are more content related and more invariant to color, brightness and contrast changes. These robust invariant embeddings enable the network to be more robust to the effects of global changes in tile statistics and results in smoother seamless WSI reconstruction despite the effects of the instance normalization module.

## 4  Discussion and Conclusion

We present a novel style transfer approach applied to the field of digital pathology where high resolution WSIs are required. In this specific application, we virtually generate FAP-CK images from real stained H&E images using tilewise processing because of hardware memory limitations. In particular, we propose a solution based on perceptual embedding consistency loss in order to obtain a substantially more homogeneous contrast in the WSIs.

We demonstrate that this targeted regularization forces the network to learn non-color and non-contrast based features for tile embedding and this in turn reduces variation of the output tiling artifact due to the instance normalization effect. While the proposed solution seems to improve the results and to solve one of the main issues we had to deal with in our stain virtualization frameworks, there is still a lot to investigate and a lot of room for improvement. For example, we plan to study the effect of the input staining biological features on the quality of the virtual images. Additionally, we noticed that, unlike CK which was very well correlated in real and virtual images, FAP reconstruction is still showing significant differences. We plan to investigate the problem to understand if it is correlated to biological constraints (i.e. lack of predictive features in the input staining) or to weaknesses in the architecture. For this reason we plan to add more constraints to the network in order to investigate the challenge and, when possible, improve the quality of FAP reconstruction.

## References

1. Bayramoglu, N., Kaakinen, M., Eklund, L., Heikkila, J.: Towards virtual h&e staining of hyperspectral lung histology images using conditional generative adversarial networks. In: ICCV, pp. 64–71 (2017)
2. Burlingame, E.A., Margolin, A., Gray, J.W., Chang, Y.H.: Shift: speedy histopathological-to-immunofluorescent translation of whole slide images using conditional generative adversarial networks. In: Medical Imaging 2018: Digital Pathology, vol. 10581, p. 1058105. SPIE (2018)
3. Chang, H., Lu, J., Yu, F., Finkelstein, A.: Pairedcyclegan: asymmetric style transfer for applying and removing makeup. In: CVPR, pp. 40–48 (2018)
4. Christiansen, E.M., et al.: In silico labeling: predicting fluorescent labels in unlabeled images. Cell 173(3), 792–803 (2018)
5. Gatys, L.A., Ecker, A.S., Bethge, M.: Image style transfer using convolutional neural networks. In: CVPR, pp. 2414–2423 (2016)
6. Giacomelli, M.G., et al.: Virtual hematoxylin and eosin transillumination microscopy using epi-fluorescence imaging. PLoS ONE 11(8), e0159337 (2016)

7. Johnson, J., Alahi, A., Fei-Fei, L.: Perceptual losses for real-time style transfer and super-resolution. In: Leibe, B., Matas, J., Sebe, N., Welling, M. (eds.) ECCV 2016. LNCS, vol. 9906, pp. 694–711. Springer, Cham (2016). https://doi.org/10.1007/978-3-319-46475-6_43

8. Lahiani, A., Gildenblat, J., Klaman, I., Albarqouni, S., Navab, N., Klaiman, E.: Virtualization of tissue staining in digital pathology using an unsupervised deep learning approach. arXiv preprint arXiv:1810.06415 (2018)

9. Lahiani, A., Klaiman, E., Grimm, O.: Enabling histopathological annotations onimmunofluorescent images through virtualization of hematoxylin and eosin. JPI 9, 1 (2018)

10. Ounkomol, C., Seshamani, S., Maleckar, M.M., Collman, F., Johnson, G.R.: Label-free prediction of three-dimensional fluorescence images from transmitted-light microscopy. Nat. Methods 15(11), 917 (2018)

11. Rana, A., Yauney, G., Lowe, A., Shah, P.: Computational histological staining and destaining of prostate core biopsy RGB images with generative adversarial neural networks. In: ICMLA, pp. 828–834. IEEE (2018)

12. Rivenson, Y., Wang, H., Wei, Z., Zhang, Y., Gunaydin, H., Ozcan, A.: Deep learning-based virtual histology staining using auto-fluorescence of label-free tissue. arXiv preprint arXiv:1803.11293 (2018)

13. Royer, A., et al.: XGAN: unsupervised image-to-image translation for many-to-many mappings. arXiv preprint arXiv:1711.05139 (2017)

14. Sampat, M.P., Wang, Z., Gupta, S., Bovik, A.C., Markey, M.K.: Complex wavelet structural similarity: a new image similarity index. IEEE Trans. Image Process. 18(11), 2385–2401 (2009)

15. Shaban, M.T., Baur, C., Navab, N., Albarqouni, S.: StainGan: stain style transfer for digital histological images. arXiv preprint arXiv:1804.01601 (2018)

16. Tao, Y.K., et al.: Assessment of breast pathologies using nonlinear microscopy. PNAS 111(43), 15304–15309 (2014)

17. Ulyanov, D., Vedaldi, A., Lempitsky, V.: Instance normalization: the missing ingredient for fast stylization. arXiv preprint arXiv:1607.08022 (2016)

18. Zhu, J.Y., Park, T., Isola, P., Efros, A.A.: Unpaired image-to-image translation using cycle-consistent adversarial networks. In: ICCV. pp. 2223–2232 (2017)

# Precise Separation of Adjacent Nuclei Using a Siamese Neural Network

Miguel Luna, Mungi Kwon, and Sang Hyun Park[✉]

Department of Robotics Engineering, DGIST, Daegu, South Korea
{miguel,mg930502,shpark13135}@dgist.ac.kr

**Abstract.** Nuclei segmentation in digital histopathology images plays an important role in distinguishing stages of cancer. Recently, deep learning based methods for segmenting the nuclei have been proposed, but precise boundary delineation of adjacent nuclei is still challenging. To address this problem, we propose a post processing method which can accurately separate the adjacent nuclei when an image and a predicted nuclei segmentation are given. Specifically, we propose a novel deep neural network which can predict whether adjacent two instances belong to a single nuclei or separate nuclei. By borrowing the idea of decision making with Siamese networks, the proposed network learns the affinity between two adjacent instances and surrounding features from a large amount of adjacent nuclei even though the training data is limited. Furthermore, we estimate the segmentation of instances through a decoding network and then use their overlapping Dice score for class prediction to improve the classification accuracy. The proposed method effectively alleviates the over-fitting problem and compatible with any cell segmentation algorithms. Experimental results show that our proposed method significantly improves the cell separation accuracy.

**Keywords:** Nuclei segmentation · Instance segmentation · Siamese neural networks · Classification · Separation

## 1 Introduction

Cellular atypism and homogeneity of nuclei in pathology images are important factors in diagnosing the grade and stage of cancers [2]. However, since there are tens of millions of nuclei in a pathology image, physicians perform the diagnosis without precise quantification. To assist the diagnosis, several nuclei segmentation methods have been proposed. The most segmentation methods first perform binary (or three-label) segmentation to separate nuclei and background (and boundary), then find markers to identify individual nuclei, and finally perform the region growing or watershed algorithms to separate them.

---

M. Luna and M. Kwon—These authors equally contributed to this work.

D. Shen et al. (Eds.): MICCAI 2019, LNCS 11764, pp. 577–585, 2019.
https://doi.org/10.1007/978-3-030-32239-7_64

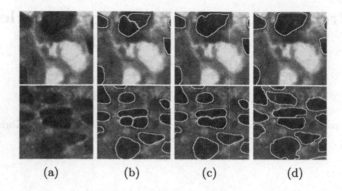

(a)              (b)              (c)              (d)

**Fig. 1.** (a) Ambiguous nuclei in pathology images, (b) segmentation generated by U-net [3], (c) post processed segmentation using our method, and (d) ground truth.

For example, Cheng et al. [1] extract the nuclei through active contour algorithm, and then estimate markers using the adaptive H-minima transform. Finally, they separate the individual nuclei through the watershed algorithm with the markers. Xing et al. [9] and Naylor et al. [7] use the convolution neural networks to predict the nuclei, and then separate them through the region growing and the watershed algorithm, respectively. To effectively separate the nuclei, Kumar et al. [6] propose the convolution neural network, which predicts each pixel as one of internal nuclei, boundary, and background labels, and then perform the region growing from the center of the predicted nuclei. Although most methods achieved good performance in extracting the nuclei from background, *i.e.*, binary segmentation, they often fail to find the accurate separation between nuclei since the boundaries between adjacent nuclei are very ambiguous.

To accurately separate the ambiguous neighboring nuclei, we propose a post processing method that can accurately separate individual nuclei when a nuclei segmentation including errors is given (see Fig. 1). Specifically, we propose a novel deep neural network that can classify whether two adjacent instances belong to a single nuclei or belong to different nuclei. Unlike the end-to-end segmentation networks, we generate instance markers from the given segmentation, and then repeat the task of merging the instances expected to be in the same nuclei through the proposed network. To improve the classification accuracy, we estimate the instance segmentation using a decoding network and then use the overlapping dice score between them to improve the class prediction. The proposed method is robust to the image characteristics and effectively avoids the overfitting problem by learning the affinity between a large number of adjacent nuclei. Moreover, the proposed is compatible with any cell segmentation algorithms.

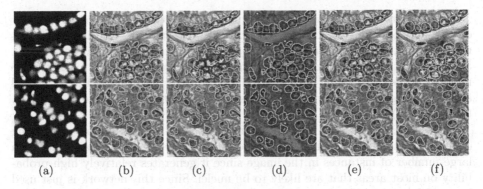

(a)      (b)      (c)      (d)      (e)      (f)

**Fig. 2.** Overall steps to extract ambiguous neighboring instances and evaluation by our proposed model: (a) Prediction map generated by a shortly trained U-Net model, (b) over-segmented prediction with instances that have multiple internal divisions, (c) under-segmented prediction that keeps only well defined inter instance divisions, (d) selected instances for affinity evaluation (red markers), (e) final result after applying our method, and (f) ground truth. (Color figure online)

## 2   Method for Nuclei Separation

The proposed method separates adjacent nuclei with ambiguous boundary from a given nuclei binary segmentation. The initial segmentation is first divided into a number of small instances (*i.e.*, segments), and then the instances, which are estimated to belong to a single nuclei, are merged until all the neighboring instances are estimated to belong to separate nuclei. In each step, two neighboring instances with ambiguous boundary are selected, and then estimated as to whether they belong to a single nuclei or not through a classifier. This procedure is repeated in similar fashion to the agglomerative clustering method [10].

To train the classifier, we propose a novel *Siamese network* that learns the affinity of various neighboring instances in training data. Even if the number of training data is small, the proposed network can learn informative features for separating the nuclei since there are many neighboring nuclei even in one training image. In the following subsections, we describe how to further divide a given segmentation into a larger number of instances, how to select neighboring instances with ambiguous boundaries, and how to classify whether adjacent instances belong to a single nuclei or not.

### 2.1   Extraction of Ambiguous Neighboring Instances

In order to predict whether two neighboring segments belong to the same nuclei or not, we generate two segmentation maps. The first map is an over-segmented prediction $S_o$ which is more likely to have nuclei instances divided into multiple fragments, while, the second prediction $S_u$ that groups several touching nuclei instances into a single segment, and thus it can be consider an under-segmented prediction.

To generate the maps, we learn a segmentation network with a small number of training epochs in the training stage. Given a test image and its initial segmentation $S_i$, we generate a probability map through the segmentation network, and then extract local maximum positions of the map as instance markers. The markers in the background of $S_i$ are excluded. Finally, we perform the watershed algorithm to generate $S_o$ by splitting instances from the foreground region of $S_i$ (see Fig. 2(b)).

Here, the segmentation network, carried out with a small number of training epochs, can not distinguish the separate nuclei correctly, but it can generate a large number of instances in the image since it generates relatively high probability on most areas that are likely to be nuclei. Since this network is just used to roughly extract the possible instance candidates, any segmentation network in early stage of training can be used. In our experiment, we used the U-Net [8] trained by Adam optimization with 10 epochs.

We perform the classification only on the neighboring instances with ambiguous boundary since classifying all combinations of small instances is time-consuming. To distinguish the ambiguity, we generate $S_u$ which separates only the clear boundaries on $S_i$, and then judge the instances which are separated in $S_o$ but included in a same cluster in $S_u$ as the ambiguous neighboring instances (see Fig. 2(c)). $S_u$ is generated by performing the distance transform from the foreground boundary of $S_i$, extracting markers above a certain threshold of the distance map, and then performing the watershed algorithm. Finally, we perform the classification task on the selected neighboring instances from $S_o$ until all the selected instances are estimated to belong to separate nuclei (see Fig. 2).

## 2.2   Proposed Network for Nuclei Separation

Our proposed network takes an image patch including two different markers from two instances. The markers are transformed into single channel images and then concatenated to the RGB image, respectively. Then, each concatenated image passes through a shared network in parallel, and then the classification (for distinguishing whether two instances belong to a single nuclei or not) is performed by comparing the feature maps generated by the shared network. Unlike the conventional Siamese network [4], we also add a decoding network to generate the segmentation of each instance, and then use the overlapping Dice score between two segmentations to improve the classification task (see Fig. 3).

Specifically, the shared network consists of 16 convolution layers for extracting informative features for the classification and segmentation tasks and 16 deconvolution layers for predicting the instance segmentations. Similar to the U-net [8], we use the skip connection between the convolution and deconvolution layers. Moreover, we perform a channel wise matrix multiplication twice in order to share information between the streams. The feature maps extracted by the convolution layers are connected to additional convolution layers and a fully connected layer to estimate the class. The estimated class is multiplied with the overlapping Dice score between the estimated segmentations generated by the deconvolution layers.

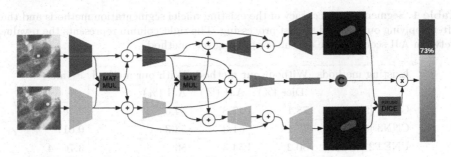

**Fig. 3.** Diagram of our proposed Siamese network. The dark and light green blocks are the same network. On the left, there are the input images with their individual markers in yellow. On the right, there are the segmentation results according to each marker and the classification result denoted by the letter C. The final instance affinity result is obtained by combining the classifier output with the pseudo dice score. (Color figure online)

The loss function $L$ of the proposed network is defined as $L = \lambda * L_c + L_s$, where the segmentation loss $L_s$ is defined as:

$$L_s = H(y_s^1, f_s(\Theta, x^1)) + H(y_s^2, f_s(\Theta, x^2)), \tag{1}$$

where $\Theta$ is a set of parameters, $x^1$ and $x^2$ are the two input features, $f_s(\Theta, \cdot)$ is the segmentation prediction for $\cdot$, and $y_s^1$ and $y_s^2$ are the segmentation ground truths for $x^1$ and $x^2$. $H(a, b)$ is the cross entropy between $a$ and $b$. The classification loss is defined as $L_c = H(y_c, Q)$, where $Q$ is the product between the classification prediction $f_c(\Theta, x^1, x^2)$ and the pseudo Dice score $D$ between segmentation predictions as:

$$Q = f_c(\Theta, x^1, x^2) \times D(f_s(\Theta, x^1), f_s(\Theta, x^2)). \tag{2}$$

The proposed $L_c$ loss allows the consistency of instance segmentations to affect the class prediction. In other words, it increases the probability that both instances are judged to be in the same nuclei if the segmentations are consistent, while it decreases the probability if inconsistent. Thus, it implicitly improves the classification and segmentation predictions compared to the method using the conventional cross entropy loss.

### 2.3 Implementation Details

In training stage, we first trained the early stage segmentation network (U-Net), and then applied it to the training data to extract the local maximum points. We constructed a list of pairs of points that are close to each other, and randomly sampled the pairs, and then extracted the image patch containing both marker points. The image patch size was determined as $128 \times 128$ so that big neighboring instances could be included in the patch. Using these data, we

**Table 1.** Segmentation accuracy of the existing nuclei segmentation methods and that after applying our method as post processing. The right column represents the p-values between AJI scores before and after applying our method.

| Existing methods | Without our method | | With our method | P-value |
|---|---|---|---|---|
| | Dice (%) | AJI (%) | AJI (%) | |
| CNN2 [9] | 78.1 | 47.8 | 54.6 | 2.4e−4 |
| CNN3 [6] | 77.1 | 51.3 | 53.3 | 0.017 |
| UNET2 [7] | 80.2 | 54.3 | 56 | 3.7e−4 |
| UNET3 [3] | 79.9 | 55.9 | 57.2 | 3.7e−4 |

learned the proposed nuclei separation network with a minibatch size of 64. The model was trained by Adam optimizer with learning rate 0.0001 and no learning rate decay for 65 thousand steps. The model was implemented in TensorFlow and trained on NVIDIA Titan XP GPUs. In inference stage, we extracted image patches of size $128 \times 128$ from the pairs of markers of ambiguous neighboring instances, and then predicted the segmentation and classification labels through the model. According to the classification prediction, we proceeded to merge the instances that belong to a single nuclei. The pairs of instances with a probability lower than 0.5 were kept separated.

## 3   Experimental Results

For evaluation, we used 30 images provided by MICCAI 2018 Monuseg challenge. A total of 30 images contained about 22,000 nuclei, and each image was extracted from seven different organs (6 breast, 6 liver, 6 kidney, 6 prostate, 2 bladder, 2 colon and 2 stomach). Among them, 4 breast, 4 liver, 4 kidney, and 4 prostate images were used for training and remaining 14 images were used for testing. The images were acquired at a magnification of 40, and the size was 1000 by 1000 per image. More information on the data can be found on the challenge webpage [5].

To demonstrate the effectiveness of our proposed method, we generated nuclei segmentation results by using four state-of-the-art deep learning based methods, *i.e.*, CNN2, CNN3, UNET2, and UNET3. We then applied our method to them to improve the segmentation separation. In CNN2, each pixel is classified to nuclei or background through a convolutional neural network (CNN), and then individual nuclei are separated through the watershed algorithm. The CNN is trained with the same way described in [9]. In CNN3, each pixel is classified to nuclei, boundary, or background, and then individual nuclei are separated through the watershed algorithm [6]. In UNET2 [7] and UNET3 [3], segmentation was predicted by U-Net instead of the pixel-level classification, and then individual nuclei are separated through the watershed algorithm.

**Separation Accuracy:** To evaluate the segmentation separation accuracy, we computed the Aggregated Jaccard Index (AJI) [6] that measures the degree of agreement between adjacent nuclei after the separation. We also computed the Dice score, that measures the degree of overlap between the binary segmentation and its label, to show the accuracy of initial segmentation generated by the existing methods. The Dice scores are not changed by our method because the separation is performed in the foreground region of the given binary segmentation.

**Table 2.** Comparison of the classification networks in terms of classification accuracy and segmentation Dice score.

| Methods | Classification (%) | Segmentation Dice (%) |
|---|---|---|
| Classifier w/o $L_s$ [4] | 75.09 | - |
| Classifier w/$L_s$, w/o Dice product | 78.95 | 67.7 |
| Classifier w/$L_s$, w/ Dice product (Ours) | 80.8 | 69.08 |

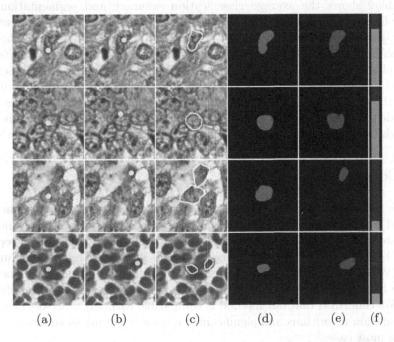

    (a)        (b)        (c)        (d)        (e)    (f)

**Fig. 4.** Segmentation and classification of markers on the same or separate nuclei. (a) First marker, (b) second marker, (c) nuclei segmentation ground truth for both markers (if they are on the same nuclei, there is one delineation), (d) predicted segmentation for the first marker, (e) predicted segmentation for the second marker, and (f) classification score.

Table 1 shows the average Dice and AJI scores of 14 testing results generated by the existing methods and the average AJI scores after our proposed method is used as a post processing. Since CNN2 performed the classification by patch unit without boundary prediction, both the Dice and AJI scores were low. On the other hand, CNN3 achieved slightly lower Dice accuracy than CNN2, but achieved better AJI by performing the boundary prediction. The U-Net based methods achieved higher accuracy than CNN2 or CNN3. For all these cases, our post processing method improved the AJI scores more than 2%, and the differences were significant ($p \leq 0.05$) when performing the two-tailed Wilcoxon signed-rank test between AJI scores before and after applying our method.

**Classification Accuracy:** The classification performance is highly related to the segmentation separation performance since a wrong merge occurs if the classification is wrong. Therefore, it is necessary to confirm how well the proposed network classifies whether two instances belong to a single nuclei or not. We compared our proposed network with a classification network that does not include a decoding network like the Siamese network [4], and the network including decoding network with the segmentation loss $L_s$, but not using the connection between classification and segmentation tasks using the Dice product $D$.

Table 2 shows the average classification accuracy and segmentation Dice scores for all testing pairs. The conventional classification model achieved the lowest performance since it cannot use any geometrical comparison between instances. The method using segmentation loss $L_s$ without product connection could obtain the instance segmentation, but both the classification and segmentation tasks are considered separately. On the other hand, our proposed method using the product between classification and segmentation tasks ensures closer dependency to each other. Thus, our method outperformed other two methods on both tasks. Figure 4 shows how the two tasks help to perform each other.

## 4   Conclusion

In this paper, we have proposed a new method for separating nuclei in H&E stained tissue slides. The main idea is to learn a deep neural network which can estimate whether neighboring two instances are in a single nuclei or in separate nuclei by learning the affinity between adjacent instances and surrounding features. We also utilize the decoding network on the shared classification network to use the consistency of instance segmentations to improve the classification task. We confirmed that our method is compatible with any state-of-the-art cell segmentation algorithms and significantly improves the nuclei separation accuracy in most cases.

**Acknowledgment.** This work was supported by the National Research Foundation of Korea (NRF) grant funded by the Korea government (MSIT) (No. 2019R1C1C1008727), and the Grant of Artificial Intelligence Bio-Robot Medical Convergence Technology funded by the Ministry of Trade, Industry and Energy, the Ministry of Science and ICT, and the Ministry of Health and Welfare (No. 20001533).

# References

1. Cheng, J., Rajapakse, J.C.: Segmentation of clustered nuclei with shape markers and marking function. IEEE Trans. Biomed. Eng. **56**, 741–748 (2009)
2. Chow, K.H., Factor, R.E., Ullman, K.S.: The nuclear envelope environment and its cancer connections. Nat. Rev. Cancer **12**, 196–209 (2012)
3. Cui, Y., Zhang, G., Liu, Z., Xiong, Z., Hu, J.: A deep learning algorithm for one-step contour aware nuclei segmentation of histopathological images. CoRR abs/1803.02786 (2018). http://arxiv.org/abs/1803.02786
4. Koch, G., Zemel, R., Salakhutdinov, R.: Siamese neural networks for one-shot image recognition. In: ICML Deep Learning Workshop, vol. 2 (2015)
5. Kumar, N., Verma, R., Anand, D., Sethi, A.: Multi-organ nuclei segmentation challenge (2018). https://monuseg.grand-challenge.org/Home/
6. Kumar, N., Verma, R., Sharma, S., Bhargava, S., Vahadane, A., Sethi, A.: A dataset and a technique for generalized nuclear segmentation for computational pathology. IEEE Trans. Med. Imaging **36**, 1550–1560 (2017)
7. Naylor, P., Laé, M., Reyal, F., Walter, T.: Nuclei segmentation in histopathology images using deep neural networks. In: 2017 IEEE 14th International Symposium on Biomedical Imaging (ISBI 2017), pp. 933–936 (2017)
8. Ronneberger, O., Fischer, P., Brox, T.: U-Net: convolutional networks for biomedical image segmentation. In: Navab, N., Hornegger, J., Wells, W.M., Frangi, A.F. (eds.) MICCAI 2015. LNCS, vol. 9351, pp. 234–241. Springer, Cham (2015). https://doi.org/10.1007/978-3-319-24574-4_28
9. Xing, F., Xie, Y., Yang, L.: An automatic learning-based framework for robust nucleus segmentation. IEEE Trans. Med. Imaging **35**, 550–566 (2016)
10. Zhang, W., Zhao, D., Wang, X.: Agglomerative clustering via maximum incremental path integral. Pattern Recogn. **46**, 3056–3065 (2013)

# PFA-ScanNet: Pyramidal Feature Aggregation with Synergistic Learning for Breast Cancer Metastasis Analysis

Zixu Zhao[1](✉), Huangjing Lin[1], Hao Chen[2], and Pheng-Ann Heng[1,3]

[1] Department of Computer Science and Engineering,
The Chinese University of Hong Kong, Hong Kong, China
zxzhao@cse.cuhk.edu.hk
[2] Imsight Medical Technology, Co., Ltd., Hong Kong, China
[3] Guangdong Provincial Key Laboratory of Computer Vision and Virtual Reality
Technology, Shenzhen Institutes of Advanced Technology,
Chinese Academy of Sciences, Shenzhen, China

**Abstract.** Automatic detection of cancer metastasis from whole slide images (WSIs) is a crucial step for following patient staging and prognosis. Recent convolutional neural network based approaches are struggling with the trade-off between accuracy and computational efficiency due to the difficulty in processing large-scale gigapixel WSIs. To meet this challenge, we propose a novel Pyramidal Feature Aggregation ScanNet (PFA-ScanNet) for robust and fast analysis of breast cancer metastasis. Our method mainly benefits from the aggregation of extracted local-to-global features with diverse receptive fields, as well as the proposed synergistic learning for training the main detector and extra decoder with semantic guidance. Furthermore, a high-efficiency inference mechanism is designed with dense pooling layers, which allows dense and fast scanning for gigapixel WSI analysis. As a result, the proposed PFA-ScanNet achieved the state-of-the-art FROC of 89.1% on the Camelyon16 dataset, as well as competitive kappa score of 0.905 on the Camelyon17 leaderboard without model ensemble. In addition, our method shows leading speed advantage over other methods, about 7.2 min per WSI with a single GPU, making automatic analysis of breast cancer metastasis more applicable in the clinical usage.

## 1 Introduction

The prognosis of breast cancer mainly focuses on grading the stage of cancer, which is measured by the tumor, node, and distant metastasis (TNM) staging system [1]. With the boosting progress in high-throughput scanning and artificial intelligence technology, automatic detection of breast cancer metastasis

**Electronic supplementary material** The online version of this chapter (https://doi.org/10.1007/978-3-030-32239-7_65) contains supplementary material, which is available to authorized users.

D. Shen et al. (Eds.): MICCAI 2019, LNCS 11764, pp. 586–594, 2019.
https://doi.org/10.1007/978-3-030-32239-7_65

in sentinel lymph nodes has great potential in cancer staging to assist clinical management. The algorithm is expected to detect the presence of metastases in five slides with lymphatic tissues dissected from a patient, and measure their extent to four metastasis categories and finally grade the pathologic N stage (pN-stage) following the TNM staging system. However, the task is challenging due to several factors: (1) the difficulty in handling large-scale gigapixel images (e.g., 1–3 GB per slide); (2) the existence of hard mimics between normal and cancerous region; (3) the significant size variance among different metastasis categories.

Recently, many deep learning based methods adopt patch-based models to directly analyze whole slide images (WSIs) [2–5]. The most common way is to extract small patches in a sliding window manner and feed them to the model for inference. For example, ResNet-101 and Inception-v3 are leveraged as the backbone of detectors in [2] and [3], bringing the detection results to 85.5% and 88.5% with regard to FROC on Camelyon16 dataset, respectively. However, the patch-based inference leads to dramatically increased computational costs when applied to gigapixel WSI analysis, which are not applicable in clinical usage. To reduce the computational burden, Kong et al. utilized a lightweight network (student network) supervised by a large capacity network (teacher network) with transfer learning [6]. Also, Lin et al. proposed a modified fully convolutional network (FCN), namely Fast ScanNet, to overcome the speed bottleneck by allowing dense scanning in anchor layers [7]. These scan-based models reduce redundant computations of overlaps for faster inference but are hampered by limited discrimination capabilities. Encoding multi-scale features is still beyond attainment for scan-based models due to their relatively simple network architectures.

Another challenging problem of lymph node classification lies in how to effectively retrieve tiny metastasis, i.e., ITC ($< 0.2$ mm) and micro-metastasis ($< 2$ mm), while rejecting most of the hard mimics. Several methods [5,7] circumvent false positives via hard negative mining, which focus on the most challenging negative patches. This seems to benefit the performance overall but decreases the sensitivity on small ITC lesions remarkably. Furthermore, it may disintegrate the prediction into pieces due to mimic patches existed in metastatic regions, leading to inaccurate evaluation on metastasis size. To tackle this issue, Li et al. proposed a neural conditional random field (NCRF) deep learning framework [4] combining with hard negative mining. Although spatial correlations is considered, it still achieved limited performance on metastasis detection. Other type of guidance, e.g., semantic guidance that helps the model distinguish hard mimics, has never been incorporated into the detections methods for cancer metastasis.

Aiming at developing a detection system as accurate as possible while maintaining the efficiency, we propose a novel Pyramidal Feature Aggregation Scan-Net (PFA-ScanNet). Our contributions are threefold: (1) We raise a novel way to aggregate pyramidal features for scan-based model which can increase its discrimination capability. Specifically, we focus on local-to-global features extracted from pyramidal features by proposed Parameter-efficient Feature Extraction (PFE) modules. (2) A high-efficiency inference mechanism is designed with dense pooling layers, allowing the detector to take large sized images as input for inference while being trained in a flexible patch-based fashion. (3) Synergistic learning is proposed to collaboratively train the detector and decoder with semantic guidance, which can improve the model's ability to retrieve metastasis with significantly different size. Overall, our method achieved the highest FROC (90.2%), competitive AUC (99.2%) and kappa score (0.905) on Camelyon16 and Camelyon17 datasets with faster inference speed.

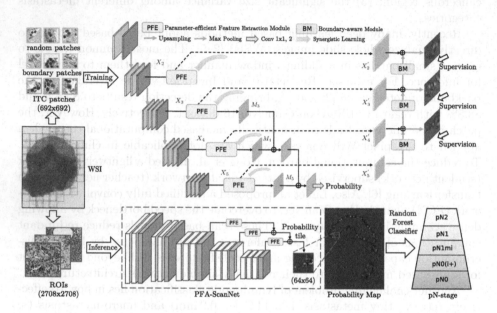

**Fig. 1.** An overview of the proposed PFA-ScanNet

## 2 Method

The proposed PFA-ScanNet is a scan-based fully convolutional network consisting of a main detector for classification and an extra decoder for segmentation. As shown in Fig. 1, Parameter-efficient Feature Extraction (PFE) modules are integrated into the detector at each feature level to extract local-to-global features with diverse receptive fields and less parameters. The extracted features are then aggregated in a top-down path (detector) and a bottom-up path (decoder).

### 2.1 Pyramidal Feature Aggregation for Accurate Classification

Inspired by the feature pyramid network [8], we propose to make full use of pyramidal features for a scan-based model. We firstly raise the Parameter-efficient Feature Extraction (PFE) module to extract local-to-global features with less parameters from pyramidal features. It also benefits the fast inference in Sect. 2.2.

Figure 2(a) shows the detailed structure of PFE. Let $\{X_i\}$ denotes the pyramidal feature generated by the detector at feature level $i$ ($i = 2, 3, 4, 5$). $X_i$ is firstly passed through a global convolution [9] with a large kernel to enlarge the receptive fields and reduce the feature map number. To further reduce the computation burden and number of parameters, we employ symmetric and separable large filters, which is a combination of $1 \times 15 + 15 \times 1$ and $15 \times 1 + 1 \times 15$ convolutions instead of directly using larger kernel of size $15 \times 15$. To formulate local-to-global features from the refined feature $X_i'$, regions with $\{1/4, 1/2, 1/1\}$ size of $\left\{X_3', X_4', X_5'\right\}$ are cropped to capture diverse receptive fields before average pooling layer. The local-to-global features $M_i$ is then added with $M_{i+1}$ from a higher feature level and finally passed through a $1 \times 1$ convolution with softmax activation to predict the probability. In this way, our detector can efficiently encode pyramidal features and present a strong discrimination capability.

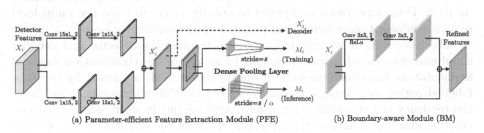

(a) Parameter-efficient Feature Extraction Module (PFE)     (b) Boundary-aware Module (BM)

**Fig. 2.** Detail structure of (a) Parameter-efficient Feature Extraction Module (PFE) and (b) Boundary-aware Module (BM) in proposed PFA-ScanNet.

## 2.2 WSI Processing with High-Efficiency Inference

To meet the speed requirement, we inherit the no-padding FCN in Fast ScanNet [7] as the trunk of our detector but remove the last three fully convolutional layers where the computation is expensive in the inference phase. Unlike the anchor layer raised in [7], we propose a dense pooling layer in PFE which allows dense scanning with little extra cost. A dense coefficient $\alpha$ is introduced in the dense pooling layer to control the pooling strides of average pooling operation. The pooling strides $\{128, 64, 32\}$ are associated with feature level $\{3, 4, 5\}$ in the training phase and will be converted to $\{128/\alpha, 64/\alpha, 32/\alpha\}$ in the inference phase. It allows dense and fast predictions when $\alpha$ increases in the form of $\alpha = 2^n \times 16$ ($n = 0, 1, 2, ...$). Accordingly, our network can take regions of interest (ROIs) with a size of $L_R$ as input for inference while being trained with small patches with a size of $L_p$ for extensive augmentation. In other words, our network inherently falls into the category of FCN architecture, which is equivalent to a patch-based CNN with input size $L_p$ and scanning stride $S_p$, but the inference speed becomes much faster by removing redundant computations of overlaps. To better understand this mechanism, we denote the scanning stride for refetching ROIs as $S_R$ and size of the predicted probability tile as $L_m$, and summarize the rules for high-efficiency inference as follows:

$$\begin{cases} L_R = L_p + (L_m - 1) \times (S_p/\alpha), \\ S_R = (S_p/\alpha) \times L_m, \end{cases} \tag{1}$$

## 2.3   Semantic Guidance with Synergistic Learning

Given that the surrounding tissue region is helpful to determine whether the small patch is metastasis or not, we develop our network with an extra decoder branch to synergistically learn the semantic information along with the detector. In the decoder, feature map $X_i'$ generated in PFE is firstly passed through a Boundary-aware Module (BM) to refine the boundary of the metastatic region. As shown in Fig. 2(b), BM models the boundary alignment in a residual structure [9] to take advantage of the local contextual information and localization cue. Afterwards, the generated feature is upsampled with deconvolutions and then added with $X_{i-1}'$ of higher resolutions to generate new score maps in a bottom-up path. Deep supervision is injected to specific layers to learn the multi-level semantic information, which can also speed up the convergence rate.

The basic idea of synergistic learning is training the detector and decoder simultaneously. Nevertheless, it is hard to minimize the classification loss and segmentation loss simultaneously in one iteration. This is caused by the mislabelled region and zigzag boundaries existed in WSI annotations, which have the tendency to overwhelm other informative regions in segmentation loss calculation and thus dominate the gradients. To solve the problem, we modify the binary cross-entropy loss into a truncated form [10] that can reduce the contribution of outliers with high confidence prediction. Our segmentation loss is shown as follows:

$$\mathcal{L}_{seg}(\mathcal{X}; \mathcal{W}) = \begin{cases} \sum\limits_{x \in \mathcal{X}} \sum\limits_{t \in \{0,1\}} (-\log(\gamma) + \frac{1}{2}(1 - \frac{p^2(t|x;\mathcal{W})}{\gamma^2})), p(t|x;\mathcal{W}) < \gamma \\ \sum\limits_{x \in \mathcal{X}} \sum\limits_{t \in \{0,1\}} -\log(p(t|x;\mathcal{W})) \qquad\quad , p(t|x;\mathcal{W}) \geqslant \gamma \end{cases} \tag{2}$$

where $\mathcal{W}$ denotes parameters of our model, $\mathcal{X}$ denotes the training patches, and $p(t|x;\mathcal{W})$ is the predicted probability for the ground truth label $t$ given the input pixel $x$. The segmentation loss will clip outliers at the truncated point $\gamma \in [0, 0.5]$ when $p(t|x;\mathcal{W}) < \gamma$, while preserving the loss value for others. Therefore, it can ease the gradient domination and benefit the learning of informative regions. When $\gamma = 0$, it will degrade into binary cross-entropy. Meanwhile, we directly employ the binary cross-entropy loss as our classification loss to train the detector. Let $\mathcal{W}_d$ denote parameters in the detector and $\lambda$ be the trade-off hyperparameter, the overall loss function for synergistic learning is defined as:

$$\mathcal{L}_{total}(\mathcal{X}; \mathcal{W}) = \mathcal{L}_{cla}(\mathcal{X}; \mathcal{W}_d) + \lambda \mathcal{L}_{seg}(\mathcal{X}; \mathcal{W}) \tag{3}$$

## 2.4   Overall Framework for pN-stage Classification

The overall pipeline of our framework contains: (1) *Data Preprocessing*. We firstly extract informative tissue regions from WSIs with Otsu algorithm [11]. Training patches and corresponding mask patches are augmented with random flipping, scaling, rotation, and cropping together. Color jittering and HSV augmentation are applied to training patches to overcome color variance. (2) *Slide-level Metastasis Detection.* We extract ITC and boundary patches at first and add them to the original training set to train the full PFA-ScanNet. Only the detector of our PFA-ScanNet is used for inference. (3) *Patient-level pN-stage Classification.* Morphological features (i.e., major axis length and metastasis area) are extracted from the probability maps to formulate feature vectors. We then utilize them to train a random forest classifier to classify the lymph nodes into four types, i.e., normal, ITC, Micro, and Macro. The patient's pN-stage is finally determined by the given rules in Chamelyon17 Challenge.

## 3    Experimental Results

**Datasets and Evaluation Metrics.** We evaluate our method on two public WSI datasets, Camelyon16[1] and Camelyon17[2] datasets. The Camelyon16 dataset contains a total of 400 WSIs (270 training and 130 testing) with lesion-level annotations for all cancerous WSIs. The Camelyon17 dataset contains 1000 WSIs with 5 slides per patient (500 training and 500 testing), providing pN-stage labels for 100 patients in the training set and lesion-level annotations for only 50 WSIs where ITC and Micro have been included. For Camelyon17 Challenge, we use the whole Camelyon16 dataset and 215 WSIs including 50 slides with lesion-level annotations from Camelyon17 training set to train the network. We adopt two metrics provided in Camelyon16 Challenge to evaluate slide-level metastasis detection, including AUC and average FROC. The latter is an average sensitivity at 6 false positive rates: 1/4, 1/2, 1, 2, 4, and 8 per WSI. For pN-stage classification, we utilize quadratic weighted Cohen's kappa provided in Camelyon17 Challenge as the evaluation metric.

**Implementation Details.** We implement our method using TensorFlow library on the workstation equipped with four NVIDIA TITAN Xp GPUs. The sizes of training patches and mask patches are $692 \times 692$ and $512 \times 512$, respectively. Our model can take ROIs with a size up to $2708 \times 2708$ (determined by the memory capacity of GPU) for inference and outputs a $64 \times 64$ sized probability tile. To maximize the performance of synergistic learning, we set the truncated point $\gamma$ in Eq. (2) as 0.04. The hyperparameter $\lambda$ is set to 0.5 in Eq. (3). SGD optimizer is used to optimize the whole network with momentum of 0.9 and learning rate is initialized as 0.0001.

**Quantitative Evaluation and Comparison.** We validate our method on Camelyon16 testing set and Camelyon17 testing set with ground truths held out. Results of Camelyon17 Challenge are provided by organizers. Table 1 compares our method with top-ranking teams as well as the state-of-the-art methods. It is observed that our method without synergistic learning (*PFA-ScanNet w/o SL*)

---

[1] http://camelyon16.grand-challenge.org/.
[2] http://camelyon17.grand-challenge.org/.

achieves striking improvements (3% in FROC and 14% in kappa score) compared with previous Fast ScanNet, demonstrating the superiority of aggregating pyramidal features in scan-based models. After introducing synergistic learning, our PFA-ScanNet without model ensemble boosts the results to 89.1% with regard to FROC (1st) and 99.2% in terms of AUC on Camelyon16 testing set. It also achieves competitive kappa score of 0.905 on Camelyon17 testing set, surpassing the Challenge winner (Lunit Inc.) who utilized model ensembles.

**Table 1.** Comparison with different approaches on Camelyon16 and Camelyon17 Challenges. Runtime per ROI and per WSI are reported (unit: minute) in this table.

| Camelyon16 challenge | | | | Camelyon17 challenge | | |
|---|---|---|---|---|---|---|
| Method | Runtime (ROI/WSI) | AUC | FROC | Team | Runtime (ROI/WSI) | Kappa score |
| Harvard & MIT [5]* | 0.668/267.2 | **99.4%** | 80.7% | IMT Inc. (Fast ScanNet) | 0.020/8.0 | 0.778 |
| NCRF [4] | 0.743/297.2 | - | 81.0% | MIL-GPAT* | 0.247/98.8 | 0.857 |
| Fast ScanNet [7] | 0.020/8.0 | 98.7% | 85.3% | VCA-TUe | 1.162/464.8 | 0.873 |
| Lunit Inc. [2] | 1.136/454.4 | 98.5% | 85.5% | HMS-MGH-CCDS | 0.067/26.8 | 0.881 |
| Kong et al. [6] | **0.014/5.6** | - | 85.6% | ContextVision* | 1.636/654.4 | 0.883 |
| LYNA [12]* | 1.155/462.0 | 99.3% | 86.1% | Lunit Inc. (2017 winner)* | 1.136/454.4 | 0.899 |
| Liu et al. [3]* | 1.155/462.0 | 97.7% | 88.5% | DeepBio Inc.* | 1.583/633.2 | **0.957** |
| PFA-ScanNet w/o SL | 0.018/7.2 | 98.3% | 87.8% | PFA-ScanNet w/o SL | **0.018/7.2** | 0.887 |
| **PFA-ScanNet** | 0.018/7.2 | 99.2% | **89.1%** | **PFA-ScanNet** | **0.018/7.2** | 0.905 |

Note: *denotes methods using model ensembles.

For the speed performance, we measure the time cost of each method on a 2708 × 2708 sized ROI with scanning stride of 32 (corresponding to the dense coefficient $\alpha = 16$) using one single GPU. Since a typical WSI consists of around 400 ROIs in average with size 2708 × 2708, the runtime can be converted from per ROI to per WSI. As illustrated in Table 1, our method shows leading speed advantages over the state-of-the-art methods on Camelyon16 and Camelyon17 Challenges. Note that the proposed PFA-ScanNet is faster than Fast ScanNet in the inference phase (7.2 min vs. 8.0 min). Our large capacity network is even on par with Kong's method (a lightweight network) [6] in terms of speed performance while achieving notably higher accuracy on detection results. Besides, our method takes only 1.1% time of the DeepBio Inc. to obtain probability maps (7.2 min vs. 633.2 min) and achieves competitive kappa score.

**Qualitative Analysis.** Figure 3 visualizes metastasis detection results of five typical cases. As we can observe, the proposed PFA-ScanNet can generate more complete results with higher probability for metastatic regions compared with the relatively sparse predictions from *PFA-ScanNet w/o SL* and *Fast ScanNet*. It thus increases the ability to detect macro- and micro-metastases, which is of great importance in clinical practice. Besides, the challenging ITC cases (see yellow boxes) can be detected by our method with few false positives, highlighting the advantage of PFA-ScanNet and proposed synergistic learning.

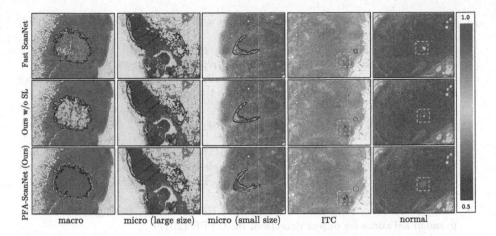

**Fig. 3.** Typical examples of probability maps. The colors ranging from blue to red denote low to high probability. The lesion-level annotation is shown in black. (Color figure online)

## 4   Conclusions

Automatic cancer metastasis analysis is essential for cancer staging and following patient's treatment. In this paper, we propose the PFA-ScanNet with synergistic learning for metastasis detection and pN-stage classification to improve the accuracy close to clinical usage while maintaining the computational efficiency. Competitive results have been demonstrated on the Camelyon16 and Camelyon17 datasets with a much faster speed. Inherently our method can be applied to a wide range of medical image classification tasks to boost the analysis of gigapixel WSIs.

**Acknowledgments.** This work was supported by 973 Program (Project No. 2015CB351706), Research Grants Council of Hong Kong Special Administrative Region (Project No. CUHK14225616), Hong Kong Innovation and Technology Fund (Project No. ITS/041/16), grants from the National Natural Science Foundation of China (Project No. U1613219).

## References

1. Sobin, L.H., Fleming, I.D.: TNM classification of malignant tumors. Cancer: Interdisc. Int. J. Am. Cancer Soc. **80**(9), 1803–1804 (1997)
2. Lee, B., Paeng, K.: A robust and effective approach towards accurate metastasis detection and pN-stage classification in breast cancer. In: Frangi, A.F., Schnabel, J.A., Davatzikos, C., Alberola-López, C., Fichtinger, G. (eds.) MICCAI 2018. LNCS, vol. 11071, pp. 841–850. Springer, Cham (2018). https://doi.org/10.1007/978-3-030-00934-2_93
3. Liu, Y., et al.: Detecting cancer metastases on gigapixel pathology images. arXiv preprint arXiv:1703.02442 (2017)

4. Li, Y., Ping, W.: Cancer metastasis detection with neural conditional random field. arXiv preprint arXiv:1806.07064 (2018)
5. Wang, D., Khosla, A., Gargeya, R., Irshad, H., Beck, A.H.: Deep learning for identifying metastatic breast cancer. arXiv preprint arXiv:1606.05718 (2016)
6. Kong, B., Sun, S., Wang, X., Song, Q., Zhang, S.: Invasive cancer detection utilizing compressed convolutional neural network and transfer learning. In: Frangi, A.F., Schnabel, J.A., Davatzikos, C., Alberola-López, C., Fichtinger, G. (eds.) MICCAI 2018. LNCS, vol. 11071, pp. 156–164. Springer, Cham (2018). https://doi.org/10.1007/978-3-030-00934-2_18
7. Lin, H., Chen, H., Graham, S., Dou, Q., Rajpoot, N., Heng, P.: Fast scannet: fast and dense analysis of multi-gigapixel whole-slide images for cancer metastasis detection. IEEE Trans. Med. Imaging 1 (2019). https://doi.org/10.1109/TMI.2019.2891305
8. Lin, T.Y., Dollár, P., Girshick, R., He, K., Hariharan, B., Belongie, S.: Feature pyramid networks for object detection. In: CVPR (2017)
9. Peng, C., Zhang, X., Yu, G., Luo, G., Sun, J.: Large kernel matters - improve semantic segmentation by global convolutional network. In: CVPR (2017)
10. Zhou, Y., Onder, O.F., Dou, Q., Tsougenis, E., Chen, H., Heng, P.A.: CIA-NET: robust nuclei instance segmentation with contour-aware information aggregation. arXiv preprint arXiv:1903.05358 (2019)
11. Otsu, N.: A threshold selection method from gray-level histograms. IEEE Trans. Syst. Man Cybern. 9(1), 62–66 (1979)
12. Liu, Y., et al.: Artificial intelligence-based breast cancer nodal metastasis detection. Archives of pathology & laboratory medicine (2018)

# DeepACE: Automated Chromosome Enumeration in Metaphase Cell Images Using Deep Convolutional Neural Networks

Li Xiao[1]([✉]), Chunlong Luo[1,3], Yufan Luo[1,3], Tianqi Yu[2], Chan Tian[2], Jie Qiao[2], and Yi Zhao[1]

[1] Key Laboratory of Intelligent Information Processing,
Advanced Computer Research Center, Institute of Computing Technology,
Chinese Academy of Sciences, Beijing, China
{xiaoli,biozy}@ict.ac.cn
[2] Peking University Third Hospital, Beijing, China
tianchan_cdc@126.com, jie.qiao@263.net
[3] School of Computer and Control Engineering,
University of Chinese Academy of Sciences (UCAS), Beijing, China

**Abstract.** Chromosome enumeration is an important but tedious procedure in karyotyping analysis. In this paper, to automate the enumeration process, we developed a chromosome enumeration framework, DeepACE, based on the region based object detection scheme. Firstly, the ability of region proposal network is enhanced by a newly proposed Hard Negative Anchors Sampling to extract unapparent but important information about highly confusing partial chromosomes. Next, to alleviate serious occlusion problems, we novelly introduced a weakly-supervised mechanism by adding a Template Module into classification branch to heuristically separate overlapped chromosomes. The template features are further incorporated into the NMS procedure to further improve the detection of overlapping chromosomes. In the newly collected clinical dataset, the proposed method outperform all the previous method, yielding an mAP with respect to chromosomes as 99.45, and the error rate is about 2.4%.

## 1  Introduction

Karyotyping is a cytogenetic experiment method used to help cytologists to observe the structures and features of chromosomes presented on metaphase images [9]. Cytologists firstly need to pay attention to the problem of numerical abnormalities of chromosomes that may result in some genetic diseases, such as Down syndrome [8]. Counting chromosomes is performed manually now on at least 20 images per patient and needs 50–100 images more when chromosome

**Electronic supplementary material** The online version of this chapter (https://doi.org/10.1007/978-3-030-32239-7_66) contains supplementary material, which is available to authorized users.

© Springer Nature Switzerland AG 2019
D. Shen et al. (Eds.): MICCAI 2019, LNCS 11764, pp. 595–603, 2019.
https://doi.org/10.1007/978-3-030-32239-7_66

mosaicism is explored. Considering that each human cell normally contains 46 chromosomes, it is tedious and time consuming, therefore it is an urgent need to develop a computer-aided system for chromosomes enumeration.

However, despite that there are some methods have been developed to solve classification [7,10] and segmentation [2,6] problems of chromosomes, very few of the researches have tried to develop automated chromosomes enumeration method. Gajendran et al. [4] presented a study by combining a variety of pre-processing methods and counting algorithm based on topological analysis, but the error rate is high. Furthermore, some segmentation method may solve the problem indirectly such as Arora et al. [2] and Minaee et al. [6], but they only focused on segmenting touching or overlapping chromosomes, and the accuracy is not high enough. The challenges of chromosome enumeration mostly rely on two aspects: chromosomes in metaphase images usually contain severe occlusion and cross overlapping problem (Fig. 1(a)); some partial chromosomes or two chromosomes connected head to head are similar to a whole chromosome (Fig. 1(b, c)). Above two problems are often occurred simultaneously (Fig. 1(d)), which make it difficult to detect all the chromosome objects accurately.

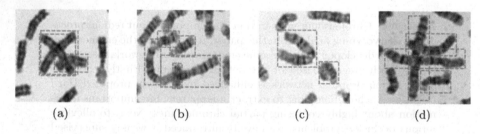

(a)                    (b)                    (c)                    (d)

**Fig. 1.** The green boxes are the ground truth bounding boxes of the chromosomes. (a) shows occlusion and cross overlapping problem, two ground truth boxes are very close to each other. (b) (c) shows self-similarity problem, the three connected chromosomes are likely to be classified as one chromosome and the deformed chromosomes are likely to be classified as two chromosomes connected to each other. (d) shows complex situation. (color figure online)

In this paper, following region based objection detection scheme, we proposed a deep learning algorithm to address chromosomes enumeration directly on the entire G-band metaphase image. We firstly introduced a Hard Negative Anchors Sampling method on RPN [11] to learn more information about highly confusing partial chromosomes to solve self-similarity problem. Secondly, in classification branch, we proposed a weakly-supervised Template Module to heuristically separate touching and overlapping chromosomes. The features generated from the Template Module is further used to guide NMS procedure in order to avoid over deletion of overlapped chromosomes. Our model is trained and validated on a newly collected dataset with thousands of labeled metaphase images from cytogenetic laboratory, and achieves higher performances than previous studies on 47.6% of WCR, 2.389% of AER, 99.45% of mAP and 98.81% of F1-Score.

## 2   Method

As shown in Fig. 2, the proposed framework consists of three main parts: (1) candidate chromosomes detection using RPN in which a Hard Negative Anchors Sampling procedure is proposed (Sect. 2.1); (2) an isolated classification branch with weakly-supervised Template Module (Sect. 2.2) and Feature-guided NMS (Sect. 2.3); (3) a parallel bounding box regression branch with $1 \times 1$ kernel for keeping identical feature map sizes.

### 2.1   Hard Negative Anchors Sampling in Region Proposal Network

The region based object detection models such as Faster R-CNN [11] firstly introduces a region proposal network(RPN) to generate candidate proposals. Typically, RPN only focus on binary classification of integrated objects (eg. IoU $\geq 0.7$) and background (eg. IoU $< 0.3$), and the selected proposals are passed to Fast R-CNN for further fine classification and regression in which partial objects (eg. $0.3 \leq$ IoU $< 0.7$) are taken care of. However, unlike natural object, chromosomes usually have various length and similar banding patterns, which confuse the network to discriminate partial and whole chromosomes, namely self-similarity problem. Meanwhile, the risk of irreversibly losing information in Fast R-CNN, such as cropping features and RoI Pooling, also make the network hard to distinguish partial chromosomes. To this end, we proposed a novel hard negative anchors sampling method during the RPN sampling procedure to better identify partial chromosomes and solve the self-similarity problem.

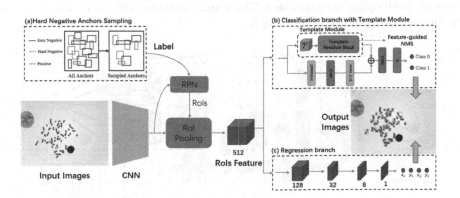

**Fig. 2.** The framework of DeepACE: (a) shows Hard Negative Anchors Sampling procedure in the first stage. (b) illustrates the classification branch containing Template Module and Feature guided NMS. (c) represents the regression branch. The details of template module is depicted in Fig. 3.

For clarity, we regard those anchors that have the IoU in the $[0.3, 0.7)$ as hard negative anchors and the original negative anchors with an IoU $< 0.3$ are named as easy negative anchors. Considering that RPN suffers from severe inter-class imbalance (positive : negative $\approx$ 1 : 2000) and intra-class imbalance (hard negative : easy negative$\approx$ 1 : 25), a new Hard Negative Anchors Sampling method inspired by stratified sampling is then proposed. As shown in Fig. 2(a), we divide all anchors into positive, hard negative and easy negative according to IoU overlap with ground truth box. We use mini-batches of size R = 256 for training RPN and take 25% of the anchors from positive. The half of remaining are uniformly sampled from hard negatives (37.5%), and the rest are sampled from easy negatives (37.5%). Finally, positive anchors are labeled with a foreground object class, both hard and easy negative anchors are labeled as background, the loss function is the same as the original RPN. In this way, feature maps generated by RPN is enhanced by hard negative anchors informations, and the following stage is improved by these features.

## 2.2 Template Module for Disentangling Occlusion Chromosomes

Touching and overlapping chromosomes bring severe intra-class occlusion, in which network is unable to localize and classify the chromosomes correctly. To alleviate this problem, we insert a weakly-supervised Template Module into the classification branch to heuristically separate the touching or overlapping chromosomes. Specifically, although chromosomes are usually displayed with bending or deformation in metaphase images, they can be summarized into some regular schemes. Therefore, it is reasonable to introduce several general template masks to represent patterns of chromosomes. When two or more chromosomes are overlapped together within a selected proposal, particular chromosome is able to be extracted by the corresponding template mask, and thus facilitate the separation of overlapping chromosomes. The implementation details of the template module can be summarized in Fig. 3.

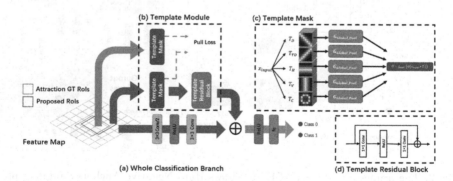

**Fig. 3.** The illustration of classification branch of DeepACE: (a) shows the whole classification branch. (b) illustrates the structure of weakly-supervised Template Module. (c) shows the Template Mask which select the most relevant template of the chromosome and output their features. (d) presents Template Residual Block.

The design of template module is essential to influence the performance. Chromosomes are usually displayed as slender strips in metaphase images.

Therefore, peak values located at the central part of feature map along the diagonal or horizontal or vertical direction, which leads to $T_D$, $T_{TD}$, $T_H$ and $T_V$. Besides, a circle-like template mask $T_C$ is introduced since there are also a few of seriously bending chromosomes as shown Fig. 1(c). The feature map size is $7 \times 7$, we introduce $ID_{row} \in \{0, 1, 2, 3, 4, 5, 6\}$ and $ID_{col} \in \{0, 1, 2, 3, 4, 5, 6\}$ to indicate the positions of feature map, all the five template masks are designed as constant tensors with Gaussian distribution, where $x_{row} = ID_{row} - 3$, $y_{col} = ID_{col} - 3$:

$$T_D(ID_{row}, ID_{col}) = e^{-\frac{(x_{row} - y_{col})^2}{3}}, \quad T_H(ID_{row}, ID_{col}) = e^{-\frac{y_{col}^2}{3}}$$

$$T_{TD}(ID_{row}, ID_{col}) = e^{-\frac{(x_{row} + y_{col})^2}{3}}, \quad T_V(ID_{row}, ID_{col}) = e^{-\frac{x_{row}^2}{3}} \tag{1}$$

$$T_C(ID_{row}, ID_{col}) = e^{-\frac{|x_{row}^2 + y_{col}^2 - 5|}{3}}$$

After RoI Pooling layer, feature maps with shape of $7 \times 7 \times 512$ are sent into template module and a shortcut pathway at the same time. The shortcut pathway is composed of one ReLU unit and two $3 \times 3$ convolutional kernel with strides equal to 2 and 1. Meanwhile, as shown in Fig. 3(b), the template module is composed of template mask and template residual block. Based on five template masks, the template mask component (as shown in Fig. 3(c)) firstly extract features of specific locations followed by global average pooling. We select the $1 \times 1 \times 512$ tensor which has the maximum mean value in the five tensors as the template feature. The template residual block (as shown in Fig. 3(d)) is composed of convolutional layers with ReLU and an identify mapping. Finally, the outputs of template module and shortcut pathway are combined together followed by ReLU layer and one 32-D fully connected layer to obtain the binary classification score.

We also design a weakly-supervised mechanism to guide the template feature selection procedure during training, in which the output of template module for ground truth is introduced as the label. The newly designed pull loss $L_{Pull}$ is composed of feature pull loss $L_{Pull_f}$ and mean pull loss $L_{Pull_m}$. The feature pull loss $L_{Pull_f}$ is to minimize the template feature distance between a proposal and its ground truth if they are fall into the same template mask, and maximize the distance if they are fall into different template mask. The square of L2 norm of the ground truth template feature is used for normalization, the definition is as:

$$L_{Pull_f} = \begin{cases} \dfrac{\|f_g - f_p\|^2}{\|f_g\|^2} & \text{, if } T_g = T_p \\[3mm] \max(0, 1 - \dfrac{\|f_g - f_p\|^2}{\|f_g\|^2}) & \text{, if } T_g \neq T_p \end{cases} \tag{2}$$

where $f_p$ and $f_g$ represent template feature vector of proposals and corresponding ground truth. Both $T_p$ and $T_g$ come from $\{T_D, T_{TD}, T_H, T_V, T_C\}$ which represent template masks of selected proposals and corresponding ground truth. For training, we apply the feature pull loss $L_{Pull_f}$ at positive candidate proposals.

The mean pull loss $L_{Pull_m}$ provides a penalty when proposals and corresponding ground truths are fell into different template masks. The $L_{Pull_m}$ is defined as:

$$L_{Pull_m} = \sum_i (\bar{f_g}^i - \bar{f_p}^i)^2 \text{ , where } i \in \{T_D, T_{TD}, T_H, T_V, T_C\} \tag{3}$$

where $\bar{f_g}$ and $\bar{f_p}$ represent the mean value of template features, respectively. Similar to feature pull loss, we only apply the mean pull loss $L_{Pull_m}$ at the positive candidate proposals. The total pull loss $L_{Pull}$ is obtained as follows:

$$L_{Pull} = L_{Pull_f} + L_{Pull_m} \tag{4}$$

### 2.3   Feature-Guided NMS

In post-processing stage, IoU based algorithms like Non Maximum Suppression(NMS) [5] and Soft-NMS [3] are widely used in recent years. They suppress redundancy according to IoU metric, in which highly overlapped predicted bounding boxes are removed directly or inhibited through decaying its detection scores. However, over deletion still exists when severe occlusion occur, which is frequently happen between chromosomes. Thus, we propose a Feature-Guided NMS based on Soft-NMS, which introduce template features to optimize the score decay function. The basic idea is that if two bounding boxes are fell into different template masks or their template features are far away, they should represents two different chromosomes. Therefore, in Feature-Guided NMS, we compute the normalized distance $d$ between template features and assign a threshold value $\Delta$ (set as 0.5). We will lighter decay score if $d > \Delta$ and heavier decay score if $d < \Delta$. The overview of the algorithm is summarized in Algorithm 1.

## 3   Experiments Results

**Data Set and Evaluation Metrics.** 1375 metaphase images with pixels of $1600 \times 1200$ containing 63026 objects were collected from the Peking University Third Hospital. All metaphase images are labeled by professional cytologists and are splited into 3(training):1(validation):1(testing). Besides mean average precision (mAP) and F1-Score, we also introduced the Whole Correct Ratio (WCR) and Average Error Ratio (AER) as the metrics to evaluate the ensemble performance which has more clinical meanings. We called images that all chromosomes are correctly detected as all right images, and WCR is defined as the percentage of all right images in the whole testing set. We regarded a predicted bounding box as a false positive if it does not have an IoU greater than a threshold with any ground truth (0.5 in this work) or it has the max IoU with a ground truth that has already been detected. A ground truth that is not detected by any bounding box is regarded as a false negative. The AER is defined as the fraction of sum of false positives and false negatives divided by the number of ground truth. For fair comparisons, we perform the ablation study on validation set and report final results on the testing set.

---

**Algorithm 1.** Feature-Guided Non Maximum Suppression

---

**Input:**

    The list of initial detection boxes $B = \{b_1, \ldots, b_N\}$;

    The list of corresponding detection scores $S = \{s_1, \ldots, s_N\}$;

    The list of corresponding template features $F = \{f_1, \ldots, f_N\}$;

**Output:**

    The list of detection boxes with new order $D'$;

    The list of corresponding detection scores which are decayed by function $S'$

1: Initialize $D' = \{\}$;

2: **while** $B \neq \{\}$ **do**

3:    Sort all the detection boxes $B$ by scores $S$ in descending order, mark the first candidate as $b_{max}$, corresponding score $s_{max}$ and template feature $f_{max}$

4:    Append the $b_{max}$ into $D'$ and pop it from $B$

5:    Append the $s_{max}$ into $S'$ and pop it from $S$

6:    **for** $b_i \in B$ **do**

7:        Measure the normalized distance $d = \frac{\|f_{max} - f_i\|}{\|f_{max}\|}$

8:        Compute new detection score $s_i$ by: $s_i = s_i e^{-\frac{iou(b_{max}, b_i)(2 - \Delta + d)}{\sigma}}$

9:    **end for**

10: **end while**

11: **return** $D'$ and $S'$

---

**Implementation Details.** During the pre-processing step, we perform one vertical and one horizontal flipping to augment data, and subtract the mean along each channel for zero centering. The $\sigma$ of Feature-Guided NMS are set as 0.2. Network is implemented on TensorFlow framework [1]. We trained the network for $100k$ iterations, with initialize learning rate set as 0.001 and decay by a factor of 10 at $60k$ iterations. Stochastic Gradient Descent (SGD) is adopted to optimize our network on a Nvidia Titan Xp GPU with momentum= 0.9.

## 3.1    Comparison

We verify the effectiveness of our proposed method by comparing with the chromosomes enumeration method proposed in [4], which is based on digital image analysis and evaluated by Cluster-Based Error criterion. The criterion only concerns the error of the chromosome number caused by cutting entire chromosome incorrectly or connecting individual chromosomes incorrectly. So, the criterion is much looser than AER criterion in this paper. Besides, some segmentation methods may also contain some potential connection with chromosomes enumeration task, which report detection accuracy about touching chromosomes $ACC_T$ and overlapping chromosomes $ACC_O$, we list some of them. Nevertheless, as shown in Table 1, our method still greatly outperform the previous method [4] and achieve an AER of 2.389% and WCR of 47.63%. Furthermore, it is worth mention that although DeepACE does not involve any pretraining, it still significantly outperforms the Faster RCNN which has been pretrained on ImageNet.

**Table 1.** The comparison of chromosomes counting methods. Avg-CB-Error means average cluster-based error, $ACC_T$ means detection accuracy for touching or partial overlapping chromosomes, $ACC_O$ means detection accuracy for overlapping chromosomes

| Method | Avg-CB-Error | $ACC_T$ | $ACC_O$ | WCR | AER | mAP | F1-Score |
|---|---|---|---|---|---|---|---|
| Gajendran et al. [4] | 6.4% | - | - | - | - | - | - |
| Minaee et al. [6] | - | 91.9% | - | - | - | - | - |
| Arora et al. [2] | - | 96.7% | 81% | - | - | - | - |
| Faster R-CNN | - | - | - | 39.64% | 2.44% | 99.03% | 98.79% |
| DeepACE | - | - | - | **47.63%** | **2.39%** | **99.45%** | **98.81%** |

## 3.2  Ablation Study

**Hard Negative Anchors Sampling.** To verify HNAS's contribution to performance, we train another network without HNAS. Table 2(a) shows that HNAS improves WCR greatly over baseline by 29.1%, AER by 2.7%, mAP by 2.18% and F1-Score by 1.37%. This is expected because self-similarity problem may happen on most of the chromosomes. Notice that the Faster R-CNN performs much better than DeepACE(w/o HNAS), this may because pretraining makes the network learn features more accurately thus the network is able to identify those subtle features which is essential to solve self-similarity problem.

**Template Module with Feature-Guided NMS.** we use features came from the second conv layer of shortcut pathway as an alternative of template feature for experiment of Table 2(b). Results show that both Template Module and Feature-Guided NMS improves the performances significantly. Table 2(c) also represents that discriminative template feature can optimize the nms procedure, which improves WCR by 2.55%, AER by 0.31%, mAP by 0.41% and F1-Score by 0.15% in condition of high benchmark.

**Table 2.** Ablation study on different component.

| | WCR | AER | mAP | F1-Score |
|---|---|---|---|---|
| (a) w/o HNAS | 15.64% | 5.03% | 98.18% | 97.46% |
| (b) w/o Template Module | 36.73% | 2.76% | **99.53%** | 98.63% |
| (c) w/o Feature-Guided NMS | 42.18% | 2.64% | 99.05% | 98.68% |
| (d) DeepACE | **44.73%** | **2.33%** | 99.46% | **98.83%** |

## 4  Conclusion

In this paper, we developed an automated chromosome enumeration algorithm, DeepACE. Hard Negative Anchors Sampling learns more about partial chromosomes and Template Module equipped with Feature-Guided NMS use weakly-supervised mechanism to heuristically identify overlapping chromosomes. Experiments on clinical datasets demonstrate its effectiveness. The future plan is to continue develop DeepACE to solve chromosomes detection and segmentation tasks on whole metaphase images.

**Acknowledgements.** This work was supported by National Natural Science Foundation of China(31900979) and CAS Pioneer Hundred Talents Program(2017-074) to Li Xiao. We thank Professor S. Kevin Zhou, Professor Yang Wu and Professor Hui Li for critical comments during manuscript preparation.

# References

1. Abadi, M., et al.: Tensorflow: a system for large-scale machine learning. OSDI **16**, 265–283 (2016)
2. Arora, T., Dhir, R.: A novel approach for segmentation of human metaphase chromosome images using region based active contours. Int. Arab J. Inf. Technol. **16**, 132–137 (2016)
3. Bodla, N., Singh, B., Chellappa, R., Davis, L.S.: Soft-NMS—improving object detection with one line of code. In: 2017 IEEE International Conference on Computer Vision (ICCV), pp. 5562–5570. IEEE (2017)
4. Gajendran, V., Rodríguez, J.J.: Chromosome counting via digital image analysis. In: 2004 International Conference on Image Processing 2004. ICIP 2004, vol. 5, pp. 2929–2932. IEEE (2004)
5. Girshick, R.: Fast R-CNN. In: Proceedings of the IEEE International Conference on Computer Vision, pp. 1440–1448 (2015)
6. Minaee, S., Fotouhi, M., Khalaj, B.H.: A geometric approach to fully automatic chromosome segmentation. In: 2014 IEEE Signal Processing in Medicine and Biology Symposium (SPMB), pp. 1–6. IEEE (2014)
7. Munot, M.V.: Development of computerized systems for automated chromosome analysis: current status and future prospects. Int. J. Adv. Res. Comput. Sci. **9**(1), 782–791 (2018)
8. Patterson, D.: Molecular genetic analysis of down syndrome. Human Genet. **126**(1), 195–214 (2009)
9. Piper, J.: Automated cytogenetics in the study of mutagenesis and cancer. In: Obe, G. (ed.) Advances in Mutagenesis Research, pp. 127–153. Springer, Heidelberg (1990)
10. Qin, Y., et al.: Varifocal-net: A chromosome classification approach using deep convolutional networks. arXiv preprint arXiv:1810.05943 (2018)
11. Ren, S., He, K., Girshick, R., Sun, J.: Faster R-CNN: towards real-time object detection with region proposal networks. In: Advances in Neural Information Processing Systems, pp. 91–99 (2015)

# Unsupervised Subtyping of Cholangiocarcinoma Using a Deep Clustering Convolutional Autoencoder

Hassan Muhammad[1,2(✉)], Carlie S. Sigel[1], Gabriele Campanella[1,2], Thomas Boerner[1], Linda M. Pak[1], Stefan Büttner[3], Jan N. M. IJzermans[3], Bas Groot Koerkamp[3], Michael Doukas[3], William R. Jarnagin[1], Amber L. Simpson[4], and Thomas J. Fuchs[1,2]

[1] Memorial Sloan Kettering Cancer Center, New York, USA
muhammah@mskcc.org
[2] Weill Cornell Medicine, New York, USA
[3] Erasmus Medical Center-Rotterdam, Rotterdam, The Netherlands
[4] Queen's University, Kingston, Canada

**Abstract.** Unlike common cancers, such as those of the prostate and breast, tumor grading in rare cancers is difficult and largely undefined because of small sample sizes, the sheer volume of time and experience needed to undertake such a task, and the inherent difficulty of extracting human-observed patterns. One of the most challenging examples is intrahepatic cholangiocarcinoma (ICC), a primary liver cancer arising from the biliary system, for which there is well-recognized tumor heterogeneity and no grading paradigm or prognostic biomarkers. In this paper, we propose a new unsupervised deep convolutional autoencoder-based clustering model that groups together cellular and structural morphologies of tumor in 246 digitized whole slides, based on visual similarity. Clusters based on this visual dictionary of histologic patterns are interpreted as new ICC subtypes and evaluated by training Cox-proportional hazard survival models, resulting in statistically significant patient stratification.

**Keywords:** Computational pathology · Cholangiocarcinoma · Clustering

# 1 Introduction

Cancer subtyping is an important tool used to determine disease prognosis and direct therapy. Commonly occurring cancers, such as those of breast and prostate, have well established subtypes, validated on large sample sizes [4]. The manual labor required to subtype a cancer, by identifying different histologic patterns and using them to stratify patients into different risk groups, is an extremely complex task requiring years of effort and repeat review of large amounts of visual data, often by one pathologist.

D. Shen et al. (Eds.): MICCAI 2019, LNCS 11764, pp. 604–612, 2019.
https://doi.org/10.1007/978-3-030-32239-7_67

Subtyping a rare cancer poses a unique set of challenges. Intrahepatic cholangiocarcinoma (ICC), a primary liver cancer emanating from the bile duct, has an incidence of approximately 1 in 160,000 in the United States, and rising [14]. Currently, there exists no universally accepted histopathology-based subtyping or grading system for ICC and studies classifying ICC into different risk groups have been inconsistent [1,12,15]. A major limiting factor to subtyping ICC is that only small cohorts are available to each institution. There is an urgent need for efficient identification of prognostically relevant cellular and structural morphologies from limited histology datasets of rare cancers, such as ICC, to build risk stratification systems which are currently lacking across many cancer types.

Computational pathology offers a new set of tools, and more importantly, a new way of approaching the historical challenges of subtyping cancers using computer vision-based deep learning, leveraging the digitization of pathology slides, and taking advantage of the latest advances in computational processing power. In this paper, we offer a new deep learning-based model which uses a unique neural network-based clustering approach to group together histology based on visual similarity. With this visual dictionary, we interpret clusters as subtypes and train a survival model, showing significant results for the first time in ICC.

## 2   Materials and Methods

Cancer histopathology images exhibit high intra- and inter-heterogeneity because of their size (as large as tens of billions of pixels). Different spatial or temporal sampling of a tumor can have sub-populations of cells with unique genomes, theoretically resulting in visually different patterns of histology [3]. In order to effectively cluster this extremely large amount of high intra-variance data into subsets which are based on similar morphologies, we propose combining a neural network-based clustering cost-function, previously shown to outperform traditional clustering techniques on images of hand-written digits [16], with a novel deep convolutional architecture. We hypothesize that a k-means style clustering cost function under the constraint of image reconstruction which is being driven by adaptive learning of filters will produce clusters of histopathology relevant to patient outcome. Finally, we assess the performance and usefulness of this clustering model by conducting survival analysis, using both Cox-proportional hazard modeling and Kaplan-Meier survival estimation, to measure if each cluster of histomorphologies has significant correlation to recurrence of cancer after resection. While other studies have performed unsupervised clustering of whole slide tiles based on image features, they have been used to address the problem of image segmentation [11] and relied on clustering a developed latent space [7,8]. Our study adjusts the latent space with each iteration of clustering.

### 2.1   Deep Clustering Convolutional Autoencoder

A convolutional auto-encoder is made of two parts, an encoder and decoder. The encoder layers project an image into a lower dimensional representation, an embedding, through a series of convolution, pooling, and activation functions. This is described in Eq. 1a, where $x_i$ is an input image or input batch of images transformed by $f_\theta()$, and $z_i$ is the resulting representation embedding. The decoder layers try to reconstruct the original input image from its embedding using similar functions. Mean-squared-error loss (MSE) is commonly used to optimize such a model, updating model weights ($\theta$) relative to the error between the original (input, $x_i$) image and the reconstruction (output, $x_i'$) image in a set of $N$ images. This is shown in Eq. 1b.

$$(a)\ z_i = f_\theta(x_i) \qquad (b)\ \epsilon = \min_\theta \frac{1}{N} \sum_{i=1}^{N} ||x_i - x_i'||^2 \qquad (1)$$

Although a convolutional auto-encoder can learn effective lower-dimensional representations of a set of images, it does not cluster together samples with similar morphology. To overcome this problem, we amend the traditional MSE-loss function by using the reconstruction-clustering error function, as proposed first by Song et al. [16]:

$$\epsilon = \min_\theta \frac{1}{N} \sum_{i=1}^{N} ||x_i - x_i'||^2 + \lambda \sum_{i=1}^{N} ||z_i - c_i^*||^2, \qquad (2)$$

where $z_i$ is the embedding as defined in Eq. 1a, $c_i^*$ is the centroid assigned to sample $x_i$ from the previous training epoch, and $\lambda$ is a weighting parameter. Cluster assignment is determined by finding the shortest Euclidean distance between a sample embedding from epoch $t$ and a centroid, across $j$ centroids from epoch $t - 1$:

$$c_i^* = \arg\min_j ||z_i^t - c_j^{t-1}||^2 \qquad (3)$$

The algorithm is initialized by assigning a random cluster to each sample. Centroid locations are calculated for each cluster class by Eq. 4. Each mini-batch is forwarded through the model and network weights are respectively updated. At the end of an epoch, defined by the forward-passing of all mini-batches, cluster assignments are updated by Eq. 3, given the new embedding space. Finally, the centroid locations are updated from the new cluster assignments. This process is repeated until convergence. Figure 1 shows a visualization of this training procedure.

$$c_j^t = \frac{\sum_{t=1}^{N} z_i}{|C_j^{t-1}|} \qquad (4)$$

## 2.2 Dataset

Whole slide images were obtained from Memorial Sloan Kettering Cancer Center (MSK) and Erasmus Medical Center with approval from each respective Institutional Review Boards. In total, 246 patients with resected ICC without neoadjuvant chemotherapy were included in the analysis. All slides were digitized at MSK using Aperio AT2 scanners (Leica Biosystems; Wetzlar Germany). Up-to-date retrospective data for recurrence free survival after resection were also obtained. Though currently a small sample size when compared to commonly occurring cancers, this collection is the largest known ICC dataset in the world.

A library of extracted image tiles was generated from all digitized slides. First, each slide was reduced to a thumbnail, where one pixel in the thumbnail represented a $224 \times 224$px tile in the slide at 20x magnification. Next, using Otsu thresholding on the thumbnail, a binary mask of tissue (positive) vs. background (negative) was generated. Connected components below 10 thumbnail pixels in tissue were considered background to exclude dirt or other insignificant masses in the digitized slide. Finally, mathematical morphology was used to erode the tissue mask by one thumbnail pixel to minimize tiles with partial background. To separate the problem of cancer subtyping, as discussed in this paper, from the problem of tumor segmentation, the areas of tumor were manually annotated using a web-based whole slide viewer. Using a touchscreen (Surface Pro 3, Surface Studio; Microsoft Inc., Redmond, WA, USA), a pathologist painted over regions of tumor to identify where tiles should be extracted. Tiles were added to the training set if they lay completely within these regions of identified tumor.

**Quality Control.** Scanning artifacts such as out-of-focus areas of an image can impact model performance on smaller datasets. A deep convolutional neural network was trained to detect blurred tiles to further reduce noise in the dataset. Training a detector on real blur data was beyond the scope of this study because obtaining annotations for blurred regions in the slide is unfeasible and would also create a strong class imbalance between blurred and sharp tiles. To prepare data for training a blur detector, we used an approach similar to a method described in [6]: To start, half of the tiles were artificially blurred by applying Gaussian-blur with a random radius ranging from 1 to 10. The other half were labeled "sharp" and no change was made to them. A ResNet18 was trained to output an image quality score by regressing over the values of the applied filter radius using MSE. A value of 0 was used for images in the sharp class. Finally, a threshold was manually selected to exclude blurred tiles based on the output value of the detector.

## 2.3 Architecture and Training

We propose a novel convolutional autoencoder architecture to optimize performance in image reconstruction. The encoder is a ResNet18 [9] pretrained on ImageNet [13]. The parameters of all layers of the encoder updated when training the full model on pathology data. The decoder is comprised of five convolutional layers, each with a padding and stride of 1, for keeping the tensor size constant with each convolution operation. Upsampling is used before each convolution step to increase the size of the feature map. Empirically, batch normalization layers did not improve reconstruction performance and thus, were excluded.

Two properties of the model need to be optimized: first, the weights of the network, $\theta$, and then locations of the cluster centers, or centroids, in the embedding space, $C_j$. In order to minimize Eq. 2 and update $\theta$, the previous training

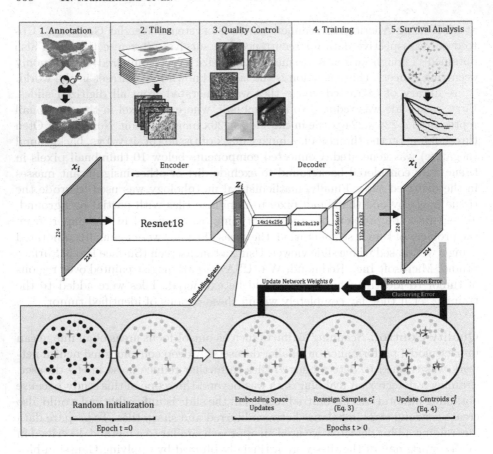

**Fig. 1.** Training the model is the fourth phase of our complete pipeline. At each iteration, the model is updated in two steps. After a each forward-pass of a minibatch, the network weights are updated. At the end of each epoch, centroid locations are updated by reassigning all samples in the newly updated embedding space to the nearest centroid from the previous epoch, as described in Eq. 3. Finally, each centroid location is recalculated using Eq. 4. All centroids are randomly initialized before training.

epoch's set of centroids, $C_j^{t-1}$, is used. In the case of the first training epoch, centroid locations are randomly assigned upon initialization. A training epoch is defined by the forward-passing of all mini-batches once through the network. After $\theta$ have been updated, all samples are reassigned to the nearest centroid using Eq. 3. Finally, all centroid locations are updated using Eq. 4 and used in the calculations of the next training epoch. Figure 1 illustrates this process and architecture.

All training was done on DGX-1 compute nodes (NVIDIA, Santa Clara, CA) using PyTorch 0.4 on Linux CentOS 7. The models were trained using Adam optimization for 150 epochs, a learning rate of $1e^{-2}$, and weight decay of

$1e^{-4}$. To save on computation time, 100,000 tiles were randomly sampled from the complete tile library to train each model, resulting in approximately 400 tiles from each slide on average. The following section describes the selection process for hyper-parameters $\lambda$ and $J$, clustering weight and number of clusters, respectively.

**Experiments.** The Calinski-Harabaz Index ($CHI$) [5], also known as the variance ratio criterion, was used to measure cluster performance, defined by measuring the ratio of between-clusters dispersion mean and within-cluster dispersion. A higher $CHI$ indicates stronger cluster separation and lower variance within each cluster.

A series of experiments were conducted to optimize $\lambda$ and $J$ for model selection. With $\lambda$ set to 0.2, five different models were trained with varying $J$ clusters, ranging from 5 to 25. Secondly, five models were trained with varying $\lambda$, from 0.2 to 1, with $J$ set to the value corresponding with the highest CHI from the previous experiment. A final model was trained with optimized $J$ and $\lambda$ to cluster all tiles in the dataset. Each slide was assigned a class based on which cluster was measured to occupy the largest area in the slide. This approach is used because it is similar to how a pathologist would classify a cancer into a subtype based on the most commonly occurring histologic pattern.

**Survival Modeling.** In order to measure the usefulness and effectiveness of the clustered morphological patterns, we conducted slide-level survival analysis, based on the assigned classes to associated outcome data. Survival data often includes right-censored time durations. This means that the time of event of interest, in our case recurrence detected by radiology, is unknown for some patients. However, the time duration of no recurrence, as measured until the patient's last follow-up date, is still useful information which can be harnessed for modeling. Cox-proportional hazard modeling is a commonly used model to deal with right-censored data:

$$H(t) = h_o e^{b_i x_i}, \tag{5}$$

where $H(t)$ is the hazard function dependant on time $t$, $h_o$ is a baseline hazard, and covariate $x_i$ is weighted by coefficient $b_i$. The hazard ratio, or relative likelihood of death, is defined by $e^{b_j}$. A hazard ratio greater than one indicates that a cluster class contributes to a worse prognosis. Conversely, a hazard ratio less than one contributes to a good prognostic factor. To measure significance in the survival model, p-values based on the Wald statistic, likelihood ratio, and log-rank test are presented for each model.

Five univariate cox models were trained, each with one cluster class held out as a reference to measure impact of survival relative to the other classes. Further, we show Kaplan-Meier curves to illustrate survival outcomes within each class by estimating the survival function $S(t)$:

$$S(t) = \prod_{t_i < t} \frac{n_i - d_i}{n_n}, \qquad (6)$$

where $d_i$ are the number of recurrence events at time $t$ and $n_i$ are the number of subjects at risk of death or recurrence prior to time $t$.

# 3  Results

Results of model selection by varying $\lambda$ and $J$ are shown in Table 1. Best performance was measured by CHI with $\lambda$ set to 0.2 and $J$ set to 5.

Cox-proportional hazard modeling showed strong significance in recurrence-free survival between patients when classifying their tissue based on clusters produced by the unsupervised model. Table 2 details the hazard ratios of each cluster, relative to the others in five different models. Each model has one clus-

**Table 1.** The Calinski-Harabaz Index (CHI) was highest when the model was set to 5 clusters $(J)$ and clustering weight $(\lambda)$ was set to 0.2 This indicates the model which best produces clusters that are dense and well-separated from each other.

| $J$ | 5 | 10 | 15 | 20 | 25 |
|---|---|---|---|---|---|
| CHI | **3863** | 2460 | 2064 | 957 | 1261 |
| $\lambda$ | 0.2 | 0.4 | 0.6 | 0.8 | 1.0 |
| CHI | **4314** | 3233 | 3433 | 3897 | 3112 |

ter held as a reference to produce the hazard ratio. Figure 2 shows a visualization of the survival model using Kaplan-Meier analysis.

**Table 2.** Hazard ratios show strong significance as measured by three different statistical tests. This indicates that the cluster classes produced by the unsupervised model suggest clinical usefulness. If each cluster class is considered a cancer subtype, five subtypes is the strongest stratification seen in the literature thus far.

| Cluster | Hazard ratio | | | | |
|---|---|---|---|---|---|
| | Dependent variable: | | | | |
| | 0 | 1 | 2 | 3 | 4 |
| 0 | Reference | 1.332*** (0.206) | 0.789*** (0.250) | 1.788*** (0.237) | 0.873*** (0.235) |
| 1 | 0.751*** (0.206) | Reference | 0.593** (0.251) | 1.342*** (0.236) | 0.655*** (0.235) |
| 2 | 1.267*** (0.250) | 1.688*** (0.251) | Reference | 2.265*** (0.277) | 1.106*** (0.272) |
| 3 | 0.559** (0.237) | 0.745*** (0.236) | 0.441 (0.277) | Reference | 0.488* (0.264) |
| 4 | 1.145*** (0.235) | 1.526*** (0.235) | 0.904*** (0.272) | 2.048*** (0.264) | Reference |
| Wald Test | 12.740** | 12.740** | 12.740** | 12.740** | 12.740** |
| LR Test | 13.183** | 13.183** | 13.183** | 13.183** | 13.183** |
| Logrank Test | 13.097** | 13.097** | 13.097** | 13.097** | 13.097** |

*Note:* *p<0.1; **p<0.05; ***p<0.01

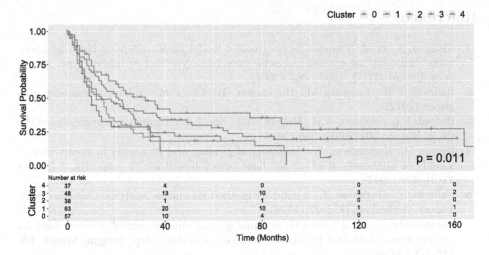

**Fig. 2.** Kaplan-Meier visualization of survival probabilities for each patient classified into one of the five cluster classes produced by the unsupervised model. Patients with high presence of tissue in cluster 3 have a better recurrence-free survival than those with clusters 2 or 4.

## 4    Conclusion

Our model offers a novel approach for identifying histological patterns of potential prognostic significance, circumventing the tasks of tedious tissue labeling and laborious human evaluation of multiple whole slides. As a point of comparison, a recent study showed that an effective prognostic score for colorectal cancer was achieved by first segmenting a slide into eight predefined categorical regions using supervised learning [10]. These kind of models limit the model to pre-defined histologic components (tumor, fat, debris, etc.) and the protocol may not extend to extra-colonic anatomic sites lacking a similar tumor specific stroma interactions [2]. In contrast, the design of our model lacks predefined tissue classes, and has the capability to analyze any number of clusters, thus removing potential bias introduced by training and increasing flexibility in application of the model. We truly hope that novel subtyping approaches like this lead to better grading of cholangiocarcinoma and improve treatment and outcome of patients.

## 5    Disclosures

T.J.F. is the Chief Scientific Officer of Paige.AI, co-founder, and equity holder of Paige.AI. H.M. and T.J.F. have intellectual property interests relevant to the work that is the subject of this paper. MSK has financial interests in Paige.AI and intellectual property interests relevant to the work that is the subject of this paper.

# References

1. Aishima, S., et al.: Proposal of progression model for intrahepatic cholangiocarcinoma: clinicopathologic differences between hilar type and peripheral type. Am. J. Surg. Pathol. **31**(7), 1059–1067 (2007)
2. Balkwill, F.R., Capasso, M., Hagemann, T.: The tumor microenvironment at a glance (2012)
3. Bedard, P.L., Hansen, A.R., Ratain, M.J., Siu, L.L.: Tumour heterogeneity in the clinic. Nature **501**(7467), 355 (2013)
4. Bloom, H., Richardson, W.: Histological grading and prognosis in breast cancer: a study of 1409 cases of which 359 have been followed for 15 years. Br. J. Cancer **11**(3), 359 (1957)
5. Caliński, T., Harabasz, J.: A dendrite method for cluster analysis. Commun. Stat. Theory Methods **3**(1), 1–27 (1974)
6. Campanella, G., et al.: Towards machine learned quality control: a benchmark for sharpness quantification in digital pathology. Comput. Med. Imaging Graph. **65**, 142–151 (2018)
7. Dercksen, K., Bulten, W., Litjens, G.: Dealing with label scarcity in computational pathology: a use case in prostate cancer classification. arXiv preprint arXiv:1905.06820 (2019)
8. Fouad, S., Randell, D., Galton, A., Mehanna, H., Landini, G.: Unsupervised morphological segmentation of tissue compartments in histopathological images. PLoS ONE **12**(11), e0188717 (2017)
9. He, K., Zhang, X., Ren, S., Sun, J.: Deep residual learning for image recognition. In: Proceedings of the IEEE Conference on Computer Vision and Pattern Recognition, pp. 770–778 (2016)
10. Kather, J.N., et al.: Predicting survival from colorectal cancer histology slides using deep learning: a retrospective multicenter study. PLoS Med. **16**(1), e1002730 (2019)
11. Moriya, T., et al.: Unsupervised pathology image segmentation using representation learning with spherical k-mean. arXiv preprint arXiv:1804.03828 (2018)
12. Nakajima, T., Kondo, Y., Miyazaki, M., Okui, K.: A histopathologic study of 102 cases of intrahepatic cholangiocarcinoma: histologic classification and modes of spreading. Hum. Pathol. **19**(10), 1228–1234 (1988)
13. Russakovsky, O., et al.: ImageNet large scale visual recognition challenge. Int. J. Comput. Vis. (IJCV) **115**(3), 211–252 (2015)
14. Saha, S.K., Zhu, A.X., Fuchs, C.S., Brooks, G.A.: Forty-year trends in cholangiocarcinoma incidence in the us: intrahepatic disease on the rise. Oncologist **21**(5), 594–599 (2016)
15. Sempoux, C., et al..: Intrahepatic cholangiocarcinoma: new insights in pathology. In: Seminars in Liver Disease, vol. 31, pp. 049–060. Thieme Medical Publishers (2011)
16. Song, C., Liu, F., Huang, Y., Wang, L., Tan, T.: Auto-encoder based data clustering. In: Ruiz-Shulcloper, J., Sanniti di Baja, G. (eds.) CIARP 2013. LNCS, vol. 8258, pp. 117–124. Springer, Heidelberg (2013). https://doi.org/10.1007/978-3-642-41822-8_15

# Evidence Localization for Pathology Images Using Weakly Supervised Learning

Yongxiang Huang[✉] and Albert C. S. Chung

Lo Kwee-Seong Medical Image Analysis Laboratory,
Department of Computer Science and Engineering,
The Hong Kong University of Science and Technology, Hong Kong, China
{yhuangch,achung}@cse.ust.hk

**Abstract.** Despite deep convolutional neural networks boost the performance of image classification and segmentation in digital pathology analysis, they are usually weak in interpretability for clinical applications or require heavy annotations to achieve object localization. To overcome this problem, we propose a weakly supervised learning-based approach that can effectively learn to localize the discriminative evidence for a diagnostic label from weakly labeled training data. Experimental results show that our proposed method can reliably pinpoint the location of cancerous evidence supporting the decision of interest, while still achieving a competitive performance on glimpse-level and slide-level histopathologic cancer detection tasks.

**Keywords:** Pathology image detection · Weakly-supervised learning · Computer-aided diagnosis

## 1 Introduction

Pathology analysis based on microscopic images is a critical task in medical image computing. In recent years, deep learning of digitalized pathology slide has facilitated the progress of automating many diagnostic tasks, offering the potential to increase accuracy and improve review efficiency. Limited by computation resources, deep learning-based approaches on whole slide pathology images (WSIs) usually train convolutional neural networks (CNNs) on patches extracted from WSIs and aggregate the patch-level predictions to obtain a slide-level representation, which is further used to identify cancer metastases and stage cancer [10]. Such a patch-based CNN approach has been shown to surpass pathologists in various diagnostic tasks [5].

Off-the-shelf CNNs have been shown to be able to accurately classify or segment pathology images into different diagnostic types in recent studies [3,9]. However, most of these methods are weak in interpretability especially for clinicians, due to a lack of evidence supporting for the decision of interest. During

© Springer Nature Switzerland AG 2019
D. Shen et al. (Eds.): MICCAI 2019, LNCS 11764, pp. 613–621, 2019.
https://doi.org/10.1007/978-3-030-32239-7_68

diagnosis, a pathologist often inspects abnormal structures (e.g., large nucleus, hypercellularity) as the evidence for determining whether the glimpsed patch is cancerous. For CAD systems, learning to pinpoint the discriminative evidence can provide precise visual assistance for clinicians. Strong supervision-based feature localization methods require a large number of pathology images annotated in pixel-level or object-level, which are very costly and time-consuming and can be biased by the experiences of the observers. In this paper, we propose a weakly supervised learning (WSL) method that can learn to localize the discriminative evidence for the class-of-interest on pathology images from weakly labeled (i.e. image-level) training data. Our contributions include: (i) proposing a new CNN architecture with multi-branch attention modules and deep supervision mechanism, to address the difficulty of localizing discrete and small objects in pathology images, (ii) formulating a generalizable approach that leverages gradient-weighted class activation map and saliency map in a complementary way to provide accurate evidence localization, (iii) designing a new attention module which allows capturing spatial attention from various context, (iv) quantitatively and visually evaluating WSL methods on large scale histopathology datasets, and (v) constructing a new dataset (HPLOC) based on Camelyon16 for effectively evaluating evidence localization performance on histopathology images.

**Related Work.** Recent studies have demonstrated that CNN can learn to localize discriminative features even when it is trained on image-level annotations [12]. However, these methods are evaluated on natural image datasets (e.g., PASCAL), where the objects of interest are usually large and distinct in color and shape. In contrast, objects in pathology images are usually small and less distinct in morphology between different classes. A few recent studies investigated WSL approaches on medical images, including lung nodule detection and placental ultrasound images [1]. These methods employ GAP-based class activation map and require CNNs ending with global average pooling, which degrades the performance of CNNs as a side effect [12].

## 2    Methods

The overview of the framework is shown in Fig. 1. The model is trained to predict the cancer score for a given image, indicating the presence of cancer metastasis. In the test phase, besides giving a binary classification, the model generates a cancerous evidence localization map and performs localization.

### 2.1    Cancerous Evidence Localization Networks (CELNet)

Given the object of interest is relatively small and discrete, a moderate number of convolutional layers is sufficient for encoding locally discriminative features. As discussed in Sect. 1, instances on pathology images are similar in morphology and can be densely distributed, the model should avoid over-downsampling in order to pinpoint the cancerous evidence from the densely distributed instances. The proposed CELNet starts with a $3 \times 3$ convolution head followed by 3

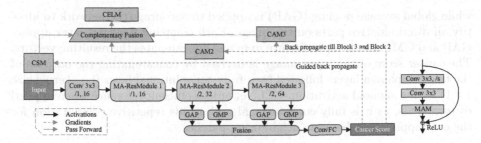

**Fig. 1.** Left: Framework overview of the proposed WSL method. The under line (e.g., /1, 16) denotes stride and number of channels. Right: A building block for the multi-branch attention based residual module (MA-ResModule).

**Multi-branch Attention-based Residual Modules (MA-ResModule)[1] [2].** Each MA-ResModule is composed of 3 consecutive building blocks integrated with the proposed attention module (MAM) as shown in Fig. 1 (Right). We use $3 \times 3$ convolution with stride of 2 for downsampling in residual connections instead of $1 \times 1$ convolution to reduce information loss. Batch normalization and ReLU are applied after each convolution layer for regularization and non-linearity.

**Multi-branch Attention Module (MAM).** To eliminate the effect of background contents and focus on representing the cancerous evidence (which can be sparse), we employ attention mechanism. Improved on Convolutional Block Attention Module (CBAM), which extracts channel attention and spatial attention of an input feature map in a squeeze and excitation manner, we propose a multi-branch attention module. MAM can better approximate the importance of each location on the feature map by looking at its context at different scales. Given a squeezed feature map $F_{sq}$ generated by the channel attention module, we compute and derive a 2D spatial attention map $A_s$ by $A_s = \sigma(\sum_{k'} f^{k' \times k'}(F_{sq}))$, where $f^{k' \times k'}$ represents a convolution operation with kernel size of $k' \times k'$, and $\sigma$ denotes the sigmoid function. We set $k' \in \{3, 5, 7\}$ in our experiments, corresponding to 3 branches. Hereby, the feature map $F_{sq}$ is refined by element-wise multiplication with the spatial attention map $A_s$.

MAM is conceptually simple but effective in improving detection and localization performance as demonstrated in our experiments.

**Deep Supervision.** Deep supervision [4] is employed to empower the intermediate layers to learn class-discriminative representations, for building the cancer activation map in a higher resolution. We achieve this by adding two companion output layers to the last two MA-ResModules, as shown in Fig. 1. Global max pooling (GMP) is applied to search for the best discriminative features spatially,

---

[1] Densely connected module is not employed considering it is comparatively speed-inefficient for WSIs application due to its dense tensor concatenation.

while global average pooling (GAP) is applied to encourage the network to identify all discriminative parts on the image. Each companion output layer applies GAP and GMP on the input feature map and concatenates the resulting vectors. The cancer score of the input image is derived by concatenating the outputs of the two companion layers followed by a fully convolutional layer (i.e., kernel size $1 \times 1$) with a sigmoid activation. CELNet enjoys efficient inference when applied to test WSIs, as it is fully convolutional and avoids repetitive computation for the overlapping part between neighboring patches.

## 2.2 Cancerous Evidence Localization Map (CELM)

**Cancer Activation Map (CAM).** Given an image $I \in \mathbb{R}^{H \times W \times 3}$, let $y^c = S_c(I)$ represent the cancer score function governed by the trained CELNet (before sigmoid layer). A cancer-class activation map $M^c$ shows the importance of each region on the image to the diagnostic value. For a target layer $l$, the CAM $M_l^c$ is derived by taking the weighted sum of feature maps $F_l$ with the weights $\{\alpha_{k,l}^c\}$, where $\alpha_{k,l}^c$ represents the importance of $k^{th}$ feature plane. The weights $\alpha_{k,l}^c$ are computed as $\alpha_{k,l}^c = Avg_{i,j}(\frac{\partial y^c}{\partial F_l^k(i,j)})$, i.e., spatially averaging the gradients of cancer score $y^c$ with respect to the $k^{th}$ feature plane $F_l^k$, which is achieved by back propagation (see Fig. 1). Thus, the CAM of layer $l$ can be derived by $M_l^c = ReLU(\sum_k \alpha_{k,l}^c F_l^k)$, where ReLU is applied to exclude the features with negative influence on the class of interest [6].

We derive two CAMs, $M_2^c$ and $M_3^c$ from the last layer of the second and the third residual module on CELNet respectively (i.e., CAM2 and CAM3 in Fig. 1). CAM3 can represent discriminative regions for identifying a cancer class in a relatively low resolution while CAM2 enjoys higher resolution and still class-discriminative under deep supervision.

**Cancer Saliency Map (CSM).** In contrast with CAM, the cancer-class saliency map shows the contribution of each pixel site to the cancer score $y^c$. This can be approximated by the derivate of a linear function $S^c(I) \approx w^T I + b$. Thus the pixel contribution is computed as $w = \frac{\partial S^c(I)}{\partial I}$. Different from [7], we derive $w$ by the guided back-propagation [8] to prevent backward flow of negative gradients. For a RGB image, to obtain its cancer saliency map $M^s \in \mathbb{R}^{H \times W \times 1}$ from $w \in \mathbb{R}^{H \times W \times 3}$, we first normalize $w$ to $[0, 1]$ range, followed by greyscale conversion and Gaussian smoothing, instead of simply taking the maximum magnitude of $w$ as proposed in [7]. Thus, the resulting cancer saliency map (see Fig. 2(b)) is far less noisy and more focus on class-related objects than the original one proposed in [7].

**Complementary Fusion.** The generated CAMs coarsely display discriminative regions for identifying a cancer class (see Fig. 2(c)), while the CSM is fine-grained, sensitive and represents pixelated contributions for the identification (see Fig. 2(b)). To combine the merits of them for precise cancerous evidence localization, we propose a complementary fusion method. First, CAM3 and CAM2 are combined to obtain a unified cancer activation map $M^c \in \mathbb{R}^{H \times W \times 1}$ as $M^c = \alpha f_u(M_3^c) + (1 - \alpha)f_u(M_2^c)$, where $f_u$ denotes a upsampling function by bilinear interpolation, and the coefficient $\alpha$ in range $[0,1]$ is confirmed by validation. The CELM is derived by complementarily fusing CSM and CAM as $M = \beta(M^c \odot M^s) + (1 - \beta)M^c$, where $\odot$ denotes element-wise product, and the coefficient $\beta$ captures the reliability of the point-wise multiplication of CAM and CSM, and the value of $\beta$ is estimated by cross-validation in experiments.

## 3   Experiments and Results

We first evaluate the detection performance of the proposed model as for clinical requirements, followed by evidence localization evaluations.

### 3.1   Datasets and Experimental Setup

The detection performance of the proposed method is validated on two benchmark datasets, PCam [9] and Camelyon16[2].

**PCam:** The PCam dataset contains 327,680 lymph node histopathology images of size $96 \times 96$ with binary class labels indicating the presence of cancer metastasis, split into 75% for training, 12.5% for validation, and 12.5% for testing as originally proposed. The class distribution in each split is balanced (1:1). For a fair comparison, following [9], we perform image augmentation by random 90-degree rotations and horizontal flipping during training.

**Camelyon16:** The Camelyon16 dataset includes 270 H&E stained WSIs (160 normal and 110 cancerous cases) for training and 129 WSIs held out for testing (80 normal and 49 cancerous cases) with average image size about $65000 \times 45000$, where regions with cancer metastasis are delineated in cancerous slides. To apply our CELNet on WSIs, we follow the pipeline proposed in [5], including WSI pre-processing, patch sampling and augmentation, heatmap generation, and slide-level detection tasks. For slide-level classification, we take the maximum tumor score among all patches as the final slide-level prediction. For tumor region localization, we apply non-suppression maximum algorithm on the tumor probability map aggregated from patch predictions to iteratively extract tumor region coordinates. We work on the WSI data at $10\times$ resolution instead of $40\times$ with the available computation resources.

In our experiments, all models are trained using binary cross-entropy loss with L2 regularization of $10^{-5}$ to improve model generalizability, and optimized by SGD with Nesterov momentum of 0.9 with a batch size of 64 for 100 epochs. The learning rate is initialized with $10^{-4}$ and is halved at 50 and 75 epochs. We select model weights with minimum validation loss for test evaluation.

---

[2] https://camelyon16.grand-challenge.org.

## 3.2    Classification Results

As Table 1 shows, CELNet consistently outperforms ResNet, DenseNet, and P4M-DenseNet [9] in histopathologic cancer detection on the PCam dataset. P4M-DenseNet uses less parameters due to parameter sharing in the p4m-equivariance. For auxiliary experiments, we perform ablation studies and visual analysis. From Table 1, we observe that our attention module brings 1.77% accuracy gain, which is larger than the gain brought by CBAM [11]. Both the CAM and CELM on CELNet are mainly activated for the cancerous regions (see Figs. 2(c) and (d)). These subfigures indicate that CELNet is effective in extracting discriminative evidence for histopathologic classification.

**Table 1.** Quantitative comparisons on the PCam test set. P4M-DenseNet [9]: current SoTA method for the PCam benchmark, CELNet: our method, ⁻: removal of the proposed multi-branch attention module, +CBAM: integration with convolutional block attention module [11].

| Methods | Acc | AUC | #Params |
|---------|-----|-----|---------|
| ResNet18 [2] | 88.73 | 95.36 | 11.2M |
| DenseNet [9] | 87.20 | 94.60 | 902K |
| P4M-DenseNet | 89.80 | 96.30 | 119K |
| CELNet | **91.87** | **97.72** | 297K |
| CELNet⁻ | 90.10 | 96.45 | 292K |
| CELNet⁻ +CBAM | 90.86 | 97.17 | 296K |

On slide-level detection tasks, as shown in Table 2, our CELNet based approach achieves higher classification performance (1.7%) in terms of AUC than the baseline method [5], and outperforms previous state-of-the-art methods in slide-level tumor localization performance in terms of FROC score. The results illustrate that instead of using off-the-shelve CNNs as the core patch-level model for histopathologic slide detection, adopting CELNet can potentially bring larger performance gain. CELNet is more parameter-efficient as shown in Table 1 and testing a slide on Camelyon16 takes about 2 min on a Nvidia 1080Ti GPU.

## 3.3    Weakly Supervised Localization and Results

Given that the trained CELNet can precisely classify a pathology image, here we aim to investigate its performance in localizing the supporting evidence based on the proposed CELM. To achieve this, based on Camelyon16, we first construct a dataset with region-level annotations for cancer metastasis, namely HPLOC, and develop the metrics for measuring localization performance on HPLOC.

**HPLOC:** The HPLOC dataset contains 20,000 images of size $96 \times 96$ with segmentation masks for cancerous region. Each image is sampled from the test

**Table 2.** Quantitative comparisons of slide-level classification performance (AUC) and slide-level tumor localization performance (FROC) on the Camelyon16 test set. *: The Challenge Winner uses 40× resolution while results of other methods are based on 10×.

| Methods | AUC | FROC |
|---------|-----|------|
| P4M-DenseNet | - | 84.0 |
| Liu [5] | 96.5 | 79.3 |
| Challenge Winner* [10] | **99.4** | 80.7 |
| Pathologist | 96.6 | 73.3 |
| CELNet | 97.2 | **84.8** |

set of Camelyon16 and contains both cancerous regions and normal tissue in the glimpse, which harbors the high quality of the Camelyon16 dataset.

**Metrics:** To perform localization, we generate segmentation masks from CELM/CAM/CSM by thresholding and smoothing (see Fig. 2(e)). If a segmentation mask intersects with the cancerous region by at least 75%[3], it is defined as a true positive. Otherwise, if a segmentation mask intersects with the normal region by at least 75%, it is considered as a false positive. Thus, we can use precision and recall score to quantitatively assess the localization performance of different WSL methods, where the results are summarized in Table 3.

**Table 3.** Quantitative comparisons for different weakly supervised localization methods on the HPLOC dataset. Ours: CELNet + CELM. MAM and DS are short for multi-branch attention module and deep supervision respectively.

| Methods | Precision | Recall |
|---------|-----------|--------|
| ResNet18 + Backprop [7] | 79.8 | 85.5 |
| ResNet18 + GradCAM [6] | 85.6 | 82.4 |
| Ours | **91.6** | 87.3 |
| Ours w/o MAM | 88.1 | 85.6 |
| Ours w/o DS | 90.5 | **87.7** |
| CELNet + GradCAM | 91.0 | 85.4 |

We observe that our WSL method based on CELNet and CELM consistently performs better than the back propagation-based approach [7] and the class activation map-based approach [6]. Note that we used ResNet18 [2] as the backbone for the compared methods because it achieves better classification performance and provides higher resolution for GradCAM (12 × 12) as compared to DenseNet

---

[3] The annotated contour in Camelyon16 is usually enlarged to surround all tumors.

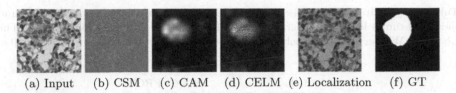

(a) Input     (b) CSM     (c) CAM     (d) CELM     (e) Localization     (f) GT

**Fig. 2.** Evidence localization results of our WSL method on the HPLOC dataset. (a) Input glimpse, (b) Cancer saliency map, (c) Cancer activation map, (d) CELM: Cancerous Evidence Localization Map, (e) Localization results based on CELM, where the localized evidence is highlighted for providing visual assistance, (f) GT: ground truth, white masks represent tumor regions and the black represents normal tissue

(3 × 3) [9]. We perform ablation studies to further evaluate the key components of our method in Table 3. We observe the effectiveness of the proposed multi-branch attention module in increasing the localization accuracy. The deep supervision mechanism effectively improves the precision in localization despite slightly lower recall score, which can be caused by the regularization effect on the intermediate layers, that is, encouraging the learning of discriminative features for classification but also potentially discouraging the learning of some low-level histological patterns. We observe that using CELM can improve the recall score and precision, which indicates that CELM allows better discovery of cancerous evidence than using GradCAM. We present the visualization results in Fig. 2, the cancerous evidence is represented as large nucleus and hypercellularity in the images, which are precisely captured by the CELM. Figure 2(e) visualizes the localization results by overlaying the segmentation mask generated from CELM onto the input image, which demonstrates the effectiveness of our WSL method in localizing cancerous evidence.

## 4  Discussion and Conclusions

In this paper, we have proposed a generalizable method for localizing cancerous evidence on histopathology images. Unlike the conventional feature-based approaches, the proposed method does not rely on specific feature descriptors but learn discriminative features for localization from the data. To the best of our knowledge, investigating weakly supervised CNNs for cancerous evidence localization and quantitatively evaluating them on large datasets have not been performed on histopathology images. Experimental results show that our proposed method can achieve competitive classification performance on histopathologic cancer detection, and more importantly, provide reliable and accurate cancerous evidence localization using weakly training data, which reduces the burden of annotations. We believe that such an extendable method can have a great impact in detection-based studies in microscopy images and help improve the accuracy and interpretability for current deep learning-based pathology analysis systems.

# References

1. Feng, X., Yang, J., Laine, A.F., Angelini, E.D.: Discriminative localization in CNNs for weakly-supervised segmentation of pulmonary nodules. In: Descoteaux, M., Maier-Hein, L., Franz, A., Jannin, P., Collins, D.L., Duchesne, S. (eds.) MICCAI 2017. LNCS, vol. 10435, pp. 568–576. Springer, Cham (2017). https://doi.org/10.1007/978-3-319-66179-7_65
2. He, K., Zhang, X., Ren, S., Sun, J.: Deep residual learning for image recognition. In: Proceedings of the IEEE Conference on Computer Vision and Pattern Recognition, pp. 770–778 (2016)
3. Huang, Y., Chung, A.C.-S.: Improving high resolution histology image classification with deep spatial fusion network. In: Stoyanov, D., et al. (eds.) OMIA/COMPAY -2018. LNCS, vol. 11039, pp. 19–26. Springer, Cham (2018). https://doi.org/10.1007/978-3-030-00949-6_3
4. Lee, C.Y., Xie, S., Gallagher, P., Zhang, Z., Tu, Z.: Deeply-supervised nets. In: Artificial Intelligence and Statistics, pp. 562–570 (2015)
5. Liu, Y., Gadepalli, K., et al.: Detecting cancer metastases on gigapixel pathology images. CoRR abs/1703.02442 (2017)
6. Selvaraju, R.R., Cogswell, M., Das, A., Vedantam, R., et al.: Grad-cam: Visual explanations from deep networks via gradient-based localization. In: Proceedings of the IEEE International Conference on Computer Vision, pp. 618–626 (2017)
7. Simonyan, K., Vedaldi, A., et al.: Deep inside convolutional networks: Visualising image classification models and saliency maps. CoRR abs/1312.6034 (2013)
8. Springenberg, J.T., Dosovitskiy, A., Brox, T., Riedmiller, M.: Striving for simplicity: The all convolutional net. arXiv preprint arXiv:1412.6806 (2014)
9. Veeling, B.S., Linmans, J., Winkens, J., Cohen, T., Welling, M.: Rotation equivariant CNNs for digital pathology. In: Frangi, A.F., Schnabel, J.A., Davatzikos, C., Alberola-López, C., Fichtinger, G. (eds.) MICCAI 2018. LNCS, vol. 11071, pp. 210–218. Springer, Cham (2018). https://doi.org/10.1007/978-3-030-00934-2_24
10. Wang, D., Khosla, A., Gargeya, R., Irshad, H., Beck, A.H.: Deep learning for identifying metastatic breast cancer. CoRR abs/1606.05718 (2016)
11. Woo, S., Park, J., Lee, J.-Y., Kweon, I.S.: CBAM: convolutional block attention module. In: Ferrari, V., Hebert, M., Sminchisescu, C., Weiss, Y. (eds.) ECCV 2018. LNCS, vol. 11211, pp. 3–19. Springer, Cham (2018). https://doi.org/10.1007/978-3-030-01234-2_1
12. Zhou, B., Khosla, A., Lapedriza, A., Oliva, A., Torralba, A.: Learning deep features for discriminative localization. In: Proceedings of the IEEE conference on computer vision and pattern recognition, pp. 2921–2929 (2016)

# Nuclear Instance Segmentation Using a Proposal-Free Spatially Aware Deep Learning Framework

Navid Alemi Koohbanani[1,3]([envelope]), Mostafa Jahanifar[2], Ali Gooya[4], and Nasir Rajpoot[1,3]

[1] University of Warwick, Coventry, UK
n.alemi-koohbanani@warwick.ac.uk
[2] NRP Co., Tehran, Iran
[3] The Alan Turing Institute, London, UK
[4] University of Leeds, Leeds, UK

**Abstract.** Nuclear segmentation in histology images is a challenging task due to significant variations in the shape and appearance of nuclei. One of the main hurdles in nuclear instance segmentation is overlapping nuclei where a smart algorithm is needed to separate each nucleus. In this paper, we introduce a proposal-free deep learning based framework to address these challenges. To this end, we propose a spatially-aware network (SpaNet) to capture spatial information in a multi-scale manner. A dual-head variation of the SpaNet is first utilized to predict the pixel-wise segmentation and centroid detection maps of nuclei. Based on these outputs, a single-head SpaNet predicts the positional information related to each nucleus instance. Spectral clustering method is applied on the output of the last SpaNet, which utilizes the nuclear mask and the Gaussian-like detection map for determining the connected components and associated cluster identifiers, respectively. The output of the clustering method is the final nuclear instance segmentation mask. We applied our method on a publicly available multi-organ data set (https://nucleisegmentationbenchmark.weebly.com/) and achieved state-of-the-art performance for nuclear segmentation.

**Keywords:** Computational pathology · Instance segmentation · Nuclear segmentation

## 1 Introduction

Nuclear segmentation is often the first step toward a detailed analysis of histology images. For instance, automatic nuclear pleomorphism scoring and cancer grading heavily rely on morphological appearance and structure of nuclei, which have

**Electronic supplementary material** The online version of this chapter (https://doi.org/10.1007/978-3-030-32239-7_69) contains supplementary material, which is available to authorized users.

© Springer Nature Switzerland AG 2019
D. Shen et al. (Eds.): MICCAI 2019, LNCS 11764, pp. 622–630, 2019.
https://doi.org/10.1007/978-3-030-32239-7_69

been verified by a wide range of studies, see for example [8]. The complexity of nuclei shape and appearance, imperfect slide preparation/staining, and scanning artifacts make the automatic instance segmentation of nuclei hardly achievable. To overcome these challenges and reduce the burden of manual segmentation, several algorithms have been proposed for nuclear segmentation and detection, ranging from simple thresholding techniques to more sophisticated approaches [14]. However, since the emergence of deep learning and its applications in segmentation, most of these methods have been replaced by Convolutions Neural Networks (CNNs) or are only used as a post/pre-processing step in conjunction with CNNs [14].

Previous methods are mainly based on region-proposal networks, like Mask-RCNN [2] and PA-Net [10], or encoder-decoder neural structures particularly U-Net model [13]. Since U-Net was not well established for separating close object in complex histology images, various methods have been introduced in the literature which concentrates on the following 4 aspects: (i) modifying the network architecture to extract richer information (like CIA-Net [15]), (ii) introducing auxiliary outputs to the network, the auxiliary output can be the nucleus contour or bounding box (like DCAN [1], BES-Net [12]), (iii) some methods proposed CNNs that predicts distance map (or other geometrical mappings) of nuclei instances (like DR-Net [11]), and (iv) taking into account different combinations of above-mentioned variations to make their deep learning platform more robust for detecting individual objects [14]. Despite these advancements, these models lack spatial awareness which can improve instance-wise segmentation of clustered nuclei, especially in advanced stages of the tumor.

Here, we introduce a novel proposal-free deep learning framework (SpaNet) that can predict spatial information of each nucleus. Outputs of SpaNet are then post-processed through a simple yet effective clustering algorithm to achieve instance-level segmentation. Our contributions can be summarized as: (i) a deep learning based proposal-free framework for nuclei instance segmentation having low computational cost and simple post-processing steps inspired by [9], (ii) a spatially-aware network architecture, which is equipped with a novel multi-scale dense convolutional unit, (iii) incorporating a nuclei detection map for estimating the number of clusters per nuclei clump, (iv) achieving state-of-the-art results on a well-known publicly available multi-organ data set.

Details for the methodology of the above-mentioned contributions are described in Sect. 2, experimental setups, results and discussion are elaborated in Sect. 3, and finally paper is concluded in Sect. 4.

## 2    Methods

Our proposed method consists of predicting positional information of each nucleus through a spatial aware CNN, and then clustering that information to construct instance-level segmentation. To achieve a reasonable spatial prediction and to estimate the number of clusters in nuclei clumps, we additionally incorporated a dual-head network for nuclei mask segmentation (semantic level)

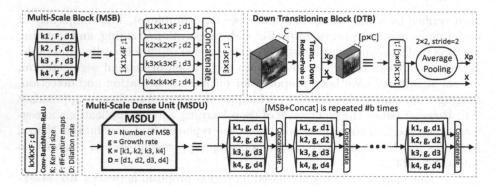

**Fig. 1.** Structuring blocks used in the SpaNet architecture.

and detection maps. In this section, we firstly describe the network architecture, which is used throughout our framework. Afterward, details of employing the proposed CNN for instance segmentation will be discussed.

### 2.1 Spatially Aware Neural Network

An essential step in our proposed nuclear instance segmentation framework is predicting the positional information of each nuclei using CNNs. Conventional CNNs cannot capture positional details due to the nature of kernels. Convolutional kernels in common CNN architectures extract local features. Hence they give no intuition about the relative position of objects (detected features) in the image. To address this issue, we propose spatial information aware CNN capable of capturing positional information in all layers. By providing the network with positional information ($x$ and $y$ image coordinates) in the input and keeping that information available to all convolutional kernels, spatial awareness is guaranteed. Details about the positional information in the input and structuring element of the network are discussed in the following sections.

**Structuring Blocks.** Preserving spatial information throughout the network is feasible using our proposed multi-scale dense unit (MSDU). MSDU is a densely connected building block inspired by [3]. Unlike the ordinary dense unit, our proposed MSDU benefits from the multi-scale convolutional block (MSB) [5]. Figure 1 demonstrates the configuration of a single MSB composed of four parallel convolutional blocks (convolution layer followed by batch-normalization and ReLU layers) with varying kernel size. Having the flexibility to stack convolutional blocks with varying kernel (dilation) rates allows us to obtain multi-resolution feature maps, leading to better performance. MSB Blocks are configured with a specific number of channels ($F$), kernel sizes ($\mathbf{k}$), and dilation rates ($\mathbf{d}$). Each MSB block has a $1 \times 1$ and a $3 \times 3$ convolutional block in its terminals to reduce the number of processed and generated feature maps.

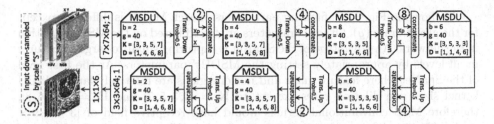

**Fig. 2.** Overview of the SpaNet architecture.

As depicted in Fig. 1, concatenation layers in the MSDU aggregate the output feature maps from their preceding MSBs. The feature aggregation property of MSDUs enables the proposed instance detection network in Fig. 2 to preserve the positional information (which were passed to the network's input) at all convolutional blocks throughout its path, making it a spatial aware network. An MSDU has four configuring parameters: growth rate $(g)$, which indicates the number of feature maps generated by every MSB inside the MSDU. $\mathbf{K}$ and $\mathbf{D}$ vectors showing the kernels' sizes and dilation rates of MSB blocks, and $b$ denotes the number of MSB and concatenation pair repetitions. It has been shown that restricting the number of extracted features in each convolutional blocks (setting small growth rates) and aggregating the feature maps instead, result in better performance while reducing the computational costs [3].

Other two structuring blocks are Down Transitioning Block (DTB) and Up Transitioning Block (UTB) which down-sample and up-sample their input feature by the scale of 2, respectively. The structure of a DTB is shown in Fig. 1, which comprises a $1 \times 1$ convolutional block that generates $[p \times C]$ feature maps $(\mathbf{X})$. The parameter $C$ is the number of input feature maps to the DTB, and $0 < p < 1$ is the reducing rate. DTB also consists of a $2 \times 2$ average pooling layer with a stride of 2, which will down-sample the size of feature maps in half $(\mathbf{Xp})$. UTB comprises a $2 \times 2 \times [p \times C]$ transposed convolution layer followed by batch-normalization and ReLU layers.

**Spa-Net Architecture.** The proposed spatial aware network for nuclei instance segmentation, SpaNet, is illustrated in Fig. 2. The main structure in SpaNet is MSDU, which is equipped with a feature aggregation property that enables positional information flows throughout the network. Feature maps in SpaNet are down-sampled three times by DTBs in the encoding path and are up-sampled accordingly by UTBs in the decoding path. Skip connections will make the feature maps in the decoding path more spatially enriched and facilitate gradient flow during training [13]. More importantly, there are some points in the network that we lose direct access to the positional information (after DTB and UTB units) where feature aggregation is not applied. As a workaround, we appropriately scaled the network input and added it in these layers via concatenation layers.

As shown in Fig. 2, configuring parameters of each MSDU is different, except for the growth rate $(g)$. Other parameters are tuned based on the MSDU position in the network. An advantage of the SpaNet is capturing small-to-large structures in all levels by appropriately setting the MSDUs' parameters. At the first level of the SpaNet where feature maps and nuclei regions are relatively large, MSDU kernel sizes and dilation rates are set to $\mathbf{K} = [3, 3, 5, 7]$ and $\mathbf{D} = [1, 4, 6, 8]$, therefore MSB convolutional kernels would have receptive field of $[3 \times 3, 9 \times 9, 25 \times 25, 49 \times 49]$ over their input feature maps. Whereas, in the final level of the encoding path where feature maps are down-sampled by a factor of 8 and are in their smallest state, MSDU kernel sizes and dilation rates are to $\mathbf{K} = [3, 5, 3, 3]$ and $\mathbf{D} = [1, 1, 4, 6]$ resulting in receptive field sizes of $[3 \times 3, 5 \times 5, 9 \times 9, 13 \times 13]$ for MSB. This means that the convolutional kernels in our proposed MSDUs can extract relevant features starting from the scale of local structures size to the scale of nucleus size. We set the parameters of MSDUs heuristically based on the nuclei diameter analysis on the available data set.

## 2.2   Proposal-Free Instance Segmentation

**Segmentation and Centroid Detection.** For predicting mask and position of each nucleus, a dual-head network with similar architecture to SpaNet is utilized (see supplementary materials Fig. 1). One head predicts the mask of nuclei, and another head predicts the centroids. The ground truth for predicting the centroids is built by considering each nucleus as a Gaussian-Shaped function where the maximum of Gaussian occurs at the center of the nucleus. The function [6] for constructing GT for each nucleus centroid on images, $\mathbf{G}_n$, is:

$$\mathbf{G}_n(x, y) = \begin{cases} \frac{1}{1 + \beta \|(c_{nx}, c_{ny}) - (x, y)\|} & \text{if} \quad \|(c_{nx}, c_{ny}) - (x, y)\| \leq r \\ 0 & \text{elsewhere,} \end{cases} \quad (1)$$

where $(c_{nx}, c_{ny})$ and $(x, y)$ are the coordinate of nuclei centroid and all possible coordinates of image pixels, respectively. In our experimentation $\beta$ and $r$ are, 0.01 and 8 respectively. Input to this network is RGB image, and we used smooth Jaccard and mean squared loss functions to minimize error for predicting mask and detection map respectively.

**Instance Segmentation.** An important part of instance segmentation is providing a GT that can reflect the separation between nuclei. To this end, we propose to use a GT tensor, $\mathbf{P}_{h \times w \times 6}$, that encompasses spatial information of all nuclei in the image. In $\mathbf{P}$, all pixels related to the $n^{\text{th}}$ nucleus, are assigned with the same feature vector of spatial information, $p_n$. This vector is in the form of [9]: $p_n = (c_{nx}/w, c_{ny}/h, l_{nx}/w, l_{ny}/h, r_{nx}/w, r_{ny}/h)$, where $(c_{nx}, c_{ny})$, $(l_{nx}, l_{ny})$, and $(r_{nx}, r_{ny})$ are the coordinates of the center, left top, and bottom right of the $n^{\text{th}}$ nucleus' bounding box, respectively. All the values are normalized by the width and height of bounding box, $(w, h)$. A smoothed $L_1$ objective function that also ignores the background region in loss computation has been incorporated for the network optimization [9]. It is expected that the network predicts similar values for pixels belonging to the same nucleus. Note that the input to SpaNet for predicting nuclei spatial information has nine channels. The first six are made by concatenating RGB and HSV color channels, since nuclei are sometimes more distinguishable in HSV color space. The remaining 3 channels are, predicted segmentation map (achieved in the previous step), $\mathbf{M}_{seg}$, and spatial coordinate maps of pixels, $(\mathbf{M}_x, \mathbf{M}_y)$. These last three channels inject the positional information to the SpaNet.

**Post-processing.** After predicting the spatial information of nuclei instances via SpaNet, we cluster them to attain the final instance segmentation. Directly clustering the predicted maps might fail due to the large spatial domain (number of pixels) and a high number of nuclei (number of clusters) in them. Therefore, we propose to apply the clustering algorithm on nuclei clumps separately. To identify these clumps, we firstly use a threshold the segmentation maps (Sect. 2.2) with a value of 0.3 and remove objects with an area smaller than 5 pixels to generate the nuclei masks. Connected components (CC) in the generated mask indicate isolated nuclei or nuclei clumps. By estimating the number of candidate nuclei (clusters) in a CC, we can start the clustering procedure. The number of clusters per CC is determined by counting the number of local maxima in the intersection of that CC with the predicted detection map (Sect. 2.2). Similar to [9] we use spectral clustering algorithm for it's effectiveness compared to other models by selecting Radial Basis Function kernel (RBF) as the affinity function.

# 3    Results and Discussion

**Dataset.** The dataset consists of 30 images (16 for training and 14 for test set) from seven different tissues. Images were obtained from The Cancer Genome Atlas (TCGA) where $1000 \times 1000$ patches were extracted from Whole Slide Images (WSIs) [7]. These seven tissues are kidney, stomach, liver, bladder, colorectal, prostate, and liver. Out of 14 test images, eight belongs to the same tissue type as the training set (seen organs), and six images are from different tissue types (unseen organs). For more details regarding dataset and test/train split refer to [7].

**Networks Setup.** To attain generalization and robust predictions, we followed stochastic weight averaging approach proposed in [4]. Cycling learning rate $(\alpha_i)$ is adopted at each iteration $i$ as follows: $\alpha_i = (1 - t_i)\alpha_1 + t_i\alpha_2$, where $t_i = (\mod(i - 1, c) + 1)/c$, initial learning rate and final learning rate for each cycle are set to $\alpha_1 = 0.01$ and $\alpha_2 = 0.0001$, respectively, and cycling length is $c = 20$ epochs. Overall the network is trained for 100 epochs and the average of weights at the end of all cycles are computed for test time prediction.

All networks in the proposed framework have been trained using the same strategy, and "SGD" has been used as an optimizer to minimize objective

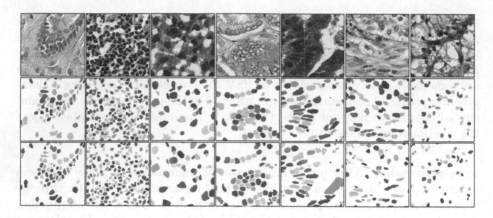

**Fig. 3.** Cropped images of seven different organs with their corresponding ground truth (second row) and prediction of our proposed method (third row).

**Table 1.** Results of different methods on the nuclei instance segmentation test sets.

| Method | AJI (%) | | F1-score (%) | |
|---|---|---|---|---|
| | Seen organ | Unseen organ | Seen organ | Unseen organ |
| CNN3 [7] | 51.54 | 49.89 | 82.26 | 83.22 |
| DR [11] | 55.91 | 56.01 | – | – |
| DCAN [1] | 60.82 | 54.49 | 82.65 | 82.14 |
| PA-Net [10] | 60.11 | 56.08 | 81.56 | 83.36 |
| Mask-RCNN [2] | 59.78 | 55.31 | 81.07 | 82.91 |
| BES-Net [12] | 59.06 | 58.23 | 81.18 | 79.52 |
| CIA-Net [15] | 61.29 | 63.06 | 82.44 | **84.58** |
| Spa-Net (ours) | **62.39** | **63.40** | **82.81** | 84.51 |

functions. The input patch size for all networks is $256 \times 256$. Networks for segmentation-detection and instance predictions are trained with a batch size of 2 and 4, respectively. Various data augmentation techniques were employed during the training of the network, their related details can be found in [5].

**Results and Comparative Analysis.** Performance of the proposed model is compared against several deep learning based methods as reported in Table 1. Except the baseline method (CNN3) [7] which categories the image pixels into three classes using a CNN-based classifier, other methods in Table 1 (DR-Net [11], DCAN [1], BES-Net [12], and CIA-Net [15]) took a dense prediction approach and used encoder-decoder like CNN.

As deduced from the results in Table 1, our proposed method based on SpaNet outperforms other state-of-the-art methods. Achieving AJI of 62.39% and F1-score of 82.81% shows an improvement of 1.10% for AJI and 0.37% for

F1-score metrics compared to the best performing method in the literature. The superiority of the proposed method performance can be observed in both seen and unseen organs. Figure 3 demonstrate the qualitative results of our method applied on all tissue types in test set.

The proposed framework offers several benefits. First, owing to the multi-scale and feature aggregation properties of MSDUs, using SpaNet architecture in this framework leads to more accurate instances' positional information. The performance of the current framework using off-the-shelf network architectures has also been shown in the supplementary material (see supplementary materials Figs. 5 and 6). Second, in our proposed framework, we used separate models for predicting positional information and nuclei detection. Based on our experiments, considering a single network for all tasks (see supplementary materials Fig. 3) results in performance drop (see supplementary materials Fig. 4). Third, our proposed model incorporates much less number of parameters ($\sim$21M) in comparison with other models ($\sim$31M for U-Net and $\sim$40M for CIA-Net); therefore it has a better chance to generalize on unseen data (see supplementary materials Fig. 6). This is an important behavior in the current application with such a small data set.

# 4    Conclusion

In this work, we presented a proposal-free framework for nuclear instance segmentation of histology images. Prediction of segmentation map, detection map, and spatial information of nuclei were aggregated in a principled manner to obtain final instance-level segmentation. To have a precise prediction, we proposed a spatial aware network which preserves the positional information throughout the network by incorporating a novel multi-scale dense unit. We showed that our method can achieve state-of-the-art performance on a multi-organ publicly available data set.

# References

1. Chen, H., Qi, X., Yu, L., Dou, Q., Qin, J., Heng, P.A.: Dcan: deep contour-aware networks for object instance segmentation from histology images. Med. Image Anal. **36**, 135–146 (2017)
2. He, K., Gkioxari, G., Dollár, P., Girshick, R.: Mask R-CNN. In: Proceedings of the IEEE International Conference on Computer Vision, pp. 2961–2969 (2017)
3. Huang, G., Liu, Z., Van Der Maaten, L., Weinberger, K.Q.: Densely connected convolutional networks. In: Proceedings of the IEEE Conference on Computer Vision and Pattern Recognition, pp. 4700–4708 (2017)
4. Izmailov, P., et al.: Averaging weights leads to wider optima and better generalization. arXiv preprint arXiv:1803.05407 (2018)
5. Jahanifar, M., Zamani Tajeddin, N., Alemi Koohbanani, N., Gooya, A., Rajpoot, N.: Segmentation of skin lesions and their attributes using multi-scale convolutional neural networks and domain specific augmentations. arXiv preprint arXiv:1809.10243 (2018)

6. Koohababni, N.A., Jahanifar, M., Gooya, A., Rajpoot, N.: Nuclei detection using mixture density networks. In: Shi, Y., Suk, H.-I., Liu, M. (eds.) MLMI 2018. LNCS, vol. 11046, pp. 241–248. Springer, Cham (2018). https://doi.org/10.1007/978-3-030-00919-9_28

7. Kumar, N., Verma, R., Sharma, S., Bhargava, S., Vahadane, A., Sethi, A.: A dataset and a technique for generalized nuclear segmentation for computational pathology. IEEE Trans. Med. Imaging **36**(7), 1550–1560 (2017)

8. Lee, G., Veltri, R.W., Zhu, G., Ali, S., Epstein, J.I., Madabhushi, A.: Nuclear shape and architecture in benign fields predict biochemical recurrence in prostate cancer patients following radical prostatectomy: preliminary findings. Eur. Urol. Focus **3**(4–5), 457–466 (2017)

9. Liang, X., Lin, L., Wei, Y., Shen, X., Yang, J., Yan, S.: Proposal-free network for instance-level object segmentation. IEEE Trans. Pattern Anal. Mach. Intell. **40**(12), 2978–2991 (2017)

10. Liu, S., Qi, L., Qin, H., Shi, J., Jia, J.: Path aggregation network for instance segmentation. In: Proceedings of the IEEE Conference on Computer Vision and Pattern Recognition, pp. 8759–8768 (2018)

11. Naylor, P., Laé, M., Reyal, F., Walter, T.: Segmentation of nuclei in histopathology images by deep regression of the distance map. IEEE Trans. Med. Imaging **38**(2), 448–459 (2018)

12. Oda, H., et al.: BESNet: boundary-enhanced segmentation of cells in histopathological images. In: Frangi, A.F., Schnabel, J.A., Davatzikos, C., Alberola-López, C., Fichtinger, G. (eds.) MICCAI 2018. LNCS, vol. 11071, pp. 228–236. Springer, Cham (2018). https://doi.org/10.1007/978-3-030-00934-2_26

13. Ronneberger, O., Fischer, P., Brox, T.: U-net: convolutional networks for biomedical image segmentation. In: Navab, N., Hornegger, J., Wells, W.M., Frangi, A.F. (eds.) MICCAI 2015. LNCS, vol. 9351, pp. 234–241. Springer, Cham (2015). https://doi.org/10.1007/978-3-319-24574-4_28

14. Vu, Q.D., et al.: Methods for segmentation and classification of digital microscopy tissue images. Front. Bioeng. Biotechnol. **7** (2019)

15. Zhou, Y., Onder, O.F., Dou, Q., Tsougenis, E., Chen, H., Heng, P.-A.: CIA-net: robust nuclei instance segmentation with contour-aware information aggregation. In: Chung, A.C.S., Gee, J.C., Yushkevich, P.A., Bao, S. (eds.) IPMI 2019. LNCS, vol. 11492, pp. 682–693. Springer, Cham (2019). https://doi.org/10.1007/978-3-030-20351-1_53

# GAN-Based Image Enrichment in Digital Pathology Boosts Segmentation Accuracy

Laxmi Gupta[1]([✉]), Barbara M. Klinkhammer[2], Peter Boor[2], Dorit Merhof[1], and Michael Gadermayr[1,3]

[1] Institute of Imaging & Computer Vision, RWTH Aachen University, Aachen, Germany
laxmi.gupta@lfb.rwth-aachen.de
[2] Institute of Pathology, University Hospital Aachen, RWTH Aachen University, Aachen, Germany
[3] Salzburg University of Applied Sciences, Salzburg, Austria

**Abstract.** We introduce the idea of 'image enrichment' whereby the information content of images is increased in order to enhance segmentation accuracy. Unlike in data augmentation, the focus is not on increasing the number of training samples (by adding new virtual samples), but on increasing the information for each sample. For this purpose, we use a GAN-based image-to-image translation approach to generate corresponding virtual samples from a given (original) image. The virtual samples are then merged with the original sample to create a multichannel image, which serves as the enriched image. We train and test a segmentation network on enriched images showing kidney pathology and obtain segmentation scores exhibiting an improvement compared to conventional processing of the original images only. We perform an extensive evaluation and discuss the reasons for the improvement.

**Keywords:** Histology · Kidney · Augmentation · Enrichment · Sensor fusion · Segmentation · Adversarial networks

## 1 Motivation

Data augmentation has become common knowledge and exhibits an indispensable method to boost the performance of state-of-the-art machine learning approaches, especially if the amount of training samples is relatively small. While data augmentation typically refers to increasing the number of samples, we introduce image enrichment for increasing the information content for every individual sample. An application, for example, is given by medical image fusion [5], where the information of one image (e.g. CT) is enriched by information obtained from another image showing the same underlying structure, but using a different imaging modality (e.g. MRI). The additional information obtained by merging the images either facilitates medical diagnosis or exhibits the basis for further computer-aided decision support systems.

© Springer Nature Switzerland AG 2019
D. Shen et al. (Eds.): MICCAI 2019, LNCS 11764, pp. 631–639, 2019.
https://doi.org/10.1007/978-3-030-32239-7_70

While in specific fields multi-modal image data is available and indispensable for reliable diagnosis, in many other areas we (need to) deal with single images and mostly do not even think about adding data from a different domain. However, recent achievements in deep-learning facilitate translations between different imaging modalities, e.g. between CT and MRI scans [8]. A conversion is obtained by the so-called image-to-image translation approaches, showing attractive and realistic output [4,9]. A specific generative adversarial network (GAN) architecture also enables translation without the need for any corresponding pairs to train the networks [9]. The proposed GANs rely on cyclic loss functions which are combined with the GAN loss. The cyclic loss ensures that after circular translations (e.g. from a domain A to a domain B and back to domain A) the final images are similar to the input image. The GAN loss ensures that the output images look real. As image pairs often cannot be obtained (or are at least difficult and/or expensive to achieve), this architecture, allowing unpaired training, opens up entirely new opportunities for the field of medical image analysis.

In the field of digital pathology, GANs can also be used for image normalization [1,3] and for domain adaptation [2]. The authors of [2] considered a scenario, where labeled samples are only available in a source stain and not in the target stain, and performed domain adaptation on image-level using image-to-image translation. They concluded that GANs can be applied to create realistic fake images showing a stain different from the input stain. They showed that the fake images can be effectively used for segmentation in a domain adaptation scenario but noticed that the direction of translation makes a clear difference. A translation to one specific stain showed higher segmentation scores than to others. They assume that certain stains are easy to segment while others more difficult. To obtain optimum results, they suggest to translate to the stain which is easier to segment (either source or target stain) before segmentation.

## Contribution

With the outlook of improving segmentation accuracy, we propose a method called 'image enrichment', whereby the information content within each sample is increased. We consider a scenario where labeled images (training and testing images) are available for a single stain only. Unlike in recent work [2], we do not consider a domain change scenario, but focus on the segmentation of samples showing the same stain as the training data. We perform image-to-image translation to generate virtual images showing stains different from the input sample. The corresponding virtual images are merged with the original samples and further utilized for training and testing the segmentation network. In an experimental study on kidney pathology data, we show that this approach is capable of increasing the segmentation accuracy and discuss the underlying causes. Related work [7] presents a similar generator-to-classifier network that jointly optimizes stain-translation and classification. In contrast, we investigate an approach based on two individual networks and focus on a segmentation task. Our two step approach allows higher flexibility at the time of application.

## 2    Methods

We consider a domain of labeled images, denoted as $S_0$, referring to one specific stain, and further domains $S_1$, ... , $S_n$ of images, each showing a specific stain different from $S_0$. For the domains $S_1$, ... , $S_n$, no labels are available. There is also no need for any corresponding image pairs. The only restriction is that all sets show similar underlying tissue (e.g. kidney tissue).

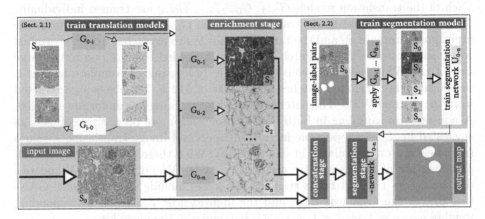

**Fig. 1.** Outline of the proposed segmentation pipeline: for an image to be segmented (input image), first corresponding virtual images are created (enrichment stage) and concatenated (concatenation stage). Finally, the resulting multi-channel image is segmented using a segmentation network (segmentation stage). The image translation and segmentation models are trained individually.

We propose a segmentation pipeline consisting of an enrichment, a concatenation, and a segmentation stage, as shown in Fig. 1. An input image of domain $S_0$ to be segmented is first passed to the enrichment stage. In this phase, several generators $G_{0-1}$, $G_{0-2}$, ... , $G_{0-n}$ are applied to the input image in order to generate a virtual sample for each of the domains $S_1$ to $S_n$. The networks $G_{0-i}$ are trained beforehand in an unpaired manner using a cycle-consistency GAN. Next, the input image is concatenated with all the virtual images generated from it. The resulting domain is referred to as $S_{0,1,...,n}$, in the following also as $S_{All}$. Supposing that the original and the $n$ virtual images consist of $M \times N$ pixels and $C$ color channels, we obtain multi-channel images exhibiting a dimensionality of $M \times N \times (C \cdot (n + 1))$. Finally, the multi-channel images so obtained are fed to a fully-convolutional network for segmentation. The rationale behind this approach is that image translation in histology effectively generates highly realistic images [2]. Here, we assess if the additional information, available from a set of different histological stains, is helpful to support the final network to learn the segmentation task. Each trained generator ($G_{0-i} : S_0 \rightarrow S_i$) is only based on the input image and does not incorporate any further information when creating virtual samples. However, additional information is created due to the learned ability of the generator to convert between the different domains. It can be argued that segmentation should be independent of the modality because the underlying image content in all the domains is the same. Nevertheless, it was shown that the domain in which segmentation is performed does influence the accuracy [2].

## 2.1  Image Translation Model

Each of the translation models $G_{0-1}$, $G_{0-2}$, ... , $G_{0-n}$ are trained individually. To train an individual image translation model $G_{0-i}$, firstly, patches from the input image domain $S_0$ and the target domain $S_i$ are extracted from the original whole slide images (WSIs). Patch extraction is needed because due to the large size of the WSIs (few gigapixels), a holistic processing of complete images is not feasible. For training, patches with a size of $512 \times 512$ pixels are extracted from the original WSIs. The patches utilized for training are uniformly sampled. A non-uniform sampling in both domains focusing more on positive objects as suggested in [2] is not possible in this unsupervised image translation scenario (as labels are only available in one domain). With these patches, a cycleGAN [9] consisting of two generative models, $F : \mathcal{X} \to \mathcal{Y}$ and $G : \mathcal{Y} \to \mathcal{X}$ and two discriminators $D_X$ and $D_Y$ is trained. The losses include the established GAN-loss $\mathcal{L}_{GAN}$, the cycle-loss $\mathcal{L}_{cyc}$, and the identity loss $\mathcal{L}_{id}$ (with corresponding weights $w_{GAN} = 1, w_{cyc} = 1, w_{id} = 1$). Particularly, the cycle-loss

$$\mathcal{L}_{cyc} = \mathbb{E}_{x \sim p_{data}(x)}[||G(F(x)) - x||_1] + \mathbb{E}_{y \sim p_{data}(y)}[||F(G(y)) - y||_1] , \quad (1)$$

forces the generator to maintain the image content without requiring paired samples. The identity-loss is applied to stabilize the training process as suggested in [9]. For training, standard data augmentation (rotation, flipping) is applied. Apart from a U-Net generator network [6], the standard configuration based on the patch-wise CNN discriminator is used [9][1]. Initial learning rate is set to 0.0002. Adam optimizer is used.

## 2.2  Segmentation Model

For segmentation, we rely on an established fully-convolutional network architecture, specifically the so-called U-Net [6] which was successfully applied for segmenting kidney pathology [2]. For taking the distribution of objects into account (the glomeruli are small, sparse objects covering only approximately 2% of the renal tissue area) training patches ($512 \times 512$ pixels) are not randomly extracted. Instead, as suggested in [2], 50% of the patches are extracted from regions containing objects (to obtain class balance) whereas the other 50% are randomly extracted (to include regions far away from the objects-of-interest). Batch-size is set to one and L2-normalization is applied. Due to the very low within-stain variability in the data set, there is no need to apply stain-normalization. Standard data augmentation (rotation, flipping) is applied. Initial learning rate is set to 0.001, and Adam optimizer is used.

---

[1] We use the PyTorch reference implementation [9].

# 3 Image Data and Experimental Settings

We investigate WSIs showing tissue of mouse kidney. The images are captured with the whole slide scanner model C9600-12, by Hamamatsu with a 40× objective lens. The overall data set comprises: 23× periodic acid Schiff (PAS), 12× Acid Fuchsin Orange G (AFOG), 12× cluster-of-differentiation (CD31) stained WSIs, and 12× images dyed with a stain focused on highlighting Collagen III (Col3).

As suggested in [2], we perform both, segmentation and image translation, on the second highest resolution (20× magnification). We consider a scenario where manually annotated PAS stained WSIs are available for training a supervised segmentation model. Therefore, PAS is considered as the $S_0$ domain. Consequently, we refer to CD31 as $S_1$, AFOG as $S_2$, and Col3 as $S_3$. Eleven of the PAS images and all of the CD31, AFOG, and Col3 images are used for training the translation model, where the three latter stains are employed for image enrichment. We train the segmentation model on patches extracted from the WSIs (400 from each WSI). However, to avoid any bias, the training and testing data is separated on WSI level. For this purpose, we randomly select ten WSIs for training and two for testing. This procedure is repeated 12 times.

# 4 Evaluation Metrics

We compute precision, recall and the Dice similarity coefficient (DSC) individually for each of 12 repetitions. We investigate the baseline setting with the original PAS images ($S_0$) and the proposed method using additionally all the virtual stains ($S_{All}$). To gain further insight, we also evaluate combinations of the PAS domain with single virtual domains ($S_{0,1}$, $S_{0,2}$, $S_{0,3}$) and also individual virtual domains without any real data ($S_1$, $S_2$, $S_3$). Two setups are investigated.

## Setup 1

Evaluation is performed for (a) randomly sampled patches representing the DSC on WSI level, and (b) patches containing (at least one pixel of) one or more objects. The latter is motivated by the fact that large regions do not contain any objects and can be easily manually "excluded".

## Setup 2

In this setting, we incorporate the fact that small objects (specifically objects with an area below 5,000 pixels) are not relevant for further analysis. These small objects occur in 2D images if a 3D glomerulus is cut marginally (i.e. the cut is close to the object's border). As it is difficult to determine the exact size during manual annotation, these objects are partly labeled in the ground truth. Consequently, we additionally compute the DSC as follows. If a small object (area < 5000 pixels) is detected but not labeled in the ground truth, it is ignored when calculating the measures (precision, recall, DSC). If a small object is marked in the ground-truth and not detected, it is also ignored.

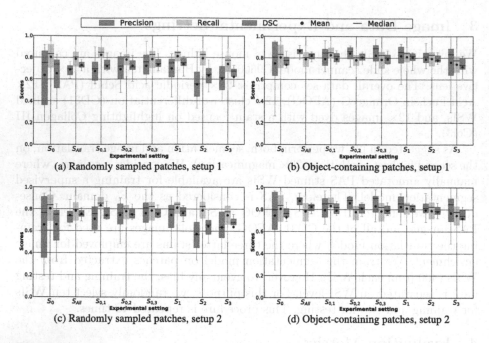

(a) Randomly sampled patches, setup 1

(b) Object-containing patches, setup 1

(c) Randomly sampled patches, setup 2

(d) Object-containing patches, setup 2

**Fig. 2.** Segmentation scores (precision, recall, DSCs) shown individually for the baseline method ($S_0$), the proposed method ($S_{All}$), the concatenation of original images with a single virtual image ($S_{0,1}$, $S_{0,2}$, $S_{0,3}$), and the individual virtual images ($S_1$, $S_2$, $S_3$). The subfigures correspond to the evaluation settings Setup 1 and Setup 2.

## 5   Results

Figure 2 shows the experimental results. The subfigures correspond to the four evaluation methods (a)–(d) explained above. Results are shown for the baseline performing segmentation on original PAS images ($S_0$), the proposed method incorporating all the available stains ($S_{All}$), combinations of real PAS and one virtual stain, and individual virtual stains. In all the four subfigures, the proposed method $S_{All}$ shows higher mean DSCs ((a): 0.73 vs. 0.65, (b): 0.82 vs. 0.74, (c): 0.75 vs. 0.66, (d): 0.82 vs 0.73) and lower standard deviations, as compared to the baseline approach $S_0$. Especially precision is increased on average while the standard deviation in clearly reduced. A similar trend is observed for the other test settings, namely $S_{0,1}$, $S_{0,2}$, and $S_{0,3}$, also showing improvements compared to $S_0$ and reaching scores similar to $S_{All}$. Regarding the settings based on a single virtual stain only, we observe divergent scores. $S_2$ and $S_3$ show partly degraded performance in case of randomly samples patches. Setting $S_1$ shows segmentation scores similar to $S_{All}$ and clearly higher than the baseline $S_0$. It is noteworthy that precision (and hence DSC) increases when we consider only object-containing patches (Fig. 2(b)). The difference is especially relevant for the settings $S_1$, $S_2$, and $S_3$. Setup 1 and setup 2 show similar trends. In Fig. 3, we see examples of the segmentation outputs for the baseline and the proposed setting in comparison with the ground truth. Figure 4 shows qualitative results of the image translation process. We do not notice any systematic differences between virtual and real images. The virtual patches also show a high correspondence (i.e. the object outlines do not change) to the real images.

# 6    Discussion

With the help of unpaired image-to-image translation, we propose a method which solves a segmentation task in two steps. In the first step the image data is enriched and in the second step, the available data is fed into a specifically trained segmentation network. Summarizing the results, we notice two core findings. Firstly, the proposed method including all available virtual stains ($S_{All}$) exhibits improved scores for all evaluation settings compared to the straight-forward segmentation of $S_0$ (PAS) images. Also experiments with subsets using only $S_0$ and one single virtual stain consistently show improved (mean) DSCs. Secondly, we notice that especially one virtual stain, namely $S_1$, exhibits scores similar to the setting $S_{All}$ with all information merged. Highly interestingly, the virtual domain $S_1$ is obviously even "easier" to segment than the original domain $S_0$. Based on these two findings, we summarize that image enrichment based on image-to-image translation can actually improve the segmentability of images. In other words, solving segmentation in two steps can be more accurate than performing a segmentation in a single step. We explain this as follows: for the first step, we train a network to perform a task on a rather low level. To perform image translation in histology, details are more important than large contextual information. In the second step, large context is required to decide if a potential object is a real object or a similar artifact. We hypothesize that two networks, individually specialized and trained for different sub-problems, are more powerful than one single network applied to one, but more difficult task. However, this requires that an appropriate intermediate domain (in our case, an appropriate histological stain) exists.

Regarding the segmentation of single (virtual or real) and combined domains, we summarize that a single highly powerful domain ($S_1$) is sufficient in our setting to show superior results. A fusion with further virtual or real stains does not show any further improvements. Interestingly, we find that the virtual domains show decreased standard deviations which is highly likely due to the lower variability within the virtual stains compared to the real PAS stain. This might be due to a naturally low variability of the histological stains (considered as virtual stains) or due to a normalizing effect of the generator network. Even though the slides have a homogeneous appearance in terms of color, we do observe intra-slide variations in texture. Another positive effect could also be introduced by the generator network which might be able to compensate for degradations in the image domain. For example, the network might remove minor artifacts and thereby generate optimized virtual domains. However, we did not notice such cases and it can also be argued that the generator is not optimized to remove artifacts, but rather to produce samples similar to those drawn from the original distribution. In order to clearly separate the effect of the individual properties of the underlying histological stain and the potentially normalizing effect of the generator network, further experiments need to be performed in the future. This requires large amounts of annotated samples for each of the stains used as virtual stains as well, for supervisedly training the segmentation network.

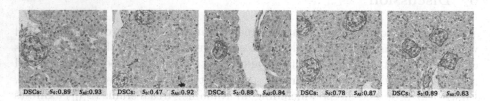

**Fig. 3.** Qualitative Results of the segmentation process: Red and blue show the segmentation outputs of the approaches based on $S_0$ and $S_{All}$, respectively. Green shows the ground truth. To improve visibility, we show two approaches only and provide an overlay with gray-scale images. (Color figure online)

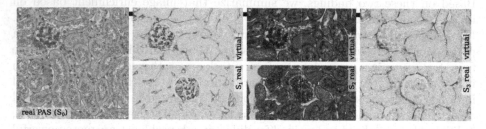

**Fig. 4.** Example images showing a real $S_0$ (PAS) patch, corresponding virtual images (top row) and similar real images (bottom row) for comparison. While the virtual images correspond to the real patch, the real ones surely do not.

To conclude, we propose the idea of image enrichment, which exploits the fact that image-to-image translation based on unpaired training can be used to improve segmentation accuracy. In a two-step approach, we firstly enrich, i.e. boost the information content on the available data using unpaired image-to-image translation, and secondly, train a segmentation network which benefits from this enriched data. We tested segmentation performance on a given stain by enriching it with three additional stains and obtained improved segmentation scores. Even with a specific single virtual stain, we achieved improved scores, similar to the DSCs obtained when merging all available data. This is expected to be due to the fact that specific histological stains are more appropriate for subsequent segmentation. Secondly, the generator might be able to improve average image quality by reducing variability (and artifacts) in the image domain. Noticing generally lower standard deviations for the virtual stains and stain specific differences, we strongly assume that both effects play a vital role. To provide a clear answer, further experiments based on additional labeled training data will be performed in the future.

**Acknowledgment.** This work was supported by the German Research Foundation (DFG) under grant no. ME3737/3-1.

# References

1. Bentaieb, A., Hamarneh, G.: Adversarial stain transfer for histopathology image analysis. IEEE Trans. Med. Imaging **37**(3), 792–802 (2018)
2. Gadermayr, M., Appel, V., Klinkhammer, B.M., Boor, P., Merhof, D.: Which way round? A study on the performance of stain-translation for segmenting arbitrarily dyed histological images. In: Frangi, A.F., Schnabel, J.A., Davatzikos, C., Alberola-López, C., Fichtinger, G. (eds.) MICCAI 2018. LNCS, vol. 11071, pp. 165–173. Springer, Cham (2018). https://doi.org/10.1007/978-3-030-00934-2_19
3. Zanjani, F.G., Zinger, S., de With, P.H.N., Bejnordi, B.E., van der Laak, J.A.W.M.: Histopathology stain-color normalization using deep generative models. In: Proceedings of the Conference on Medical Imaging with Deep Learning, MIDL 2018, pp. 1–11 (2018)
4. Isola, P., Zhu, J.Y., Zhou, T., Efros, A.A.: Image-to-image translation with conditional adversarial networks. In: Proceedings of the International Conference on Computer Vision and Pattern Recognition, CVPR 2017 (2017)
5. James, A.P., Dasarathy, B.V.: Medical image fusion: a survey of the state of the art. Inf. Fusion **19**, 4–19 (2014)
6. Ronneberger, O., Fischer, P., Brox, T.: U-Net: convolutional networks for biomedical image segmentation. In: Navab, N., Hornegger, J., Wells, W.M., Frangi, A.F. (eds.) MICCAI 2015. LNCS, vol. 9351, pp. 234–241. Springer, Cham (2015). https://doi.org/10.1007/978-3-319-24574-4_28
7. Wu, B., et al.: G2C: a generator-to-classifier framework integrating multi-stained visual cues for pathological glomerulus classification. ArXiv abs/1807.03136 (2019)
8. Zhao, Y., et al.: Towards MR-only radiotherapy treatment planning: synthetic CT generation using multi-view deep convolutional neural networks. In: Frangi, A.F., Schnabel, J.A., Davatzikos, C., Alberola-López, C., Fichtinger, G. (eds.) MICCAI 2018. LNCS, vol. 11070, pp. 286–294. Springer, Cham (2018). https://doi.org/10.1007/978-3-030-00928-1_33
9. Zhu, J.Y., Park, T., Isola, P., Efros, A.A.: Unpaired image-to-image translation using cycle-consistent adversarial networks. In: Proceedings of the International Conference on Computer Vision, ICCV 2017 (2017)

# IRNet: Instance Relation Network for Overlapping Cervical Cell Segmentation

Yanning Zhou[1], Hao Chen[2(✉)], Jiaqi Xu[1], Qi Dou[3], and Pheng-Ann Heng[1,4]

[1] Department of Computer Science and Engineering,
The Chinese University of Hong Kong, Hong Kong SAR, China
{ynzhou,hchen}@cse.cuhk.edu.hk
[2] Imsight Medical Technology, Co., Ltd., Hong Kong SAR, China
[3] Department of Computing, Imperial College London, London, UK
[4] Guangdong Provincial Key Laboratory of Computer Vision and Virtual Reality
Technology, Shenzhen Institutes of Advanced Technology,
Chinese Academy of Sciences, Shenzhen, China

**Abstract.** Cell instance segmentation in Pap smear image remains challenging due to the wide existence of occlusion among translucent cytoplasm in cell clumps. Conventional methods heavily rely on accurate nuclei detection results and are easily disturbed by miscellaneous objects. In this paper, we propose a novel Instance Relation Network (IRNet) for robust overlapping cell segmentation by exploring instance relation interaction. Specifically, we propose the Instance Relation Module to construct the cell association matrix for transferring information among individual cell-instance features. With the collaboration of different instances, the augmented features gain benefits from contextual information and improve semantic consistency. Meanwhile, we proposed a sparsity constrained Duplicate Removal Module to eliminate the misalignment between classification and localization accuracy for candidates selection. The largest cervical Pap smear (CPS) dataset with more than 8000 cell annotations in Pap smear image was constructed for comprehensive evaluation. Our method outperforms other methods by a large margin, demonstrating the effectiveness of exploring instance relation.

## 1 Introduction

Pap smear test is extensively used in cervical cancer screening to assist premalignant and malignant grading [11]. By estimating the shape and morphology structure, e.g., nuclei to cytoplasm ratio, cytologists can give a preliminary diagnosis and facilitate the subsequent treatment. Given that this work is time-consuming and has large intra-/inter-observer variability, designing automatic cell detection and segmentation methods is a promising way towards accurate, objective and efficient diagnosis. However, it remains challenging because the multiple layers of cells partially occlude each other in the Pap smear image, while in H&E image cells do not have multiple layers of translucent overlap. The widely existence of cell clumps along with the translucent cytoplasm raises obstacles to accurately

© Springer Nature Switzerland AG 2019
D. Shen et al. (Eds.): MICCAI 2019, LNCS 11764, pp. 640–648, 2019.
https://doi.org/10.1007/978-3-030-32239-7_71

find the cell boundary. In addition, apart from the target cervical cells, other miscellaneous instances such as white blood cells, mucus and other artifacts are also scattered in the image, which requires an algorithm robust enough to identify them from targets.

Previously, most of the overlapping cell segmentation methods in Pap smear image utilize the shape and intensity information and can be divided into the following steps: cell clump segmentation, nuclei detection and cytoplasm boundary refinement [3,10,13]. However, they demand the precise nuclei detection results as the seeds for the further cytoplasm partition and refinement, which is easily disturbed by the mucus, blood and other miscellaneous instances in clinical diagnosis. Many deep learning based methods have been proposed for gland/nuclei instance segmentation tasks [2,7,12]. Raza et al. proposed Micro-Net for general segmentation task and achieved good results for cell, nuclei and gland segmentation [12]. But it cannot tackle overlapping instances where one pixel could be assigned to multiple instance IDs. On the other hand, the proposal based method can assign multiple labels to a single pixel, which has shown promising results in general object segmentation task. [4] firstly extended the detection method with a segmentation head for instance segmentation, [9] proposed a powerful feature aggregation network backbone. Akram et al. presented the CSPNet consisting of two sub-nets for proposal generation and segmentation nuclei respectively in microscopic image [1]. However, in the Pap smear image, directly extracting in-box features from cell clumps for further processing is not informative enough to distinguish the foreground/background cytoplasm fragment. Meanwhile, the large appearance variance between the single cell and clumps make features semantically inconsistent, which eventually leads to the ambiguous boundary prediction. Besides, it is easy for greedy Non-Maximum Suppression (NMS) to reject true positive predictions in heavy cluster regions due to the misalignment between classification and localization accuracy. Motivated by clinical observation that the appearance of each independent cervical cell in Pap smear image has strong similarity, it shows the potential of leveraging relation information which has been shown effectiveness in other tasks [5,6,14] for better feature representation. For the first time we introduce relation interaction to instance segmentation task and present the Instance Relation Network (IRNet) for overlapping cervical cell segmentation. A novel Instance Relation Module (IRM) is introduced which computes the class-specific instance association for feature refinement. By transferring information among instances using self-attention mechanism, the augmented feature takes merit of contextual information and increase semantic consistency. We also proposed the Duplicate Removal Module (DRM) with the sparsity constraint to benefit proposal selection by calibrating the misalignment between classification score and localization accuracy. To the best of our knowledge, the IRNet is the first end-to-end deep learning method for overlapping cell segmentation in Pap smear image.

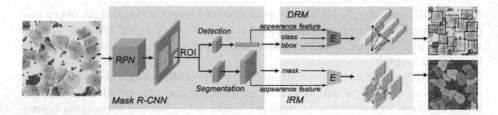

**Fig. 1.** Overview of the proposed IRNet.

# 2 Method

As shown in Fig. 1, the proposed IRNet conforms to the two-stage proposal based instance segmentation paradigm [4]. The input image is firstly fed into the Region Proposal Network (RPN) to generate object candidates. Then the candidate features are extracted by the RoIAlign layer [4] and passed through two branches for detection and segmentation. To strengthen the network's ability of candidate selection in cell clumps and improve the semantic consistency among in-box features, we leverage the contextual information among different cells by adding Duplicate Removal Module (DRM) and Instance Relation Module (IRM) after detection and segmentation head.

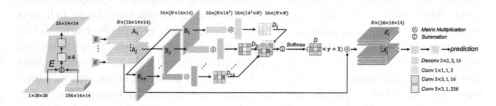

**Fig. 2.** Detail structure of the Instance Relation Module in IRNet.

## 2.1 Instance Relation Module

Utilizing in-box features to generate each mask independently is susceptible for cell clumps due to the low foreground contrast and the overlapping boundaries, which eventually leads to ambiguous predictions. Directly enlarging the anchor size to add context won't help a lot in the overlapping region since the surroundings are cells with low contrast. Given that nuclei share the strong appearance similarity so as the cells (shape, texture), we hypothesize that utilizing contextual information from other instance as guidance can increase semantic consistency, especially from those well-differentiated cells. Therefore, we propose the Instance Relation Module (IRM) to exploit the collaborative interaction of instances. Generally speaking, the IRM takes embedded features from each instance to calculate the instance association matrix, then parses message among features according to their instance relations.

Specifically, the encoder (denotes as $\mathbf{E}$ in Fig. 2) takes the combination of the predicted mask and deep features as the input to generate the fused features for each candidate. Let $n$ denotes the number of instances in the image, the self-attention mechanism [14]is used to build the association among $n$ instances. As can be seen in Fig. 2, the IRM firstly aggregated the fused features in channel-wise to construct 16 features, denoted as $B_j$, $j = 1, 2 \ldots 16$, with the shape of $n \times 14 \times 14$. For each $B_j$, it is reshaped to $\mathbb{R}^{c \times hw}$ and multiplied with its transpose matrix to calculate the channel-wise instance associations, $D_j = B_j B_j^T$. The overall instance association matrix is finally obtained by averaging among all the channel-wise association matrices followed by a Softmax layer for normalization, $D = Softmax(avg(D_1, D_2 \ldots D_c))$. Therefore, the impact of the $q$-th instance to the $p$-th instance is computed as $w_{pq} = \frac{exp(d_{pq})}{\sum_k exp(d_{pk})}$, where $d_{pq}$ represents the $p$-th row, $q$-th column entry. Let $A_p$ and $A_q$ denotes the $p$-th and the $q$-th instance features, $A_p'$ denotes the $p$-th instance features after relation interaction, the message parsing process can be formulated as:

$$A_p' = \gamma \sum_{q=1}^{n} w_{pq} A_q + A_p, \tag{1}$$

where $\gamma$ denotes a learnable scalar factor.

By associating with all the instances, the augmented feature takes merit of contextual information from other instance areas to increase semantic consistency. It is then passed through one $2 \times 2$ deconvolution layer with a stride of two, followed by a convolution layer serving as the classifier to output the predicted masks. During training, the Binary Cross-Entropy (BCE) loss is calculated on the ground truth class of masks ($\mathcal{L}_{IRM}$).

## 2.2   Sparsity Regularized Duplicate Removal Module

Directly utilizing objectness score for NMS leads to sub-optimal results due to the misalignment between classification and localization accuracy, which is more severe for proposals in cell clumps. To calibrate the misalignment, [5] proposed the Duplicate Removal Module (DRM) which takes appearance and location features as input and then utilizes transformed features after relation interaction to directly predict the proposal be *correct* or the *duplicate* using BCE loss ($\mathcal{L}_{DRM}$). The motivation for adding DRM is that the cells and corresponding nuclei have highly correlated spatial distribution.

Based on the observation that cells in Pap smear image gather in several local small clusters instead of one large clump, we propose to add a sparsity constraint on DRM to let the module focus on interaction among the subset of proposals. Specifically, for each target, it only takes proposals with relation weight ranked in the top $k$ for message parsing, where we set $k = 40$ in the experiments. Meanwhile, instead of directly utilizing predicted probability for duplicate removal, we use the multiplication of classification score and predicted probability for NMS to give a hard constraint of overlapping ratio. Notice that the DRM also exploits the relation information. The proposed IRM is significantly different to adapt to instance segmentation by utilizing a fully convolutional encoder to combine features and predicted masks which effectively preserves the location information and strengthens the effort of shape information.

### 2.3  Overall Loss Function and Optimization

A multi-task loss is defined as $\mathcal{L} = \mathcal{L}_{cls} + \mathcal{L}_{reg} + \mathcal{L}_{seg} + \alpha\mathcal{L}_{DRM} + \beta\mathcal{L}_{IRM}$, where $\mathcal{L}_{cls}$ and $\mathcal{L}_{reg}$ denote the BCE loss and smooth L1 loss for classification and regression in detection head, and $\mathcal{L}_{seg}$ denotes pixel-wise BCE loss in segmentation head, which are identical as those defined in [4]. $\mathcal{L}_{DRM}$ denotes the BCE loss for *correct* or *duplicate* classification in DRM, where we define the *correct* as the predicted bounding box with the maximum Intersection over Union to the corresponded grounding truth, while others are *duplicate*. $L_{IRM}$ is the pixel-wise BCE loss for refined masks after IRM. $\alpha$ and $\beta$ are hyper-parameters term for balancing loss weights.

## 3    Experiments and Results

**Dataset and Evaluation Metrics.** The liquid-based Pap test specimen was collected from 82 patients to build the CPS dataset. The specimen was imaged in $\times 40$ objective to give the image resolution of around 0.2529 μm per pixel. Then they were cropped into 413 images with the resolution of $1000 \times 1000$. In all, 4439 cytoplasm and 4789 nuclei were annotated by the cytologist. To the best of our knowledge, there is no public cervical cell dataset with the annotations on the same order of magnitude to the CPS dataset. To evaluate the proposed method, we split the dataset in patient-level with the ratio of 7:1:2 into the train, valid and test set.

For quantitative evaluation, Average Jaccard Index (AJI) is used which considers in both pixel and object level [7]. AJI= $\frac{\sum_{i=1}^{n} G_i \bigcap S_j}{\sum_{i=1}^{n} G_i \bigcup S_j + \sum_{k \in N} S_k}$ , where $G_i$ is the $i$-th ground truth, $S_j$ is the $j$-th prediction, $j = \text{argmax}_k \frac{G_i \bigcap S_k}{G_i \bigcup S_k}$. It measures the ratio of the aggregated intersection and aggregated union for all the predictions and ground truths in the image. F1-score (F1) is used to measure the detection accuracy for reference [2].

**Implementation Details.** We implemented the proposed IRNet with PyTorch 1.0. The network architecture is the same as [8] in the condition of Feature Pyramid Network with 50-layer ResNet (ResNet-50-FPN). One NVIDIA TITIAN Xp graphic card with CUDA 9.0 and cuDNN 6.0 was used for the computation. During training, we used SGD with 0.9 momentum as the optimizer. The initial learning rate was set as 0.0025 with a factor of 2 for the bias, while the weight decay was set 0.0001. We linear warmed up the learning rate in the first 500 iterations with a warm-up factor of $\frac{1}{3}$.

**Effectiveness of the Proposed IRNet.** Firstly, we conducted experiments to compare different algorithms for overlapping cell segmentation. (1). *JOMLS* [10]: an improved joint optimization of multiple level set functions for the segmentation of cytoplasm and nuclei from clumps of overlapping cervical cells. (2). *CSPNet* [1]: a cell segmentation proposal network with two CNNs for cell proposal prediction and cell mask segmentation respectively. To give a fair comparison, we reproduce the ResNet-50-FPN instead of the original 6-layer CNN for candidates prediction in the first stage. (3). *Mask R-CNN* [4]: IRNet without Duplicate Removal Module and Instance Relation Module, which can be considered as a standard mask-rcnn structure with ResNet-50-FPN as the backbone. (4). *IRNet w/o IRM*: IRNet without Instance Relation Module. (5). *IRNet w/o DRM*: IRNet without Duplicate Removal Module. (6). *IRNet*: The proposed IRNet.

**Table 1.** Quantitative comparison against other methods on the test set.

| Method | AJI | | F1 | |
|---|---|---|---|---|
| | Cyto | Nuclei | Cyto | Nuclei |
| JOMLS [10] | 0.1974 | 0.3167 | 0.3794 | 0.3618 |
| CSPNet [1] | 0.4607 | 0.3891 | 0.5307 | 0.5942 |
| Mask R-CNN [4] | 0.6845 | 0.5169 | 0.6664 | 0.7192 |
| IRNet w/o IRM | 0.6887 | 0.5342 | 0.7266 | 0.7424 |
| IRNet w/o DRM | 0.6995 | 0.5471 | 0.7010 | 0.7501 |
| IRNet | **0.7185** | **0.5496** | **0.7497** | **0.7554** |

As can be seen in Table 1, all the deep learning based methods achieve better performance compared with the level-set based method [10]. The reason is that our dataset has more complicated background information including white blood cells and other miscellaneous instances compared with that used in [10], which requires the algorithm to be more robust for the noise. Apart from CSPNet [1] that uses a separate CNN to extract multi-level features in ROI-pooling, our baseline model extracts features from the shared FPN backbone in specific resolution according to the box size, which effectively improves cytoplasm AJI from 0.4607 to 0.6845 and nuclei AJI from 0.3891 to 0.5169. In addition, adding the DRM (*IRNet w/o IRM*) gives a striking 9.03% and 3.23% improvement of F1 score for cytoplasm and nuclei, which proves that the duplicated boxes can be effectively suppressed by parsing message among boxes, especially for the cytoplasm in cell clumps. Compared with baseline model (*Mask R-CNN*), adding IRM after segmentation branch (*IRNet w/o DRM*) gains 2.19% and 5.84% AJI improvements for cytoplasm and nuclei, demonstrates that by leveraging instance association for transferring information, the augmented features are more consistent and discriminative for semantic representation. By combining DRM and IRM in our framework, the proposed IRNet (*Ours*) outperforms other methods by a large margin, with 4.97% and 6.33% improvements of AJI as well as 12.5% and 5.03% improvements of F1 score for cytoplasm and nuclei comparing with the baseline model (*Mask R-CNN*).

**Ablation Study for the Instance Relation Module.** We then conduct the ablation study for the design of the proposed IRM. (1). *DF* (Deep Feature): Using deep features before the deconvolution layer in segmentation branch with the shape of $256 \times 14 \times 14$ for further process. (2). *MSK* (Mask): Using predicted mask from segmentation branch for further process. We keep the masks from the predicted class in detection branch only and remove the other class. (3). *RL* (Relation Learning): Conducting channel-wise instance relation learning. Results are shown in Table 2.

We first add the same number of convolution layers as that in IRM encoder and remove the relation interaction part (*DF + MSK*). Adding more parameters to build deeper layers do improve the results, but all the methods with relation learning have better performance. Compared with *IRNet w/o IRM*, directly utilizing deep features for relation interaction (*DF+RL*) yields the results of 0.7097 and 0.5367 in AJI, which brings 3.05% and 0.47% improvement for cytoplasm and nuclei. Meanwhile, directly using predicted masks (*MSK+RL*) outperforms *IRNet w/o IRM* by 2.67% AJI for cytoplasm. The nuclei class does not improve in *MSK+RL* because the shape of masks are almost the same so that it does not contain enough information for message parsing. Furthermore, when we adopt deep features with selected masks simultaneously, it significantly improves the performance over the (*DF+RL*) by 4.33% and 2.88% for cytoplasm and nuclei, which shows the effectiveness of the IRM design.

**Table 2.** Ablation study for the Instance Relation Module.

| DF | MSK | RL | AJI | | F1 | |
|----|-----|-----|------|--------|--------|--------|
| | | | Cyto | Nuclei | Cyto | Nuclei |
| | | | 0.6887 | 0.5342 | 0.7266 | 0.7424 |
| ✓ | ✓ | | 0.7042 | 0.5283 | 0.7355 | 0.7306 |
| ✓ | | ✓ | 0.7097 | 0.5367 | 0.7350 | 0.7442 |
| | ✓ | ✓ | 0.7071 | 0.5299 | 0.7324 | 0.7366 |
| ✓ | ✓ | ✓ | **0.7185** | **0.5496** | **0.7497** | **0.7554** |

**Qualitative Comparison.** Figure 3 shows representative samples in the test set with challenging cases such as the heavily occlusion of cytoplasm and the scatted white blood cells. Conventional method (*JOMLS*) fails on identifying the miscellaneous instance and the nucleus (see the third row and fourth row). Compared with *Mask R-CNN*, adding IRM mitigates the ambiguous cytoplasm boundary prediction in cell clumps (see (a) and (e)), which is important for further accurate cell classification by morphology analysis. Moreover, combining DRM further suppresses the duplicated predictions successfully (see (e) and (f)).

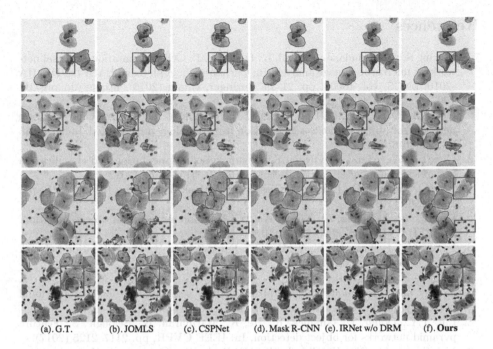

(a). G.T.        (b). JOMLS        (c). CSPNet        (d). Mask R-CNN        (e). IRNet w/o DRM        (f). **Ours**

**Fig. 3.** Qualitative results of overlapping cervical cell segmentation in Pap smear image on the test set (each closed curve denotes an individual instance). Rectangles show the main differences among different methods.

# 4    Conclusion

Accurately segmenting the cytoplasm and nucleus instance in Pap smear image is pivotal for further cell morphology analysis and cervical cancer grading. In this paper, we proposed a novel IRNet which leverages the instance relation information for better semantic consistent feature representation. By aggregating the features from other instances, they tend to generate masks with more consistent boundary shape. Quantitative and qualitative results demonstrate the effectiveness of our method. Notice the proposed IRM is inherently general and can be complementary for various proposal-based instance segmentation methods.

**Acknowledgement.** This work was supported by 973 Program (Project No. 2015CB351706) grants from the National Natural Science Foundation of China with Project No. U1613219, Research Grants Council of Hong Kong Special Administrative Region under Project No. CUHK14225616, Hong Kong Innovation and Technology Fund under Project No. ITS/041/16, and Shenzhen Science and Technology Program (No. JCYJ20180507182410327).

# References

1. Akram, S.U., Kannala, J., Eklund, L., Heikkilä, J.: Cell segmentation proposal network for microscopy image analysis. In: Carneiro, G., et al. (eds.) LABELS/DLMIA -2016. LNCS, vol. 10008, pp. 21–29. Springer, Cham (2016). https://doi.org/10.1007/978-3-319-46976-8_3
2. Chen, H., Qi, X., Yu, L., Dou, Q., Qin, J., Heng, P.A.: Dcan: deep contour-aware networks for object instance segmentation from histology images. Med. Image Anal. **36**, 135–146 (2017)
3. GençTav, A., Aksoy, S., ÖNder, S.: Unsupervised segmentation and classification of cervical cell images. Pattern Recogn. **45**(12), 4151–4168 (2012)
4. He, K., Gkioxari, G., Dollár, P., Girshick, R.: Mask R-CNN. In: IEEE CVPR, pp. 2961–2969 (2017)
5. Hu, H., Gu, J., Zhang, Z., Dai, J., Wei, Y.: Relation networks for object detection. In: IEEE CVPR, pp. 3588–3597 (2018)
6. Fu, J., Liu, J., Tian, H., Li, Y., Bao, Y., Fang, Z., Lu, H.: Dual attention network for scene segmentation (2019)
7. Kumar, N., Verma, R., Sharma, S., Bhargava, S., Vahadane, A., Sethi, A.: A dataset and a technique for generalized nuclear segmentation for computational pathology. IEEE Trans. Med. Imaging **36**(7), 1550–1560 (2017)
8. Lin, T.Y., Dollár, P., Girshick, R., He, K., Hariharan, B., Belongie, S.: Feature pyramid networks for object detection. In: IEEE CVPR, pp. 2117–2125 (2017)
9. Liu, S., Qi, L., Qin, H., Shi, J., Jia, J.: Path aggregation network for instance segmentation. In: IEEE CVPR, pp. 8759–8768 (2018)
10. Lu, Z., Carneiro, G., Bradley, A.P.: An improved joint optimization of multiple level set functions for the segmentation of overlapping cervical cells. IEEE Trans. Image Proc. **24**(4), 1261–1272 (2015)
11. Papanicolaou, G.N.: A new procedure for staining vaginal smears. Science **95**(2469), 438–439 (1942)
12. Raza, S.E.A., et al.: Micro-Net: A unified model for segmentation of various objects in microscopy images. Med. Image Anal. **52**, 160–173 (2019)
13. Song, Y., et al.: Accurate cervical cell segmentation from overlapping clumps in pap smear images. IEEE Trans. Med. Imaging **36**(1), 288–300 (2017)
14. Vaswani, A., et al.: Attention is all you need. In: NIPS. Curran Associates, Inc. (2017)

# Weakly Supervised Cell Instance Segmentation by Propagating from Detection Response

Kazuya Nishimura[1]([✉]), Dai Fei Elmer Ker[2], and Ryoma Bise[1]

[1] Kyushu University, Fukuoka, Japan
kazuya.nishimura@human.ait.kyushu-u.ac.jp
[2] The Chinese University of Hong Kong, Hong Kong, China

**Abstract.** Cell shape analysis is important in biomedical research. Deep learning methods may perform to segment individual cells if they use sufficient training data that the boundary of each cell is annotated. However, it is very time-consuming for preparing such detailed annotation for many cell culture conditions. In this paper, we propose a weakly supervised method that can segment individual cell regions who touch each other with unclear boundaries in dense conditions without the training data for cell regions. We demonstrated the efficacy of our method using several data-set including multiple cell types captured by several types of microscopy. Our method achieved the highest accuracy compared with several conventional methods. In addition, we demonstrated that our method can perform without any annotation by using fluorescence images that cell nuclear were stained as training data. Code is publicly available in https://github.com/naivete5656/WSISPDR.

**Keywords:** Microscopy · Cell segmentation · Weakly supervised learning

## 1 Introduction

Noninvasive microscopy imaging techniques, such as phase contrast and differential interference contrast microscopy, have been widely used to capture cell populations for their appearance (shape) analysis and behavior analysis without staining. Segmentation of individual cells is an essential task for such cell image analysis. However, phase contrast microscopy images contain artifacts such as the halo and shade-off due to the optical principle as shown in Fig. 1(a). This makes segmentation difficult. To address the difficulties, many CNN-based machine learning methods have been proposed. In general, CNN requires a large amount of supervised data for each cell boundary. Because cell shapes are complex,

**Electronic supplementary material** The online version of this chapter (https://doi.org/10.1007/978-3-030-32239-7_72) contains supplementary material, which is available to authorized users.

© Springer Nature Switzerland AG 2019
D. Shen et al. (Eds.): MICCAI 2019, LNCS 11764, pp. 649–657, 2019.
https://doi.org/10.1007/978-3-030-32239-7_72

annotating individual cell shapes is very time-consuming. We should annotate cell regions under many situations such as types of cells, density, and microscopy. In addition, the techniques for staining an entire cell region are not suitable for generation ground-truth of instance cell segmentation in dense conditions since it is difficult to separate the cell regions from such data. We thus need to recognize cell shape from the simpler annotation.

Our aim is to develop a weakly supervised segmentation method that can segment individual cells in dense cell conditions by only using simple annotation, such as the centroid positions of individual cells, which does not include the cell shape (boundary) information. The key assumptions of this study are as follows:

1. The rough centroid positions of individual cells (weak labels) are useful for an instance cell segmentation task that is difficult for direct segmentation methods without any training data; such weak label information makes segmentation easy. In addition, such rough centroid positions can be easily collected using fluorescent images in which the nuclei of cells are stained.
2. In the process of deep learning for "detecting the center of individual cells", the networks use "cell shape" information and thus the analysis of contributing pixels for detection is useful for the instance segmentation task.

Based on the assumptions, we propose a weakly supervised instance cell segmentation method that first learns cell detection by CNN using centroid cell positions and segment individual cell regions by effectively using the contribution pixels for detection. The main contributions of this paper are summarized as follows:

- To address the challenging task for segmenting individual cells, who touch each other with unclear boundaries, without the training data for cell regions, we propose a weakly supervised method that first detects the cell centroids using the weak label, and then uses the contribution pixel analysis in the trained detection network for instance cell segmentation.
- For the contribution pixel analysis of detection, we use guided backpropagation (GB) [7], which was developed to visualize pixels contributing to classification. GB backpropagates the responses from a class label node in the network. Instead, our method backpropagates the signals only from the particular regions of the output feature image in U-Net [6]. Our method can extract the contributed pixels respectively.
- We demonstrated the efficacy of our method using several microscopic images including multiple cell types captured by several types of microscopy techniques. Our method achieved the highest accuracy compared with several conventional methods. In addition, we demonstrated that our method can perform without any annotation by using fluorescence images in which cell nuclei were stained as training data[1].

---

[1] In the test, the stained image is not required.

## 2  Related Work

Many cell segmentation methods have been proposed for non-invasive microscopy images such as those taken with phase contrast microscopy using image processing methods based on intensity features [2], Graph-cut optimization [1], and optical model-based method [8]. These methods often do not work due to the differences in intensity distribution that arise from the difference in cell types (shape and thickness). Many deep learning-based methods such as U-Net have been proposed. However, these methods require sufficient training data that contains individual cell boundaries annotated by experts and such annotation is time consuming.

On the other hand, weakly supervised object segmentation methods for a general object have been proposed that use weak labels such as class labels and bounding boxes. Zhou *et al.* [9] proposed an instance segmentation method using only class labels as training data. This method implicitly supposes that objects to be segmented appear sparsely in an image. Therefore, it does not work for our target, in which many cells touch each other. Li *et al.* [4] uses faster R-CNN [5] to detect the bounding boxes of the target objects, and segment individual object regions using a conditional random field (CRF), where they do not use network analysis. Their loss function is designed to exclude the region that the intersect regions of bounding boxes of nearby objects; this is a key for their method to succeed. However, cells have a non-rigid and complex shape and they touch each other. Thus, the intersect regions of bounding boxes become much larger than those of general objects.

Unlike these methods, we effectively use a network analysis that can extract contributed pixels for each cell from a U-Net trained for cell detection in order to segment individual cell regions in dense conditions.

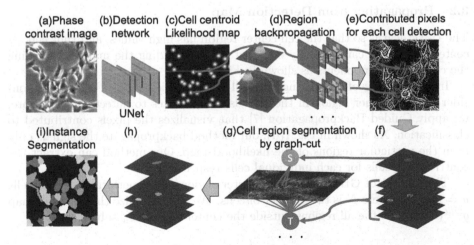

**Fig. 1.** Outline of proposed method.

# 3   Method

Figure 1 shows an overview of the proposed method. The proposed method first roughly detects the centroid positions of cells by a U-Net that is trained to output the likelihood map of cell positions (Fig. 1(c)). For each detected cell, the method performs back propagation from the center regions of a detected cell to extract the pixels that contributed to detecting the cell centroid (Fig. 1(d)). Then, the information is used for graph-cut segmentation to segment individual cells, where the corresponding channel is used for the foreground seeds and the other channels are used for the background seeds (Fig. 1(g)).

## 3.1   Cell Detection with Likelihood Map

A Bounding box has been widely used as a ground-truth of object detection. As discussed above, however, a cell has non-rigid and complex shape and they often touch each other. In this case, a bounding box often contains multiple cell regions. Therefore, we use cell centroid positions as training data. This annotation is easier than annotating bounding boxes. The annotation may be off the cell centroid since the human annotations are not generally strict. To represent the gap between the human annotation and the true position, we use the cell position likelihood map as training data, where an annotated cell position becomes a peak and the value gradually decreases with a Gaussian distribution (Fig. 1(c)). To train the U-Net from the input of the original microscopy image, we use the mean of squared error loss function (MSE) between the estimated image by the U-Net and the ground-truth likelihood map. The output of U-Net defines $\mathbf{y}$.

## 3.2   Propagating from Detection Map

The U-Net learns so that the cell center region has high values, and thus cell $u$'s center regions $S_u$ can be easily detected by thresholding the map and labeling the connected components as shown in Fig. 2(c).

In the process of estimating the cell center region $S_u$ by U-Net, we consider that the other region in the cell also contributes to detection. Therefore, we apply Guided Backpropagation [7] that visualizes the pixels contributed to classification. As shown in Fig. 1(d), our method backpropagate the signals only from the particular regions of the likelihood map. Our method can extract the contributed pixels for each individual cells respectively.

The process of GB from the cell center regions $S_u$ is performed for all cells $u = 1, ..., N$, where $N$ is the number of cells. We first initialize the response map $g^{Out}(u)$ so that the all regions outside the center regions $S_u$ substitute 0.

$$g_i^{Out}(u) = \begin{cases} y_i & if\ i \in S_u \\ 0 & if\ i \notin S_u, \end{cases} \tag{1}$$

where $i$ denotes the pixel coordinates. The GB is back propagating the signals from the output layer to the input layer using the trained parameters in the network. The GB is similar to compute the gradient of output to input.

A difference of normal gradient is the propagation at a ReLU function that uses both forward and backward pass information, where a forward pass in the estimation is recorded in the estimation process. We consider a case in which a ReLU function is at the $l + 1$-th layer, where $g^{l+1}$ is the backward propagated value of the $l + 1$-th layer, and $f^l$ is the forward propagated value of the $l$-th layer. The signal is propagated to the $l$-th layer only if the both propagations are positive; otherwise, the backward propagation is to 0, formulated as:

$$g_i^l(u) = I(f_i^l) \cdot I(g_i^l(u)) \cdot g_i^{l+1}(u) \tag{2}$$

$$I(x), = \begin{cases} 1 & \text{if } x > 0 \\ 0 & \text{otherwise,} \end{cases} \tag{3}$$

where $I$ is an indicator function. Finally, the back propagated signal $g^0(u)$ is the map of the pixels that contributed to detecting the $u$-th cell. For each detected cell, this process is respectively performed to obtain the contribution map of each cell.

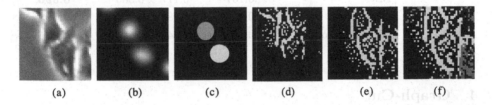

(a)             (b)             (c)             (d)             (e)             (f)

**Fig. 2.** (a) Enlarged phase contrast image, (b) likelihood map, (c) each cell region, (d) and (e) each back propagation, (f) fused contribution map aggregating all cells in the image, where color indicates an individual cell. (Color figure online)

However, the outside regions of the target cell also have values in the contribution map for each cell. Figure 2 shows the examples of the extracted contribution map from the touching cells. Figure 2(d) is obtained from the blue region in Figs. 2(c) and (e) is obtained from the yellow region. We can observe that the regions on the other cell also have positive values in each map. That adversely affects the individual cell segmentation if we simply use this information for segmenting each cell. To address this problem, we compared the values with the other channel (*i.e.*, cell) based on the basic of the fact that the pixel value $g_i^0(u)$ on the $u$-th cell in the $u$-th (cell's) contribution map tends to be larger than the values of the same pixel on the other cell's maps $g_N^0(\forall N \neq u)$. The maximum projection contribution map $C(u)$ for the $u$-th cell can be formalized as:

654    K. Nishimura et al.

$$C_i(u) = \phi_i(\arg\max_k g_i^0(k), u). \tag{4}$$

$$\phi_i(k, u) = \begin{cases} g_i(k) & if \ (k = u) \\ 0 & \text{otherwise.} \end{cases} \tag{5}$$

This indicates that the value of the $i$-th pixel of the $u$-th map takes value only if the value is larger than the value of the same pixel $i$ on any other channels. This process is also done for each cell. These maps are registered as channels (Fig. 1(f)). Figure 1(e) shows the fusion image of all channels, where each color indicates an individual cell.

**Table 1.** Performance of compared methods.

| Metric | Data | Zhou [9] | Bensch [1] | Yin [8] | Chalfoun [2] | Ours |
|--------|------|----------|------------|---------|--------------|------|
| F-measure | C2C12 [3] | 0.513 | 0.407 | 0.613 | 0.707 | **0.948** |
| | NSC | - | 0.645 | 0.559 | 0.818 | **0.911** |
| | B23P17 | - | 0.209 | 0.719 | 0.679 | **0.887** |
| | No annotation | - | 0.669 | 0.403 | 0.836 | **0.951** |
| mDice | C2C12 [3] | 0.244 | 0.380 | 0.421 | 0.556 | **0.638** |
| | NSC | - | 0.167 | 0.177 | 0.385 | **0.596** |
| | B23P17 | - | 0.061 | 0.487 | 0.354 | **0.598** |
| | No annotation | - | 0.165 | 0.343 | 0.500 | **0.625** |

## 4  Graph-Cut

We segment the individual cells independently by using graph-cut. To segment the $u$-th cell, the proposed method uses the $u$-th contribution map $C(u)$ as a foreground seed and the maximum intensity projection image from all the other channels as a background seed. The saliency map of the original image is used for the data term. We simply use the inverse image of the original image for phase contrast microscopy images. Then the final instance segmentation result is obtained by fusing all the segmented images as shown in Fig. 1(i).

## 5  Experiments

In the experiments, we evaluated the effectiveness of the proposed method compared with several methods in four challenging data-sets. In the comparison, we selected three methods; Bensch [1], Chalfoun [2], and Zhou [9].

The state-of-the-art method proposed by Li [4], which detects the bounding box using faster R-CNN, and then each object is segmented, is one of the most related works with our method. However, it totally did not work since the bounding boxes of nearby cells often overlap. Instead, we selected the method proposed by Zhou [9] that estimates the instance object regions by a deep neural network trained only using the class label. To train their network, we prepared images to belong to the foreground (cell) that contains cells or background that does not contain by clipping the original images. We prepared a small validation data for instance segmentation to tune the parameters of the methods of Bensch and Chalfoun since their methods require a small amount of annotation data about cell region boundaries as a validation data.

## 5.1  Dataset

We evaluated our methods by using three challenging data-set with annotation that cells were cultured in dense and captured by different microscopy as shown in Fig. 3(a); (1) C2C12: myoblast cells captured by phase contrast microscopy [3] at the resolution of 1040 × 1392 pixels, (2) B23P17: bovine epithelial cells captured by phase contrast microscopy at the resolution of 1040 × 1392 pixels, (3) NSC: neural stem cells captured by differential interference microscopy at the resolution of 512 × 512 pixels. For ground-truth, cell centroids were roughly annotated in 880, 124, 120 images, respectively. In addition, the individual cell regions were annotated as the test data, where the total number of cells are 796, 711, and 416 cells. The images were divided into 320 × 320 patches to train our U-Net.

Furthermore, we evaluated our method using a dataset without any annotation; (4) No annotation: myoblast cells captured by phase contrast microscopy with the fluorescence images, where cell nuclear were stained as training data, where the number of images is 86 pairs, and the resolution is 1360 × 1024. For the test data, the boundaries of 1306 individual cells were annotated.

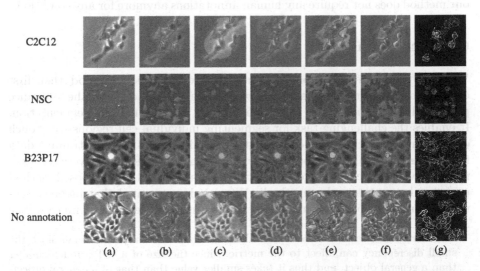

**Fig. 3.** (a) Original image, (b) ground-truth, (c) Bensch, (d) Yin, (e) Chalfoun, (f) ours, and (g) fused contribution map.

## 5.2   Evaluation

We first evaluated the performance of cell detection, where we use F-measure as the performance metric with the three-fold cross-validations. Table 1 shows the average of the metrics for each data-set. The proposed method outperformed the other methods in all data-set. In particular, our method worked well from the dataset without human annotation (*i.e.*, instead, using fluorescence images).

Next, we evaluated the performance of the instance segmentation task. We use the mean of Dice-coefficient (mDice) as the performance metrics. To compute Dice, we first assigned the estimated cell regions and the regions of ground-truth. The mDice is defined as $mDice = \frac{1}{M} \sum_{u=0}^{M} \frac{2 \times tp^u}{2 \times tp^u + fn^u + fp^u}$. $tp^u$ is the number of true positive pixels of cell $u$ (overlap regions), $fn^u$, $fp^u$ are the number of false negative and false positive pixels, respectively, where $M$ is the number of cells[2].

Table 1 summarizes the performance metrics[3]. In the results, our method outperformed other methods under all the dataset. Figure 3 shows the examples of cell segmentation results of the compared methods. Bensh's method, which uses the modified graph-cut, works for a cell that is located sparsely, but it did not work in dense conditions. Yin's method, which uses the optical principle of phase contrast microscopy, did not work for cells that often change the thickness due to mitosis or differentiation. Chalfoun's method, which first segments the cell cluster regions and then separates the individual cell regions, is sensitive to the intensity values, and thus it also did not work well. Contrast to these methods, our method worked robustly under the various images since our method is based on the contribution map, where the contribution map showed good results Fig. 3. In particular, our method produced good results even under the totally different images captured by different microscopy. In addition, our method worked well using fluorescent images as training data. It demonstrated the possibility that our method does not require any human annotations anymore for any conditions.

## 6   Conclusion

We proposed a weakly supervised instance segmentation method that first detects the cell centroids using the weak label, and then uses the relevance pixel analysis in the trained detection network for instance cell segmentation. It enables the challenging task for segmenting individual cell regions who touch each other with unclear boundaries in dense conditions without the training data for cell regions. Evaluation for instance segmentation tasks using several types of noninvasive microscopy image data-set demonstrated that the proposed method performs better than other methods. We also demonstrated that instance segmentation is possible without annotations by using nuclei-stained images. The

---

[2] In general, Dice takes a small value when the size of the object is small since the small discrepancy can affect to the metric. Since the size of a cell is much smaller than a general object, and thus it takes smaller value than that of a general object.

[3] Zhou's method requires the training images that do not contain any cell. However, we could not make enough training data except (1) C2C12 due to the dense cells.

very thin thickness regions around the boundaries of the cell were not correctly segmented by all the methods. It still remains challenges to segment such detailed regions in various conditions. This is our future work.

**Acknowledgement.** This work was supported by JSPS KAKENHI Grant Number JP18H05104 and JP19K22895.

# References

1. Bensch, R., Ronneberger, O.: Cell segmentation and tracking in phase contrast images using graph cut with asymmetric boundary costs. In: ISBI (2015)
2. Chalfoun, J., Majurski, M., Dima, A., et al.: Fogbank: a single cell segmentation across multiple cell lines and image modalities. BMC Bioinform. **15**(1), 431 (2014)
3. Ker, D.F.E., Eom, S., Sanami, S., et al.: Phase contrast time-lapse microscopy datasets with automated and manual cell tracking annotations. In: Scientific data (2018)
4. Li, Q., Arnab, A., Torr, P.H.S.: Weakly- and semi-supervised panoptic segmentation. In: Ferrari, V., Hebert, M., Sminchisescu, C., Weiss, Y. (eds.) ECCV 2018. LNCS, vol. 11219, pp. 106–124. Springer, Cham (2018). https://doi.org/10.1007/978-3-030-01267-0_7
5. Ren, S., He, K., Girshick, R., Sun, J.: Faster R-CNN: towards real-time object detection with region proposal networks. In: NIPS, pp. 91–99 (2015)
6. Ronneberger, O., Fischer, P., Brox, T.: U-Net: convolutional networks for biomedical image segmentation. In: Navab, N., Hornegger, J., Wells, W.M., Frangi, A.F. (eds.) MICCAI 2015. LNCS, vol. 9351, pp. 234–241. Springer, Cham (2015). https://doi.org/10.1007/978-3-319-24574-4_28
7. Selvaraju, R.R., Cogswell, M., Das, A., et al.: Grad-CAM: visual explanations from deep networks via gradient-based localization. In: ICCV, pp. 618–626 (2017)
8. Yin, Z., Kanade, T., Chen, M.: Understanding the phase contrast optics to restore artifact-free microscopy images for segmentation. Med. Image Anal. **16**, 1047–1062 (2012)
9. Zhou, Y., Zhu, Y., Ye, Q., et al.: Weakly supervised instance segmentation using class peak response. In: CVPR (2018)

# Robust Non-negative Tensor Factorization, Diffeomorphic Motion Correction, and Functional Statistics to Understand Fixation in Fluorescence Microscopy

Neel Dey[1]([✉]), Jeffrey Messinger[2], R. Theodore Smith[3], Christine A. Curcio[2], and Guido Gerig[1]

[1] Department of Computer Science and Engineering,
New York University, Brooklyn, NY 11201, USA
neel.dey@nyu.edu
[2] Department of Ophthalmology and Visual Sciences,
University of Alabama at Birmingham, Birmingham, AL 35294, USA
[3] Department of Ophthalmology, Icahn School of Medicine at Mount Sinai,
New York, NY 10029, USA

**Abstract.** Fixation is essential for preserving cellular morphology in biomedical research. However, it may also affect spectra captured in multispectral fluorescence microscopy, impacting molecular interpretations. To investigate fixation effects on tissue, multispectral fluorescence microscopy images of pairs of samples with and without fixation are captured. Each pixel might exhibit overlapping spectra, creating a blind source separation problem approachable with linear unmixing. With multiple excitation wavelengths, unmixing is intuitively extended to tensor factorizations. Yet these approaches are limited by nonlinear effects like attenuation. Further, light exposure during image acquisition introduces subtle Brownian motion between image channels of non-fixed tissue. Finally, hypothesis testing for spectral differences due to fixation is non-trivial as retrieved spectra are paired sequential samples. To these ends, we present three contributions, (1) a novel *robust* non-negative tensor factorization using the $\beta$-divergence and $L_{2,1}$-norm, which decomposes the data into a low-rank multilinear and group-sparse non-multilinear tensor without making *any* explicit nonlinear modeling choices or assumptions on noise statistics; (2) a diffeomorphic atlas-based strategy for motion correction; (3) a non-parametric hypothesis testing framework for paired sequential data using functional principal component analysis. PyTorch code for robust non-negative tensor factorization is available at https://github.com/neel-dey/robustNTF.

---

**Electronic supplementary material** The online version of this chapter (https://doi.org/10.1007/978-3-030-32239-7_73) contains supplementary material, which is available to authorized users.

© Springer Nature Switzerland AG 2019
D. Shen et al. (Eds.): MICCAI 2019, LNCS 11764, pp. 658–666, 2019.
https://doi.org/10.1007/978-3-030-32239-7_73

# 1    Introduction

Imaging spectroscopy is a ubiquitous tool to investigate the chemical nature of biological samples. Each pixel contains an entire spectrum in a desired modality (e.g., reflectance) whose multivariate nature allows for rich applications in image analysis such as segmentation and unmixing. However, prior to any form of imaging, fixation is performed to protect tissue from postmortem decay and improve mechanical strength. Doing so allows for the preparation of thin and storable tissue sections, a universal requirement. However, as fixation changes the chemistry of a sample to prevent decay, it may further alter its spectra and confound its interpretation. In image analysis applications where the spectra are of interest (e.g., detecting malignancy in surgical biopsies), it is imperative to verify whether fixation changes their shape characteristics [5].

Towards understanding this effect for applications in retinal biology and pathology, we perform a self-controlled experiment. Human eyes were obtained in pairs from deceased donors, and tissue sections from corresponding locations in both eyes were imaged. Sections from the right and left eyes were fixed and not fixed, respectively. Imaging was performed with multispectral fluorescence microscopy with multiple light sources (excitation wavelengths), allowing for the high-dimensional analysis of spectral differences in these paired samples. However, several image analysis challenges arise from this experimental design.

First, compound co-localization leads to pixels containing mixed spectra. To separate constituent spectra and retrieve their spatial distributions in the image, non-negative matrix and tensor factorizations are used when there are one or more light sources, respectively [2,8]. Non-negative data analysis is required as physical spectra cannot be negative. However, these models are deficient when there are nonlinear effects present like absorption and scattering within tissue. A nonlinear matrix/tensor factorization was proposed in [6] which incorporated attenuation but required reference spectra, precluding several applications.

Second, without fixation, tissue heating during image acquisition causes subtle Brownian motion of organelles between image channels. Thus, the observed spectrum at a pixel may be erroneous and can be a source of noise to analysis. Third, our measurements are paired *sequential* observations. This precludes the use of standard paired hypothesis tests to test for differences caused by fixation as they assume normality and ignore the sequential nature of spectral curves.

Therefore, our image and statistical analysis contributions are threefold. First, we propose a novel robust non-negative tensor factorization (rNTF) that decomposes the tensor of multi-excitation multispectral images into a low-rank multilinear tensor and an additional group-sparse tensor which contains the non-linearities. Existing methods for tensor factorization often make strong assumptions on noise statistics, whereas fluorescence microscopy is affected by a mixture of Poisson and Gaussian noise [12]. Therefore, we minimize the $\beta$-divergence, an information geometric metric which allows us to interpolate between noise statistics assumptions [3]. Group-sparsity is enforced on the resulting nonlinear tensor via $L_{2,1}$-norm regularization. We iteratively impute missing values common in fluorescence measurements via expectation maximization [11]. The algorithm has element-wise updates and is thus executed on GPUs for fast execution.

Second, we propose a granular motion correction strategy in fluorescence microscopy using unbiased diffeomorphic atlas building [7], where all images in the stack are nonlinearly registered to an estimated template, minimizing subtle intra-stack motion without tearing the image due to the diffeomorphic constraint. Third, inspired by the functional testing of fractional anisotropy along axonal tracts between groups in diffusion tensor imaging [9], we propose a framework for *paired* hypothesis testing of spectra using functional principal component analysis [10] and the Wilcoxon signed-rank test.

## 2   Methods

**Preliminaries.** We use the notation of $\mathbf{x}$ for a vector, $\mathbf{X}$ for a matrix, and $\mathcal{X}$ for a tensor. The tensor columns are mode-1 fibers, rows are mode-2 fibers and so on. Mode-$i$ matricization refers to taking the mode-$i$ fibers of a tensor and arranging them as columns of a matrix. The rank-$P$ factorization of a tensor $\mathcal{L} \in \mathbb{R}^{I \times J \times K}$ can be formulated as the sum of $P$ rank-one tensors, such that $\mathcal{L} \approx \sum_{i=1}^{P} \mathbf{a}_i \circ \mathbf{b}_i \circ \mathbf{c}_i$ where $\mathbf{a}_i \in \mathbb{R}^I$, $\mathbf{b}_i \in \mathbb{R}^J$, and $\mathbf{c}_i \in \mathbb{R}^K$. Factor matrices $\mathbf{A}$, $\mathbf{B}$ and $\mathbf{C}$ are generated from $\mathcal{L}$ by concatenating vectors from the rank-one components, such that $\mathbf{A} = [\mathbf{a}_1, \ldots, \mathbf{a}_P]$, $\mathbf{B} = [\mathbf{b}_1, \ldots, \mathbf{b}_P]$, and $\mathbf{C} = [\mathbf{c}_1, \ldots, \mathbf{c}_P]$.

**Robust Non-negative Tensor Factorization.** Robust tensor factorizations have a rich recent history in machine learning and computer vision [13]. Given a tensor $\mathcal{M}$ corrupted with gross outliers, it is possible to recover a low rank and sparse combination of tensors ($\mathcal{L}$ and $\mathcal{S}$, respectively) such that $\mathcal{M} \approx \mathcal{L} + \mathcal{S}$. Recently, there has been interest in replacing the squared Euclidean distance error term with other metrics and divergences which may accommodate other forms of data and noise statistics [4]. Further, there is interest in detecting structured outliers (common in medical imaging), motivating the replacement of $L_1$-norm regularization with the $L_{2,1}$-norm which induces group sparsity [13].

Consider a rank-$P$ robust tensor factorization of $\mathcal{M} \approx \sum_{i=1}^{P} \mathbf{a}_i \circ \mathbf{b}_i \circ \mathbf{c}_i + \mathcal{S}$, where $\mathbf{A}, \mathbf{B}, \mathbf{C}, \mathcal{S} \geq 0$. Block coordinate descent using various tensor matricizations is the workhorse algorithm for calculating tensor factorizations and is adopted here by iteratively fixing three out of four quantities $\mathbf{A}, \mathbf{B}, \mathbf{C}, \mathcal{S}$ and solving for the remaining one. Using the formulation of factor matrices, the factorization can be written as, $\mathbf{M}_{(1)} \approx \mathbf{A}(\mathbf{C} \odot \mathbf{B})^T + \mathbf{S}_{(1)}$, $\mathbf{M}_{(2)} \approx \mathbf{B}(\mathbf{C} \odot \mathbf{A})^T + \mathbf{S}_{(2)}$ and $\mathbf{M}_{(3)} \approx \mathbf{C}(\mathbf{B} \odot \mathbf{A})^T + \mathbf{S}_{(3)}$ where $\mathbf{M}_{(i)}$ and $\mathbf{S}_{(i)}$ are the mode-$i$ matricized representation of the tensors $\mathcal{M}$ and $\mathcal{S}$ respectively, and $\odot$ is the matrix Khatri-Rao product. Given the above considerations, we propose to solve the following model alternating between all matricizations, where $k$ is the matricization mode,

$$\min_{\mathbf{A}, \mathbf{B}, \mathbf{C}, \mathcal{S}} \mathbf{E}(\mathbf{A}, \mathbf{B}, \mathbf{C}, \mathcal{S}) = \mathbf{D}_\beta(\mathbf{M}_{(k)}, \mathbf{L}_{(k)} + \mathbf{S}_{(k)}) + \lambda \|\mathbf{S}_{(k)}\|_{2,1},$$

such that $\mathbf{A}, \mathbf{B}, \mathbf{C}, \mathbf{S} \geq 0$, where $\mathbf{D}_\beta(\cdot, \cdot)$ is the beta divergence, and $\| \cdot \|_{2,1}$ is the $L_{2,1}$-norm, such that $\|\mathbf{S}_{(k)}\|_{2,1} = \sum_{i=1}^{G} \|\mathbf{s}_i\|_2$ where $\mathbf{S}_{(k)}$ has $G$ columns. The $\beta$-divergence is an information-geometric measure of fit parameterized by a scalar

$\beta$, which takes the squared Euclidean, Kullback-Leibler and Itakura-Saito divergences (corresponding to Gaussian, Poisson or Gamma noise assumptions) as limiting cases corresponding to $\beta = 2, 1, 0$ and all interpolating cases in between.

Consider the matricization $\mathbf{M}_{(1)} \approx \mathbf{A}(\mathbf{C} \odot \mathbf{B})^T + \mathbf{S}_{(1)}$ to solve for $\mathbf{A}$ and $\mathbf{S}_{(1)}$. As derived in [3] for robust NMF, fixing $\mathbf{B}, \mathbf{C}$ and $\mathcal{S}$ allows us to multiplicatively update $\mathbf{A}$ such that $\mathbf{A}, \mathbf{B}, \mathbf{C}, \mathcal{S} \geq 0$ in a majorization-minimization framework. Using a convex-concave decomposition of the $\beta$-divergence, majorizing the convex and concave parts by the Jensen and Tangent inequalities respectively and minimizing in closed form w.r.t. to $\mathbf{A}$, we get,

$$\mathbf{A} \to \mathbf{A} * \left( \frac{(\mathbf{M}_{(1)} * \hat{\mathbf{M}}_{(1)}^{.(\beta-2)})(\mathbf{C} \odot \mathbf{B})}{\hat{\mathbf{M}}_{(1)}^{.(\beta-1)}(\mathbf{C} \odot \mathbf{B})} \right),$$

where the numerator and denominator undergo element-wise division, $\hat{\mathbf{M}}_{(1)}$ denotes the mode-1 matricization of the current low-rank approximation $\hat{\mathcal{M}}$, '$*$' denotes the element-wise (Hadamard) product, and the '.' operator in the exponents indicates element-wise power. To estimate $\mathbf{S}_{(1)}$, given fixed $\mathbf{A}, \mathbf{B}, \mathbf{C}$ and an $L_{2,1}$ penalty term on $\mathbf{S}_{(1)}$, a similar optimization yields the following update,

$$\mathbf{S}_{(1)} \to \mathbf{S}_{(1)} * \left( \frac{\mathbf{M}_{(1)} * \hat{\mathbf{M}}_{(1)}^{.(\beta-2)}}{\hat{\mathbf{M}}_{(1)}^{.(\beta-1)} + \lambda \mathbf{S}_{(1)} \mathrm{diag}(\|\mathbf{s}_1\|_2, \ldots, \|\mathbf{s}_G\|_2)^{-1}} \right),$$

where $\lambda$ is the regularization weight on the $L_{2,1}$-norm and $G$ is the number of columns in $\mathbf{S}_{(1)}$. The $\mathbf{S}_{(1)} \mathrm{diag}(\|\mathbf{s}_1\|_2, \ldots, \|\mathbf{s}_G\|_2)^{-1}$ term in the denominator is the columnwise normalized matrix $\mathbf{S}_{(1)}$ which we compute by looping through the columns instead of direct evaluation for numerical stability. For brevity, we analogously update $\mathbf{B}, \mathbf{S}_{(2)}$ and $\mathbf{C}, \mathbf{S}_{(3)}$, as shown in the supplementary material.

If the input data tensor $\mathcal{M}$ has missing entries (as in our application), we can iteratively estimate the missing values by single imputation [11]. This involves generating an indicator tensor $\mathcal{W}$ with $w_{ijk} = 0$ if $m_{ijk}$ is missing and vice-versa. During the iterations, we impute the missing entries of $\mathcal{M}$ via $\mathcal{M} \leftarrow \mathcal{W} * \mathcal{M} + (1 - \mathcal{W}) * \hat{\mathcal{M}}$ where $\hat{\mathcal{M}}$ is the current estimate of the reconstruction. As $\mathcal{W}$ is binary, the imputation reduces to expectation maximization [11].

**Atlas-Based Motion Correction.** Subtle Brownian motion of organelles across image channels in a multispectral image must be corrected such that the organelles are stationary across the spectral sequence. Particle tracking methods can track individual particles across multiple images and obtain displacement fields, yet they are inapplicable for our registration-based correction as the fields need not be invertible (thus tearing the image) and assume constant intensity or require pre-segmentation. Further, a spectral channel must be arbitrarily chosen as the reference image towards registration, thus inducing user bias.

We propose to use a large deformation diffeomorphic metric mapping-based atlas building framework towards this correction. Unbiased atlas building [7] is

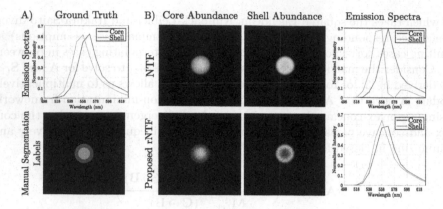

**Fig. 1. rNTF validation.** A bead with two concentric fluorescent chemicals with similar spectra imaged in a confocal microscope with two excitation wavelengths. Bovine hemoglobin was added to simulate attenuation in tissue imaging, thus creating non-linearities. As shown in B, the spectrum of the shell recovered by NTF is significantly distorted, and NTF is unable to spatially resolve the two substances due to the extrinsically added attenuation. rNTF recovers spectra which are undistorted, while also being able to spatially separate the two fluorophores on the bead as shown in the abundances images.

used to generate a deformable template image by minimizing its distance to every channel in the spectral image. Symmetric diffeomorphic registrations and atlas estimation are performed using cross-correlation as a metric [1]. This approach has the following advantages: (1) the diffeomorphic constraint ensures invertible deformation fields and prevents tearing, (2) this does not require constant intensity due to the use of cross-correlation as a matching metric and (3) it removes user bias in picking a registration target.

**Paired Hypothesis Testing for Spectra.** The differences in retrieved spectra from each fixed/unfixed pair are difficult to interpret and necessitate a hypothesis testing framework. Here, our features are the spectral channels. Paired multivariate tests should not be directly used as they do not account for the sequential nature of these features and the number of features are comparable to the sample size. We start by noticing that spectra are discrete realizations of continuous curves (i.e. functional data). Inspired by [9], we use functional PCA to reduce dimensionality while accounting for the sequential nature of features and further extend their work to the case of paired samples.

Once we retrieve constituent spectra from all the tissue sections, corresponding length-$m$ spectra from $n$ tissue sections (i.e. the same spectral component in each donor identified by spatial localization) are stacked into a matrix of size $m \times n$. Applying functional PCA with rank-$k$, we get $k$ functional eigenbases and their coefficients $\xi$. We wish to test whether the difference in distribution of these coefficients for paired samples (fixed/unfixed) are significantly different. We state our $k$ null hypotheses as $H_0^k : [\xi_j^1 - \xi_j^2]_{j=1}^k$ comes from a symmetric distribution with zero

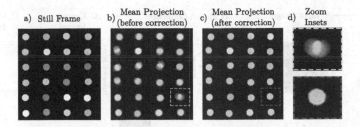

**Fig. 2. Toy Example for Motion Correction.** A grid of circles with random intensity changes and conditional deformations and are used to simulate the changing intensities and motion over image channels, respectively. With Brownian motion, the framework corrects the motion with some minor artefacts. (a) A still frame from a sequence of images of circles on a randomly deforming grid. (b) Mean projection of the raw image sequence. Note the blurry edges due to movement. (c) Mean projection of the image sequence after correction. The circles are not returned to their initial positions due to our assumption of zero-mean motion. However, they are stationary which is sufficient for our application. (d) Insets showing a sample circle with (bottom) and without (top) motion correction. Readers are encouraged to view supplementary material for videos of both synthetic and real examples.

median, where the coefficient superscript indicates group membership. Rejecting this null hypothesis implies significant differences between fixed and unfixed pairs. All $k$ hypotheses are tested with the Wilcoxon signed-rank test which is a nonparametric test for paired samples. As there are $k$ hypotheses, we apply the Bonferroni multiple comparisons correction. If we apply rank-$r$ rNTF (i.e., $r$ spectra from each section), we have $r$ such matrices and repeat this for each matrix.

## 3   Experiments and Results

**Experimental Dataset.** 24 pairs of tissue sections are used here. Tissue sections from corresponding locations in human donors from both eyes (one fixed, one not) were imaged with a multispectral fluorescence microscope, capturing multiple channels per image. Four excitation light sources were used, thus acquiring four multi-channel images per tissue section. After atlas-based motion correction, the images are preprocessed similarly to [2]. Each channel in an image is vectorized and treated as a row of a matrix. Repeating this across the four images and stacking the matrices, we get a 3D tensor (channels × pixels × light sources). This is illustrated in Fig. 3A, B, C, D and E. The multispectral images each have a different number of channels and therefore, when the images are stacked into a tensor, unavailable channels are treated as missing data.

**Implementation Details.** The four multispectral images are first affinely aligned. To build an image-specific atlas, 12 iterations of atlas building are computed with ANTs [1] for each channel in a stack with 80 iterations of diffeomorphic registration per iteration. Another atlas building step is done to create an atlas of atlases for each tissue section, to which each of the original images is mapped. Linear interpolation is used so as to not create values outside data range.

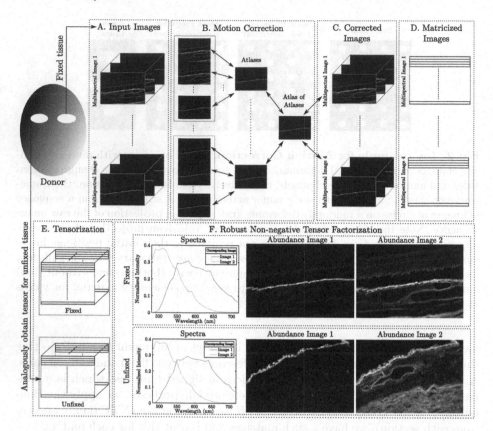

**Fig. 3.** An overview of the proposed pipeline and sample results. Panels A, B, C and D are only shown for the fixed tissue for brevity, with the unfixed tissue undergoing the same procedure. **Pipeline:** Fixed and unfixed images are obtained from the same donor. The images are motion corrected (A, B and C show the process for two out of four total images outlined in blue and red for each fixed tissue section). The images are then flattened into a matrix (D) and stacked into a tensor for each set (E). The two tensors undergo rNTF to reveal constituent spectra and spatial distributions (sample results shown in F). The spectra from all 24 pairs are used for functional statistics. See supplementary material for an expanded view of sample results. (Color figure online)

We implement rNTF on GPUs for fast execution using PyTorch at fp64 precision. A rank-2 tensor factorization model is chosen using the CORCONDIA heuristic [11] and all factors were initialized uniformly at random. Parameters $\beta = 1.6$ (corresponding to mixed Poisson-Gaussian noise) and $\lambda = 2.5$ were chosen heuristically and a tolerance of $10^{-6}$ was used for all of the optimization. Sample tensor factorization results for a fixed/unfixed pair are shown in Fig. 3F.

**Hypothesis Testing.** Once constituent spectra are retrieved from all 24 pairs of tissues, a matrix is created with the spectrum from the blue curve in Fig. 3F (lipofuscin, in retinal biology terminology) from each tissue section. All spectra are normalized to unit 2-norm to only consider shape changes. Functional PCA is then performed with model selection using the Bayesian Information Criterion. Two eigenbases are retrieved, with two sets of coefficients. The pairs of coefficients are given to the Wilcoxon signed-rank test for testing. After Bonferroni correction for two comparisons, we find no statistically significant differences between the pairs. The procedure is repeated for the red curves in Fig. 3F from each donor and finds no statistically significant difference between them, either.

## 4  Discussion

To our application, we provide image and statistical analysis methodologies and find no significant differences between the fluorescence spectra of fixed and unfixed tissue. This finding informs applications in multispectral retinal microscopy. Further validation is required as two limitations exist: (1) in this specific application, rNTF results are not guaranteed to be unique due to the additional need for data imputation; (2) the motion correction cannot retrieve the original positions and instead moves structures to the nonlinear mean of their movement.

The methods presented are general and amenable to several applications. rNTF is suitable for applications in machine learning to handle grossly corrupted measurements (outliers and nonlinearities), making only mild assumptions on the outliers being sparse. The motion correction framework can be applied to any spectral image displaying nonlinear deformations between channels. Finally, when samples are paired functional observations, we develop a non-parametric hypothesis testing framework. E.g., this statistical framework can be applied to a longitudinal analysis of fiber tracts in diffusion MRI by registering fiber tracts from the same subjects across a baseline and followup visit to test for differences in fractional anisotropy.

**Acknowledgments.** Author support and HPC provided by NIH R01EY027948 and NSF MRI-1229185, respectively. Validation data provided by Hayato Ikoma.

## References

1. Avants, B.B., Epstein, C.L., Grossman, M., Gee, J.C.: Symmetric diffeomorphic image registration with cross-correlation: evaluating automated labeling of elderly and neurodegenerative brain. Med. Image Anal. **12**(1), 26–41 (2008)
2. Dey, N., et al.: Tensor decomposition of hyperspectral images to study autofluorescence in age-related macular degeneration. Med. Image Anal. **56**, 96–109 (2019)
3. Févotte, C., Dobigeon, N.: Nonlinear hyperspectral unmixing with robust nonnegative matrix factorization. IEEE Trans. Image Process. **24**(12), 4810–4819 (2015)
4. Hong, D., Kolda, T.G., Duersch, J.A.: Generalized canonical polyadic tensor decomposition. arXiv preprint arXiv:1808.07452 (2018)
5. Huang, Z., et al.: Effect of formalin fixation on the near-infrared raman spectroscopy of normal and cancerous human bronchial tissues. Int. J. Oncol. **23**(3), 649–655 (2003)

6. Ikoma, H., Heshmat, B., Wetzstein, G., Raskar, R.: Attenuation-corrected fluorescence spectra unmixing for spectroscopy and microscopy. Opt. Express **22**(16), 19469–19483 (2014)
7. Joshi, S., Davis, B., Jomier, M., Gerig, G.: Unbiased diffeomorphic atlas construction for computational anatomy. NeuroImage **23**, S151–S160 (2004)
8. Neher, R.A., Mitkovski, M., Kirchhoff, F., Neher, E., Theis, F.J., Zeug, A.: Blind source separation techniques for the decomposition of multiply labeled fluorescence images. Biophys. J. **96**(9), 3791–3800 (2009)
9. Pomann, G.M., Staicu, A.M., Ghosh, S.: A two-sample distribution-free test for functional data with application to a diffusion tensor imaging study of multiple sclerosis. J. Roy. Stat. Soc.: Ser. C (Appl. Stat.) **65**(3), 395–414 (2016)
10. Ramsay, J.O.: Functional Data Analysis. Springer, New York (2005). https://doi.org/10.1007/b98888
11. Smilde, A., Bro, R., Geladi, P.: Multi-way Analysis: Applications in the Chemical Sciences. Wiley, Hoboken (2005)
12. Waters, J.C.: Accuracy and precision in quantitative fluorescence microscopy. Rockefeller University Press (2009)
13. Zhou, P., Feng, J.: Outlier-robust tensor PCA. In: Proceedings of the IEEE Conference on Computer Vision and Pattern Recognition, pp. 2263–2271 (2017)

# ConCORDe-Net: Cell Count Regularized Convolutional Neural Network for Cell Detection in Multiplex Immunohistochemistry Images

Yeman Brhane Hagos[1], Priya Lakshmi Narayanan[1], Ayse U. Akarca[2], Teresa Marafioti[2], and Yinyin Yuan[1(✉)]

[1] Division of Molecular Pathology, The Institute of Cancer Research, London, UK
Yinyin.Yuan@icr.ac.uk
[2] Department of Cellular Pathology, University College London, London, UK

**Abstract.** In digital pathology, cell detection and classification are often prerequisites to quantify cell abundance and explore tissue spatial heterogeneity. However, these tasks are particularly challenging for multiplex immunohistochemistry (mIHC) images due to high levels of variability in staining, expression intensity, and inherent noise as a result of preprocessing artefacts. We proposed a deep learning method to detect and classify cells in mIHC whole-tumor slide images of breast cancer. Inspired by inception-v3, we developed Cell COunt RegularizeD Convolutional neural Network (ConCORDe-Net) which integrates conventional dice overlap and a new cell count loss function for optimizing cell detection, followed by a multi-stage convolutional neural network for cell classification. In total, 20447 cells, belonging to five cell classes were annotated by experts from 175 patches extracted from 6 whole-tumor mIHC images. These patches were randomly split into training, validation and testing sets. Using ConCORDe-Net, we obtained a cell detection F1 score of 0.873, which is the best score compared to three state of the art methods. In particular, ConCORDe-Net excels at detecting closely located and weakly stained cells compared to other methods. Incorporating cell count loss in the objective function regularizes the network to learn weak gradient boundaries and separate weakly stained cells from background artefacts. Moreover, cell classification accuracy of 96.5% was achieved. These results support that incorporating problem specific knowledge such as cell count into deep learning based cell detection architectures improves robustness of the algorithm.

**Keywords:** Cell detection · Convolutional neural network · Multiplex immunohistochemistry · Cell counter · Deep learning · Breast cancer

© Springer Nature Switzerland AG 2019
D. Shen et al. (Eds.): MICCAI 2019, LNCS 11764, pp. 667–675, 2019.
https://doi.org/10.1007/978-3-030-32239-7_74

# 1   Introduction

Cell detection and classification are often the first key steps in a wide range of histology image analysis tasks, such as investigating the interplay of the tumor and immune cells [1]. Multiplex Immunohistochemistry (mIHC) is a multi-parametric protocol that allows simultaneous examination of expression of multiple markers in a single section [2,3]. Combined with robust cell detection and classification techniques, mIHC has the potential to allow detailed investigation of cells spatial interaction and signalling for the study of tumor heterogeneity [2].

The field of digital pathology has recently witnessed a surge of interest in the application of deep learning for cell classification [4], cell detection [5,6], and cell counting [7–10]. However, automated cell detection and classification remain challenging due to variation in slide preparation and cell morphological diversity in shape and size. For example, closely located cells with weak boundaries are often difficult to discern [5–8]. Moreover, often a parameter such as a kernel size needed to be fixed [5], which cannot cater for cells with a range of size and shape. Furthermore, the need to differentiate cells with a subtle difference in marker expression intensity, as exemplified in Fig. 1a, adds another layer of complexity in mIHC image analysis.

In this paper, to address the above stated challenges, we developed a new cell detection method followed by multi-stage CNN to analyse mIHC images of breast cancer. Our work has the following main contributions: (1) We developed Cell Count RegularizeD Convolutional neural Network (ConCORDe-Net) inspired by inception-v3 which incorporates cell counter and designed for cell detection without the need of pre-specifying parameters such as cell size. (2) The parameters of ConCORDe-Net were optimized using an objective function that combines conventional Dice overlap and a new cell count loss function which regularizes the network parameters to detect closely located cells. (3) Our quantitative experiments support that ConCORDe-Net outperformed the state of the art methods at detecting closely located as well as weakly stained cells.

# 2   Materials

The dataset used in this paper were mIHC whole-tumor slide images from patients with breast cancer, and the images were scanned at 40X resolution. A total of 175 regions/patches were annotated from different parts of 6 whole tumor images by experts. The patches were extracted from different regions of the slides to incorporate the variation in the data. The patches were then randomly split into training (120), validation (28), and testing (27). Inside these patches 20477 cells were annotated and these belonged to five different types of cells as depicted in Table 1. Illustrative example of patches are shown in Fig. 1a. The distribution of the data for each cell is presented in Table 1.

**Table 1.** Distribution of dataset

| Cell type | Training | Validation | Test |
|---|---|---|---|
| CD8 | 2971 | 653 | 624 |
| GAL8+ pSTAT− | 4118 | 881 | 903 |
| GAL8+ pSTAT+ strong | 919 | 183 | 200 |
| GAL8+ pSTAT+ moderate | 1558 | 295 | 279 |
| GAL8+ pSTAT+ weak | 4770 | 1038 | 1102 |

# 3  Methodology

## 3.1  Dot Annotation to Cell Pseudo-segmentation

The reference ground truth obtained was a dot annotation at the center of a cell instead of cell spatial extent segmentation which is generally tedious task. However, to train the proposed cell detection pipeline, cells mask $(G)$ and the number of cells $(C_t)$ were needed as a target. $C_t$ is simply the number of annotated cells in the input patch. Cell pseudo-segmentation was generated from dot annotation using Eq. (1).

$$G(i,j) = \begin{cases} 1 & \text{if } d < r \\ 0 & otherwise \end{cases} \tag{1}$$

where $G(i,j)$ is pixel intensity value at $(i,j)$ of pseudo-segmentation image $(G)$, $d$ is an Euclidean distance between pixel location $(i,j)$ and any of cell dot annotations, and $r$ is threshold distance. $r$ was empirically set to 4 pixels to guarantee pseudo-segmentation of cells do not touch each other.

## 3.2  Cell Counter

Our proposed cell counter network is shown in Fig. 1b. It is a mapping function, $f : \mathbb{R}^{nxn} \rightarrow \mathbb{R}^1$, where $n$ is the size of the input patch, which is 224 in our case. It consists of feature extraction and regression parts. The feature extraction part is composed of four consecutive convolutional layers of $3 \times 3$ filter size, and *"same"* padding. The number of neurons in these layers are $\{16, 32, 64, 128\}$ respectively. Every convolutional layer was followed by max-pooling layer of size $(2 \times 2)$ with stride 2 to reduce the dimensionality of features in the previous layer. The regressor part has a series of two dense layers of $\{200, 1\}$ neurons. The output dense layer has one neuron which computes estimated number of cells in the input tensor or image. The activation of all convolutional and dense layers was set to rectified linear unit (ReLU).

Parameters of all layers were randomly initialized using uniform glorot initialization [11]. Optimization of the parameters was done using Adam [12], learning rate of $10^{-4}$. Initially, we have experimented with Euclidean loss [10] and exponential loss functions. However, these suffer from loss explosion during the initial epochs and we came up with a new cell count loss $(C_l)$ function in Eq. (2).

$$C_l = (1 - \frac{1}{1 + \frac{1}{B}\sum_{j=1}^{B}|C_{pj} - C_{tj}|}) \tag{2}$$

where the summation is over $B$ mini-batch images, $C_{pj}$ and $C_{tj}$ are predicted and true number of cells in the $j^{th}$ image, respectively. Figure 2a shows profile of $C_l$ as a function of cell count difference $(C_p - C_t)$ and it is bounded between 0 and 1.

Before integrating the cell counter model to cell detection pipeline, it was trained and evaluated using pseudo-segmentation and number of cells as an input and output, respectively. To increase the amount of data, horizontal and vertical flipping were applied to all input training patches. The pseudo-segmentation is a binary image, however, when it is integrated with the cell detection model, a tensor of floating value will be fed. Thus, morphological and intensity deformation was applied as follows; Morphological erosion using rectangular structuring element of width $w = 2$ was performed to every patch with a probability $p = 0.4$, where $p$ and $w$ were empirically chosen. Then, the images were multiplied by a random matrix of the same size as the image with an empirically chosen probability $p = 0.4$. All elements in the random matrix were in range $[0.7, 1]$ to set pixel values between 0.7 and 1.

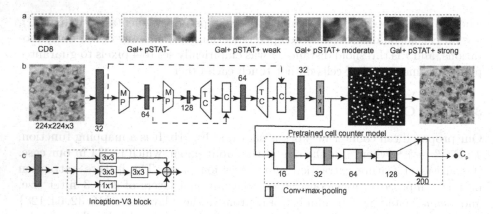

**Fig. 1.** (a) Sample patches representing different types of cells. (b) Schematics of ConCORDe-Net architecture. $3 \times 3$ and $1 \times 1$ indicate filter size of convolutional layers. TC = Transposed Convolution, MP = Max-pooling, C = Concatenate. The network has two outputs, probability map and predicted number of cells $(C_p)$. The probability map was thresholded using an empirically optimized threshold $T = 0.85$ to convert to binary image. The center of every binary object represents center of a cell. (c) Schematics of inception module.

## 3.3   Cell Detection

Figure. 1b shows the proposed ConCORDe-Net cell detection convolutional neural network. The input is $224 \times 224 \times 3$ size patch. The network has three parts; encoder, decoder and cell counter. The encoder-decoder section is extended version U-Net [13]. The standard U-Net architecture [13] uses VGG-style in its encoder and decoder section. We have proposed to use inception-v3 module shown in Fig. 1c instead of VGG block. The parallel and varying size filters in inception block enables the network to extract multi-scale features in a given layer. The encoder contains three inception modules and the first two modules were followed by 2D max-pooling layers. The decoder is composed of transposed convolution, concatenation, and inception modules. The $1 \times 1$ filter size convolutional layer at the end of the decoder is used to reduce the dimension of the tensor from $224 \times 224 \times 32$ to $224 \times 224 \times 1$. The output of the decoder was taken as cell location prediction map (P) and connected to the pretrained cell counter model (explained in Sect. 3.2), which generates predicted number of cells $(C_p)$. Activation of all layers was set to ReLU, but sigmoid for the last layer in the decoder section. Therefore, the cell detection architecture has two outputs, cell location prediction map and predicted number of cells.

The parameters of cell counter model were transfer learned from cell pseudo-segmentation as explained in Sect. 3.2. Parameters of the other layers were randomly initialized using uniform glorot initialization [11], and optimized using Adam [12], learning rate $= 10^{-4}$ and an objective function shown in Eq. (3). Cell detection loss $(D_l)$ in Eq. (3) has two parts. The first part is Dice overlap loss, and the second part is cell count loss.

$$D_l = (1 - 2\frac{\sum_{j=1}^{B}\sum_{i=1}^{N} p_{ij} g_{ij}}{1 + \sum_{j=1}^{B}\sum_{i=1}^{N} p_{ij} + \sum_{j=1}^{B}\sum_{i=1}^{N} g_{ij}}) + K(1 - \frac{1}{1 + \frac{1}{B}\sum_{j=1}^{B} |C_{pj} - C_{tj}|})$$

$$(3)$$

where summations in the first part is over batch size $(B)$ images, and $N$ pixels of the ground truth image, $g_i \in G$ and prediction map, $p_i \in P$. The second part is same as Eq. (2), but weighted by empirically optimized constant $K = 0.3$.

Horizontal and vertical flipping was applied to training patches to increase the amount and diversity of our data.

## 3.4   Cell Classification

In our dataset, there were five types of cells: CD8, GAL8+ pSTAT−, GAL8+ pSTAT+ strong, GAL8+ pSTAT+ moderate, and GAL8+ pSTAT+ weak. GAL8+ pSTAT+ cells were divided based on the expression level of pSTAT into strong, moderate, and weak. However, discriminating among GAL8+ pSTAT+ cells is challenging, even for experts. Inspired by the principle of divide and conquer algorithm, we convert the problem into multi-stage classification. The first classifier (**classifier1**) differentiates between CD8, Gal8+ pSTAT−, and all GAL8+ pSTAT+ cells. Then, a second classifier (**classifier2**) was trained to further divide GAL8+ pSTAT+ cells in to GAL8+ pSTAT+ strong, GAL8+ pSTAT+ moderate, and GAL8+ pSTAT+ weak.

Both classifiers were trained using $28 \times 28 \times 3$ patches which can cover the whole cell area for the majority of the cells. Similar network architecture was used for both classifiers. The classifier has feature extraction and classification sections. The feature extraction part is a modified version of VGG architecture [14] consisting of four convolutional layers of $\{32, \ 64 \ 128 \ 128\}$ neurons with filters size $3 \times 3$, stride 1 and *"same"* padding. Each convolutional layers were followed by $2 \times 2$ max-pooling. The classification layer consisted of two dense layers of $\{200, \ 3\}$ neurons with dropout layer, rate $= 0.3$ in between. Softmax activation was applied to the last dense layer and ReLU for the other layers. Categorical cross-entropy objective function was applied. Uniform glorot [12] was applied to initialize parameters of the layers and optimized using Adam [12], learning rate $= 10^{-4}$. To handle class imbalance, in each mini-batch, an equal number of patches from all cell types were fed to the network and the number of iterations were determined by the number of patches in the most underestimated class. Moreover, runtime augmentation of flipping, and zooming with scale $s = [0.85 \ 1.15]$ was applied with a probability of $p = 0.4$, where $s$ and $p$ were empirically optimized.

## 4   Results and Discussion

The proposed deep learning based unified cell detection and classification pipeline was evaluated on mIHC whole-tumor slide images. Implementation of the proposed approach was done in Python, and we used Keras API [15] for development of the deep learning pipeline.

To investigate if convolutional neural networks (CNN) can regress the number of cells from an input image, the proposed cell counter model was trained and then, evaluated on a test patches pseudo-segmentation image before integrating to ConCORDe-Net. Pearson correlation $r = 0.999$ was obtained between the true and predicted number of cells. The high correlation supports that the proposed cell counter network can be used as a cell count approximation function.

Quantitatively, we evaluated ConCORDe-Net using standard metrics: precision, recall and F1-score. A detection was considered true positive if it lies with in an Euclidean distance of 8 pixels ($2r$, where $r$ is in Eq. (1)) to a ground truth annotation.

Moreover, we compared ConCORDe-Net with state of the art methods, MapDe [5] and U-Net [13] as shown in Table 2. The same data augmentation as explained in Sect. 3.3 was applied to all models depicted in the Table. U-Net [13] was trained to regress pseudo-segmentation explained in Sect. 3.1. The output of CNN models in Table 2 is probability map that approximates pseudo-segmentation. The center of cells was regressed as follows from the probability map. Firstly, a global threshold maximizing F1-score was applied for each model to generate binary image. Secondly, hole filling morphological operation was applied to remove holes created after thresholding. Finally, the center of every connected component was computed which corresponds to center of a cell. ConCORDe-Net achieved the highest recall and F1-score compared to state of

**Table 2.** Cell detection performance comparison. Model1 is a model after cell counter is removed from ConCORDe-Net. U-Net [13] + Cell Counter is a CNN after integrating cell counter CNN to the original U-Net [13] architecture.

| Method | Precision | Recall | F1-score |
|--------|-----------|--------|----------|
| **ConCORDe-Net** | 0.854 | **0.892** | **0.873** |
| U-Net [13] + Cell Counter | 0.872 | 0.837 | 0.854 |
| Model1 | **0.908** | 0.80 | 0.845 |
| U-Net [13] | **0.908** | 0.785 | 0.841 |
| MapDe [5] | 0.804 | 0.876 | 0.838 |

the art methods, MapDe [5] and U-Net [13]. Moreover, in both ConCORDe-Net and U-Net [13], integrating cell counter CNN has improved cell detection F1-score. For MapDe [5], we used the parameters that were specified in the paper and tuning the dimensions of *"mapping filter"* might improve the result.

Precision of ConCORDe-Net was lower than the three other methods due to the following reasons: (1) ConCORDe-Net identifies weakly stained cells that were missed by other methods, which could be missed by expert too. (2) Over-detection of large cells when there are more than one intensity peaks within the cell. We believe that these limitations could be improved by training and validating on a large cohort.

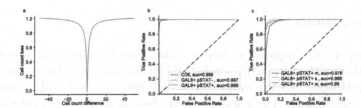

**Fig. 2.** (a) Cell count loss profile. ROC and AUC evaluation of (b) classifier1 (c) classifier2 on test data. Where s = strong, m = moderate, w = weak

Performance of the proposed classifier models was qualitatively evaluated using receiver characteristic curve (ROC), area under the curve (AUC), accuracy, precision, recall, and F1-score on test data shown in Table 1. ROC and AUC of **classifier1** are presented in Fig. 2b. AUC value of greater than 0.99 was achieved for all cell types. Overall accuracy computed on the original distribution of data was found around 98%. Moreover, precision, recall and F1-score were all 0.98. Figure 2c shows ROC and AUC of this **classifier2**. For all cell types, AUC value was higher than 0.97 and overall accuracy of around 93% was obtained. After cascading the two classifiers, overall accuracy of 96.5% was achieved.

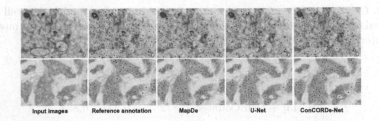

Input images     Reference annotation     MapDe     U-Net     ConCORDe-Net

**Fig. 3.** Illustrative examples of the proposed unified cell detection and classification on test data, and comparison with state-of-the-art method, MapDe [5] and U-Net [13]. White, red, yellow, cyan and dark green colored points represent CD8, GAL8+ pSTAT-, GAL8+ pSTAT+ strong, GAL8+ pSTAT+ moderate, and GAL8+ pSTAT+ weak cells, respectively. The red circles on the top left input images highlights cells that were missed by MapDe [5] and U-Net [13], but detected using ConCORDe-Net. (Color figure online)

Figure 3 shows a visual output of ConCORDe-Net followed by cell classification and comparison with MapDe [5] and U-Net [13] which uses Dice overlap loss as an objective function. ConCORDe-Net is better in discerning touching cells with weak boundary gradient and weakly stained GAL8+ pSTAT- cells compared to MapDe [5] and U-Net [13]. By regularizing the objective function with cell count, the network was able to learns patterns that can separate closely located cells and identify weakly stained cells.

## 5   Conclusions

In this paper, we proposed a deep learning based unified cell detection and classification method in mIHC whole-tumor slide images of breast cancer. Cell count regularized CNN was employed for cell detection followed by multi-stage CNN to classify cells. The parameters in the cell detection architecture were learnt using a new objective function which optimizes dice overlap and cell count. F1 score of 0.873 was achieved on test data which outperformed state of the art methods MapDe [5] and U-Net [13]. Our proposed approach is better in detecting closely located and weakly stained cells compared to MapDe [5] and U-Net [13]. Moreover, 96.5% classification accuracy was achieved. Our experiment shows that incorporating problem specific knowledge such as cell count improves robustness of the cell detection algorithm.

**Acknowledgement.** This project was funded by the European Union's Horizon 2020 research and innovation programme under the Marie Sklodowska-Curie grant agreement No 766030.

# References

1. Yuan, Y.: Spatial heterogeneity in the tumor microenvironment. Cold Spring Harb. Perspect. Med. **6**(8), a026583 (2016)
2. Blom, S., et al.: Systems pathology by multiplexed immunohistochemistry and whole-slide digital image analysis. Sci. Rep. **7**(1), 15580 (2017)
3. Kalra, J., Baker, J.: Multiplex immunohistochemistry for mapping the tumor microenvironment, pp. 237–251 (2017)
4. Sirinukunwattana, K., Raza, S.E.A., Tsang, Y.-W., Snead, D.R.J., Cree, I.A., Rajpoot, N.M.: Locality sensitive deep learning for detection and classification of nuclei in routine colon cancer histology images. IEEE Trans. Med. Imaging **35**(5), 1196–1206 (2016)
5. S.E.A., Raza: Deconvolving convolution neural network for cell detection, June 2018
6. Yang, G., Sau, C., Lai, W., Cichon, J., Li, W.: Efficient and robust cell detection: a structured regression approach. **344**(6188), 1173–1178 (2018)
7. Weidi, X., Noble, J.A., Zisserman, A.: Microscopy cell counting with fully convolutional regression networks. In: MICCAI 1st Workshop on Deep Learning in Medical Image Analysis (2015)
8. Rad, R.M., Saeedi, P., Au, J., Havelock, J.: Blastomere cell counting and centroid localization in microscopic images of human embryo. In: 2018 IEEE 20th International Workshop on Multimedia Signal Processing, MMSP 2018, pp. 1–6 (2018)
9. Paul Cohen, J., Boucher, G., Glastonbury, C.A., Lo, H.Z., Bengio, Y.: Countception: counting by fully convolutional redundant counting. In: Proceedings - 2017 IEEE International Conference on Computer Vision Workshops, ICCVW 2017, 2018, pp. 18–26, January 2018
10. Xue, Y., Ray, N., Hugh, J., Bigras, G.: Cell counting by regression using convolutional neural network. In: Hua, G., Jégou, H. (eds.) ECCV 2016. LNCS, vol. 9913, pp. 274–290. Springer, Cham (2016). https://doi.org/10.1007/978-3-319-46604-0_20
11. Glorot, X., Bengio, Y.: Understanding the difficulty of training deep feedforward neural networks. Technical report
12. Kingma, D.P., Ba, J.: Adam: a method for stochastic optimization, December 2014
13. Ronneberger, O., Fischer, P., Brox, T.: U-Net: convolutional networks for biomedical image segmentation. In: Navab, N., Hornegger, J., Wells, W.M., Frangi, A.F. (eds.) MICCAI 2015. LNCS, vol. 9351, pp. 234–241. Springer, Cham (2015). https://doi.org/10.1007/978-3-319-24574-4_28
14. Simonyan, K., Zisserman, A.: Very deep convolutional networks for large-scale image recognition, September 2014
15. Chollet, F., et al.: Keras (2015)

# Multi-task Learning of a Deep K-Nearest Neighbour Network for Histopathological Image Classification and Retrieval

Tingying Peng[1,3], Melanie Boxberg[2], Wilko Weichert[2], Nassir Navab[1,4(✉)], and Carsten Marr[3(✉)]

[1] Computer Aided Medical Procedures (CAMP),
Technical University of Munich, Munich, Germany
nassir.navab@tum.de

[2] Institute for Pathology, School of Medicine,
Technical University of Munich, Munich, Germany

[3] Institute of Computational Biology, Helmholtz Zentrum München – German Research Center for Environmental Health, Munich, Germany
carsten.marr@helmholtz-muenchen.de

[4] Computer Aided Medical Procedures (CAMP),
Johns Hopkins University, Baltimore, USA

**Abstract.** Deep neural networks have achieved tremendous success in image recognition, classification and object detection. However, deep learning is often criticised for its lack of transparency and general inability to rationalise its predictions. The issue of poor model interpretability becomes critical in medical applications: a model that is not understood and trusted by physicians is unlikely to be used in daily clinical practice. In this work, we develop a novel multi-task deep learning framework for simultaneous histopathology image classification and retrieval, leveraging on the classic concept of k-nearest neighbours to improve model interpretability. For a test image, we retrieve the most similar images from our training databases. These retrieved nearest neighbours can be used to classify the test image with a confidence score, and provide a human-interpretable explanation of our classification. Our original framework can be built on top of any existing classification network (and therefore benefit from pretrained models), by (i) combining a triplet loss function with a novel triplet sampling strategy to compare distances between samples and (ii) adding a Cauchy hashing loss function to accelerate neighbour searching. We evaluate our method on colorectal cancer histology slides and show that the confidence estimates are strongly correlated with model performance. Nearest neighbours are intuitive and useful for expert evaluation. They give insights into understanding possible model failures, and can support clinical decision making by comparing archived images and patient records with the actual case.

TP and NN acknowledge support from the DFG funded CRC SFB824(Z2). CM acknowledges support from SFB1243 (A09) and the "MicMode-I2T" project (FKZ#017x1710D) funded by the Federal Ministry of Education and Research of Germany (BMBF), DLR project management, in the "e:Med" framework program.

D. Shen et al. (Eds.): MICCAI 2019, LNCS 11764, pp. 676–684, 2019.
https://doi.org/10.1007/978-3-030-32239-7_75

# 1    Introduction

Since the overwhelming success of deep learning in the ImageNet challenge in 2012 [1], image recognition techniques are now based on deep learning. This is also true for histopathological image analysis, with deep learning based methods developed for mitosis detection [2], cancer classification [3], mutation prediction [4] and survival prediction [5].

Despite the breakthroughs they have made, the adoption of deep neural networks in daily clinical practice is slow. One bottleneck is that deep neural networks are often perceived as 'black-box' models, as it is very difficult to understand how networks make their predictions with their millions of model parameters. This issue becomes critical in computational pathology, as pathologists need to understand the rationale of a network's decision to use it for diagnostic purpose. Moreover, recent studies have found that deep neural networks are particularly vulnerable to adversarial examples [6]: with a small amount of image pixel permutations that are imperceptible to human, adversarial inputs can easily fool deep neural network and result in completely wrong classification, which suggests that it is dangerous to use deep neural networks without expert control.

In this paper, we aim to improve model interpretability of deep neural networks to pathologists without the need of a computational background. Inspired by the decision making process of pathologists, i.e. relating the current case to similar cases stored in their brains, we design a multi-task learning framework for simultaneous image classification and retrieval. In addition to cross-entropy loss used for the classification task, we add a triplet loss function to compare the distance between samples [7] and a Cauchy hashing loss function to accelerate nearest neighbour search in Hamming space [8]. Through deeply retrieved nearest neighbour images, we can provide pathologists with intuitive explanations of model predictions by visualizing the embedding space that is close to human perception, and calculate confidence by measuring the variations of the retrieved neighbours. This approach pushes classification networks in histopathology for the first time towards confident, interpretable and efficient image retrieval and hence will have a big impact on the quickly growing field of computational pathology.

# 2    Method

A schematic of our proposed multi-task learning framework for k-nearest neighbour retrieval is shown in Fig. 1. Each compartment of the framework is explained in the following subsections.

## 2.1    Triplet Loss with Batch-Hard Sampling

The triplet loss has been first introduced for face recognition [7]. In contrast to Siamese networks that measure pairwise distance, triplet loss considers the triangular relationship between three samples: an anchor instance $x$, a positive instance $x^+$ that is similar to $x$ (usually belonging to the same class), and a negative instance $x^-$ that is different from $x$ (usually belonging to a different class). The network is then trained to learn an embedding function $f(.)$, with a loss function defined in [9]:

$$L_a(d^+, d^-) = \|(d^+, d^- - 1)\|^2 \tag{1}$$

where:

$$d^+ = \frac{e^{\|f(x)-f(x^+)\|_2}}{e^{\|f(x)-f(x^+)\|_2} + e^{\|f(x)-f(x^-)\|_2}}, d^- = \frac{e^{\|f(x)-f(x^-)\|_2}}{e^{\|f(x)-f(x^+)\|_2} + e^{\|f(x)-f(x^-)\|_2}}. \tag{2}$$

Fundamental to triplet networks is the right sampling strategy. Random sampling is usually not sufficient as most random negative images radically differ from the anchor image in the embedding space and no longer contribute to the gradients in the optimisation process. Hence, [7] proposed a batch-hard strategy which selects for each anchor sample the most distant positive (hard-positive) sample and the closest negative (hard-negative) sample. Here we propose an improved batch-hard strategy: (1) sample a balanced data set of $k$ samples from each of the $n$ classes; (2) compute embedding for each sample; (3) choose each sample to be an anchor, and match it with all $k - 1$ positive samples; (4) for

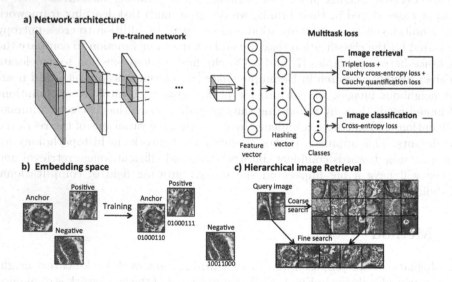

**Fig. 1.** A multi-task learning framework for simultaneous image classification and retrieval. (a) Our network consists of a convolutional neural network backbone for learning a deep representation of each image as a feature vector and a multi-loss function for simultaneous image retrieval and classification. (b) During training, we use a triple loss function which brings close samples from same class and push apart samples from different classes and Cauchy loss function to encoder every image into a binary code. (c) During testing, for each query image, we first make a rapid image retrieval based on binary codes and then make a finer retrieval based on feature vectors.

each anchor sample, choose $k$ closest negative (hard-negative) samples, hence matching all anchor-positive pairs. This strategy results in $n * k * (k-1)$ triplets when computing $n * k$ embeddings only, which is more computational efficient than the original strategy where three embeddings were computed for one triplet. Moreover, sampling $k$ hard-negative samples instead of one makes our approach more robust against outliers.

## 2.2   Cauchy Loss for Efficient Image Retrieval in Hamming Space

Although the triplet network can train an efficient embedding function that preserves similarity, the resulted embedding vectors are continuous and need a $L2$ distance comparison for neighbour searching. A more efficient searching method is hashing, which compares binary codes in hamming space [10]. Recent works have focused on combining convolutional neural network with hashing methods, yielding an end-to-end framework that jointly preserves pairwise similarity and controls the quantization error [10]. Here we use the Deep Cauchy Hashing proposed in [8], which achieves superior performance over other state-of-the-art hashing approaches such as Hashnet [11]. In combination with our triplet sampling, we write the Cauchy loss function as:

$$L_b(x, x^+, x^-) = \log \frac{\|f(x)-f(x^+)\|_2}{\gamma} + \log \left(1 + \frac{\gamma}{\|f(x)-f(x^+)\|_2}\right) + \log \left(1 + \frac{\gamma}{\|f(x)-f(x^-)\|_2}\right) \quad (3)$$

$$L_c(x, x^+, x^-) = \log \left(1 + \frac{\|f(x)-1\|_2}{\gamma}\right) + \log \left(1 + \frac{\|f(x^+)-1\|_2}{\gamma}\right) + \log \left(1 + \frac{\|f(x^-)-1\|_2}{\gamma}\right) \quad (4)$$

where $L_b$ is the cross-entropy term that preserves similarities and $L_c$ measures the quantification error before and after discretization, where we generate a binary hashing code by taking the sign of each neuron of the hashing vector. The scale parameter $\gamma$ controls the decaying speed of the probability of the Cauchy distribution: a smaller $\gamma$ will impose more force to concentrate similar samples into a small Hamming radius. Here we choose $\gamma$ to be $K/2$, where $K$ is the bit number of our hashing code.

## 2.3   Cross-entropy Loss as an Auxiliary Classification Task

To enable our framework for classification, we add a classification layer after the hashing layer, in which a cross-entropy loss is used to minimize the discrepancy between prediction and ground-truth labels. The addition of a classification function also allows us to compare the performance of our framework to previous work of [5], which use standard classification networks.

## 2.4   Hierarchical Image Retrieval

In the testing phase, for each query image, we adopt a coarse-to-fine search strategy for rapid and accurate image retrieval (see Fig. 1c). We first retrieve a candidate pool with similar binary hashing codes after discretisation within a small Hamming radius (e.g. of 1) from the query image. To further filter images with similar appearance, we extract the feature vector (one layer before the hashing vector, see Fig. 1a) and rank the retrieved samples using a $L_2$ distance of the feature vector. In our implementation, we use the built-in functions *Ball-Tree* and *cKDTree* of the *Scikit-learn* toolbox for nearest neighbour searching in Hamming space and Euclidean space, respectively. As one important purpose of our image retrieval is for expert evaluation, we limit the number of retrieved images for each query image to be 10.

### 2.5   Confidence Measure

The retrieved nearest neighbours of a given query image also provide a straight-forward confidence measure of our prediction on that image by simply counting the frequency of the predicted class in the retrieved neighbourhood.

## 3   Results and Discussions

### 3.1   Experimental Data

To evaluate our framework we use the colorectal cancer (CRC) histology dataset [5]. It contains more than 100,000 hematoxylin-eosin (HE)-stained image patches from 86 CRC tissue slides from the NCT biobank and the UMM pathology archive (NCT-CRC-HE-100K) and a testing data set of 7,180 image patches from 25 CRC patients from an independent cohort (CRC-VAL-HE-7K). Both datasets are created by pathologists by manually delineating tissue regions in whole slide images into the following nine tissue classes: adipose tissue, background, cellular debris (comedonecrosis), lymphocytes, extracellular mucus, smooth muscle (lamina muscularis mucosae), normal colon mucosa, cancer-associated stroma, and neoplastic cell population (CRC epithelium). CRC epithelium was exclusively derived from human CRC specimen (primary and metastatic). Normal tissue such as smooth muscle and adipose tissue was mostly derived from CRC surgical specimen, but also from upper gastrointestinal tract specimen (including smooth muscle from gastrectomy) in order to maximize variability in this training set. The created non-overlapping image patches are $224 \times 224$ px ($112 \times 112\,\mu$m) and have a approximately equal distribution among the nine tissue classes. [5] trained a classification network on NCT-CRC-HE-100K and reach 98.8% accuracy on the test split of the dataset and 94.3% accuracy on the independent test set (CRC-VAL-HE-7K).

### 3.2   Evaluation of Image Classification

To train our framework we split the training data (NCT-CRC-HE-100K) into 70% training set, 15% validation set and 15% test set. The independent cohort (CRC-VAL-HE-7K) is used for testing purpose only. We choose convolutional neural networks of different architectures and replace the last layer of each network with our hashing and classification layers (see Sect. 2 and Fig. 1). To train each network, we initiate it with ImageNet pretrained weights, train our added layers first and then fine tuning the entire network. In addition to different network architectures, we also examine the influence of multi-task learning by comparing the classification performance when training with multi-task loss vs. training with cross-entropy loss for classification only. The classification accuracy we achieve is comparable to the results reported in [5], suggesting our networks are properly trained (see Table 1). Moreover, we demonstrate that the multi-task learning improves the classification performance on an unseen test set, suggesting the advantage of using our multi-task loss combination. It also illustrates that there is a domain shift between the histology images from the two different cohorts, so the network that achieves the best performance on the internal test set of NCT-CRC-HE-100K does not generalize best on the independent CRC-VAL-HE-7K test set.

## 3.3    Evaluation of Image Retrieval

To evaluate image retrieval, we use the entire NCT-CRC-HE-100K set as our database and the independent CRC-VAL-HE-7K set as query images. As explained in Sect. 2.4, for a query image, we use the coarse-to-fine strategy to retrieve its nearest neighbours. To make a comparison, we formulate a baseline neighbour searching method for our classification network: we amend our coarse search to compare hashing vectors without discretisation using $L_2$ distance and to retrieve 100 neighbours as the candidate pool for the next fine search. We measure our retrieval precision for each query image by counting the number of true neighbours, i.e. belonging to the same class, among the top 10 retrieved samples, as proposed in [8,11]. Over 6000 images out of our 7180 query images reach a perfect retrieval precision of 10 true neighbours by using our multi-task network (Fig. 2), which is around 30% higher than that achieved by the baseline classification network (4697 images). This suggests that the embedding space created by the multi-task framework is more compact, i.e. a sample is surrounded predominantly by neighbours of its own class. By contrast, in the embedding space created by the baseline classification, a sample is more mixed with neighbours of different classes. A dispersed embedding could be one reason that classification networks are vulnerable to attacks of adversarial samples [6].

Figure 4 shows exemplary results of our image retrieval. The first query image is a patch of the cancer-associated stroma. While the classification network confuses it with patches of smooth muscle in healthy tissue due to their similar

**Table 1.** Evaluation of classification accuracy on both test set of NCT-CRC-HE-100K and an independent test set of CRC-VAL-HE-7K.

| Testing accuracy | Multitask Resnet18 | Resnet18 | Resnet34 | Resnet50 | VGG19[a] |
|---|---|---|---|---|---|
| NCT-CRC-HE-100K (%) | 98.6 | 98.5 | 98.8 | **99.4** | 98.8 |
| CRC-VAL-HE-7K (%) | **95.0** | 94.4 | 94.2 | 93.6 | 94.3 |

[a]The results of VGG19 is directly quoted from [5] and are shown here as a comparison.

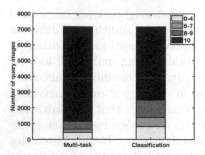

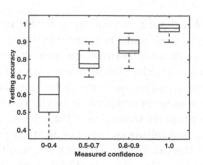

**Fig. 2.** Multi-task learning retrieves more correct images than simple classification.

**Fig. 3.** Our confidence measure is highly correlated with their testing accuracy (variations come from multiple testing of batches of size 50).

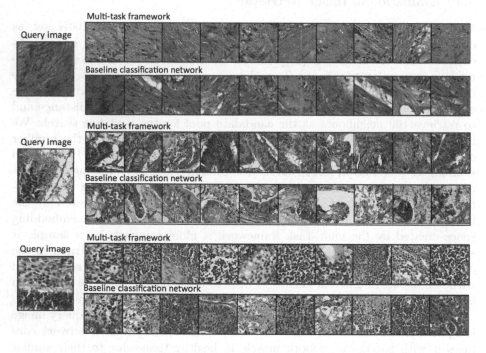

**Fig. 4.** The top 10 retrieved images returned by our multi-task framework as compared to a baseline classification network for exemplary cases. See text for explanation.

colour appearance, our multi-task network, by contrast, is not fooled by the colour variations and is able to reach perfect retrieval. The second query image is a patch of colorectal adenocarcinoma epithelium, which is mixed with normal colon mucosa by the classification network but not by the multi-task network.

Figure 3 shows that the confidence measurement of our framework is highly correlated with the actual performance of our classification on the testing set. One exemplary low confident retrieval case captured by our framework is shown in the last row of Fig. 4, the query image is annotated as normal colon mucosa yet is considered to be mostly lymphocytes, debris, cancer-associated stroma and colorectal adenocarcinoma epithelium by our framework. An expert pathologist also reviewed the case and did not agree with its original annotation as normal colon mucosa, though a more definite conclusion could not be reached due to the limited context provided by this patch. Our framework can be used to highlight these uncertain cases for review by more than one pathologists.

## 4    Conclusion

We propose a novel multi-task learning framework for simultaneous image classification and retrieval. Our objective function is composed of a triplet loss function to compare distance between samples, a Cauchy hashing loss function to accelerate nearest neighbour search in Hamming space and a classic cross-entropy loss to assess classification performance. We demonstrate that such a multi-task learning framework learns a more compact and accurate embedding space as compared to classic classification networks and allows medical experts to explore and check the embedding space without the need of in-depth machine learning knowledge. Moreover, we illustrate that the confidence measure provided by the variations of the retrieved neighbourhood is highly correlated with the model performance and hence can be used to select low confident predictions for expert review. Our framework can be turned into a very useful tool to support clinical decision making of pathologists by comparing archived images and patient records with the actual case.

## References

1. Krizhevsky, A., et al: ImageNet classification with deep convolutional neural networks. In: NIPS, pp. 1097-1105 (2012)
2. Cireşan, Dan C., Giusti, Alessandro, Gambardella, Luca M., Schmidhuber, Jürgen: Mitosis detection in breast cancer histology images with deep neural networks. In: Mori, Kensaku, Sakuma, Ichiro, Sato, Yoshinobu, Barillot, Christian, Navab, Nassir (eds.) MICCAI 2013. LNCS, vol. 8150, pp. 411–418. Springer, Heidelberg (2013). https://doi.org/10.1007/978-3-642-40763-5_51
3. Esteva, A., et al.: Dermatologist-level classification of skin cancer with deep neural networks. Nature **542**(7639), 115–118 (2017)
4. Coudray, N., et al.: Classification and mutation prediction from non small cell lung cancer histopathology images using deep learning. Nat. Med. **24**(10), 1559–1567 (2018)
5. Kather, J.N., et al.: Predicting survival from colorectal cancer histology slides using deep learning: a retrospective multicenter study. PLOS Med. **16**(1), e10027300 (2019)

6. Paschali, M., Conjeti, S., Navarro, F., Navab, N.: Generalizability *vs.* robustness: investigating medical imaging networks using adversarial examples. In: Frangi, A.F., Schnabel, J.A., Davatzikos, C., Alberola-López, C., Fichtinger, G. (eds.) MICCAI 2018. LNCS, vol. 11070, pp. 493–501. Springer, Cham (2018). https://doi.org/10.1007/978-3-030-00928-1_56

7. Shroff, F., et al.: FaceNet: a unified embedding for face recognition and clustering. In: CVPR, pp. 815–823 (2015)

8. Cao, Y., et al.: Deep cauchy hashing for hamming space retrieval. In: CVPR, pp. 1229–1237 (2018)

9. Hoffer, E., et al.: Deep metric learning using triplet network. In: ICLR, pp. 84–92 (2015)

10. Wang, J., et al.: A survey on learning to hash. IEEE Trans. Pattern Anal. Mach. Intell. **40**(4), 769–790 (2018)

11. Cao, Z., et al.: HashNet: deep learning to hash by continuation. In: ICCV, pp. 5609–5618 (2017)

# Multiclass Deep Active Learning for Detecting Red Blood Cell Subtypes in Brightfield Microscopy

Ario Sadafi[1,2,3], Niklas Koehler[1], Asya Makhro[4], Anna Bogdanova[4],
Nassir Navab[2,5], Carsten Marr[1(✉)], and Tingying Peng[1,2(✉)]

[1] Institute of Computational Biology,
Helmholtz Zentrum München – German Research Center for Environmental Health,
Munich, Germany
carsten.marr@helmholtz-muenchen.de

[2] Computer Aided Medical Procedures, Technische Universität München,
Munich, Germany
tingying.peng@tum.de

[3] Arivis AG, Munich, Germany

[4] Red Blood Cell Research Group, Institute of Veterinary Physiology,
Vetsuisse Faculty and the Zurich Center for Integrative Human Physiology,
University of Zurich, Zurich, Switzerland

[5] Computer Aided Medical Procedures, Johns Hopkins University, Baltimore, USA

**Abstract.** The recent success of deep learning approaches relies partly on large amounts of well annotated training data. For natural images object annotation is easy and cheap. For biomedical images however, annotation crucially depends on the availability of a trained expert whose time is typically expensive and scarce. To ensure efficient annotation, only the most relevant objects should be presented to the expert. Currently, no approach exists that allows to select those for a multiclass detection problem.

Here, we present an active learning framework that identifies the most relevant samples from a large set of not annotated data for further expert annotation. Applied to brightfield images of red blood cells with seven subtypes, we train a faster R-CNN for single cell identification and classification, calculate a novel confidence score using dropout variational inference and select relevant images for annotation based on (i) the confidence of the single cell detection and (ii) the rareness of the classes contained in the image. We show that our approach leads to a drastic increase of prediction accuracy with already few annotated images.

Our original approach improves classification of red blood cell subtypes and speeds up the annotation. This important step in diagnosing blood diseases will profit from our framework as well as many other clinical challenges that suffer from the lack of annotated training data.

This project has received funding from the European Union's Horizon 2020 research and innovation programme under grant agreement No 675115 – RELEVANCE – H2020-MSCA-ITN-2015/H2020-MSCA-ITN-2015. CM acknowledges support from the BMBF (Project MicMode).

© Springer Nature Switzerland AG 2019
D. Shen et al. (Eds.): MICCAI 2019, LNCS 11764, pp. 685–693, 2019.
https://doi.org/10.1007/978-3-030-32239-7_76

**Keywords:** Active learning · Multiclass annotation · Single cell
microscopy

# 1   Introduction

A typical human red blood cell can be morphologically described as a bicon-
cave discoid, called a discocyte [11]. Changes in the volume of the cell change
its appearance: as the volume decreases, it shrivels into a star-like shape
called echinocyte with distinguishable convex rounded protrusions. As volume
increases, the cell expands into a shape with single- or multi-concave invagina-
tions, called a stomatocyte. In physiological conditions, seven different morphological subtypes can be distinguished by hematologists (see Fig. 1) and appear
in a particular frequencies, which change upon environmental challenges or in a
course of a number of diseases [8].

Detection and classification of the red blood cell subtypes is a crucial step
for blood sample analysis and the diagnosis of blood diseases [11]. Earlier on,
morphological analysis was always performed on blood smears. However, more
and more 2D and 3D images of living, often moving, red blood cells are produced
for research and clinical needs with different modalities, illumination conditions
and zoom levels. Classification of red bloods cells nowadays still relies on manual
annotation by an expert.

Deep learning approaches are known to be versatile and adaptive to new
environments and excel on a couple of recent biomedical challenges, like the
classification of skin cancer [4] or the prediction of mutations from histopathological slides [2]. A first approach to the classification of red bloods cells has
been recently also proposed [14]. However in general, the application of powerful
deep learning algorithms in clinical applications is heavily limited by the need of
large amounts of well annotated data, since expert time is typically scarce and
expensive. We thus want to significantly reduce redundancy in manual annotation by developing uncertainty based scores that allow us to involve expensive
expert knowledge only where necessary.

One promising approach to break the bottleneck of data annotation is active
learning, which uses a learning algorithm to interactively query experts for new
annotations. This expert-in-the-loop process has been demonstrated to achieve
similar or even greater performance as compared to a fully labelled data-set,
with a fraction of the cost and time that it takes to label all the data [9].
Here, we combine active learning with object detection and develop a novel
active learning annotation tool to guide expert annotation. Although different
active learning methods have been proposed to accelerate the annotation process
for classification problems, e.g. [5], few approach exist that allow for object
detection, and none for a multiclass detection problem with clinical relevance.

Our active learning annotation approach interactively selects a candidate
annotation set by measuring the uncertainty of classification and detection of
single cells, and by considering rare classes in data set. Our approach is the first
to calculate relevance for the goal of active learning in multiclass object detection
and the first to come up with intelligent data selection for expert annotation for
biomedical images.

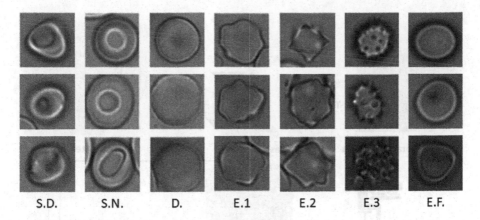

S.D.        S.N.        D.        E.1        E.2        E.3        E.F.

**Fig. 1.** Red bloods cells change their morphology due to microenvironmental changes or in the course of a disease. They can be classified into seven subtypes, from left to right: dehydrated stomatocyte (S.D.), normal stomatocyte (S.N.), discocyte (D), primary, secondary, tertiary and final echinocyte (E.1, E.2, E.3, E.F.). We show three exemplary cells for each class from our brightfield dataset containing 208 images and near 8000 cells.

## 2    Method

Our proposed active learning annotation approach starts from a Faster R-CNN model with an annotated training set (see Fig. 2). We apply the trained model on not annotated images and select the most relevant images based on a novel uncertainty analysis in order to ask for expert annotations. With these additional annotations, we update our model and select new images for more annotations. We keep iterating this annotation process until all cells above a particular uncertainty are annotated or a desired classification performance is achieved.

### 2.1    Object Detection with Faster R-CNN

Faster R-CNN is an advanced version of Fast R-CNN [6] and R-CNN [7] and was first proposed in [12]. In this approach a Fast R-CNN is coupled with a Region Proposal Network (RPN) and both networks are trained together: convolutional layers extract features from the input image, the RPN generates object proposals based on the feature map, and each proposal is classified into one of the defined classes. We used a VGG-16 network [13] pretrained on ImageNet [3] as the backbone. More formally, considering $F_\theta$ a Faster R-CNN model with weights $\theta$ and $I$ an input image we have

$$p, t^k = F_\theta(I) \tag{1}$$

where $p$ is discrete probability distribution over all classes (as is normally computed with soft-max over the last fully connected layer) and $t^k$ is the bounding

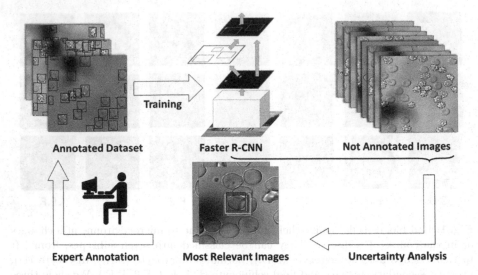

**Fig. 2.** Overview of the proposed active learning annotation tool. First, a Faster R-CNN model is trained on an annotated dataset. Not annotated images are then analyzed with the trained model, the uncertainty of detection and classification is determined, and the most relevant images are passed to the expert for annotation. With the new annotations, a new cycle starts.

box regression for every class. The multi-task loss $L$ of the Fast R-CNN can be defined as:

$$L = L_{cls}(p, u) + \lambda[u > 0]L_{loc}(t^u, v) \tag{2}$$

where $u,v$ are annotations of bounding boxes and their classes from the dataset respectively and $t^u$ is the bounding box regression corresponding to the ground truth $u$. Brackets are Iverson brackets that yield 0 for the background class ($u = 0$) and 1 for the rest. $\lambda$ is a balancing parameter between classification loss $L_{cls}$ and localization loss $L_{loc}$ [6]. The localization loss is defined as

$$L_{loc}(t_i, v) = \sum_{m \in \{x,y,w,h\}} \text{smooth}_{L1}(t_i^m - v^m). \tag{3}$$

The classification loss $L_{cls}$ is calculated with softmax cross entropy:

$$L_{cls} = -\log p_u. \tag{4}$$

For training we used an approximate joint training method [12].

## 2.2   Uncertainty Score per Cell

For each cell, we measure the uncertainty of our model prediction with three scores: (i) the detection uncertainty, (ii) the classification uncertainty and (iii) a binary score for the possibility of the object belonging to a rare class. We explain each score in the following subsections.

**Detection Uncertainty.** For each non-annotated image, we apply our model $N$ times and quantify uncertainty using dropout variational inference [10]. To evaluate the certainty of the model in detecting cells, we compare bounding boxes of each cell across $N$ inferences. For every inference, we only keep the bounding box of the class that has the highest probability in $p$. We call this bounding box $d$. Our uncertainty score of detection $U^d$ is thus defined as

$$U^d = \frac{1}{N-1} \sum_{i=2}^{i=N} \text{IoU}(d_1, d_i) \tag{5}$$

where $d_i$ is bounding box $d$ in the $i^{th}$ inference and IoU measures intersection over union between two given bounding boxes. It is clear that $U^d \in [0,1]$.

**Classification Uncertainty.** For each detected cell, the most probable class $c$ from $p$ is picked. Having $N$ inferences we have the set $c = \{c_1, c_2, ..., c_N\}$. Hence, we measure the uncertainty of classification using

$$U^c = \frac{1}{N} \sum_{i=1}^{N} [c_i = c_m] \tag{6}$$

where $c_m$ is the mode, i.e. the item with the most frequency, in set $c$ and $U^c$ is its frequency. Similar to $U^d$, $U^c$ is also in $[0,1]$.

**Rare Class Prediction.** The red blood cell dataset has a strong class unbalance: cells belonging to the discocyte (D.) or primary echinocyte (E.1, see Fig. 1) class are much more frequent compared to dehydrated stomatocytes (S.D.) or final echinocytes (E.F.). Blood cells of rare classes are clinically interesting yet detecting them is extremely challenging due to the small number of samples and large variations in appearance. In order to boost the precision of detection in rare classes, we introduce a metric $U^r$ to prioritize annotation of those cells that are likely to belong to a rare class.

$$\forall j \in R : U^r = \begin{cases} 0 & p^j \leq 0.2 \\ 1 & p^j > 0.2 \end{cases} \tag{7}$$

where $R$ is the set of rare classes and $p^j$ is the probability of class $j$ in the Faster R-CNN discrete class probability.

## 2.3   Relevance Score per Image

We rank every non-annotated image with a relevance score defined as

$$R_{\text{img}} = \sum_{j=1}^{M}(U_j^c \leq \alpha) + \sum_{j=1}^{M}(U_j^d \leq \beta) + \gamma \times \sum_{j=1}^{M} U_j^r \tag{8}$$

where $M$ is the number of detected cells in the image, and $\alpha$ and $\beta$ are thresholds defined for detection and classification uncertainties. Images having a higher uncertainty are selected for the analysis of the expert. $\gamma$ weights the contribution of cells that are suspected to be rare classes. In our experiments, we chose $\alpha = 0.80$, $\beta = 0.90$ and $\gamma = 10$.

## 3 Experiment and Results

### 3.1 Data

Our dataset consists of 208 brightfield images with $572 \times 572$ pixel obtained from human blood samples by an Axiocam mounted on Axiovert 200 m Zeiss microscope with a 100x objective. Cells are not stained and no preprocessing is performed. Each image contains 30–40 cells, with a total of 7669 cells in the dataset. Each red blood cell belongs to one out of seven classes according to the morphology classification shown in Fig. 1. Class frequency is highly unbalanced: While we find 3803 (=50%) discocytes, but only 36 (=0.5%) dehydrated stomatocytes. From the 208 images, we use 30 expert annotated images ($\approx$1100 cells) to train our initial Faster R-CNN model and hold out 20 annotated images ($\approx$720 cells) to evaluate the model accuracy. The remaining images are used for experiments of either active-learning guided expert annotation or randomly selected annotation.

### 3.2 Cell Uncertainty

Our approach is able to determine the uncertainty of each single cell, calculate the relevance of each image and rank images for annotation accordingly. Figure 3 shows three exemplary images with different types of cells selected by our strategy: cells associated with high detection uncertainty (Fig. 3a), cells associated with high classification uncertainty (Fig. 3b), and cells that are predicted to belong to a rare class (Fig. 3c). We highlight these cells in red boxes. In contrary, cells in green boxes are considered to be less informative for the model and do not require expert review. Images containing many or highly uncertain cells are ranked as highly relevant and presented to the expert for annotation.

### 3.3 Evaluation

We evaluate our active learning annotation approach systematically by comparing its performance with a baseline method where the expert is asked to annotate randomly selected images. In Fig. 4a we show the object detection precision for all seven classes, weighted by the number of cells in each class:

$$\text{Precision}_{\text{all}} = \frac{\sum_{k=1}^{K} N_k \times AP_k}{\sum_{k=1}^{K} N_k} \tag{9}$$

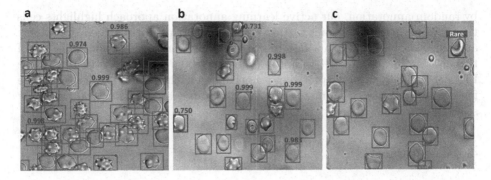

**Fig. 3.** Exemplary cells (marked with a red box) that are considered to need expert annotation by our uncertainty assessment due to uncertain classification (a), uncertain detection (b) and association to a rare class (c). In (a) and (b), numbers above boxes indicate the measured certainty per instance and red boxes are below the acceptable threshold. (Color figure online)

where $N_k$ is number of detected cells in class $k$. This value increases by 5% as we add 1000 newly annotated cells using active learning. In contrast, the performance boost with the same number of randomly annotated cells is slower and around only 2% for 1000 additionally annotated cells. The difference between the two methods is even more pronounced in the detection precision of blood cells of a rare class. The peculiar morphology of dehydrated stomatocytes and a potential over-representation has been linked to disease mutations [1]. Hence an accurate detection of this subtype is clinically highly important but impeded by the rareness of the cells. While dehydrated stomatocytes can be hardly captured

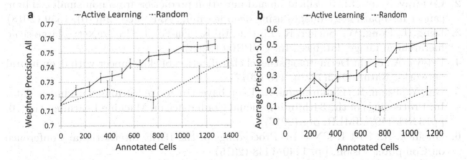

**Fig. 4.** Active learning based annotation boosts the precision in cell detection and classification. (a) Weighted detection precision of all classes increases more rapidly with active learning (solid line) as compared to a random selection of cells (dashed) (b) Average precision for the rare class of dehydrated stomatocytes (S.D.), a rare subtype with high clinical relevance, increases sharply when active learning is used. We show the mean and standard deviation from 10 experiments, where we order the images to be newly annotated either randomly, or by sorting 50 randomly selected images according to their relevance score.

by random annotation, our active learning annotation approach highlights cells that are predicted to belong to this rare class and prioritizes them for expert annotations. This leads to a fast increase of the average detection precision of this class from around 15% to around 50% for 1000 newly annotated cells (see Fig. 4b), while the average precision is unchanged in the random approach, where few if any dehydrated stomatocytes are annotated among the 1000 randomly selected new annotations.

## 4   Conclusion

Our original active learning annotation approach is able to speed up annotation and improve classification of red blood cell sub-types. This is an important task in diagnosis and prognosis of many blood diseases. Efficient annotation is urgently required for other biomedical data sets, and in particular for digital pathology applications. An extension of our framework into a software prototype will boost annotated data sets and open new avenues for computational pathology solutions.

**Acknowledgements.** CM acknowledges support from the DFG funded SFB1243 (A09) and the "MicMode-I2T" project (FKZ#017x1710D) funded by the Federal Ministry of Education and Research of Germany (BMBF), DLR project management, in the "e:Med" framework program

## References

1. Andolfo, I., et al.: Multiple clinical forms of dehydrated hereditary stomatocytosis arise from mutations in piezo1. Blood **121**(19), 3925–3935 (2013)
2. Coudray, N., et al.: Classification and mutation prediction from non-small cell lung cancer histopathology images using deep learning. Nat. Med. **24**(10), 1559 (2018)
3. Deng, J., Dong, W., Socher, R., Li, L.J., Li, K., Fei-Fei, L.: ImageNet: a large-scale hierarchical image database. In: CVPR09 (2009)
4. Esteva, A., et al.: Dermatologist-level classification of skin cancer with deep neural networks. Nature **542**(7639), 115 (2017)
5. Gal, Y., Islam, R., Ghahramani, Z.: Deep bayesian active learning with image data. In: Proceedings of the 34th International Conference on Machine Learning, vol. 70, pp. 1183–1192. JMLR. org (2017)
6. Girshick, R.: Fast R-CNN. In: Proceedings of the IEEE International Conference on Computer Vision, pp. 1440–1448 (2015)
7. Girshick, R., Donahue, J., Darrell, T., Malik, J.: Rich feature hierarchies for accurate object detection and semantic segmentation. In: Proceedings of the IEEE Conference on Computer Vision and Pattern Recognition, pp. 580–587 (2014)
8. Hw, G.L., Wortis, M., Mukhopadhyay, R.: Stomatocyte-discocyte-echinocyte sequence of the human red blood cell: evidence for the bilayer-couple hypothesis from membrane mechanics. Proc. Natl. Acad. Sci. **99**(26), 16766–16769 (2002)
9. Ilhan, H.O., Amasyali, M.F.: Active learning as a way of increasing accuracy. Int. J. Comput. Theory Eng. **6**(6), 460 (2014)

10. Kendall, A., Gal, Y.: What uncertainties do we need in bayesian deep learning for computer vision? In: Advances in Neural Information Processing Systems, pp. 5574–5584 (2017)
11. Minetti, G., et al.: Red cell investigations: art and artefacts. Blood Rev. **27**(2), 91–101 (2013)
12. Ren, S., He, K., Girshick, R., Sun, J.: Faster R-CNN: towards real-time object detection with region proposal networks. In: Advances in Neural Information Processing Systems, pp. 91–99 (2015)
13. Simonyan, K., Zisserman, A.: Very deep convolutional networks for large-scale image recognition. arXiv preprint arXiv:1409.1556 (2014)
14. Xu, M., Papageorgiou, D.P., Abidi, S.Z., Dao, M., Zhao, H., Karniadakis, G.E.: A deep convolutional neural network for classification of red blood cells in sickle cell anemia. PLoS Comput. Biol. **13**(10), e1005746 (2017)

# Enhanced Cycle-Consistent Generative Adversarial Network for Color Normalization of H&E Stained Images

Niyun Zhou, De Cai, Xiao Han, and Jianhua Yao[✉]

Tencent AI Lab, Shenzhen 518057, China
{niccozhou,daviddecai,haroldhan,jianhuayao}@tencent.com

**Abstract.** Due to differences in tissue preparations, staining protocols and scanner models, stain colors of digitized histological images are excessively diverse. Color normalization is almost a necessary procedure for quantitative digital pathology analysis. Though several color normalization methods have been proposed, most of them depend on selection of representative templates and may fail in regions not matching the templates. We propose an enhanced cycle-GAN based method with a novel auxiliary input for the generator by computing a stain color matrix for every H&E image in the training set. The matrix guides the translation in the generator, and thus stabilizes the cycle consistency loss. We applied our proposed method as a pre-processing step for a breast metastasis classification task on a dataset from five medical centers and achieved the highest performance compared to other color normalization methods. Furthermore, our method is template-free and may be applied to other datasets without finetuning.

**Keywords:** Color normalization · Stain color matrix · Generative adversarial network

## 1 Introduction

Computer-aided diagnosis of H&E stained images is a tendency in digital pathology. With the help of dedicated algorithms, doctors can be much more efficient to finish quantitative tasks such as counting mitosis and detecting cancerous regions. However, tissue preparation, staining protocol, and even digital scanner have significant influences on the color appearance of H&E images, and thus affect the performance of image analysis algorithms. Therefore, it is necessary to pre-process the input images before quantitative analysis. One solution is to normalize all H&E stained images to similar color patterns and minimize the impact of color variation on subsequent computational process.

**Electronic supplementary material** The online version of this chapter (https://doi.org/10.1007/978-3-030-32239-7_77) contains supplementary material, which is available to authorized users.

D. Shen et al. (Eds.): MICCAI 2019, LNCS 11764, pp. 694–702, 2019.
https://doi.org/10.1007/978-3-030-32239-7_77

Several color normalization methods have been proposed, which can be categorized in three sub-classes: histogram matching, color deconvolution and deep learning. The histogram-matching based methods aim to transfer the color statistics of the target image to the input image. Reinhard et al. [11] converted images to $l\alpha\beta$ space and scaled the input image by factors related to the standard deviation of color distribution of both images. The quality of transfer highly depends on the histogram similarity of the two images.

Color deconvolution methods first decompose light absorbing stain colors and then apply stain color components of the target image onto the input image. Ruifrok and Johnston [12] manually selected representative pixels to estimate the color deconvolution matrix. Rabinovich et al. [10] employed non-negative matrix factorization (NMF) to perform color deconvolution. However, this method cannot guarantee a global optimum since the problem is non-convex. Macenko et al. [9] used singular value decomposition (SVD) to achieve a closed-form solution. Vahadane et al. [14] added sparseness to restrict the solution space for NMF optimization. Besides, other methods were also proposed, such as blind color decomposition (BCD) [3] and stain color descriptor (SCD) [8].

More recent methods utilized deep learning models for image encoding or feature extraction. An unsupervised sparse autoencoder (StaNoSA) [6] was trained to subdivide the input image into sub-type tissue regions and independent color normalization was performed to match each tissue type with a single template. BenTaieb and Hamarneh [2] used generative adversarial network (GAN) to train a task-specific network and a generative model to learn image-specific color translation. Zanjani et al. [15] employed GAN in CIELab color space with prior latent variables with an auxiliary network used to estimate image noise after transformation.

Most of the aforementioned methods are template based, which extract a translation matrix from given target images. However, the template may not represent all input images. For example, in the region containing lots of adipocytes, nucleuses are scarce and the tissue appearance is vastly different from other tissue regions, which may result in mismatch and poor performance in template-based color normalization.

In this paper, we propose a template-free method based on cycle consistency GAN (named color normalization GAN, CNGAN) for color normalization of H&E stained images. We add a novel auxiliary input for the generator to guide the color translation. We also propose an approach to automatically generate a stable stain color domain from the training set so that template is not needed.

## 2   Method

We formulate the color normalization problem as translating the color pattern of images from one domain (domain $A$) to the color pattern in another domain (domain $B$), where domain $A$ has a wide spectrum of color patterns and domain $B$ has a relatively uniform color pattern. Our proposed method is summarized as follow: given a training set of images with various color patterns (domain $A$), we first extract a subset of images to be domain $B$. We then train an enhanced cycle-GAN to translate color patterns in domain $A$ to domain $B$ and backward. A stain color matrix is designed to facilitate training. The trained model allows us to normalize all H&E images within the color pattern of domain $B$.

## 2.1    Stain Color Matrix for H&E Stain Images

The hematoxylin and eosin dyes bind to specific cell structures and tissues and absorb different spectrum of lights. This procedure can be described by Beer-Lambert law. Let $A$ be the absorbance matrix of the stains appearing in the image. Let $I_0$ be the incident light intensity, and let $I_t$ be the transmission light intensity. Then $A$ can be written as

$$A = \log \frac{I_0}{I_t}. \tag{1}$$

$I_t \in R^{m \times n}$ is the matrix representing a H&E stain image, where $m = 3$ for RGB channels, and $n$ is number of pixels in the image. Let $W \in R^{m \times s}$ be the stain color matrix, where $s = 2$ is the number of stains, and let $H \in R^{s \times n}$ be the stain density maps. $I_t$ can be written as [3]

$$I_t = I_0 \exp(-WH). \tag{2}$$

Combine Eqs. (1) and (2)

$$A = WH. \tag{3}$$

$A$ can be calculated from original H&E stained images. We use sparse non-negative matrix factorization (SNMF) to solve $W$ and $H$, which significantly outperforms NMF in color deconvolution [14].

Stain color matrix $W$ is a $3 \times 2$ matrix. Each row of $W$ represents one RGB channel, and two columns represent hematoxylin and eosin stain appearance, respectively. $W$ describes the stain statistics of a H&E image. We visualize stain color matrices by drawing vectors starting with its first column and ending with the second column in a 3-D coordinate space (see Fig. 1 and Supplementary Fig. 1 for details). The matrices are used as an auxiliary input in our model to guide the color translation.

## 2.2    Stain Color Matrix Enhanced Cycle-GAN

It is not trivial to compute the color translation between two domains, especially when the data are not paired. We enhance the original cycle-GAN and apply it to color normalization of histopathological H&E stained images.

Domain $A$ has images from multiple sources with various stain styles. In order to form a domain $B$ with relatively uniform stain style, we apply a k-means clustering technique on the stain color matrices of images in domain $A$ and retrieve a tight cluster as domain $B$. Figure 1 shows the visualization of stain color matrices in domain $A$ and $B$ and the color translation operation between them. The visualization of stain color matrices from domain $A$ indicates that the stain styles are highly diversified, whereas domain $B$ demonstrates uniform stain style.

In the original architecture of cycle-GAN, we can translate images from domain $A$ to domain $B$ but not reversely since it is an $n$-to-1 mapping from domain $A$ to domain $B$. In order to make the cycle-GAN work both ways, we use the stain color matrix as an auxiliary input to the network.

As shown in Fig. 2, our proposed CNGAN contains two cycles: domain $A \rightarrow$ domain $B$ (forward cycle consistency, green arrows) and domain $B \rightarrow$ domain $A$ (backward cycle consistency, blue arrows). In forward cycle consistency, one image from domain $A$ (denoted as $a$) is translated to domain $B$ (denoted as $\hat{b}$) by generator $G_A$, expressed as $\hat{b} = G_A(a)$. Image $\hat{b}$ is translated back to domain $A$ (denoted as $\hat{a}$), combined with pre-calculated stain color matrix $W_A$ of the original image and generator $G_B$, i.e. $\hat{a} = G_B(\hat{b}, W_A)$. Cycle consistency loss between $a$ and $\hat{a}$ is calculated as (Fig. 2 black dashed arrows)

$$\mathcal{L}_{cycle}(G_A, G_B, A, W_A) = \mathbb{E}_{a \sim p_{data}(a)}[\|a - G_B(G_A(a), W_A)\|_1]. \quad (4)$$

In addition, discriminator $D_B$ is employed to distinguish between real image $b$ and generated image $\hat{b}$ where the adversarial loss in forward cycle $\mathcal{L}_{adv}$ can be written as

$$\mathcal{L}_{adv}(G_A, D_B, A, B) = \mathbb{E}_{b \sim p_{data}(b)}[\log D_B(b)]$$
$$+ \mathbb{E}_{a \sim p_{data}(a)}[\log(1 - D_B(G_A(a)))]. \quad (5)$$

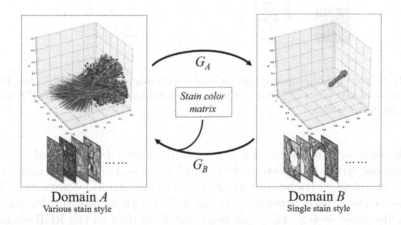

**Fig. 1.** Data distribution of domain $A$ and domain $B$. The vectors in 3-D coordinate represent stain color matrix of H&E stained images (a vector from column 1 to column 2 of stain color matrix $W$). Our method learns the mapping between these two domains.

The backward consistency cycle behaves similarly as the forward cycle. Real image from domain $B$ (denoted as $b'$) is translated to domain $A$ by generator $G_B$ with corresponding stain color matrix $W_A$ calculated in Eq. 3. Output image $\hat{a}'$ is then used to generate $\hat{b}'$ by $G_A$ to calculate cycle consistency loss $\mathcal{L}_{cycle}(G_A, G_B, B, W_A)$. Meanwhile, $\hat{a}'$ and real image $a$ are used to train discriminator $D_A$. Adversarial loss in backward cycle $\mathcal{L}_{adv}(G_B, D_A, A, B)$ is calculated in a similar way as the forward cycle. The overall loss of our CNGAN expressed as

$$\mathcal{L}(G_A, G_B, D_A, D_B, W_A) = \mathcal{L}_{adv}(G_A, D_B, A, B) + \mathcal{L}_{adv}(G_B, D_A, A, B)$$
$$+ \lambda(\mathcal{L}_{cycle}(G_A, G_B, A, W_A) + \mathcal{L}_{cycle}(G_A, G_B, B, W_A)).$$
(6)

The objective of our CNGAN is to maximize the loss in $D_A$ and $D_B$ and minimize the loss in $G_A$ and $G_B$. The full objective of CNGAN is

$$G_A^*, G_B^* = \arg \min_{G_A, G_B} \max_{D_A, D_B} \mathcal{L}(G_A, G_B, D_A, D_B, W_A).$$
(7)

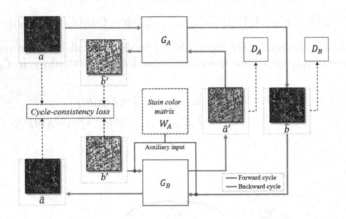

**Fig. 2.** An overview of proposed approach for color normalization of H&E stain images. Stain color matrix plays important role in translating image from domain $B$ to domain $A$. (Color figure online)

The architecture of generator $G_A$ is modified from Johnson et al. [7], which contains one stride-1 and two stride-2 convolutions and followed by nine residual blocks, two stride-2 transpose convolutions and one stride-1 convolution. Batch normalization is used between each layers. Network architecture of generator $G_B$ is the same as $G_A$. The stain color matrix is tiled to the RGB channel of input image. For discriminators, $70 \times 70$ PatchGAN [5] is used: three stride-2 and two stride-1 convolutions with leaky ReLU activation functions and batch normalization layers. Shrivastava et al.'s strategy [13] is used: 50 previously generated images are buffered and imported into discriminator instead of one latest generated image, which is effective to stabilize adversarial loss.

The training procedure proceeds as follow: first, stain color matrix $W_A$ of input images from domain $A$ is calculated and the forward cycle is run ($a \rightarrow$

$\hat{b} \to \hat{a}$). Next, the backward cycle is executed to translate real images $b'$ from domain $B$ to domain $A$ and back to domain $B$ ($b' \to \hat{a}' \to \hat{b}'$) using the stain color matrix $W_A$. Due to the guidance of $W_A$, the translated color in both cycles are the same, which limits the diversity of color and thus reduces the oscillation of the loss function.

After model is trained, the generator $G_A$ is capable of normalizing any stain color image to the color pattern in domain $B$.

## 3   Experiments

We evaluate the performance of our proposed color normalization method by using it as a preprocessing step for tumor classification and examine whether it improves the classification accuracy. The goal of a tumor classification task is to classify whether there are tumor cells in an H&E stained image. Methods from Reinhard et al. [11], Macenko et al. [9] and Vahadane et al. [14] were select as baseline methods for comparison.

CAMELYON16 [1] and CAMELYON17 [4] are challenges for automated classification and segmentation of breast cancer metastases in WSI of histological lymph node sections. CAMELYON16 contains WSIs from 2 independent medical centers and CAMELYON17 contains WSIs from 5 independent medical centers.

### 3.1   Training Setup

We used 270 WSIs from CAMELYON16 dataset to train the CNGAN for color normalization. Overall, 200,000 $256 \times 256$ patches were randomly cropped from the original WSIs at level 0. All patches in the training set made up domain $A$. Next, a k-means clustering technique is applied on the stain color matrices, dividing all patches in domain $A$ into 20 clusters. Top 10,000 patches closest to the cluster center in the largest cluster were selected as domain $B$. Our proposed model was trained from scratch with Adam optimizer and learning rate 0.0002. The weights were initialized with Xavier initialization and biases were initialized as zero. $\lambda$ was set to 10 in Eq. 6. Total number of training epochs was 200 and the training batch size was 4.

### 3.2   Evaluation Setup

CAMELYON17 [4] was used for evaluating our color normalization methods. Since this data set came from 5 independent medical centers, the staining style variations degrade the classification results without color normalization. Area under curve (AUC) was used as the classification performance metric.

In CAMELYON17 dataset, only 50 positive WSIs have mask level label. We randomly split these positive WSIs and all negative WSIs into training (about 80%) and test (about 20%) sets for the classification task with the following distribution (training/test): center1: 59/15, center2: 54/14, center3: 67/18, center4: 55/15, center5: 56/15. From the training set, 30% WSIs were used as validation set. Resnet50 model was used as the classifier. The batch size was 32 and Adam optimizer was used with learning rate of 0.001. All models were trained for 50 epochs. We trained a model on data from one center and evaluate it on data from the other centers. The mean AUC of all five centers with or without color normalization was used to evaluate our normalization method.

### 3.3    Result and Discussion

We applied the baseline methods and our proposed model in the pre-processing step of tumor classification task. The mean AUCs of tumor classification are listed in Table 1 and the AUC distributions are shown in Supplementary Fig. 2. Our proposed method achieved highest mean AUC in 4 out of 5 test datasets.

**Table 1.** Mean AUC of tumor classification with different color normalization methods.

| Methods | Center1 | Center2 | Center3 | Center4 | Center5 | Average |
|---|---|---|---|---|---|---|
| W/O normalization | 0.8300 | 0.7099 | 0.7211 | 0.8450 | 0.8017 | 0.7815 |
| Reinhard [11] | 0.7810 | 0.7729 | 0.8202 | 0.7962 | 0.7608 | 0.7862 |
| Macenko [9] | 0.7407 | 0.7035 | 0.8495 | 0.7151 | 0.7263 | 0.7470 |
| Vahadane [14] | 0.9266 | 0.7169 | **0.9145** | 0.8797 | 0.8044 | 0.8484 |
| Proposed | **0.9575** | **0.7878** | 0.7897 | **0.9505** | **0.9113** | **0.8794** |

By applying our model to data from five different medical centers, it demonstrates strong generalizability (Fig. 3 first two rows). We also applied our model trained on CAMELYON16 to TUPAC, MITOS-ATYPIA14 and GlaS15 datasets (Fig. 3 last two rows) without finetuning. The staining style from these datasets were translated successfully and nearly no artifacts were observed. It suggests that our model have potential to be trained as a general color normalization tool for any H&E stained images.

Our proposed method is template-free. The normalized color space is determined by domain $B$ which is formed through an unsupervised clustering step. It is much robust to different situations compared to template-dependent methods. Besides, the stain color matrix plays an essential role in our method. In data preparation stage, the pre-calculated stain color matrices are utilized to cluster images to construct domain $B$ with homogeneous color patterns. In the training step, the stain color matrix is used as an auxiliary input for generator $G_B$ which guides the direction of color translation and stabilize cycle consistency loss.

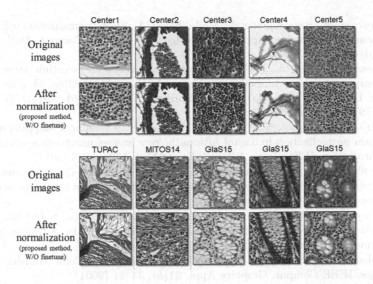

**Fig. 3.** H&E stained images from 5 medical centers of CAMELYON17, TUPAC, MITOS14 and GlaS15 datasets with or without color normalization of proposed method.

# 4 Conclusion

Color normalization is an important pre-processing step in processing H&E stained images. Most previously proposed methods rely on a normalization template which is unlikely to represent all kinds of images. We proposed an enhanced cycle-GAN method for color normalization of H&E images. It calculates stain color matrices of training images and uses them to guide the translation. The superiority and strong generalizability of our method are confirmed by comparing with other methods in metastasis classification datasets from multiple centers.

# References

1. Bejnordi, B.E., van der Laak, J.: Camelyon16: grand challenge on cancer metastasis detection in lymph nodes 2016 (2017)
2. BenTaieb, A., Hamarneh, G.: Adversarial stain transfer for histopathology image analysis. IEEE Trans. Med. Imaging **37**(3), 792–802 (2018)
3. Gavrilovic, M., et al.: Blind color decomposition of histological images. IEEE Trans. Med. Imaging **32**(6), 983–994 (2013)
4. Geessink, O., Bándi, P., Litjens, G., van der Laak, J.: Camelyon17: grand challenge on cancer metastasis detection and classification in lymph nodes (2017)
5. Isola, P., Zhu, J.Y., Zhou, T., Efros, A.A.: Image-to-image translation with conditional adversarial networks. In: Proceedings of the IEEE Conference on Computer Vision and Pattern Recognition, pp. 1125–1134 (2017)

6. Janowczyk, A., Basavanhally, A., Madabhushi, A.: Stain normalization using sparse autoencoders (stanosa): application to digital pathology. Comput. Med. Imaging Graph **57**, 50–61 (2017)
7. Johnson, J., Alahi, A., Fei-Fei, L.: Perceptual losses for real-time style transfer and super-resolution. In: Leibe, B., Matas, J., Sebe, N., Welling, M. (eds.) ECCV 2016. LNCS, vol. 9906, pp. 694–711. Springer, Cham (2016). https://doi.org/10.1007/978-3-319-46475-6_43
8. Khan, A.M., Rajpoot, N., Treanor, D., Magee, D.: A nonlinear mapping approach to stain normalization in digital histopathology images using image-specific color deconvolution. IEEE Trans. Biomed. Eng. **61**(6), 1729–1738 (2014)
9. Macenko, M., et al.: A method for normalizing histology slides for quantitative analysis. In: Proceedings of IEEE International Symposium on Biomedical Imaging, pp. 1107–1110 (2009)
10. Rabinovich, A., Agarwal, S., Laris, C., Price, J.H., Belongie, S.J.: Unsupervised color decomposition of histologically stained tissue samples. In: Advances in Neural Information Processing Systems, pp. 667–674 (2004)
11. Reinhard, E., Adhikhmin, M., Gooch, B., Shirley, P.: Color transfer between images. IEEE Comput. Graphics Appl. **21**(5), 34–41 (2001)
12. Ruifrok, A.C., Johnston, D.A., et al.: Quantification of histochemical staining by color deconvolution. Anal. Quant. Cytol. Histol. **23**(4), 291–299 (2001)
13. Shrivastava, A., Pfister, T., Tuzel, O., Susskind, J., Wang, W., Webb, R.: Learning from simulated and unsupervised images through adversarial training. In: Proceedings of the IEEE Conference on Computer Vision and Pattern Recognition, pp. 2107–2116 (2017)
14. Vahadane, A., et al.: Structure-preserving color normalization and sparse stain separation for histological images. IEEE Trans. Med. Imaging **35**(8), 1962–1971 (2016)
15. Zanjani, F.G., Zinger, S., Bejnordi, B.E., van der Laak, J.A., de With, P.H.: Stain normalization of histopathology images using generative adversarial networks. In: 2018 IEEE 15th International Symposium on Biomedical Imaging, pp. 573–577 (2018)

# Nuclei Segmentation in Histopathological Images Using Two-Stage Learning

Qingbo Kang[✉], Qicheng Lao, and Thomas Fevens

Department of Computer Science and Software Engineering, Concordia University,
Montréal, QC, Canada
{qi_kang,qi_lao,fevens}@encs.concordia.ca

**Abstract.** Nuclei segmentation is a fundamental and important task in histopathological image analysis. However, it still has some challenges such as difficulty in segmenting the overlapping or touching nuclei, and limited ability of generalization to different organs and tissue types. In this paper, we propose a novel nuclei segmentation approach based on a two-stage learning framework and Deep Layer Aggregation (DLA). We convert the original binary segmentation task into a two-step task by adding nuclei-boundary prediction (3-classes) as an intermediate step. To solve our two-step task, we design a two-stage learning framework by stacking two U-Nets. The first stage estimates nuclei and their coarse boundaries while the second stage outputs the final fine-grained segmentation map. Furthermore, we also extend the U-Nets with DLA by iteratively merging features across different levels. We evaluate our proposed method on two public diverse nuclei datasets. The experimental results show that our proposed approach outperforms many standard segmentation architectures and recently proposed nuclei segmentation methods, and can be easily generalized across different cell types in various organs.

**Keywords:** Nuclei segmentation · Convolutional neural network · Deep Layer Aggregation · Two-stage learning

## 1 Introduction

Since histopathological images provide extensive information regarding cell morphology and tissue architecture, they are used in a broad range of applications in clinical practice, e.g., medical diagnosis [8], cancer malignancy grading [4] and treatment effectiveness prediction [7]. However, the manual assessment of histopathological images by a Pathologist is time-consuming and subjective. Digital histopathological image analysis aims to automatically analyze histopathological images, which can significantly improve the reproducibility and objectivity of diagnosis [8]. In particular, segmenting each nucleus in histopathological images is a fundamental and important task. Many techniques have been proposed; an extensive review is presented in [18]. However, this task still has several challenges such as difficulty in segmenting the overlapping or touching nuclei, and limited generalization ability to different organs and tissue types.

© Springer Nature Switzerland AG 2019
D. Shen et al. (Eds.): MICCAI 2019, LNCS 11764, pp. 703–711, 2019.
https://doi.org/10.1007/978-3-030-32239-7_78

Recently, many approaches have introduced the nuclei-boundary prediction as part of nuclei segmentation to help segment overlapping or touching nuclei. Chen *et al.* [3] design a deep contour-aware network (DCAN) by utilizing contours to separate clustered objects in gland segmentation task. Kumar *et al.* [10] present a Convolutional Neural Network (CNN) model that predicts nuclei and boundary segmentation map based on a patch-wise approach. Naylor *et al.* [13] convert the binary segmentation task into a regression task by predicting the distance map of nuclei. Although these methods have lead to some performance improvements, they still have some disadvantages such as needing complex post-processing and excessive redundant computation.

U-Net [15] is an architecture based on Fully Convolutional Network (FCN) that has been widely adopted and has obtained superior performance for medical image segmentation. Among many works [2,5,6,16] that attempt to improve the original U-Net, stacking or cascading multiple U-Nets have attracted intensive research. For example, Sevastopolsky *et al.* [16] stack two kinds of building blocks, U-Net or Res-U-Net, for optic disc and cup image segmentation, while Christ *et al.* [5] cascade two U-Nets for liver and lesion segmentation in CT images. However, these approaches do not design different tasks or outputs for the sub-networks, i.e., in each case, their stacked networks perform exactly the same task with the same single output. The network designed by Bi *et al.* [2] has multiple outputs but again performs the same task.

Inspired by the core idea of curriculum learning [1] and the aforementioned segmentation approaches, we propose a novel nuclei segmentation approach based on a two-stage learning framework to solve the above-mentioned challenges in nuclei segmentation. The core idea of curriculum learning is that a complex task can be solved by dividing it into numerous sub-tasks, and one can start with the easiest one, followed by subsequent tasks that have increased level of difficulty. Specifically, in order to tackle the overlapping or touching nuclei, we convert the original binary segmentation task into a two-step task by adding the prediction of nuclei-boundary (3-classes) as an intermediate step. Along with this two-step task, we design a two-stage FCN by stacking two U-Nets that have two different outputs. The coarse boundary from the first stage acts like auxiliary information to guide the segmentation of overlapping or touching nuclei in the second stage, therefore decreases the difficulty of segmenting nuclei from scratch. Along with this two-step task, we design a two-stage FCN by stacking two U-Nets that has two different outputs. In addition, we extend our U-Net with Deep Layer Aggregation (DLA) proposed by Yu *et al.* [19], which has been demonstrated to have superior performance in many visual applications.

Consequently, this paper proposes a novel nuclei segmentation approach with two main contributions:

1. Converting the binary nuclei segmentation task into a two-step task by introducing nuclei-boundary prediction as the intermediate step. Along with the two-step task, we design a two-stage FCN by stacking two U-Nets.
2. Extending the U-Net with DLA to better fuse features across different levels and learn better semantic representations for nuclei segmentation.

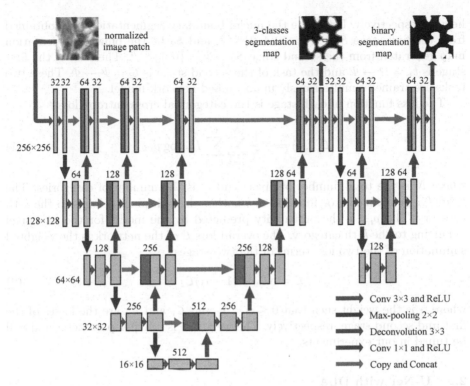

**Fig. 1.** The architecture of our proposed network. Blue boxes correspond to feature maps. The number of features is indicated on top of the box. The dimension of each level (features have the same dimension) is indicated at the bottom left of each level. (Color figure online)

## 2   Methodology

In this section, we give more details of our proposed approach for nuclei segmentation.

### 2.1   Two-Stage Learning Framework

The architecture of our proposed network is illustrated in Fig. 1. In the first stage, a U-Net with DLA is utilized to predict the 3-classes nuclei-boundary segmentation map from color-normalized image patches. For the second stage, a shallow U-Net with DLA is used to refine the coarse nuclei-boundary segmentation map generated from the first stage for the final binary segmentation map. Based on our experiments, we did not notice considerable performance difference between deep and shallow architectures for the second stage, so for the consideration of computation cost and efficiency, the shallower one is used.

Formally, let $I$ be the input color-normalized image patch, $I$ belongs to RGB image domain, $I \in \Omega = \mathbf{R}^{w \times h \times 3}$, where $w$ and $h$ represent image width and height, respectively. Let $S_1$ be the nuclei-boundary segmentation map obtained from the first stage $S_1 \in \Psi = \{0,1,2\}^{w \times h}$, and $S_2$ be the binary segmentation map generated from the second stage $S_2 \in \Phi = \{0,1\}^{w \times h}$. The task of the first stage is $t_1 = \Omega \rightarrow \Psi$ and the task of the second stage is $t_2 = \Psi \rightarrow \Phi$. These two tasks are trained simultaneously in an unified network model.

The loss function of each stage is the categorical cross entropy loss:

$$\mathcal{L}(\hat{y}, y) = -\frac{1}{N} \sum_{i=1}^{N} \sum_{k=1}^{C} I_{i,k} \log p_{i,k} \tag{1}$$

where $N$ is the total number of pixels and $C$ is the number of categories. The term $I_{i,k}$ is the indicator function of whether the $i$-th pixel belongs to the $k$-th category. The $p_{i,k}$ is the probability predicted by the model for the $i$-th pixel belonging to the $k$-th category. The overall loss $\mathcal{L}$ of the network is the weighted summation of the two loss terms of the two stages,

$$\mathcal{L} = \alpha \mathcal{L}_1 + (1 - \alpha) \mathcal{L}_2 \tag{2}$$

where $\alpha$ is the weight such that $0 \leq \alpha < 1$, and $\mathcal{L}_1$ and $\mathcal{L}_2$ are the losses of the first and second stage, respectively. The weight $\alpha$ is a hyper-parameter and will be tuned in our experiments.

## 2.2    U-Net with DLA

Originally, U-Net has skip connections to fuse low-level and high-level features. However, these connections are still linear and shallow [19]. Yu *et al.* [19] introduce two kinds of DLA: Iterative Deep Aggregation (IDA) and Hierarchical Deep Aggregation (HDA). We extend the original U-Net with IDA in this paper. Following [19], IDA is defined as

$$I(x_1, ..., x_n) = \begin{cases} x_1 & \text{if } n = 1 \\ I(N(x_1, x_2), ..., x_n) & \text{otherwise} \end{cases} \tag{3}$$

where the aggregation node is denoted as $N$. In our case, $N$ is defined as

$$N(x_1, x_2) = \text{Conv}(\text{Concat}(x_1, x_2)) \tag{4}$$

where Conv is a $3 \times 3$ convolution operation followed by ReLU activation, and Concat represents the concatenation operation.

## 3    Experiments and Results

### 3.1    Datasets

We evaluate our proposed nuclei segmentation approach on two publicly available nuclei datasets: TCGA [10] and TNBC [12]. The TCGA dataset contains 30

Hematoxylin and Eosin(H&E) stained images with $1000 \times 1000$ resolution. It's a highly diverse dataset since images are taken from seven different organs (breast, liver, kidney, prostate, bladder, colon and stomach). In total, more than 21000 nuclei are annotated in this dataset. The TNBC dataset consists of 50 H&E stained images with $512 \times 512$ resolution and 4022 nuclei have been annotated. All the images of TNBC are taken from 11 triple negative breast cancer patients, and include different cell types such as myoepithelial breast cells, endothelial cells and inflammatory cells.

### 3.2    Evaluation Metrics

Two types of metrics are used to evaluate the performance of different approaches in this paper: object-level and pixel-level metrics.

The Aggregated Jaccard Index (AJI) presented in [10] is used as an object-level evaluation metric. Basically, the AJI is an extension of the Jaccard Index. Specifically, the AJI is defined as

$$AJI = \frac{\sum_{i=1}^{K} |GT_i \cap PD_j^*(i)|}{\sum_{i=1}^{K} |GT_i \cup PD_j^*(i)| + \sum_{l \in U} |PD_l|} \tag{5}$$

where $GT = \cup_{i=1,2,\cdots,K} GT_i$ are the pixels of whole ground truth nuclei objects, and $PD = \cup_{j=1,2,\cdots,L} PD_j$ are the pixels of whole predicted nuclei objects. $PD_j^*(i)$ is the connected component object from the predicted result that has the maximum Jaccard Index with the ground truth objects, and $U$ is the union of predicted nuclei objects that does not correspond to any ground truth objects (also known as ghost objects).

For pixel-level evaluation metrics, we use precision, recall and $F_1$ score. These 3 metrics are defined as

$$precision = \frac{TP}{TP + FP}, \ recall = \frac{TP}{FN + TP}, \ F_1 = 2 \cdot (\frac{precision \cdot recall}{precision + recall}) \tag{6}$$

where $TP$ is true positives, $FP$ is false positives and $FN$ is false negatives.

### 3.3    Implementation Details

The only pre-processing preformed is color normalization and no post-processing is needed. H&E stained histopathological images in general have diverse color variations due to differences in scanners, materials and staining process. Therefore we adopt the color normalization technique proposed by Vahadane *et al.* [17] to eliminate color variations. After color normalization, image patches are seamlessly extracted by the overlap-tile strategy which was introduced by Ronneberger *et al.* [15]. For the consideration of performance and GPU memory limitation, we set the size of image patches to $256 \times 256$. The nuclei-boundary mask images for training are obtained by morphological operations on the ground truth of segmentation maps.

**Table 1.** Results by choosing different loss weight $\alpha$

| $\alpha$ | 0.0 | 0.1 | 0.2 | 0.3 | 0.4 | 0.5 | 0.6 | 0.7 | 0.8 | 0.9 |
|---|---|---|---|---|---|---|---|---|---|---|
| $F_1$ Score | 0.793 | 0.797 | 0.800 | 0.800 | 0.801 | 0.804 | 0.804 | 0.805 | **0.808** | 0.806 |
| AJI | 0.567 | 0.571 | 0.571 | 0.575 | 0.578 | 0.581 | 0.581 | 0.586 | **0.590** | 0.586 |

Since we propose two different types of improvements in our approach compared to other segmentation methods, in order to validate each of them, we implement three models in this paper, i.e., **U-Net (DLA)** which is a U-Net extended with DLA, **Ours** which is our two-stage learning model with the original U-Net and **Ours (DLA)** which combines two-stage learning and DLA. We use an ADADELTA [20] optimizer with the default values suggested by Zeiler [20] to train all the three models, with the same configuration.

### 3.4    Results and Discussions

In order to determine the loss weight $\alpha$ in Eq. 2, we perform experiments on the TCGA dataset using **Ours (DLA)** model and the results are shown in Table 1. From Table 1, we can observe that when $\alpha$ is set to 0.8, both $F_1$ score and AJI achieve the highest value. Therefore, for the rest of our experiments, the loss weight $\alpha$ is set to 0.8.

For the TCGA dataset, in order to make a comparison with other methods, we follow the same training and testing split suggested by Kumar et al. [10]. We compare our methods with numerous standard segmentation architectures such as FCN-8 [11], Mask R-CNN [9], U-Net [15] and other state-of-the-art nuclei segmentation methods like DIST [13] and CNN3 [10]. In addition, we also stack two U-Nets, where both sub-nets have the same binary segmentation task, which we call Stacked U-Net. Table 2 and Table 3 show the AJI and $F_1$ scores for different organs of different methods on the test set, respectively.

For the TNBC dataset, we follow the same leave-one-patient-out scheme used by Naylor et al. [12] to evaluate our method. Table 4 shows the experimental

**Table 2.** AJI of different methods on the TCGA test set

| Aggregated Jaccard Index (AJI) ↑ | | | | | | | | |
|---|---|---|---|---|---|---|---|---|
| Organ | Bladder | Colorectal | Stomach | Breast | Kidney | Liver | Prostate | Overall |
| FCN-8 [11] | 0.5376 | 0.4018 | 0.5279 | 0.5509 | 0.5267 | 0.5045 | 0.5709 | 0.5171 |
| Mask R-CNN [9] | 0.5011 | 0.3814 | 0.6151 | 0.4913 | 0.5182 | 0.4622 | 0.5322 | 0.5002 |
| U-Net [15] | 0.5403 | 0.4061 | 0.6529 | 0.4681 | 0.5426 | 0.4284 | 0.5888 | 0.5182 |
| CNN3 [10] | 0.5217 | 0.5292 | 0.4458 | 0.5385 | 0.5732 | **0.5162** | 0.4338 | 0.5083 |
| DIST [13] | 0.5971 | 0.4362 | 0.6479 | 0.5609 | 0.5534 | 0.4949 | **0.6284** | 0.5598 |
| Stacked U-Net | 0.6138 | 0.5188 | 0.5845 | 0.5605 | 0.5647 | 0.4594 | 0.5300 | 0.5474 |
| U-Net (DLA) | 0.6215 | 0.5322 | 0.5938 | 0.5747 | 0.5624 | 0.4642 | 0.5602 | 0.5584 |
| Ours | 0.6263 | 0.5346 | 0.6352 | 0.6037 | 0.5928 | 0.4961 | 0.5606 | 0.5784 |
| Ours (DLA) | **0.6285** | **0.5376** | **0.6620** | **0.6096** | **0.6024** | 0.5142 | 0.5720 | **0.5895** |

results of the different methods. We make a comparison with DeconvNet [14], FCN-8 [11], Ensemble method [12], U-Net [15] and Stacked U-Net.

**Table 3.** $F_1$ scores of different methods on the TCGA test set

| $F_1$ Score ↑ | | | | | | | | |
|---|---|---|---|---|---|---|---|---|
| Organ | Bladder | Colorectal | Stomach | Breast | Kidney | Liver | Prostate | Overall |
| FCN-8 [11] | 0.8084 | 0.6934 | 0.7982 | 0.8113 | 0.7597 | **0.7589** | **0.8367** | 0.7809 |
| Mask R-CNN [9] | 0.7610 | 0.6820 | 0.8269 | 0.7481 | 0.7554 | 0.7157 | 0.7401 | 0.7470 |
| U-Net [15] | 0.7953 | 0.7360 | 0.8638 | 0.7818 | 0.7913 | 0.6981 | 0.7904 | 0.7795 |
| CNN3 [10] | 0.7808 | 0.7399 | **0.8948** | 0.7181 | 0.7222 | 0.6881 | 0.7922 | 0.7623 |
| DIST [13] | 0.8196 | 0.7286 | 0.8534 | 0.8071 | 0.7706 | 0.7281 | 0.7967 | 0.7863 |
| Stacked U-Net | 0.8249 | 0.7685 | 0.8498 | 0.7990 | 0.7986 | 0.7276 | 0.7829 | 0.7930 |
| U-Net (DLA) | 0.8296 | 0.7756 | 0.8530 | 0.8025 | 0.7994 | 0.7296 | 0.7895 | 0.7970 |
| Ours | 0.8213 | 0.7773 | 0.8700 | 0.8068 | **0.8066** | 0.7437 | 0.7890 | 0.8021 |
| Ours (DLA) | **0.8360** | **0.7808** | 0.8629 | **0.8183** | 0.8022 | 0.7513 | 0.8037 | **0.8079** |

**Table 4.** Quantitative comparison of different methods on the TNBC dataset

| Method | Recall↑ | Precision↑ | $F_1$ ↑ | AJI↑ |
|---|---|---|---|---|
| DeconvNet [14] | 0.773 | **0.864** | 0.805 | – |
| FCN-8 [11] | 0.752 | 0.823 | 0.763 | – |
| Ensemble [12] | **0.900** | 0.741 | 0.802 | – |
| U-Net [15] | 0.800 | 0.820 | 0.810 | 0.578 |
| Stacked U-Net | 0.802 | 0.830 | 0.816 | 0.580 |
| U-Net (DLA) | 0.812 | 0.826 | 0.818 | 0.586 |
| Ours | 0.818 | 0.824 | 0.821 | 0.595 |
| Ours (DLA) | 0.833 | 0.826 | **0.829** | **0.611** |

These experimental results indicate that our model with two improvements (**Ours (DLA)**) performs significantly better and achieved the highest overall AJI and $F_1$ scores compared with other segmentation methods both on the TCGA and TNBC datasets. Even the performance of our model with just one improvement (**U-Net (DLA) or Ours**) is better than the majority of the other methods. In addition, the results on the two datasets indicate that our proposed approach has an excellent generalization ability since these images in the two datasets are come from different organs, tissue and cell types.

## 4    Conclusion

In this paper, we propose a two-stage learning framework based on stacking two U-Nets with DLA for nuclei segmentation. We convert the binary segmentation task into a two-step task inspired by the idea of curriculum learning.

The difficulty of segmenting overlapping or touching nuclei directly from histopathological images is addressed by introducing nuclei-boundary prediction as the intermediate step. Furthermore, along with the two-step task, we design a two-stage learning framework by stacking two U-Nets, where the task of each U-Net is different but highly-related and trained simultaneously. Finally, DLA is adopted to extend the skip connections in U-Net to better fuse features across different levels for nuclei segmentation. The experimental results on two public and diverse nuclei datasets demonstrate that our proposed approach outperforms many standard segmentation architectures and the most recently proposed nuclei segmentation methods and can be easily generalized to different organs, tissue and cell types.

# References

1. Bengio, Y., Louradour, J., Collobert, R., Weston, J.: Curriculum learning. In: ICML, pp. 41–48. ACM (2009)
2. Bi, L., et al.: Dermoscopic image segmentation via multistage fully convolutional networks. IEEE Trans. Biomed. Eng. **64**(9), 2065–2074 (2017)
3. Chen, H., Qi, X., Yu, L., Heng, P.A.: DCAN: deep contour-aware networks for accurate gland segmentation. In: Proceedings of the IEEE Conference on Computer Vision and Pattern Recognition, pp. 2487–2496 (2016)
4. Chow, K.H., Factor, R.E., Ullman, K.S.: The nuclear envelope environment and its cancer connections. Nat. Rev. Cancer **12**(3), 196 (2012)
5. Christ, P.F.: Automatic liver and lesion segmentation in CT using cascaded fully convolutional neural networks and 3d conditional random fields. In: Ourselin, S., Joskowicz, L., Sabuncu, M.R., Unal, G., Wells, W. (eds.) MICCAI 2016. LNCS, vol. 9901, pp. 415–423. Springer, Cham (2016). https://doi.org/10.1007/978-3-319-46723-8_48
6. Drozdzal, M., Vorontsov, E., Chartrand, G., Kadoury, S., Pal, C.: The importance of skip connections in biomedical image segmentation. In: Carneiro, G., et al. (eds.) LABELS/DLMIA -2016. LNCS, vol. 10008, pp. 179–187. Springer, Cham (2016). https://doi.org/10.1007/978-3-319-46976-8_19
7. Filipczuk, P., Fevens, T., Krzyżak, A., Monczak, R.: Computer-aided breast cancer diagnosis based on the analysis of cytological images of fine needle biopsies. IEEE Trans. Med. Imaging **32**(12), 2169–2178 (2013)
8. Gurcan, M.N., Boucheron, L., et al.: Histopathological image analysis: a review. IEEE Rev. Biomed. Eng. **2**, 147 (2009)
9. He, K., Gkioxari, G., et al.: Mask R-CNN. In: ICCV, pp. 2961–2969 (2017)
10. Kumar, N., et al.: A dataset and a technique for generalized nuclear segmentation for computational pathology. IEEE Trans. Med. Imaging **36**(7), 1550–1560 (2017)
11. Long, J., Shelhamer, E., Darrell, T.: Fully convolutional networks for semantic segmentation. In: CVPR, pp. 3431–3440 (2015)
12. Naylor, P., Lae, M., Reyal, F., Walter, T.: Nuclei segmentation in histopathology images using deep neural networks. In: ISBI 2017, pp. 933–936. IEEE (2017)
13. Naylor, P., Laé, M., Reyal, F., Walter, T.: Segmentation of nuclei in histopathology images by deep regression of the distance map. IEEE Trans. Med. Imaging **38**(2), 448–459 (2019)
14. Noh, H., Hong, S., Han, B.: Learning deconvolution network for semantic segmentation. In: ICCV, pp. 1520–1528 (2015)

15. Ronneberger, O., Fischer, P., Brox, T.: U-Net: convolutional networks for biomedical image segmentation. In: Navab, N., Hornegger, J., Wells, W.M., Frangi, A.F. (eds.) MICCAI 2015. LNCS, vol. 9351, pp. 234–241. Springer, Cham (2015). https://doi.org/10.1007/978-3-319-24574-4_28

16. Sevastopolsky, A., et al.: Stack-u-net: refinement network for image segmentation on the example of optic disc and cup. arXiv preprint arXiv:1804.11294 (2018)

17. Vahadane, A., et al.: Structure-preserving color normalization and sparse stain separation for histological images. IEEE Trans. Med. Imaging **35**(8), 1962–1971 (2016)

18. Xing, F., Yang, L.: Robust nucleus/cell detection and segmentation in digital pathology and microscopy images: a comprehensive review. IEEE Rev. Biomed. Eng. **9**, 234–263 (2016)

19. Yu, F., et al.: Deep layer aggregation. In: CVPR, pp. 2403–2412 (2018)

20. Zeiler, M.D.: Adadelta: an adaptive learning rate method. arXiv preprint arXiv:1212.5701 (2012)

# ACE-Net: Biomedical Image Segmentation with Augmented Contracting and Expansive Paths

Yanhao Zhu[1], Zhineng Chen[2($\boxtimes$)], Shuai Zhao[2], Hongtao Xie[3], Wenming Guo[1], and Yongdong Zhang[3]

[1] Beijing University of Posts and Telecommunications, Beijing, China
[2] Institute of Automation, Chinese Academy of Sciences, Beijing, China
zhineng.chen@ia.ac.cn
[3] University of Science and Technology of China, Hefei, China

**Abstract.** Nowadays U-net-like FCNs predominate various biomedical image segmentation applications and attain promising performance, largely due to their elegant architectures, e.g., symmetric contracting and expansive paths as well as lateral skip-connections. It remains a research direction to devise novel architectures to further benefit the segmentation. In this paper, we develop an ACE-net that aims to enhance the feature representation and utilization by augmenting the contracting and expansive paths. In particular, we augment the paths by the recently proposed advanced techniques including ASPP, dense connection and deep supervision mechanisms, and novel connections such as directly connecting the raw image to the expansive side. With these augmentations, ACE-net can utilize features from multiple sources, scales and reception fields to segment while still maintains a relative simple architecture. Experiments on two typical biomedical segmentation tasks validate its effectiveness, where highly competitive results are obtained in both tasks while ACE-net still runs fast at inference.

## 1 Introduction

Biomedical image segmentation aims at partitioning an image into multiple regions corresponding to anatomical objects of interest. It is an essential technique that allows the quantification of shape related clinical parameters. Recently fully convolution networks (FCNs) have shown compelling advantages compared with traditional methods like Otsu thresholding, watershed segmentation, etc.

Among the developed architectures in this field, U-net [14] is probably the most famous one. It consists of a contracting path and a symmetric expansive path that enable multi-scale feature extraction and successive feature aggregation, respectively. Moreover, there are skip-connections from contracting to

Yanhao Zhu: This work was performed at Institute of Automation, Chinese Academy of Sciences.

expansive path at each scale to compensate the loss caused by downsampling. They are important for biomedical images whose differences are typically subtle [8]. In various biomedical segmentation tasks, U-net outperforms several FCN architectures that achieve promising results on natural image segmentation thanks to this elegantly designed architecture.

Following the success of U-net, a number of research efforts have been devoted to further enhance the segmentation performance. We can broadly categorize them into three types. The first one emphasizes on extracting more discriminative features by employing advanced deep modules. For example, residual and dense blocks were leveraged by FusionNet [13] and FC-DenseNet [10]. The second type is deep supervision that utilizes the groundtruth to guide model learning at intermediate layers of a CNN. It yielded better performance on several segmentation tasks, as demonstrated in [9,19,22]. The third type is devising architectures that stack or concatenate multiple U-net-like FCNs. For example, cascade-FCN [6] was proposed for liver and tumor segmentation. It consisted of two U-nets. The first U-net aimed to segment liver from a CT slice while the second learned to segment lesions from the liver mask given by the first U-net. Zeng et al. [21] also developed the RIC-Unet that segmented the contour mask and foreground of nuclei by using different branches. Despite satisfactory performance attained, these architectures are typically dataset-specific thus need to be modified when migrating to other tasks.

Standing on the shoulders of these studies, in this paper we develop a novel ACE-Net that aims to improve the performance of general biomedical segmentation. ACE-net inherits an u-shape architecture. It is also featured by applying the recently proposed ASPP module [5] to strengthen the contrasting path, which robustly extracts features covering multiple scales and reception fields. Meanwhile, the expansive path receives information from multiple sources including the raw image, features combined with detailed and global context from both the contrasting and expansive sides through different ways. They are densely connected to generate a comprehensive feature representation that is critical to the identification of boundary pixels. In addition, deep supervision on side response [19] is applied to both paths to further facilitate the segmentation. By leveraging the augmented paths, ACE-net can intensively utilize the features to segment while still maintains a relative simple architecture. We apply ACE-net to two typical biomedical segmentation tasks, i.e., the segmentation of neuronal structures in electron microscopic stacks (EM segmentation) [1] and the segmentation of digital retinal images for vessel extraction (DRIVE) [16] which is quite different with the previous one. Experiments demonstrate that ACE-net achieves highly competitive results in both tasks while still runs fast at inference.

## 2 Proposed Method

The proposed ACE-net is presented in Fig. 1, which is an augmented u-shape architecture with intensive connections among blocks. Specifically, on the contrasting path, four augmented contrasting blocks (ACBs) with size decreased

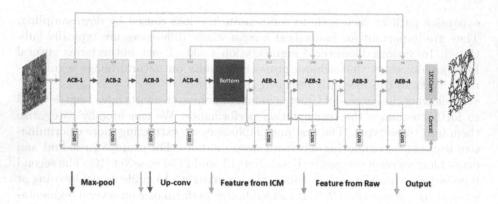

**Fig. 1.** An overview of the proposed ACE-net for biomedical image segmentation.

progressively are stacked to extract discriminative features combined with context of multiple scales and reception fields. While on the expansive path, the same number of augmented expansive blocks (AEBs) are developed to integrate features from multiple sources to better localize. Besides, side output is applied to give deep supervision in every block.

## 2.1 Augmented Contrasting Block with Intensive Context Modeling

To effectively explore the feature locally and holistically, an intensive context modeling (ICM) module is introduced to augment the contrasting block (see Fig. 2 (a)). In particular, besides the same contrasting block as in U-net, an ICM is added for feature enhancement. It separably takes as input the two $3 \times 3$ convolutions from the contrasting block, each first followed by another $3 \times 3$ convolution for feature abstraction and then concatenated. The generated feature maps are fed into a $1 \times 1$ convolution for dimension regularization. Then, an ASPP module with different rates is carried out for context modeling at multiple reception fields. A $1 \times 1$ convolution is followed by and the resulted feature maps are concatenated with the corresponding expansive block via a skip-connection. Parallel to this, another $1 \times 1$ convolution is also applied for the purpose of dimension reduction, and a side output is calculated on this branch.

Two kinds of augmentation are obtained from the ACB. First, by employing ASPP, a block can model context at multiple reception fields rather than a single one as in U-net. It significantly enriches the feature passed to the expansive side and thus can alleviate the intra-class inconsistency problem which is elaborated in [20]. Second, deep supervision on the side branch is carried out. It is beneficial to extracting more targeted features and improving the segmentation.

## 2.2 Multi-source Aggregation for Augmented Expansive Block

We also devise a multi-source aggregation (MSA) module to augment the expansive block (See Fig. 2(b)). It is combined with the raw expansive block to

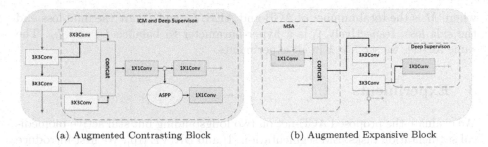

(a) Augmented Contrasting Block          (b) Augmented Expansive Block

**Fig. 2.** Detail structures of (a) Augmented contrasting block and (b) Augmented expansive block in the proposed ACE-net.

generate a comprehensive feature representation for better segmentation. To be specific, let MSA-$i$ be the MSA of the $i$-th AEB in the expansive path, it can concatenate up to four kinds of input from different sources: feature from the bottleneck layer (for $i = 1$) or previous AEB (for the rest), the $i$-th ACB feature, the resized raw image, and densely connective features from previous AEBs except for its direct ancestor, e.g., AEB-1 and AEB-2 for MSA-4. Before feeding into the MSA, the latter two kinds of features experience a $1 \times 1$ convolution for dimension alignment, i.e., making different inputs have an equal number of feature maps. Then, two $3 \times 3$ convolutions the same as the raw expansive block are applied to generate features for the following stacked AEBs. Meanwhile, to establish deep supervision, the two $3 \times 3$ convolutions are followed by a $1 \times 1$ convolution, whose output is utilized to calculate the side loss. Note that the deep supervision in AEB undergoes less convolutions, as its features are deeper and more abstract compared with those in ACB.

The augmentation of AEB is threefold. First, it receives rich features from different sources covering multiple scales and reception fields, which are critical for resolving the challenging edge ambiguity. Second, explicit supervision from the raw image is obtained. It contains the most accurate location information and is helpful to the segmentation especially for those small-sized convolutional layers. It is also one peculiar feature of ACE-net as existing work seldom directly supervises in this way. Third, deep supervision is again carried out at every block, which serves as both learner and regularizer to the whole network.

### 2.3   Loss Function

Following U-net, ACE-net employs the sparse softmax cross-entropy as loss function, which is computed by a pixel-wise softmax over the feature maps combined with the cross-entropy. We calculate it for the final output and the eight side outputs. The overall loss function is given by

$$L = L_p(\omega) + \lambda \sum_{n=1}^{M} L_s^{(n)}(\omega)$$

where $M$ is the total number of ACB and AEB, $L_p$ and $L_s$ are the final loss and the side loss, respectively, $\lambda$ is a hyper-parameter to balance $L_p$ and $L_s$. The same as [19], we set $\lambda = 1$ in all experiments.

## 3    Experiments

We evaluate the proposed ACE-net on two longstanding but still active biomedical segmentation tasks: EM segmentation [1] and DRIVE [16]. We first introduce our implementation details, followed by the ablation study and experimental results on EM segmentation. Finally, we show the result on DRIVE.

### 3.1    Implementation Details

We implemented ACE-net by using TensorFlow (version 1.4.0). Data augmentations including flip, zoom and rotate were employed. The network was trained on one NVIDIA TITAN Xp GPU with a mini-batch size of one. Adam optimizer was used to optimize the whole network and the learning rate was fixed to 1e-4. It took approximate 10 h and 14 h to train ACE-net from scratch on the EM segmentation and DRIVE datasets, respectively. Besides, ACE-net runs fast on both datasets at inference. It took 0.53 s to segment a $512 \times 512$ EM neuronal image, and 0.83 s to segment a $592 \times 576 \times 3$ retinal image on average.

### 3.2    Experiments on EM Segmentation

The segmentation of neural EM images is an important task in observing the structure and function of brain. The EM segmentation dataset has 30 training images with publicly available groundtruth and 30 test images with annotations kept private for the assessment of segmentation accuracy. Website of the task remains open for submission although the competition is in year 2012. The evaluation metric is $Vrand$, which is elaborated in [1].

**Table 1.** Performance of ACE-net under different settings. CP(**C**): the contrasting path. EP(**E**): the expansive path. ICM(**I**): the intensive context modeling module. MSA(**M**): the multi-source aggregation module. DS(**D**): deep supervision.

| Method | $Vrand$ | Method | $Vrand$ |
|---|---|---|---|
| C+E+I+D | 0.9725 | C+E+M+D | 0.9723 |
| C+E+I+D+M(1) | 0.9774 | C+E+M+D+I(1) | 0.9730 |
| C+E+I+D+M(1,2) | **0.9797** | C+E+M+D+I(1,2) | 0.9760 |
| C+E+I+D+M(1,2,3) | 0.9746 | C+E+M+D+I(1,2,3) | 0.9769 |
| C+E+I+D+M(1,2,3,4) | 0.9726 | C+E+M+D+I(1,2,3,4) | **0.9797** |

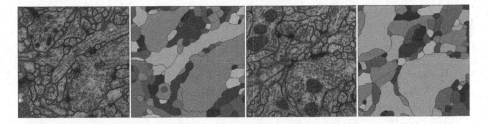

**Fig. 3.** Segmentation instances on ISBI 2012 EM segmentation (slice 7 and 30).

**Ablation Study.** To better understand ACE-net, we execute controlled experiments on the EM dataset. All the experiments are under the same setting except for the specified difference.

As explained, the ICM and MSA modules are important w.r.t ACE-net. To assess their effects, we first equip all the ACBs with the ICM module and stepwisely add the MSA module to AEB. Specifically, we test the absence/existance of the resized raw image only, as the effectiveness of skip-connections and dense connections have been proven in [4,8]. As shown in Table 1, the best result is obtained when the raw image is available for the first two MSAs. This is reasonable as the subsequent AEBs are connected with shallow ACBs, which convey rich location information such that supplement from the raw image is less meaningful. We then keep the raw image seen by the first two AEBs and evaluate the ICM module. It is seen that the incorporation of all the four ICM modules yields the best performance, indicating the effectiveness of applying ASPP to extract features. In view of the study above, we determine the final architecture of ACE-net, as depicted in Fig. 1.

**Results.** We submit the result of ACE-net to the website of EM segmentation, and list several top-ranked results and their papers as well as ours. The challenge lasted seven years and the leader board accumulated over 180 different submissions. From Table 2, we can seen that a performance gain of 0.007 was obtained when compared U-net with ACE-net without post-processing, which yielded a prominent difference of over 30 rankings in the leader board. It indicates that ACE-net is suitable for biomedical segmentation. We also presented the results with the post-processing of [3], which were used by all the four methods listed in the right of Table 2. Two images segmented by ACE-net are shown in Fig. 3. Our result is highly competitive compared with the state-of-the-arts.

### 3.3    Experiments on DRIVE

The DRIVE dataset includes 40 color fundus photographs divided into two parts: 20 training images and 20 test images with manual segmentation of the vasculature and binary masks of FOV. As for the evaluation metrics, we use sensitivity,

**Table 2.** Results of published entries on the EM segmentation task [1]. The full leader board is available at: http://brainiac2.mit.edu/isbi_challenge/leaders-board-new

| Method (without post-process) | $Vrand$ | Method (with post-process) | $Vrand$ |
|---|---|---|---|
| ACE-net (ours) | **0.9797** | SFCNN [17] | **0.9868** |
| M2FCN [15] | 0.9780 | ACE-net (ours) | 0.9850 |
| FusionNet [13] | 0.9780 | M2FCN [15] | 0.9838 |
| U-net [14] | 0.9727 | IAL LMC [3] | 0.9822 |

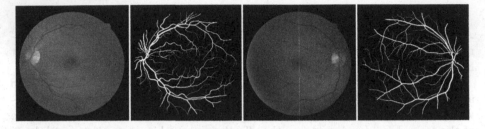

**Fig. 4.** Results on DRIVE (image 1 and 19). For the segmented images, correct detections are white, misses are red, and false positives are blue. (Color figure online)

specificity, accuracy and the area under the ROC curve (AUC). The measurements are calculated only for pixels inside the FOV area. Table 3 lists several top results as well as ours.

**Table 3.** Comparison to start-of-the-art methods on DRIVE dataset.

| Method | Sensitivity(%) | Specificity(%) | Accuracy(%) | AUC(%) |
|---|---|---|---|---|
| Azzopardi et al. [2] | 76.55 | 97.04 | 94.42 | 96.14 |
| Li et al. [11] | 75.69 | 98.16 | 95.27 | 97.38 |
| Orlando et al. [12] | 78.97 | 96.84 | N.A | 95.07 |
| Dasgupta et al. [7] | 76.91 | 98.01 | 95.33 | 97.44 |
| Wu et al. [18] | 78.44 | 98.19 | 95.67 | **98.07** |
| Zhang et al. [22] | **87.23** | 96.18 | 95.04 | 97.99 |
| ACE-net (ours) | 77.25 | **98.42** | **95.69** | 97.42 |

It is seen that ACE-net also gets competitive results on DRIVE without any modification in architecture or training settings. It attains the highest values on specificity and accuracy while the values for the other two metrics are still competitive except for the sensitivity of [22]. The prominent higher sensitivity of [22] is largely attributed to a dedicated pre-processing, which enhances the segmentation of the capillaries significantly. However, the pre-processing is network-independent. It also can be combined with ACE-net to seek for a better sensitivity although we have not implemented it now. Besides, ACE-Net performs similar to [18], but it is likely to run 10x faster on a similar server due to a simpler architecture. Two instances segmented by ACE-net are shown in Fig. 4.

## 4    Conclusion

Aiming at improving the performance on different biomedical segmentation applications, we devise ACE-net with augmented contracting and expansive paths, where advanced modules and novel connections are introduced to enhance the feature representation from multiple sources, scales and reception fields. The experiments conducted on EM segmentation and DRIVE datasets basically validate our proposal, where competitive results to state-of-the-arts are obtained in both tasks while ACE-net still maintains a fast inference speed.

**Acknowledgement.** This work is supported by the National Natural Science Foundation of China under grant no. 61772526

## References

1. Arganda-Carreras, I., et al.: Crowdsourcing the creation of image segmentation algorithms for connectomics. Front. Neuroanat. **9**, 142 (2015)
2. Azzopardi, G., Strisciuglio, N., et al.: Trainable cosfire filters for vessel delineation with application to retinal images. Med. Image Anal. **19**(1), 46–57 (2015)
3. Beier, T., Pape, C., Rahaman, N., et al.: Multicut brings automated neurite segmentation closer to human performance. Nat. Methods **14**(2), 101 (2017)
4. Bilinski, P., Prisacariu, V.: Dense decoder shortcut connections for single-pass semantic segmentation. In: Proceedings of the IEEE Conference on Computer Vision and Pattern Recognition, pp. 6596–6605 (2018)
5. Chen, L.C., Papandreou, G., Schroff, F., Adam, H.: Rethinking atrous convolution for semantic image segmentation. arXiv preprint arXiv:1706.05587 (2017)
6. Christ, P.F., Ettlinger, F., Grün, F., Elshaera, M.E.A., Lipkova, J., et al.: Automatic liver and tumor segmentation of CT and MRI volumes using cascaded fully convolutional neural networks. arXiv preprint arXiv:1702.05970 (2017)
7. Dasgupta, A., Singh, S.: A fully convolutional neural network based structured prediction approach towards the retinal vessel segmentation. In: IEEE 14th ISBI 2017, pp. 248–251 (2017)
8. Drozdzal, M., Vorontsov, E., Chartrand, G., Kadoury, S., Pal, C.: The importance of skip connections in biomedical image segmentation. In: Deep Learning and Data Labeling for Medical Applications, pp. 179–187 (2016)
9. Hu, K., Zhang, Z., Niu, X., et al.: Retinal vessel segmentation of color fundus images using multiscale convolutional neural network with an improved cross-entropy loss function. Neurocomputing **309**, 179–191 (2018)
10. Jégou, S., et al.: The one hundred layers tiramisu: Fully convolutional densenets for semantic segmentation. In: IEEE CVPR Workshops, pp. 11–19 (2017)
11. Li, Q., Feng, B., Xie, L., et al.: A cross-modality learning approach for vessel segmentation in retinal images. IEEE Trans. Med. Imaging **35**(1), 109–118 (2016)

12. Orlando, J.I., Prokofyeva, E., Blaschko, M.B.: A discriminatively trained fully connected conditional random field model for blood vessel segmentation in fundus images. IEEE Trans. Biomed. Eng. **64**(1), 16–27 (2017)
13. Quan, T.M., et al.: Fusionnet: a deep fully residual convolutional neural network for image segmentation in connectomics. arXiv preprint arXiv:1612.05360 (2016)
14. Ronneberger, O., Fischer, P., Brox, T.: U-Net: convolutional networks for biomedical image segmentation. In: Navab, N., Hornegger, J., Wells, W.M., Frangi, A.F. (eds.) MICCAI 2015. LNCS, vol. 9351, pp. 234–241. Springer, Cham (2015). https://doi.org/10.1007/978-3-319-24574-4_28
15. Shen, W., et al.: Multi-stage multi-recursive-input fully convolutional networks for neuronal boundary detection. In: IEEE ICCV, pp. 2391–2400 (2017)
16. Staal, J., et al.: Ridge-based vessel segmentation in color images of the retina. IEEE Trans. Med. Imaging **23**(4), 501–509 (2004)
17. Weiler, M., Hamprecht, F.A., Storath, M.: Learning steerable filters for rotation equivariant CNNs. In: IEEE CVPR, pp. 849–858 (2018)
18. Wu, Y., Xia, Y., Song, Y., Zhang, Y., Cai, W.: Multiscale network followed network model for retinal vessel segmentation. In: Frangi, A.F., Schnabel, J.A., Davatzikos, C., Alberola-López, C., Fichtinger, G. (eds.) MICCAI 2018. LNCS, vol. 11071, pp. 119–126. Springer, Cham (2018). https://doi.org/10.1007/978-3-030-00934-2_14
19. Xie, S., Tu, Z.: Holistically-nested edge detection. In: IEEE ICCV, pp. 1395–1403 (2015)
20. Yu, C., Wang, J., Peng, C., et al.: Learning a discriminative feature network for semantic segmentation. In: IEEE CVPR, pp. 1857–1866 (2018)
21. Zeng, Z., Xie, W., Zhang, Y., Lu, Y.: RIC-Unet: an improved neural network based on Unet for nuclei segmentation in histology images. IEEE Access **7**, 21420–21428 (2019)
22. Zhang, Y., Chung, A.C.S.: Deep supervision with additional labels for retinal vessel segmentation task. In: Frangi, A.F., Schnabel, J.A., Davatzikos, C., Alberola-López, C., Fichtinger, G. (eds.) MICCAI 2018. LNCS, vol. 11071, pp. 83–91. Springer, Cham (2018). https://doi.org/10.1007/978-3-030-00934-2_10

# CS-Net: Channel and Spatial Attention Network for Curvilinear Structure Segmentation

Lei Mou[1,2], Yitian Zhao[2(✉)], Li Chen[1], Jun Cheng[2], Zaiwang Gu[2],
Huaying Hao[2], Hong Qi[3], Yalin Zheng[4], Alejandro Frangi[2,5], and Jiang Liu[2,6]

[1] School of Computer Science and Technology,
Wuhan University of Science and Technology, Wuhan, China
[2] Cixi Institute of Biomedical Engineering,
Chinese Academy of Sciences, Ningbo, China
yitian.zhao@nimte.ac.cn
[3] Department of Ophthalmology, Peking University Third Hospital, Beijing, China
[4] Department of Eye and Vision Science, University of Liverpool, Liverpool, UK
[5] School of Computing, University of Leeds, Leeds, UK
[6] Department of Computer Science and Engineering,
Southern University of Science and Technology, Shenzhen, China

**Abstract.** The detection of curvilinear structures in medical images,
e.g., blood vessels or nerve fibers, is important in aiding management of
many diseases. In this work, we propose a general unifying curvilinear
structure segmentation network that works on different medical imaging
modalities: optical coherence tomography angiography (OCT-A), color
fundus image, and corneal confocal microscopy (CCM). Instead of the
U-Net based convolutional neural network, we propose a novel network
(CS-Net) which includes a self-attention mechanism in the encoder and
decoder. Two types of attention modules are utilized - spatial attention
and channel attention, to further integrate local features with their global
dependencies adaptively. The proposed network has been validated on
five datasets: two color fundus datasets, two corneal nerve datasets and
one OCT-A dataset. Experimental results show that our method outperforms state-of-the-art methods, for example, sensitivities of corneal
nerve fiber segmentation were at least 2% higher than the competitors.
As a complementary output, we made manual annotations of two corneal
nerve datasets which have been released for public access.

**Keywords:** Curvilinear structure · Segmentation · Encoder and
decoder

## 1 Introduction

Accurate detection of curvilinear structures, such as retinal vasculature from
color fundus image [1], optical coherence tomography angiography (OCT-A),

© Springer Nature Switzerland AG 2019
D. Shen et al. (Eds.): MICCAI 2019, LNCS 11764, pp. 721–730, 2019.
https://doi.org/10.1007/978-3-030-32239-7_80

and corneal nerve fiber from corneal confocal microscopy (CCM), are essential for many clinical applications [2]. Manual labeling the curvilinear structures is an exhausting, subjective and tedious tasks for human operators, and practically impossible in high-throughput analysis settings like screening programs or high-throughput microscopy. In consequence, an automatic segmentation method for general curvilinear structures is indispensable to overcome time constraints, scale-up to big data analysis, and avoid human error. However, computer-aided systems under development have yet to solve the segmentation problems as posed by high anatomical variation across the population, and the varying scales of curvilinear structures within an image. Noise, poor contrast and low resolution, exacerbate these problems.

Extensive work has been carried out towards automatic vessel segmentation or fiber tracing (see [3] for extensive review). As vasculatures or fibers are curvilinear structures distributed across different orientations and scales, various filtering methods have been proposed, include Hessian matrix-based filters [4], symmetry filter [2], and tensor-based filter [5], to name only the most widely used ones. These approaches aim to remove undesired intensity variations in the image, and suppress background structures and image noise, thereby easing the subsequent segmentation problem. Recently, several deep learning-based methods have been proposed for vessel segmentation and nerve fiber tracing in color fundus and CCM, respectively. Liskowski et al. [6] introduced a retinal vessel segmentation method based on Convolutional Neural Network (CNN), and Fu et al. [7] further applied the CNN along with Conditional Random Field to detect retinal vessels. Alom et al. [8] adopted recurrent residual convolution block as the backbone of the U-shaped network (R2U-Net) to segment the vessels. Colonna et al. [9] used the U-Net-based CNN [10] to trace the corneal nerve. However, deep learning-based method has yet to be used to segment retinal vessels in OCT-A.

Most of these models were designed for segmentation of vessels or fibers from specific biomedical imaging modalities. In this work, we proposed a Channel and Spatial Attention Network (CS-Net) based on U-Net that has proven to be effective to extract curvilinear structures from three biomedical imaging modalities. This paper makes four contributions: (1) a new segmentation method was proposed with self-attention mechanism; (2) CS-Net can deal with multiple types of curvilinear structure segmentation in a unified manner; (3) results on 5 datasets demonstrate state-of-the-art performance; (4) we made manual annotations of two corneal nerve datasets which have been released for public access.

## 2    Proposed Method

The proposed CS-Net consists of three phases: the encoder module, the channel and spatial attention module (CSAM), and the decoder module, as shown in Fig. 1. The feature encoder module includes four encoder blocks, and the residual network (ResNet) block was employed as the backbone for each block, and then followed by a max-pooling layer to increase the receptive field for better extraction of global features. Then the features from the encoder are fed into

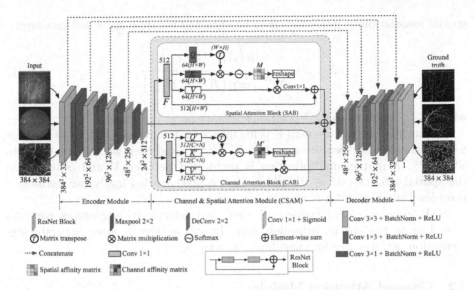

**Fig. 1.** CS-Net structure diagram. It comprises of three phases: the feature encoder module, the channel and spatial attention module and the feature decoder module. (Color figure online)

two parallel attention blocks - the channel attention block (CAB) and a spatial attention block (SAB), as shown in the red and blue rectangles in Fig. 1. Finally, the decoder module was used to reconstruct depth feature.

## 2.1 Spatial Attention Module

Many recent works have shown the local feature representation produced by traditional fully convolutional networks (FCNs) may lead to object mis-classification [11,12]. To model rich contextual dependencies over local feature representations, the first step is to generate a spatial attention matrix, which models spatial relationships between features of any two pixels. In practice, tree-like structures always are distributed throughout the biomedical image [13]. In consequence, we introduce the SAB to encode a wider range of contextual information into local features, to increase their representative capability.

We first feed the input features $F \in \mathbb{R}^{C \times H \times W}$ with batch normalization and ReLU layers or channel transformation, where $C$ indicates the number of input channels, $H$ and $W$ are the height and width of $F$, respectively. Then a $1 \times 3$ and a $3 \times 1$ kernel convolution layer is to generate two new feature maps $Q \in \mathbb{R}^{C \times H \times W}$, and $K \in \mathbb{R}^{C \times H \times W}$, respectively, to capture edge information of tree-like structures in horizontal and vertical orientations. These two new feature maps are then reshaped to $\mathbb{R}^{C \times N}$, where $N = H \times W$ is the number of features. The transpose of $Q$ and $K$ is further fused by a matrix multiplication, and the spatial association of intra-class may be obtained by applying a softmax layer:

$$\mathcal{S}_{(x,y)} = \frac{\exp\left(K_{(x)} \cdot Q^{\mathrm{T}}{}_{(y)}\right)}{\sum_{x=1}^{N} \exp\left(K_{(x)} \cdot Q^{\mathrm{T}}{}_{(y)}\right)}, \tag{1}$$

where $\mathcal{S}_{(x,y)}$ denotes the $x^{th}$ position's impact on $y^{th}$ position.

Meanwhile, the feature map $F$ is fed into a $1 \times 1$ convolution layer to produce a dimension-reduced feature map $V \in \mathbb{R}^{C \times H \times W}$, and then we reshape the $\mathcal{S}$ to $\mathbb{R}^{C \times H \times W}$. A matrix multiplication is performed between $V$ and $\mathcal{S}$ to obtain the spatial affinities $M \in \mathbb{R}^{C \times H \times W}$ at the pixel level. Finally, we perform a pixel-level summation of $F$ and $M$.

SAB gains a global contextual view and selectively aggregates contexts according to the spatial attention map. It will achieve a more accurate segmentation performance for curvilinear structures.

## 2.2 Channel Attention Module

Each channel of a high-level feature can be regarded as a specific-class response [13]. Therefore, we further exploit the interdependencies of channel maps in this section. Feature representation may be improved by emphasizing interdependent feature maps.

Three channel attention maps $Q' \in \mathbb{R}^{C \times H \times W}$, $K' \in \mathbb{R}^{C \times H \times W}$, and $V' \in \mathbb{R}^{C \times H \times W}$ are calculated directly by a $1 \times 1$ convolution layer on the input feature maps $F \in \mathbb{R}^{C \times H \times W}$. Similar to SAB, we reshape $F$ to $\mathbb{R}^{C \times N}$. We then perform a multiplication between $F$ and its transpose. The channel affinities map $M' \in \mathbb{R}^{C \times C}$ is then obtained by applying a softmax layer:

$$\mathcal{C}_{(x,y)} = \frac{\exp\left(F_{(x)} \cdot F_{(y)}\right)}{\sum_{x=1}^{C} \exp\left(F_{(x)} \cdot F_{(y)}\right)}, \tag{2}$$

where $\mathcal{C}_{(x,y)}$ denotes the similarity between the $x^{th}$ channel and the $y^{th}$ channel. A matrix multiplication between the transpose of $\mathcal{C}$ and $V'$ is added to obtain the final output. The result is reshaped as $\mathbb{R}^{C \times H \times W}$. Such operations emphasize class-dependent feature mapping and help improve feature discriminability.

Instead of directly upsampling the features of the CSAM to the original image dimensions, we introduce a feature decoder module that restores the dimensions of the high level semantic features layer by layer. In each layer, we use ResNet block as the backbone of the decoder block which is followed by a $2 \times 2$ deconvolution layer. Similar to U-Net [10], we add a skip connection between each layer of the encoder and decoder. At the end of the CS-Net, we apply a $1 \times 1$ convolution layer and a sigmoid layer on the output of the feature encoder module to gain the final segmentation map.

# 3   Experiment Results

The proposed CS-Net was implemented on PyTorch library with a single NVIDIA GPU (GeForce GTX 1080Ti). We choose adaptive moment estimation (Adam) optimization. The initial learning rate is set to 0.0001 and a weight decay of 0.0005. We use poly learning rate policy where the learning rate is multiplied by $\left(1 - \frac{iter}{max\_iter}\right)^{power}$ with power 0.9. All training images are rescaled to $384 \times 384$. We use the k-fold (k = 4 for STARE; and k = 5 for CCM-1, CCM-2, and OCT-A) cross-validation method to divide the images. The reported values are the mean values across all the folds.

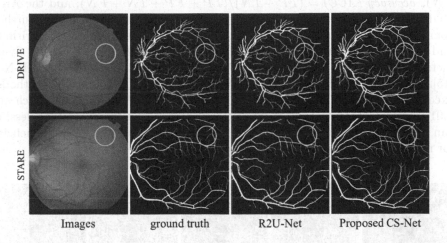

| | Images | ground truth | R2U-Net | Proposed CS-Net |

**Fig. 2.** Retinal vessel segmentation results for two randomly selected images by R2U-Net and our CS-Net.

**Table 1.** Performance of vessel segmentation methods on color fundus datasets.

| Methods | DRIVE | | | | STARE | | | |
|---|---|---|---|---|---|---|---|---|
| | ACC | SE | SP | AUC | ACC | SE | SP | AUC |
| BCOSFIRE [14] | 0.9442 | 0.7655 | 0.9704 | 0.9614 | 0.9497 | 0.7716 | 0.9701 | 0.9563 |
| WSF [2] | 0.9580 | 0.7740 | 0.9790 | 0.9750 | 0.9570 | 0.7880 | 0.9760 | 0.9590 |
| DeepVessel [7] | 0.9533 | 0.7603 | 0.9776 | 0.9789 | 0.9609 | 0.7412 | 0.9701 | 0.9790 |
| U-Net [10] | 0.9531 | 0.7537 | 0.9639 | 0.9601 | 0.9409 | 0.7675 | 0.9631 | 0.9705 |
| R2U-Net [8] | 0.9556 | 0.7792 | 0.9813 | 0.9784 | 0.9712 | 0.8298 | **0.9862** | 0.9914 |
| CE-Net [15] | 0.9545 | **0.8309** | 0.9747 | 0.9779 | 0.9583 | 0.7841 | 0.9725 | 0.9787 |
| CS-Net | **0.9632** | 0.8170 | **0.9854** | **0.9798** | **0.9752** | **0.8816** | 0.9840 | **0.9932** |

### 3.1   Vessel Segmentation in Color Fundus Image

We evaluated the proposed method for retinal blood vessel segmentation on two color fundus datasets: DRIVE[1] and STARE[2]. We chose the first manual annotation of both datasets as the groundtruth. Figure 2 demonstrates the retinal vessel segmentation performance by applying one of the state-of-the art methods (named R2U-Net) and the CS-Net. It is clear from visual inspection that CS-Net achieved better performance than the R2U-Net, as more small vessels were extracted from regions of poor contrast.

To facilitate better observation and objective performance evaluation of the proposed method, these metrics were calculated: *sensitivity (SE)* $= TP/(TP + FN)$, *accuracy (ACC)* $= (TP + TN)/(TP + FP + TN + FN)$, and the Area Under the ROC Curve (AUC). In addition, the segmentation results were further compared with those of state-of-the-art retinal vessel segmentation algorithms and deep learning networks: Bar-COSFIRE (BCOSFIRE) [14], Weighted Symmetry Filter (WSF) [2], DeepVessel [7], U-Net [10], R2U-Net [8], and CE-Net [15]. Table 1 shows the proposed CS-Net outperforms all competing methods, except for SE in the DRIVE dataset and SP in the STARE dataset, which are 0.91% and 0.22% lower than those of [15] and [8], respectively. Nevertheless, it can be confirmed that the spatial and channel attention modules are beneficial for retinal vessel detection in color fundus image.

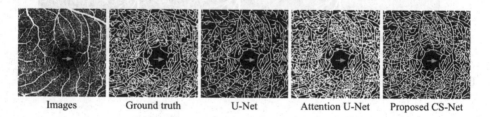

Images          Ground truth          U-Net          Attention U-Net          Proposed CS-Net

**Fig. 3.** Visualization results of vessel segmentation in OCT-A.

### 3.2   Vessel Segmentation in OCT-A Image

We then evaluate the proposed CS-Net on one in-house OCT-A dataset to further validate its segmentation performance. All the 30 OCT-A images were acquired using Heidelberg Spectralis device (Heidelberg, Germany) and all the vessels within the superficial vascular plexus (SVP) were manually traced using an in-house program written in Matlab (Mathworks R2018, Natwick) by a clinical expert as the ground truth.

To our best knowledge, it is the first attempt to use deep learning approach to extract the vessels for OCT-A image. We compared the proposed network with

---

[1] http://www.isi.uu.nl/Research/Databases/DRIVE/.

[2] http://www.ces.clemson.edu/ahoover/stare/.

**Table 2.** Performance of compared methods on OCT-A dataset.

| Methods | ACC | SE | SP | AUC |
|---|---|---|---|---|
| U-Net [10] | 0.8422 | 0.7867 | 0.8780 | 0.9108 |
| Deep ResUNet [16] | 0.8659 | 0.8032 | 0.8863 | 0.9175 |
| UNet++ [17] | 0.8965 | 0.8309 | 0.9101 | 0.9203 |
| Attention U-Net [18] | 0.9125 | 0.8274 | 0.9007 | 0.9290 |
| CS-Net | **0.9183** | **0.8631** | **0.9192** | **0.9453** |

other state-of-the-art segmentation networks: U-Net [10], Deep ResUNet [16], UNet++ [17], and Attention U-Net [18]. Figure 3 presents for visual comparison the vessel segmentation results of the competing methods on an example image. Overall, all methods demonstrated similar performance on vessel with large diameters. The Attention U-Net is able to detect most larger vessels, but also falsely enlarges background features where elongated intensity inhomogeneities are presented. U-Net misses vessels with small diameters, which leads to a relative lower sensitivity. In contrast to these networks, the proposed CS-Net integrates local features with global dependencies adaptively, hence, it demonstrated superior performance in detecting small vessels, indicated by the green arrow, and provided relatively higher sensitivity. These findings were also confirmed by the evaluation measures reported in Table 2: the CS-Net shows this superior segmentation performance in terms of all metrics, since it considers the attention mechanism to build the association among features.

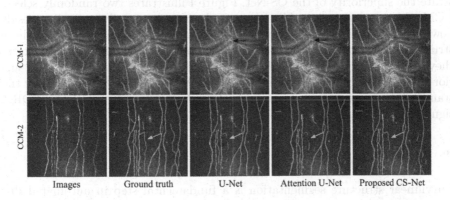

**Fig. 4.** Illustrative results of corneal nerve fiber tracing by different networks. (Color figure online)

### 3.3  Corneal Nerve Fiber Tracing in CCM Image

Finally, the proposed CS-Net was verified by the corneal nerve fiber tracing on two CCM datasets. **CCM-1** has 1578 CCM, which were acquired from Peking

**Table 3.** Fiber tracing performance of different methods on two CCM datasets (mean ± standard deviation).

| Methods | CCM-1 | | CCM-2 | |
|---|---|---|---|---|
| | SE | FDR | SE | FDR |
| U-Net [10] | 0.7856 ± 0.0096 | 0.3257 ± 0.0238 | 0.7657 ± 0.0193 | 0.3365 ± 0.0178 |
| Deep ResUNet [16] | 0.8067 ± 0.0056 | 0.2873 ± 0.0210 | 0.8009 ± 0.0221 | 0.2949 ± 0.0217 |
| UNet++ [17] | 0.8290 ± 0.0077 | 0.2685 ± 0.0134 | 0.8257 ± 0.0177 | 0.2744 ± 0.0101 |
| Attention U-Net [18] | 0.8231 ± 0.0031 | 0.2717 ± 0.0145 | 0.8101 ± 0.0231 | 0.2806 ± 0.0094 |
| CS-Net | **0.8415 ± 0.0030** | **0.2521 ± 0.0044** | **0.8345 ± 0.0165** | **0.2591 ± 0.0011** |

University Third Hospital; **CCM-2** includes 120 CCM, which were obtained from University of Padova[3]. All the images were acquired at size 384 × 384. The fiber ground truths of these two datasets were segmented manually by our ophthalmologist, who traced the centerlines of all visible nerves, and we made these manual annotations available online[4].

To validate the nerve fiber tracing performance, we computed the sensitivity and *false discovery rate* (FDR) [19] between the predicted centerlines and groundtruth. FDR is defined as the fraction of the total of pixels incorrectly detected as nerve segments over the total of pixels of the traced nerves in groundtruth. As customary in the evaluating methods extracting one pixel-wide curves [19], a three-pixel tolerance region around the manually traced nerves is considered a true positive.

In a similar fashion to the vessel segmentation in OCT-A, we also used U-Net [10], Deep ResUNet [16], UNet++ [17], and Attention U-Net [18] to demonstrate the superiority of the CS-Net. Figure 4 illustrates two randomly selected CCMs from two datasets. All the methods present visually appealing results, however, both U-Net and Attention U-Net have falsely detect part of the K-structures [20] (indicated by red arrows) as nerve fibers, due to the fact that they share similar morphological characteristics. Table 3 demonstrates this superior tracing performance in terms of SE and FDR, and is accompanied by their standard deviations: demonstrating both higher sensitivity and lower FDR by significant margins.

# 4    Conclusion

Curvilinear structure segmentation is a fundamental step in automated diagnosis of many diseases, and it remains a challenging medical image analysis problem despite considerable efforts in research. In this paper, we developed a new channel and spatial attention network named CS-Net for curvilinear structure segmentation. It considers the attention mechanism to build the associates among features, and aggregate the global contextual information, as thus to improve the inter-class discrimination and intra-class aggregation abilities by

---

[3] http://bioimlab.dei.unipd.it/.
[4] http://imed.nimte.ac.cn/.

applying a self-attention mechanism to high level features in the channel and spatial dimension. Our experimental results show that the proposed method can improve the segmentation of curvilinear structure for color fundus, OCT-A and CCM images. Its superior performance confirms it as a powerful tool for wide healthcare applications and beyond.

**Acknowledgement.** This work was supported by National Science Foundation Program of China (61601029, 61773297), Zhejiang Provincial Natural Science Foundation (LZ19F0 10001), and Ningbo Natural Science Foundation (2018A610055).

# References

1. Zhao, Y., et al.: Automated vessel segmentation using infinite perimeter active contour model with hybrid region information with application to retinal images. IEEE Trans. Med. Imag. **34**(9), 1797–1807 (2015)
2. Zhao, Y., et al.: Automatic 2D/3D vessel enhancement in multiple modality images using a weighted symmetry filter. IEEE Trans. Med. Imag. **37**(2), 438–450 (2018)
3. Fraz, M., et al.: Blood vessel segmentation methodologies in retinal images - a survey. Comput. Meth. Prog. Bio. **108**, 407–433 (2012)
4. Frangi, A.F., Niessen, W.J., Vincken, K.L., Viergever, M.A.: Multiscale vessel enhancement filtering. In: Wells, W.M., Colchester, A., Delp, S. (eds.) MICCAI 1998. LNCS, vol. 1496, pp. 130–137. Springer, Heidelberg (1998). https://doi.org/10.1007/BFb0056195
5. Cetin, S., Unal, G.: A higher-order tensor vessel tractography for segmentation of vascular structures. IEEE Trans. Med. Imag. **34**, 2172–2185 (2015)
6. Liskowski, P., Krawiec, K.: Segmenting retinal blood vessels with deep neural networks. IEEE Trans. Med. Imag. **35**, 2369–2380 (2016)
7. Fu, H., Xu, Y., Lin, S., Kee Wong, D.W., Liu, J.: DeepVessel: retinal vessel segmentation via deep learning and conditional random field. In: Ourselin, S., Joskowicz, L., Sabuncu, M.R., Unal, G., Wells, W. (eds.) MICCAI 2016. LNCS, vol. 9901, pp. 132–139. Springer, Cham (2016). https://doi.org/10.1007/978-3-319-46723-8_16
8. Alom, M., et al.: Recurrent residual convolutional neural network based on U-net (R2U-Net) for medical image segmentation. arXiv:1802.06955 (2018)
9. Colonna, A., Scarpa, F., Ruggeri, A.: Segmentation of corneal nerves using a U-Net-based convolutional neural network. In: Stoyanov, D., et al. (eds.) OMIA/COMPAY -2018. LNCS, vol. 11039, pp. 185–192. Springer, Cham (2018). https://doi.org/10.1007/978-3-030-00949-6_22
10. Ronneberger, O., Fischer, P., Brox, T.: U-Net: convolutional networks for biomedical image segmentation. In: Navab, N., Hornegger, J., Wells, W.M., Frangi, A.F. (eds.) MICCAI 2015. LNCS, vol. 9351, pp. 234–241. Springer, Cham (2015). https://doi.org/10.1007/978-3-319-24574-4_28
11. Zhao, H., et al.: Pyramid scene parsing network. In: CVPR 2017, pp. 2281–2890 (2017)
12. Peng, C., et al.: Large kernel matters-improve semantic segmentation by global convolutional network. In: CVPR 2017, pp. 4353–4361 (2017)
13. Jun, F., et al.: Dual attention network for scene segmentation. In: CVPR 2019, pp. 3146–3154 (2019)
14. Azzopardi, G., et al.: Trainable cosfire filters for vessel delineation with application to retinal images. Med. Image Anal. **19**(1), 46–57 (2015)

15. Gu Z., et al.: CE-NET: context encoder network for 2D medical image segmentation. IEEE Trans. Med. Imaging (2019)
16. Zhang, Z., Liu, Q., Wang, Y.: Road extraction by deep residual U-NET. IEEE Geosci. Remote Sens. Lett. **15**(5), 749–753 (2018)
17. Zhou, Z., Rahman Siddiquee, M.M., Tajbakhsh, N., Liang, J.: UNet++: a nested U-Net architecture for medical image segmentation. In: Stoyanov, D., et al. (eds.) DLMIA/ML-CDS -2018. LNCS, vol. 11045, pp. 3–11. Springer, Cham (2018). https://doi.org/10.1007/978-3-030-00889-5_1
18. Oktay, O., et al.: Attention U-NET: learning where to look for the pancreas. arXiv:1804.03999 (2018)
19. Guimarães, P., et al.: A fast and efficient technique for the automatic tracing of corneal nerves in confocal microscopy. Trans. Vis. Sci. Technol. **5**(5), 7 (2016)
20. Yokogawa, H., et al.: Mapping of normal corneal K-structures by in vivo laser confocal microscopy. Cornea **27**, 879–883 (2008)

# PseudoEdgeNet: Nuclei Segmentation only with Point Annotations

Inwan Yoo, Donggeun Yoo, and Kyunghyun Paeng[✉]

Lunit Inc., Seoul, South Korea
{iwyoo,dgyoo,khpaeng}@lunit.io

**Abstract.** Nuclei segmentation is one of the important tasks for whole slide image analysis in digital pathology. With the drastic advance of deep learning, recent deep networks have demonstrated successful performance of the nuclei segmentation task. However, a major bottleneck to achieving good performance is the cost for annotation. A large network requires a large number of segmentation masks, and this annotation task is given to pathologists, not the public. In this paper, we propose a weakly supervised nuclei segmentation method, which requires only point annotations for training. This method can scale to large training set as marking a point of a nucleus is much cheaper than the fine segmentation mask. To this end, we introduce a novel auxiliary network, called PseudoEdgeNet, which guides the segmentation network to recognize nuclei edges even without edge annotations. We evaluate our method with two public datasets, and the results demonstrate that the method consistently outperforms other weakly supervised methods.

**Keywords:** Nuclei segmentation · Weakly supervised learning · Point annotation

## 1 Introduction

With the advent of digital pathology [2], extracting information of biological components from whole slide images (WSIs) is attracting more attention since the statistics can be utilized for biomarker development as well as accurate diagnosis [3]. However, it is infeasible for human experts (e.g. pathologists) to manually extract the statistics due to the huge dimensions of WSI space. A WSI can comprise up to $100k \times 100k$ pixels [12]. Despite its huge dimensions, the area of a target instance is usually small, such as a tumor cell. In order to automate this process, a variety of visual recognition methods from computer vision has been applied to WSIs [8,11,14,18]. Among the various recognition tasks, this paper focuses on the nuclei segmentation problem [14].

During the last few years, we have witnessed drastic progress in segmentation tasks on WSIs [8,14] with deep learning. Despite its successful performance, the cost for annotations is still worrisome. Drawing fine masks of target instances is much more labor-intensive than drawing bounding boxes or tagging class labels.

© Springer Nature Switzerland AG 2019
D. Shen et al. (Eds.): MICCAI 2019, LNCS 11764, pp. 731–739, 2019.
https://doi.org/10.1007/978-3-030-32239-7_81

Furthermore, only experts such as pathologists, not the public, can conduct this annotation task. The situation gets much worse when we choose a deep network as a segmentation model which can be learned with a large number of training samples. These factors make it difficult to create a large-scale segmentation dataset in the WSI domain.

This paper aims at cutting the annotation cost for nuclei segmentation. The quickest and easiest way to annotate a nucleus is to mark a point on it. A point does not contain fine boundary information of a nucleus, but we can obtain a much larger amount of training samples than segmentation masks, given a fixed budget for annotation. This strategy is scalable for learning a large network, and it is also expected that a large amount of training samples will contribute to the generalization performance [13] of the network.

To this end, we propose a novel weakly-supervised model, which is composed of a segmentation network and an auxiliary network, called PseudoEdgeNet. The segmentation network produces nuclei segments while the auxiliary network helps the main network learn to recognize nuclei boundaries with point annotations only. We evaluate this model over two public datasets [8,14] and the results demonstrate successful segmentation performance compared to other recent methods [9,15] for weakly-supervised segmentation.

## 2    Related Research

**Nuclei Segmentation.** There have been several works for nuclei segmentation based on deep learning, but all of the methods use a fully-supervised learning model that requires nuclei segmentation masks. [8] makes a public nuclei dataset containing full segmentation masks and introduces a segmentation model based on a pixel-level classification approach. [14] approaches the nuclei segmentation task as a regression problem. The work done by [19] is also a regression method but a sparsity constraint is introduced. [1] adopts a two-step approach where the model produces cell proposals first and then segments the nuclei.

**Cell Detection with Points.** Cell detection methods are related to ours since these often utilize point annotations [5,16,18]. One popular family casts cell detection as a regression problem, such as [5] and [16] adopt a regression Random Forest and a CNN regressor, respectively. Another approach is pixel-level classification with point annotations [18], which is similar to the typical semantic segmentation approach. However, these methods use the point annotations to learn a detection model which predicts the cell locations as points, not a segmentation model.

**Weakly-Supervised Segmentation.** To the best of our knowledge, there has been no weakly-supervised method for nuclei segmentation. However, in the natural image domain, a long line of works has been presented to reduce the cost of pixel-level annotations. An object segmentation model is learned with bounding-boxes [6] or scribbles [10,15], which are much cheaper to obtain than the pixel-level masks. The work presented by [9] is similar to ours in that it also uses point annotations. However, their target task is to find "rough blobs" on objects while we have to predict "fine boundaries" of nuclei.

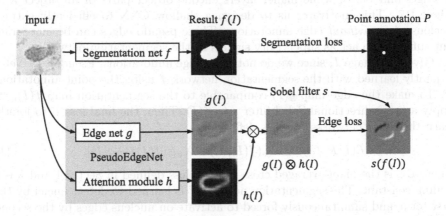

**Fig. 1.** The overall architecture for weakly-supervised nuclei segmentation. The segmentation network $f$ is jointly learned with PseudoEdgeNet $\{g, h\}$. In edge maps, the gray color represents zero while the white and black colors encode positive and negative pixel values, respectively.

## 3    Method

The proposed architecture is composed of a segmentation network and PseudoEdgeNet. The segmentation network is our target model that segments nuclei from inputs. PseudoEdgeNet, only introduced for training phase, encourages the segmentation network to recognize nucleus edges without edge annotations. Figure 1 is illustrating the proposed architecture.

### 3.1    Segmentation Network

To learn a segmentation network with point annotations, we follow the label assignment scheme presented by [9]. In this scheme, positive labels are given to the pixels corresponding to point annotations, while negative labels are assigned to pixels on Voronoi boundaries that can be obtained by distance transform with point annotations. Then, binary cross-entropy losses are evaluated and averaged over the labels and corresponding pixel outputs.

The segmentation network learned with this loss can successfully localize nuclei as blobs. However, it fails to segment along the edges of nuclei since there is no direct supervision for edges. For this reason, we introduce an auxiliary network that can provide fine boundary information with that the segmentation network is supervised to segment along the nucleus edges.

## 3.2 Learning with PseudoEdgeNet

In CNNs, it is well known that lower layers extract low-level information such as edges and blobs, while higher layers encode object parts or an object as a whole [17]. This motivates us to design a shallow CNN to efficiently extract nucleus edges *without* edge annotations. These pseudo edges can be inaccurate but sufficient to act as supervisory signals to the segmentation network.

Given an image $I$, since we do not have edge annotations, PseudoEdgeNet $g$ is jointly learned with the segmentation network $f$ using the point annotations $P$. To make the edge map $g(I)$ comparable to the segmentation map $f(I)$, we apply a $(x, y)$-directional Sobel filter $s$ to $f(I)$. Then, the final loss $\mathcal{L}$ to jointly learn these two networks $\{f, g\}$ is defined as

$$\mathcal{L}(I, P, f, g) = \mathcal{L}_{ce}(f(I), P) + \lambda \cdot |s(f(I)) - g(I)|, \tag{1}$$

where $\mathcal{L}_{ce}$ is the pixel-averaged cross-entropy loss defined in Sect. 3.1 and $\lambda$ is a scaling constant. The segmentation network $f$ is learned to detect nuclei by the first term, and simultaneously forced to activate on nucleus edges by the second term. PseudoEdgeNet $g$ is used only to learn $f$ with this loss, and unnecessary at inference time.

What is noteworthy here is the capacity gap between $f$ and $g$. If $g$ is as large as $f$, then $g$ will be learned just like $f$, except that the outputs are edges. However, since we design $g$ to be much smaller than $f$, $g$ is able to encode low/mid-level edges, not the high-level information, which only $f$ can cope with. Empirical analysis on this will be discussed later with Table 2 in Sect. 4.3.

## 3.3 Attention Module for Edge Network

According to our experiment in Table 1, the method presented up to Sect. 3.2 shows clear performance gains. However, there is still much room for improving the quality of edges used for auxiliary supervision. Due to the low capacity of $g$, a significant portion of edges originates from irrelevant backgrounds. To suppress these, we add an attention module $h$ inside PseudoEdgeNet, which produces an attention map $h(I)$, that indicates where to extract edges. Since this task requires high-level understanding of nuclei, we use a large architecture for this module. The attention map $h(I)$ is applied to the raw edge $g(I)$, and then the loss function is re-defined as

$$\mathcal{L}(I, P, f, g, h) = \mathcal{L}_{ce}(f(I), P) + \lambda \cdot |s(f(I)) - g(I) \otimes h(I)|, \tag{2}$$

where $\otimes$ means element-wise multiplication. We jointly learn parameters in $\{f, g, h\}$, and only use the segmentation network $f$ at inference time. Figure 2(b, c, d) shows how attention improves quality of edges.

## 4 Evaluation

### 4.1 Datasets

We evaluate our method with two major nuclei segmentation datasets: MoNuSeg [8] and *TNBC* [14]. MoNuSeg comprises 30 images in which each image size is $1,000 \times 1,000$. TNBC is composed of 50 images with $512 \times 512$ size. These two datasets provide full nuclei masks, that enable us to automatically generate point annotations and to evaluate segmentation results with full masks. To construct a training set composed of images and point annotations, we extract nuclei points by calculating the center of mass of each nucleus instance mask. We conduct $k$-fold cross-validation with $k = 10$ for thorough evaluation. Among 10 folds of data, we use two folds as a validation set and a test set, and the rest as a training set.

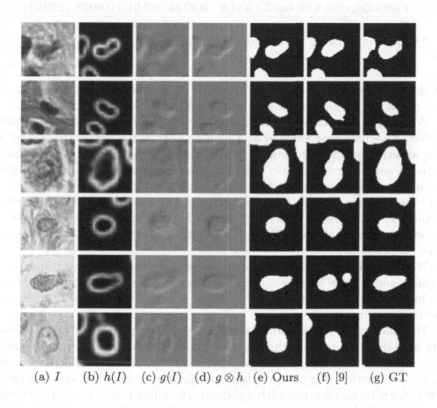

(a) $I$     (b) $h(I)$     (c) $g(I)$     (d) $g \otimes h$     (e) Ours     (f) [9]     (g) GT

**Fig. 2.** Qualitative examples and comparisons: (a) inputs, (b) attention maps, (c) $(x, y)$-directional raw edge maps, (d) final edge maps in which attentions are multiplied, (e) final segmentation results from our segmentation network, (f) segmentation results from the baseline method [9], and (g) ground-truth masks. In (c, d), each map is averaging the $x$- and $y$-directional edge maps. The gray color represents zero while the white and black colors encode positive and negative pixel values, respectively.

## 4.2   Implementation Details

We choose [9] as a baseline method, which is the most recent work for learning with point annotations. Among the loss terms in [9], we do not use the

**Table 1.** Nuclei segmentation performance comparison between methods. The mean and standard deviation of 10-fold cross-validation results (10 IoU scores) are reported.

| Methods | MoNuSeg | TNBC |
|---|---|---|
| Baseline [9] | 0.5710 ($\pm$0.02) | 0.5504 ($\pm$0.04) |
| DenseCRF* [15] | 0.5813 ($\pm$0.03) | 0.5555 ($\pm$0.04) |
| PseudoEdgeNet with large $g$ | 0.5786 ($\pm$0.04) | 0.5787 ($\pm$0.04) |
| PseudoEdgeNet with small $g$ | 0.6059 ($\pm$0.04) | 0.5853 ($\pm$0.03) |
| PseudoEdgeNet with small $g$ and $h$ | **0.6136** ($\pm$0.04) | **0.6038** ($\pm$0.03) |
| Fully supervised (upper bound) | 0.6522 ($\pm$0.03) | 0.6619 ($\pm$0.04) |

*Authors' open source is used: https://github.com/meng-tang/rloss

image-level classification loss since almost of image patches contain nuclei, but only adopt the pixel-averaged cross-entropy loss $\mathcal{L}_{ce}$ described in Sect. 3.1.

We employ a Feature Pyramid Network (FPN) for segmentation [7] with a ResNet-50 [4] backbone followed by a sigmoid layer as the segmentation network $f$ in all experiments. We compose $g$ of PseudoEdgeNet with four convolution layers to make it much smaller than the segmentation network $f$. Each of the convolution layers contains 64 filters and is followed by batch normalization and ReLU, except for the last layer, which produces a two-channel output representing $(x, y)$-directional Sobel edge maps. For the attention module $h$ inside PseudoEdgeNet, we use an FPN with a Resnet-18 backbone and stack a sigmoid as an output layer.

We set the label weights applied to the cross-entropy loss as 0.1 and 1.0 for negative and positive labels respectively since much more negatives are given to the loss function compared to the positives. The scaling constant $\lambda$ in Eqs. (1) and (2) is set to 1.0.

To achieve high generalization performance, we apply a lot of data augmentation methods to inputs including color jittering, Gaussian blurring, Gaussian noise injection, rotation, horizontal or vertical flip, affine transformation, and elastic deformation. We use an Adam optimizer with an initial learning rate of 0.001. We train all networks with a plateau scheduling policy where the learning rate is halved when the average loss per epoch does not decrease for the current five epochs.

The threshold to determine positive pixels from $f(I)$ is 0.5. We evaluate the model on the validation set for each epoch and choose the best model to evaluate that on the test set. We choose the intersection over union (IoU), which is the most common metric for semantic segmentation, as an evaluation metric.

### 4.3    Results

Table 1 is summarizing the experimental results. The most recent weakly supervised segmentation method [15] noted by DenseCRF marginally beats the baseline [9]. However, PseudoEdgeNet with small $g$ significantly improves the baseline by a large margin of +3.49% for both of the datasets. When PseudoEdgeNet is equipped with the attention module $h$, the performance gains increase to +4.26% and +5.34%. These results clearly demonstrate the effectiveness of $g$ and $h$. Compared to small $g$, the worse performance of large $g$ proves the importance of the capacity of $g$. For large $g$, we use the same architecture of $f$, so $g$ is learned just like $f$, resulting in a small improvement to the baseline.

To take a closer look at the importance of capacity, we try to densely change the depth of $g$. Table 2 is summarizing the results. For the family of small networks, the depth change from 2 to 8 does not make any significant difference in performance. However, when $g$ is equipped with large ResNets, the performance significantly drops. The depth variation within the large architecture also shows minor performance changes.

**Table 2.** Nuclei segmentation performance to the size of edge networks. The mean and standard deviation of 10-fold cross-validation results (10 IoU scores) are reported.

| Edge networks ($g$) | | MoNuSeg | TNBC |
|---|---|---|---|
| Small | CNN with 2 conv layers | 0.6117 ($\pm$0.03) | 0.5928 ($\pm$0.04) |
| | CNN with 4 conv layers | **0.6136** ($\pm$0.04) | **0.6038** ($\pm$0.03) |
| | CNN with 6 conv layers | 0.6105 ($\pm$0.04) | 0.5896 ($\pm$0.03) |
| | CNN with 8 conv layers | 0.6119 ($\pm$0.02) | 0.5934 ($\pm$0.04) |
| Large | FPN-ResNet18 | 0.6005 ($\pm$0.03) | 0.5795 ($\pm$0.04) |
| | FPN-ResNet34 | 0.6069 ($\pm$0.03) | 0.5796 ($\pm$0.03) |
| | FPN-ResNet50 | 0.5786 ($\pm$0.04) | 0.5787 ($\pm$0.04) |

## 5 Conclusion and Future Work

We have presented a novel nuclei segmentation method only with point supervision. Our auxiliary network, PseudoEdgeNet, can find object edges without edge annotations as it has low capacity, which acts as a strong constraint for weakly-supervised learning. Our method can scale to large-scale segmentation problem for better performance, as point annotations are much cheaper than segmentation masks.

However, given the same amount of data, the performance of weakly-supervised learning is bounded to that of supervised learning. It will be a promising future work to annotate a small number of segmentation masks, and use both mask and point annotations to achieve performance comparable to supervised learning, while greatly saving the annotation cost.

## References

1. Akram, S.U., Kannala, J., Eklund, L., Heikkilä, J.: Cell segmentation proposal network for microscopy image analysis. In: Carneiro, G., et al. (eds.) LABELS/DLMIA

-2016. LNCS, vol. 10008, pp. 21–29. Springer, Cham (2016). https://doi.org/10.1007/978-3-319-46976-8_3

2. Al-Janabi, S., Huisman, A., Van Diest, P.J.: Digital pathology: current status and future perspectives. Histopathology **61**(1), 1–9 (2012)

3. Beck, A.H., et al.: Systematic analysis of breast cancer morphology uncovers stromal features associated with survival. Sci. Transl. Med. **3**(108), 108ra113 (2011)

4. He, K., Zhang, X., Ren, S., Sun, J.: Deep residual learning for image recognition. In: Proceedings of the IEEE Conference on Computer Vision and Pattern Recognition (2016)

5. Kainz, P., Urschler, M., Schulter, S., Wohlhart, P., Lepetit, V.: You should use regression to detect cells. In: Navab, N., Hornegger, J., Wells, W.M., Frangi, A.F. (eds.) MICCAI 2015. LNCS, vol. 9351, pp. 276–283. Springer, Cham (2015). https://doi.org/10.1007/978-3-319-24574-4_33

6. Khoreva, A., Benenson, R., Hosang, J., Hein, M., Schiele, B.: Simple does it: weakly supervised instance and semantic segmentation. In: Proceedings of the IEEE Conference on Computer Vision and Pattern Recognition, pp. 876–885 (2017)

7. Kirillov, A., He, K., Girshick, R., Dollár, P.: A unified architecture for instance and semantic segmentation

8. Kumar, N., Verma, R., Sharma, S., Bhargava, S., Vahadane, A., Sethi, A.: A dataset and a technique for generalized nuclear segmentation for computational pathology. IEEE Trans. Med. Imaging **36**(7), 1550–1560 (2017)

9. Laradji, I.H., Rostamzadeh, N., Pinheiro, P.O., Vazquez, D., Schmidt, M.: Where are the blobs: counting by localization with point supervision. In: Proceedings of the European Conference on Computer Vision (ECCV), pp. 547–562 (2018)

10. Lin, D., Dai, J., Jia, J., He, K., Sun, J.: ScribbleSup: scribble-supervised convolutional networks for semantic segmentation. In: Proceedings of the IEEE Conference on Computer Vision and Pattern Recognition, pp. 3159–3167 (2016)

11. Litjens, G., et al.: Deep learning as a tool for increased accuracy and efficiency of histopathological diagnosis. Sci. Rep. **6** (2016). Article number: 26286

12. Liu, Y., et al.: Detecting cancer metastases on gigapixel pathology images. arXiv preprint arXiv:1703.02442 (2017)

13. Mahajan, D., et al.: Exploring the limits of weakly supervised pretraining. In: The European Conference on Computer Vision (ECCV), September 2018

14. Naylor, P., Laé, M., Reyal, F., Walter, T.: Segmentation of nuclei in histopathology images by deep regression of the distance map. IEEE Trans. Med. Imaging **38**(2), 448–459 (2018)

15. Tang, M., Perazzi, F., Djelouah, A., Ben Ayed, I., Schroers, C., Boykov, Y.: On regularized losses for weakly-supervised CNN segmentation. In: Proceedings of the European Conference on Computer Vision (ECCV), pp. 507–522 (2018)

16. Weidi, X., Noble, J.A., Zisserman, A.: Microscopy cell counting with fully convolutional regression networks. In: 1st Deep Learning Workshop, Medical Image Computing and Computer-Assisted Intervention (MICCAI) (2015)

17. Zeiler, M.D., Fergus, R.: Visualizing and understanding convolutional networks. In: Fleet, D., Pajdla, T., Schiele, B., Tuytelaars, T. (eds.) ECCV 2014. LNCS, vol. 8689, pp. 818–833. Springer, Cham (2014). https://doi.org/10.1007/978-3-319-10590-1_53

18. Zhou, Y., Dou, Q., Chen, H., Qin, J., Heng, P.A.: SFCN-OPI: detection and fine-grained classification of nuclei using sibling FCN with objectness prior interaction. In: Thirty-Second AAAI Conference on Artificial Intelligence (2018)

19. Zhou, Y., Chang, H., Barner, K.E., Parvin, B.: Nuclei segmentation via sparsity constrained convolutional regression. In: 2015 IEEE 12th International Symposium on Biomedical Imaging (ISBI), pp. 1284–1287. IEEE (2015)

# Adversarial Domain Adaptation and Pseudo-Labeling for Cross-Modality Microscopy Image Quantification

Fuyong Xing[1,2(✉)], Tell Bennett[2,3], and Debashis Ghosh[1,2]

[1] Department of Biostatistics and Informatics,
University of Colorado Anschutz Medical Campus, Aurora, USA
fuyong.xing@ucdenver.edu
[2] Data Science to Patient Value, University of Colorado Anschutz Medical Campus,
Aurora, USA
[3] Department of Pediatrics, University of Colorado Anschutz Medical Campus,
Aurora, USA

**Abstract.** Cell or nucleus quantification has recently achieved state-of-the-art performance by using convolutional neural networks (CNNs). In general, training CNNs requires a large amount of annotated microscopy image data, which is prohibitively expensive or even impossible to obtain in some applications. Additionally, when applying a deep supervised model to new datasets, it is common to annotate individual cells in those target datasets for model re-training or fine-tuning, leading to low-throughput image analysis. In this paper, we propose a novel adversarial domain adaptation method for cell/nucleus quantification across multimodality microscopy image data. Specifically, we learn a fully convolutional network detector with task-specific cycle-consistent adversarial learning, which conducts pixel-level adaptation between source and target domains and then completes a cell/nucleus detection task. Next, we generate pseudo-labels on target training data using the detector trained with adapted source images and further fine-tune the detector towards the target domain to boost the performance. We evaluate the proposed method on multiple cross-modality microscopy image datasets and obtain a significant improvement in cell/nucleus detection compared to the reference baselines and a recent state-of-the-art deep domain adaptation approach. In addition, our method is very competitive with the fully supervised models trained with all real target training labels.

## 1 Introduction

Convolutional neural networks (CNNs) have recently produced excellent cell detection performance [14]. Due to domain shifts, CNNs trained on one

**Electronic supplementary material** The online version of this chapter (https://doi.org/10.1007/978-3-030-32239-7_82) contains supplementary material, which is available to authorized users.

D. Shen et al. (Eds.): MICCAI 2019, LNCS 11764, pp. 740–749, 2019.
https://doi.org/10.1007/978-3-030-32239-7_82

microscopy image dataset (e.g., bright-field microscopy) might not be applicable to another (e.g., phase-contrast microscopy). It is common to annotate images in the target domain for model re-training. However, individual cell annotations are very expensive. Although one can fine-tune a pretrained CNN, it may still be difficult to collect enough annotated target data for proper fine-tuning in real applications [21]. Thus, it is necessary to design methods that can transfer learned knowledge from one to another domain without additional target data annotations.

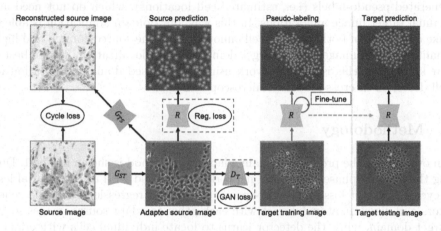

**Fig. 1.** The overview of the proposed adversarial domain adaptation method for cell detection. $G_{ST}$ and $D_T$ are the source-to-target generator and its associated discriminator, respectively. $G_{TS}$ is the target-to-source generator, and $R$ is the regression-based cell detector. The GAN loss is used to learn the adversarial networks, and the cycle loss ensures that adapted source images can translate into the original images. The detector $R$ is learned with adapted source images and then further fine-tuned with pseudo-labels on target images. The dashed gray arrow represents the transition from the training to testing stage. Here source and target images are generated using bright-field and phase-contrast microscopy, respectively. For clarity, we do not draw the target cycle.

Unsupervised domain adaptation is one type of method to address domain shifts without target data labeling [2,4]. Many previous unsupervised deep domain adaptation methods align feature distributions from source and target domains [4,16,21]. In particular, adversarial domain adaptation has been applied to medical image segmentation and classification [12,17]. However, these approaches that conduct deep feature matching might not effectively capture low-level image appearance variance. Additionally, it might be difficult to fully align feature distributions for structured output tasks [8] such as cell detection. On the other hand, some recent work [7,19] focuses on pixel-space adaptation for general image analysis using generative adversarial networks (GANs) [5]. These methods work well only for limited domain shifts, which might not hold in cross-modality microscopy image datasets, or formulate a pixel-wise classification model, which might not be optimal for cell detection [11,23].

In this paper, we propose a novel adversarial domain adaptation method for cross-modality cell/nucleus detection (see Fig. 1). Instead of conducting feature-space adaptation, we directly translate raw source images to target ones and learn a cell detector with task-specific cycle-consistent adversarial learning. In order to encode topological information in the label space, cell detector is modeled with structured regression in a fully convolutional network (FCN). In addition, we further fine-tune the detector using real target training images with generated pseudo-labels (i.e., estimated cell locations), which do not need any manual target image annotations. In this way, our domain adaptation is able to take advantage of both accurate cell annotations in the source domain and high-quality training images in the target domain for cell localization. To the best of our knowledge, this is the first work using GAN-based domain adaptation for cell detection in cross-modality microscopy images.

## 2 Methodology

An overview of the proposed domain adaptation method is shown in Fig. 1. During the training phase, the neural networks are learned with an adversarial loss, a cycle-consistent loss and a task-specific structured regression loss. The generators and discriminators interact with each other to adapt source images to the target domain, while the detector learns to locate individual cells with adapted source images, which appear as if drawn from the target domain. Next, we apply the detector to target training data for pseudo-label generation and then further fine-tune the detector with these *artificial annotations on real target images*. During the testing phase, for each new target image, the detector predicts one heat map, where local maxima indicate the locations of cell centers.

### 2.1 Task-Specific Cycle-Consistent Adversarial Learning

**Problem Definition.** Let $(\boldsymbol{X}^s, \boldsymbol{Y}^s) = \{(\boldsymbol{x}_i^s, \boldsymbol{y}_i^s)\}_{i=1}^{N^s}$ denote source training data with $N^s$ images $\boldsymbol{x}_i^s \in \mathbb{R}^{w \times h \times c}$ and corresponding structured labels $\boldsymbol{y}_i^s \in \mathbb{R}^{w \times h}$ ($w, h$ and $c$ are the width, height and channel of images or labels), and $\boldsymbol{X}^t = \{\boldsymbol{x}_i^t\}_{i=1}^{N^t}$ represent target training data with $N^t$ unannotated images $\boldsymbol{x}_i^t \in \mathbb{R}^{w' \times h' \times c'}$. With $(\boldsymbol{X}^s, \boldsymbol{Y}^s)$ and $\boldsymbol{X}^t$, our goal is to learn mappings between source $S$ and target $T$ domains such that source images $\boldsymbol{X}^s$ can be translated to target-style ones $\hat{\boldsymbol{X}}^s$, and build a cell detector $R$ based on these translated source images, which is applicable to real target data.

**Pixel-Level Domain Adaptation Modeling.** To close the gap between source and target domains, we need to map data from one domain to the other such that a discriminator fails in differentiating the two domains. Instead of relying on feature-matching adaptation, we conduct pixel-space adaptation by directly translating raw images between source and target domains. The reason is that feature-space adaptation assumes there exists a shared, cross-domain feature space, but this might not hold for structured prediction tasks [8], such as cell detection. Additionally, in order to preserve the content of source images during image translation, we apply a cycle-consistent constraint [24] to our generative adversarial learning for domain adaptation. This cycle-consistent adversarial learning has two generator-discriminator pairs, which enable the model to convert adapted images back into the domain where they come from. Meanwhile, it does not require paired source-target training images, which are generally not available in cross-modality cell detection.

Formally, given unpaired training data from source $S$ and target $T$ domains, our generative adversarial domain adaptation model learns two generators, $G_{ST}$ : $S \rightarrow T$ and $G_{TS} : T \rightarrow S$. Generator $G_{ST}$ adapts source images to the target domain so that its associated discriminator $D_T$ is unable to distinguish between adapted source images and real target images. Similarly, $G_{TS}$ maps data from the target to source domain, aiming to fool its corresponding discriminator $D_S$. This is achieved by using the adversarial loss [5] in both directions

$$\mathcal{L}_{GAN}(G_{ST}, D_T) = \mathbb{E}_{\boldsymbol{x}^t \sim \boldsymbol{X}^t}[\log D_T(\boldsymbol{x}^t)] + \mathbb{E}_{\boldsymbol{x}^s \sim \boldsymbol{X}^s}[\log(1 - D_T(G_{ST}(\boldsymbol{x}^s)))], (1)$$
$$\mathcal{L}_{GAN}(G_{TS}, D_S) = \mathbb{E}_{\boldsymbol{x}^s \sim \boldsymbol{X}^s}[\log D_S(\boldsymbol{x}^s)] + \mathbb{E}_{\boldsymbol{x}^t \sim \boldsymbol{X}^t}[\log(1 - D_S(G_{TS}(\boldsymbol{x}^t)))], (2)$$

where $\boldsymbol{x}^s / \boldsymbol{x}^t$ is a sample from the source/target domain. Differing from the vanilla GAN taking random noise as input [5], our generator $G_{ST}/G_{TS}$ synthesizes realistic target/source images from source/target images, i.e., adapting source/target data to the target/source domain. In order to enforce the cycle consistency [24] such that the reconstruction of adapted images is identical to their original versions, i.e., $G_{TS}(G_{ST}(\boldsymbol{x}^s)) \approx \boldsymbol{x}^s$ and $G_{ST}(G_{TS}(\boldsymbol{x}^t)) \approx \boldsymbol{x}^t$, we adopt an $\ell_1$ penalty on the reconstruction error

$$\mathcal{L}_{cycle}(G_{ST}, G_{TS}) = \mathbb{E}_{\boldsymbol{x}^s \sim \boldsymbol{X}^s}[\|G_{TS}(G_{ST}(\boldsymbol{x}^s)) - \boldsymbol{x}^s\|_1]$$
$$+ \mathbb{E}_{\boldsymbol{x}^t \sim \boldsymbol{X}^t}[\|G_{ST}(G_{TS}(\boldsymbol{x}^t)) - \boldsymbol{x}^t\|_1]. \tag{3}$$

In addition to the generators and discriminators, our framework also contains a structured regressor $R$, which maps input images into the label space for individual cell detection. Compared to pixel-wise classification, structured regression is able to exploit additional context information during training for more robust prediction [11,23]. Due to lack of data annotations in the target domain, we train this regressor with the adapted source images $G_{ST}(\boldsymbol{x}^s)$. Because the cycle-consistent adversarial learning preserves the content of source images during image translation, while making the adapted source images look similar to those from the target domain, we expect that a regressor trained with $G_{ST}(\boldsymbol{x}^s)$ and corresponding labels $\boldsymbol{y}^s$ can be applicable to the target domain. Specifically, this task-specific regression loss is chosen as a weighted mean squared error

$$\mathcal{L}_{reg}(G_{ST}, R) = \mathbb{E}_{(x^s, y^s) \sim (X^s, Y^s)}[\| (y^s + \alpha \bar{y}^s 1)^{1/2} \odot (R(G_{ST}(x^s)) - y^s) \|_F^2$$
$$+ \| (y^s + \alpha \bar{y}^s 1)^{1/2} \odot (R(x^s) - y^s) \|_F^2], (4)$$

where the label $y^s$ is a continuous-valued, non-negative proximity map and each pixel value measures the proximity of this pixel to its closest real cell center [23], higher values for closer positions. $\bar{y}^s$ is the mean value of $y^s$ and $1$ is a matrix with all entries equal to one. $\alpha$ controls the contributions from different image regions and $\odot$ denotes the element-wise multiplication. Note that we train this cell detector with both adapted and original source images [3].

With the loss functions defined above, our full objective is formulated as

$$\mathcal{L}(G_{ST}, G_{TS}, D_S, D_T, R) = \mathcal{L}_{GAN}(G_{ST}, D_T) + \mathcal{L}_{GAN}(G_{TS}, D_S)$$
$$+ \lambda \mathcal{L}_{cycle}(G_{ST}, G_{TS}) + \gamma \mathcal{L}_{reg}(G_{ST}, R), \quad (5)$$

where $\lambda$ and $\gamma$ weight the importance of cycle consistency and regression, respectively. We aim to learn the detector $R$ by solving the following problem

$$\arg \min_{\{G_{ST}, G_{TS}, R\}} \max_{\{D_S, D_T\}} \mathcal{L}(G_{ST}, G_{TS}, D_S, D_T, R). \quad (6)$$

In our implementation, $G_{ST}$ and $G_{TS}$ are FCNs [10] with 9 residual blocks [6]. $D_S$ and $D_T$ are chosen as the $70 \times 70$ PatchGAN network [9], which is computationally efficient. For regressor $R$, we use the fully residual convolutional network [23] that has 9 residual blocks [6] and 4 long-range skip connections [18].

## 2.2   Learning with Pseudo-Labels

With pixel-space domain adaptation, we are able to translate source images into target-style ones in terms of color and texture, and the detector trained with these translated images would be applicable to real target data. However, it might be difficult for cycle-consistent adversarial learning to effectively handle very large domain shifts between source and target domains. We believe that the detector can be further improved by using real target training images. Because individual cell annotations are not available in the target domain, we propose to fine-tune the detector with pseudo-labels, which are generated by applying the detector to cell location estimation/prediction on target training images.

For each target training image $x^t$, the detector $R$ predicts one identical-sized heat map $\hat{y}^t$, where larger values mean these pixels are more close to cell centers. In order to mitigate the effects of image noise, we suppress the pixels with values less than $\eta \cdot max(\hat{y}^t)$, where $\eta \in [0, 1]$, by assigning them zeros and then locate cell centers by seeking local maxima on the suppressed prediction map. With these detected centers, we follow [23] to generate (pseudo) labels $\tilde{y}^t$ for images

$x^t$ by using a function of the distance transform, and fine-tune the detector $R$ using the regression loss with $(x^t, \tilde{y}^t)$ pairs. During the testing phase, we apply the final detector to cell detection on target images and locate cells by seeking local maxima in the corresponding predicted maps, where the low-valued pixels are also suppressed.

## 3    Experiments

**Datasets.** We extensively evaluate the proposed method on three microscopy image datasets, which are acquired using different staining techniques or imaging protocols/modalities. The first dataset [20] consists of 100 hematoxylin and eosin (H&E) stained colon cancer histology images, each of which is acquired with bright-field microscopy at 20× magnification and has a dimension of 500 × 500 × 3. The second dataset contains 114 pancreatic neuroendocrine tumor bright-field microscopy images (at 20× magnification), and they use immunohistochemical (IHC) Ki67 staining and have a dimension of 500 × 500 × 3. The third dataset [1] is composed of 22 cervical cancer HeLa cell line images, which are generated with phase-contrast (PC) microscopy. This dataset does not use either H&E or IHC staining and each image has size 400 × 400 × 3. All the datasets provide gold-standard annotations of cell/nucleus centers. Following [1,23], we randomly split each dataset into two halves, one for training and the other for testing. We use the metrics [23] for detection evaluation, i.e., precision, recall and $F_1$ score.

**Table 1.** $F_1$ score (%) of domain adaptation (source → target) on different datasets. The last row denotes the fully supervised models trained with all target training data only, and the last column represents the average across all six settings in each row.

| Method | H&E → IHC | H&E → PC | IHC → H&E | IHC → PC | PC → H&E | PC → IHC | Avg. |
|---|---|---|---|---|---|---|---|
| ADDA [21] | 79.4 | 56.9 | 66.9 | 84.9 | 51.3 | 69.9 | 68.2 |
| Baseline | 77.8 | 16.7 | 54.0 | 33.7 | 60.0 | 70.7 | 52.2 |
| PL | 78.7 | 26.9 | 57.0 | 40.2 | 62.5 | 71.9 | 56.2 |
| PSA | 78.9 | 83.4 | 68.9 | 88.6 | 55.4 | 72.5 | 74.6 |
| Ours | **83.1** | **92.5** | **70.5** | **89.3** | **63.0** | **78.5** | **79.5** |
| Target only | 87.4 | 96.1 | 81.4 | 96.1 | 81.4 | 87.4 | 88.3 |

**Implementation Details.** We empirically set the parameter values as: $\alpha = 5$ in Eq. (4), $\lambda = 10, \gamma = 1$ in Eq. (5) and $\eta = 0.4$ for pixel suppression during model inference. We closely follow [24] to set the other hyperparameters and use the Adam solver [13] with a learning rate of $2 \times 10^{-4}$ for adversarial model training. We apply a stage-wise training strategy to model learning [7]. With pseudo-labels, we fine-tune the detector with $10^5$ iterations. We use data augmentation such as randomly cropping, rotation and mirroring during model training.

**Domain Adaptation Evaluation.** Table 1 lists the $F_1$ score of domain adaptation on cross-modality microscopy image datasets. The reference baselines are the regression detector models directly trained with source data only. For a comparison, we evaluate two variants of our method: (1) pseudo-labeling (PL), which fine-tunes the baseline models with estimated cell locations (i.e., pseudo-labels) obtained by running the baselines on target training data, and (2) pixel-space adaptation (PSA), which is trained with adapted source images but no further fine-tuning with pseudo-labels. We also report the results of a recent state-of-the-art deep adversarial domain adaptation method, ADDA [21], and it is outperformed by our method on all the datasets, particularly in the H&E $\rightarrow$ PC experiment, where there is a large dataset shift between the source and target domains. We note that both PL and PSA outperform the baselines, and PSA provides a significant improvement by increasing the average $F_1$ score from 52.2% to 74.6%. Our method (i.e., PSA + PL) achieves the best performance for all the domain adaptation settings, further improving the average score to 79.5% and closing the gap to the supervised models trained with all real target data labels only. In particular, our method approaches the ideal performance for H&E $\rightarrow$ IHC and H&E $\rightarrow$ PC. This indicates that our method is effective at adapting the H&E stained microscopy images to other modality domains. Qualitative results of cell detection are provided in Figures S1–S3 at the Supplementary Material.

We also extend and evaluate the proposed method by using an additional subset of real target training annotations for model training. Figure 2 shows that using only a subset of target annotations, our method further improves cell detection and provides equivalent performance to the supervised models trained with the full target annotations only. In this scenario, it can significantly reduce human effort for target data labeling. Additionally, we further notice that the improvement grows slowly when more real target training labels are used, probably because the detector approaches its model capacity with more real data.

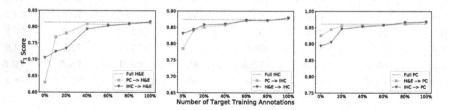

**Fig. 2.** $F_1$ score of cell detection with respect to different numbers (percentage) of real target training annotations. Red dashed lines represent the supervised models trained with the full (i.e. 100%) target training annotations only. (Color figure online)

**Comparison with State-of-the-Art Fully Supervised Methods.** We compare the proposed method to several recent fully supervised deep learning models, FCN-8s [15], U-Net [18] and FCRNA/FCRNB [22], which are trained with all real target training annotations, as shown in Table 2. We see that our method outperforms the classification models, i.e. FCN-8s and U-Net, on all the three datasets. In addition, our method is very competitive with the fully supervised regression models, i.e. FCRNA/FCRNB, especially for the IHC and PC datasets. This confirms the effectiveness of our method that requires no real target labels.

**Table 2.** Comparison with state-of-the-art fully supervised methods in terms of precision (P), recall (R), and $F_1$ score (%). For our method that does not use any real target annotations, we report the performance of the experimental settings, IHC $\rightarrow$ H&E, H&E $\rightarrow$ IHC and H&E $\rightarrow$ PC for the H&E, IHC and PC datasets, respectively.

| Method | H&E | | | IHC | | | PC | | |
|---|---|---|---|---|---|---|---|---|---|
| | P | R | $F_1$ | P | R | $F_1$ | P | R | $F_1$ |
| FCN-8s [15] | 57.3 | 79.5 | 66.6 | 97.0 | 55.0 | 70.2 | 70.2 | 93.1 | 80.0 |
| U-Net [18] | 39.5 | 85.2 | 54.0 | 88.5 | 64.0 | 74.3 | 82.7 | 80.4 | 81.5 |
| FCRNA [22] | 72.4 | 87.7 | 79.3 | 83.1 | 89.5 | 86.2 | 97.3 | 94.5 | 95.9 |
| FCRNB [22] | 68.8 | 97.0 | 80.5 | 82.4 | 92.6 | 87.2 | 98.0 | 91.5 | 94.6 |
| Ours | 81.2 | 62.3 | 70.5 | 73.9 | 94.8 | 83.1 | 92.7 | 92.3 | 92.5 |

## 4   Conclusion

We propose a novel deep generative adversarial domain adaptation method for cell/nucleus detection in cross-modality microscopy image data. It adapts raw source images to a target domain with cycle-consistent adversarial learning and trains a structured regression-based object detector with the adapted source images. Additionally, it further fine-tunes the detector with pseudo-labels of target training data. Extensive experiments on multiple microscopy image datasets demonstrate the effectiveness of the proposed method.

**Acknowledgement.** This research was supported by the National Cancer Institute of the National Institutes of Health under Award Number R21CA237493.

## References

1. Arteta, C., Lempitsky, V., Noble, J.A., Zisserman, A.: Learning to detect cells using non-overlapping extremal regions. In: Ayache, N., Delingette, H., Golland, P., Mori, K. (eds.) MICCAI 2012. LNCS, vol. 7510, pp. 348–356. Springer, Heidelberg (2012). https://doi.org/10.1007/978-3-642-33415-3_43
2. Bermúdez-Chacón, R., Becker, C., Salzmann, M., Fua, P.: Scalable unsupervised domain adaptation for electron microscopy. In: Ourselin, S., Joskowicz, L., Sabuncu, M.R., Unal, G., Wells, W. (eds.) MICCAI 2016. LNCS, vol. 9901, pp. 326–334. Springer, Cham (2016). https://doi.org/10.1007/978-3-319-46723-8_38

3. Bousmalis, K., et al.: Unsupervised pixel-level domain adaptation with generative adversarial networks. In: CVPR, pp. 3722–3731 (2017)
4. Ganin, Y., et al.: Domain-adversarial training of neural networks. JMLR **17**(1), 2096-2030 (2016)
5. Goodfellow, I., et al.: Generative adversarial nets. In: NIPS, pp. 2672–2680 (2014)
6. He, K., Zhang, X., Ren, S., Sun, J.: Deep residual learning for image recognition. In: CVPR, pp. 770–778 (2016)
7. Hoffman, J., et al.: CyCADA: cycle-consistent adversarial domain adaptation. In: ICML, pp. 1989–1998 (2018)
8. Hong, W., Wang, Z., Yang, M., Yuan, J.: Conditional generative adversarial network for structured domain adaptation. In: CVPR, pp. 1335–1344 (2018)
9. Isola, P., Zhu, J., Zhou, T., Efros, A.A.: Image-to-image translation with conditional adversarial networks. In: CVPR, pp. 5967–5976 (2017)
10. Johnson, J., Alahi, A., Fei-Fei, L.: Perceptual losses for real-time style transfer and super-resolution. In: Leibe, B., Matas, J., Sebc, N., Welling, M. (eds.) ECCV 2016. LNCS, vol. 9906, pp. 694–711. Springer, Cham (2016). https://doi.org/10.1007/978-3-319-46475-6_43
11. Kainz, P., Urschler, M., Schulter, S., Wohlhart, P., Lepetit, V.: You should use regression to detect cells. In: Navab, N., Hornegger, J., Wells, W.M., Frangi, A.F. (eds.) MICCAI 2015. LNCS, vol. 9351, pp. 276–283. Springer, Cham (2015). https://doi.org/10.1007/978-3-319-24574-4_33
12. Kamnitsas, K., et al.: Unsupervised domain adaptation in brain lesion segmentation with adversarial networks. In: Niethammer, M., et al. (eds.) IPMI 2017. LNCS, vol. 10265, pp. 597–609. Springer, Cham (2017). https://doi.org/10.1007/978-3-319-59050-9_47
13. Kingma, D.P., Ba, J.: Adam: a method for stochastic optimization. In: ICLR, pp. 1–15 (2015)
14. Litjens, G., et al.: A survey on deep learning in medical image analysis. MIA **42**, 60–88 (2017)
15. Long, J., Shelhamer, E., Darrell, T.: Fully convolutional networks for semantic segmentation. In: CVPR, pp. 3431–3440 (2015)
16. Long, M., Cao, Y., Wang, J., Jordan, M.: Learning transferable features with deep adaptation networks. In: ICML, pp. 97–105 (2015)
17. Ren, J., Hacihaliloglu, I., Singer, E.A., Foran, D.J., Qi, X.: Adversarial domain adaptation for classification of prostate histopathology whole-slide images. In: Frangi, A.F., Schnabel, J.A., Davatzikos, C., Alberola-López, C., Fichtinger, G. (eds.) MICCAI 2018. LNCS, vol. 11071, pp. 201–209. Springer, Cham (2018). https://doi.org/10.1007/978-3-030-00934-2_23
18. Ronneberger, O., Fischer, P., Brox, T.: U-Net: convolutional networks for biomedical image segmentation. In: Navab, N., Hornegger, J., Wells, W.M., Frangi, A.F. (eds.) MICCAI 2015. LNCS, vol. 9351, pp. 234–241. Springer, Cham (2015). https://doi.org/10.1007/978-3-319-24574-4_28
19. Shrivastava, A., et al.: Learning from simulated and unsupervised images through adversarial training. In: CVPR, pp. 2242–2251 (2017)
20. Sirinukunwattana, K., Raza, S.E.A., Tsang, Y.W., Snead, D.R.J., Cree, I.A., Rajpoot, N.M.: Locality sensitive deep learning for detection and classification of nuclei in routine colon cancer histology images. IEEE TMI **35**(5), 1196–1206 (2016)
21. Tzeng, E., Hoffman, J., Saenko, K., Darrell, T.: Adversarial discriminative domain adaptation. In: CVPR, pp. 2962–2971 (2017)

22. Xie, W., Noble, J.A., Zisserman, A.: Microscopy cell counting with fully convolutional regression networks. In: DLMIA Workshop, pp. 1–8 (2015)
23. Xie, Y., Xing, F., Shi, X., Kong, X., Su, H., Yang, L.: Efficient and robust cell detection: a structured regression approach. MIA **44**, 245–254 (2018)
24. Zhu, J.Y., Park, T., Isola, P., Efros, A.A.: Unpaired image-to-image translation using cycle-consistent adversarial networks. In: ICCV, pp. 2223–2232 (2017)

# Progressive Learning for Neuronal Population Reconstruction from Optical Microscopy Images

Jie Zhao, Xuejin Chen(✉), Zhiwei Xiong, Dong Liu, Junjie Zeng, Yueyi Zhang, Zheng-Jun Zha, Guoqiang Bi, and Feng Wu

National Engineering Laboratory for Brain-inspired Intelligence Technology and Application, University of Science and Technology of China, Hefei, China
xjchen99@ustc.edu.cn

**Abstract.** Reconstruction of 3D neuronal populations from optical microscopy images is essential to investigate neural pathways and functions. This task is challenging because of the low signal-to-noise ratio and non-continuous intensities of neurite segments in optical microscopy images. Recently, significant improvement has been made on neuron reconstruction due to the development of deep neural networks (DNNs). Training such a DNN usually relies on a large number of images with voxel-wise annotations, and annotating these 3D images is very costly in terms of both finance and labor. In this paper, we propose a progressive learning strategy to take advantages of both traditional neuron tracing methods and deep learning techniques. Traditional neuron tracing techniques, which do not require expensive manual annotations for dense neurites, are employed to produce pseudo labels for neuron voxels. With the pseudo labels, a deep segmentation network is trained to learn discriminative and comprehensive features for neuron voxel extraction from noisy backgrounds. The neuron tracing module and the segmentation network can be mutually complemented and progressively improved to reconstruct more complete neuronal populations without using manual annotations. Moreover, we build a dataset called "VISoR-40" that consists of 40 optical microscopy 3D images from mouse cortical regions to demonstrate the superior performance of our progressive learning method. This dataset will be available at https://braindata.bitahub.com to support further study of deep learning techniques for brain exploration.

**Keywords:** Deep learning · Neuronal population reconstruction · 3D image segmentation · Optical microscopy

**Electronic supplementary material** The online version of this chapter (https://doi.org/10.1007/978-3-030-32239-7_83) contains supplementary material, which is available to authorized users.

# 1  Introduction

Reconstruction of 3D neuronal population is essential in brain studies as it supports precise identification of neuronal pathways and functions. Recently, many efforts have been devoted to develop neuron reconstruction algorithms based on optical microscopy (OM) images. However, this task is still one of the main challenges in computational neuroscience. The challenges of 3D neuronal population reconstruction from OM images mainly come from the low quality of imaging and complex neuron structures. For example, due to the unevenly distributed fluorescence markers in neurons and complicated processes of imaging acquisition, the intensities of voxels that are occupied by neurons vary dramatically in highly inhomogeneous and noisy environments. It is highly expensive to manually extract and analyze neuron morphology from these noisy images. Therefore, an effective and automatic or semi-automatic algorithm of neuronal population reconstruction under various situations could substantially facilitate comprehensive analysis of neuron structures.

Many techniques have been proposed for 3D neuron reconstruction from OM images by combining computer vision algorithms and neuron morphological knowledge. Most traditional algorithms [5,8,12,13] consist of two stages. Typically, the first stage is to detect neuron voxels from OM images, which is essentially an foreground-background segmentation problem. The following stage is to trace neuronal trajectories from the extracted neuron voxels by integrating local searching strategies, global trajectory characteristics and pruning techniques. Most of existing methods solve neuron segmentation problem with simple hand-crafted features. While this strategy works well for high-quality images, it has difficulty in separating weak neuron voxels from an inhomogeneous background. With respect to more challenging and complex images, these methods degrade in performance and become time-consuming. Moreover, a number of parameters have to be carefully tuned to obtain satisfying performance.

Recently, significant progress has been made by learning-based methods [1, 4,15], which bring the power of machine learning to improve the performance of neuron segmentation. By extracting handcrafted features and classifying image voxels with a support vector machine classifier [1], the performance of neuron segmentation is improved, which leads to better neuron reconstruction. Later on, more comprehensive features were exploited by deep neural networks (DNNs) [4,15]. Though more accurate segmentation of neuron voxels could be achieved on a specific dataset, these learning-based methods rely on strong supervision for training, i.e., manual annotations for dense voxels. Unfortunately, due to the dense distribution of neuronal population in images, such annotations are extremely time-consuming and require expensive labor to obtain.

While traditional techniques do not need manual annotations, and learning-based methods could learn more complicated features with extensive annotated data, we propose to leverage these two techniques in a progressive learning manner. We observe that reconstruction maps inferred from existing traditional algorithms can effectively provide approximate locations of neurons. Although these voxels may not cover all neurons, they provide important cues for obtaining complicated patterns of neurons. Therefore, we take advantages of traditional techniques to produce pseudo labels to train a segmentation network to predict neuron voxels from images. We propose an iterative framework to train a segmentation network progressively without using manual annotations. The deep segmentation network is expected to learn more comprehensive features for neurons from noisy labels. With more powerful segmentation network for neuron voxels, the neuron reconstruction could be improved. We progressively refine the segmentation network with better neuron reconstruction results as pseudo labels, and produce more complete neurons with better segmentation.

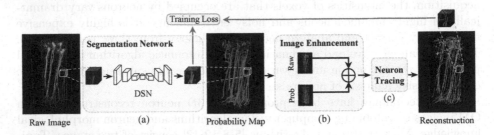

**Fig. 1.** Diagram of our method for neuronal population reconstruction.

## 2   Proposed Method

### 2.1   Progressive Learning Without Annotations

To reconstruct neurons from an image, our method consists of three key components: a segmentation network, an image enhancement module, and a neuron tracing module, as Fig. 1 shows. The segmentation network is designed to extract neuron voxels from noisy and complex backgrounds. In order to train the segmentation network to learn representative and distinctive features for extracting neuron voxels, strong supervision of dense voxel-wise annotations are required for existing deep learning-based methods. Instead of acquiring manual annotations with huge efforts, we progressively train the segmentation network with the reconstructed neurons as labels using traditional neuron tracing methods. Here, we utilize the NGPST [8] to reconstruct a neuronal population. The neuron tracing block can be replaced by any tracing technique that does not require voxel-wise annotations for training. Then the raw image is enhanced by fusing the predicted probability map of neuron voxels with the raw intensities in order to preserve both global structures and local signals simultaneously. By feeding the enhanced image to the neuron tracing module, more complete neuronal population can be reconstructed.

Our system progressively improves the neuron reconstruction performance by combining traditional tracing methods and DNNs without any manual annotations. As shown in Fig. 2(a), neurites are subtle because of the low contrast and noises in the raw image. At the beginning, the reconstructed neurons are incomplete and many neurites are missing, as Fig. 2(g) shows, compared to the ground truth (GT) shown in Fig. 2(k). Then trained by the pseudo labels derived from non-perfect reconstruction, the segmentation network is able to learn features for global trajectories, and the predicted probability maps demonstrate the enhanced trajectories, as Fig. 2(b) shows. With more iterations of network training and neuron reconstruction, our segmentation network captures more distinctive and long-range trajectory features progressively, as shown in Fig. 2(c), (d) and (e). By combining the probability map with the raw image intensities, both global trajectories and local signal details are well preserved. Figure 2(f) shows the enhanced image. Iteration by iteration, the reconstruction of neuronal population becomes more and more complete and accurate, as shown in Fig. 2(h), (i) and (j).

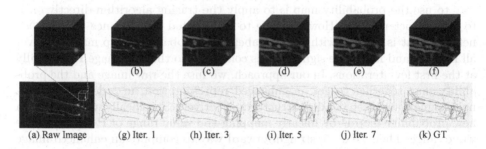

(a) Raw Image     (g) Iter. 1     (h) Iter. 3     (i) Iter. 5     (j) Iter. 7     (k) GT

**Fig. 2.** Our progressive learning technique gradually improves the segmentation network to more accurately extract neuron voxels from raw images (b–f). With better extraction of neuron voxels, more and more complete neuronal population can be reconstructed (g–j). Individual neurons are delineated in different colors. (Color figure online)

## 2.2 Segmentation Network and Training

Since neurons vary significantly in size, morphology, and intensity, we adopt a 3D segmentation network to exploit the neuron structures in 3D. The segmentation network can be any end-to-end trainable 3D segmentation network, such as 3D U-Net [2], 3D DSN [3], and DenseVoxNet [14]. In this paper, we adopt the 3D DSN as our neuron segmentation network to balance the performance and memory cost. Although DSN has demonstrated its excellent performance in volumetric medical image segmentation [3], it is still prone to overfitting in our case, with limited training data. We employ the dropout technique [9] for training our network and the dropout layer is implemented following each convolutional layer with a dropout rate of 0.5.

Moreover, the volume of non-neuron voxels is typically much larger than that of neurons in images. This data imbalance could suppress the performance of the segmentation network. We use a data balancing technique to address this issue. Specifically, for each cube, we randomly select a certain portion of background voxels as non-neuron samples, while the rest background voxels are not included in the loss computation. The number of background voxels for training is set as 10 times that of neuron voxels. Last but not the least, voxel intensities along the axial dimension in OM images are interpolated to the same resolution with the lateral dimension after the imaging process. Due to the inhomogeneity of imaging quality of different dimensions, a random transposition process of each cube is employed as data augmentation for training.

### 2.3  Image Enhancement

By using the trained segmentation network, a probability cube of the corresponding input cube is predicted. Then all probability cubes are stitched together to obtain a probability map $\mathbf{P}$ for the entire image stack. Each element of $\mathbf{P}(x)$ indicates the probability of the corresponding voxel $x$ as a neuron. A natural way to use the probability map is to apply the tracing algorithm directly on it to reconstruct neurons. However, due to the limited performance of the DNN network that is trained with pseudo labels, the probability map may not cover all neurons and lose some signal details compared to the raw image $\mathbf{I}$, especially at the first few iterations. In our approach, we fuse the raw image and the probability map together to get an enhanced representation, in order to suppress noise signals and keep detailed structures effectively. Specifically, we construct a new probability map $\widetilde{\mathbf{P}}$ by linearly mapping the value range of $\mathbf{P} \in [0, 1]$ to the value range. Then we use a straightforward way to compute an enhanced image $\mathbf{A}$ from the probability map $\widetilde{\mathbf{P}}$ and the raw image $\mathbf{I}$ as

$$\mathbf{A}(x) = \alpha\widetilde{\mathbf{P}}(x) + (1 - \alpha)\mathbf{I}(x), \tag{1}$$

where $\alpha$ is a weight to control the contributions the probability and the original intensity. We empirically select $\alpha = 0.1$. Experiment results with different values of $\alpha$ are reported in the supplementary materials to demonstrate the robustness of our method. When the enhanced images are used as input to the neuron tracing module, more complete neurites can be reconstructed.

## 3  Experiments and Results

### 3.1  Datasets and Settings

In order to validate our approach, and more importantly, to support further studies on the dense neuronal population reconstruction, we construct an OM image dataset called **VISoR-40**, which consists of 40 volumetric images from mouse cortical regions. These images were captured by the VISoR imaging system [10], with image sizes that range from $419 \times 1197 \times 224$ to $869 \times 1853 \times 575$ and the physical resolution of $0.5 \times 0.5 \times 0.5 \,\mu m^3$ per voxel. At this scale, identification of every individual neuron is feasible for neuron morphology analysis. The raw volumetric data has 16-bit dynamic range of intensity that preserves enough neurite details. We randomly pick 4/5 of the entire dataset for progressively training the segmentation network. Then the remaining images were used as the testing data to evaluate our method. To get manual annotations of the testing data, we ask two experts to manually annotate individual neurons using the 3D Virtual Finger plugin in Vaa3D [6]. Their agreed annotations are set as the ground truth for evaluation.

The **BigNeuron** [7] dataset is a well-known neuron dataset which includes about 20,000 OM images. These OM images are captured from different species and imaging pipelines, and a small part of them have the corresponding manual annotations. Unlike our VISoR-40 dataset which is built for dense neuronal population reconstruction, each image in BigNeuron dataset contains a single neuron or disconnected neurite segments which is suitable for evaluation of single neuron reconstruction. For further comparison, we adopt the same training data and testing data applied in Li2017 [4] as additional data.

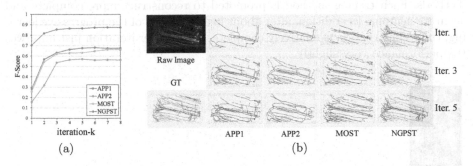

(a)       (b)

**Fig. 3.** Comparisons of neuronal population reconstruction performance on the VISoR-40 test dataset at different iterations using four neuron tracing methods.

Pytorch is adopted to implement the DSN model. At each iteration of our progressive learning, the DSN model is trained from random initialization with Gaussian distribution with zero-mean and variance of 0.01. The optimization is realized with the stochastic gradient descend algorithm (batch size of 1, weight decay of 0.0005, momentum of 0.9). The base learning rate was set to 0.001 and descended with "poly" learning rate policy (power of 0.9 and the maximum iteration number of 24000). The cube size is selected as $160 \times 160 \times 160$ considering the memory limitation on a GTX 1080Ti GPU.

## 3.2 Results and Discussions

To quantitatively evaluate our method, four commonly used metrics defined in [8], including Precision, Recall, F-Score, and Jaccard, are computed to measure the fidelity between a reconstruction and the ground truth.

**Progressive Learning.** Our key idea is to progressively learn features to extract neuron voxels from noisy backgrounds by utilizing a deep segmentation network with pseudo labels obtained by traditional tracing methods. This progressive learning strategy greatly improves neuronal population reconstruction performance without any annotations. We test four widely used techniques as the neuron tracing module in our framework. They are NGPST [8], MOST [11], APP1 [5] and its variant APP2 [12], respectively. Their implementations are available in the software Vaa3D [6]. Each neuron tracing method is tested to produce pseudo labels for the training of the segmentation network on our VISoR-40 dataset. Eight iterations are tested, and the improvement of reconstruction performance using different neuron tracing methods is shown in Fig. 3(a). Here, we only show the F-Score, which is commonly used to reflect the overall performance of the reconstruction results. Accordingly, Fig. 3(b) shows the reconstructed neurons on a test image at different iterations. More quantitative and qualitative results are reported in the supplementary materials. It can be seen that our progressive learning framework effectively facilitates traditional neuron tracing methods. Each tracing method is promoted to reconstruct more complete and accurate neurons. In addition, after about five iterations of the progressive learning, the reconstruction is relatively complete, and further iteration just improves the performance very slightly.

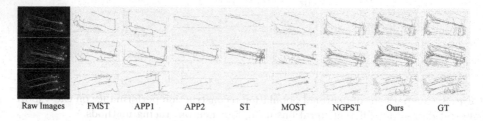

Raw Images    FMST    APP1    APP2    ST    MOST    NGPST    Ours    GT

**Fig. 4.** Comparisons of neuron reconstruction results by different methods on three test images from the VISoR-40 dataset.

**Comparisons on VISoR-40 Dataset.** In order to validate the effectiveness of our method on reconstructing dense neuronal population, we compare our results with six widely used methods on our VISoR-40 dataset, including FMST [13], APP1 [5], APP2 [12], MOST [11], SmartTracing (ST) [1], and NGPST [8]. Table 1 shows the quantitative results of our method, compared with the six methods. "Ours" means that we use NGPST with DSN enhancement after progressive learning on VISoR-40 dataset. It can be observed that our approach makes a significant improvement compared with the second best result [8]. Figure 4 shows the reconstructed neurons using different methods on three test images. It can be seen that our method outperforms others in both sparse and dense neurites. APP1, APP2, ST, MOST tend to extract the main trunk of the neurons while a large portion of subtle neurites are missing. Therefore, these methods lead to very high precision but significantly lower recall. NGPST works better to identity dense neurites. However, subtle neurites are still hard to extract by using hand-crafted features. In comparison, our method benefits from the progressively trained DSN, and reconstructs more complete and precise neurites for challenging OM images, even there exhibit low contrast, noises, and blending of fluorescence in the images.

**Comparisons on BigNeuron Dataset.** To further validate the effectiveness of our method, we also compare our results with six methods on a public BigNeuron [7] dataset, including FMST, MOST, APP2, SmartTracing, NGPST and Li2017 [4]. For a fair comparison with deep learning-based method, we use the test dataset and three evaluation metrics the same as Li2017 [4]. Specifically, these metrics are "entire structure average" (ESA), "different structure average" (DSA) and "percentage of different structures" (PDS). The weighted average of the ESA, DSA and PDS on all test images of different methods are reported in Table 2. The weights are proportional to the neuron lengths identified in the ground truth. "Ours" means that we use NGPST with DSN enhancement after progressive learning on the VISoR-40 dataset first and then finetuned on the BigNeuron dataset using pseudo labels rather than using the provided annotations. It can be seen that our method outperforms others in both ESA and PDS metrics and also achieves comparable performance in DSA metric with the best one. In particular, different from the supervised deep learning-based method [4], our progressive learning algorithm gets even better performance without using any manual annotations. As more and more unlabeled datasets are collected, our method can easily utilize these datasets to further improve the performance.

**Table 1.** Comparison on VISoR-40 dataset of neuronal population reconstruction.

| Methods | Precision | Recall | F-Score | Jaccard |
|---|---|---|---|---|
| ST [1] | 0.961 | 0.133 | 0.205 | 0.128 |
| APP1 [5] | 0.935 | 0.169 | 0.284 | 0.167 |
| APP2 [12] | **0.980** | 0.091 | 0.157 | 0.091 |
| MOST [11] | 0.969 | 0.151 | 0.258 | 0.151 |
| FMST [13] | 0.884 | 0.179 | 0.296 | 0.176 |
| NGPST [8] | 0.978 | 0.557 | 0.703 | 0.549 |
| Ours | 0.971 | **0.801** | **0.875** | **0.781** |

**Table 2.** Comparison on BigNeuron dataset of single neuron reconstruction.

| Methods | ESA | DSA | PDS |
|---|---|---|---|
| ST [1] | 8.532 | 11.609 | 0.543 |
| APP2 [12] | 13.457 | 17.923 | 0.562 |
| MOST [11] | 31.730 | 38.211 | 0.633 |
| FMST [13] | 17.878 | 23.459 | 0.558 |
| NGPST [8] | 10.168 | 14.880 | 0.542 |
| Li2017 [4] | 4.917 | **7.972** | 0.461 |
| Ours | **4.784** | 8.309 | **0.451** |

## 4 Conclusions

In this paper, we propose a progressive learning framework to utilize a deep segmentation network to extract neuron voxels for neuronal population reconstruction from noisy and low-contrast OM images. Without any manual annotations on neurons, we take the advantage of neuron tracing techniques, which reconstruct individual neurons with hand-crafted features and global cues. The reconstructed neurons from neuron tracing provide pseudo labels to train a deep segmentation network, which thereby models more distinctive and global features for extracting neuron voxels. From the extracted neuron voxels using the deep segmentation network, more complete and accurate reconstruction of neurons is obtained from neuron tracing. Therefore, the DNN-based segmentation and neuron tracing techniques could mutually complement and promote each other progressively. Compared with existing methods, our method shows its superiority on reconstruction of dense neuronal population. We also build the VISoR-40 dataset to evaluate neuronal population reconstruction. The dataset will be published to support further study on brain research, including but not limited to neuron reconstruction, neuron counting, neuron morphology analysis, and so on.

**Acknowledgment.** We acknowledge funding from Natural Science Foundation of China under Grant 61632006 and 91732304, and the Fundamental Research Funds for the Central Universities under Grant WK2380000002 and WK3490000003.

# References

1. Chen, H., et al.: SmartTracing: self-learning-based neuron reconstruction. Brain Inform. **2**(3), 135 (2015)
2. Çiçek, Ö., Abdulkadir, A., Lienkamp, S.S., Brox, T., Ronneberger, O.: 3D U-Net: learning dense volumetric segmentation from sparse annotation. In: Ourselin, S., Joskowicz, L., Sabuncu, M.R., Unal, G., Wells, W. (eds.) MICCAI 2016. LNCS, vol. 9901, pp. 424–432. Springer, Cham (2016). https://doi.org/10.1007/978-3-319-46723-8_49
3. Dou, Q., et al.: 3D deeply supervised network for automated segmentation of volumetric medical images. IEEE Trans. Med. Imaging **41**, 40–54 (2017)
4. Li, R., et al.: Deep learning segmentation of optical microscopy images improves 3-D neuron reconstruction. IEEE Trans. Med. Imaging **36**(7), 1533–1541 (2017)
5. Peng, H., et al.: Automatic 3D neuron tracing using all-path pruning. Bioinformatics **27**(13), 239–247 (2011)
6. Peng, H., et al.: Virtual finger boosts three-dimensional imaging and microsurgery as well as terabyte volume image visualization and analysis. Nat. Commun. **5**, Article ID 4342 (2014)
7. Peng, H., et al.: BigNeuron: large-scale 3D neuron reconstruction from optical microscopy images. Neuron **87**(2), 252–256 (2015)
8. Quan, T., et al.: NeuroGPS-Tree: automatic reconstruction of large-scale neuronal populations with dense neurites. Nat. Methods **13**, 51–54 (2015)
9. Srivastava, N., et al.: Dropout: a simple way to prevent neural networks from overfitting. J. Mach. Learn. Res. **15**, 1929–1958 (2014)
10. Wang, H., et al.: Scalable volumetric imaging for ultrahigh-speed brain mapping at synaptic resolution. Natl. Sci. Rev. (2019)
11. Wu, J., et al.: 3D BrainCV: simultaneous visualization and analysis of cells and capillaries in a whole mouse brain with one-micron voxel resolution. NeuroImage **87**, 199–208 (2014)
12. Xiao, H., et al.: APP2: automatic tracing of 3D neuron morphology based on hierarchical pruning of a gray-weighted image distance-tree. Bioinformatics **29**(11), 1448–1454 (2013)
13. Yang, J., et al.: FMST: an automatic neuron tracing method based on fast marching and minimum spanning tree. Neuroinformatics **17**, 1–12 (2018)

14. Yu, L., et al.: Automatic 3D cardiovascular MR segmentation with densely-connected volumetric ConvNets. In: Descoteaux, M., Maier-Hein, L., Franz, A., Jannin, P., Collins, D.L., Duchesne, S. (eds.) MICCAI 2017. LNCS, vol. 10434, pp. 287–295. Springer, Cham (2017). https://doi.org/10.1007/978-3-319-66185-8_33

15. Zhou, Z., et al.: DeepNeuron: an open deep learning toolbox for neuron tracing. Brain Inform. 5(2), 3 (2018)

# Whole-Sample Mapping of Cancerous and Benign Tissue Properties

Lydia Neary-Zajiczek[1,2]([✉]), Clara Essmann[2], Neil Clancy[1], Aiman Haider[3],
Elena Miranda[4], Michael Shaw[2,5], Amir Gander[6], Brian Davidson[1],
Delmiro Fernandez-Reyes[2], Vijay Pawar[2], and Danail Stoyanov[1]

[1] Wellcome/EPSRC Centre for Surgical and Interventional Sciences (WEISS),
Charles Bell House, London W1W 7TS, UK
[2] UCL TouchLab, Malet Place Engineering Building, London WC1E 7JE, UK
lydia.zajiczek.17@ucl.ac.uk
[3] Department of Cellular Pathology, UCLH,
Shropshire House, London WC1E 6JA, UK
[4] UCL Cancer Research Biobank, Rockefeller Building, London WC1 6JJ, UK
[5] National Physical Laboratory, Hampton Road, Teddington TW11 0LW, UK
[6] UCL Department of Surgical Biotechnology,
Gower Street, London WC1E 6BT, UK

**Abstract.** Structural and mechanical differences between cancerous and healthy tissue give rise to variations in macroscopic properties such as visual appearance and elastic modulus that show promise as signatures for early cancer detection. Atomic force microscopy (AFM) has been used to measure significant differences in stiffness between cancerous and healthy cells owing to its high force sensitivity and spatial resolution, however due to absorption and scattering of light, it is often challenging to accurately locate where AFM measurements have been made on a bulk tissue sample. In this paper we describe an image registration method that localizes AFM elastic stiffness measurements with high-resolution images of haematoxylin and eosin (H&E)-stained tissue to within $\pm 1.5\,\mu$m. Color RGB images are segmented into three structure types (lumen, cells and stroma) by a neural network classifier trained on ground-truth pixel data obtained through $k$-means clustering in HSV color space. Using the localized stiffness maps and corresponding structural information, a whole-sample stiffness map is generated with a region matching and interpolation algorithm that associates similar structures with measured stiffness values. We present results showing significant differences in stiffness between healthy and cancerous liver tissue and discuss potential applications of this technique.

**Keywords:** Digital pathology · Whole-slide imaging · Cancer diagnostics · Tissue stiffness

## 1 Introduction

The development of cancer in otherwise healthy tissue can be detected in numerous ways, however a final diagnosis can only be made after a tissue biopsy or

© Springer Nature Switzerland AG 2019
D. Shen et al. (Eds.): MICCAI 2019, LNCS 11764, pp. 760–768, 2019.
https://doi.org/10.1007/978-3-030-32239-7_84

smear, whereby a pathologist inspects stained tissue sections and confirms the presence of cancerous cells. While histopathological analysis remains the "gold standard" for diagnosis, the macroscopic properties of tumorous tissue are widely known, with surgeons using tactile stiffness information when palpating to locate masses during biopsies or resection surgeries. Attempts have been made to quantify these differences using elastography [1] and tactile sensing [2]. Differences have also been measured in the elastic stiffness of single cells cultured from cancerous and healthy tissue using atomic force microscopy (AFM) [3,4], which arise from interactions between cells and the extra-cellular matrix (ECM) [5,6]. Given that extra-cellular components contribute significantly to the mechanical properties of the tissue, thicker tissue sections show more significant variation between cancerous and healthy tissue. While AFM measurements are highly sensitive, measuring the stiffness of an entire tissue sample using this method is wholly impractical due to time constraints, and using a small number of measurement sites to characterize bulk tissue properties is problematic as such significant extrapolation is susceptible to sampling errors. Furthermore, accurately localizing where AFM measurements have been made can be difficult as thick unstained tissue sections are highly scattering, resulting in low contrast images when using conventional light microscopy; post-measurement imaging as done in [7] does not allow for any meaningful comparison between measurements and underlying tissue structure.

In this paper we present a combined image registration and propagation method that localizes AFM measurements and hence the estimation of the Young's modulus of thick tissue sections with high-resolution haematoxylin and eosin (H&E)-stained images of the same section, revealing detailed tissue structure information. Measured tissue properties are propagated through the sample by comparing regions of similar structural content, resulting in whole-sample maps that can be used to draw larger conclusions about relevant nanomechanical differences between cancerous and healthy tissue rather than relying on a small number of measurement sites that are highly localized relative to the size of the sample and not necessarily representative of the tissue as a whole. The tissue property maps generated through this technique allow for detailed analysis of the underlying cellular structure that contributes to measurable changes in macroscopic tissue properties; such information would be of great use in further understanding how cancer develops or in identifying measurable signatures, with implications for early detection of cancerous tissue [7].

## 2   Methods

### 2.1   Sample Preparation

Clinical liver tissue samples were obtained, with healthy and cancerous tissue sections acquired from each patient. Malignancy was confirmed through examination of H&E -stained and fixed thin sections (5 μm) prior to AFM data acquisition. For each sample undergoing AFM measurements (healthy and cancerous), a thick cryosection (40 μm) was freshly thawed, adhered to the slide using tissue glue and immersed into physiological buffer for the duration of the measurements, with the buffer solution held in place with a customized 3D printed structure. A custom-built whole slide imaging (WSI) system was used to take a series of low-magnification (4X, 0.16 NA) images of each unstained sample. The low contrast of the thick tissue necessitated the use of a low numerical aperture microscope objective. The WSI consisted of an Olympus BX63 upright microscope, motorized stages and a large sensor sCMOS RGB camera (PCO edge 3.1c) with a sensor size of $2048 \times 1536$ pixels, 16-bit (27,000:1) dynamic range and $6.5\,\mu m$ square pixel size. Images of the unstained samples were combined using a stitching algorithm employing a Fourier transform-based phase correlation method to find translational offsets followed by small affine transformations and linear blending [8]. A typical sized sample ($6\,mm \times 4\,mm$) required between 5 and 10 low-magnification images to be stitched together.

## 2.2 Stiffness Measurement and Registration

After determining suitable measurement sites (i.e. areas of the tissue without significant voids or areas that were not firmly affixed to the slide), a JPK Nanowizard 3 Atomic Force Microscope was used in "force mapping mode" to extract a grid of force-displacement curves over a $10 \times 10\,\mu m$ area of the sample. Measurements were taken with tipless, soft cantilevers having a $10\,\mu m$ borosilicate bead attached ($0.03-8\,N/m$; NSC12 $\mu$Masch). The elastic modulus of the tissue was calculated from the acquired force curves based on the Hertz-Sneddon contact mechanic model [9] using JPK analysis software. The same camera and microscope objective from the WSI system was attached to the AFM system for capturing a FOV of the cantilever in place immediately prior to each scan (Fig. 1a). The high dynamic range and large sensor area of the camera allowed for capture of high-contrast detail that greatly improved the robustness of the feature matching and image registration procedures compared to images captured with the camera supplied with the AFM system (sensor size of $1024 \times 768$ pixels and 8-bit dynamic range).

To accurately locate the tissue contact point of the cantilever on the AFM FOVs, two images of the cantilever were taken: one at 40X magnification (0.6 NA) with the cantilever bead sharply in focus, where the tissue contact point was visible as the brightest point in the image, and a second at 4X magnification of the cantilever in the same position. These two images were registered using normalized cross correlation. The occlusion of the AFM assembly indicated in Fig. 1a resulted in very dark regions which could be thresholded to generate a binary mask showing only the assembly and cantilever, removing all detail of the sample. The cantilever template image with tissue contact point overlaid was also converted to a binary mask, and a feature-matching technique based on speeded up robust features (SURF) was used to estimate any geometric rotation between the cantilever template and AFM FOV masks. Maximum normalized cross correlation was used to register the AFM FOV (Fig. 1a) with the unstained image (Fig. 1b), localizing the tissue contact point from the cantilever template image of each measurement site to within several microns (Fig. 1c).

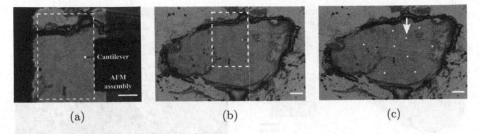

(a)             (b)             (c)

**Fig. 1.** (a) AFM image with tissue contact point of cantilever indicated by white box (not to scale). Registration FOV indicated by dashed red box. (b) AFM FOV registered and overlaid on whole sample image. (c) Localized measurement sites (white boxes). Scale bars are all 500 μm. (Color figure online)

The sample was then fixed and stained with H&E immediately after measurement and imaged with the WSI system at higher magnification (20X, 0.45 NA). Since the samples were significantly thicker than normal tissue sections (40 μm compared with 5 μm for regular H&E stained sections), a volumetric whole-slide scan was carried out, with a 14-plane z-stack spaced by 3 μm for a total of 42 μm in focal depth at each field position. A wavelet-based image fusion method was used to generate extended depth of field (EDOF) images containing in-focus structures from all focal planes [10]. The high-resolution EDOF images were stitched together, the resulting tiled H&E image was scaled to the same size as the unstained image and the feature-matching normalized cross correlation method described previously was used to register the two whole-sample images. Figures 2a and c show localized measurement sites for a healthy and cancerous tissue sample from the same patient overlaid on the corresponding high-resolution tiled H&E image.

## 2.3 Stiffness Propagation

A combination of methods were used to propagate elastic modulus measurements throughout the sample. The tiled high-resolution H&E images were first segmented into structural information using a technique based on [11]. First, 18 color images (each just over 3 megapixels) from both cancerous and benign tissue samples were manually selected that contained all three relevant structure types: cell nuclei and surrounding cytoplasm, stroma, and lumen or background. These RGB images were converted into HSV color space and all pixel color values (represented as a location in three dimensional space) were grouped into 10 clusters using $k$-means clustering with 10 replicates [12]. The distance metric used was squared Euclidean distance, with the $k$ seeds chosen using the $k$-means++ algorithm. Every pixel in each cluster was assigned the cluster centroid as its HSV color value, and the pseudo-color images were displayed for manual structural assignment. Of the 10 pseudo colors, 1 corresponded to lumen, 4 corresponded to cell nuclei and cytoplasm and the remaining 5 were classified as stroma.

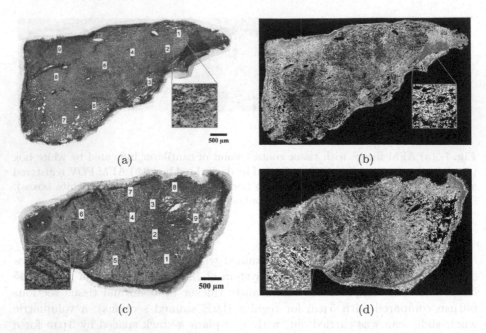

**Fig. 2.** Stitched high-resolution H&E images of (a) healthy and (c) cancerous samples with measurement sites overlaid. (b) and (d) are corresponding structural information maps of (a) and (b), where white pixels represent stroma, orange represent cells and black represent lumen. Insets are 250 × 250 μm. (Color figure online)

This color assignment generated a training set of approximately 150 million pixels with three input variables (position in 3D HSV space) and three classification labels (lumen, cell or stroma) which was used to train a fully connected neural network classifier in Keras using a Tensorflow backend. The fully connected layer contained 8 hidden nodes and used a rectified linear unit (ReLU) activation function while the output layer used a softmax activation function. The model was compiled using the Adam optimization algorithm with a categorical crossentropy (logarithmic) loss function and accuracy as a performance metric. It was trained with a batch size of 4 times the largest dimension of each image (8192 pixels total) for 20 epochs, achieving maximum training and validation accuracies of 94.5%. The trained model then predicted the structure type represented by each pixel in the tiled H&E whole-sample images (Figs. 2b and d). For each measurement location, regions of interest (ROIs) were extracted from both the H&E and structural images (Figs. 3a and b) that were slightly larger than the AFM scan area (Fig. 3c) to account for small errors during registration; ROIs were 13 μm square in size while the scan areas were 10 μm square in size.

The structural information map corresponding to each 10 × 10 μm AFM measurement site (Fig. 3b) was compared with the structural information map of the entire sample (Fig. 2b), using normalized cross correlation (NCC), where NCC was calculated between the structural information ROIs of all $k$ measurement

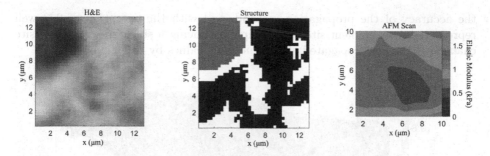

**Fig. 3.** (a) H&E image and (b) corresponding structural information map of AFM measurement site #1 of healthy sample, with (c) showing the measured elastic modulus values of the site. In (b), white pixels represent stroma, orange represent cells and black represent lumen. (Color figure online)

sites $s_k(x, y)$ and the rest of the structural information map $S(i, j)$, with an arg max selection along $k$ resulting in a maximum correlation map $C(i, j)$:

$$C(i, j) = \arg \max_k \frac{1}{n} \sum_{x,y} \frac{s_k(x, y) S(i - x, j - y)}{\sigma_{s_k} \sigma_S}$$

where $i > x$, $j > y$, $n$ is the number of pixels in $(x, y)$ and $\sigma$ denotes standard deviation over $(x, y)$. Note that $C$ is the same size as $S$, i.e. zero padding is not applied at the edges. The correlation map $C$ was then thresholded to identify regions of the sample that are structurally similar to the measurement sites. Each of the thresholded pixels was assigned the average elastic modulus value of the measurement site it is structurally most similar to, resulting in a propagated stiffness map. To better visualize the distribution of stiffness values across the sample, elastic modulus values of unassigned pixels were interpolated using a moving window least-squares approach, but interpolated values were not used in any statistical comparisons.

## 3   Results

The resulting propagated and interpolated tissue property maps are shown in Fig. 4. The cancerous sample overall shows a larger average elastic modulus than the healthy sample, with regions of high variation throughout. The average propagated elastic modulus for healthy tissue was $239 \pm 15$ Pa, while the cancerous sample's average was $440 \pm 136$ Pa. The average of all measured values for each sample was $369 \pm 18$ Pa and $659 \pm 171$ Pa for healthy and cancerous tissue, respectively. A t-test performed on 50 randomly selected data points from each measurement set showed a statistically significant difference between propagated elastic modulus values of normal and cancerous tissue ($\bar{p} = 0.004$), however for directly measured values the results of the t-test did not consistently show statistically significant differences. Leave-one-out cross validation was used to test the accuracy of the propagation method, and with the exception of 2–3 well represented measurement sites per sample, removing a single measurement site changed the mean propagated elastic modulus values by less than 5%.

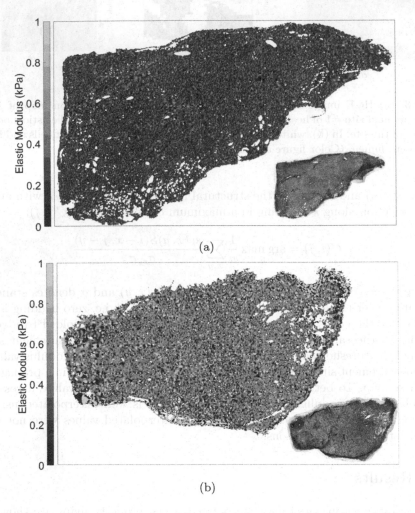

(a)

(b)

**Fig. 4.** Whole-sample propagated and interpolated maps of (a) healthy and (b) cancerous tissue properties. Maximum values have been truncated to improve visualization. Insets are H&E stained whole-sample images.

## 4   Discussion and Future Work

The whole-sample tissue property maps presented here are consistent with well-known qualitative observations that cancerous tissue is stiffer and less homogeneous than healthy tissue. The described propagation method is robust, with cross validation results demonstrating that propagation reduces the influence of measured values that may not be representative of the whole sample's structure. Future work will extract quantitative information from the structural maps, such as relative fractions of structural material and nuclear size, and investigate correlations with observed tissue properties. Refinement of the sample mounting technique is also a future consideration, as occasionally AFM measurements can be affected by the sample becoming detached from the slide, reducing the number of valid measurements per sample. Measuring additional samples will result in additional training data for increasing the sensitivity of the structural information classification algorithm, i.e. classifying pixels into more than 3 classes for more detailed and accurate propagation of tissue properties. Finally, the image registration techniques presented here could be applicable in validating potential intraoperative methods for quantitatively measuring the presence of cancer during tissue resectioning for example, using a more robust and scalable stiffness measurement technique than AFM such as direct indentation of tissue using a capacitive force sensor as described in [6].

**Acknowledgements.** This work was supported by the Wellcome/EPSRC Centre for Interventional and Surgical Sciences (WEISS) at UCL (203145Z/16/Z), EPSRC (EP/N027078/1, EP/P012841/1, EP/P027938/1, EP/R004080/1) and the European Commission Project-H2020-ICT-24-2015 (Endoo EU Project-G.A. number: 688592).

# References

1. Rouvière, O., et al.: Stiffness of benign and malignant prostate tissue measured by shear-wave elastography: a preliminary study. Eur. Radiol. **27**(5), 1858–1866 (2017)
2. Åstrand, A.P., Andersson, B.M., Jalkanen, V., Ljungberg, B., Bergh, A., Lindahl, O.A.: Prostate cancer detection with a tactile resonance sensor-measurement considerations and clinical setup. Sensors **17**(11), 2453 (2017)
3. Lekka, M., et al.: Cancer cell detection in tissue sections using AFM. Arch. Biochem. Biophys. **518**(2), 151–156 (2012)
4. Hayashi, K., Iwata, M.: Stiffness of cancer cells measured with an AFM indentation method. J. Mech. Behav. Biomed. Mater. **49**, 105–111 (2015)
5. Huang, S., Ingber, D.E.: Cell tension, matrix mechanics, and cancer development. Cancer Cell **8**(3), 175–176 (2005)
6. Zajiczek, L., et al.: Nano-mechanical single-cell sensing of cell-matrix contacts. Nanoscale **8**(42), 18105–18112 (2016)
7. Plodinec, M., et al.: The nanomechanical signature of breast cancer. Nat. Nanotechnol. **7**(11), 757–765 (2012)
8. Preibisch, S., Saalfeld, S., Tomancak, P.: Globally optimal stitching of tiled 3D microscopic image acquisitions. Bioinformatics **25**(11), 1463–1465 (2009)
9. Hertz, H.R.: Uber die beruhrung fester elastischer korper und uber die harte. Verhandlung des Vereins zur Beforderung des Gewerbefleißes, Berlin, p. 449 (1882)
10. Forster, B., Van De Ville, D., Berent, J., Sage, D., Unser, M.: Complex wavelets for extended depth-of-field: a new method for the fusion of multichannel microscopy images. Microsc. Res. Tech. **65**(1–2), 33–42 (2004)

11. Zarella, M.D., Yeoh, C., Breen, D.E., Garcia, F.U.: An alternative reference space for H&E color normalization. PLoS ONE **12**(3), e0174489 (2017)
12. Arthur, D., Vassilvitskii, S.: k-means++: the advantages of careful seeding. In: Proceedings of the Eighteenth Annual ACM-SIAM Symposium on Discrete Algorithms. Society for Industrial and Applied Mathematics (2007)

# Multi-task Neural Networks with Spatial Activation for Retinal Vessel Segmentation and Artery/Vein Classification

Wenao Ma[1,2], Shuang Yu[1(✉)], Kai Ma[1], Jiexiang Wang[1,2], Xinghao Ding[2], and Yefeng Zheng[1]

[1] Youtu Lab, Tencent, Shenzhen, China
shirlyyu@tencent.com
[2] School of Information Science and Engineering, Xiamen University, Xiamen, China

**Abstract.** Retinal artery/vein (A/V) classification plays a critical role in the clinical biomarker study of how various systemic and cardiovascular diseases affect the retinal vessels. Conventional methods of automated A/V classification are generally complicated and heavily depend on the accurate vessel segmentation. In this paper, we propose a multi-task deep neural network with spatial activation mechanism that is able to segment full retinal vessel, artery and vein simultaneously, without the pre-requirement of vessel segmentation. The input module of the network integrates the domain knowledge of widely used retinal preprocessing and vessel enhancement techniques. We specially customize the output block of the network with a spatial activation mechanism, which takes advantage of a relatively easier task of vessel segmentation and exploits it to boost the performance of A/V classification. In addition, deep supervision is introduced to the network to assist the low level layers to extract more semantic information. The proposed network achieves pixel-wise accuracy of 95.70% for vessel segmentation, and A/V classification accuracy of 94.50%, which is the state-of-the-art performance for both tasks on the AV-DRIVE dataset. Furthermore, we have also tested the model performance on INSPIRE-AVR dataset, which achieves a skeletal A/V classification accuracy of 91.6%.

**Keywords:** Retinal vessel segmentation · Artery/vein classification · Deep learning · Spatial activation

## 1 Introduction

Many systemic and cardiovascular diseases have manifestations in the retinal vessels and affect the arteries and veins (A/V) differently [1]. For example, it has been reported that the asymmetrical change of retinal A/V is associated with several cardiovascular diseases [15]. In addition, clinical research has also found that the narrowing of retinal arteriolar caliber is related to the risk of

© Springer Nature Switzerland AG 2019
D. Shen et al. (Eds.): MICCAI 2019, LNCS 11764, pp. 769–778, 2019.
https://doi.org/10.1007/978-3-030-32239-7_85

hypertension [3]. Therefore, there is a significant clinical interest in the accurate and automatic A/V classification.

Conventionally, the automated A/V classification in the related literature was performed in a two-stage approach [4,5,11,17,19]. Retinal vessels were first segmented from the background, based on which, vessels were further classified into A/V, using pure hand-crafted features or incorporating the connection information with a graph-based method. Representative works of using a pure feature-based method include [11,17], which extracted the handcrafted features from vessel centerlines and then classified each pixel into artery or vein. Graph based research [4,5,19], on the other hand, first reconstructed the vascular graph from vessel centerline via node analysis or graph estimation, and then classified individual graph trees into arteries or veins.

The above mentioned two-step methods share the same limitation that the performance of A/V classification heavily depends on the accurate vessel segmentation, especially for the graph reconstruction methods. Defects in the vessel segmentation, e.g., broken or wrongly segmented vessels, will be propagated to the subsequent graph reconstruction step, and further influence the performance of A/V classification. Similarly, pure feature-based methods heavily rely on the complex hand-crafted features extracted from the vessel centerline.

Very recently, there has been several emerging works using a Fully Convolutional Network (FCN) to segment and classify retinal A/V at the same time. AlBadawi and Fraz [2] adopted the FCN with an encoder-decoder structure for the pixel-wise classification of A/V. Meyer *et al.* [9] also used FCN for the task of A/V classification and reported performance on major vessels thicker than three pixels. The deep learning based methods have demonstrated the potential to segment A/V in an end-to-end approach. However, the overall vessel segmentation performance of the existing methods using direct A/V segmentation is affected when A/V pixels are classified as background. There is still a research gap of how to improve the vessel segmentation performance together with A/V classification, especially for the capillary vessels.

In this paper, we propose a deep network with a spatial activation mechanism that performs full vessel segmentation and A/V classification simultaneously, so as to improve the accuracy of both tasks. In particular, we design a multi-task output block with an activation mechanism which utilizes the result of vessel segmentation, a relatively easier task, to enhance that of the A/V classification, especially for capillary vessels. The input module of the network integrates the domain knowledge of widely used retinal image processing and filter-based vessel enhancement techniques. In addition, deep supervision modules are attached to the early stages of the encoder section, which can assist the low-level features to extract more semantic information. The proposed framework achieves state-of-the-art performance for both A/V classification and vessel segmentation tasks on AV-DRIVE database, and skeletal A/V classification for INSPIRE-AVR dataset.

## 2    Method

The system workflow of the proposed algorithm is described as below: the color fundus image is firstly processed through modules of illumination correction (IC) and vessel enhancement (VE). Then, patches extracted from those three different sources (original, IC and VE processed) are fed to the proposed deep learning architecture, which further generates three segmentation maps of artery, vein and full vessels simultaneously. The final segmentation and classification maps are generated by stitching the corresponding patches together.

### 2.1    Multi-input Module

The multi-input module of the proposed method integrates the domain knowledge of how the vessel segmentation task is performed conventionally in the non deep learning based methods. In order to remove the non-uniformly distributed brightness across the image, the illumination correction is generally adopted as the pre-processing step for retinal images. In addition, we enhance the vessel map using two conventional vessel segmentation techniques, e.g. the multi-scale Gabor filtering [14] and line detector [10], as auxiliary inputs to the network.

### 2.2    Network Architecture with Spatial Activation

The network architecture of the proposed framework is shown on Fig. 1. We adopt the classic U-Net architecture initialized by a pretrained ResNet as the encoder. In order to accommodate the multi-input channels, we insert an expanding-compressing layer before the ResNet, which first expands the input to a high-dimension space and then compresses the feature maps to three channels, so as to match the input channel number of the ResNet model.

We specifically design a multi-task output block for the effective full vessel segmentation and A/V classification simultaneously. In order to get more accurate results for A/V classification, the network is expected to learn more discriminative features between artery and vein. However, if the network focuses only on A/V classification, it may fail to segment finer capillary vessels. Therefore, it is necessary for the network to learn more common features between A/V, i.e., vessel features. In our proposed framework, we design two parallel branches at the end of the network. One branch focuses on extracting common features between A/V, and generates the probability map of vessel segmentation. Meanwhile, the other one focuses on the discriminative A/V features. Output feature maps of the two branches are then concatenated and further used to generate the final result of A/V classification.

In order to utilize the result of a relatively easier task, i.e. the vessel segmentation in this case, to facilitate the performance of a more complicated task of A/V classification, especially for the capillary vessels, a customized activation block is proposed, as in Eq. (1):

$$m(x) = \sigma(e^{-(x-0.5)^2} - e^{-\frac{1}{4}}) + 1, \tag{1}$$

where $\sigma$ is the activation factor and set as one in our network. The activation block is designed based on the observation that capillary vessels and boundary pixels generally have a value around 0.5 in the obtained vessel probability map generated by our algorithm, while thick vessels and background pixels have a value near 1 or 0. In order to emphasize the importance of capillary vessels, we adopt a Gaussian function to enhance the weights of pixel values around 0.5. In addition, a bias is added to the activation function to constrain the weight within a range between $[1, 1 + \sigma(1 - e^{-\frac{1}{4}})]$. Then, the activation map is used to adjust each feature map spatially for the A/V classification task, by assigning higher weights for capillary vessel pixels (close to $1 + \sigma(1 - e^{-\frac{1}{4}})$), and lower weights for background and thick vessel pixels (close to 1). In other words, potential capillary vessels can be activated through this process. An example of the activation map can be seen in Fig. 2(E).

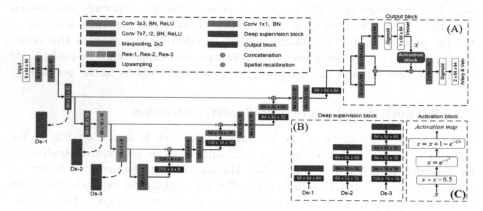

**Fig. 1.** Architecture of the proposed network. (A) Multi-task output block; (B) Deep supervision block; (C) Spatial activation block.

## 2.3   Deep Supervision

As pointed out by Zhang *et al.* [18], a simple fusion of low-level and high-level features, as generally used in U-Net, could be less effective, as there is a gap between the two features in terms of semantic level and spatial resolution. Thus, learning more "semantic" low-level features can help the network to achieve better performance for the U-Net architecture. In addition, the presence of vanishing gradients also makes the loss back-propagation less effective for layers close to the input layer. Considering the two limitations of the network, we introduce deep supervision to the architecture by adding extra side output layers at the encoder section after each ResNet block, as shown in Fig. 1, so as to assist the low-level layers to extract more semantic features and accelerate the convergence.

We also specifically design the loss function accordingly, which contains three elements, including binary cross-entropy loss of the final output, losses of deep supervision blocks and a weight decay regularization term, as in Eqs. (2) and (3):

$$Loss = BCE(output, GT) + \frac{1}{3} \sum_{i=1}^{3} BCE(side_i, GT) + \frac{\lambda}{2}\|\Theta\|_2^2 \qquad (2)$$

$$BCE(pred, target) = - \sum_{c=1}^{3} \mu_c \cdot target_c \cdot \log(pred_c) \qquad (3)$$

where $\Theta$ represents the network parameters; $i$ represents the $i^{th}$ deep supervision block; $c$ denotes the $c^{th}$ class of the output; the weight of each class is denoted as $\mu_c$ with $\frac{3}{7}$, $\frac{2}{7}$ and $\frac{2}{7}$ for vessel, artery and vein, respectively.

## 3    Experimental Results

Our model was primarily trained and evaluated on the publicly available AV-DRIVE database [7]. The AV-DRIVE database contains 20 training and 20 test retinal color fundus images with dimension of $584 \times 565$ pixels, with pixel-wise labeling of vessel segmentation and A/V classification provided. Apart from this, we have also evaluated the model performance on INSPIRE-AVR dataset [12], which contains 40 color images with dimension of $2048 \times 2392$. Since INSPIRE-AVR provides only A/V labels for centerline, without pixel-wise vessel segmentation, thus it cannot be used to train the model. In order to enrich the usable training data for the model, we have also manually labeled the A/V classification for publicly available High Resolution Fundus (HRF) dataset [13], where the original database contains only pixel-wise vessel segmentation.

In the training stage, patches with size of $64 \times 64$ were randomly extracted from the retinal images and fed to the network. Whereas in the test stage, ordered patches were extracted at the stride of 10 and final result was obtained by stitching the corresponding patch predictions together. Stochastic gradient descent with momentum was adopted to optimize the model for a maximum of 60,000 iterations with batch size of 16. The initial learning rate was set as 0.05 and halved every 7500 iterations. The training process tooks around 2 h on a NVIDIA Tesla P40 GPU and it takes around 8 s to segment one image during the test phase.

Figure 2 shows a representative performance for vessel segmentation and A/V classification result for an image from the AV-DRIVE test set. Note the enlarged view of two representative patches deemed as challenging for the conventional methods, with the upper one being complex crossovers and lower one being two close-by parallel vessels. Under the multi-task framework, our model is able to accurately segment the overlapping vessels and classify the complex vessels.

### 3.1    Ablation Studies

Comprehensive ablation studies have been performed to evaluate the contribution of different modules of the proposed model, including the multi-task (MTs),

Multi-input (MIs) and spatial activation mechanism (AC). The baseline model was built by removing the above mentioned three modules and direct segmenting A/V pixels from the background. We adopt four metrics for the evaluation of vessel segmentation: the average accuracy (Acc), sensitivity (Sen), specificity (Sp), and area under curve (AUC). A/V classification performance is evaluated using pixel-wise Acc, Sen and Sp for the ground-truth artery vein pixels. By taking arteries as positives and veins as negatives, Sen reflects the model's capability of detecting arteries and Sp for veins.

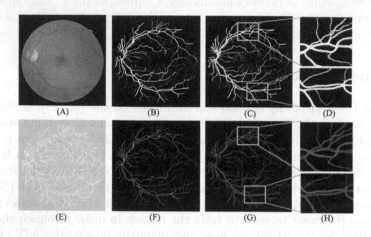

**Fig. 2.** Representative performance of vessel segmentation and A/V classification result. (A) original image from the AV-DRIVE test set; (E) activation map; (B)(F) manual label of vessel segmentation and A/V classification; (C)(G) model segmentation result; (D)(H) enlarged view of two representative challenging regions for the conventional method.

**Table 1.** The ablation study results of vessel segmentation and A/V classification.

| Combination | | | Vessel segmentation | | | | A/V classification | | |
|---|---|---|---|---|---|---|---|---|---|
| MTs | MIs | AC | Acc(%) | Sen(%) | Sp(%) | AUC(%) | Acc(%) | Sen(%) | Sp(%) |
| | | | 94.98 | 68.86 | **98.79** | 97.60 | 91.25 | 89.68 | 92.55 |
| ✓ | | | 95.61 | 78.50 | 98.10 | 98.01 | 91.63 | 90.46 | 92.63 |
| ✓ | ✓ | | 95.66 | 78.30 | 98.19 | 98.08 | 91.98 | 90.36 | **93.42** |
| ✓ | ✓ | ✓ | **95.70** | **79.16** | 98.11 | **98.10** | **92.58** | **92.18** | 92.98 |

As listed in Table 1, by using the multi-task module in the model, both vessel segmentation and A/V classification performances are improved, by 0.6% and 0.4% respectively. This indicates the necessity of a multi-task solution to the problem, which improves the performance for both tasks. The integration of domain knowledge from conventional methods increases the A/V classification performance by 0.3%. In particular, when we add the activation mechanism

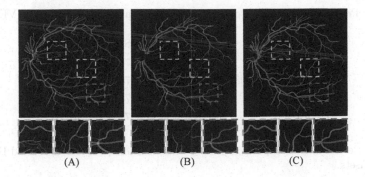

(A)                                (B)                                (C)

**Fig. 3.** Comparison of model performance for baseline and proposed method. (A) Ground truth; (B) Baseline model performance; (C) Proposed method.

to the network, the A/V classification performance is further boosted by 0.6%. Compared with A/V classification, the vessel segmentation task is a relatively easier task. The special design of the multi-task out block and activation mechanism takes advantage of the performance of the easier task to enhance that of a more complicated one. And ablation study has proved the effectiveness of this approach. At last, the proposed network achieves a pixel-wise accuracy of 95.70% for vessel segmentation and 92.58% for A/V classification.

Figure 3 visualizes the performances of the proposed model against that of the baseline. As marked on the enlarged views, the proposed method has remarkably improved the segmentation and classification of A/Vs over the baseline. More capillary vessels are segmented and correctly classified by the proposed method where the baseline model fails to.

## 3.2   Comparison to Existing Methods

Tables 2 and 3 list the performance comparison between existing methods and our proposed model on the AV-DRIVE database. Note in Table 3, existing methods evaluated the A/V classification performance on the segmented vessels only. In contrast, we evaluate the performance on all the ground truth artery/vein pixels, which is relatively more strict than that on the segmented vessels, since the classification of major vessels is comparatively an easier task if capillary vessels are not segmented. When evaluating under the same criteria with existing methods, our model achieves a pixel-wise accuracy of 94.50%, which surpasses the current best A/V classification method by a noticeable margin.

In addition, we have tested our model on the INSPIRE-AVR dataset. The training set contains 20 images from AV-DRIVE and 45 images from HRF dataset, which contains publicly available vessel segmentation label and we manually labeled the A/V class. The skeletal A/V classification of INSPIRE-AVR achieved 91.6% without fine-tuning, which is the state-of-the-art performance.

**Table 2.** Performance comparison of vessel segmentation on the AV-DRIVE dataset.

| Methods | Acc(%) | Sp(%) | Sen(%) | AUC(%) |
|---|---|---|---|---|
| Fu *et al.* [6] | 94.70 | - | 72.94 | - |
| Liskowski *et al.* [8] | 95.35 | 98.07 | 78.11 | 97.90 |
| Wu *et al.* [16] | 95.67 | **98.19** | 78.44 | 98.07 |
| **Proposed** | **95.70** | 98.11 | **79.16** | **98.10** |

**Table 3.** Performance comparison of A/V classification on AV-DRIVE and INSPIRE-AVR datasets.

| Methods | AV-DRIVE | | | INSPIRE | | |
|---|---|---|---|---|---|---|
| | Acc(%) | Sen(%) | Sp(%) | Acc(%) | Sen(%) | Sp(%) |
| Dashtbozorg *et al.* [4] | 87.4 | 90.0 | 84.0 | 84.9 | 91.0 | 86.0 |
| Estrada *et al.* [5] | 93.5 | 93.0 | 94.1 | 90.9 | 91.5 | 90.2 |
| Xu *et al.* [17] | 92.3 | 92.9 | 91.5 | - | - | - |
| Zhao *et al.* [19] | - | 91.9 | 91.5 | 91.0 | 91.8 | 90.2 |
| **Proposed (GT)** | 92.6 | 92.2 | 93.0 | 90.3 | 91.4 | 89.7 |
| **Proposed** | **94.5** | **93.4** | **95.5** | **91.6** | **92.4** | **91.3** |

## 4    Conclusion

In this paper, we proposed a novel multi-tasking neural network with spatial activation mechanism that enables the end-to-end segmentation of artery, vein and full vessel maps simultaneously. We evaluated our method on the AV-DRIVE dataset and compared it to the other existing research. The result shows that our method outperforms the existing methods, achieving state-of-the-art performance for both vessel segmentation and A/V classification tasks.

The proposed framework has significantly improved the accuracy and efficiency of A/V classification, which lays the foundation for quantitative vessel parameterization. In the near future, fully automatic vascular parameter generation modules will be implemented and validated on the basis of the current work, so as to facilitate the clinical retinal vascular biomarker study.

**Acknowledgment.** This work was funded by the Key Area Research and Development Program of Guangdong Province, China (No. 2018B010111001).

## References

1. Abràmoff, M.D., Garvin, M.K., Sonka, M.: Retinal imaging and image analysis. IEEE Rev. Biomed. Eng. **3**, 169–208 (2010)
2. AlBadawi, S., Fraz, M.M.: Arterioles and venules classification in retinal images using fully convolutional deep neural network. In: Campilho, A., Karray, F., ter Haar Romeny, B. (eds.) ICIAR 2018. LNCS, vol. 10882, pp. 659–668. Springer, Cham (2018). https://doi.org/10.1007/978-3-319-93000-8_75

3. Chew, S.K., Xie, J., Wang, J.J.: Retinal arteriolar diameter and the prevalence and incidence of hypertension: a systematic review and meta-analysis of their association. Curr. Hypertens. Rep. **14**(2), 144–151 (2012)
4. Dashtbozorg, B., Mendonça, A.M., Campilho, A.: An automatic graph-based approach for artery/vein classification in retinal images. IEEE Trans. Image Process. **23**(3), 1073–1083 (2014)
5. Estrada, R., Allingham, M.J., Mettu, P.S., Cousins, S.W., Tomasi, C., Farsiu, S.: Retinal artery-vein classification via topology estimation. IEEE Trans. Med. Imaging **34**(12), 2518–2534 (2015)
6. Fu, H., Xu, Y., Wong, D.W.K., Liu, J.: Retinal vessel segmentation via deep learning network and fully-connected conditional random fields. In: 2016 IEEE 13th International Symposium on Biomedical Imaging (ISBI), pp. 698–701. IEEE (2016)
7. Hu, Q., Abràmoff, M.D., Garvin, M.K.: Automated separation of binary overlapping trees in low-contrast color retinal images. In: Mori, K., Sakuma, I., Sato, Y., Barillot, C., Navab, N. (eds.) MICCAI 2013. LNCS, vol. 8150, pp. 436–443. Springer, Heidelberg (2013). https://doi.org/10.1007/978-3-642-40763-5_54
8. Liskowski, P., Krawiec, K.: Segmenting retinal blood vessels with deep neural networks. IEEE Trans. Med. Imaging **35**(11), 2369–2380 (2016)
9. Meyer, M.I., Galdran, A., Costa, P., Mendonça, A.M., Campilho, A.: Deep Convolutional artery/vein classification of retinal vessels. In: Campilho, A., Karray, F., ter Haar Romeny, B. (eds.) ICIAR 2018. LNCS, vol. 10882, pp. 622–630. Springer, Cham (2018). https://doi.org/10.1007/978-3-319-93000-8_71
10. Nguyen, U.T., Bhuiyan, A., Park, L.A., Ramamohanarao, K.: An effective retinal blood vessel segmentation method using multi-scale line detection. Pattern Recognit. **46**(3), 703–715 (2013)
11. Niemeijer, M., van Ginneken, B., Abràmoff, M.D.: Automatic classification of retinal vessels into arteries and veins. In: Medical Imaging 2009: Computer-Aided Diagnosis, vol. 7260, p. 72601F (2009)
12. Niemeijer, M., et al.: Automated measurement of the arteriolar-to-venular width ratio in digital color fundus photographs. IEEE Trans. Med. Imaging **30**(11), 1941–1950 (2011)
13. Odstrcilik, J., et al.: Retinal vessel segmentation by improved matched filtering: evaluation on a new high-resolution fundus image database. IET Image Process. **7**(4), 373–383 (2013)
14. Soares, J.V.B., Leandro, J.J.G., Cesar, R.M., Jelinek, H.F., Cree, M.J.: Retinal vessel segmentation using the 2-d gabor wavelet and supervised classification. IEEE Trans. Med. Imaging **25**(9), 1214–1222 (2006)
15. Wong, T.Y., et al.: Retinal arteriolar narrowing and risk of coronary heart disease in men and women: the atherosclerosis risk in communities study. JAMA **287**(9), 1153–1159 (2002)
16. Wu, Y., Xia, Y., Song, Y., Zhang, Y., Cai, W.: Multiscale network followed network model for retinal vessel segmentation. In: Frangi, A.F., Schnabel, J.A., Davatzikos, C., Alberola-López, C., Fichtinger, G. (eds.) MICCAI 2018. LNCS, vol. 11071, pp. 119–126. Springer, Cham (2018). https://doi.org/10.1007/978-3-030-00934-2_14
17. Xu, X., Ding, W., Abràmoff, M.D., Cao, R.: An improved arteriovenous classification method for the early diagnostics of various diseases in retinal image. Comput. Methods Programs Biomed. **141**, 3–9 (2017)

18. Zhang, Z., Zhang, X., Peng, C., Xue, X., Sun, J.: ExFuse: enhancing feature fusion for semantic segmentation. In: Ferrari, V., Hebert, M., Sminchisescu, C., Weiss, Y. (eds.) ECCV 2018. LNCS, vol. 11214, pp. 273–288. Springer, Cham (2018). https://doi.org/10.1007/978-3-030-01249-6_17

19. Zhao, Y., et al.: Retinal artery and vein classification via dominant sets clustering-based vascular topology estimation. In: Frangi, A.F., Schnabel, J.A., Davatzikos, C., Alberola-López, C., Fichtinger, G. (eds.) MICCAI 2018. LNCS, vol. 11071, pp. 56–64. Springer, Cham (2018). https://doi.org/10.1007/978-3-030-00934-2_7

# Fine-Scale Vessel Extraction in Fundus Images by Registration with Fluorescein Angiography

Kyoung Jin Noh[1], Sang Jun Park[1(✉)], and Soochahn Lee[2(✉)]

[1] Department of Ophthalmology, Seoul National University College of Medicine, Seoul National University Bundang Hospital, Seongnam, Korea
sangjunpark@snu.ac.kr
[2] School of Electrical Engineering, Kookmin University, Seoul, Korea
sclee@kookmin.ac.kr

**Abstract.** We present a new framework for fine-scale vessel segmentation from fundus images through registration and segmentation of corresponding fluorescein angiography (FA) images. In FA, fluorescent dye is used to highlight the vessels and increase their contrast. Since these highlights are temporally dispersed among multiple FA frames, we first register the FA frames and aggregate the per-frame segmentations to construct a detailed vessel mask. The constructed FA vessel mask is then registered to the fundus image based on an initial fundus vessel mask. Postprocessing is performed to refine the final vessel mask. Registration of FA frames, as well as registration of FA vessel mask to the fundus image, are done by similar hierarchical coarse-to-fine frameworks, both comprising rigid and non-rigid registration. Two CNNs with identical network structures, both trained on public datasets but with different settings, are used for vessel segmentation. The resulting final vessel segmentation contains fine-scale, filamentary vessels extracted from FA and corresponding to the fundus image. We provide quantitative evaluation as well as qualitative examples which support the robustness and the accuracy of the proposed method.

**Keywords:** Fundus images · Fine-scale vessel segmentation ·
Fluorescein angiography · Registration · Filamentary vessels

## 1 Introduction

Retinal fundus images are the only type of medical image that directly observes the blood vessels to generate clear, high resolution visualizations. They are simple, noninvasive, relatively cheap, and require no radiation or pharmaceuticals.

This work was supported by the National Research Foundation of Korea (NRF) grants funded by the Korean government (MoE) (NRF-2018R1D1A1A09083241 and NRF-2019R1F1A1063656).

© Springer Nature Switzerland AG 2019
D. Shen et al. (Eds.): MICCAI 2019, LNCS 11764, pp. 779–787, 2019.
https://doi.org/10.1007/978-3-030-32239-7_86

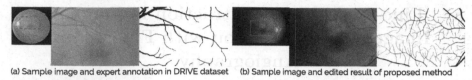

(a) Sample image and expert annotation in DRIVE dataset    (b) Sample image and edited result of proposed method

**Fig. 1.** Qualitative comparison between (a) manual expert annotations of DRIVE [14] and (b) the results of the proposed method with minimal manual editing of minor errors. Our goal is to construct a foundational dataset for achieving superhuman accuracy in deep learning based retinal vessel segmentation.

They are used to diagnose various retinal diseases including diabetic retinopathy, age-related macular degeneration, epiretinal membrane, and glaucoma. They can also be used for early diagnosis and prevention of chronic diseases including diabetes and hypertension.

Chronic diseases can damage vessels and also cause new vessels to be formed [15]. Clinicians require highly accurate detection and measurement of vessels, including fine, filamentary vessels with thin complex shapes and low contrast, for better diagnoses. Thus, this problem has been extensively researched [1].

Public retinal image datasets including DRIVE [14], STARE [9], CHASE_DB1 [6], and HRF [3] have been vital to the research. These datasets all include vessel region masks achieved by manual expert annotations. While they are assumed as the ground truth, it is actually very difficult to measure their accuracy. Comparison with a second expert actually show the limitations of human annotations. The accuracy of recent automatic vessel segmentation methods [11,13] are higher than the annotations by the second expert. This is because inter-observer differences inevitably occur at ambiguous regions. Filamentary vessels are often barely visible in the retinal fundus image, even with zooming and contrast enhancement. If we can provide consistent and detailed annotations at these regions, ground truth expert annotations can be improved, which in turn can improve machine learning based methods.

In this paper we present a new framework for retinal vessel extraction from fundus images through registration and segmentation of corresponding fluorescein angiography (FA) images. In FA, a fluorescent dye is injected into the bloodstream to highlight the vessels by increasing contrast. But the highlights are temporally dispersed among the multiple FA frames while the dye flows through the vessels from arterioles to venules. Thus we must first align the FA frames and aggregate the per-frame segmentations to construct a detailed vessel mask. Here, alignment is done by keypoint based registration, and vessel segmentation is done using a convolutional neural net (CNN) [11]. The constructed FA vessel mask is then registered to the fundus image based on an initial vessel segmentation for the fundus image, again using a CNN. Postprocessing is performed to refine the final fundas image vessel mask based on the FA vessel mask. We believe the proposed method is the first method to successfully elevate the level of detail and accuracy in automatic vessel segmentation of filamentary vessels for fundus images by incorporating FA. Moreover, it can be used to generate more detailed and consistent ground truth vessel masks as shown in Fig. 1.

## 2   Methods

The proposed method can be compartmentalized into three subprocesses, corresponding to (1) registration of FA frames and their vessel extraction, (2) multimodal registration of aggregated FA vessels to the fundus image, (3) postprocessing for fine refinement of the vessel mask. We describe the details of each subprocess in the following subsections.

### 2.1   Registration and Vessel Extraction of FA Frames

Here, the objective is to extract a mask of all vessels including the filamentary ones. We thus extract all vessels from all FA frames and aggregate them in a combined registered frame. In contrast to methods based on registration of extracted vessels [12], vessels are extracted after registration, since the highlighted vessels change considerably due to blood flow. Moreover, registration actually helps the vessel extraction, since false positives can be avoided through the aggregation of vessel regions. Thus, we propose a three step hierarchical process, combining coarse rigid registration in the pixel domain and fine non-rigid registration in the vessel mask domain to ensure robustness against appearance changes of the frames and its vessels. A visual summary of the framework is given in Fig. 2. We note that this process is iteratively performed for all adjacent frame pairs with the initial frame as the reference frame.

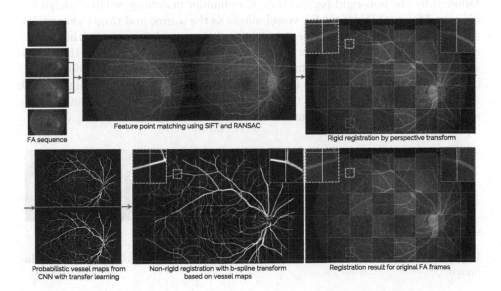

**Fig. 2.** The registration framework for a pair of FA frames.

In the first step, feature point matching is performed in the pixel domain. We use the SIFT descriptor on local maxima in the difference of Gaussians [10]. Keypoint matching is performed using RANSAC (random sample consensus) with the perspective transform matrix [8]. The source image is then rigidly registered to the target image using the transform matrix determined by the keypoint matches.

We next refine the rigid registration by non-rigid registration of vessel probability maps. Here, we leverage recent developments in deep learning by using a recently proposed convolutional neural network (CNN) called the retinal SSANet [11]. Since no training data is available for supervised learning of the network for the FA frames, we utilize the public datasets DRIVE [14] and HRF [3] comprising fundus images and expert annotated ground truth vessel maps. To account for the differences in image characteristics, we convert to greyscale and then invert intensity before training. We also resize the images to match FA resolution.

Given the vessel probability maps, we then perform pixel-wise non-rigid registration. We assume a b-spline transform model with similarity measured by normalized cross-correlation and optimization with the gradient based L-BFGS-B [4] algorithm.

## 2.2   Registration of FA and Fundus Image

To register the aggregated probabilistic vessel map of FA, we generate a similar map for the fundus image. Again, we train a retinal SSANet [11], this time without any preprocessing on images of DRIVE and HRF images. The vessel maps are generated from inference of this network. Based on the vessel maps, we again perform coarse rigid registration, this time using chamfer matching, followed by fine non-rigid registration. For chamfer matching, we first assign the binarized fundus image and FA vessel masks as the source and target shapes. We then find the global displacement vector and the rotation angle (within a $\pm 5°$ range) that minimizes the sum of distances between each point on the source shape and the target shape by brute force search on the distance transform (DT) of the target shape. We use the inverse of the obtained transform to align the FA map to the fundus image. For non-rigid registration, we use the same specifics as in Subsect. 2.1. A visual summary of the framework is given in Fig. 3

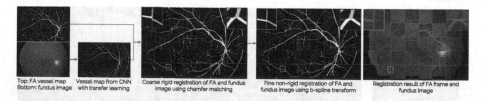

Top: FA vessel map    Vessel map from CNN    Coarse rigid registration of FA and fundus    Fine non-rigid registration of FA and    Registration result of FA frame and
Bottom: fundus image    with transfer learning    image using chamfer matching    fundus image using b-spline transform    fundus image

**Fig. 3.** The registration framework for the aggregated FA vessel mask and fundus image.

## 2.3  Postprocessing

Here, we aim to generate an accurate binary vessel mask of the fundus image, from the aligned probabilistic vessel map of the FA. The postprocessing comprises binarization and refinement. A visual summary is given in Fig. 4.

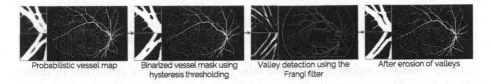

| Probabilistic vessel map | Binarized vessel mask using hysteresis thresholding | Valley detection using the Frangi filter | After erosion of valleys |

**Fig. 4.** The postprocessing framework comprising binarization and refinement.

To avoid discontinuities that may occur at the filamentary vessels from simple thresholding, we apply hysteresis thresholding for binarization. Pixels over a higher threshold $\tau_h$ are used as seeds for region growing pixels with probability higher than a lower threshold $\tau_l$. Here, we empirically set $\tau_h = 0.75$ and $\tau_l = 0.1$.

Furthermore, we refine the vessel mask to align the vessel boundaries to the image gradients in the fundus image. Specifically, we utilize the Frangi filter [5], in an inverted manner with sigma values 1 to 3, to detect the valleys between vessels and the outer boundaries, and then erode these regions.

## 3  Experimental Results

### 3.1  Dataset and Experimental Environment

The dataset comprises 200 cases of FA and fundus image pairs from 153 patients. They were acquired using Canon CF60Uvi, Kowa VX-10, and Kowa VX-10a cameras. The number of FA frames was on average 7.14, with minimum 2 to maximum 24. Image resolutions originally varying from 1604 × 1216 to 2144 × 1424 were all normalized to 1536 × 1024.

Computation times for the FA registration per frame pair, FA-fundus registration, and postprocessing averaged 57, 28, and 3 s, respectively, running on a 2.2 GHz Intel Xeon CPU and a nVidia Titan V GPU. Most of the computation was due to feature point matching (over 40 of the 57 s), and non-rigid registration took 15–16 s on average. OpenCV [2] was used for feature point matching and SimpleITK [16] was used for non-rigid registration.

### 3.2  Qualitative Evaluation

Figure 5 shows qualitative results of six sample cases. Here, we provide the vessel segmentation results generated by a CNN, namely, the SSANet [11] trained on the HRF [3] dataset, as a reference point for comparison. Although we are aware that this comparison maybe unfair, we were unable to establish an alternative comparative reference. Here, we can see that many filamentary vessels are indeed visible in the fundus images, but only with close visual inspection. Figure 6 shows a particular example of this case.

## 3.3   Quantitative Evaluation

Ground truth (GT) segmentation masks are required for quantitative evaluation. But we cannot rely on expert annotation for filamentary vessels. We thus generate GT masks by manually editing the results from the proposed method. Editing mostly comprised removal of false positives near the optic disk by direct annotation. The average duration was 53 s per image.

We compared the results of the proposed method with the aforementioned SSANet [11] trained with different public training datasets including DRIVE [14], STARE [9], CHASE_DB1 [6], and HRF [3], in Table 1. The networks were trained on the resolution of the images in each dataset, and fundus images of our FA-fundus image set were resized accordingly and given as input images. Measures were computed based on the aforementioned GT. We present these results as a reference for understanding the performance of the proposed method.

**Table 1.** Quantitative results of proposed method compared to results obtained by a CNN (SSANet [11]) trained on public fundus image datasets with expert annotated ground truth. Sensitivity (Se), specificity (Sp), accuracy (Acc), area-under-curve of the receiver operating characteristic curve (AUC-ROC) are presented.

| Method | Se | Sp | Acc | AUC-ROC |
|---|---|---|---|---|
| SSANet trained on DRIVE | 0.693 | 0.981 | 0.958 | 0.944 |
| SSANet trained on STARE | 0.697 | 0.985 | 0.962 | 0.936 |
| SSANet trained on CHASE_DB1 | 0.723 | 0.984 | 0.963 | 0.949 |
| SSANet trained on HRF | 0.720 | 0.985 | 0.964 | 0.950 |
| **Proposed method** | **0.894** | **0.983** | **0.976** | **0.982** |

## 4   Discussion

We present a new method to generate fine-scale vessel segmentation masks for fundus images by registration with FA. We have shown that the obtained results contain a considerable amount of filamentary vessels that are virtually indiscernible to the naked eye with only the color fundus image. We believe that these results conversely show the limitations of expert annotations as ground truth, which is the standard of all previously released public datasets. Nonetheless, since the proposed method may still contain errors, the requirement of expert annotation remains in order to designate data as ground truth.

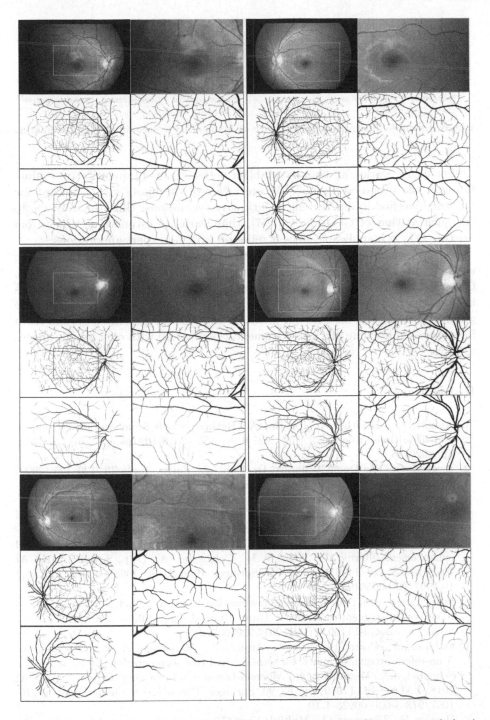

**Fig. 5.** Qualitative results. Six sample cases are shown in 3 × 2 formation, with (top) the original image, (middle) the results of the proposed method, and (bottom) vessel segmentation results of the SSANet [11] trained on the public HRF [3] dataset. Left and right columns shows the images in full and zoomed resolution, respectively.

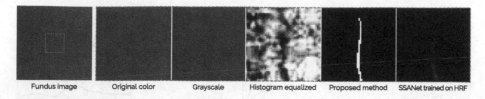

Fundus image     Original color     Grayscale     Histogram equalized     Proposed method     SSANet trained on HRF

**Fig. 6.** Example illustrating the visibility of filamentary vessels in the fundus images.

For future works, we plan to establish better means of quantitative evaluations for the proposed method. We are aware of the biases of GT toward the proposed method in our current quantitative evaluations. Unfortunately, methods such as that of Galdran et al. [7], that learns to estimate accuracy from existing GT, is inapplicable since it relies on existing expert annotations.

Also, we plan to construct a new dataset for filamentary vessels that can be used for improving deep learning based methods for retinal vessel segmentation. Our ultimate aim is to construct a dataset that can be the foundation for achieving superhuman accuracy. Particularly, although we utilize FA to construct the ground truth for this dataset, our intention is to use the generated ground truth for supervised learning of a vessel segmentation method with only fundus images as input.

# References

1. Almotiri, J., Elleithy, K., Elleithy, A.: Retinal vessels segmentation techniques and algorithms: a survey. Appl. Sci. **8**(2), 155 (2018). https://doi.org/10.3390/app8020155
2. Bradski, G.: The OpenCV library. Dr. Dobb's J. Softw. Tools **25**, 120–125 (2000)
3. Budai, A., Bock, R., Maier, A., Hornegger, J., Michelson, G.: Robust vessel segmentation in fundus images. Int. J. Biomed. Imaging **2013**, 154860 (2013)
4. Byrd, R.H., Lu, P., Nocedal, J., Zhu, C.: A limited memory algorithm for bound constrained optimization. SIAM J. Sci. Comput. **16**(5), 1190–1208 (1995)
5. Frangi, A.F., Niessen, W.J., Vincken, K.L., Viergever, M.A.: Multiscale vessel enhancement filtering. In: Wells, W.M., Colchester, A., Delp, S. (eds.) MICCAI 1998. LNCS, vol. 1496, pp. 130–137. Springer, Heidelberg (1998). https://doi.org/10.1007/BFb0056195
6. Fraz, M.M., et al.: An ensemble classification-based approach applied to retinal blood vessel segmentation. IEEE Trans. Biomed. Eng. **59**(9), 2538–2548 (2012). https://doi.org/10.1109/TBME.2012.2205687
7. Galdran, A., Costa, P., Bria, A., Araújo, T., Mendonça, A.M., Campilho, A.: A no-reference quality metric for retinal vessel tree segmentation. In: Frangi, A.F., Schnabel, J.A., Davatzikos, C., Alberola-López, C., Fichtinger, G. (eds.) MICCAI 2018. LNCS, vol. 11070, pp. 82–90. Springer, Cham (2018). https://doi.org/10.1007/978-3-030-00928-1_10
8. Hartley, R., Zisserman, A.: Multiple View Geometry in Computer Vision, 2nd edn. Cambridge University Press, New York (2003)

9. Hoover, A.D., Kouznetsova, V., Goldbaum, M.: Locating blood vessels in retinal images by piecewise threshold probing of a matched filter response. IEEE Trans. Med. Imaging **19**(3), 203–210 (2000). https://doi.org/10.1109/42.845178

10. Lowe, D.G.: Distinctive image features from scale-invariant keypoints. Int. J. Comput. Vis. **60**(2), 91–110 (2004). https://doi.org/10.1023/B:VISI.0000029664.99615.94

11. Noh, K.J., Park, S.J., Lee, S.: Scale-space approximated convolutional neural networks for retinal vessel segmentation. Comput. Methods Programs Biomed. **178**, 237–246 (2019). https://doi.org/10.1016/j.cmpb.2019.06.030

12. Perez-Rovira, A., Trucco, E., Wilson, P., Liu, J.: Deformable registration of retinal fluorescein angiogram sequences using vasculature structures. In: International Conference of the IEEE Engineering in Medicine and Biology (EMBS), pp. 4383–4386, August 2010. https://doi.org/10.1109/IEMBS.2010.5627094

13. Son, J., Park, S.J., Jung, K.H.: Towards accurate segmentation of retinal vessels and the optic disc in fundoscopic images with generative adversarial networks. J. Digit. Imaging **32**, 499–512 (2018). https://doi.org/10.1007/s10278-018-0126-3

14. Staal, J., Abramoff, M.D., Niemeijer, M., Viergever, M.A., van Ginneken, B.: Ridge-based vessel segmentation in color images of the retina. IEEE Trans. Med. Imaging **23**(4), 501–509 (2004). https://doi.org/10.1109/TMI.2004.825627

15. Viswanath, K., McGavin, D.D.M.: Diabetic retinopathy: clinical findings and management. Community Eye Health **16**(46), 21–24 (2003). https://www.ncbi.nlm.nih.gov/pubmed/17491851

16. Yaniv, Z., Lowekamp, B.C., Johnson, H.J., Beare, R.: SimpleITK image-analysis notebooks: a collaborative environment for education and reproducible research. J. Digit. Imaging **31**(3), 290–303 (2018). https://doi.org/10.1007/s10278-017-0037-8

# DME-Net: Diabetic Macular Edema Grading by Auxiliary Task Learning

Xiaodong He[✉][iD], Yi Zhou, Boyang Wang, Shanshan Cui, and Ling Shao

Inception Institute of Artificial Intelligence (IIAI), Abu Dhabi, United Arab Emirates
{xiaodong.he,yi.zhou,boyang.wang,shanshan.cui,ling.shao}@inceptioniai.org

**Abstract.** Diabetic macular edema (DME) is a consequence of diabetic retinopathy (DR), characterized by the abnormal accumulation of fluid and protein deposits in the macular region of the retina. Early detection and grading of DME is of great clinical significance, yet remains a challenging problem. In this work, we propose a highly accurate DME grading model by exploiting macular and hard exudate detection results in an auxiliary learning manner. Specifically, we adopt XGBoost [4] as the classifier, which allows us to use different types of multi-scale features that are extracted by the multi-scale feature extraction models from the image, hard exudate mask, macula mask, and macula image. Experiments have been conducted on the IDRiD and Messidor datasets. Our model achieves a large improvement over previous methods. Our method yields an accuracy of 0.9417 on IDRiD and beats the champion method of the "Diabetic Retinopathy: Segmentation and Grading Challenge" [1]. Our method also produces a high overall performance on Messidor, obtaining scores of 0.9591, 0.9712, 0.9824 and 0.9633 in terms of sensitivity, specificity, AUC and accuracy, respectively.

## 1 Introduction

Diabetic macular edema (DME) is the most common complication of diabetic retinopathy (DR), which can cause a serious loss of vision. Therefore, early intervention therapy for DR patients is particularly important for retarding DR progression and preventing vision loss [5]. DME can be diagnosed either by the presence of exudates (glossy lesions) in the retinal fundus images or optical coherence tomography (OCT) [8]. According to the International Clinical Diabetic Macular Edema Disease Severity Scale [14], DME grading on fundus images (which is less expensive and easier to operate than OCT) is mainly based on the appearance of the macular region and the location of hard exudates relative to the macular. With this in mind, we propose a deep learning model that fully exploits features from fundus images, as well as macular and hard exudates to perform DME grading.

**Electronic supplementary material** The online version of this chapter (https:// doi.org/10.1007/978-3-030-32239-7_87) contains supplementary material, which is available to authorized users.

© Springer Nature Switzerland AG 2019
D. Shen et al. (Eds.): MICCAI 2019, LNCS 11764, pp. 788–796, 2019.
https://doi.org/10.1007/978-3-030-32239-7_87

Deep learning has became increasingly popular in many fields, and it is gradually being applied by medical image processing to solve problems such as medical image segmentation, detection, and classification [9,10,15]. For example, several researchers have begun to apply deep learning methods for analyzing fundus images to solve problems that only OCT has been able to explore until now. Arcadu et al. used transfer learning from Inception-v3 trained on a DR grading dataset to predict diabetic macular thickness from color fundus photographs [3].

As for DME grading, Deepak et al. used traditional feature extraction to capture the global characteristics of the fundus images, and then used these to distinguish between normal and DME images, achieving an AUC value of 0.96 [7]. Akram et al. proposed a medical system based on image processing and pattern recognition to solve DME grading [2]. They extracted region features (including area, compactness, mean hue, entropy, energy, etc.) as inputs, then used a Gaussian mixture classifier for DME grading. The proposed system achieved average values of 97.3%, 95.9% and 96.8% in terms of sensitivity, specificity, and accuracy, respectively, on the Messidor dataset [6].

In this paper, we use a deep learning model to extract features from fundus images, the model combines multi-scale features from a fundus image, hard exudate masks, macular mask and macular image as input data, and then uses XGBoost as the classifier for DME grading. The main contributions of our method are highlighted as follows:

(1) A mask segmentation model is proposed to generate the pixel-wise hard exudates and macular masks. We design a segmentation model based on the U-net framework and use a supervised segmentation loss for training.
(2) For image-level inputs, we devise a multi-scale feature integration model that can extract multi-scale features, which contribute more to DME grading than original image inputs.
(3) XGBoost - a scalable tree boosting system - is introduced as the classifier for DME grading. XGBoost can fuse different scale features from different types of input, and improve the DME grading accuracy.

## 2   Proposed Methods

### 2.1   Macular and Hard Exudate Segmentation

Our model introduces the U-net segmentation model $G(\cdot)$ to segment macular and hard exudate masks [12]. Since the segmentation model requires pixel-level annotated training data, we use the Indian Diabetic Retinopathy Image Dataset [11](IDRiD), which is the only diabetic retinopathy dataset that contains pixel-level annotations of hard exudates and macular (the mask generation method are clarified in the supplementary file). Our model takes original fundus images $X^S$ from IDRiD as inputs, hard exudates and macular masks $M^T$ as the labels for segmentation. We aim to minimize the distance between the predicted and ground-truth masks by using the mean square error loss function:

$$Loss_{seg} = \min \left\| G(X^S), M^T \right\|_2. \tag{1}$$

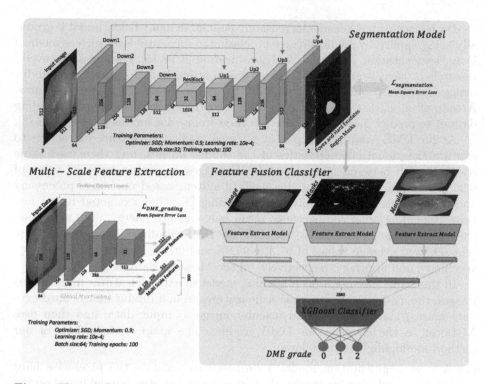

**Fig. 1.** The pipeline of the proposed method. The input data consists of pixel-level annotated lesion images and DME grading images. The segmentation model is proposed for learning the hard exudate and macular masks.

## 2.2   Multi-scale Feature Extraction Model

We adopt the VGG-16 [13] framework as the encoder to extract features, then use global max-pooling to squeeze features from different layers and combine them as multi-scale features (**MS Features**). As shown in Fig. 1, we use the original image, hard exudates, macular masks, and macular image to train our feature extraction model separately.

To obtain low-level and high-level features from the input data, we adopt global max-pooling to squeeze features from different layers in the encoder and then integrate them as multi-scale features $F^m$. We will compare the effectiveness between using the feature from the last layer and using the multi-scale features in Sect. 3.3.

As shown in Fig. 1, we use different types of images $X^F$ as inputs, fully-connected layers as the classifier $C(\cdot)$, and DME grades as the ground-truth $Y^c$. To extract features that contribute to DME grading from the input images, we introduce the mean square error loss function to minimize the distance between predictions and DME grading labels:

$$Loss_{DME_{grading}} = \min \left\| C(\boldsymbol{X}^F), \boldsymbol{Y}^c \right\|_2. \tag{2}$$

## 2.3 Multi-feature Fusion Classifier

We use XGBoost as the classifier for DME grading. To verify the generalizability of different features, we train different classifiers for each type of feature and compare their performance in terms of accuracy and AUC. We conduct experiments on last layer features ($512 \times n$), multi-scale features ($960 \times n$), all last layer features ($1536 \times n$) and all multilayer features ($2880 \times n$) to compare the generalizability of different features. We also compare the classifier of the fully-connected layer, SVM and XGBoost to the three classifiers trained on the extracted features. The experimental results are shown in Sect. 3.3. Details on the multi-scale feature fusion classifier are shown in Fig. 1.

## 3 Experiments

To evaluate our method, we conduct experiments on the IDRiD dataset to assess segmentation performance for the segmentation model, and use the IDRiD and Messidor datasets for DME grading, we also compare our method with other state-of-the-art DME grading models.

### 3.1 Datasets and Evaluation

**IDRiD Dataset.** To the best of our knowledge, the Indian Diabetic Retinopathy Image Dataset (IDRiD) [11] is the only Fundus Image set providing pixel-level annotations of hard exudates as well as image-level DME grading labels. The pixel-level annotations contain 54 color fundus images for training and 27 images for testing. The masks, including microaneurysms, hemorrhages, hard exudates, soft exudates, and optical discs, are annotated by medical experts as binary images. Moreover, the image-level grading dataset contains 413 training images and 103 testing images, which have DME and DR grading labels. We use hard exudate masks and generated macular masks to train our segmentation model. Then, the grading dataset is used to train our multi-scale feature extraction model and feature fusion classifier.

**Messidor Dataset.** The Messidor dataset contains 1200 fundus images with DME and DR grades. Its grading scale is the same as that of the IDRiD dataset, with 0, 1, 2 grades [6,14]. Since there are no hard exudate or macular masks in the Messidor dataset, we only use this dataset for training and testing our multi-scale feature extraction model and feature fusion classifier for DME grading.

**Data Preprocessing and Augmentation.** Since the grading image sets have a strong imbalance(Detailed in the supplementary document), we introduce a data pre-processing method(Detailed in the supplementary document) and data augmentation strategy (Detailed in the supplementary document), which can mitigate the imbalance of samples across different classes while increasing data diversity.

**Evaluation Metrics.** In our segmentation model, for macular and hard exudate segmentation evaluation, we adopt average precision (AP), intersection over union (IOU) and dice index. In our multi-scale feature extraction model, we compute the accuracy of DME grading in the training set and testing set to compare the accuracy and generalization of different models. The higher the accuracy of the testing set is, the higher the accuracy of the model is; the smaller the accuracy gap between the training set and testing set is, the stronger the generalizability of the model is. For our multi-feature fusion classifier, the specificity and sensitivity are introduced to evaluate the model's ability to handle unbalanced samples. We use the accuracy and AUC of the testing dataset to evaluate our model's performance and compare it with the results of other models.

## 3.2  Ablation Studies

**Macular and Hard Exudate Segmentation.** We use the segmentation training and testing sets of IDRiD to train and test our segmentation model. The image pre-processing method and data augmentation strategy mentioned in Sect. 3.1 is conducted during segmentation model training. The dice indices of our segmentation model are 0.9619 (hard exudate) and 0.9497 (macula). All the segmentation results for macula and hard exudates are shown in Table 1 and Fig. 2.

**Table 1.** Results of hard exudate and macular segmentation.

| Mask | AP | IOU | Dice Index |
|---|---|---|---|
| Hard exudate | 0.9459 | 0.9784 | 0.9619 |
| Macular | 0.9254 | 0.9741 | 0.9497 |

**Multi-scale Feature Extraction** We employ VGG-16 as the multi-scale feature extraction model and train it using DME classification training and testing sets. We use different types of input data (original fundus image, hard exudate and macular masks, macular image), and conduct experiments with six different models. We compare the accuracy of these different models on the training and testing sets and find the VGG-16 model performs best. The image pre-processing method and data augmentation strategy mentioned in Sect. 3.1 are conducted

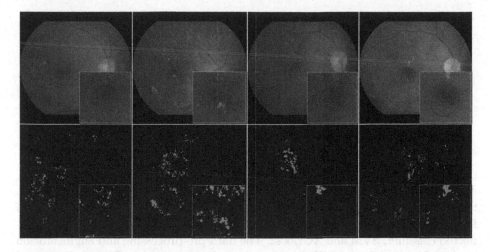

**Fig. 2.** Segmentation mask of the macula and hard exudates. Red contours in the images of the first row are macula predictions, green contours are ground-truths. The masks in the second row are ground-truths and hard exudate predictions, yellow areas show overlap between prediction and ground-truth, green areas are ground-truths, red areas are predictions (Color figure online)

during model training and testing. Detailed experimental results are shown in Table 2 and Fig. 3. They indicate that, compared with other models, in terms of the accuracy and generalizability, the VGG-16 model is the best feature extraction model.

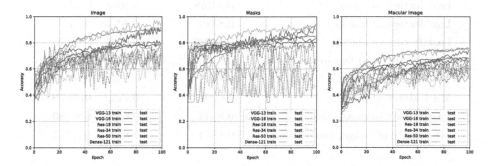

**Fig. 3.** The accuracy of different models

**Effectiveness of Feature Fusion Classifier.** We use XGBoost as the feature fusion classifier of our final grading model. The accuracy of our model on the testing set is 0.9417, which beats the top-performing method on the leaderboard [1]. We train the classifier with features from the 413 training images in IDRiD and

**Table 2.** The DME grading accuracy of different models.

| Model | Image(test/train) | Masks(test/train) | Macular(test/train) |
|-------|-------------------|-------------------|---------------------|
| VGG13 | 0.7859/0.7915 | 0.7968/0.8159 | 0.6564/0.6865 |
| VGG16 | **0.7904**/0.8202 | **0.8294**/0.8502 | **0.6758**/0.6859 |
| ResNet18 | 0.7857/0.9027 | 0.7970/0.8560 | 0.6692/0.7590 |
| ResNet34 | 0.7764/0.9198 | 0.7954/0.9383 | 0.6487/0.6724 |
| ResNet50 | 0.7442/0.9187 | 0.7512/0.9357 | 0.6162/0.7423 |
| DenseNet121 | 0.7231/**0.9709** | 0.7447/**0.9430** | 0.6011/**0.7642** |

test it on the testing sets of IDRiD and Messidor datasets. Different kinds of features are introduced as input data, to three different classifiers: the fully connected classifier, SVM and XGBoost. The data pre-processing and augmentation are mentioned in Sect. 3.1. Experimental results are shown in Table 3. Compared with the other two classifiers(the fully connected classifier, SVM), XGBoost is the best classifier for fusing all features, and the highest accuracy of XGBoost on the IDRiD DME testing set is 0.9417. No matter which classifier do we use, multi-scale features of the image, masks and macula achieve the best performance. This indicates that our feature extraction method can extract the most generalized features.

**Table 3.** The DME grading Accuracy of IDRiD testing set.

| Input feature | Fully-connected | SVM | XGBoost |
|---------------|-----------------|-----|---------|
| Last feature of image | **0.8058** | 0.8058 | 0.7961 |
| Last feature of masks | 0.8349 | **0.8543** | 0.8447 |
| Last feature of macula | **0.6796** | 0.6796 | 0.6796 |
| Multi-Scale (MS) features of image | 0.8155 | 0.8349 | **0.8447** |
| MS features of masks | 0.8447 | 0.8543 | **0.8741** |
| MS features of macula | 0.6990 | 0.7282 | **0.7379** |
| Last feature of image, masks & macula | 0.8543 | 0.8640 | **0.9080** |
| MS feature of image, masks & macula | 0.8543 | 0.8741 | **0.9417** |

## 3.3   DME Grading Results and Comparison with State-of-the-arts

Compared with the 1st and 2nd places on the leaderboard [1], a large improvement is obtained by our method. DME grading evaluation is based on metrics that include sensitivity, specificity, AUC and accuracy. Details of our experimental results are listed in Table 4. The specificity and sensitivity of our model are 0.9384 and 0.9553, respectively. According to these experimental results, our model did not overfit. This indicates that our classifier contributes to the full use of the extracted features for DME grading.

**Table 4.** Comparision with State-of-the-arts.

| Model & dataSet | Specificity | Sensitivity | AUC | Accuracy |
|---|---|---|---|---|
| Mammoth [1] in IDRiD | - | - | - | **0.9322** |
| SDNU [1] in IDRiD | - | - | - | 0.8789 |
| HarangiM1 [1] in IDRiD | - | - | - | 0.8741 |
| Fundus Image (Ours) in IDRiD | 0.8352 | 0.8568 | 0.8715 | 0.8447 |
| All Features (Ours) in IDRiD | 0.9384 | 0.9553 | 0.9637 | **0.9417** |
| Deepak et al. in Messidor | - | - | 0.96 | - |
| Akram et al. in Messidor | 0.9730 | 0.9590 | - | **0.9680** |
| All Features (Ours) in Messidor | 0.9591 | 0.9712 | 0.9824 | **0.9633** |

## 4    Conclusion

In this paper, we extract multi-scale features from fundus images, masks, and macula images to assist DME grading. The grading accuracy of our final model is 94.17%, which is 13.59% higher than that of the baseline only trained on original images. Our experiments show that our multi-scale feature extraction method and feature fusion classifier can combine relevant features from multiple sources to improve the accuracy of our model. Furthermore, compared with the accuracy of the winner and other participants in the IDRiD online challenge [1], large improvements are obtained by our model. This indicates that the combination of hard exudate and macular segmentation results contributes to the improvement of DME grading.

## References

1. Diabetic retinopathy: Segmentation and grading challenge. https://idrid.grand-challenge.org/Leaderboard/. Accessed 27 Mar 2019
2. Akram, M.U., Tariq, A., Khan, S.A., Javed, M.Y.: Automated detection of exudates and macula for grading of diabetic macular edema. Comput. Methods Programs Biomed. **114**(2), 141–152 (2014)
3. Arcadu, F., et al.: Deep learning predicts oct measures of diabetic macular thickening from color fundus photographs. Invest. Ophthalmol. Vis. Sci. **60**(4), 852–857 (2019)
4. Chen, T., Guestrin, C.: Xgboost: a scalable tree boosting system. In: Proceedings of the 22nd ACM SIGKDD International Conference on Knowledge Discovery and Data Mining, pp. 785–794. ACM (2016)

5. Ciulla, T.A., Amador, A.G., Zinman, B.: Diabetic retinopathy and diabetic macular edema: pathophysiology, screening, and novel therapies. Diabetes Care **26**(9), 2653–2664 (2003)
6. Decencière, E., et al.: Feedback on a publicly distributed image database: the Messidor database. Image Anal. Stereol. **33**(3), 231–234 (2014)
7. Deepak, K.S., Sivaswamy, J.: Automatic assessment of macular edema from color retinal images. IEEE Trans. Med. Imaging **31**(3), 766–776 (2012)
8. Hee, M.R., et al.: Topography of diabetic macular edema with optical coherence tomography. Ophthalmology **105**(2), 360–370 (1998)
9. Lee, J.G., et al.: Deep learning in medical imaging: general overview. Korean J. Radiol. **18**(4), 570–584 (2017)
10. Liu, H., Wong, D.W.K., Fu, H., Xu, Y., Liu, J.: DeepAMD: detect early age-related macular degeneration by applying deep learning in a multiple instance learning framework. In: Jawahar, C.V., Li, H., Mori, G., Schindler, K. (eds.) ACCV 2018. LNCS, vol. 11365, pp. 625–640. Springer, Cham (2019). https://doi.org/10.1007/978-3-030-20873-8_40
11. Porwal, P., et al.: Indian diabetic retinopathy image dataset (IDRiD): a database for diabetic retinopathy screening research. Data **3**(3), 25 (2018)
12. Ronneberger, O., Fischer, P., Brox, T.: U-Net: convolutional networks for biomedical image segmentation. In: Navab, N., Hornegger, J., Wells, W.M., Frangi, A.F. (eds.) MICCAI 2015. LNCS, vol. 9351, pp. 234–241. Springer, Cham (2015). https://doi.org/10.1007/978-3-319-24574-4_28
13. Simonyan, K., Zisserman, A.: Very deep convolutional networks for large-scale image recognition. Comput. Sci. (2014)
14. Wilkinson, C., et al.: Proposed international clinical diabetic retinopathy and diabetic macular edema disease severity scales. Ophthalmology **110**(9), 1677–1682 (2003)
15. Zhou, Y., et al.: Collaborative learning of semi-supervised segmentation and classification for medical images. In: The IEEE Conference on Computer Vision and Pattern Recognition (CVPR), June 2019

# Attention Guided Network for Retinal Image Segmentation

Shihao Zhang[1], Huazhu Fu[2], Yuguang Yan[1], Yubing Zhang[4], Qingyao Wu[1],
Ming Yang[4], Mingkui Tan[1,3(✉)], and Yanwu Xu[5(✉)]

[1] South China University of Technology, Guangzhou, China
mingkuitan@scut.edu.cn
[2] Inception Institute of Artificial Intelligence, Abu Dhabi, UAE
[3] Peng Cheng Laboratory, Shenzhen, China
[4] CVTE Research, Guangzhou, China
[5] Cixi Institute of Biomedical Engineering,
Ningbo Institute of Materials Technology and Engineering,
Chinese Academy of Sciences, Ningbo, China
ywxu@ieee.org
https://github.com/HzFu/AGNet

**Abstract.** Learning structural information is critical for producing an
ideal result in retinal image segmentation. Recently, convolutional neural
networks have shown a powerful ability to extract effective representations. However, convolutional and pooling operations filter out some useful structural information. In this paper, we propose an Attention Guided
Network (AG-Net) to preserve the structural information and guide the
expanding operation. In our AG-Net, the guided filter is exploited as
a structure sensitive expanding path to transfer structural information
from previous feature maps, and an attention block is introduced to
exclude the noise and reduce the negative influence of background further. The extensive experiments on two retinal image segmentation tasks
(i.e., blood vessel segmentation, optic disc and cup segmentation) demonstrate the effectiveness of our proposed method.

## 1 Introduction

Retinal image segmentation plays an important role in automatic disease diagnosis. Compared to general natural images, retinal images contain more contextual
structures, e.g., retinal vessel, optic disc and cup, which often provide important
clinical information for diagnosis. As the main indicators for eye disease diagnosis, the segmentation accuracy of these information is important. Recently,
convolutional neural networks (CNNs) have shown the strong ability in retinal

---

This work was done when S. Zhang is intern at CVTE Research.

---

**Electronic supplementary material** The online version of this chapter (https://
doi.org/10.1007/978-3-030-32239-7_88) contains supplementary material, which is
available to authorized users.

© Springer Nature Switzerland AG 2019
D. Shen et al. (Eds.): MICCAI 2019, LNCS 11764, pp. 797–805, 2019.
https://doi.org/10.1007/978-3-030-32239-7_88

image segmentation with remarkable performances [1–4]. Existing CNN based models learn increasingly abstract representations by cascade convolutions and pooling operations. However, these operations may neglect some useful structural information such as edge structures, which are important for retinal image analysis. To address this issue, one possible solution is to add extra expanding paths to merge features skipped from the corresponding resolution levels. For example, FCN [5] sums up the upsampled feature maps and the feature maps skipped from the contractive path. And U-Net [6] concatenates them and add convolutions and non-linearities. However, these works can not effectively leverage these structural information, which may hamper the segmentation performance. Therefore, it is desirable to design a better expanding path to preserve structural information.

To address this, we introduce guided filter [7] as a special expanding path to transfer structural information extracted from low-level feature maps to high-level ones. Guided filter [7] is an edge-preserving image filter, and has been demonstrated to be effective for transferring structural information. Different from existing works which use the guided filter at the image level, we incorporate the guided filter into CNNs to learn better features for segmentation. We further design an attention mechanism in guided filter, called attention guided filter, to remove the noisy components, which are introduced from the complex background by original guided filter. Finally, we propose **Attention Guided Network (AG-Net)** to preserve the structural information and guide the expanding operation. The experiments on vessel segmentation and optic disc/cup segmentation demonstrate the effectiveness of our proposed method.

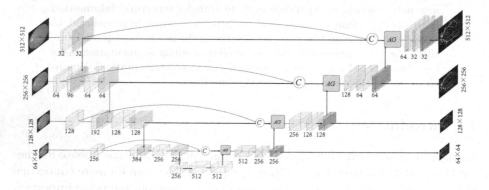

**Fig. 1.** Architecture of proposed AG-Net. Our AG-Net is based on M-Net [3], which is a multi-scale multi-label segmentation network. The block $AG$ represents our attention guided filter and the operator $C$ is the concatenation. In our AG-Net, the attention guided filter is used as a structural sensitive skip-connection to replace the skip-connection and upsampling layer for better information fusion.

## 2    Methodology

Figure 1 shows the architecture of proposed AG-Net, where M-Net [3] is utilized as the backbone to learn hierarchical representations. We propose attention guided filter into the network, which contains the guided filter and attention block to filter out the noise from the background and address the boundary blur problem caused by upsampling. The details of our AG-Net are illustrated as follows.

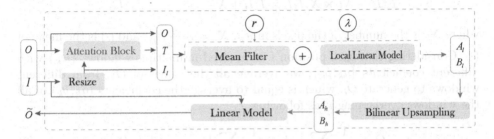

**Fig. 2.** Illustration of the attention guided filter. The attention guided filter first produces the attention map $T$ through the attention block, then calculates $A_l, B_l$ with the attention map $T$, resized guidance feature map ($I_l$), filtering feature map ($O$) and hyperparameter $r, \epsilon$. By using bilinear upsampling $A_l$ and $B_l$, we obtain $A_h$ and $B_h$ for producing the final output $\tilde{O}$ with $I$.

### 2.1    Attention Guided Filter

The attention guided filter recovers spatial information and merges structural information from the various resolution levels by filtering the low-resolution feature maps with high-resolution feature maps. The inputs include a guidance feature map ($I$), and a filtering feature map ($O$). The output is a high-resolution feature map $\tilde{O}$. The attention feature map $T$ is produced by an attention block. As shown in Fig. 2, the attention guided filter firstly downsamples the guidance feature map $I$ to obtain a low-resolution feature map $I_l$, which has the same size of the filtering feature map $O$. Then we minimize the reconstruction error between $I_l$ and $O$ to obtain the coefficients of the attention guided filter $A_l, B_l$, which correspond to $I_l$. After that, by upsampling $A_l$ and $B_l$, the coefficients $A_h$ and $B_h$ are obtained to generate the final high-resolution output $\tilde{O}$ of the attention guided filter. Concretely, the attention guided filter constructs a squared window $w_k$ with a radius $r$ for each position $k$. Let $I_{l_i}$ be a pixel of $I_l$, its output with respect to $w_k$ is obtained by a linear transformation: $\hat{O}_{ki} = a_k I_{l_i} + b_k, \forall i \in w_k$, where $a_k$ and $b_k$ are the linear coefficients of the window $w_k$.

To determine the linear coefficients $(a_k, b_k)$, we minimize the difference between $\hat{O}_{ki}$ and $O_i$ for all the pixels in the window $w_k$, which is formulated as the following optimization problem:

$$\min_{a_k, b_k} E(a_k, b_k) := \sum_{i \in w_k} (T_i^2(a_k I_{l_i} + b_k - O_i)^2 + \lambda a_k^2), \qquad (1)$$

where $\lambda$ is a regularization parameter, and $T_i$ is the attention weight at the position $i$. The closed-form solution to Problem (1) is given as:

$$a_k = \frac{\overline{T_i^2 I_i O_i} - N_k \times \overline{X_i T_i I_i} \times \overline{T_i O_i}}{\overline{T_i^2 I_i^2} - N_k \times \overline{X_i T_i I_i} \times \overline{T_i I_i} + \lambda}, \qquad b_k = \frac{\overline{T_i O_i} - a_k \times \overline{T_i I_i}}{\overline{T_i}}, \qquad (2)$$

where $N_k$ is the number of the pixels in $w_k$, $X_i = \frac{T_i}{\sum_{i \in w_k} T_i}$, and $\overline{(\cdot)}$ is the mean of $(\cdot)$. Considering that each position $i$ is involved in multiple windows $\{w_k\}$ with different coefficients $\{a_k, b_k\}$, we average all the values of $\hat{O}_{ki}$ from different windows to generate $\hat{O}_i$, which is equal to average the coefficients $(a_k, b_k)$ of all the windows overlapping $i$, as following,

$$\hat{O}_i = \frac{1}{N_k} \sum_{k \in \Omega_i} a_k I_i + \frac{1}{N_k} \sum_{k \in \Omega_i} b_k = A_l * I_l + B_l, \qquad (3)$$

where $\Omega_i$ is the set of all the windows including the position $i$, and $*$ is the element-wise multiplication. After upsampling $A_l$ and $B_l$ to obtain $A_h$ and $B_h$, respectively, the final output is calculated as $\tilde{O} = A_h * I + B_h$.

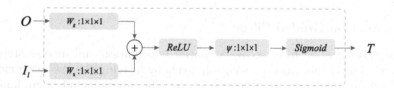

**Fig. 3.** Schematic of the attention block. $O$ and $I$ are the inputs of attention guided filter and $T$ is the calculated attention map.

**Attention Block** is very essential in our method. Specially, the attention block is used to highlight the foreground and reduce the effect of background. As shown in Fig. 3, the attention block consists of three steps: (1) given the feature maps $O, I_l \in \mathbb{R}^{C \times H \times W}$, a channel-wise $1 \times 1 \times 1$ convolution is used to do a linear transformation. Note that this can be referred to as the vector concatenation-based attention [8], where the concatenated features are linearly mapped into a latent space. (2) two transformed feature maps are combined with element-wise addition with a ReLU layer. (3) a $1 \times 1 \times 1$ convolution is applied as a additional linear transformation with a Sigmoid activation to produce the final attention map $T$.

# 3    Experiments

In this paper, we evaluate our method in two major tasks of vessel segmentation, and optic disc/cup segmentation from retina fundus images.

## 3.1    Vessel Segmentation on DRIVE Dataset

We conduct vessel segmentation experiments on DRIVE to evaluate performance of our proposed AG-Net. The DRIVE [9] (Digital Retinal Images for Vessel Extraction) dataset contains 40 colored fundus images, which are obtained from a diabetic retinopathy screening program in Netherlands. The 40 images are divided into 20 training images and 20 testing images. All the images are made by a 3CCD camera and each has size of $565 \times 584$. We apply gamma correction to improve the image quality, and resize the preprocessed images into $512 \times 512$ as inputs. In the experiment, we train our AG-Net from scratch using Adam with the learning rate of 0.0015. The batch size is set to 2. The radius of windows $r$ and the regularization parameter $\lambda$ in attention guided filter are set to 2 and 0.01 respectively. Following the previous work [10], we employ Specificity (Spe), Sensitivity (Sen), Accuracy (Acc), intersection-over-union(IOU) and Area Under ROC (AUC) as measurements.

We compare our AG-Net with several state-of-the-art methods, including Li [11], Liskowski [12], and Zhang [10]. Li [11] remolded the task of segmentation as a problem of cross-modality data transformation from retinal image to vessel map, and outputted the label map of all pixels instead of a single label of the center pixel. Liskowski [12] trained a deep neural network on sample of examples preprocessed with global contrast normalization, zero-phase whitening, and augmented using geometric transformations and gamma corrections. MS-NFN [13] generates multi-scale feature maps with an 'up-pool' submodel and a 'pool-up' submodel. To verify the efficacy of attention in guided filter and transfer structural information, we replaced the attention guided filter in AG-Net with the original guided filter, named GF-Net.

**Table 1.** Quantitative comparison of segmentation results on DRIVE

| Method | Acc | AUC | Sen | Spe | IOU |
|--------|-----|-----|-----|-----|-----|
| Li [11] | 0.9527 | 0.9738 | 0.7569 | 0.9816 | – |
| Liskowski [12] | 0.9535 | 0.9790 | 0.7811 | 0.9807 | – |
| MS-NFN [13] | 0.9567 | 0.9807 | 0.7844 | 0.9819 | – |
| U-Net [6] | 0.9681 | 0.9836 | 0.7897 | 0.9854 | 0.6834 |
| M-Net [3] | 0.9674 | 0.9829 | 0.7680 | **0.9868** | 0.6726 |
| GF-Net | 0.9682 | 0.9837 | 0.7895 | 0.9856 | 0.6839 |
| AG-Net | **0.9692** | **0.9856** | **0.8100** | 0.9848 | **0.6965** |

Table 1 shows the performances of different methods on DRIVE. Form the results, we could have several interesting observations: Firstly, GF-Net performs better than original M-Net, which demonstrates the superiority of the guided filter compared to the skip connection for transferring structural information. Secondly, AG-Net outperforms GF-Net by 0.0010, 0.0019, 0.0205 and 0.0126 in terms of Acc, AUC, Sen and IOU respectively. This demonstrates the effectiveness of the attention strategy in attention guided filter. Lastly, unlike other deep learning methods which crop images into patches, our method achieves the best performance with the original preprocessed 20 images. We draw similar observations from the results on the CHASE_DB1 dataset, which are shown in Table 2.

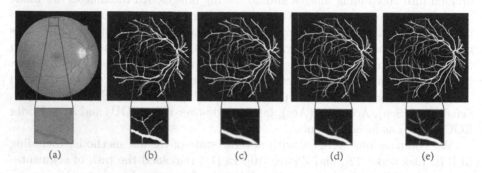

(a)                (b)                (c)                (d)                (e)

**Fig. 4.** (a) A test image from DRIVE dataset; (b) Ground truth segmentation; (c) Segmentation result by M-Net; (d) Segmentation result by GF-Net; (e) Segmentation result by AG-Net. From (c), M-Net neglect some edge structures which are very similar to choroidal vessels. On the contrary, by exploiting attention guided as a special expanding path, AG-Net gains better discrimination power and is able to distinguish objects from similar structures. Moreover, GF helps to obtain clearer boundaries.

Figure 4 shows an example test, including the ground truth vessel and the segmentation results obtained by M-Net, M-Net+GF and the proposed AG-Net. M-Net+GF produces clearer boundaries than M-Net, which demonstrates the effectiveness of the guided filter to better leverage structure information. Compared with M-Net+GF, our proposed AG-Net produces more precise segmentation boundaries, which verifies that the attention mechanism is able to highlight the foreground and reduce the effect of background.

In terms of time consumption, we compare our AG-Net with M-Net which is the backbone of our method. In our experiment, both algorithms are implemented with Pytorch and tested on a single NVIDIA Titan X GPU (200 iterations on DRIVE dataset). The running time is shown in Table 3.

### 3.2 Optic Dice/Cup Segmentation on ORIGA Dataset

Optic Dice/Cup Segmentation is another important retinal segmentation task. In this experiment, we use ORIGA dataset, which contains 650 fundus images with

**Table 2.** Quantitative comparison of segmentation results on CHASE_DB1

| Method | Acc | AUC | Sen | Spe | IOU |
|---|---|---|---|---|---|
| Li [11] | 0.9581 | 0.9716 | 0.7507 | 0.9793 | – |
| Liskowski [12] | 0.9628 | 0.9823 | 0.7816 | 0.9836 | – |
| MS-NFN [13] | 0.9637 | 0.9825 | 0.7538 | 0.9847 | – |
| U-Net [6] | 0.9723 | 0.9837 | 0.7715 | **0.9858** | 0.6366 |
| M-Net [3] | 0.9729 | 0.9845 | 0.7922 | 0.9851 | 0.6483 |
| GF-Net | 0.9734 | 0.9853 | 0.8089 | 0.9845 | 0.6572 |
| AG-Net | **0.9743** | **0.9863** | **0.8186** | 0.9848 | **0.6669** |

**Table 3.** Quantitative comparison of the time consumption

| Method | Train time (s) | Test time (s/image) |
|---|---|---|
| M-Net | 1800 | 0.0691 |
| AG-Net | 2800 | 0.0158 |

168 glaucomatous eyes and 482 normal eyes. The 650 images are divided into 325 training images (including 73 glaucoma cases) and 325 testing images (including 95 glaucoma cases). We crop the OD area and resize it into $256 \times 256$ as the input. The training setting of our AG-Net is as same as in vessel segmentation task. We compare AG-MNet with several state-of-the-art methods in OD and/or OC segmentation, including ASM [14], Superpixel [15], LRR [16], U-Net [6], M-Net [3], and M-Net with polar transformation (M-Net + PT). ASM [14] employs the circular hough transform initialization to segmentation. Superpixel method in [15] utilizes superpixel classification to detect the OD and OC boundaries. The methods in LRR [16] obtain good results, but it only focus on OC segmentation.

Following the setting in [3], we firstly localize the disc center, and then crop $640 \times 640$ pixels to obtain the input images. Inspired by M-Net+PT [3], we provide the results of AG-Net with polar transformation, called AG-MNet+PT. Besides, to reduce the impacts of changes in the size of OD, we construct a method AG-MNet+PT*, which enlarges 50 pixels of bounding-boxes in up, down, right and left, where the bounding boxes are obtained from pretrained LinkNet [17]. We employ overlapping error (OE) as the evaluation metric, which is defined as $OE = 1 - \frac{A_{GT} \bigcap A_{SR}}{A_{GT} \bigcup A_{SR}}$, where $A_{GT}$ and $A_{SR}$ denote ground truth area and segmented mask, respectively. In particular, $OE_{disc}$ and $OE_{cup}$ are the overlapping error of OD and OE. $OE_{total}$ is the average of $OE_{disc}$ and $OE_{cup}$.

Table 4 shows the segmentation results, where the overlapping errors of other approaches come directly from the published results. Our method outperforms all the state-of-the-art OD and/or OC segmentation algorithms in terms of the aforementioned two evaluation criteria, which demonstrates the effectiveness of our model. Besides, Our AG-Mnet performs much better than original M-Net under the same situation, which further demonstrates our attention guided filter

**Table 4.** Quantitative comparison of segmentation results on ORIGA

| Method | $OE_{disc}$ | $OE_{cup}$ | $OE_{total}$ |
|---|---|---|---|
| ASM [14] | 0.148 | 0.313 | 0.231 |
| SP [15] | 0.102 | 0.264 | 0.183 |
| LRR [16] | – | 0.244 | – |
| U-Net [6] | 0.115 | 0.287 | 0.201 |
| M-Net [3] | 0.083 | 0.256 | 0.170 |
| M-Net+PT [3] | 0.071 | 0.230 | 0.150 |
| AG-Net (ours) | 0.069 | 0.227 | 0.148 |
| AG-Net+PT (ours) | 0.067 | 0.217 | 0.142 |
| AG-Net+PT* (ours) | **0.061** | **0.212** | **0.137** |

is beneficial for the segmentation performance. More visualization results could be found in Supplementary Material.

## 4  Conclusions

In this paper, we propose an attention guided filter as a structure sensitive expanding path. Specially, we employ M-Net as the main body and exploit our attention guided filter to replace the skip-connection and upsampling, which brings better information fusion. In addition, by introducing the attention mechanism into the guided filter, the attention guided filter can highlight the foreground and reduce the effect of background. Experiments on two tasks demonstrate the effectiveness of our method.

**Acknowledments.** This work was supported by National Natural Science Foundation of China (NSFC) 61602185 and 61876208, Guangdong Introducing Innovative and Enterpreneurial Teams 2017ZT07X183, and Guangdong Provincial Scientific and Technological Fund 2018B010107001, 2017B090901008 and 2018B010108002, and Pearl River S&T Nova Program of Guangzhou 201806010081, and CCF-Tencent Open Research Fund RAGR20190103.

## References

1. Fu, H., Xu, Y., Lin, S., Kee Wong, D.W., Liu, J.: DeepVessel: retinal vessel segmentation via deep learning and conditional random field. In: Ourselin, S., Joskowicz, L., Sabuncu, M.R., Unal, G., Wells, W. (eds.) MICCAI 2016. LNCS, vol. 9901, pp. 132–139. Springer, Cham (2016). https://doi.org/10.1007/978-3-319-46723-8_16
2. Gu, Z., et al.: CE-Net: context encoder network for 2D medical image segmentation. IEEE TMI (2019)
3. Fu, H., et al.: Joint optic disc and cup segmentation based on multi-label deep network and polar transformation. IEEE TMI **37**, 1597–1605 (2018)

4. Yan, Z., Yang, X., Cheng, K.-T.: A skeletal similarity metric for quality evaluation of retinal vessel segmentation. IEEE TMI **37**, 1045–1057 (2017)
5. Long, J., Shelhamer, E., Darrell, T.: Fully convolutional networks for semantic segmentation. In: CVPR (2015)
6. Ronneberger, O., Fischer, P., Brox, T.: U-net: convolutional networks for biomedical image segmentation. In: Navab, N., Hornegger, J., Wells, W.M., Frangi, A.F. (eds.) MICCAI 2015. LNCS, vol. 9351, pp. 234–241. Springer, Cham (2015). https://doi.org/10.1007/978-3-319-24574-4_28
7. He, K., Sun, J., Tang, X.: Guided image filtering. IEEE TPAMI **35**, 1397–1409 (2013)
8. Wang, X., et al.: Non-local neural networks. In: CVPR (2018)
9. Staal, J., et al.: Ridge-based vessel segmentation in color images of the retina. IEEE TMI **23**, 501 (2004)
10. Zhang, Y., Chung, A.C.S.: Deep supervision with additional labels for retinal vessel segmentation task. In: Frangi, A.F., Schnabel, J.A., Davatzikos, C., Alberola-López, C., Fichtinger, G. (eds.) MICCAI 2018. LNCS, vol. 11071, pp. 83–91. Springer, Cham (2018). https://doi.org/10.1007/978-3-030-00934-2_10
11. Li, Q., et al.: A cross-modality learning approach for vessel segmentation in retinal images. IEEE TMI **35**, 109–118 (2016)
12. Liskowski, P., Krawiec, K.: Segmenting retinal blood vessels with deep neural networks. TMI **35**, 2369–2380 (2016)
13. Wu, Y., et al.: Multiscale network followed network model for retinal vessel segmentation. In: Frangi, A., Schnabel, J., Davatzikos, C., Alberola-Lopez, C., Fichtinger, G. (eds.) MICCAI 2018. LNCS, vol. 11071, pp. 119–126. Springer, Heidelberg (2018). https://doi.org/10.1007/978-3-030-00934-2_14
14. Yin, F., et al.: Model-based optic nerve head segmentation on retinal fundus images. In: EMBC. IEEE (2011)
15. Cheng, J., et al.: Superpixel classification based optic disc and optic cup segmentation for glaucoma screening. TMI **32**, 1019–1032 (2013)
16. Xu, Y., et al.: Optic cup segmentation for glaucoma detection using low-rank superpixel representation. In: Golland, P., Hata, N., Barillot, C., Hornegger, J., Howe, R. (eds.) MICCAI 2014. LNCS, vol. 8673, pp. 788–795. Springer, Cham (2014). https://doi.org/10.1007/978-3-319-10404-1_98
17. Chaurasia, A., Culurciello, E.: Linknet: exploiting encoder representations for efficient semantic segmentation. In: VCIP. IEEE (2017)

# An Unsupervised Domain Adaptation Approach to Classification of Stem Cell-Derived Cardiomyocytes

Carolina Pacheco[✉] and René Vidal

Center for Imaging Science, Mathematical Institute for Data Science,
Department of Biomedical Engineering, Johns Hopkins University, Baltimore, USA
cpachec2@jhu.edu

**Abstract.** The use of human embryonic stem cell-derived cardiomy-ocytes (hESC-CMs) in applications such as cardiac regenerative medicine requires understanding them in the context of adult CMs. Their classification in terms of the major adult CM phenotypes is a crucial step to build this understanding. However, this is a challenging problem due to the lack of labels for hESC-CMs. Adult CM phenotypes are easily distinguishable based on the shape of their action potentials (APs), but it is still unclear how these phenotypes are expressed in the APs of hESC-CM populations. Recently, a metamorphosis distance was proposed to measure similarities between hESC-CM APs and adult CM APs, which led to state-of-the-art performance when used in a 1 nearest neighbor scheme. However, its computation is prohibitively expensive for large datasets. A recurrent neural network (RNN) classifier was recently shown to be computationally more efficient than the metamorphosis-based method, but at the expense of accuracy. In this paper we argue that the APs of adult CMs and hESC-CMs intrinsically belong to different domains, and propose an unsupervised domain adaptation approach to train the RNN classifier. The idea is to capture the domain shift between hESC-CMs and adult CMs by adding a term to the loss function that penalizes their maximum mean discrepancy (MMD) in feature space. Experimental results in an unlabeled 6940 hESC-CM dataset show that our approach outperforms the state of the art in terms of both clustering quality and computational efficiency. Moreover, it achieves state-of-the-art classification accuracy in a completely different dataset without retraining, which demonstrates the generalization capacity of the proposed method.

**Keywords:** Domain adaptation · LSTM · Embryonic cardiomyocytes

## 1 Introduction

The insufficient supply of oxygen-rich blood to the heart, known as Ischaemic Heart Disease (IHD), has remained the global leading cause of death for more than 15 years, taking the lives of almost 18 million people in 2016 [1]. Along with

© Springer Nature Switzerland AG 2019
D. Shen et al. (Eds.): MICCAI 2019, LNCS 11764, pp. 806–814, 2019.
https://doi.org/10.1007/978-3-030-32239-7_89

prevention, there is a need for innovative approaches to treat IHD. In particular, cardiomyocyte (CM) transplantation has shown favorable results of remuscularization in animals [2], which is promising for post-myocardial infarction patients.

Human embryonic stem cell-derived cardiomyocytes (hESC-CMs) successfully resemble embryonic CMs in terms of structure and function [3]. Thus, they are an important source of CMs not only for regenerative medicine, but also for other applications such as drug screening. However, any application requires to understand hESC-CM characteristics relative to the ones of adults CMs, which remain unclear. A first step in that direction is to study the presence of the major adult CM phenotypes (atrial, ventricular, etc.) in hESC-CM populations.

Initial approaches to classification of hESC-CMs like [4] or [5] were based on handcrafted action potential (AP) features with ad-hoc thresholds in small datasets, which made them subjective and difficult to transfer to other datasets. New electrophysiological recording techniques increased the size of the datasets from dozens and hundreds to several thousand samples [6], which required automatic methods for their classification. However, the lack of ground truth labels for hESC-CMs makes this problem challenging. Gorospe et al. [7,8] proposed to leverage the existence of electrophysiological models of adult CMs to build a 1 nearest neighbor classifier based on a minimum deformation distance called metamorphosis. Their method, 1NN-M, achieved good performance in hESC-CM populations but it is computationally expensive because it requires to solve 20 optimization problems for each new sample to be classified. To overcome this drawback, a recurrent neural network (RNN) based classifier was proposed in [9]. They trained the RNN in a semi-supervised way using labeled adult CM APs and unlabeled hESC-CM APs, showing significant computational advantages with respect to 1NN-M and reaching similar, but not better, clustering quality. Although its computational advantages are undeniable, the approach presented in [9] lacks in a fundamental aspect: the classifier is not aware of the existence of two different domains. Classical machine learning algorithms rely on the assumption that training and testing data are sampled from the same distribution. Unfortunately, this assumption does not hold in the case of adult CMs and hESC-CMs, and therefore we argue that a domain adaptation approach is needed to appropriately train the RNN.

Domain adaptation addresses the problem of optimizing the performance in one domain (called target domain), given training data in a different domain (called source domain). We propose to use the RNN architecture presented in [9], but train it in a different way. We consider the output of its hidden layer as a feature space shared by adult CMs and hESC-CMs. The domain shift between their distributions in the feature space is then reduced by adding their maximum mean discrepancy (MMD) to the loss function. The RNN classifier is trained using a subset of 1600 samples from an unlabeled 6940 hESC-CM APs dataset and 1600 adult CM APs from electrophysiological models. Experimental results confirm that the addition of a domain adaptation term to the loss function improves with respect to the state of the art in terms of clustering quality, and at the same time keeps the computational advantages of previous RNN-based approaches. Moreover, it also reaches state-of-the-art classification accuracy in a completely different dataset without retraining (outperforming previous RNN-based methods), which further demonstrate the advantages of our approach.

## 2   Methods

### 2.1   Problem Formulation

Let $\Omega_e = \{\mathbf{x}_j^e\}_{j=1}^{N_e}$ be an *unlabeled* hESC-CM APs dataset from the target domain, where the sequence $\mathbf{x}_j^e = \{x_j^e(k) \in \mathbb{R}\}_{k=1}^K$ represents the $j$th hESC-CM AP and $K$ is the total number of samples in one cycle length. Hereafter we will refer to this dataset as *embryonic* because of its resemblance of embryonic CM APs. Let $\Omega_a = \{(\mathbf{x}_i^a, y_i^a)\}_{i=1}^{N_a}$ be a *labeled* adult dataset from the source domain, where $\mathbf{x}_i^a = \{x_i^a(k) \in \mathbb{R}\}_{k=1}^K$ is the $i$th adult AP and $y_i^a \in \{0,1\}$ is its ground truth label ($y_i^a = 0$ denotes atrial and $y_i^a = 1$ denotes ventricular). We consider the problem of assigning a label $\hat{y}_j^e$ to each $\mathbf{x}_j^e \in \Omega_e$, where $\hat{y}_j^e = 0$ denotes atrial-like and $\hat{y}_j^e = 1$ denotes ventricular-like. Let $\delta \in \{e, a\}$ indicate the embryonic or adult domain. $\mathbb{P}\{\mathbf{x}|\delta = e\}$ denotes the probability density function of APs in embryonic domain and $\mathbb{P}\{\mathbf{x}|\delta = a\}$ denotes the probability density function of APs in the adult domain. We assume: (i) $\mathbb{P}\{\mathbf{x}|\delta = e\} \neq \mathbb{P}\{\mathbf{x}|\delta = a\}$, and (ii) $\mathbb{P}\{y|\mathbf{x}, \delta = e\} = \mathbb{P}\{y|\mathbf{x}, \delta = a\}$ (covariate shift assumption).

Classifying samples from $\Omega_e$ using training data from $\Omega_a$ corresponds to unsupervised domain adaptation, which according to [10] can be addressed via: instance weighting, self-labeling approaches, clustering-based methods, or feature representation methods. Instance weighting approaches require shared support between both distributions, which does not hold in our case because there are embryonic APs never observed in adult data. On the other hand, self-labeling approaches as well as clustering-based methods often rely on computing similarities between samples, which can be computationally expensive for APs. Thus, we use a feature representation approach in which probability distribution functions of both domains are forced to be similar in a learned feature space $\varphi(\mathbf{x})$.

### 2.2   Maximum Mean Discrepancy

Maximum mean discrepancy [11] corresponds to the distance between the mean of two probability distribution functions mapped into a reproducing kernel Hilbert space (RKHS), embedding their samples via $\psi(\cdot)$. An estimation of the MMD between two datasets $\Omega_a = \{\mathbf{x}_i^a\}_{i=1}^{N_a}$ and $\Omega_e = \{\mathbf{x}_j^e\}_{j=1}^{N_e}$ is given by

$$\widehat{\mathcal{MMD}}^2(\Omega_a, \Omega_e) = \sum_{i=1}^{N_a}\sum_{i'=1}^{N_a} \frac{\mathcal{K}(\mathbf{x}_i^a, \mathbf{x}_{i'}^a)}{N_a^2} + \sum_{j=1}^{N_e}\sum_{j'=1}^{N_e} \frac{\mathcal{K}(\mathbf{x}_j^e, \mathbf{x}_{j'}^e)}{N_e^2} - \sum_{i=1}^{N_a}\sum_{j=1}^{N_e} \frac{2\mathcal{K}(\mathbf{x}_i^a, \mathbf{x}_j^e)}{N_a N_e},$$
(1)

where $\mathcal{K}(x,y)$ is a positive semidefinite kernel such that $\mathcal{K}(x,y) = \psi(x)^\top \psi(y)$. The Gaussian kernel $\mathcal{K}(\mathbf{x}_i, \mathbf{x}_j) = \exp\left(\frac{-\|\mathbf{x}_i - \mathbf{x}_j\|^2}{2\sigma_k^2}\right)$ is commonly used.

The equation in (1) allows us to estimate how different the distributions are based on their samples. The MMD estimator has been successfully applied to learn appropriate kernels for cross-domain SVM-based classification, regression and video concept detection, among others [12,13]. This estimator has also been recently applied with fixed kernels as a metric to learn the parameters of generative networks [14], and the parameters of feature extraction layers for multi-task learning in multiple domains [15], which is closely related to our task.

## 2.3   Network Architecture

As shown in Fig. 1, we use the architecture proposed in [9]: one input layer, one hidden LSTM layer of dimension $p = 3$, and a single sigmoid unit as output layer. The LSTM layer is explicitly considered as a feature extractor, such that $\mathbf{x} \mapsto \varphi_{W_{\mathcal{F}}}(\mathbf{x}) = h(\mathbf{x}, K) \in \mathbb{R}^3$. Note that $h(\mathbf{x}, K)$

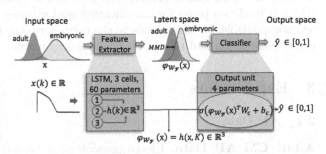

**Fig. 1.** Domain adapted classification approach.

emphasizes that the output cell at time $K$ depends on the entire input sequence. The feature vector $\varphi_{W_{\mathcal{F}}}$ depends on the parameters of the feature extractor $W_{\mathcal{F}}$, and thus it is learnable. For a given set of parameters $W = \{W_{\mathcal{F}}, W_c, b_c\}$, we represent the classifier as the function $f_W(\mathbf{x}) = \hat{y}$ that maps an action potential $\mathbf{x}$ to a predicted label $\hat{y}$.

## 2.4   Domain Adaptation Objective Function

We aim to enforce similarity between the probability density functions of both domains in feature space, i.e. $\mathbb{P}\{\varphi_{W_{\mathcal{F}}}(\mathbf{x})|\delta = a\} \approx \mathbb{P}\{\varphi_{W_{\mathcal{F}}}(\mathbf{x})|\delta = e\}$, while training a classifier with source domain data. In that sense, the network learns to classify samples in a space in which embryonic and adult data "are similar". We propose an objective function that builds on top of the semisupervised loss presented in [9] as follows

$$\frac{1-\lambda}{N_a}\left(\sum_{i=1}^{N_a} \ell\left(y_i^a, f_W(\mathbf{x}_i^a)\right)\right) + \frac{\lambda}{N_e(N_e-1)}\left(\sum_{j=1}^{N_e}\sum_{j'\neq j} \ell_u\left(f_W(\mathbf{x}_j^e), f_W(\mathbf{x}_{j'}^e)\right)\right)$$

$$+ \gamma\widehat{\mathcal{MMD}}^2\left(\{\varphi_{W_{\mathcal{F}}}(\mathbf{x}_i^a)\}_{i=1}^{N_a}, \{\varphi_{W_{\mathcal{F}}}(\mathbf{x}_j^e)\}_{j=1}^{N_e}\right),$$

$$(2)$$

where $\gamma \geq 0$ and $\lambda \in [0,1]$ modulate the relative importance given to the domain adaptation term and unsupervised term, respectively. The first two terms of (2) correspond to the supervised and unsupervised losses presented in [9]. $\ell(\cdot, \cdot)$ is the crossentropy loss, and $\ell_u(\cdot, \cdot)$ is an unsupervised contrastive loss that depends on the similarity between the samples. The domain adaptation term is the square of the empirical estimator of MMD in feature space using a Gaussian kernel.

### 2.5   Metrics

**Classification Accuracy.** When ground truth labels are available, it is the ratio between correctly classified samples and the total number of samples.

**Davies-Bouldin Index (DBI)** [16]. The DBI is a measure of clustering quality, which is used as a proxy for classification performance when ground truth labels are not available. It corresponds to the ratio between the intra-cluster and inter-cluster dispersion and should be as small as possible.

## 3   Experiments

### 3.1   AP Data

**Adult CM AP Data.** Electrophysiological models of adult atrial [17] and ventricular [18] CMs were paced at 1.5 Hz to generate 800 APs of each class by randomizing their parameters as described in [9]. Figure 2(a) shows their normalized version (maximum value 1 and resting membrane potential 0).

**hESC-CM AP Data: Optical Recording Dataset** [6]. Large *unlabeled* dataset composed of 6940 APs optically recorded from 9 cell aggregates paced at 1.5 Hz. Figure 2(b) shows the normalized hESC-CM APs from this dataset.

**hESC-CM AP Data: Single Cell Recording Dataset** [4]. Small *labeled* dataset composed of 52 APs recorded from spontaneously beating hESC-CMs. The nonlinear mapping proposed in [19] was used to adjust them to 1.5 Hz pacing rate. As shown in Fig. 2(c), 16 of them are atrial-like (blue) and 36 of them are ventricular-like (red). This dataset is only used for testing purposes.

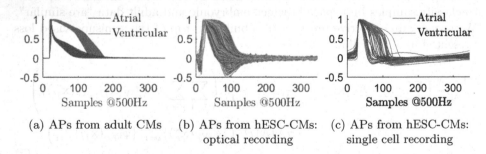

(a) APs from adult CMs    (b) APs from hESC-CMs:    (c) APs from hESC-CMs:
optical recording             single cell recording

**Fig. 2.** Action potentials: (a) 1600 adult CMs, (b) 6940 unlabeled hESC-CMs, and (c) 52 labeled hESC-CMs. (Color figure online)

## 3.2 Implementation Details

The classifier was implemented in Keras [20] with TensorFlow backend and trained using the RMSprop optimizer ($\epsilon = 0.003$). The weights were initialized from the Sup-LSTM network presented in [9]: a network trained for 100 epochs in a fully supervised way using 300 adult atrial and ventricular APs.

$N_e = 1600$ embryonic APs from the optical recording dataset and $N_a = 1600$ adult APs are used for training and validation in balanced batches of 32 samples. The data was split into 10 folds, and the average performance of 10-fold crossvalidation experiments is reported. Once the network is trained, a forward pass in the optical recording dataset is performed to compute the clustering quality (DBI) of the output. Similarly, a forward pass in the single cell recording dataset is done to compute the classification accuracy.

Four cases are studied: (i) Supervised learning $\lambda = 0$ and $\gamma = 0$ (Sup-LSTM); (ii) Semisupervised learning with metamorphosis distances $\lambda = 0.1$ and $\gamma = 0$ (Semi-M-LSTM), (iii) Supervised learning with domain adaptation $\lambda = 0$ and $\gamma = 1$ (DA-Sup-LSTM); and (iv) Semisupervised learning with metamorphosis distances and domain adaptation $\lambda = 0.1$ and $\gamma = 5$ (DA-Semi-M-LSTM). They are trained for 100 epochs, except Sup-LSTM which converges in 15 epochs.

## 3.3 Results

Classification results for the 9 cell aggregates of the optical recording dataset are depicted in Fig. 3 along with the mean clustering quality index (DBI). In all cases the LSTM network suggests heterogeneity in the cell clusters and generates smooth classification boundaries, which coincides with previous findings [6,8]. As reported in [9], Sup-LSTM results are easily distinguishable from all the other approaches and lead to significantly worse clustering quality, which supports the idea that adult CMs and hESC-CMs intrinsically belong to different domains. In that sense, the simple addition of the domain adaptation term to the loss function (DA-Sup-LSTM) improves the mean clustering quality from 0.2793 to 0.2412, which makes it comparable to Semi-M-LSTM (0.2449), but with significant compu-

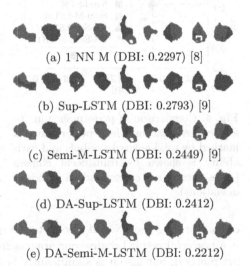

(a) 1 NN M (DBI: 0.2297) [8]

(b) Sup-LSTM (DBI: 0.2793) [9]

(c) Semi-M-LSTM (DBI: 0.2449) [9]

(d) DA-Sup-LSTM (DBI: 0.2412)

(e) DA-Semi-M-LSTM (DBI: 0.2212)

**Fig. 3.** LSTM classification results (each pixel corresponds to one hESC-CM AP). Blue indicates atrial-like phenotype and red indicates ventricular-like phenotype. (Color figure online)

tational advantages since it does not require any computation of metamorphosis distances. However, the addition of the unsupervised term along with the domain

**Table 1.** Performance comparison in the 10-fold crossvalidation experiments.

| | Accuracy ↑ | | | DBI ↓ | | |
|---|---|---|---|---|---|---|
| | Mean | Median | (Std) | Mean | Median | (Std) |
| 1NN M [8] | 0.9615 | 0.9615 | (0.0000) | 0.2297 | 0.2297 | (0.0000) |
| Sup-LSTM [9] | 0.3269 | 0.3269 | (0.0000) | 0.2793 | 0.2795 | (0.0009) |
| Semi-M-LSTM [9] | 0.7154 | 0.7596 | (0.1301) | 0.2449 | 0.2420 | (0.0059) |
| DA-Sup-LSTM (ours) | 0.8385 | 0.9135 | (0.1339) | 0.2412 | 0.2408 | (0.0047) |
| DA-Semi-M-LSTM (ours) | **0.9673** | **0.9904** | (0.0472) | **0.2212** | **0.2197** | (0.0072) |

adaptation (DA-Semi-M-LSTM) leads to the best performance, outperforming the state-of-the-art method (1NN-M) in terms of clustering quality. Therefore, the effects of the semi-supervised term and the domain adaptation term seem to be complementary.

Table 1 and Fig. 4 summarize the results for the studied cases in terms of the clustering quality achieved in the optical recording dataset as well as the classification accuracy obtained in the single cell recording dataset.

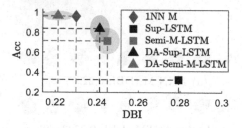

**Fig. 4.** Comparison of performance in 10-fold crossvalidation. Mean performance is marked by solid-colored symbols and variability is shown by translucent ellipses (whose semi-axes correspond to standard deviations).

Whereas Semi-M-LSTM and DA-Sup-LSTM are comparable in terms of clustering quality, the domain adaptation approach performs significantly better in terms of classification accuracy (0.8385 vs 0.7154). Note that this corresponds to a forward pass on the single cell recording dataset, so it shows that the the domain adaption method provides better generalization across datasets. However, their classification accuracy is still far from the one achieved by 1NN-M (0.9615). Again it is the complementary action of semisupervised and domain adaptation terms (DA-Semi-M-LSTM) that succeeds in outperforming the 1NN-M also in terms of classification accuracy (0.9673). This is a powerful result because our approach not only outperforms the state-of-the-art method, but also it is significantly faster. The classification of the single cell recording dataset is reported to take approximately 12 s with the most efficient algorithm for 1NN-M in 2 8-core computer nodes with 8 hyperthreaded 2.3 GHz CPUs per node [8], whereas in our case it takes less than 0.4 s in one 2.2 GHz CPU with 2 cores, 4 threads.

The first row of Fig. 5 shows the distribution of adult samples and unlabeled hESC-CM samples in latent space in the four cases studied. Noticeably, atrial and ventricular samples are located in different areas of the feature space, and the hESC-CMs form a one dimensional path between them. The second row of Fig. 5

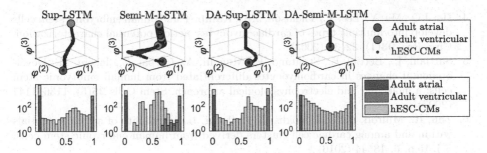

**Fig. 5.** Distribution of adult CMs and hESC-CMs in latent space (first row) and histogram of their projection on the one dimensional path (second row).

represents the histogram of samples along this path. The effect that the domain adaptation term has in the data distribution in the feature space is subtle for the supervised case (DA-Sup-LSTM vs Sup-LSTM): it induces a more balanced distribution of hESC-CMs samples in the location of atrial and ventricular adult CMs. In the semisupervised case however, Semi-M-LSTM generates a high concentration of embryonic samples far from adult CM data, and the addition of the domain adaptation term significantly reduces this effect (DA-Semi-M-LSTM).

## 4    Conclusion

We have applied for the first time the concept of domain adaptation to address discrepancies related to the stem cell differentiation process. Moreover, the proposed approach has proven to be useful, since it outperforms the state-of-the-art method for classification of hESC-CM APs not only in terms of clustering quality, but also in terms of computational efficiency and inter-dataset generalization.

**Acknowlegement.** This work has been supported by NIH #5R01HD87133. The authors thank Dr. Giann Gorospe for insightful discussions, and Dr. Renjun Zhu and Prof. Leslie Tung for providing the hESC-CMs dataset.

## References

1. World Health Organization: World Health Statistics 2018: Monitoring health for the Sustainable Development Goals (2018)
2. Hartman, M.E., Chong, J.J.H., Laflamme, M.A.: State of the art in cardiomyocyte transplantation. In: Ieda, M., Zimmermann, W.-H. (eds.) Cardiac Regeneration. CVB, pp. 177–218. Springer, Cham (2017). https://doi.org/10.1007/978-3-319-56106-6_9
3. Kehat, I., et al.: Human embryonic stem cells can differentiate into myocytes with structural and functional properties of cardiomyocytes. J. Clin. Invest. **108**(3), 407–414 (2001)

4. He, J.Q., Ma, Y., Lee, Y., Thomson, J.A., Kamp, T.J.: Human embryonic stem cells develop into multiple types of cardiac myocytes: action potential characterization. Circ. Res. **93**(1), 32–39 (2003)
5. Sartiani, L., Bettiol, E., Stillitano, F., Mugelli, A., Cerbai, E., Jaconi, M.: Developmental changes in cardiomyocytes differentiated from human embryonic stem cells: a molecular and electrophysiological approach. Stem Cells **25**(5), 1136–1144 (2007)
6. Zhu, R., Millrod, M.A., Zambidis, E.T., Tung, L.: Variability of action potentials within and among cardiac cell clusters derived from human embryonic stem cells. Sci. Rep. **6**, 18544 (2016)
7. Gorospe, G., Younes, L., Tung, L., Vidal, R.: A metamorphosis distance for embryonic cardiac action potential interpolation and classification. In: Mori, K., Sakuma, I., Sato, Y., Barillot, C., Navab, N. (eds.) MICCAI 2013. LNCS, vol. 8149, pp. 469–476. Springer, Heidelberg (2013). https://doi.org/10.1007/978-3-642-40811-3_59
8. Gorospe, G., Zhu, R., He, J.Q., Tung, L., Younes, L., Vidal, R.: Efficient metamorphosis computation for classifying embryonic cardiac action potentials. In: 5th Workshop on Mathematical Foundations of Computational Anatomy (2015)
9. Pacheco, C., Vidal, R.: Recurrent neural networks for classifying human embryonic stem cell-derived cardiomyocytes. In: Frangi, A.F., Schnabel, J.A., Davatzikos, C., Alberola-López, C., Fichtinger, G. (eds.) MICCAI 2018. LNCS, vol. 11070, pp. 581–589. Springer, Cham (2018). https://doi.org/10.1007/978-3-030-00928-1_66
10. Margolis, A.: A literature review of domain adaptation with unlabeled data. Technical report, pp. 1–42 (2011)
11. Gretton, A., Borgwardt, K.M., Rasch, M., Schölkopf, B., Smola, A.J.: A kernel method for the two-sample-problem. In: Advances in Neural Information Processing Systems, pp. 513–520 (2007)
12. Pan, S.J., Kwok, J.T., Yang, Q.: Transfer learning via dimensionality reduction. In: AAAI Conference on Artificial Intelligence, vol. 8, pp. 677–682 (2008)
13. Duan, L., Tsang, I.W., Xu, D., Maybank, S.J.: Domain transfer SVM for video concept detection. In: IEEE Conference on Computer Vision and Pattern Recognition, pp. 1375–1381 (2009)
14. Dziugaite, G., Roy, D., Ghahramani, Z.: Training generative neural networks via maximum mean discrepancy optimization. In: The Conference on Uncertainty in Artificial Intelligence, pp. 258–267 (2015)
15. Chen, H.Y., Chien, J.T.: Deep semi-supervised learning for domain adaptation. In: IEEE International Workshop on Machine Learning and Signal Processing, pp. 1–6. IEEE (2015)
16. Davies, D.L., Bouldin, D.W.: A cluster separation measure. IEEE Trans. Pattern Anal. Mach. Intell. (2), 224–227 (1979)
17. Nygren, A., et al.: Mathematical model of an adult human atrial cell: the role of K+ currents in repolarization. Circ. Res. **82**(1), 63–81 (1998)
18. O'Hara, T., Virág, L., Varró, A., Rudy, Y.: Simulation of the undiseased human cardiac ventricular action potential: model formulation and experimental validation. PLoS Comput. Biol. **7**(5), e1002061 (2011)
19. Iravanian, S., Tung, L.: A novel algorithm for cardiac biosignal filtering based on filtered residue method. IEEE Trans. Biomed. Eng. **49**(11), 1310–1317 (2002)
20. Chollet, F., et al.: Keras (2015). https://keras.io

# Author Index

Printed in the United States
By Bookmasters